t

D1349136

Diabetic Neuropathy

Diabetic Neuropathy

$2nd$ *Edition*

Peter James Dyck, MD

Professor of Neurology
Department of Neurology
Mayo Clinic
Rochester, Minnesota

P. K. Thomas, MD, DSC

Professor Emeritus
Department of Clinical Neurosciences
Royal Free Hospital School of Medicine
University of London
London, England

W.B. SAUNDERS COMPANY

A Division of Harcourt Brace & Company
Philadelphia London Toronto Montreal Sydney Tokyo

W.B. SAUNDERS COMPANY
A Division of Harcourt Brace & Company

The Curtis Center
Independence Square West
Philadelphia, Pennsylvania 19106

Library of Congress Cataloging-in-Publication Data

Diabetic neuropathy / [edited by] Peter James Dyck, P. K. Thomas.—2nd ed.

p.   cm.

Includes bibliographical references and index.

ISBN 0–7216–6182–3

1. Diabetic neuropathies.   I. Dyck, Peter James.   II. Thomas, P. K. (Peter Kynaston).
  [DNLM: 1. Diabetic Neuropathies.   WK 835 D5358 1999]

RC422.D52D53 1999   616.8—dc21

DNLM/DLC   97–39762

DIABETIC NEUROPATHY   ISBN 0–7216–6182–3

Printed in the United States of America.

Last digit is the print number: 9   8   7   6   5   4   3   2   1

Contributors

Andrew J. M. Boulton, MD, FRCP
Professor of Medicine, University of Manchester, Manchester; Professor of Medicine, Department of Medicine, Manchester Royal Infirmary, Manchester, England
Peripheral Vascular Disease

William E. Bradley, MD
Clinical Professor of Urology and Neurology, University of Washington School of Medicine, Seattle, Washington
Assessment of Diabetic Sexual Dysfunction and Cystopathy; Treatment of Diabetic Sexual Dysfunction and Cystopathy

S. Brimijoin, PhD
Professor of Pharmacology, Mayo Medical School, Rochester, Minnesota
Axonal Transport in Diabetic Neuropathy

Robert D. Brown, Jr., MD
Associate Professor of Neurology, Mayo Medical School, Rochester; Consultant in Neurology, Mayo Clinic, Rochester, Minnesota
Cardiovascular Disease and Diabetes

Michael Brownlee, MD
Anita and Jack Saltz Professor of Diabetes Research, Professor of Medicine and Pathology, Co-Director Diabetes Research Center, Albert Einstein College of Medicine, Bronx, New York
Advanced Glycation End Products and Diabetic Peripheral Neuropathy

Norman E. Cameron, BSc, DPhil
Senior Lecturer, Department of Biomedical Sciences, University of Aberdeen, Aberdeen, Scotland
Role of Linolenic Acid in Diabetic Polyneuropathy

Michael Camilleri, MD, MPhil(Lond.), FRCP(Lond.), FRCP(Edin.), FACG, FACP
Professor of Medicine and Physiology and Consultant in Gastroenterology and Physiology, Mayo Clinic and Mayo Foundation, Rochester, Minnesota
Assessment of Gastrointestinal Function; Treatment of Diabetic Gastroparesis and Diarrhea

Mary A. Cotter, BSc, PhD
Senior Lecturer, Department of Biomedical Sciences, University of Aberdeen, Aberdeen, Scotland
Role of Linolenic Acid in Diabetic Polyneuropathy

Regis Coutant, MD
The Research Institute for Children, New Orleans, Louisiana; Fellowship, The Fondation pour la Recherche Medicale
Prediction and Prevention of Immune-Mediated Diabetes

Jasper R. Daube, MD
Professor of Neurology, Mayo Medical School, Rochester, Minnesota
Electrophysiologic Testing in Diabetic Neuropathy

P. James B. Dyck, MD
Peripheral Nerve Research Fellow, Mayo Clinic, Rochester, Minnesota
Diabetic Polyneuropathy

Peter James Dyck, MD
Professor of Neurology, Department of Neurology, Mayo Clinic, Rochester, Minnesota
Neuropathy Tests and Normative Results; Quantitative Sensory Assessment; Epidemiology; Diabetic Polyneuropathy; Pathologic Alterations in Human Diabetic Polyneuropathy; Classification of the Diabetic Neuropathies; Differential Diagnosis of Diabetic Neuropathies; Hypoglycemic Polyneuropathy; Pathophysiology of Nerve Compression

M. E. Edmonds, MD
King's Diabetes Centre, King's College Hospital, London, England
Plantar Neuropathic Ulcer and Charcot Joints: Risk Factors, Presentation, and Management

Robert D. Fealey, MD
Assistant Professor of Neurology, Mayo Medical School, Rochester; Consultant in Neurology, Mayo Clinic, Rochester, Minnesota
Sudomotor Neuropathy

Eva L. Feldman, MD, PhD
Associate Professor of Neurology, Department of Neurology, University of Michigan Medical School, Ann Arbor, Michigan
Glycemic Control; Growth Factors and Peripheral Neuropathy

Caterina Giannini, MD, PhD
Consultant in Pathology, Department of Pathology, Regional Hospital of Treviso, Treviso, Italy
Pathologic Alterations in Human Diabetic Polyneuropathy; Pathophysiology of Nerve Compression

Ian A. Grant, MD, FRCP(C)
Assistant Professor, Division of Neurology, Dalhousie University, Halifax; Staff Neurologist, Queen Elizabeth II Health Sciences Centre, Halifax, Nova Scotia, Canada
Neuropathy Tests and Normative Results; Differential Diagnosis of Diabetic Neuropathies

Douglas A. Greene, MD
Chief, Division of Endocrinology and Metabolism, Professor of Internal Medicine, Department of Internal Medicine, University of Michigan Medical School, Ann Arbor, Michigan
Glycemic Control

Jeffrey B. Halter, MD
Professor of Internal Medicine, Chief, Division of Geriatric Medicine, Director, University of Michigan Geriatric Center, University of Michigan Medical School, Ann Arbor; Director, GRECC, Ann Arbor Veterans Administration Medical Center, Ann Arbor, Michigan
The Clinical Syndrome of Diabetes Mellitus

Johannes Jakobsen, MD
Arbus Kommunehopital, Universitehospital Arbus Amt, Denmark
Hypoglycemic Polyneuropathy

Ryuichi Kikkawa, MD
Professor, Third Department of Medicine, Shiga University of Medical Science, Otsu, Shiga, Japan
Role of Antiprostaglandins in Diabetic Neuropathy

Phillip A. Low, MD
Professor of Neurology, Mayo Medical School, Rochester; Consultant in Neurology, Chairman, Division of Clinical Neurophysiology, Mayo Clinic, Rochester, Minnesota
Sudomotor Neuropathy; Role of Hypoxia, Oxidative Stress, and Excitatory Neurotoxins in Diabetic Neuropathy

Noel K. Maclaren, MD
Professor, Pediatrics and Genetics, Louisiana State University School of Medicine, New Orleans; Director, Research Institute for Children, New Orleans, Louisiana
Prediction and Prevention of Immune-Mediated Diabetes

Allison Malcolm, MD
Department of Gastroenterology, Royal North Shore Hospital, St Leonards, Sydney; Department of Medicine, University of Sydney, Sydney, Australia
Assessment of Gastrointestinal Function; Treatment of Diabetic Gastroparesis and Diarrhea

L. Joseph Melton III, MD
Michael M. Eisenberg Professor of Epidemiology, Mayo Medical School, Rochester, Minnesota
Epidemiology

K. R. Mills, PhD, MB, BS, FRCP
University Lecturer in Clinical Neurophysiology, University of Oxford, Oxford; Honorary Consultant in Clinical Neurophysiologist; The Radcliffe Infirmary, Oxford, England
Quantitative Motor Assessment

Kim K. Nickander, BA
Research Associate, Mayo Foundation, Rochester, Minnesota
Role of Hypoxia, Oxidative Stress, and Excitatory Neurotoxins in Diabetic Neuropathy

Peter O'Brien, PhD
Professor of Biostatistics, Mayo Medical School, Rochester, Minnesota
Neuropathy Tests and Normative Results

John M. Pach, MD
Assistant Professor of Ophthalmology, Mayo Medical School, Rochester, Minnesota
Diabetic Retinopathy

Michael Pfeifer, MD, MS, CDE, FACE
Professor and Chief of Endocrinology and Metabolism, East Carolina University School of Medicine, Greenville, North Carolina
Cardiovascular Assessment

Daniel Porte, Jr., MD
Professor of Medicine, University of Washington School of Medicine, Seattle; Associate Chief of Staff for Research and Development, VA Puget Sound Health Care System, Seattle, Washington
The Clinical Syndrome of Diabetes Mellitus

Gerard Said, MD
Professor of Neurology, Universite Paris-Sud,
Paris; Chief, Service de Neurologie, Centre
Hospitalo-Universitaire de Bicetre, Le
Kremlin-Bicetre, France
Proximal Diabetic Neuropathy

Luciano Scionti, MD
Assistant Professor of Endocrinology,
University of Perugia Medical School,
Perugia, Italy
*Role of Hypoxia, Oxidative Stress, and
Excitatory Neurotoxins in Diabetic Neuropathy*

Benn E. Smith, MD
Assistant Professor of Neurology, Mayo
Medical School, Rochester, Minnesota;
Consultant in Neurology, Mayo Clinic
Scottsdale, Scottsdale, Arizona
Cranial Neuropathy in Diabetes Mellitus

Shirley A. Smith, PhD
Principal Physiologist, Diabetes Day Centre,
St. Thomas' Hospital, London, England
Assessment of Pupil Function

Stephen E. Smith, DM, PhD
Emeritus Professor of Applied Pharmacology
and Therapeutics, University of London;
Senior Research Fellow, Department of
Neuroophthalmology, National Hospital for
Neurology and Neurosurgery, London,
England
Assessment of Pupil Function

Peter C. Spittell, MD
Assistant Professor of Medicine, Mayo
Medical School, Rochester; Consultant,
Department of Internal Medicine and Division
of Cardiovascular Diseases, Mayo Medical
Center, Rochester, Minnesota
Cardiovascular Disease and Diabetes

Martin J. Stevens, MD
Assistant Professor of Internal Medicine,
Department of Internal Medicine, Division of
Endocrinology and Metabolism, University of
Michigan Medical School, Ann Arbor,
Michigan
Glycemic Control

Guillermo A. Suarez, MD
Associate Consultant in Neurology, Mayo
Clinic, Rochester, Minnesota
Quantitative Sensory Assessment

Bruce V. Taylor, MBBS, FRACP
Clinical Lecturer, University of Tasmania,
Tasmania; Staff Neurologist, Royal Hobart
Hospital, Hobart, Tasmania, Australia
Classification of the Diabetic Neuropathies

P. K. Thomas, MD, DSC
Professor Emeritus, Department of Clinical
Neurosciences, Royal Free Hospital School of
Medicine, University of London, London,
England
*Mechanisms and Treatment of Pain; Diabetic
Truncal Radiculoneuropathy; Proximal Diabetic
Neuropathy*

David R. Tomlinson, PhD, DSc
Professor and Chairman of Pharmacology,
St. Bartholomew's and the London School of
Medicine, London, England
*Role of Aldose Reductase Inhibitors in the
Treatment of Diabetic Polyneuropathy*

Frank Vinicor, MD, MPH
Director, Division of Diabetes Translation,
Centers for Disease Control and Prevention,
Atlanta; Clinical Associate Professor of
Medicine, Emory University School of
Medicine, Atlanta, Georgia
Primary Prevention of Type 2 Diabetes Mellitus

P. J. Watkins, MD, FRCP
Honorary Senior Lecturer, King's College
School of Medicine and Dentistry, London;
Consultant Physician, King's Diabetes Centre,
King's College Hospital, London, England
*Plantar Neuropathic Ulcer and Charcot Joints:
Risk Factors, Presentation, and Management;
Diabetic Truncal Radiculoneuropathy*

Asa J. Wilbourn, MD
Associate Clinical Professor of Neurology,
Case-Western Reserve School of Medicine,
Cleveland; Director, EMG Laboratory,
Cleveland Clinic, Cleveland, Ohio
*Diabetic Entrapment and Compression
Neuropathies*

David M. Wilson, MD
Director, Renal Laboratory and Consultant,
Department of Medicine, Division of
Nephrology, and Department of Laboratory
Medicine, Mayo Clinic School of Medicine,
Rochester, Minnesota
Diabetic Nephropathy

Anthony J. Windebank, MA, FRCP(UK)
Professor of Neurology, Mayo Medical School, Rochester; Dean, Mayo Graduate School and Director, Molecular Neuroscience PhD Program, Mayo Clinic and Mayo Foundation, Rochester, Minnesota
Growth Factors and Peripheral Neuropathy

Claire C. Yang, MD
Assistant Professor of Urology, University of Washington, Seattle; Staff Urologist, VA Puget Sound Health Care System, Seattle, Washington
Assessment of Diabetic Sexual Dysfunction and Cystopathy; Treatment of Diabetic Sexual Dysfunction and Cystopathy

Shunji Yasaki, MD, PhD, FACP
Assistant Professor, Third Department of Internal Medicine, St. Marianna University School of Medicine, Kawasaki, Japan
Hypoglycemic Polyneuropathy

Hitoshi Yasuda, MD, PhD
Assistant Professor, Third Department of Medicine, Shiga University of Medical Science, Otsu, Shiga, Japan
Role of Antiprostaglandins in Diabetic Neuropathy

Matthew J. Young, MD, MRCP(UK)
Consultant Physician, Department of Diabetes, Royal Infirmary, Edinburgh, England
Peripheral Vascular Disease

Foreword

Abnormality of peripheral nerve was formally recognized as an accompaniment of diabetes mellitus well over a century ago, although the symptoms were known for much longer. In the first half of this century, studies of diabetic peripheral neuropathy were relatively infrequent. Emphasis was, by necessity, placed on clinical descriptions, because few other approaches could be brought to bear. What little pathological study that was reported, performed as it was on autopsy tissue or on amputated limbs, established the occurrence of breakdown and loss of peripheral nerve fibers in association with diabetes, but it did not advance our knowledge much further. The second half of this century has witnessed a remarkable surge of research on diabetic neuropathies, and much of that has been stimulated and pioneered by the principal editors of this volume, Peter James Dyck and P. K. Thomas.

The first edition of *Diabetic Neuropathy* was published in 1987. Previously only individual journal articles and occasional monographs of proceedings of conferences on diabetic neuropathy comprised our information base. A growing sense of the magnitude of the problem and of the progress being made by studying it prompted the first edition. That first comprehensive effort to summarize knowledge of diabetic neuropathy has served admirably as the standard reference on the subject.

In the 12 years since publication of the first edition, the tide of new information on diabetic neuropathy has reached flood stage. The capacity to measure accurately the various aspects of diabetic neuropathy, including subclinical neuropathy, quantitative sensory deficit, and autonomic dysfunction, has developed steadily. The massive Diabetes Control and Complications Trial (DCCT) in the United States has come to completion and has demonstrated to a startling degree the positive effect of strict glycemic control on suppressing the appearance of diabetic complications including neuropathy. Numerous clinical trials of many agents selected for their potential for preventing or controlling diabetic neuropathy are underway around the world.

While the press of investigative activity in the field of diabetic neuropathy is heartening and cause for optimism, there are some stark facts to keep in mind. Notably, the capacity to control diabetic neuropathic pain is still far from adequate. Further, strict glycemic control is quite difficult to sustain, and frequent hypoglycemia attends such efforts. Closed-loop systems of glycemic control that can maintain normal blood sugar levels on a continuous basis are still a dream for the future. Effective adjunct therapy for the prevention of diabetic complications, such as later-generation aldose reductase inhibitors, is still not at hand.

The challenges to manage and prevent diabetic neuropathy are still with us. With these considerations in mind, this second edition of *Diabetic Neuropathy* is welcome indeed. Drs. Dyck and Thomas have assembled an outstanding group of authors to summarize their experience, covering all aspects of diabetic neuropathy. The update is badly needed, and this second edition does a superb job of meeting that need.

Arthur K. Asbury, M.D.
University of Pennsylvania
Philadelphia, PA

Preface

The first edition of *Diabetic Neuropathy* was published in 1987 with the purpose of providing a comprehensive overview of the clinical features, pathophysiology, causation, and treatment of this highly troublesome complication of diabetes mellitus. Since then there have been many new developments so that a second edition has become necessary. Further epidemiologic studies have provided more detailed information as to the prevalence of diabetic neuropathy, both from clinic-based and community-based surveys. The heterogeneity of the clinical manifestations has become increasingly obvious, emphasizing that there is no single diabetic neuropathy but a wide range of neuropathy syndromes that must reflect correspondingly complex pathogenetic mechanisms. The American Diabetes Control and Complications Trial (DCCT) has provided unequivocal evidence that hyperglycemia or factors connected with it are responsible for the occurrence of neuropathy in insulin-dependent diabetes. Strict diabetic control from continuous subcutaneous insulin infusion can prevent the development of neuropathy. Unfortunately, this form of treatment is only feasible in a minority of patients with diabetes.

It is general experience in diabetic clinics that good glycemic control can only be achieved in about 25% of patients overall. It is therefore vital that the underlying causes of peripheral nerve damage are established so that appropriate treatment can be given despite imperfect control. The relative contributions of direct metabolic and indirect vascular mechanisms are still a source of lively debate. Since the first edition of *Diabetic Neuropathy*, new pathogenetic mechanisms have emerged and others have achieved greater prominence. For the common predominantly distal sensory polyneuropathy, the possibility that neurotrophic agents may be implicated has attracted considerable attention, and vasculitic or other inflammatory changes have been shown to be involved in focal and multifocal neuropathies.

The assessment of new therapies has demanded the development of informative and validated criteria for the detection and staging of neuropathy. Such evaluations have been modified in the light of experience gained during treatment trials. Although valuable in earlier trials, the use of nerve biopsy is now no longer considered to be a requirement; clinical and electrophysiologic measures are adequate. Disappointingly, apart from the DCCT, treatment regimes that have held promise have largely failed to fulfill their initial expectations. The assessment of treatment regimes for diabetic polyneuropathy poses particular problems in view of the slow evolution of the neuropathy and the fact that, once established, it is substantially irreversible. Therefore, prevention of deterioration may be the appropriate goal of therapy.

In the first edition, we emphasized use of standard tests to characterize and quantitate symptoms, impairments, attributes of nerve conduction, sensory tests, and autonomic tests. We also emphasized use of rigorous abnormal limits. We proposed minimal criteria for diabetic polyneuropathy. We also outlined recently proposed staging of diabetic polyneuropathy. In this edition, we extend this effort to defining minimal criteria for diabetic polyneuropathy more comprehensively, using composite scores and abnormality based on percentile (e.g., 97.5th) as obtained from a healthy subject cohort without neurologic disease, neuropathy, or diseases predisposing to polyneuropathy. We have further refined the classification of diabetic neuropathies into specific types. This is in agreement in general, but not in specific detail or name, about classification. To illustrate, diabetic lumbosacral radiculoplexus neuropathy is also called diabetic amyotrophy, proximal diabetic neuropathy, Bruns-Garland syndrome, or femoral neuropathy. The latitude we, as editors, have provided the contributors is deliberate to encourage them to state their preference and to reveal different facets of what is known. We hope that this does not produce confusion. We take the position that the quality of many of the reports of the frequency and severity of diabetic neuropathies remains poor. Much more attention needs to be given to studying patients prospectively, based on population-based cohorts and using only controlled instruments and appropriate normative abnormal limits.

We are still handicapped by the lack of a suitable animal model. The changes observed in chemically-induced and genetic diabetes in rodents probably reflect the abnormalities seen in early diabetes in humans, and it is as yet uncertain whether they are informative as to the causation of degenerative human neuropathy. A convincing animal counterpart of the human disorder would constitute a major advance.

These and other themes are taken up in this second edition of *Diabetic Neuropathy*. As before we are most grateful to the contributors for their industry and expertise. We are also grateful to their personal secretaries for their help, and to the editorial and production staffs at W.B. Saunders.

Peter James Dyck
P. K. Thomas

Contents

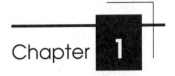

Chapter 1

The Clinical Syndrome of Diabetes Mellitus

Daniel Porte, Jr. • *Jeffrey B. Halter*

INTRODUCTION

Diabetes mellitus is a clinical syndrome characterized by abnormal carbohydrate metabolism leading to an increased risk for atherosclerosis and development of specific microvascular and neurologic complications. The primary mechanism for diagnosing diabetes is based on an excessive plasma glucose level during fasting or after a standard glucose challenge. It has been separated into two major and distinct syndromes that differ etiologically and clinically. Type 1 diabetes is due to an autoimmune destruction of the pancreatic beta cells, usually requiring insulin treatment. Type 2 diabetes is a nonautoimmune disorder with varying degrees of insulin resistance and impaired insulin secretion usually associated with obesity. Both have strong genetic predisposing factors. Hyperglycemia secondary to other diseases is called diabetes associated with other conditions. Long-term management requires adjusting calories to maintain weight in type 1 diabetes and reducing calories and increasing exercise to lower weight in type 2 diabetes. This basic therapy is augmented by insulin in type 1 diabetes and oral agents or insulin in type 2 diabetes to bring plasma glucose to as near normal levels as possible to reduce the risk of specific complications. Oral agents include sulfonylureas, metformin, thiazolidinediones, and α-glucosidase inhibitors alone or in combination with insulin. Major microvascular complications occur in the eye (retinopathy), in the kidney (nephropathy), and in peripheral nerves (neuropathy). Each has risk factors in addition to hyperglycemia that require identification and treatment. Despite present treatment approaches, diabetes remains the leading cause of new end-stage renal disease, new cases of blindness in adults 20–74 years, and amputations. Direct health costs were estimated at 45 billion dollars in 1992.

DEFINITION

Diabetes mellitus is a common disease that has devastating consequences for many individuals and for society as a whole. It is estimated that more than 7 million people in the United States have diabetes mellitus and that this number is growing by approximately 5% per year.[46] Diabetes with its vascular complications is a major contributing cause of myocardial infarction and cerebrovascular and peripheral vascular disease. It is the leading cause of new end-stage renal disease in the United States and the leading cause of new cases of blindness in Americans 20 to 74 years of age. The total yearly direct health care cost related to diabetes mellitus was estimated to be nearly $45 billion in 1992. Indirect costs related to loss of productive years of work capacity are estimated at $46 billion.[46, 82] These costs have risen rapidly since 1985.[18]

Diabetes mellitus is a disease that has been recognized for centuries by the presence of high levels of sugar in body fluids. However, we now recognize that diabetes mellitus is a much more complex condition than simply an abnormality of glucose regulation. Diabetes continues to be defined by glucose measurements primarily because abnormalities of glucose metabolism have been easiest to measure and were the first discovered. It has been difficult, however, to strictly define the normal limits of glucose metabolism because carbohydrate tolerance is distributed as a continuous function. The lack of a clear separation of normal from abnormal carbohydrate tolerance most likely results from the distance of the measurement from the underlying genetic abnormalities, from multigenetic regulation of carbohydrate metabolism, and from the variable interaction of hereditary with environmental factors.

Therefore, diabetes mellitus should be viewed as a clinical syndrome that is characterized by abnormal carbohydrate metabolism. It

is also associated with altered regulation of fat and protein metabolism. A complete review of the syndrome, with coverage of basic and clinical aspects, has recently been edited by one of the authors.[93] There are three other features of the diabetes syndrome that are present in many patients. Thus, the syndrome of diabetes mellitus includes:

1. *Hyperglycemia.* This abnormality probably contributes to the other features but seems unlikely to be their sole cause.
2. *Large vessel disease.* There is an increased risk of atherosclerosis and medial calcification of medium and large arteries.
3. *Microvascular disease.* There is a generalized abnormality of retina and kidney capillaries. Capillary basement membranes are characterized by thickness and abnormal function. These capillary-related lesions, often termed the *microvascular* or *small-vessel concomitants of diabetes*, have been shown to be in part a consequence of hyperglycemia.
4. *Neuropathy.* There are peripheral sensory and motor defects, autonomic nervous system dysfunction, axonal loss, segmental demyelination, and abnormalities of Schwann cell function, which are also in part related to hyperglycemia.

None of these findings is absolutely specific for diabetes, because each is also found in other diseases and syndromes. It is likely that more than one mechanism can produce each of these four abnormal findings. Because the primary defect or defects for most patients with diabetes is unknown, a patient with any of these abnormalities may have diabetes. Because plasma glucose can be measured simply and accurately, it remains the standard for establishing a diagnosis.

CLINICAL CLASSIFICATION

For many years, clinicians have recognized differences in the presentation and clinical course of patients with diabetes mellitus. In some cases, hyperglycemia is associated with diseases of other endocrine systems, such as Cushing's syndrome and acromegaly, or with extensive damage to the pancreas caused by trauma, surgical intervention, or chronic pancreatitis. After eliminating these various underlying causes for hyperglycemia, one is left with a large group of patients with varying degrees of hyperglycemia without an obvious explanation who have an increased likelihood of ath-

TABLE 1.1   CLINICAL CHARACTERISTICS OF THE TWO MAJOR TYPES OF DIABETES MELLITUS

National Diabetes Data Group Terminology	Type 1 Diabetes Mellitus Insulin-dependent Diabetes Mellitus (IDDM)	Type 2 Diabetes Mellitus Non–insulin-dependent Diabetes Mellitus (NIDDM)
Previous Clinical Terminology	*Juvenile Onset Diabetes (JOD) Brittle Diabetes*	*Maturity Onset Diabetes (MOD) Adult Onset Diabetes (AOD) Stable Diabetes*
Age of onset	Usually younger than 45 years	Usually older than 30 years
Genetics	Less than 10% of first-degree relatives affected	More than 20% of first-degree relatives affected
HLA	Associated with HLA-DR-3, DR-4, DQB-DQA	No HLA association
Immunity	Increased incidence of autoimmune phenomena, particularly islet cell antibodies (ICA) and glutamic acid decarboxylase antibodies (GAD-65)	No increase in autoimmune phenomena
Body weight	Usually lean	Usually obese
Metabolism	Ketosis prone	Ketosis resistant
Treatment	Insulin	Weight loss, oral agent, or insulin

From Porte D Jr, Halter JB. The endocrine pancreas and diabetes mellitus. *In* Williams RH (ed): Textbook of Endocrinology, ed 6. Philadelphia, WB Saunders, 1981, pp 716–843.

erosclerosis, microvascular disease, and neuropathy. Even within this group there are obvious clinical differences that led to use of terms such as juvenile diabetes and maturity diabetes, separating patients on the basis of the age of diagnosis. A summary of the differences in the two most common clinical types of diabetes is given in Table 1.1.

Although it is true that diabetics with an early age of onset tend to have more difficulty managing hyperglycemia, age at onset does not really segregate the clinical types of diabetes. Furthermore, a classification system based on age of diagnosis does not take into account information available about genetic markers and modes of inheritance that is now available.

To address this problem, the National Diabetes Data Group of the National Institutes of Health organized an international workshop in 1978. The result was a new classification system for diabetes that has been widely adopted.[81] Although the system is descriptive rather than based on specific etiologic entities, it does take into account current information about genetic markers and modes of inheritance. It is simple to apply and limits use of the diagnosis of diabetes mellitus to those patients whose degree of hyperglycemia puts them at high risk for development of major diabetes complications. In addition to diabetes associated with other conditions, two clinical types of diabetes are defined based on the need for insulin therapy: type 1 or insulin-dependent

diabetes mellitus and type 2 or non–insulin-dependent diabetes mellitus. Unfortunately, at the present time there are no absolute criteria for distinguishing type 1 from type 2. Because insulin treatment is often given to patients who are not prone to development of ketoacidosis, in individual cases, particularly in the older age group, it may be difficult to correctly place a specific patient into the appropriate syndrome category.

Patients with abnormalities of glucose metabolism identified by glucose tolerance test, who are at increased risk for the development of diabetes mellitus, fall into the impaired glucose tolerance category. Pregnant patients with impaired glucose tolerance who are at risk for pregnancy complications have gestational diabetes. This system also recognizes that there are some patients with normal glucose metabolism who may be at risk for developing diabetes in the future. The criteria for each of these categories are presented in Table 1.2.[37]

Type 1 Diabetes Mellitus

Severe insulin deficiency is the most characteristic finding of type 1 diabetes mellitus (DM). It is the classical type that has been described for more than 2000 years, with sudden onset, severe hyperglycemia, rapid progression to ketoacidosis, and death unless treated with insulin. About 50% of these patients are diagnosed before age 21 years, with a peak incidence near

TABLE 1.2 DIAGNOSTIC CRITERIA FOR DIABETES MELLITUS

Category	Fasting Plasma Glucose	Oral Glucose Tolerance Test*		
		1 Hour	*2 Hour*	*3 Hour*
Diabetes mellitus†	1. Random hyperglycemia plus classic diabetes symptoms *or* 2. ≥126 mg/dL (7.0 mmol/L) (2 occasions)‡ *or* 3. <126 mg/dL (7.0 mmol/L)	≥200 mg/dL§ (11.1 mmol/L)	≥200 mg/dL (11.1 mmol/L)	—
Impaired fasting glucose	110–125 mg/dL (6.1–7.0 mmol/L)			
Impaired glucose tolerance		≥200 mg/dL§ (11.1 mmol/L)	140–200 mg/dL (7.8–11.1 mmol/L)	—
Gestational diabetes mellitus†	1. >105 mg/dL (5.8 mmol/L) (2 occasions) 2. <105 mg/dL (5.8 mmol/L)	≥190 mg/dL‖ (10.6 mmol/L)	≥165 mg/dL (9.2 mmol/L)	≥145 mg/dL (8.05 mmol/L)

*Criteria are based on 75-g glucose load, except for gestational diabetes, for which 100 g is used. All values are venous plasma glucose.
†Patients meeting any one of these criteria have diabetes mellitus or gestational diabetes mellitus.
‡Recent ADA recommendation is >126 mg/dL (7.0 mmol/L) for diagnosis of diabetes.
§One additional value ≥200 mg/dL (11.1 mmol/L) at 30, 60, or 90 minutes needed to meet the criterion.
‖Two or more values abnormal for diagnosis.

puberty. Patients with type 1 DM are usually lean, and even after treatment there is little tendency for obesity. These patients do not respond to sulfonylurea drugs, and at autopsy they have gross beta-cell destruction. There may be a period after diagnosis during which insulin treatment is not essential, the so-called honeymoon phase, but this is almost always transient.

Studies of monozygotic twins indicate that the concordance rate for type 1 DM is only about 50%.[95] Thus, although there is a clear genetic factor involved in the pathogenesis, there must also be an important environmental influence. The genetic factor appears to be associated with the HLA-D region of the major histocompatibility complex. The HLA-DR4 allele is strongly associated with type 1 DM in all ethnic groups, and the HLA-DR3 allele is associated with type 1 DM in Caucasians. Heterozygous individuals who have both HLA-DR3 and HLA-DR4 alleles are at highest risk for type 1 DM, suggesting that different mechanisms may be associated with each of these genes.[127] DQ and DP region genes are also involved in susceptibility, but the specific alleles appear to vary among populations and may depend on combinations of protective and risk haplotypes. Because an HLA association is not found in type 2 DM, it is clear that the syndromes must be genetically different. Although 95% of Caucasians with type 1 DM have either HLA-DR3 or HLA-DR4 types, these HLA types are also quite common in the nondiabetic population. Thus, it is clear that other factors are important in type 1 DM. This hypothesis is strengthened by the fact that siblings with type 1 DM almost always have at least one HLA tissue antigen haplotype in common. In siblings completely matched for tissue type who share both parental gene sets, the frequency of type 1 DM is similar to that of monozygotic twins. This is true whether the diabetic subjects have or do not have any of the diabetes-related HLA antigens.

The finding that susceptibility genes for type 1 DM are linked to the major HLA complex that controls the immune response system has suggested that the genetic factor involved in type 1 DM confers increased sensitivity to an environmental event leading to immunologically mediated beta-cell destruction.[89] Consistent with this idea is the demonstration of circulating antibodies to human islet cell antigens, including insulin and islet glutamic acid decarboxylase (GAD-65), at the time of diagnosis in nearly all patients with type 1 DM.[89] Furthermore, islet cell antibodies have been demonstrated in persons at high risk for the development of type 1 DM, such as siblings of patients with type 1 DM, and in conjunction with metabolic studies and HLA typing have a strong predictive value for the subsequent development of overt type 1 DM.[89] The presence of islet cell antibodies is also a good predictor of future need for insulin treatment in older patients with recent onset of hyperglycemia who appear to have type 2 DM clinically,[44] suggesting that they in fact have type 1. The absence of such antibodies in patients with type 2 DM is consistent with a separation of these syndromes into two disease types.

Type 2 Diabetes Mellitus

Type 2 DM is characterized by the presence of fasting hyperglycemia and markedly impaired glucose tolerance (see Table 1.2). Like type 1, type 2 DM is associated with retinopathy, nephropathy, microvascular disease, neuropathy, and atherosclerosis. Type 2 DM usually has a slow onset, and in the beginning it is often asymptomatic, making it difficult to date the onset of the metabolic abnormality. These patients do not develop ketoacidosis in the absence of insulin therapy and do not need insulin therapy to survive. However, many patients with type 2 DM are treated with insulin to control hyperglycemia, and some develop ketoacidosis during severe stress. Thus, insulin treatment per se does not differentiate between types 1 and 2 DM.

There is a strong genetic component to type 2 DM, because the concordance rate for type 2 in identical twins is at least 40%, and in some studies, it approaches 100%.[101] Despite the clear genetic character of type 2 DM, the presence of this disease is frequently not detected until late in life, and the prevalence rate of type 2 DM is greatest in patients older than age 65 years. Although only 20% of family members are usually found to have type 2 DM, families have been described in which the prevalence of type 2 DM approximates 50% over several generations, compatible with autosomal dominant inheritance in this group. However, the genetic factors involved differ from type 1 DM because there is no known association with HLA antigens or evidence of autoimmune phenomena. In these families, type 2 DM also occurs in children, adolescents, and young adults. The syndrome present in these families has been termed *maturity-onset type diabetes of the young* (MODY).[37] Although initially some MODY families appeared to have a low incidence of diabetes complications, subsequent studies have established that this is a heterogenous syndrome, and other families have a rate of diabetes complications similar to families with the usual type 2 DM. Therefore, they are clinically similar to older type 2 patients without a dominant genetic inheritance pattern. Recently, mutations in glucokinase (MODY-2) and two nuclear transcription factors, hepatocyte nuclear factor (HNF) 1α (MODY-3) and HNF 4α (MODY-1), have been found in families with the MODY syndrome.[41, 129, 130] Thus, we now have three distinctly different genetic defects causing three genetically different MODY diseases.

A major clinical characteristic of type 2 DM is obesity. At least 80% of these patients are greater than 15% over ideal weight at the time of diagnosis.[14, 101] Type 2 DM has been subclassified into obese and nonobese types, although no major differences in pathophysiology have been demonstrated thus far between type 2 DM in obese and nonobese persons. Socioeconomic factors seem to be important to the age of onset and frequency of type 2 DM, probably because of the important role of nutrition and body weight in its clinical presentation.

Diabetes Mellitus Associated with Other Conditions

In a number of circumstances, the presence of diabetes mellitus may be caused by another disease process or medical problem. Table 1.3 summarizes some of the conditions associated with hyperglycemia. These include conditions associated with damage to the pancreas, with alterations of other hormones that affect glucose homeostasis, and with a variety of genetic syndromes that tend to be associated with hyperglycemia. In most of these syndromes, patients have stable hyperglycemia similar to that seen in type 2 DM. Because the frequency of type 2 DM is so high, the independent occurrence of two diseases in the same individual often cannot be excluded. Thus, particularly in conditions such as chronic pancreatitis, acromegaly, and Cushing's syndrome, in which the degree of hyperglycemia may vary considerably from individual to individual, it is possible that those patients who are most hyperglycemic have underlying type 2 DM that is simply aggravated by the superimposed illness.

A number of drugs have also been associated with the development of hyperglycemia, although again it is often unclear whether they simply bring out hyperglycemia in patients with the genetic defect of type 2 DM or whether they are independent causes. These drugs include diuretics, phenothiazines, tricyclic antidepressant drugs, diphenylhydantoin,

TABLE 1.3 DISEASES AND SYNDROMES WITH HYPERGLYCEMIA

Pancreatic diseases
  Neonatal
    Congenital absence of islets
  Postnatal
    Pancreatitis (calcific, alcoholic relapsing, infections, nutritional)
    Pancreatic neoplasia
    Cystic fibrosis
    Toxic destruction—Vacor (rat poison)
    Iron overload (hemochromatosis)
    Trauma
    Pancreatectomy
Hormonal
  Counterregulatory hormone excess
    Glucosteroid excess—Cushing's syndrome
    Catecholamine excess—pheochromocytoma
    Growth hormone excess—acromegaly
    Glucagon excess—glucagonoma syndrome
  Other endocrine-metabolic syndromes
    Mineralocorticoid excess (hypokalemia)
    Congenital growth hormone deficiency—Laron dwarfism or ateliotic dwarfism (growth failure)
    Hypoparathyroidism (hypocalcemia)
    Carcinoid syndrome (hyperserotoninemia)
    Somatostatinoma (hypersomatostatinemia)
    Hyperthyroidism
    Prolactinoma
    Hepatic cirrhosis (hypokalemia?)
Genetic syndromes
  Acute intermittent porphyria
  Alström syndrome
  Ataxia telangiectasia
  Cockayne's syndrome
  Diabetes insipidus, nerve deafness, hyperglycemia
  Down syndrome
  Friedreich's ataxia
  Glycogen storage disease
  Herrmann's syndrome
  Huntington's chorea
  Klinefelter's syndrome
  Laurence-Moon-Biedl syndrome
  Lipoatrophic diabetes
  Azorean disease
  Mendenhall's syndrome
  Myotonic dystrophy
  Optic atrophy with hyperglycemia
  Prader-Willi syndrome
  Refsum's disease
  Turner's syndrome
  Werner's syndrome

From Porte D Jr, Halter JB. The endocrine pancreas and diabetes mellitus. *In* Williams RH (ed): Textbook of Endocrinology, ed 6. Philadelphia, WB Saunders, 1981, pp 716–843.

a variety of analgesics including nonsteroidal anti-inflammatory drugs, several antineoplastic agents, and several antibiotics. The adverse effect of diuretics on carbohydrate metabolism is thought to be primarily a result of the inhibitory effect of hypokalemia on insulin secretory mechanisms.

Another group of patients has hyperglyce-mia associated with a clinical syndrome of severe insulin resistance in the presence of the skin lesion acanthosis nigricans.[54, 55, 118] In some cases, this is a familial disorder in young females who have associated hirsutism, polycystic ovaries, and accelerated growth. These patients usually have a genetic mutation leading to marked decrease in the number of insulin receptors or receptors with reduced function on cells, thereby impairing the ability of insulin to increase glucose uptake. These patients have variable degrees of hyperglycemia, and usually require massive doses of insulin to overcome the decrease in cellular insulin receptor function. Another group of patients with insulin resistance and acanthosis nigricans have features suggestive of autoimmune disease. These patients have circulating antibodies directed against insulin receptors as the cause of insulin resistance. This syndrome is generally not familial, and it appears to represent an unusual manifestation of an autoimmune process.

In a few instances, a clinically typical patient with type 2 DM has been found to produce abnormal insulin because of the presence of one abnormal structural insulin gene.[117] Because two genes are present, there is also normal insulin circulating. Not all family members with the abnormal insulin are hyperglycemic, implying either a second genetic or environmental factor for the hyperglycemia of the clinically affected individuals. In general, these patients have hyperinsulinemia because of the reduced clearance of the biologically impaired insulin, but not insulin resistance.

Type 1 DM is also observed in families with autoimmune endocrine diseases.[89] Autoimmune destruction of the thyroid, parathyroid, adrenal, and pituitary glands may be present in association with autoimmune destruction of the endocrine pancreas and hyperglycemia. Family members may have one, two, or all the manifestations of this process. In these families, diabetes is often associated with diabetes-related autoantibodies. Although the pathogenesis of diabetes in these patients appears to be similar to that in type 1 DM, the presence of other autoimmune endocrine deficiencies suggests potential differences in underlying etiology.

Impaired Glucose Tolerance

Subtle abnormalities of glucose metabolism can be detected in many individuals who do not meet the criteria for diabetes mellitus. Such abnormalities are generally demonstrated during an oral glucose challenge, with the abnormality defined statistically in relation to population studies. Thus, individuals whose glucose levels during an oral glucose tolerance test fall outside of the normal range, but who do not meet the criteria for diabetes mellitus, are currently given the diagnosis of impaired glucose tolerance (IGT).[37, 81] The main reason for separating overt diabetes from IGT and the criteria used for this separation are based on long-term follow-up studies of patients with IGT. Such individuals have an increased risk of developing overt diabetes over time compared with patients with normal glucose tolerance. In these individuals, IGT can be considered to be an early stage in the development of diabetes mellitus. However, during a 10-year follow-up period, fewer than 50% of patients with IGT developed overt diabetes, and some reverted to normal glucose tolerance.[81] Furthermore, patients with IGT do not appear to be at risk for microvascular and neuropathic complications of diabetes, although there appears to be some increased risk for cardiovascular disease in these patients. At the present time, it is not usually warranted to diagnosis IGT because treatment is not currently recommended. However, as more is learned about the relationship between the metabolic abnormality of diabetes and its complications, indications for the diagnosis and treatment of patients with this more subtle abnormality of glucose metabolism may be developed.

Gestational Diabetes Mellitus

Abnormalities of glucose metabolism that appear for the first time during pregnancy establish a diagnosis of gestational diabetes mellitus (GDM). Aggressive detection and intervention for even mild abnormalities of glucose metabolism are warranted during pregnancy because of the increased risk for perinatal morbidity and mortality as well as for fetal loss in patients with GDM.[75] Gestational DM is diagnosed using an oral glucose tolerance test, during which two or more values meet or exceed the following: fasting venous plasma glucose, 105 mg/dL (5.8 mmol/L); 1-hour value, 190 mg/dL (10.6 mmol/L); 2-hour value, 165 mg/dL (9.2 mmol/L); and 3-hour value, 145 mg/dL (8.0 mmol/L) (see also Table 1.2). Using these criteria, approximately 1 to 2% of all pregnancies will be complicated by GDM. Indications for performing a glucose tolerance test during pregnancy include previous complicated pregnancy, presence of glycosuria, family history of diabetes, obesity, high maternal age, and parity of 5 or more. In many clinics, all pregnancies are now screened for abnormal glucose tolerance. Although all but 2% of patients with GDM revert to normal glucose tolerance post partum, up to 60% of such women go on to develop overt diabetes during long-term follow-up, particularly those with obesity and GDM.[85] Intensive management of hyperglycemia in these patients and careful pregnancy monitoring can markedly reduce the associated perinatal morbidity and mortality.[24, 60, 106]

EPIDEMIOLOGY

The overall prevalence of diabetes mellitus in the United States has been estimated to be between 2 and 3% of the population. However, the prevalence of diabetes varies considerably with age.[9, 46, 82] About 10% of persons older than age 64 years have overt diabetes, whereas only about 0.8% of persons younger than age 45 years have this disease. The vast majority of patients with diabetes mellitus have type 2 DM. Type 1 DM represents 5 to 10% of the total diabetic population. Estimated incidence rates are approximately 29,000 new cases of type 1 DM per year in the United States and 625,000 cases of type 2 DM per year. The incidence of new cases of diabetes is more than 10 times greater in people older than age 64 than in people younger than age 45. There is no influence of sex on the occurrence of type 1 DM, but females have about a 40% greater risk of developing type 2 DM than males. The prevalence of type 2 DM is highest in several Native American populations, and it is also higher in Hispanics than in other groups of European origin. Obesity is associated with a threefold increased risk for the development of type 2 DM and a twofold increased risk for the development for GDM.[14, 58]

Patients with diabetes mellitus have an increased mortality rate compared with nondiabetics.[82] It has been estimated that 11 to 12% of diabetics older than age 64 die each year.[46] It has also been estimated that at the time of diagnosis, a person with diabetes has about one-third less life expectancy than a nondiabetic of the same age. Excess mortality related to diabetes has been estimated to be twofold to threefold for people older than age 40 and as high as 11-fold for diabetics younger than age 15. Renal disease is the major cause of death among patients with type 1 DM, whereas cardiovascular disease is by far the major cause of death in patients with type 2 DM. Diabetes is associated with increased risk for adverse outcomes of pregnancy, cerebrovascular disease, coronary heart disease, peripheral vascular disease, end-stage renal disease, and neuropathy.

PATHOPHYSIOLOGY OF GLUCOSE REGULATION

Normal Glucose Regulation

Interpretation of alterations of glucose regulation requires an understanding of the relationship between pancreatic islet hormones and circulating glucose levels. This relationship can be described by a closed-loop feedback system (Fig. 1.1). The glucose level is an important regulator of insulin and glucagon secretion. Glucose directly affects the secretion of both hormones and also serves to modulate the effects of a variety of neural, hormonal, and other substrate influences on these important islet hormones.[26] Insulin and glucagon, in turn, control glucose production by the liver. Insulin also affects glucose disposal by some tissues, such as fat and muscle, but other tissues, most

notably the brain, do not depend on insulin to regulate glucose uptake.

The key feature of this feedback system is that in the presence of a responsive islet secretory mechanism, any factor affecting glucose production or used to cause an increase in glucose level will result in a compensatory increase of insulin secretion and decrease in glucagon secretion. Such changes will tend to counterbalance the hyperglycemic influence, resulting in maintenance of plasma glucose at a near-normal level. For this reason, conditions associated with insulin resistance, such as uncomplicated obesity, result in hyperinsulinemia but relatively normal glucose regulation.

Glucose Intolerance

Glucose tolerance is determined primarily by the rate of glucose use after glucose ingestion. Therefore, the major emphasis in understanding the pathophysiology of glucose intolerance has been on factors affecting glucose storage and metabolism by tissues. Because insulin is a key regulator of glucose use, much work has focused on the question of inadequate supply of insulin to peripheral tissues (i.e., decreased

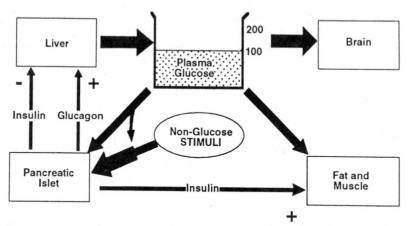

■ **Figure 1.1** A model for the normal steady-state regulation of the plasma glucose level. Plasma glucose has direct effects on the pancreas to modulate insulin and glucagon secretion and interacts with nonglucose stimuli to modify alpha-cell and beta-cell responses to these stimuli. During hyperglycemia, insulin secretion is increased and glucagon secretion is reduced. When hypoglycemia prevails, glucagon secretion is enhanced and insulin secretion is diminished. Glucagon stimulates hepatic glucose production. Insulin inhibits glucose release by the liver and stimulates glucose use in insulin-sensitive tissues. Glucose uptake by the brain is insulin independent, but in the peripheral tissues, glucose uptake by fat and muscle is enhanced by insulin. Any change in hormone or substrate concentration or glucose use will be modulated by the loop so that glucose use and production remain balanced. The plasma glucose level at which this occurs is determined by the efficiency with which the peripheral tissues take up glucose, the rate of hepatic glucose production, and islet alpha-cell and beta-cell responsiveness to glucose. (Adapted from Porte D Jr. B-cells in type II diabetes mellitus. Diabetes 1991; 40:166–180.)

insulin secretion) versus tissue insensitivity to insulin action. The mechanisms underlying glucose intolerance have been particularly well studied in normal aging.

A number of studies have clearly established that the effect of insulin on glucose use is impaired in healthy, nondiabetic elderly persons compared with young controls. Similarly, a defect in insulin-mediated suppression of hepatic glucose production has been described.[38] Because measurements of insulin binding to cells have generally revealed no defect in elderly persons, the insulin resistance observed has been ascribed to a defect in the cellular effects of insulin action beyond the insulin receptor. One potential site of such a defect is the glucose transport system, because there is evidence of diminished insulin-stimulated glucose transport in isolated adipocytes from elderly subjects compared with young controls.[39]

Impaired insulin secretion in aging has also been found. Studies in experimental animals have clearly demonstrated an age-related impairment of beta-cell function.[19, 97, 98] The problem has been that insulin levels during oral glucose tolerance tests tend to be relatively normal in elderly humans.[30] Interpretation of such responses is difficult because of differences of glucose levels during the test. Interpretation of plasma insulin levels in the elderly is also complicated by an apparent age-related decrease in the clearance rate of insulin from the circulation.[40, 76, 99] Other insulin resistance states, such as obesity or glucocorticoid excess, are accompanied by an adaptive hyperinsulinemia that appears to be in part the result of enhanced beta-cell sensitivity to glucose.[7, 8] In contrast, elderly subjects with insulin resistance appear to have diminished beta-cell sensitivity to glucose.[20] When matched for similar degrees of insulin sensitivity, the beta-cell abnormality becomes easier to identify.[57] Thus, a lack of beta-cell adaptation to the increased insulin need from insulin resistance also plays an important role in the age-related deterioration of glucose tolerance. Reduced responsiveness to dietary carbohydrate may play a role in this phenomenon.[21]

As summarized in Table 1.4, a number of factors can contribute to glucose intolerance by affecting insulin secretion or tissue sensitivity to insulin. Damage to pancreatic beta-cells or the presence of inhibitors of insulin secretion can result in impaired insulin secretion and hyperglycemia. A period of reduced carbohydrate intake in the diet or a reduced responsiveness to dietary carbohydrate can also result

TABLE 1.4 POTENTIAL MECHANISMS FOR GLUCOSE INTOLERANCE

Decreased insulin secretion
  Beta-cell damage or dysfunction
  Low carbohydrate diet
  Starvation
  Inhibitor of insulin release
    Catecholamines
    Somatostatin
    ? Other
Resistance to insulin action
  Aging
  Obesity
  Decreased physical activity
  Starvation
  Stress hormones
  Decreased insulin secretion

in impaired insulin secretion and contribute to carbohydrate intolerance.

A number of environmental factors can contribute to insulin resistance and glucose intolerance. Increased adiposity can be a factor, because there is a close association between adiposity and insulin resistance.[14, 87] Conversely, starvation and low carbohydrate diets can cause insulin resistance and may play a role in the carbohydrate intolerance of some subjects. Diminished physical activity is also associated with insulin resistance. Insulin resistance can result from the release of catabolic hormones such as the catecholamines and glucocorticoids during stressful illness. Finally, the ability of insulin treatment to improve insulin sensitivity in diabetes[42] suggests that diminished insulin secretion per se is also a cause of insulin resistance.

Type 2 Diabetes Mellitus

The presence of hyperglycemia in the fasting state is a characteristic feature of type 2 DM and is currently a major diagnostic criterion for the presence of this disease.[81] In contrast to glucose intolerance, in which inefficient peripheral glucose use seems to be important, the major contributing factor to hyperglycemia in the fasting state appears to be increased glucose production. The close positive correlation between the fasting plasma glucose level and the basal rate of hepatic glucose production in patients with type 2 DM is illustrated in Figure 1.2.[10] Further support for the importance of the rate of glucose production as a determinant of fasting hyperglycemia in type 2 DM comes from studies demonstrating that various regimens for type 2 DM that result in a fall in the

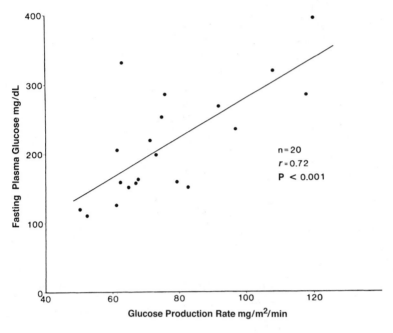

■ **Figure 1.2** Correlation between fasting plasma glucose and glucose production rate in 20 patients with untreated type 2 diabetes. Despite the suppressive effect of hyperglycemia per se on glucose production, those patients with the highest glucose levels had the highest production rates. (From Best JD, Judzewitsch RG, Pfeifer MA, et al. The effect of chronic sulfonylurea therapy on hepatic glucose production in diabetes. Diabetes 1982; 31:333–338.)

fasting plasma glucose level are associated with a concomitant reduction in glucose production.[10, 16, 63, 107] Furthermore, the degree of fall of the fasting glucose level has correlated with the magnitude of the fall of the glucose production rate.[10, 63, 107]

The mechanism for increased glucose production rates in type 2 DM has received considerable attention. Altered regulation of glucagon secretion by glucose level has been demonstrated in patients with type 2 DM and may contribute to enhanced glucose production.[88, 125] A role for increased mobilization of free fatty acids from fat tissue to stimulate glucose production in type 2 DM has been suggested by the close relationship between free fatty acid levels, lipid oxidation rate, and basal glucose production in Pima Indians with type 2 DM.[15] However, the major emphasis in studies of regulation of glucose production in type 2 DM has focused on the roles of impaired insulin secretion and diminished hepatic sensitivity to insulin.

Impaired pancreatic beta-cell sensitivity to glucose is characteristic of type 2 DM and is an important contributing factor to the increased glucose production and fasting hyperglycemia in this disease. Although some aspects of insulin secretion appear to be maintained well in these patients, the direct effect of intravenous glucose to stimulate insulin secretion is markedly impaired in patients with fasting hyperglycemia.[56, 92] In addition, there is a marked impairment of the role of glucose to

potentiate insulin secretory responses to a variety of nonglucose signals that are important in the maintenance of basal insulin secretion and in the insulin secretory response to a meal. This impairment has been demonstrated by studying the dose-response relationship between glucose level and the insulin secretory response to nonglucose secretagogues.[125] As illustrated in Figure 1.3, patients with type 2 DM have lower insulin responses to arginine than normal subjects at any matched glucose level. Mathematical analysis of these dose-response curves has demonstrated a defect in responsiveness to maximal glucose levels, suggesting that impaired beta-cell secretory capacity is characteristic of type 2 DM.[125]

Several studies have also addressed the role of decreased sensitivity of the liver to insulin's suppressive effect on glucose production in type 2 DM. Hyperinsulinemic glucose clamp studies have demonstrated a shift to the right of the dose-response curve for suppression of glucose production by insulin in patients with type 2 DM, but full suppression of glucose production occurs at high insulin levels.[15, 63] Such a decrease of hepatic sensitivity to insulin would tend to lead to an increased rate of glucose production. Because of the feedback loop between plasma glucose level and beta-cell function, increased glucose production, leading to an increased plasma glucose level, would normally result in increased insulin secretion, which would tend to overcome the hepatic insensitivity. However, because patients with type 2 DM have impaired beta-cell function, they cannot compensate normally for increased insulin resistance. As a result of beta-cell insensitivity to glucose, the plasma glucose level may have to increase considerably to augment insulin secretion sufficiently to compensate for the insulin resistance present. Thus, in type 2 DM, the plasma glucose level and the rate of glucose production will be determined by the degree of impaired beta-cell function and the degree of hepatic insensitivity to insulin. An understanding of this interaction between impaired beta-cell function and insulin resistance in type 2 DM is important as one considers therapeutic options for patients that may affect one or both of these important factors contributing to the degree of hyperglycemia.[56]

Type 1 Diabetes Mellitus

Type 1 DM is characterized by destruction of pancreatic beta-cells and severe insulin deficiency. In long-standing type 1 DM, not only is basal insulin secretion lower than normal, but insulin secretory responses to stimuli are virtually absent. This severe deficiency of insulin responses to all stimuli in type 1 DM contrasts with type 2 DM, in which there is some preservation of insulin secretion. Although pancreatic beta-cells in patients with long-standing type 1 DM respond poorly to all stimuli, the situation in the prediabetic period or during remission ("honeymoon phase") appears to be different. As the beta-cells deteriorate during the 2 to 5 years before the onset of overt hyperglycemia, the insulin secretory response to glucose declines, particularly the first-phase, glucose-induced insulin response, which becomes nonexistent.[34, 111, 112] However, some small amount of endogenous insulin secretion is often present for years after the diagnosis of overt type 1 DM.

Considerable attention has been given to methods of preserving beta-cell function in newly diagnosed patients with type 1 DM. For example, strict glycemic control has been reported to improve beta-cell function[71] and to increase the frequency and duration of remissions[77] as compared with conventional treatment. The use of immunosuppressive therapy, such as cyclosporine at the time of diagnosis, may also increase the frequency of remissions in type 1 DM, but such responses were limited,[36] and subsequent studies with other general suppressants have been disappointing.[89]

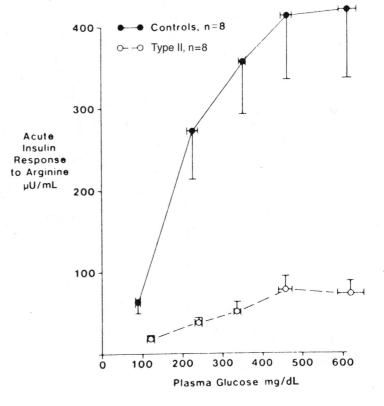

■ **Figure 1.3** A comparison of the acute insulin responses to arginine (5 g intravenous bolus) at five plasma glucose levels in eight patients with type 2 diabetes and in eight control subjects. The insulin responses to arginine were greater in the control group than in the diabetic group at all matched glucose levels ($P < 0.001$ at all levels). Data are mean ± SEM. (From Ward WK, Bolgiano DC, McKnight B, et al. Diminished B cell secretory capacity in patients with noninsulin-dependent diabetes mellitus. J Clin Invest 1984; 74:1318–1328.)

Thus, there is no therapy to prevent ultimate development of type 1 DM at present.

Secretion of glucagon is also abnormal in type 1 DM. Basal levels are particularly high during ketoacidosis or in patients with very poorly controlled disease. When tested with arginine, these subjects have increased glucagon levels.[91] When such patients are injected with glucose, there is impaired suppression of the elevated glucagon level. Insulin treatment will usually minimize the abnormality and restore basal glucagon concentration to the normal range.

If sufficient insulin is given to produce hypoglycemia, the normal glucagon elevation to this hypoglycemic stimulus is not observed in patients with type 1 DM. Thus, glucose is perceived poorly when it is elevated and not at all when it is lowered by insulin, whereas nonglucose stimuli such as arginine produce super-normal glucagon responses. During mixed meal feeding, the usual balance between stimulatory and inhibitory forces in normal subjects is converted into a hyperglucagonemic response in the patient with type 1 DM. Thus, glucagon levels are often inappropriately high for the metabolic state and contribute significantly to hyperglycemia in type 1 DM.

Elevations of other counterregulatory hormones, such as epinephrine, norepinephrine, cortisol, and growth hormone, have also been reported in type 1 DM patients at the time of diagnosis and during ketoacidosis or periods of poor metabolic control. Because all these hormones are elevated during stress states and are important to stress hyperglycemia, they must have a role in the hyperglycemia and metabolic abnormalities found in type 1 DM. Because uncontrolled diabetes leads to glycosuria and volume depletion, which results in baroreceptor-mediated activation of the sympathetic nervous system, at least some of the neuroendocrine hormone abnormalities in type 1 DM may be secondary to the insulin deficiency. A vicious circle continues their stimulation and maintains the metabolic abnormality. However, even during periods of exceedingly good diabetes control, subtle abnormalities of growth hormone and glucagon secretion may remain. Because the normal response to these stress hormones is hyperglycemia, which then feeds back to the normal pancreatic islet to stimulate insulin secretion in a modulatory way, the inability to respond with an increase in insulin also exaggerates the hyperglycemic response to stress in the patient with type 1 DM.

LONG-TERM MANAGEMENT OF DIABETES
General Principles

Long-term treatment of diabetes has been generally directed toward control of the glucose level in the hope of preventing or reversing the microvascular, atherosclerotic, and neuropathic changes found in diabetes mellitus.[109] The Diabetes Complications and Control Trial (DCCT)[33] showed that intensified insulin treatment of type 1 DM was capable of improving metabolic control, reducing microvascular complications of the eye and kidney, and reducing the progression of neuropathy. Macrovascular disease was reduced, but this was not statistically significant in this young, still relatively low-risk population. Side effects were an increased risk of hypoglycemia and weight gain. However, it is still not clear whether this goal can be achieved in ordinary clinical practice. As a result of this trial, there is general agreement that treatment of overt diabetes should therefore be directed toward control of the measurable metabolic abnormalities to normalize fat, protein, and carbohydrate metabolism. The physician usually sets two goals in relation to the known metabolic effects of relative or absolute insulin deficiency present in overt diabetes: (1) control of excessive fatty acid mobilization and oxidation (i.e., treatment and prevention of ketoacidosis); and (2) control of excessive protein catabolism and muscle wasting, carbohydrate wastage, and urinary caloric loss (symptomatic hyperglycemia). After these goals have been reached, the patient is asymptomatic, but often still has hyperglycemia. Recommendations to attempt to achieve normal glucose homeostasis are based largely on two major intensified treatment trials: the DCCT[33] and the Stockholm trials,[100] of type 1 DM, which have been augmented by a similar trial in type 2 diabetes patients in Japan.[86]

Dietary Therapy

Diet interventions are an essential part of all therapeutic programs for diabetes. However, the focus of diet treatment may be different in types 1 and 2 DM.[124] Because the fundamental physiologic abnormality in diabetes is the inability to store calories properly for later use, dietary therapy should stress caloric control and regularity. In general, sufficient calories should be provided to achieve and maintain ideal body weight (in children and adolescents, this includes normal growth and development). Thus, patients with type 1 DM, who are often malnourished and underweight, must be provided with additional calories to restore weight. Patients with type 2 DM, who are often obese, must be encouraged to restrict calories to lose excess weight.

Although major emphasis in the past had been placed on the proportion of carbohydrate, fat, and protein calories of the diet, many studies suggest that this proportional distribution is not very important to carbohydrate metabolism. In fact, clinicians over the years have prescribed diets varying from 10 to 65% carbohydrate, and all have claimed therapeutic successes. As far as glucose control is concerned, the percent carbohydrate content of the diet does not usually seem to have much influence on hyperglycemia and glycosuria, provided that calories remain constant and caloric distribution is unchanged.[84] Thus, calories rather than carbohydrate content per se appear to be most crucial. In view of the desire of many to use low animal-fat and low cholesterol diets in the hope of preventing atherosclerosis, the American Diabetes Association recommends a relatively low-fat, high-carbohydrate diet (50 to 60% carbohydrate, 30% fat).[2]

Having decided on the total caloric content, distribution, and type of diet to be prescribed, the physician is faced with the necessity of educating the patient to achieve these therapeutic goals. The further the prescribed diet deviates from the average American diet, the greater the need for precise and careful dietary instruction. Therefore, the time spent in education should be proportional to the complexity of the diet. In general, it is best to work closely with a nutritionist or educator who will implement the plan. Dietary goals and emphasis are generally different for insulin treated and non–insulin treated patients, reflecting the metabolic differences of the two clinical types of diabetes.

Patients with type 1 DM are generally lean and quite active. Because there is little tendency to obesity, caloric restriction is less usually indicated. However, the DCCT experience indicates that a careful matching of insulin treatment to metabolic need is necessary during intensified insulin treatment regimens that seem to increase the risk of excess weight gain.[124] Thus, the major focus must be to match caloric intake to the timing and quantity of exercise, insulin, and food calories. A broad range of foods are usually suitable to maintaining weight and nutrition; however, a knowledge of caloric values is necessary to maintain the same caloric equivalence of meals taken at the same time each day. Some knowledge of the glycemic response to individual foods may also be helpful, because this response may vary considerably among foods similar in caloric and carbohydrate content.[3] Because of the long-acting insulin preparations often used, most patients will require three meals per day and an evening snack. In children, the number of meals may be increased to six. Caloric values of foods can be learned by weighing foods or using the food exchange system developed by the American Diabetes Association. The system was devised to simplify dietary prescription by segregating foods into exchange lists, each food group on the list containing about the same amount of carbohydrate, protein, and fat as any other food on the list. It allows for reasonable variety in the meals and yet does not require the accurate weighing of food before preparation, although it is still essential for the patient to be aware of the caloric value of foods. Frequent glucose monitoring will be necessary the more one attempts to normalize glucose levels.

In most patients with type 2 DM, obesity is the major problem; therefore, caloric control should be instituted. Again, a balanced diet is explained and provided, but the total number of calories is reduced. Because caloric restriction reduces the ability to respond to sudden nutrient ingestion, it is important that dietary regulation is instituted in such patients and that intermittent periods of fasting and feasting are avoided as the obese diabetic patient attempts to regulate body weight. Because this group of patients may respond to caloric restriction alone with significant improvement in glycosuria and hyperglycemia, insulin and oral therapeutic agents are not given until the effectiveness of dietary control can be evaluated. At the present time, it is our practice to instruct patients in the caloric value of foods, to prescribe total caloric levels to be adhered to by each patient, and to attempt to achieve this without a complex dietary program. Unfortunately, reduction of body weight is a goal that is difficult to achieve and even harder to maintain. Nevertheless, because caloric restriction with even modest weight reduction is often associated with marked improvement in carbohydrate metabolism, caloric restriction and weight loss should be a major focus for the patient with newly diagnosed disease.

Exercise

Exercise increases glucose use by a mechanism that does not depend on increased secretion of insulin. This increased use is balanced by an increased output of glucose by the liver in normal individuals. Therefore, plasma glucose levels are not changed. The mechanism for the compensation is not completely clear, but activation of the sympathetic nervous system to increase hepatic glucose output is important.[22, 48] Insulin release is suppressed in the normal individual by this activation, which allows the increase in hepatic glucose output to occur. In the insulin-treated diabetic patient, increased blood flow to the subcutaneous tissues during exercise has been shown to increase circulating insulin levels by mobilization of the injected depot.[62, 132] Under these conditions, hepatic glucose production is restrained and muscle glucose uptake accelerates even more, leading to a rather precipitous decline in plasma glucose and frank hypoglycemia. The risk of hypoglycemia can be minimized by reducing insulin in anticipation of exercise, by food ingestion immediately before the exercise,[80] or by instituting a plan that will include regular amounts of exercise at specified times. The patient with diabetes treated with diet or an oral agent has no subcutaneous exogenous insulin depot to mobilize, and sympathetic suppression of insulin secretion is intact. Therefore, hypoglycemia during exercise does not occur.

Chronic exercise training has been shown to increase tissue sensitivity to the effects of insulin on glucose metabolism in experimental animals[27, 78] and in humans.[45, 62] Exercise training is also associated with a decrease in plasma triglyceride concentration and an increase in high-density lipoprotein cholesterol levels,[49, 115] both of which tend to be associated with a decreased risk of macrovascular disease. These beneficial effects of exercise take some time to appear (1 to 2 weeks), but they may be lost very quickly (within days). Although exercise training is often part of the overall plan for diabetes treatment, beneficial metabolic effects of chronic exercise (i.e., blood glucose reduction) have not been clearly demonstrated.[51]

Patient Education and Glucose Monitoring

The insulin-treated patient with diabetes must substitute external control of diet and insulin, for which he or she is responsible, for internal control of insulin, which in the normal individual keeps plasma glucose levels relatively constant. Therefore, education in the physiology of normal metabolism and in the external controls

that will be prescribed by the physician is an essential part of the treatment program. In general, it is probably best to think of the diabetic patient as caring for his or her own disease with the advice and consultation of the physician rather than as a patient for whom all therapeutic decisions are made by the physician. The patient should be aware of the effects of diet and exercise on metabolic control and be aware of methods of measuring the degree of metabolic control as reflected in the urine and blood. In particular, modern management of diabetes requires that most patients become familiar with methods for doing estimation of blood glucose in the home. The frequency with which such measurements are made depends on the complexity of the treatment regimen. The patient also should be able to make adjustments in the treatment program, depending on his or her physiologic and pathophysiologic state as it changes from day to day. Much of this information can be imparted through formal classwork, but the physician should use the routine clinic visit for continuing education of the diabetic patient. In general, it is preferable for the formal education programs to be coordinated in a community or area so that there may be interaction between the patient, other people with diabetes, and the instructor. There is a growing tendency for this work to be done by a team of allied health professionals as part of a teaching unit.

Sulfonylureas

Until the past few years, sulfonylureas were the mainstay of the oral drugs available in the United States for treatment of hyperglycemia in type 2 DM. They are derivatives of sulfur-containing antibiotics, with a sulfonylurea radical as the active site, that are ineffective as antimicrobial agents. Although the potency, metabolism, and side effects of each of the sulfonylureas differ, their major mechanism of action appears to be the same. Potential advantages of these drugs (compared with the use of insulin) include the ease with which they are administered and the low incidence of adverse side effects. The two major side effects are a low risk of hypoglycemia, when used appropriately, and a tendency for weight gain during treatment, particularly when compared with metformin.

When these oral agents first became available, there was much hope that their use in patients with mild, overt type 2 DM would improve longevity by inhibiting progression of atherosclerosis, microvascular disease, and neuropathy. However, the report of the University Group Diabetes Program (UGDP) indicated that patients with impaired glucose tolerance or mild hyperglycemia treated with tolbutamide for 8 years had a higher, rather than lower, incidence of death from cardiovascular disease than did untreated control patients.[121] Although other investigators have reported net benefits from these drugs,[66] their observations have been less carefully controlled and have been made in different types of patients. The UGDP report has created a persistent controversy concerning not only the use of tolbutamide, but also the use of other sulfonylureas. We do not yet know to what extent the long-range advantages of other sulfonylureas outweigh their disadvantages. Therefore, when deciding on treatment, the patient should share in the decision, if possible, and be aware of the inherent risks of each form of treatment.

MECHANISMS OF ACTION

In general, it appears that the mechanism of action of all sulfonylurea drugs is similar. The presence of responsive islets is necessary for these compounds to lower plasma glucose, and all have been shown to increase the secretion of insulin.[90] The mechanism by which sulfonylureas increase insulin release is related to a specific class of protein molecules that bind adenosine triphosphate (ATP) and combine with specific K^+ channels to regulate K^+ conductance as inward rectifiers. The combination is called a K-ATP channel. The K-ATP channels normally are open until ATP levels increase and adenosine diphosphate (ADP) levels decrease during glucose metabolism, thus leading to a reduced K^+ conductance and depolarization of the beta-cell. This in turn activates voltage sensitive Ca^{2+} channels that permit Ca^{2+}

entry to trigger insulin secretion. The ATP binding protein also binds sulfonylurea drugs and closes the K^+ channel through an unknown mechanism. The net result is the same as glucose-membrane depolarization and activation of the beta-cell secretory mechanism.[26]

Although enhanced pancreatic beta-cell function is the primary mechanism of action, under certain circumstances it is possible to demonstrate some increase in the sensitivity of peripheral tissues and liver to the effects of insulin during sulfonylurea administration. Therefore, some of the plasma glucose lowering may also be related to an improvement of insulin action. However, this is most likely caused by the increase in insulin secretion.

CLINICAL PHARMACOLOGY

There are major differences in the potency, rates of absorption, degradation, and methods of excretion of the sulfonylureas. As a result, their daily dosage and duration of action differ considerably[65] (Table 1.5). Tolbutamide, glyburide, and glipizide are metabolized by the liver to inert products. Tolazamide and acetohexamide are metabolized to active products, which are excreted by the kidney. Chlorpropamide is metabolized very slowly by the liver, so urine excretion plays a prominent role in its elimination. Because chlorpropamide is dependent on renal excretion for the termination of its activity, it is contraindicated for individuals with significantly reduced renal function. The newer agents, glyburide, glipizide, and glimepiride, are about 20 to 100 times more potent than the older sulfonylurea drugs; however, a maximally effective dose produces about the same glucose lowering.

The potency or efficacy of any sulfonylurea may be altered by other drugs. One of the most common effects reported consists of augmentation of the hypoglycemic effect of the sulfo-

TABLE 1.5 SULFONYLUREA DRUGS

Generic Name	Brand Name	Daily Dosage Range (mg)	Approx. Duration of Action (hr)
Tolbutamide	Orinase	500–3000	6–12
Chlorpropamide	Diabinese	100–750	40–72
Acetohexamide	Dymelor	250–1250	12–18
Tolazamide	Tolinase	100–1000	12–16
Glyburide	DiaBeta, Micronase	2.5–20	24
Glipizide	Glucotrol	5–40	8–12
Glimepiride	Amaryl	1–8	24

nylureas. Hypoglycemia may be reported more frequently because it is clinically obvious and important, whereas a diminution in the effect of the agent and hyperglycemia may erroneously be attributed to some other factor. Drugs such as probenecid, salicylate, coumadin, alcohol, sulfisoxazole, and monoamine oxidase inhibitors have been implicated in severe hypoglycemia associated with sulfonylurea administration.[67, 105] It is likely that these compounds either decrease sulfonylurea excretion or reduce its binding to plasma proteins. Because of potentially prolonged hypoglycemic activity of sulfonylureas in these clinical settings, observation and treatment may be required for more than 24 hours. Compounds that may antagonize the hypoglycemic action of sulfonylureas include thiazides, corticosteroids, chloramphenicol, furosemide, oral contraceptives, and propranolol.

TOXICITY

Sulfonylureas may have a variety of side effects independent of their hypoglycemic properties. The magnitude of these effects may vary considerably depending on the specific drug, but, in general, differences in their effects are quantitative and not qualitative.

Hypoglycemia is rare with moderate doses of sulfonylureas given to patients who are in relatively good health and who do not have significant impairment of renal or liver function.[105] However, sulfonylurea-induced hypoglycemia may occur without any other drug therapy, generally the result of dosages that are clinically inappropriate. Thus, more than 90% of reported episodes of severe sulfonylurea-induced hypoglycemia have occurred in acutely or chronically starved patients or in patients who have demonstrable hepatic or renal impairment or both. This is often compounded by the intake of alcohol, which by itself causes hypoglycemia in the starved individual.

Weight gain has usually been found in carefully controlled clinical trials whether used alone or in conjunction with other oral agents. Although usually modest, it can be severe (10 kg or more). The mechanisms are unknown, but may relate to subclinical hypoglycemia, a "side effect" of better metabolic control, or the anabolic properties of the extra secreted insulin.[119]

Some patients treated with chlorpropamide have developed symptomatic hyponatremia and water intoxication.[53] Chlorpropamide appears to have an effect on renal tubules similar to that of antidiuretic hormone and to increase release of the hormone. No other sulfonylurea has been reported to significantly potentiate antidiuretic hormone secretion or action. A reaction to alcohol similar to that seen after disulfiram treatment, with a clinical syndrome of headache, flushing, and tachycardia, may be seen in patients treated with a sulfonylurea, almost exclusively chlorpropamide.[94] Intestinal symptoms such as anorexia, nausea, vomiting, diarrhea, and abdominal pain are observed in about 5% of patients treated with sulfonylureas, but this incidence is not much higher than that associated with placebo ingestion.

Hepatic reactions to these drugs are less frequent, but mild to severe cholestatic jaundice has been reported. The greater the hypoglycemic potency of the drug, the more likely it is to cause liver impairment. This toxic effect is dose related, especially with chlorpropamide. Hepatocellular damage has been suggested at times, but liver biopsies usually have shown only canalicular bile stasis, similar to that reported for chlorpromazine. Maculopapular skin eruptions have been reported often with pruritus and are probably symptoms of allergic hypersensitivity. Hematologic toxicity has been reported rarely; it includes agranulocytosis and pancytopenia.

DOSAGE AND PRACTICAL USE

The choice of sulfonylurea depends on its potency, biologic half-life, cost, and side effects. In a diabetic patient taking insulin, it is not possible to predict with certainty whether a sulfonylurea can be used satisfactorily as a substitute. In general, individuals who have had episodes of ketoacidosis or who use more than 40 U of insulin per day, unless there is significant obesity, are unlikely to be responsive to sulfonylureas. The dosage used is that necessary to maintain blood sugar at the desired level up to the maximum recommended for each compound. The incidence of secondary failures is not established but appears to be about 5% per year. Patients who have failed on one sulfonylurea drug may be tried on another. However, the majority of such patients will require the addition of another oral agent or insulin therapy to achieve treatment goals.[65] Sulfonylureas are rarely used for pregnant women in the United States, but in some investigations in Scotland and South Africa, no ill effects were reported. During elective surgery, minor infections, and other minor illnesses, it is not necessary to substitute insulin unless ketosis appears. During emergency surgery or severe infections, it is best to substitute insulin. Because of reports of prolonged hypoglycemia in some diabetic patients using chlorprop-amide, this drug is less frequently used in older patients.

Metformin

Available as a second oral drug since the 1960s in Europe and Canada, metformin was marketed as Glucophage in 1996 in the United States.[5] This agent does not stimulate insulin secretion. Its mechanism of action is unknown. It is chemically a biguanide and had been developed to accelerate glucose use independent of insulin. The first of this class, phenformin, was removed from the market because of an increase in the frequency of lactic acidosis. Although controversial, worldwide experience has not demonstrated a significant risk of lactic acidosis with metformin, although a rare case has occurred in association with impaired renal function. Early studies suggested an improvement in peripheral insulin action and increased glucose use,[4] but more recent studies show reduction of hepatic glucose production as the predominant effect of treatment.[32] Metformin can be used alone or in combination with a sulfonylurea. It has been combined with insulin in patients with difficult-to-manage disease. Because of a reduced tendency for weight gain despite better metabolic control, its use in younger obese patients with normal renal function has been particularly attractive. The secondary failure rate is not well described, but it appears to be similar to sulfonylureas.[120] An improvement in the lipid profile and a lower plasma insulin are potential beneficial side effects of treatment.[65] The major side effects are gastrointestinal symptoms, including anorexia, nausea, and diarrhea, and a decrease in vitamin B_{12} levels. Because lactic acidosis is a theoretical possibility, the drug is contraindicated in patients with significant renal or cardiopulmonary disease. A rare case of pernicious anemia has been reported.

Acarbose

Released in Germany in the 1980s and approved in the United States in 1996 as Precose,[65] acarbose is an inhibitor of intestinal α-glucosidase. Its action is to impair the hydrolysis of sucrose and other disaccharides so that the absorption of their constituent monosaccharides is delayed. When acarbose is taken long-term, the normally restricted upper small intestinal location of the enzyme becomes more generalized to include the jejunum and even the ileum. Thus, eventually almost all the carbohydrate is absorbed in the small bowel, although some is fermented in the lower ileum and colon, leading to an increase in short-chain fatty acids and intestinal gas. Postprandial glucose tolerance is flattened and somewhat more prolonged. In clinical trials, the drug was also associated with a decline in fasting plasma glucose and a decrease in glycohemoglobin. At maximum therapeutic levels, it is about half as effective as sulfonylurea or metformin in reducing glycohemoglobin or mean plasma glucose.[25] It can be added to either of these other oral agents, leading to the possibility of double or even triple therapy. The major side effects, abdominal fullness, diarrhea, and flatulence, have limited its acceptability. It may be most appropriate in obese subjects early in the course of their diabetes. The greatest experience with its use has been in Germany, where it was developed.

Troglitazone

This most recently approved oral agent (1997) represents yet another class of therapeutic agents. It was marketed as Romozin in the United Kingdom, but was withdrawn because of hepatotoxicity. Discovered during routine screening of experimental animals for hypoglycemic agents, it represents the first of a class of chemicals called thiazolidinediones to be released as Rezulin. The mechanism of action appears to involve an increase in peripheral glucose use, which requires insulin; therefore, this class of drugs is often referred to as "insulin-sensitizing" agents. The insulin required can either be exogenous or endogenous. The associated increase in glucose uptake and decrease in hepatic glucose production leads to lower glucose values and lower endogenous insulin secretion.[52, 83, 116] Approved first only in insulin-treated patients, its use was associated with a reduction in insulin dose required for control, a decline in glucose level, or both.[35] This class of drugs has been shown to bind to a specific nuclear transcription factor called PPARγ (peroxisome proliferator activator receptor gamma), which changes gene expression. This particular receptor is found in highest quantities in adipose tissue and lesser amounts in liver and muscle. Therefore, the primary site(s) of action are not clear at present, i.e., why a primary adipocyte-acting drug would lower plasma glucose by decreasing hepatic glucose output and increasing muscle glucose uptake.[103] Other members of this class are under development. In late 1997 monotherapy and combination therapy with sulfonylurea agents was approved because they have different mechanisms of action. Because many patients with type 2 DM are insulin resistant, it is expected that this group of patients would be particularly appropriate for troglitazone treatment. While clinical trials have been limited, the drug appears to be as effective as sulfonylurea and metformin, but variably so. Recent reports indicate a significant incidence (2%) of abnormal liver enzymes and several cases of jaundice and hepatic failure. Monthly hepatic enzyme monitoring for 6 months after initiation of therapy is recommended.

The rapid development of new oral agents for the treatment of diabetes has entered an extremely complex and challenging era, with many possibilities for improving blood glucose control. The challenge will be to chose among them wisely and efficiently.

Insulin Treatment

Insulin secretion in the normal individual is regulated by the nature and amount of exogenous foodstuffs needed to maintain normal metabolism of ingested carbohydrate, fat, and protein. In contrast, the diabetic patient treated with insulin receives fixed doses of insulin to which he must match his food intake, because there will not be the normal peaks of insulin in association with food ingestion. Therefore, even with insulin therapy, diabetic patients are unable to store foodstuffs as efficiently as a normal individual who responds to a challenge by suddenly secreting insulin. Because exogenous insulin treatment is an inadequate physiologic replacement, the attainment of reasonable metabolic control requires an understanding of the properties of the various insulin preparations, the nature of the interaction of injected insulin with basic metabolic processes, and the potential complications of insulin therapy.

INSULIN PREPARATIONS

Many insulin products are now available, differing in manufacturer, species of origin, and duration of action after injection.[12] These preparations consist of recrystallized extracts of beef or pork pancreas or of synthetic products identical to human insulin. At the present time, all commercial insulins are chromatographed on Sephadex and are at least 99% pure. Because beef insulin has different antigenic properties, a number of manufacturers also prepare pure pork insulin. However, the increasing availability and declining cost of human insulin made by recombinant DNA technology or through a semisynthetic process have largely replaced animal insulins. Although the antigenicity of these products is much lower than previously available, insulin antibodies are generally still developed during therapy, even though human insulin is used.

Nearly all insulin preparations now contain 100 international units/mL (U100). These preparations can be thought of as being either short acting (Semilente or crystalline zinc), intermediate acting (Lente or NPH), or long acting (Ultralente). However, the action of the human insulin-Ultralente product is shorter than the comparable beef product. In practice, combinations of insulins of different duration of action are often administered as multiple injections to achieve the goals of the treatment program.

CLINICAL PHARMACOLOGY

Insulin injected subcutaneously must be absorbed into the bloodstream and distributed to insulin-sensitive tissues to be effective. Therefore, differences in the rates of absorption from different sites contribute to variations in response.[13] In general, all types of commercial insulin are stable, even when stored for moderate intervals at room temperature. Although it is desirable to keep insulin refrigerated to maintain full potency, during periods of traveling there is no appreciable loss of activity at room temperature—even up to a month. Insulin put into intravenous fluids, as is sometimes done during surgery, has caused problems, one of which is the binding of insulin to the intravenous tubing. As much as 50% of the insulin can bind to glass and plastic surfaces when the fluid contains no protein, but this occurs only at very low concentrations.[64]

A number of other factors determine responses to insulin. The larger the dose of any insulin, the longer is its duration of action, and the later is its maximal effect.[13] Therefore, in an insulin-resistant patient who requires more than 200 U of insulin per day, regular crystalline zinc insulin may be effective for as long as NPH or Lente insulin is in other patients. Important factors that are determinants of the insulin "requirement" are hormones that antagonize insulin action; insulin-resistant states, such as bacterial or viral infections; and the amount of circulating insulin antibodies. The catecholamines, estrogens, growth hormone, and corticosteroids induce insulin resistance. Therefore, with all other factors remaining equal, excess of any of these hormones increases the need for insulin. Certain physiologic and pathophysiologic states will have the same effect. The most important of these, obesity, induces insulin-resistance in proportion to the degree of adiposity and necessitates larger amounts of insulin for maintaining metabolic control. Chronic liver disease and uremia may also produce an insulin-resistant state.[87]

CLINICAL INSULIN USE

Research into insulin secretion using the C-peptide assay and the development of a variety of mechanical systems to infuse insulin have radically changed our understanding of the therapeutic use of insulin. The management of a patient with type 1 DM who has very little residual endogenous insulin secretion may be quite different from the insulin treatment of a patient with type 2 DM who failed to respond to diet or a sulfonylurea. However, the major goals for these patients are the same: (1) to give enough insulin to free the diabetic patient of symptoms of hyperglycemia and glycosuria; (2) to avoid hypoglycemia; and (3) to control the hyperglycemia as physiologically as possible in the hope of reducing the frequency and severity of the neural and microvascular complications. Conflict arises between these last two goals because as plasma glucose levels become more normal, hypoglycemia may become more frequent.

Type 1 Diabetes Mellitus. Patients with type 1 DM require replacement of basal insulin secretion and insulin responses to meal ingestion. Because about half of normal total insulin secretion is basal (i.e., not a response to nutrient stimulation), the use of one injection of insulin per day is rarely effective in type 1 DM. Therefore, we usually begin with two injections per day, each containing a mixture of short- and intermediate-acting insulin. The first injection is given before breakfast, and the second one is given before the evening meal.

With the availability of home self-monitoring of blood glucose, it is now possible to strive for normalization of the blood glucose level in the suitably motivated and educated patient.[114]

The key to such a regimen is to provide enough intermediate- to long-acting insulin to meet ongoing basal insulin needs. Increased insulin needs related to meals can then be met by multiple injections of short-acting insulin with frequent blood glucose monitoring to help determine frequency and dose of the injections. An alternative to this conventional, but intensive, multiple injection regimen is to use a portable infusion pump to administer insulin subcutaneously. Basal insulin needs can be met by a continuous infusion. Meal-related increases in insulin infusion rate can be programmed into these devices.

A number of studies have demonstrated the feasibility of achieving excellent metabolic control with either of these intensive regimens.[74, 102, 114] However, it must be emphasized that patient motivation is crucial to the success of such a program and that there are risks for significant hypoglycemia. Thus, patients must be carefully selected for participation.

Other routes of insulin may also be used. In the acutely decompensated diabetic or the postsurgical patient, insulin may be given by intravenous infusion to allow predictable maintenance of insulin levels. Diabetics with renal failure who are treated with peritoneal dialysis can often be managed well with intraperitoneal insulin.[1] This approach is actually more physiologic because insulin given this way enters predominantly via the portal system and reaches the liver before peripheral tissues.

Hypoglycemia continues to be a major concern in patients treated intensively with insulin.[28] Hypoglycemia may be a particular problem in diabetics with autonomic neuropathy who may not get the normal warning signals resulting from adrenergic activation.[17] In such patients, impaired cognition may be the first sign of a drop in glucose level. In recent years, it has become apparent that many patients develop a similar constellation of symptoms and lack of hypoglycemia awareness, but without significant clinical autonomic neuropathy. This constellation has been termed *hypoglycemia-associated autonomic failure* (HAAF) because it seems to be caused by hypoglycemia itself. Cryer and Gerich have shown that one episode of hypoglycemia leads to a reduced epinephrine, norepinephrine, growth hormone, and cortisol response to a second episode of hypoglycemia 24 hours later.[29] In patients with type 1 DM who do not have a normal glucagon response to insulin-induced hypoglycemia, this phenomenon can lead to reduced counterregulation and less awareness of the hypoglycemia. This feed-forward concept may explain why intensified diabetes control has been difficult to implement. On the other hand, if HAAF is a common contributor to the problem of hypoglycemia, attempts to minimize it should improve glycemic awareness and improve outcome.

Some patients have difficult-to-manage disease regardless of attempts by the physician to understand the problem. Experience has focused on a number of potential causes to explain the etiology of *brittle diabetes*. The following are some common findings: (1) severe insulin deficiency (total lack of C peptide secretion); (2) errors in management (a deficiency of patient education or knowledge); (3) intercurrent illness; (4) factors influencing the dynamics of insulin action (injection site, exercise, insulin antibodies; and (5) psychosocial factors that interfere with the maintenance of a diabetic regimen, such as conflicts with the treatment goal, anxiety about the disease, frustration, parental rebellion, and emotional stress. The latter has been emphasized by Schade.[104]

Type 2 Diabetes Mellitus. Insulin continues to be used often in the management of type 2 DM.[79] Many of these patients are either lean to begin with or are obese and have reached stable weight. Until recently, physicians had to choose between sulfonylurea drugs and insulin for these patients. We were more likely to use insulin in patients who were young and lean. In the obese patient and in the older patient, we are now more conservative in beginning nondietary treatment, and new drugs that can be added provide more possibilities. Insulin treatment in these patients may be simpler than in patients with type IDM because they have sufficient residual insulin secretion to prevent ketoacidosis. Therefore, one injection of intermediate-acting insulin may sometimes restore reasonable control of hyperglycemia. If hyperglycemia occurs in the morning after breakfast, short-acting insulin is added. If hyperglycemia is present on arising or if more than 30 U of insulin per day is needed, then a second long-lasting insulin dose is added in the evening. Because exercise and site of injection are important modifiers of insulin delivery in this group, we either adjust the dose of insulin on exercise days or add calories before exercise and advise the use of the abdominal site. Because many patients with type 2 DM are also obese, considerable resistance to insulin action may be present. To have a significant impact on diabetes management, such patients may require very large doses of insulin (1 to 2 U/kg/d) if used alone.

Summary of Diabetes Management

Despite major scientific advances in the past 50 years, there is insufficient knowledge of the basic etiology and pathogenesis of the long-term complications of diabetes. Therefore, treatment directed toward the vascular and neuropathic effects of the disease has been inadequate. Insulin treatment for severe insulin deficiency in patients with type 1 DM is obviously necessary. Deciding about treatment for milder carbohydrate abnormalities is more complex. Treatment of obese patients who have type 2 DM should begin with caloric restriction; an oral drug or insulin treatment should be started when there are indications that diet (caloric control) is not achieving control of the hyperglycemia. The choice of therapy between insulin and the oral antidiabetic agents in this group can be made only after the possible problems and benefits from all forms of therapy are considered and discussed with the patient. A long-term program must be developed. The recent availability of metformin, acarbose, and troglitazone provides many choices for therapy and many combinations whose usefulness will be important to define. Despite the limited information currently available about the precise relationships between degree of hyperglycemia and diabetes complications, a general goal for treatment is a glycosylated hemoglobin value within 1% of the upper limit of normal ($HbA_{1C} < 7.1$). This goal can be modified by a variety of factors, including patient preference, life expectancy, other coexisting illnesses, and the patient's ability to adhere to a prescribed regimen.

The therapy of carbohydrate intolerance remains a controversial issue. In view of the difficulties with insulin therapy and the potential hazards of the oral antidiabetic agents, many physicians treat such patients only with diet (caloric restriction). At the present time, we are not inclined to treat with pills or insulin a patient who does not have an abnormal fasting glucose. We will usually treat anyone with an elevated fasting plasma unless there is some specific contraindication. We are less inclined to be aggressive with older patients who have shortened life spans (<15 years) and more aggressive with younger ones.

MAJOR NONNEUROPATHIC COMPLICATIONS OF DIABETES

There are no specific pathologic findings associated with diabetes mellitus. However, degenerative changes occur in many organ systems and lead to considerable morbidity and mortality. The following pathophysiologic changes can be thought of as complications of the disease. Although they may not be solely caused by the direct effects of insulin deficiency (either relative or absolute) or hyperglycemia, older literature linked these complications directly to the degree of hyperglycemia,[96, 108, 110, 128] and the recent clinical trials strongly support this view.[109] These complications of diabetes appear to be produced by the interaction of other risk factors with hyperglycemia and insulin deficiency in diabetes mellitus in ways that are not well understood.

Macrovascular Disease—Arteriosclerosis

Arteriosclerosis involving the entire vascular system can be present. Findings in the larger arteries and coronary circulation are identical to those in nondiabetic subjects but seem to be more frequent and to occur at an earlier age in the diabetic population.[68] Thus, there appears to be no specific large vessel morphologic lesion related to diabetes. Cardiovascular lesions account for 75 to 80% of the total mortality in diabetes and have assumed great importance as the cause of premature death in this syndrome.[50] Coronary artery disease is the single most common cause of death in diabetics.[18] The degree of vascular disease does not appear to be proportional to the alterations in carbohydrate metabolism, but correlates best with the duration of the disease and the age of the patient.

Arteriolosclerosis is an entirely separate pathologic process that is prominent in diabetics but undistinguishable from that found in patients with essential hypertension. It appears as a concentric hyaline thickening of the arterioles, widening of the endothelium, and eventual encroachment on the vascular lumen by a plaque that stains with periodic acid–Schiff (PAS).[68] There is some evidence that this material is related to or resembles basement membrane, because it is PAS-positive and presumably contains glycoprotein. However, the exact nature of the deposit is unknown. The most prevalent site in the diabetic patient is the kidney, particularly if the individual has had clinical nephropathy, but other organs, including the pancreas, are frequently involved.

For reasons that are not completely clear, advanced vascular disease in the lower legs is common in diabetics and can be particularly severe, leading to gangrene or death of the affected extremity.[68] The concomitant neuropathy and loss of pain and touch sensation may explain the high frequency of lower-leg vascular complications seen in the diabetic population; however, there may be an interaction between capillary microangiopathy and arteriosclerosis that is also important.[70] Diabetics may develop atherosclerotic complications in the cerebral circulation and in the renal and mesenteric circulations, leading to occlusive disease and complications in these organs as well.

A major goal of diabetes management is prevention of gangrene by avoiding trauma and infection and by not restricting blood flow. The patient can accomplish this to some extent by keeping the feet clean; applying lanolin or some other bland ointment to hard, dry areas on the feet; wearing clean footwear; avoiding garters; and wearing only properly fitting shoes. The patient should also avoid undue exposure to cold and heat, trim the toenails carefully, insert a wedge of cotton under ingrowing toenails, remove calluses by soaking in warm water, rub off surplus skin with a coarse towel, avoid the use of adhesive on the skin, and treat associated dermatophytoses.

To attempt to influence the rate of development of atherosclerosis complications in diabetics, an effort should be made to reduce other risk factors for atherosclerosis.[6, 18] Weight reduction is instituted when there is obesity. Smoking should be omitted, and hypertension should be treated aggressively when present. Regular exercise of moderate degree is encouraged. Control of carbohydrate abnormalities is discussed earlier in this chapter. Hyperlipidemia should be considered and treated as necessary.

Kidney Disease

Two nephropathies occur almost exclusively in diabetes: nodular glomerulosclerosis and tubular nephrosis.[31] There are, in addition, several other renal lesions that are less specific for diabetes but that occur with increased frequency: diffuse glomerulosclerosis, atherosclerosis, arteriosclerosis, pyelonephritis, necrotizing papillitis, and acute tubular necrosis.

Renal disease may be expected clinically in

50% of all diabetics who survive more than 20 years. Diabetes is now the leading cause of end-stage renal disease in the United States.[18, 82] Consequently, the physician should measure creatinine clearance every 1 to 2 years in all diabetics and follow the serum creatinine level. The urine characteristically shows proteinuria, white blood cells, and granular casts. These alterations increase in intensity as the process becomes advanced, but may be detected early in the course of the disease using a sensitive immunoassay for urinary albumin.[123] Eventually, hypoalbuminemia with the nephrotic syndrome, nitrogen retention, and hypertension may be observed. The degree of these changes is an indication, at least in part, of the intensity of the glomerulosclerosis. As renal impairment becomes severe, a decrease in glycosuria may be noted. This is partly caused by the decrease in glomerular filtration and the relatively greater impairment of glomerular function than tubular function, permitting reabsorption of a greater proportion of the filtered glucose. This decrease in glycosuria may also occur because the degradation of insulin, which normally occurs to a significant extent in the kidneys, is reduced so that a given amount of insulin is more effective.

It is important to be sure that renal disease in patients who have only minimal hyperglycemia is really the result of diabetes rather than some primary renal condition. The physician should ascertain whether other evidence of microangiopathy is present and attempt to eliminate other nephropathies that might account for the renal changes under observation. Evidence for renal infection should be sought. It should be emphasized, however, that pyelonephritis is very commonly associated with diabetes and, indeed, often coexists with glomerulosclerosis. Occasionally, renal biopsy is indicated, because it is usually not difficult to establish the diagnosis when the tissue can be studied.

Unfortunately, the disease process tends to be progressive and irreversible once it has become advanced. Because a significant number (about 40%) of deaths in patients with type 1 DM can be related to renal failure after 20 to 30 years of diabetes, when many of the patients are still young, an increasing number of patients are referred for dialysis or renal transplantation. However, uremia increases the risk of serious atherosclerosis, even after dialysis or transplantation. Therefore, treatment with either modality has had a high complication rate, particularly in males.[131] Follow-up of the transplanted kidney has demonstrated evidence of asymptomatic vascular lesions within 2 to 3 years.[31, 72, 73]

Frequently, infection develops in the kidney or urinary tract or both. It is important to detect such developments promptly and to eliminate them. The infection intensifies the manifestations of the diabetes and may also eventually lead to significant impairment in kidney function. The most important considerations are to look for and correct obstructions, select the most appropriate antibiotic, and give it in sufficiently large doses to eliminate the infection completely. Catheterization should be avoided as much as possible. Carefully collected, clean, voided specimens can be used for immediate direct examination and urine cultures.

Necrotizing renal papillitis is a relatively rare form of acute pyelonephritis associated with severe infection, which produces ischemic necrosis of the renal papillae. It occurs in diabetics much more often than in nondiabetics. It is characterized by fever, hematuria, renal colic, and rapidly advancing azotemia. Characteristic pyelographic changes are observed, and sloughed portions of the renal papillae may be found in the urine. The bacteria involved should be identified, and treatment should be based on their drug sensitivity.

Acute tubular necrosis can occasionally occur as a complication of diabetic coma, usually when there are prolonged periods of hypotension and shock. Acute renal failure can also be precipitated in diabetic patients with elevated serum creatinine levels who receive injections of iodinated contrast material for diagnostic purposes.[122, 126] Thus, such diagnostic procedures should be performed only for clear indications, and these patients should be followed very carefully after the procedure for evidence of acute renal failure.

Because of the progressive nature of renal failure in diabetic nephropathy, preventative efforts are important. In addition to controlling the degree of hyperglycemia, meticulous control of coexisting hypertension is very important. In those patients with early nephropathy and increased albumin excretion, treatment with an angiotensin-converting enzyme inhibitor slows the rate of progression.

Eye Disease

RETINOPATHY

Changes in the retina of diabetics are common and among the most characteristic findings in patients with diabetes. Because of the opportunity for direct observation, the changes in the eyes may be followed more easily than those in the kidneys and other tissues. The pathologic retinal alterations may be classified as two types: (1) background retinopathy with edema, microaneurysms, exudates, and hemorrhages; and (2) retinitis proliferans.[61]

Microaneurysms tend to be among the earliest and most specific lesions in the retina. Minute aneurysmal dilation of the capillaries, arterioles, or occasionally the venules occurs. These aneurysms average 30 to 90 μm in diameter. The exact mechanism for their production is not known. Many hypotheses have been advanced to explain this lesion, including venous stasis, hyaline deposition, capillary basement membrane thickening, a disorder of polysaccharide metabolism, and loss of mural pericytes; none has been established as the sole etiologic mechanism. Such aneurysms may occasionally occur with conditions other than diabetes, such as malignant hypertension, pernicious anemia, obstruction of the central vein, sickle cell anemia, and hypercorticosteroidism (iatrogenic or endogenous). However, they tend to be much more numerous and to occur with much greater frequency in diabetes.

In time, the microaneurysms become more numerous. After they have been present for several months, they may even seem to be disappearing. This may be the result of rupture, hemorrhage, or leakage of plasma proteins. These hemorrhages are small, localized, blot- and dot-shaped lesions with well-defined, relatively deep margins, or they may be larger, more superficial, flame-shaped lesions. Eventually, the proteins are organized into deposits that consist chiefly of hyalinized material and lipids that stain heavily with PAS. The exudates are close to the microaneurysms, beginning on the vitreous side of the retina but eventually including all layers. Cotton-wool spots are sometimes visualized as white fluffy exudates even in the absence of hypertension. It has been suggested that these represent accumulation of axoplasmic debris as the result of interruption of axoplasmic transport by ischemia. Edema may be an important associated finding, particularly if the macula is involved. This causes a fuzzy or hazy appearance and is a result of an incompetent endothelial cell barrier.

Diabetic maculopathy is a condition in which severe edema or a plaque of hard exudate impairs macula function.[47] Usually there are associated microaneurysms and hemor-

rhage. It is difficult to see with the ophthalmoscope, but it can be suspected when a large number of surrounding hard exudates are seen or when a sudden deterioration of vision occurs without an obvious explanation. This lesion is almost exclusively found in patients with type 2 DM, often after less than 10 years of known duration of diabetes.[47] It can be diagnosed by fluorescein angiography and careful slit-lamp examination.

In about 25% of diabetics with retinopathy, a proliferative change occurs. This is observed as small vessels arising from the disk or elsewhere in the retina growing along the surface of the retina or into the vitreous. Usually such patients have microaneurysms, hemorrhages, and exudates, but it is not clear whether these are causative or associated lesions. Retinitis proliferans has been assumed to begin with retinal hemorrhage into the vitreous, although recent evidence suggests that vessel growth precedes such an event. Whatever the initial event, it is followed by an ingrowth of blood vessels and invasion with fibrous tissue. With contraction of the resulting scar tissue, separation of the retina and hemorrhage may occur. The hemorrhages and the neovascularization may occur anywhere in the retina, but tend to be more numerous in the vicinity of the optic disk. A decrease or total loss of vision may result.

The proliferative changes tend to be more frequent in patients with type 1 DM,[47] but this may be related to the length of time required for the changes in the retina to develop. On the average, retinitis proliferans is found 15 years from the time of the diagnosis in younger diabetics, compared with about 6 to 10 years in older diabetics. The prognosis for vision depends on the site of the new vessels. Eyes with new vessels on the disk have a 40% chance of losing vision in 1 year. Those with peripheral lesions do better, but this complication is the major cause of vision loss in diabetes. Although it is particularly likely to be associated with glomerulosclerosis and other chronic manifestations of diabetes, in one third of patients albuminuria and hypertension are absent. Retinitis proliferans is not absolutely specific for diabetes. It is found occasionally with retinal vein occlusion and sickle cell anemia.

The treatment of ocular complications of diabetes is a major therapeutic problem. Diabetic retinopathy now stands as the primary cause of new blindness in adults.[82] The development of photocoagulation therapy has had a dramatic effect on the treatment of diabetic retinopathy.[61, 69] The light energy of xenon, and more recently that of ruby or argon lasers, has been used to produce first a burn and then a scar in the retina by absorption of light energy by the retinal pigment epithelium. At first, photocoagulation was directed toward specific abnormal areas of neovascularization and suspected bleeding sites. Most recently, retinal lesions have not been treated alone, but instead, 300 to 1100 small retinal scars have been made throughout the retina. The mechanism by which such scars should reduce proliferative retinopathy is unknown, but it has been hypothesized to be related to a reduction in retinal oxygen demand to reduce new vessel growth. Results from double blind trials have carefully documented maintenance of vision, with a 60% reduction in blindness in patients with new vessels on the disk in the first 2 years. The present recommendations are for treatment of high-risk eyes, if there are (1) moderate or severe new vessels on or within one disk diameter of the optic disk; (2) mild new vessels on or within one-disk diameter of the optic disk if fresh hemorrhage is present; or (3) moderate or severe new vessels elsewhere if fresh hemorrhage is present.[61] Because of the success of these interventions, regular screening for early retinopathy is recommended for all patients with diabetes.

Vitrectomy is another useful procedure for some patients with diabetic retinopathy. It is a procedure requiring special technical skill in which vitreous is removed from the eye and replaced with saline. It has been used to remove blood or fibrous bands in the vitreous after retinal hemorrhage. However, vitrectomy has potential serious complications, including retinal tears, glaucoma, and additional retinal hemorrhage. Therefore, this procedure has generally been reserved for eyes that have already had persistent major visual loss caused by vitreous hemorrhage.

CATARACTS

Abnormalities of lens function and structure are very common in diabetics.[47] Two types of cataracts have been described in diabetics: metabolic (or snowflake) and senile. The metabolic type tends to occur particularly in the insulin-treated diabetic and may be related to the degree of glucose control. These cataracts have a snowflake appearance and start in the subcapsular region of the lens. The senile type appears more often in the elderly patient and is similar to the cataracts in nondiabetic elderly subjects.[113] The presence of this type of cataract appears to be no more frequent in the diabetic than in the nondiabetic population, but they are said to mature more rapidly in the diabetic and lead to an increase in cataract extraction rate. Hyperglycemia alone can induce cataracts in experimental animals that are probably similar to the metabolic cataracts of the diabetic.[59]

The mechanism by which cataracts occur in diabetics has been clarified by studies of lens metabolism. These studies have indicated that the sugar alcohol sorbitol is present in high concentrations when cataracts have been induced by high extracellular glucose levels. Aldose reductase, the enzyme responsible for the reduction of glucose to sorbitol, is known to be present in lens tissue. A role for the aldose reductase system in the development of diabetic cataracts has been strengthened by the dramatic effect of inhibitors of aldose reductase to prevent cataracts in experimental animals with diabetes.[11, 23, 43]

References

1. Amair P, Khanna R, Leibel B, et al. Continuous ambulatory peritoneal dialysis in diabetics with end-state renal disease. N Engl J Med 1982; 306:625–630.
2. American Diabetes Association. Nutrition recommendations and principles for people with diabetes mellitus. Diabetes Care 1994; 17:519–522.
3. American Diabetes Association Council on Nutrition. Glycemic effects of carbohydrates. Diabetes Care 1984; 7:607–608.
4. Bailey CJ. Biguanides and NIDDM. Diabetes Care 1992; 15(6):755–772.
5. Bailey CJ, Turner RC. Drug therapy: Metformin. N Engl J Med 1996; 334:574–579.
6. Beach KW, Strandness DEJ. Arteriosclerosis obliterans and associated risk factors in insulin-dependent and non-insulin-dependent diabetes. Diabetes 1980; 29:882–889.
7. Beard JC, Halter JB, Best JD, et al. Dexamethasone-induced insulin resistance enhances B-cell responsiveness to glucose level in normal men. Am J Physiol 1984; 247:E592–E596.
8. Beard JC, Ward WK, Halter JB, et al. Relationship of islet function to insulin action in human obesity. J Clin Endocrinol Metab 1987; 65:59–64.
9. Bennett PH, Rewers MJ, Knowler WC. Epidemiology of diabetes mellitus. In Porte D Jr, Sherwin RS (eds): Ellenberg & Rifkin's Diabetes Mellitus, ed 5. Stamford, CT, Appleton & Lange, 1996, pp 373–400.
10. Best JD, Judzewitsch RG, Pfeifer MA, et al. The effect of chronic sulfonylurea therapy on hepatic glucose production in diabetes. Diabetes 1982; 31:333–338.
11. Beyer-Mears A, Cruz E. Reversal of diabetic cataract by sorbinil, an aldose reductase inhibitor. Diabetes 1985; 34:15–21.
12. Binder C, Brange J. Insulin chemistry and pharmacokinetics. In Porte D Jr, Sherwin RS (eds): Ellenberg & Rifkin's Diabetes Mellitus, ed 5. Stamford, CT, Appleton & Lange, 1996, pp 689–708.

13. Binder C, Lauritzen T, Faber O, et al. Insulin pharmacokinetics. Diabetes Care 1984; 7:188–199.
14. Bjorntorp P. Obesity and diabetes mellitus. *In* Porte D Jr, Sherwin RS (eds): Ellenberg & Rifkin's Diabetes Mellitus, ed 5. Stamford, CT; Appleton & Lange, 1996, pp 553–563.
15. Bogardus C, Lillioja S, Howard BV, et al. Relationships between insulin secretion, insulin action, and fasting plasma glucose concentration in non-diabetic and non-insulin-dependent diabetic subjects. J Clin Invest 1984; 74:1238–1246.
16. Bogardus C, Ravussin E, Robbins DC, et al. Effects of physical training and diet therapy on carbohydrate metabolism in patients with glucose intolerance and non-insulin-dependent diabetes mellitus. Diabetes 1984; 33:311–318.
17. Bolli GB, Dimitriadis GD, Pehling GB, et al. Abnormal glucose counterregulation after subcutaneous insulin in insulin-dependent diabetes mellitus. N Engl J Med 1984; 310:1706–1711.
18. Carter Center of Emory University. Closing the gap: The problem of diabetes mellitus in the United States. Diabetes Care 1985; 8:391–406.
19. Chaudhuri M, Sartin JL, Adelman RC. A role for somatostatin in the impaired insulin secretory response to glucose by islets from aging rats. J Gerontol 1983; 38:431–435.
20. Chen M, Bergman RN, Pacini G, et al. Pathogenesis of age-related glucose intolerance in man. J Clin Endocrinol Metab 1985; 60:13–20.
21. Chen M, Halter JB, Porte D Jr. The role of dietary carbohydrate in the decreased glucose tolerance of the elderly. J Am Geriatr Soc 1987; 35:417–424.
22. Christensen NJ, Galbo H. Sympathetic nervous activity during exercise. Ann Rev Physiol 1983; 45:139–153.
23. Cohen MP. Aldose reductase. *In* Porte D Jr, Sherwin RS (eds): Ellenberg & Rifkin's Diabetes Mellitus, ed 5. Stamford, CT, Appleton & Lange, 1996, pp 217–228.
24. Combs CA, Gunderson E, Kitzmiller JL, et al. Relationship of fetal macrosomia to maternal postprandial glucose control during pregnancy. Diabetes Care 1992; 15:1251–1257.
25. Coniff RF, Sharpiro JA, Seaton TB, et al. Multicenter, placebo controlled trial comparing acarbose (Bay g 5421) with placebo, tolbutamide and tolbutamide-plus-acarbose in non-insulin-dependent diabetes mellitus. Am J Med 1995; 98(5):443–451.
26. Cook DL, Taborsky GJ. B-cell function and insulin secretion. *In* Porte D Jr, Sherwin RS (eds): Diabetes Mellitus, ed 5. Stamford, CT, Appleton & Lange, 1997, pp 49–73.
27. Craig BW, Hammons GT, Garthwaite SM, et al. Adaptation of fat cells to exercise: Response of glucose uptake and oxidation to insulin. J Appl Physiol 1981; 51:1500–1506.
28. Cryer PE, Gerich JE. Glucose counterregulation, hypoglycemia, and intensive insulin therapy in diabetes mellitus. N Engl J Med 1985; 313:232–241.
29. Cryer PE, Gerich JE. Hypoglycemia in insulin dependent diabetes mellitus: Interplay of insulin excess and compromised glucose counterregulation. *In* Porte D Jr, Sherwin RS, (eds): Ellenberg & Rifkin's Diabetes Mellitus, ed 5. Stamford, CT, Appleton & Lange, 1996, pp 745–760.
30. Davidson MB. The effect of aging on carbohydrate metabolism: A review of the English literature and a practical approach to the diagnosis of diabetes mellitus in the elderly. Metabolism 1979; 28:688–705.
31. DeFronzo R. Diabetic nephropathy. *In* Porte D Jr, Sherwin RS (eds): Ellenberg & Rifkin's Diabetes Mellitus, ed 5. Stamford, CT, Appleton & Lange, 1996, pp 971–1008.
32. DeFronzo RA, Barzilai N, Simonson DC. Mechanism of metformin action in obese and lean noninsulin-dependent diabetic subjects. J Clin Endocrinol Metab 1991; 73(6):1294–1301.
33. Diabetes Control and Complications Trial Research Group. The effect of intensive treatment of diabetes on the development and progression of long-term complications in insulin dependent diabetes mellitus. N Engl J Med 1993; 329:683–689.
34. Drucker D, Zinman B. Pathophysiology of beta-cell failure after prolonged remission of insulin-dependent diabetes mellitus. Diabetes Care 1984; 1:83–87.
35. Edelman S. Troglitazone: A new and unique oral antidiabetic agent for the treatment of type II diabetes and the insulin resistance syndrome. Clin Diabetes 1997; 15:60–65.
36. Eisenbarth GS. Immunotherapy of type 1 diabetes (editorial). Diabetes Care 1983; 6:521–523.
37. Fajans SS. Classification and diagnosis of diabetes. *In* Porte D Jr, Sherwin RS (eds): Ellenberg & Rifkin's Diabetes Mellitus, ed 5. Stamford, CT, Appleton & Lange, 1996, pp 357–372.
38. Fink RI, Kolterman OG, Griffin J, et al. Mechanisms of insulin resistance in aging. J Clin Invest 1983; 71:1523–1535.
39. Fink RI, Kolterman OG, Kao M, et al. The role of the glucose transport system in the postreceptor defect in insulin action associated with human aging. J Clin Endocrinol Metab 1984; 58:721–725.
40. Fink RI, Revers RR, Kolterman OG, et al. The metabolic clearance of insulin and the feedback inhibition of insulin secretion are altered with aging. Diabetes 1985; 34:275–280.
41. Froguel P, Zouali H, Vionnet N, et al. Familial hyperglycemia due to mutations in glucokinase: Definition of a subtype of diabetes mellitus. N Engl J Med 1993; 328:697–702.
42. Garvey WT, Olefsky JM, Griffen J, et al. The effect of insulin treatment on insulin secretion and insulin action in type II diabetes. Diabetes 1985; 34:222–234.
43. Gonzalez A-M, Sochor M, McLean P. The effect of an aldose reductase inhibitor (sorbinil) on the level of metabolites in lenses of diabetic rats. Diabetes 1983; 32:482–485.
44. Hagopian WA, Karlsen AE, Gottsater A, et al. Quantitative assay using recombinant human islet glutamic acid decarboxylase (GAD-64) showed 64K autoantibody positivity at onset predicts diabetes type. J Clin Invest 1997; 91:368–374.
45. Henriksson J. Effects of physical training on the metabolism of skeletal muscle. Diabetes Care 1992; 15:1701.
46. Herman WH, Sinnock P, Brenner E, et al. An epidemiologic model for diabetes mellitus: Incidence, prevalence, and mortality. Diabetes Care 1984; 7(4):367–371.
47. Herman WH, Teutsch SM, Sepe SJ, et al. An approach to the prevention of blindness in diabetes. Diabetes Care 1983; 6:608–613.
48. Hoelzer DR, Dalsky GP, Clutter WE, et al. Glucoregulation during exercise: Hypoglycemia is prevented by redundant glucoregulatory systems, sympathochromaffin activation, and changes in islet hormone secretion. 1986; 77:212–221.
49. Huttenen JK, Lansimies E, Voutilainen E, et al. Effect of moderate physical exercise on serum lipoproteins. Circulation 1979; 60:1220–1229.

50. Jarrett J. Diabetes and the heart: Coronary heart disease. Clin Endocrinol Metab 1977; 6:389–402.
51. Jenkins DJA. Dietary fibre, diabetes and hyperlipidaemia. Lancet 1979; 2:1287–1290.
52. Johnson DG, Bressler R. New pharmacologic approaches. In Porte D Jr, Sherwin RS (eds): Ellenberg & Rifkin's Diabetes Mellitus, ed 5. Stamford, CT, Appleton & Lange, 1996, pp 1293–1305.
53. Kadowaki T, Hagura R, Kajinuma H. Chlorpropamide-induced hyponatremia: Incidence and risk factors. Diabetes Care 1983; 6(5):468–471.
54. Kahn CR, Flier JS, Bar RS, et al. The syndromes of insulin resistance and acanthosis nigricans: Insulin-receptor disorders in man. N Engl J Med 1976; 294:739–745.
55. Kahn CR, Folli F. Molecular determinants of insulin action. Horm Res 1993; 39:93.
56. Kahn SE, Porte D Jr. The pathophysiology of type II (noninsulin dependent) diabetes mellitus: Implications for treatment. In Porte D Jr, Sherwin RS (eds): Ellenberg & Rifkin's Diabetes Mellitus, ed 5. Stamford, CT, Appleton & Lange, 1996, pp 487–512.
57. Kahn SE, Larson VG, Schwartz RS, et al. Exercise training delineates the importance of B-cell dysfunction to the glucose intolerance of aging. J Clin Endocrinol Metab 1992; 74:1336–1342.
58. Kenny SJ, Aubert AE, Geiss LS. Prevalence and incidence of noninsulin-dependent diabetes. In Harris M, (ed): Diabetes in America, ed 2. Washington, DC, National Institutes of Health, 1995, pp 47–67.
59. Kinoshita JH. Mechanisms initiating cataract formation. Invest Ophthalmol Vis Sci 1974; 13:713–724.
60. Kitzmiller JL, Gavin LA, Gin GD, et al. Preconception care of diabetes: Glycemic control prevents congenital anomalies. JAMA 1991; 265:731–736.
61. Klein R. Retinopathy and other ocular complications in diabetes. In Porte D Jr, Sherwin RS, (eds): Ellenberg & Rifkin's Diabetes Mellitus, ed 5. Stamford, CT, Appleton & Lange, 1996, pp 991–969.
62. Koivisto V, Felig P. Effects of leg exercise on insulin absorption in diabetic patients. N Engl J Med 1978; 298:79.
63. Kolterman OG, Gray RS, Griffin J. Receptor and postreceptor defects contribute to the insulin resistance of non–insulin-dependent diabetes mellitus. J Clin Invest 1981; 68:957–969.
64. Kraegen EW, Lazarus L, Meler H, et al. Carrier solutions for low-level intravenous insulin infusion. Br Med J 1975; 3:464–466.
65. Lebovitz H. The oral hypoglycemic agents. In Porte D Jr., Sherwin RS, (eds.): Ellenberg & Rifkin's Diabetes Mellitus, ed 5. Stamford, CT, Appleton & Lange, 1996, pp 761–788.
66. Lebovitz HE. Oral hypoglycemic agents. In Rifkin H, Porte D Jr, (eds): Diabetes Mellitus: Theory and Practice, ed 4. New York, Elsevier, 1990, pp 554–574.
67. Lefebvre PJ, Scheen AJ. Hypoglycemia. In Porte D Jr, Sherwin RS (eds): Ellenberg & Rifkin's Diabetes Mellitus, ed 5. Stamford, CT, Appleton & Lange, 1996, pp 761–788.
68. Levin ME, Sicard GA, Rubin BG. Peripheral vascular disease in the diabetic patient. In Porte D Jr., Sherwin RS, (eds): Ellenberg & Rifkin's Diabetes Mellitus, ed 5. Stamford, CT, Appleton & Lange, 1996, pp 1127–1158.
69. Liang JC, Goldberg MF. Treatment of diabetic retinopathy. Diabetes 1980; 29:841.
70. LoGerfo FW, Coffman JD. Vascular and microvascular disease of the foot in diabetes. N Engl J Med 1984; 311:1615–1619.
71. Madsbad S, Krarup T, Faber OK, et al. The transient effect of strict glycemic control on B-cell function in newly-diagnosed type 1 diabetic patients. Diabetologia 1982; 22:16–20.
72. Mauer SM, Barbosa J, Vernier RL, et al. Development of diabetic vascular lesions in normal kidneys transplanted into patients with diabetes mellitus. N Engl J Med 1976; 295:916–920.
73. Mauer SM, Steffes MW, Connett J, et al. The development of lesions in the glomerular basement membrane and mesangium after transplantation of normal kidneys to diabetic patients. Diabetes 1983; 32:948–952.
74. Mecklenburg RS, Benson EA, Benson JWJ, et al. Long-term metabolic control with insulin pump therapy: Report of experience with 127 patients. N Engl J Med 1985; 313:465–468.
75. Metzger BE, Phelps RL, Dooley SL. The mother in pregnancies complicated by diabetes mellitus. In Porte D Jr, Sherwin RS, (eds): Ellenberg & Rifkin's Diabetes Mellitus, ed 5. Stamford, CT, Appleton & Lange, 1996, pp 887–915.
76. Minaker KL, Rowe JW, Tonino R, et al. Influence of age on clearance of insulin in man. Diabetes 1982; 31:851–855.
77. Mirouze J, Selam JL, Pham TC, et al. Sustained insulin-induced remissions of juvenile diabetes by means of an external pancreas. Diabetologia 1978; 14:223–227.
78. Mondon CE, Dolkas CB, Reaven GM. Site of enhanced insulin sensitivity in exercise-trained rats at rest. Am J Physiol Endocrinol Metab 1980; 239:E169–E177.
79. Nathan DM. Insulin treatment of non–insulin-dependent diabetes. In Porte D Jr, Sherwin RS (eds): Ellenberg & Rifkin's Diabetes Mellitus, ed 5. Stamford, CT, Appleton & Lange, 1996, pp 735–744.
80. Nathan DM, Madnek SF, Delahanty L. Programming pre-exercise snacks to prevent post-exercise hypoglycemia in intensively treated insulin-dependent diabetics. Ann Intern Med 1985; 102:483–486.
81. National Diabetes Data Group. Classification and diagnosis of diabetes mellitus and other categories of glucose intolerance. Diabetes 1979; 28:1039–1057.
82. National Diabetes Data Group. In Harris M (ed): Diabetes in America, ed 2. Washington, DC, National Institutes of Health, 1995.
83. Nolan JJ, Ludvik B, Beerdsen P, et al. Improvement in glucose tolerance and insulin resistance in obese subjects treated with troglitazone. N Engl J Med 1994; 331:1188–1193.
84. Nuttal FQ, Maryniuk MD, Kaufman M. Individualized diets for diabetic patients. Ann Intern Med 1983; 99:204–207.
85. O'Sullivan JB. Body weight and subsequent diabetes mellitus. JAMA 1982; 248:949–952.
86. Ohkubo Y, Kishikawa H, Araki E, et al. Intensive insulin therapy prevents the progression of diabetic microvascular complications in Japanese patients with non–insulin-dependent diabetes mellitus: A randomized prospective 6-year study. Diabetes Res Clin Pract 1995; 28:103–117.
87. Olefsky JR. Insulin resistance. In Porte D Jr, Sherwin RS, (eds): Ellenberg & Rifkin's Diabetes Mellitus, ed 5. Stamford, CT, Appleton & Lange, 1996, pp 513–552.
88. Palmer JP, Benson JW, Walter RM, et al. Arginine-stimulated acute phase of insulin and glucagon secretion in diabetic subjects. J Clin Invest 1976; 58:565–570.

89. Palmer JP, Lernmark A. Pathophysiology of Type I (insulin dependent) diabetes. *In* Porte D Jr, Sherwin RS (eds.): Ellenberg & Rifkin's Diabetes Mellitus, ed 5. Stamford, CT, Appleton & Lange, 1996, pp 455–486.

90. Pfeifer MA, Halter JB, Judzewitsch RG, et al. Acute and chronic effects of sulfonylurea drugs on pancreatic islet function in man. Diabetes Care 1984; 7:25–34.

91. Pfeifer MA, Halter JB, Porte D Jr. Insulin secretion in diabetes mellitus. Am J Med 1981; 70:579–588.

92. Porte D Jr. β-cells in type II diabetes mellitus. Diabetes 1991; 40(2):166–180.

93. Porte D Jr, Sherwin RS (eds). Ellenberg & Rifkin's Diabetes Mellitus ed 5. Stamford, CT, Appleton & Lange, 1996.

94. Pyke DA, Leslie RDG. Chlorpropamide alcohol flushing: A definition of its relation to non-insulin dependent diabetes. Br Med J 1978; 2:1521.

95. Raffel L, Scheuner MT, Rotter JI. The genetics of diabetes. *In* Porte D Jr, Sherwin RS (eds): Ellenberg & Rifkin's Diabetes Mellitus, ed 5. Stamford, CT, Appleton & Lange, 1996, pp 401–454.

96. Raskin P, Pietri AO, Unger R, et al. The effect of diabetic control on the width of skeletal-muscle capillary basement membrane in patients with type 1 diabetes mellitus. N Engl J Med 1983; 309:1546–1550.

97. Reaven E, Curry D, Moore J, et al. Effect of age and environmental factors on insulin release from the perfused pancreas of the rat. J Clin Invest 1983; 71:345–350.

98. Reaven E, Reaven GM. Structure and function changes in the endocrine pancreas of aging rats with reference to the modulating effects of exercise and caloric restriction. J Clin Invest 1981; 68:75–84.

99. Reaven GM, Greenfield MS, Mondon CE, et al. Does insulin removal rate from plasma decline with age? Diabetes 1982; 31:670–673.

100. Reichard P, Pihl M. Mortality and treatment side effects during long-term intensified conventional insulin treatment in the Stockholm Diabetes Intervention Study (SDIS). Diabetes 1994; 43:313–317.

101. Rewers M, Hamman RF. Risk factors for non–insulin-dependent diabetes. *In* Harris M (ed): Diabetes in America, vol 95-1468. Washington, DC, National Institutes of Health, 1995, pp 179–220.

102. Rizza RA, Gerich JE, Haymond MW, et al. Control of blood sugar in insulin-dependent diabetes: Comparison of an artificial endocrine pancreas, continuous subcutaneous insulin infusion, and intensified conventional insulin therapy. N Engl J Med 1980; 303:1313–1318.

103. Saltiel AR, Olefsky JM. Thiazolidinediones in the treatment of insulin resistance and type II diabetes. Diabetes 1996; 45:1661–1669.

104. Schade DS. Brittle diabetes: Pathogenesis and therapy. *In* Porte D Jr, Sherwin RS (eds): Ellenberg & Rifkin's Diabetes Mellitus, ed 5. Stamford, CT, Appleton & Lange, 1996, pp 789–810.

105. Seltzer HS. Drug-induced hypoglycemia: A review based on 473 cases. Diabetes 1972; 21:955–966.

106. Silverman BL, Ogata ES, Metzger BE. The offspring of the mother with diabetes. *In* Porte D Jr, Sherwin RS, (eds): Ellenberg & Rifkin's Diabetes Mellitus, ed 5. Stamford, CT, Appleton & Lange, 1996, pp 917–929.

107. Simonson DC, Ferrannini E, Bevilacqua S, et al. Mechanism of improvement in glucose metabolism after chronic glyburide therapy. Diabetes 1984; 33:838–845.

108. Skyler JS. Complications of diabetes mellitus: Relationship to metabolic dysfunction. Diabetes Care 1979; 2:499–509.

109. Skyler JS. Relationship of glycemic control to diabetic complications. *In* Porte D Jr, Sherwin RS, (eds): Ellenberg & Rifkin's Diabetes Mellitus, ed 5. Stamford, CT, Appleton & Lange, 1996, pp 1235–1254.

110. Sosenko JM, Miettinen OS, Williamson JR, et al. Muscle capillary basement-membrane thickness and long-term glycemia in type 1 diabetes mellitus. N Engl J Med 1984; 311:694–698.

111. Srikanta S, Ganda OP, Gleason RE, et al. Linear loss of beta cell response to intravenous glucose. Diabetes 1984; 33:717–720.

112. Srikanta S, Ganda OP, Jackson RA, et al. Type 1 diabetes mellitus in monozygotic twins: Chronic progressive beta cell dysfunction. Ann Intern Med 1983; 99:320–326.

113. Straatsma BR, Foos RY, Horwitz J, et al. Aging-related cataract: Laboratory investigation and clinical management. Ann Intern Med 1985; 102:82–92.

114. Strowig S, Raskin P. Intensive management of insulin dependent diabetes. *In* Porte D Jr, Sherwin RS, (eds): Ellenberg & Rifkin's Diabetes Mellitus, ed 5. Stamford, CT, Appleton & Lange, 1996, pp 709–734.

115. Stubbe I, Hansson P, Gustafson A, et al. Plasma lipoproteins and lipolytic enzyme activities during endurance training in sedentary men: Changes in high density lipoprotein subfractions and composition. Metabolism 1983; 32:1120–1128.

116. Suter SL, Nolan JJ, Wallace P, et al. Metabolic effects of new oral hypoglycemic agent CS-045 in NIDDM subjects. Diabetes Care 1992; 15:193–203.

117. Tager HS. Abnormal products of the human insulin gene. Diabetes 1984; 33:693–699.

118. Taylor SI, Kadowaki T, Kadowaki H, et al. Mutations in insulin-receptor patients. Diabetes Care 1990; 13:257–279.

119. U.K. Prospective Diabetes Study Group. Study 13: Relative efficacy of randomly allocated diet, sulphonylurea, insulin, or metformin in patients with newly diagnosed non-insulin dependent diabetes followed for three years. Br Med J 1995; 310:83–88.

120. U.K. Prospective Diabetes Study Group. Study 16: Progressive nature of type 2 diabetes. Diabetes 1995; 44:1249–1258.

121. University Group Diabetes Program. A study of the effects of hypoglycemic agents on vascular complications of patients with adult-onset diabetes. I. Design. II. Mortality results. Diabetes 1970; 19:747.

122. VanZee BE, Hoy WE, Talley TE, et al. Renal injury associated with intravenous pyelography in nondiabetic and diabetic patients. Ann Intern Med 1978; 89:51–54.

123. Viberti G, Keen H. The patterns of proteinuria in diabetes mellitus: Relevance to pathogenesis and prevention of diabetic nephropathy. Diabetes 1984; 33:686–692.

124. Vinik AI, Wing RR, Lauterio TJ. Nutritional management of the person with diabetes. *In* Porte D Jr, Sherwin RS, (eds): Ellenberg & Rifkin's Diabetes Mellitus, ed 5. Stamford, CT, Appleton & Lange, 1996, pp 609–652.

125. Ward WK, Bolgiano DC, McKnight B, et al. Diminished B cell secretory capacity in patients with noninsulin-dependent diabetes mellitus. J Clin Invest 1984; 74:1318–1328.

126. Weinrauch LA, Healy RW, Leland OSJ, et al. Coronary angiography and acute renal failure in diabetic azotemic nephropathy. Ann Intern Med 1977; 86:56.

127. WHO Study Group. Diabetes Mellitus. Geneva, World Health Organization, 1985.

128. Wiseman MJ, Saunders AJ, Keen H, et al. Effect of blood glucose control on increased glomerular filtration rate and kidney size in insulin-dependent diabetes. N Engl J Med 1985; 312:617–621.

129. Yamagata K, Furuta H, Oda N, et al. Mutations in the hepatocyte nuclear factor-4alpha gene in maturity-onset diabetes of the young (MODY1). Nature 1996; 384:458–460.

130. Yamagata K, Oda N, Kaisaki PJ, et al. Mutations in the hepatocyte nuclear factor-1 alpha gene in maturity-onset diabetes of the young (MODY 3). Nature 1996; 384:455–458.

131. Zincke H, Woods JE, Palumbo PJ, et al. Renal transplantation in patients with insulin-dependent diabetes mellitus. JAMA 1977; 237(11):1101–1103.

132. Zinman B, Murray FT, Vranic M, et al. Glucoregulation during moderate exercise in insulin treated diabetics. J Clin Endocrinol Metab 1977; 45:641.

Chapter 2

Prediction and Prevention of Immune-Mediated Diabetes

Regis Coutant • Noel K. Maclaren

INTRODUCTION

Immune-mediated (type 1) diabetes is a multifactorial autoimmune disease for which susceptibility is determined by environmental and genetic factors.[7] Major effector cells are T lymphocytes, and lymphocytic infiltration of islets (insulitis) is the hallmark of the disease.[79, 83]

Susceptibility to immune-mediated diabetes is inherited, and marked differences in risk have been found according to the familial relationship with the diabetic proband (Table 2.1).[51, 242] Relatives of patients with immune-mediated diabetes are at a 5- to 15-fold increased risk of developing diabetes themselves, and more in multiplex families.[194, 241] About 20 loci have been implied in genetic susceptibility.[60, 97] The major histocompatibility complex is the strongest genetic determinant, explaining about 30% of the total genetic contribution to immune-mediated diabetes. Susceptibility to diabetes correlates with several specific HLA class II DR and DQ alleles.[18, 223] The insulin gene minisatellite is also a strong genetic determinant,[20, 108] explaining about 15% of the genetic contribution to diabetes. Among the other loci, some contain genes involved in the immunologic regulation, such as CTLA-4 gene, although the way by which they act is currently hypothetical.[145, 165] Although there appears to be a gene-dose effect in susceptibility to im-

TABLE 2.1 LIFELONG RISKS OF IMMUNE-MEDIATED DIABETES

Group	Absolute Risk (%)
Normal subjects	0.4
Nondiabetic relatives of patients with immune-mediated diabetes	
Parent	3
Offspring	6
With affected father	8
With affected mother	3
Sibling	
Identical twin	30–50
Brother or sister	5

mune-mediated diabetes involving as many as 10 to 20 separate possible interacting genes (epistasis), environmental triggers appear to be required also.

The concordance rate in monozygotic twins is only 34 to 50%,[19, 124] and 90% of patients with newly diagnosed immune-mediated diabetes do not have an affected first-degree relative.[51] The incidence of diabetes has increased over the past three decades and shows temporal variations.[115] Hence, combined genetic and epidemiologic evidence has been interpreted to mean that unknown environmental factors may play a role in either inducing the autoimmunity or shaping its course in genetically susceptible individuals. Viral infection, such as enterovirus,[8] congenital rubella[174] or endogenous retrovirus infection,[55] have all been proposed or implied as important environmental factors in the development of immune-mediated diabetes. Dietary factors, such as early exposure to cow's milk, have also been suggested to be important influences.[32] Three mechanisms, not necessarily mutually exclusive, have been proposed to account for the activation of peripheral autoreactive T lymphocytes by environmental factors. First, an immune response against an exogenous protein that shares an amino acid sequence with a beta cell protein could result in the appearance of cytotoxic CD8 T lymphocytes that react with a self-protein on the beta cells. Molecular mimicry between the beta cell glutamate decarboxylase (GAD) peptide $GAD_{250-273}$ and coxsackie protein P2-C has been shown.[117] Furthermore, peripheral blood mononuclear cells of diabetic patients or patients at high risk reactive to GAD_{65} peptide cross-reacted with viral protein P2-C.[8] Second, an environmental insult of beta cells (infection with a beta-cell tropic virus) may generate cytokines and other inflamma-

tory mediators that induce the expression of adhesion molecules in the vascular endothelium of the pancreatic islets. This results in increased extravasation of circulating leukocytes and the presentation of beta-cell antigens from the damaged beta cells by infiltrating macrophages to lymphocytes. Third, a viral or bacterial superantigen may trigger the polyclonal activation of a T lymphocyte subset, within which autoreactive T lymphocytes initiate organ-specific tissue destruction. A human endogenous retrovirus has been recently isolated from islets and spleen leukocytes from new-onset diabetic patients, which encodes such a superantigen.[55]

The infiltration of islets proceeds very slowly and has been occurring for years before diagnosis.[194, 217, 220] Inflammatory infiltrate of islets consists mostly of CD8+ T lymphocytes plus variable numbers of CD4+ T lymphocytes, B lymphocytes, macrophages, and natural killer cells.[79] Studies suggest that the autoimmune process usually begins during the first few years of life.[198, 260] Although the beta-cell destruction is believed to be mediated by T lymphocytes, it is accompanied by circulating islet-cell antibodies (ICAs),[34] and less often by anti-insulin autoantibodies.[171] The antibodies can be used to predict onset of the chemical disease, even though their pathogenic role, if any, must be small.

As the disease progresses toward clinical manifestations, there is a reduction in the normal early response of insulin to the intravenous administration of glucose.[235] However, massive beta-cell destruction could be a late event in the process.[83] Histology studies suggest that an 80% reduction in the volume of beta cells is required before symptomatic immune-mediated diabetes appears.[79]

Progress in the understanding of the pathogenesis of immune-mediated diabetes, mainly through rodent models of the disease, has led to successful disease prevention in rodents, suggesting that such an approach may have applicability in man. Nonspecific immunosuppressive therapies were first used, then beta-cell antigens as immunomodulatory agents, and more recently specific beta-cell antigen peptides given as therapy.

In humans, the prospective follow-up of first-degree relatives with circulating ICAs and the discovering of new beta cell antigens targeted by the immune system led to a better accuracy to predict the disease. As a consequence, diabetes prevention trials, based on animal studies and empirical human observations, are ongoing. These once aimed at stopping the autoimmune process at the earliest stage. In the near future, antigen-specific immunotherapy appears to be a promising way to prevent immune-mediated diabetes, which should soon be evaluated in clinical trials.

In this review, we will discuss the prediction of immune-mediated diabetes and review the immunologic, genetic, and metabolic data involved in disease prediction. We will then focus on the prevention of the disease, reviewing the animal studies, the human trials at diabetes onset, and the diabetes prevention trials at earlier (preclinical) stages of the autoimmune process.

PREDICTION OF THE DISEASE

Immunologic Prediction of the Disease

Prediction in First-Degree Relatives. The detection of islet-cell autoantibodies and antibodies against islet autoantigens, which accompany the insulitis, is the cornerstone of immunologic prediction and is, at present, the most accurate way to predict the disease. Islet-cell antibodies are likely to be directed against the same antigens as beta-cell–specific pathogenic T lymphocytes. Furthermore, antigen-specific B lymphocytes may play an important role in

presentation of beta-cell autoantigens to maintain a chronic autoimmune response.

Islet-cell antibodies are detected by indirect immunofluorescence staining of frozen sections of human pancreas.[34] Seventy percent to 80% of new-onset immune-mediated diabetic patients are ICA-positive.[37, 127, 194] Results are expressed in Juvenile Diabetes Foundation (JDF) units (JDF U) using the international JDF reference serum.[86] Several studies have shown the predictive value of ICAs in first-degree relatives of diabetic probands.[49, 133, 147, 194, 221, 222, 261] Islet-cell antibodies are detected in 2 to 4% of first-degree relatives. The 5-year risk for those with ICA-positive at titers $\geq$20 JDF U is about 40 to 50%.[23, 194, 238] Risk factors for the development of immune-mediated diabetes in ICA-positive relatives include younger age[41] and higher titers of ICAs (Figs. 2.1 and 2.2).[123] Relatives positive for ICA ($\geq$10 JDF U) and less than 10 years old, or with titers >40 JDF U, have a near 80% risk of contracting diabetes in the following 5 years. The risk falls to 20% when the subject's age is 10 or more years or the titers are $\leq$40 JDF U.

Insulin autoantibodies (IAA), usually determined by radioimmunoassay, are detected in 30 to 50% of new-onset immune-mediated diabetic patients, and more frequently (about 70%) in children younger than 5 years old.[111, 236] They are the first to appear in children of diabetic

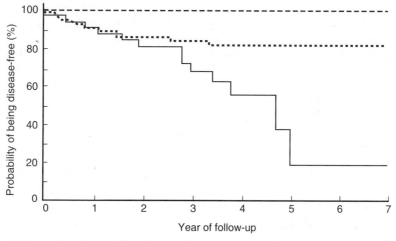

■ **Figure 2.1** Probability of remaining free of type 1 DM in three groups of relatives of probands with type 1 DM, according to islet-cell–antibody status and age at initial testing. *Dashed line,* relatives negative for antibodies; *dotted line,* relatives positive for antibodies and more than 10 years old at initial testing; *solid line,* relatives positive for antibodies and less than 10 years old at initial testing. (From Riley WJ, Maclaren NK, Krisher J, et al. A prospective study of the development of diabetes in relatives of patients with insulin-dependent diabetes. N Engl J Med 1990; 323:1167–1172. Copyright 1990 Massachusetts Medical Society. All rights reserved.)

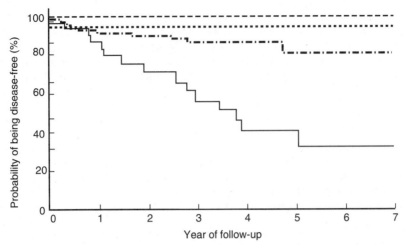

■ **Figure 2.2** Probability of remaining free of type 1 DM in four groups of relatives of probands with type 1 DM, according to islet-cell–antibody status expressed as JDF units. *Dashed line,* relatives negative for antibodies; *dotted line,* relatives with titers of 10 JDF units; *dashed and dotted line,* relatives with titers of 20 or 40 JDF units; *solid line,* relatives with titers of more than 40 JDF units. (From Riley WJ, Maclaren NK, Krisher J, et al. A prospective study of the development of diabetes in relatives of patients with insulin-dependent diabetes. N Engl J Med 1990; 323:1167–1172. Copyright 1990 Massachusetts Medical Society. All rights reserved.)

mothers or fathers.[198] Insulin autoantibodies are detected in 2 to 4% of first-degree relatives. The 5-year positive predictive value of IAAs alone was much less studied than ICAs, but it can vary from low[123] to as high as 50 to 60%, especially in young subjects.[238] First-degree relatives positive for both ICAs and IAAs have twice the risk to develop diabetes than those who are ICA positive and IAA negative.[23, 261] Proinsulin autoantibodies have been reported at a higher prevalence than IAA in new-onset immune-mediated diabetes patients.[29] However, their value in diabetes prediction has not been studied.

A series of islet proteins have been identified as targeted by the immune system in the disease, usually by immunoprecipitating islet lysates or by screening expression libraries with diabetic sera. These are GAD,[12, 17, 216] insulinoma associated antigen 2 (IA-2) and IA-2β,[52, 125, 126, 136, 138] carboxypeptidase H,[45] a 52-kD protein with homology to rubella virus capsid protein,[114] a 69-kD protein with homology to bovine serum albumin,[112, 180] pancreatic glucose transporter GLUT-2,[107] a sialoglycolipid termed GM2-1 ganglioside,[54, 63] and a membrane glycoprotein named Glima 38.[1]

To date, only antibodies to GAD_{65} and IA-2 of the above are currently detected in the purpose of diabetes prediction. They represent most of the reactivity of ICAs with pancreatic islet cell.[13, 126, 160]

Glutamate decarboxylase is a protein with two isoforms of molecular weight 65 kD and 67 kD, located in islets and brain. The GAD_{65}, encoded by a gene located on chromosome 10, is the predominant form found in human islets.[90] Glutamate decarboxylase catalyses the formation of the inhibitory neurotransmitter GABA from glutamine. Within the islet, GAD may have a role in the inhibition of somatostatin and glucagon secretion as well as regulating proinsulin synthesis and insulin secretion. The diabetes-associated epitopes in GAD_{65} are predominantly conformational.[193] Glutamate decarboxylase antibodies are best detected by radiobinding assay.[206] Seventy to 90% of new-onset immune-mediated diabetic patients are GAD antibodies positive.[17] Glutamate decarboxylase antibodies appeared after IAA in children of a diabetic mother or father.[198] They are at least as prevalent as ICAs in first-degree relatives[238] and improve the prediction of diabetes when used in combination with other autoantibodies (ICAs, IAA, IA-2) (see below).[23, 238]

IA-2 and IA-2β are members of the transmembrane protein tyrosine phosphatase family. These genes are located on chromosomes 2q35 and 7q36, respectively.[125, 126, 138] IA-2 and IA-2β are the precursors of the previously described 40 kD and 37 kD beta-cell peptide autoantigens.[52, 176] A truncated form of IA-2, named ICA 512 antigen, can be recognized by

ICA 512 radioimmunoassay.[186] Both molecules are expressed in islets and brain tissue and in cells of the neuroendocrine system.[250] Their roles in islets are currently unknown. The intracellular domains of IA-2 and IA-2β share 74% homology and are almost exclusively targeted by immune-mediated diabetes sera.[258] The diabetes-associated internal domain epitopes in IA-2 and IA-2β are predominantly conformational.[251] IA-2 and IA-2β autoantibodies are detected in about 70% and 40% of new onset immune-mediated diabetic patients, using the most sensitive radioimmunoassay (recombinant intracellular domain of the protein).[126, 136] Some 40% of such patients have ICA 512 autoantibodies.[85] The prevalence of ICA 512 in first-degree relatives seems to be somewhat less than ICA,[238] but the exact percentage remains to be determined with more sensitive IA-2 autoantibody radioimmunoassay. The 5-year risk of developing diabetes in first-degree relatives is near 80% when two autoantibodies are identified (among ICA ≥10 JDF U, IAA, GAD, or IA-2 antibodies), and near 100% with three or more positive autoantibodies.[23, 238]

Prediction in the General Population. Because immune-mediated diabetes occurs most often sporadically in patients who have no affected family member, the detection of ICAs or any of the autoantibodies in the sera of relatives cannot predict more than 10% of diabetes cases. Some studies have tested the feasibility of using ICAs to screen the general school-age population to determine their risk of developing immune-mediated diabetes. Islet-cell antibodies were found in 0.59 to 4% of children, higher than the expected prevalence of diabetes, depending on the level of ICA considered positive.[24, 28, 37, 91, 113, 128, 134, 199, 205] However, children with high ICA titers carrying the predisposing HLA class II susceptibility alleles DR3/DQB1 0201 and/or DR4/DQB1 0302 haplotypes are at high risk of developing diabetes.[28, 134, 205] In the only study with enough immune-mediated diabetes cases during the follow-up period, the 7-year estimated risk of developing diabetes in ICA-positive (≥10 JDF U) children has been found to be 45%, as high as in ICA-positive first-degree relatives.[205] Determination of additional immune markers may improve the prediction. Detection of at least two markers selected from GAD antibodies (≥97.5th percentile) and/or IA-2 antibodies (≥99.5th percentile) and/or ICA (≥5 JDF U) could give an estimated risk of about 70%,[2, 25, 91] raising the question of inclusion of such children in prevention trials.

Detection of T-cell Reactivity? Because pancreatic beta cells are thought to be destroyed by T lymphocytes, several studies have reported the detection of T lymphocyte responses to islet-cell proteins in persons with or at increased risk for immune-mediated diabetes. However, autoreactive T lymphocytes were also less frequently detectable in healthy non-diabetic control subjects.

Peripheral blood mononuclear cells showed a proliferative response to islet-cell extracts,[94] insulin-secretory granules,[47, 195] GAD$_{65}$,[14, 95] insulin,[162] IA-2,[72] the 69-kD protein,[196] and a 38-kD islet autoantigen named Imogen 38.[5] T-lymphocyte responses to GAD$_{65}$ peptides,[18, 73, 137, 172] and proinsulin peptides[201] were also studied to determine the immunodominant epitopes.

To date, the full characterization of naturally processed T-lymphocyte epitopes of GAD or other beta-cell antigen, including definition of the minimal peptides and identification of the HLA class II/class I molecules required for peptide presentation to CD4+/CD8+ T lymphocytes, and the investigation of T lymphocyte response in different disease stages, have not been available. Evaluation of T-lymphocyte autoreactivity is hampered by several factors. The precursor frequency of autoreactive T lymphocytes in peripheral blood is low; the presence of multiple HLA molecules in each individual makes the determination of MHC restriction elements difficult; and T-lymphocyte assays are not standardized.[197]

The use of mice transgenic for human major histocompatibility complex (MHC) alleles allows for the determination of MHC restricted human T-lymphocyte epitopes from GAD$_{65}$ and could be used for reactivities to other beta-cell antigens.[173, 247] Alternatively, synthetic peptide libraries allow for the identification of epitopes for autoreactive T-lymphocyte clones.[101]

To date, three different studies have established that human GAD$_{65}$ 270–285 peptide is a naturally processed T-lymphocyte epitope presented in the context of HLA-DR 0401 molecules.[73, 173, 247] Although determination of T-lymphocyte reactivity cannot be used for prediction purposes, it is essential for understanding the pathogenesis of the disease and for the development of epitope-specific immune interventions.

Genetic Prediction of the Disease

CMH II Region. The HLA class II region in the MHC on chromosome 6 (IDDM 1) encodes the most important genetic factors, counting for at least 30% of the familial aggregation of immune-mediated diabetes. Susceptibility or resistance to the disease is associated with different HLA-DR and more strongly with certain HLA-DQ genotypes, with apparent inter-racial discrepancies (Table 2.2).[18, 169, 211, 223, 229]

A molecule is considered to be predisposing or protective when its frequency is significantly higher or lower respectively in diabetic patients than in normal controls. HLA class II molecules present antigenic peptides to CD4 T lymphocytes. The interaction between an antigen-presenting cell bearing an HLA molecule associated with an antigenic peptide and a T lymphocyte bearing a receptor capable of recognizing the HLA-peptide complex triggers the activation and proliferation of those T lymphocytes. Susceptible HLA class II molecules may affect the degree of immune responsiveness to a pancreatic beta-cell autoantigen.[163, 212]

These molecules are heterodimers comprising one α chain and one β chain, encoded by α and β chain genes, respectively. There is only one monomorphic DRA gene, but several polymorphic DRB, DQA, and DQB genes. Thus, the functional properties of DR molecules are solely determined by the variable DRB genes. Functional DQ molecules are determined by the product of the polymorphic DQA1 and DQB1 genes, through *cis* or *trans* complementation. *Cis*-dimers comprise α and β chains encoded by DQA1 and DQB1 genes of the same chromosome or haplotype, and *trans*-dimers are encoded by genes on homologous chromosomes (Fig. 2.3). Thus, there are two DRB1 and four DQ molecules expressed in any individual, which act in concert to determine the overall HLA-encoded susceptibility to immune-mediated diabetes.

TABLE 2.2 HIGH-RISK AND PROTECTIVE HLA DR/DQ GENES

DR/DQ	Effect		
	Highly Susceptible (RR 5-30)	*Susceptible (RR 4-10)*	*Highly Protective (RR 0.2)*
DRB1	0405	0401	0403–0406
	0402		1501
	0301		
DQA1	0301	0501	
DQB1	0302		0602
	0201		

RR, relative risk.

TABLE 2.3 HIGH-RISK AND PROTECTIVE HLA DR/DQ HAPLOTYPES

Effect	DRB1	DQA1	DQB1
Highly susceptible (RR 5-30)	0405	0301	0302
	0402	0301	0302
	0301	0501	0201
Highly protective (RR 0.2)	0403	0301	0302
	0406	0301	0302
	1501	01	0602
	1301	0103	0603

RR, relative risk.

DQB1 alleles with an alanine at DQβ residue 57 (DQB1 0201 and DQB1 0302) confer strong susceptibility to immune-mediated diabetes.[229] Conversely, all DQB1 alleles with an aspartic acid at this position confer neutral (DQB1 0303) to protective (DQB1 0602) effects. The other susceptible or protective molecules are shown in Tables 2.2 and 2.3. Generally, highly protective DR or DQ molecules act in a dominant manner, whereas most or all DR and DQ molecules have to be susceptible factors in a predisposing genotype. One protective molecule (such as DRB1 0403) can counteract the predisposing effect of the DQB1 0201/DQB1 0302 molecules if also present.

It is unlikely that the effect of the same HLA molecule on immune-mediated diabetes varies across ethnic groups. Apparent inter-racial discrepancies of HLA associations with immune-mediated diabetes can be mainly explained by different DR-DQ linkage disequilibria and DQ$\alpha\beta$ *trans*-complementation.[211] In caucasian populations, the genotype associated with the highest relative risk (RR 20 to 50) is DRB1 03-DQA1 0501-DQB1 0201 on one chromosome, and DRB1 04-DQA1 0301-DQB1 0302 on the other. *Trans*-complementation leads to susceptible DQ *trans*-dimer DQA1 0301-DQB1 0201. In blacks, the haplotype associated with susceptibility is DRB1 07-DQA1 0301-DQB1 0201, leading to the same susceptible DQ molecule, by *cis*-complementation (Fig. 2.3).[164] In addition, other loci in the MHC region, such as tumor necrosis factor-α (TNF-α), could modulate the susceptibility or protection associated with the DR/DQ alleles.[153] HLA-associated susceptibility or protection seems to be age-dependent, because adult-onset, immune-mediated diabetic patients show lower percentages of susceptible DR3-DQB1 0201/DR4-DQB1 0302 genotypes,[38] and a higher percentage of protective DQB1 0602 than found in childhood-onset diabetes.

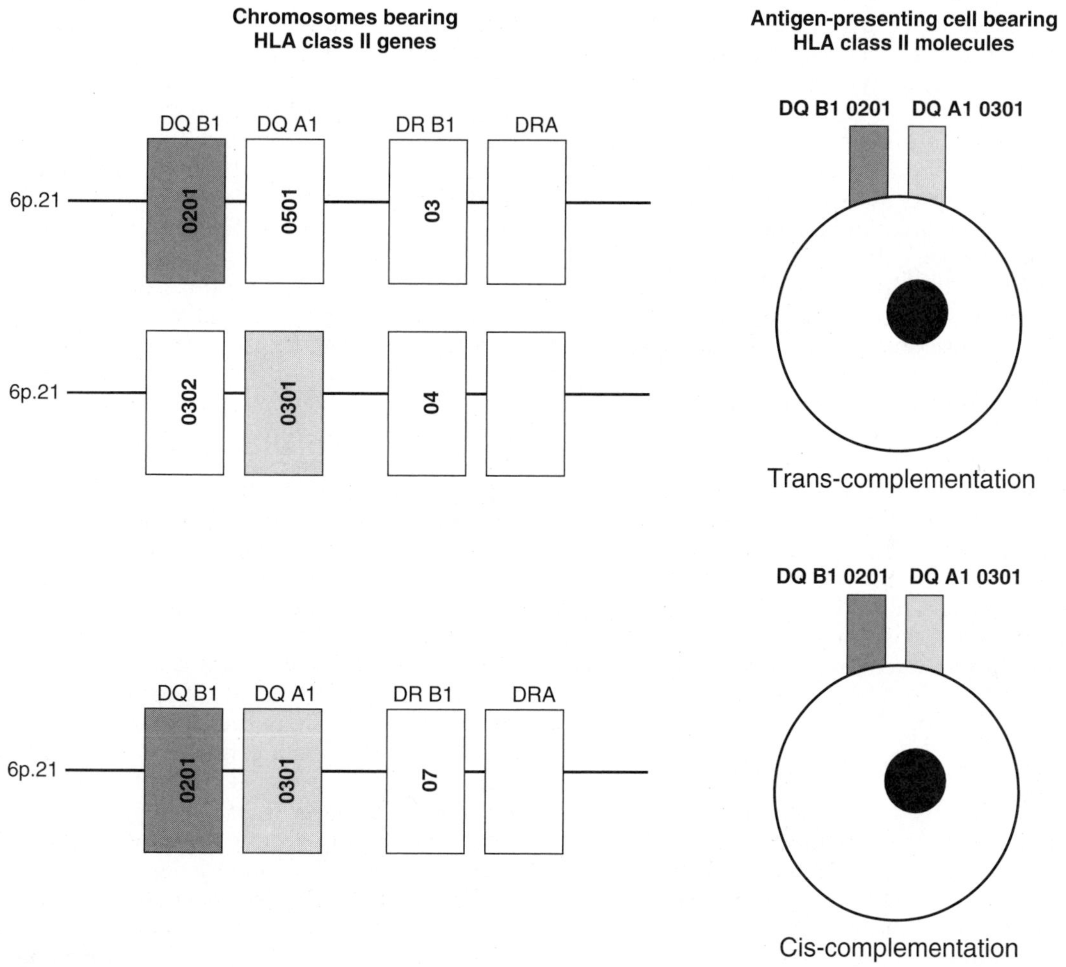

**Chromosomes bearing
HLA class II genes**

**Antigen-presenting cell bearing
HLA class II molecules**

■ **Figure 2.3** DQαβ cis- and trans-complementation.

Therefore, the determination of DR and DQ typing in first-degree relatives increases the ability of prediction, with a maximum predictive value of 20% (except in monozygotic twins) (Table 2.4).[223] In the general population, the absolute risk of individuals carrying the highest risk genotype (DRB1 03-DQA1 0501-DQB1 0201 and DRB1 04-DQA1 0301-DQB1 0302) is estimated to be about 6%.[192] These values are considerably less than those provided by immunologic prediction based on presence of autoantibody markers. Thus, determination of HLA class II genotype is only helpful in individuals who are also positive for diabetes-associated autoantibodies.

Other Loci. The insulin gene minisatellite (IDDM 2) is also a strong genetic determinant of diabetes susceptibility.[20, 108, 139] It is located on chromosome 11p15.5 in the 5' flanking region of the human insulin gene 365 bp from the transcription site. The short Variable Number of Tandem Repeats (VNTR) alleles predispose to immune-mediated diabetes, whereas the long VNTR alleles have a dominant protective effect.

However, the class of the alleles only mar-

TABLE 2.4 LIFELONG RISKS OF IMMUNE-MEDIATED DIABETES, ACCORDING TO HLA TYPING

Group	Absolute Risk (%)
Normal subjects	0.4
Nondiabetic relatives of patients with immune-mediated diabetes	
Sibling	5
HLA-identical	13
DR3/DR4 HLA-identical	20
HLA haploidentical	5
No HLA identity	1.8
Identical twins	30–50

ginally affects the insulin mRNA levels in human pancreas, which cannot explain diabetes susceptibility.[120, 140] Conversely, long alleles are reported to be associated with 2- to 3-fold higher insulin mRNA levels than short alleles in human fetal thymus.[185, 233] This mechanism is thought to ensure immune tolerance by a central (intrathymic) deletion of autoreactive thymocytes (negative selection). Expression of antigens in the thymus results in tolerance development, a process shown to be dose-dependent, because changes in the concentration of a selecting peptide in thymic organ cultures can have quantitative effects on positive selection and even induce negative rather than positive selection. Insulin VNTR alleles are currently only determined for research purposes and not for prediction programs.

Several other loci associated with the disease have been reported. The contribution of those to susceptibility to the disease is far less than the insulin gene minisatellite, and confirmation is required for most of them (Table 2.5).[56, 59, 62, 75, 76, 142, 145, 149, 154, 165, 191]

Metabolic Prediction of the Disease

The assessment of metabolic risk is based on intravenous glucose tolerance. The test can be done according to a standardized protocol.[22] First-phase insulin secretion (FPIR, $1+3$ minute insulin level) is extremely low in new-onset immune-mediated diabetes. In first-degree relatives, low first-phase insulin secretion (FPIR <300 pmol/L), together with ICA positivity, is associated with a 70 to 90% risk of progressing toward diabetes in the following 5 years in

first-degree relatives.[235] In normal children population, FPIR is positively correlated with age, rising sharply as children pass 8 years of age. In ICA-negative relatives who don't progress toward diabetes, FPIR is significantly lower than in normal children. This could be related to a genetic defect of pancreatic beta cells, independent of the autoimmune process.[42]

Thus, the intravenous glucose tolerance test is currently used in first-degree relatives positive for immunologic markers of immune-mediated diabetes.

PREVENTION OF THE DISEASE

Approximately 1 in 200 children dies at the time of diagnosis. The diabetes-associated vascular complications have a major impact on the well-being of diabetic patients and burden their lives. The diabetes health care expenditures in the United States constitute about one in every seven health care dollars spent, and immune-mediated diabetes accounts for a disproportionate share of these costs.[200] The development of therapeutic means to prevent immune-mediated diabetes would thus be highly desirable. Progress in diabetes prediction allows identifying about one high-risk individual (risk >70%) among every 100 to 150 relatives screened. Identification of such individuals is costly, but has made possible the design of preventive trials.[65] Approximately 15,000 relatives shall be screened to detect 100 high-risk subjects, and the achievement of such trials demands several years. Thus, national or multinational trials are highly desirable and are currently under way in Europe and the United States.

Several steps must be accomplished before large human prevention trials can begin.

First, animal studies provide most of the knowledge about immune-mediated diabetes pathogenesis and thus allow for the identification of potential treatments. These are essential models for studying efficacy and toxicity of preventive strategies.

Second, therapeutic trials in other human autoimmune diseases (such as multiple sclerosis or rheumatoid arthritis) together with studies in their animal models provide potentially useful information for developing immune intervention programs in the diabetes field.

Third, safety of the intervention must be assessed in animals before they are tested in diabetic and nondiabetic persons at risk.

Fourth, randomized double-blind controlled

TABLE 2.5 LOCI ASSOCIATED WITH IMMUNE-MEDIATED DIABETES SUSCEPTIBILITY

Loci		Main Genes in the Locus
6p21	(IDDM 1)	MHC II, TNF-α
11p15.5	(IDDM 2)	Insulin gene VNTR
15q26	(IDDM 3)	IGF-1 receptor gene
11q13	(IDDM 4)	Fibroblast growth factor 3
6q25	(IDDM 5)	Estrogen receptor
18q21	(IDDM 6)	
2q31	(IDDM 7)	
6q27	(IDDM 8)	
10p11-10q11	(IDDM 10)	
14q24.3-q31	(IDDM 11)	
2q33	(IDDM 12)	CTLA4/CD28
2q33-35	(IDDM 13)	
6q	(IDDM 15)	

Bold indicates confirmed loci.

trials in new-onset diabetic patients with residual insulin secretion allow for the assessment of preservation of C peptide and change in autoantibodies and T-lymphocyte autoreactivities. Overt immune-mediated diabetes is defined by absolute insulin deficiency, often leading to insulin dependence. The objective of immunotherapies at this stage is limited to preservation of the remaining pancreatic beta-cell mass. One cannot expect a complete and long-term recovery of beta-cell function, because beta cells are thought to be end-stage cells with limited regenerative capacities. Immunointervention may still be efficacious, in as much as it is started within a few days after the initiation of insulin therapy, in subjects free of ketoacidosis whose diabetes-related symptoms are recent (<4–8 weeks).[35, 214] A significant improvement of metabolic control may result because of the better efficacy of endogenously produced insulin. Beta-cell function is assessed by plasma C-peptide measurements in response to stimulation tests (standardized meal or glucagon test), and the benefits of its preservation can be determined by comparison of insulin doses and glycated hemoglobin measurements between treated and control patients. Secondary end points of such studies are to determine changes in serologic and cellular immune responses to treatment. Finally, they are essential to determine feasibility of immunotherapies in prediabetic patients.

Fifth, pilot studies in first-degree relatives to test the efficacy of treatment, measuring the occurrence of diabetes as primary end point and change in autoimmune markers as secondary end point, will be the ultimate goal.

Last, large trials sharing same outcomes as pilot studies can be initiated in first-degree relatives. As the number of the subjects receiving the therapy who would never have developed the disease grows, these trials shall carefully assess the risks and benefits of treatment. If possible, those should be ideally randomized placebo-controlled double-blind multicenter trial format. Several preventive trials are now under way in first-degree relatives. If these prove safe and therapeutically successful, prediction of the disease in the general population, which provides about 90% of diabetes cases, will become feasible. Prevention therapies would then allow for the implementation of programs to eradicate the disease.

Animal Studies

Two major models of spontaneous immune-mediated diabetes are mainly used: the non-obese diabetic (NOD) mouse[144] and the Bio Breeding (BB) rat.[161] Diabetes usually develops between 3 and 6 months in 70 to 90% of NOD female mice, and from about 4 months in BB rats, preceded by beta-cell inflammation or insulitis. Diabetes susceptibility is closely dependent on the MHC locus, and beta-cell destruction is mediated by T lymphocytes. The inciting antigen, like in human immune-mediated diabetes, is uncertain or unidentified, and the autoimmune response is spreading to a number of epitopes within a single antigen and also targeting to other autoantigens. Insulin, GAD_{65}, and GAD_{67} were the first antigens to which T-lymphocyte reactivity was demonstrated.[58, 116, 190, 227] Ganglioside GM2-1, carboxypeptidase H, hsp 65, and peripherin were also reported as autoantigens in NOD mice. T-lymphocyte clones have been derived from spleen, lymph nodes, and pancreatic infiltrates of NOD mice and are currently in use for studying the respective roles of CD4 positive and CD8 positive T-lymphocyte subsets, the antigenic peptide specificities, and the mechanisms for autoimmunity development and beta-cell destruction.[98]

These animal models provide means for genetic and immunologic manipulations that are inaccessible in man and for evaluation of various immunointervention procedures (Tables 2.6 and 2.7).[15] We will focus here in on therapies significant for pathogenesis understanding or those possibly relevant for human trials.

IMMUNOSUPPRESSIVE TREATMENTS

Early attempts to suppress immune-mediated diabetes relied on nonspecific immunosuppressive drugs. Cyclosporin, FK 506, or antilymphocyte serum efficiently prevented diabetes in NOD mice or BB rats.[16, 143, 152, 157] However, their therapeutic use in humans were limited by potential side effects and inadvisability of chronic administration.

MONOCLONAL ANTIBODIES AND CYTOKINES

Studies have focused on targeting those T lymphocytes involved in the disease process, using monoclonal antibodies that interfere with antigen recognition,[31, 50, 104, 121, 208, 219] cellular activation,[119, 132] and homing to the pancreas.[96, 253] Elsewhere, administration of antibodies targeting cytokines associated with Th1 activity (anti-interferon-γ)[39, 254] or administration of cytokines associated with Th2 activity and in-

TABLE 2.6 IMMUNOLOGIC MANIPULATIONS AND IMMUNOTHERAPY EFFICACIOUS FOR PREVENTION OF DIABETES IN ANIMAL MODELS OF IMMUNE DIABETES (NOD MICE OR BB RATS)

Strategy	Interpretation
Immune Manipulation	
Neonatal thymectomy[167]	No deletion of autoreactive T-cells
Intrathymic islet grafting[84]	Tolerization to islet
Transgenic mice expressing:	
MHC class II # from NOD[141]	Affecting presentation of antigens
Pancreatic IL 4[158]	Cytokine involved in regulation
TNFα[88]	
Proinsulin II in MHC class II cells[81]	Tolerization to proinsulin
Transgenic mice lacking:	
Perforin[109]	Lack of perforin-dependent cytotoxicity
CD4 T cells transfer[30]	Some CD4 cells can be protective
β cells deprivation-partial pancreatectomy[129]	Target cells required for autoimmunity
Bone marrow transplantation[131]	Cells involved in regulation process
Immune Suppression	
Cyclosporin[157]	Suppression of cell-specific immunity
Rapamycin[16]	
FK 506[152]	
Antilymphocyte serum[143]	
Monoclonal Antibodies Interfering With Immune Process	
Anti CD3,[50] anti CD4,[121] anti CD8,[104] anti TCR,[208] anti class I,[219] anti class II[31]	Affecting antigen recognition
Anti CD28, anti B7-2,[132] anti IL-2-R[119]	Affecting cellular activation
Anti L-selectin, anti integrin α4,[253] anti ICAM-1[96]	Affecting homing to the pancreas
Cytokines	
Antibodies anti γ interferon, anti IL-6,[39] anti TNFα[254]	Targeting cytokines generally associated with Th1 activity
IL-2,[209] IL-4,[189] IL-10[177]	Cytokines generally involved in regulation
IL-1,[77] TNFα[105]	
IL-2 coupled with toxin[170]	Destruction of activated T-cells
Immune Modulation or Miscellaneous	
Complete Freund Adjuvant[202]	Promoting Th2 response
BCG[213]	Promoting Th2 response
Diets[69, 130]	Environmental factor triggering?
Nicotinamide[252]	Free radicals scavenger
Linomide[89]	Interfering with TCR mediated activation
MHC class II binding peptide[103, 237]	Interfering with antigen presentation (and/or cellular activation)
Gangliosides[248]	
Aminoguanidine[57]	Interfering with NO production
Vitamin D3 and analogs[146]	Promoting Th2 response?
Immunoglobulins[78]	
Virus infection[168]	
Androgen treatment[80]	

Adapted from Bach JF. Insulin-dependent diabetes mellitus as an autoimmune disease. Endocr Rev 1994; 15:516–542. © The Endocrine Society.

volved in regulation process (interleukin[IL]-4) also successfully prevented diabetes.[177, 189, 209] Alternatively, administration of a toxin IL-2 fusion protein (DAB$_{486}$-IL-2), which targeted activated T lymphocytes expressing IL-2 receptor, reduced the incidence of diabetes in NOD mice.[170] It is generally admitted that effector cells of diabetes are Th1 cells that secrete IL-2, IFN-γ, TNF-α,[99] and that the regulatory cells are Th2 cells that secrete IL-4, IL-5, IL-6, and IL-10.[228] However, to view the regulation of the disease process strictly in terms of imbalance between Th1 and Th2 subsets is probably an oversimplification, even in mice. In that line, the role of certain cytokines in diabetes patho-

genesis is uncertain. Interleukin-1 and TNF-α may be cytotoxic to islet-beta cells in vitro, whereas they may prevent diabetes in NOD mice. Conversely, IL-10 administration seems to protect NOD mice,[177] whereas transgenic expression of IL-10 in islet beta cells of NOD mice was found to accelerate the onset of diabetes.[187, 249] Further, CD4 + Th1 autoreactive T-lymphocyte clones have been established from NOD mice that can actually suppress the diabetes.[3] It is likely that beta-cell destruction and T-lymphocyte suppression of autoimmunity may each involve a more complex interplay between Th1 and Th2 cells than is currently conceived. These approaches gave new insight

TABLE 2.7 ANTIGEN-SPECIFIC IMMUNOTHERAPIES EFFICACIOUS FOR PREVENTION OF DIABETES IN ANIMAL MODELS OF IMMUNE DIABETES (NOD MICE OR BB RATS)

Strategy	Interpretation
Antigen-Specific Immunotherapies	
Insulin	Promoting Th2 response
subcutaneous (0.25 to 2 U/day)[9]	
subcutaneous (6 U = 220 μg/4 or 8 weeks in IFA)[159]	
oral (1 mg/twice a week)[256]	
aerosol (during 3 to 10 days)	
Insulin B chain	
subcutaneous (140 μg/4 to 8 weeks)[93]	
subcutaneous (100 μg/4 weeks)[188]	
oral[92]	
Insulin B: 9–23	
subcutaneous (100 μg, once)[58]	
nasal (40 μg, 3 days)[58]	
GAD$_{65}$	
intrathymic (10 μg, once)[227]	
intravenous (50 μg, once)[116]	
intraperitoneal (100 μg, once)[178, 225]	
subcutaneous (100 μg/4 weeks)[188]	
GAD$_{67}$	
intraperitoneal (200 μg, once)[70]	
GAD peptides	
nasal (50 μg, once)[226]	
Hsp 65	
intraperitoneal (50 μg, once)[66]	
Hsp 65 peptide	
intraperitoneal (50 μg, once)[67]	
Glucagon[257]	
Therapies Involving β-cell Rest and/or Antigen-Specific Immunotherapies	
Insulin (subcutaneous) (0.25 to 2 U/d)[9]	Promoting Th2 response
Somatostatin (0.2 μg, twice a day)[36]	Decreasing β-cell antigens exposure?
Diazoxide[240]	

Adapted from Bach JF. Insulin-dependent diabetes mellitus as an autoimmune disease. Endocr Rev 1994; 15:516–542. © The Endocrine Society.

into pathogenesis, but their therapeutic applications in humans are limited by potential side effects, lack of selectivity, and the compromise of overall immune responses.

ANTIGEN-SPECIFIC TOLERANCE

Subsequently, specific antigen/peptides, such as insulin, insulin peptide, or GAD, have been used to induce selective immunomodulation (Table 2.7). In general, antigen-specific tolerance is mediated by clonal anergy, deletion of autoreactive T lymphocytes, or induction of regulatory T lymphocytes. Anergy induction is effective in diseases where the inciting antigen is known. It demands a high degree of specificity, thus limiting this approach in immune-mediated diabetes in which the first antigen is unknown. Further, there are T-lymphocyte responses to several autoantigens in the disease. The induction of antigen-specific regulatory Th2 T lymphocytes is thought to actively suppress the effects of nearby diabetogenic Th1 T lymphocytes through secretion of anti-inflammatory cytokines IL-4, IL-10, and transforming growth factor [TGF]-β. The suppressive effect of the regulatory T lymphocytes is termed "antigen-driven bystander suppression" and can be induced even when the inciting antigen is unknown.[150, 228, 243]

A single intravenous,[116] intrathymic,[227] or intraperitoneal[178] injection of GAD$_{65}$; monthly subcutaneous administration of GAD$_{65}$;[188] or single intraperitoneal administration of GAD$_{67}$[70] prevented diabetes in NOD mice, through generation of autoantigen specific anti-inflammatory Th2 responses.[225] A single intraperitoneal administration of a 65-kDa heat shock protein (hsp 65), a known islet-cell autoantigen in NOD mice, or of a hsp 65 peptide, was reported to prevent diabetes also.[66, 67] Repeated prophylactic administration of subcutaneous insulin to NOD mice reduced the incidence of insulitis and diabetes.[9] The possible mechanisms include reduced immunogenicity of pancreatic beta cells from "beta-cell rest" and induced active immunoregulation to insulin. Insulin administration, like diazoxide,[240] or somatostatin[36] has prevented diabetes in NOD mice or BB rats, through a putative inhibition of beta-cell function and thereby decreased antigen presentation. Alternatively, exogenous administration of insulin may trigger an active immunoregulatory process. According to this hypothesis, subcutaneous immunization with metabolically inactive insulin B-chain, but not A-chain, diminished intra-islet interferon-γ transcription and protected NOD mice from diabetes. Adoptive transfer of splenocytes from B-chain insulin-immunized mice prevented diabetes in recipients co-infused with spleen cells from acutely diabetic donors, suggestive of an active suppressive response.[159] The active epitope was the B chain peptide 8–18 (NKM, personal communication). A single subcutaneous administration of peptide B:9–23 of insulin protected NOD mice also.[58] Peptide B:9–23 acts as a dominant epitope among insulin-specific CD4+ T lymphocytes isolated from islets of NOD mice. However, it is unclear whether it associates with class II molecules through the peptide-binding groove, or through a site outside the peptide-binding-groove of the CMH II molecule, acting as a superantigen.[230]

Oral administration of antigen successfully induced active tolerance and protected animals in a number of autoimmune diseases, such as experimental autoimmune encephalomyelitis,[102] adjuvant arthritis,[255] uveitis,[166] or diabetes. It appears to be nontoxic, but requires quantities of purified antigen to induce and maintain tolerance. Oral insulin (dose 1 mg), given twice a week, prevented diabetes in NOD mice. Splenic T lymphocytes from animals orally treated adoptively transfer protection against diabetes.[21, 256] It is thought that regulatory cells generated from the gut-associated lymphoid tissue by feeding insulin migrate to the pancreas and are triggered by insulin to exert an antigen-driven bystander suppression. Oral administration of insulin shifts the balance from a Th1 to a Th2 pattern of cytokine expression in the pancreas.[92] Oral administration of insulin peptides or glucagon suppressed insulitis in NOD mice also.[257] Intranasal administration of insulin peptide B:9–23,[58] or insulin aerosol administration prevented diabetes in NOD mice, demonstrating the efficacy of mucosa-mediated tolerance.[93] Similarly, a single intranasal administration of GAD_{65} peptides induced Th2 responses and prevented diabetes in NOD mice.[226]

In most of these studies, treatment was begun between birth and 4 to 5 weeks after birth (at time of onset of insulitis), or at the latest in 8-week old mice.[225] Later treatments were generally less or not effective.[36]

The dose of the antigen to be used is important, because effects of its oral administration are variable and dose specific. Such does not appear to be the case with systemically administered antigen.[228] Low doses of antigen (µg/kg per day) can lead to the production of Th2 cells, whereas high doses (mg/kg per day) may result in anergy, as it was shown in the experimental autoimmune encephalomyelitis model.[244] Intrathymic administration of some GAD_{65} peptides accelerated diabetes onset in NOD mice.[46] Otherwise, oral administration of autoantigen has been able to induce diabetes in one study involving a murine transgenic model of autoimmune diabetes.[27]

Although it is still unclear whether antigen-specific immunotherapy effectively induces a long lasting form of active suppression with no deleterious side effects, it appears to be a promising method to prevent diabetes in humans.

MISCELLANEOUS TREATMENTS

Numerous therapies have successfully prevented diabetes in rodents (see Table 2.6). We only focus on those that were applicable to humans because of presumed safety.

Therapies thought to promote Th2 responses, such as bacille Calmette-Guérin (BCG)[213] or complete Freund's adjuvant,[202] decreased the incidence of diabetes in NOD mice.

Nicotinamide, which is a free-radical scavenger and inhibits nitric oxide synthesis,[4] has been shown to decrease the incidence of diabetes in NOD mice at doses as high as 500 mg/kg of body weight.[252]

Diet has been related to immune-mediated diabetes incidence, both in humans and rodents. Early dietary exposure to cow's milk proteins has been proposed as an important environmental factor in the development of diabetes. Cow's milk–free diet may[10, 53, 69, 110] or may not[175] prevent diabetes in BB rats or NOD mice.

Human Studies at Onset of Immune-Mediated Diabetes and in Prediabetes

IMMUNOSUPPRESSIVE TREATMENTS

In humans, cyclosporine[6, 35, 40, 74, 218] and azathioprine in association with steroids[214] induced significant remission in human immune-mediated diabetes of recent clinical onset in controlled studies. However, the remission was not indefinite, lasting less than 1 year on average,[61] but the drugs were not used for long periods of time.

In a pilot, controlled study of immunosuppression with low-dose cyclosporine in 6 young high-risk first-degree relatives of diabetic patients (ICA ≥20 JDF U and low first-phase insulin response), treatment delayed diabetes for 2 years on average, but did not prevent the disease.[43]

Because of their potential toxicity and transitory effects, immunosuppressive drugs did not undergo large therapeutic development in prediabetic patients.

NICOTINAMIDE

Several randomized controlled trials evaluated the effect of the vitamin nicotinamide on metabolic control in recent-onset diabetic patients, at doses 10 to 30 times less than the dose observed to prevent diabetes in rodents. Results were conflicting, because nicotinamide may[148, 181, 182, 234] or may not[48, 135, 183] preserve residual beta-cell function, suggesting that its effectiveness if real would be modest. Addition of steroids[184] or cyclosporine[182] to nicotinamide did not improve the results.

Nicotinamide is inexpensive and usually considered safe, even if concerns have been raised about its potential toxicity on growth at higher doses,[179] or about its ability to decrease insulin sensitivity.[87] Thus, it is currently being investigated for the prevention of immune-mediated diabetes.

In a pilot, controlled study in 14 very high-risk first-degree relatives of diabetic patients with ICA ≥80 JDF U and low first-phase insulin response,[68] 3 of 14 treated subjects and 8 of 8 controls had become insulin dependent after 2 to 57 months of follow-up. However, another pilot study had reported that 3 of 3 nicotinamide-treated patients had become diabetic.[100]

A population-based diabetes prevention trial tested nicotinamide in school children positive for ICA. Of 81,993 school children, 20,195 were screened, and 185 were found to be ICA positive. Of these, 173 received nicotinamide. After an average follow-up of 7.1 years, the diabetes incidence was 7.1/100,000 per year in this treatment group, versus 16.1/100,000 per year in the unscreened population, corresponding to a 50% delay of diabetes.[71]

Two randomized placebo-controlled trials—one a German national trial (DEutsche NIcotinamide Study: DENIS), the other a European multinational trial (European Nicotinamide Diabetes Intervention Trial: ENDIT)—are under way to evaluate the efficacy of nicotinamide in first-degree relatives of patients with immune-mediated diabetes.

PARENTERAL INSULIN

A controlled study in new-onset immune-mediated diabetes has shown that "intensive continuous intravenous therapy," delivered by an external artificial pancreas (3.8 ± 0.3 U/kg per day) during the first 2 weeks after diagnosis of diabetes, preserved pancreatic beta-cell function for 1 year, by comparison with "conventional treatment" (0.92 ± 0.04 U/kg per day in two divided doses).[210] In another controlled study, the use of an external artificial pancreas to infuse insulin at more than 1.5 U/kg per day produced prolonged remission in 9 of 14 treated subjects versus 3 of 11 conventionally treated controls.[151] "High-dose intravenous insulin infusion" (1.2 ± 0.4 U/kg per day) during the first 2 weeks after diagnosis of immune-

mediated diabetes and "intensive insulin treatment" (0.4 ± 0.1 U/kg per day, in four divided doses) equally preserved beta-cell function during the first year of insulin therapy, whereas the doses used were considerably less than in the previous studies.[207] The reduction of immunogenicity of pancreatic beta cells from "beta-cell rest" and/or induction of active immunoregulation to insulin have been proposed to explain the effects of insulin administration.

A pilot, controlled study evaluated the effect of the administration of daily subcutaneous regular and Lente insulins (0.22 ± 0.04 U/kg per day), combined with 5-day courses of intravenous insulin every 9 months (0.54 ± 0.04 U/kg per day), in 5 young first-degree relatives of diabetic patients ICA positive. One of 5 treated subjects and 7 of 7 controls developed diabetes after 0.7 to 3.7 years.[118] Additional individuals were subsequently included in the trial, totaling 3 of 9 treated subjects and 8 of 8 controls who have developed diabetes.[215] In another pilot study combining daily subcutaneous insulin with 7-days courses of intravenous insulin every 12 months in 5 high-risk first-degree relatives of diabetic patients (ICA ≥20 JDF U and low first-phase insulin secretion), 0 of 5 treated individuals versus 2 of 5 untreated controls developed diabetes after 1 to 39 months of follow-up.[155, 259]

A large multicenter diabetes prevention trial using insulin, termed DPT-1, has been initiated in the United States and is sponsored by National Institutes of Health. The study will randomize about 350 first- (4–45 years), second-, and third-degree (4–20 years) relatives at high risk for immune-mediated diabetes, whose immunologic (ICA ≥10 JDF U), genetic (not DQA1 0102, DQB1 0602), and metabolic (low first phase of insulin secretion) evaluations indicate a greater than 50% risk of developing diabetes within 5 years. Approximately a third of ICA positive subjects will meet these criteria. Treated subjects receive subcutaneous Lente insulin twice a day (0.25 U/kg per day), combined with 4-days courses of intravenous insulin once a year. The major outcome parameter of the study is the development of diabetes. By 11/30/96, 40,381 samples were analyzed for ICA, 3.4% were positive, 141 subjects were eligible, and 131 subjects were randomized.[64]

A double-blind, randomized placebo-controlled trial using insulin has been initiated in Europe (European Pediatric Prediabetes Subcutaneous Insulin Trial [EPP-SCIT]). The study will randomize 54 first-degree relatives (3–17 years), at high risk for immune diabetes, whose immunologic (ICA ≥40 JDF U or ICA ≥10 JDF U and IAA positive), genetic (not DQA1 0102, DQB1 0602), and metabolic screening (low first phase of insulin secretion) indicate a greater than 75% risk of developing diabetes within 5 years. Treated subjects receive subcutaneous Lente insulin once a day (0.20 U/kg per day). By 09/01/97, 27 subjects were so randomized.[44]

ORAL INSULIN

Several clinical trials in humans use oral tolerance for the treatment of autoimmune diseases, namely multiple sclerosis, rheumatoid arthritis, autoimmune uveitis, and diabetes.

In a double-blind, randomized pilot trial of oral tolerization with 300 mg bovine myelin antigens in relapsing-remitting multiple sclerosis, 6 of 15 treated individuals versus 12 of 15 controls had an attack during the year of the study.[245] Moreover, it has been shown that daily oral administration of bovine myelin induced TGF-β1-secreting cells and did not induce INF-γ-secreting cells in multiple sclerosis patients.[82] In a double-blind, randomized pilot trial with oral chicken type II collagen involving 60 patients with severe active rheumatoid arthritis, a decrease in the number of swollen joints and tender joints occurred in treated subjects.[231] A large trial is ongoing in multiple sclerosis,[246] and an open trial is continuing in autoimmune uveitis.[224]

Two randomized double-blind, placebo-controlled studies using oral insulin (Lilly) are ongoing in human immune-mediated diabetes. One, initiated in the United States, will randomize 150 adults (20–60 years) with latent autoimmune diabetes (not requiring insulin at time of enrollment), 75 children (5–20 years), and 75 adults (20–60 years) with immune-mediated diabetes of new onset. Treated subjects receive 1 or 10 mg of oral insulin during 1–2 years. Preservation of C peptide and changes in serologic and cellular immune responses will be assessed. By 11/30/97, 150 patients had been enrolled in the first year. The other study, initiated in France, will randomize 75 children (7–20 years) and 75 adults (20–40 years) with immune-mediated diabetes of new onset. Treated subjects will receive 2.5 or 7.5 mg of oral insulin during 1 year, and outcomes are the same as the American study. By 11/30/97, 80 patients had been enrolled. In both studies, doses were empirically determined, on the basis of low doses inducing Th2 cells response in animal studies.

A second DPT-1 study has been evaluating the efficacy of oral insulin. The study will randomize about 500 first- (3–45 years), second-, and third-degree (3–20 years) relatives of patients with immune-mediated diabetes at medium-risk of diabetes, whose immunologic (ICA ≥10 JDF U), genetic (not DQA1 0102, DQB1 0602), and metabolic (normal first phase of insulin secretion) evaluations indicate a 20 to 50% risk of developing diabetes within 5 years. Approximately 40% of the ICA-positive patients will meet these criteria. Treated subjects receive oral insulin once a day (7.5 mg/d). The major outcome parameter is development of diabetes. By 11/30/96, 28 subjects were eligible, and 26 subjects were randomized.[64]

DIET

Epidemiologic studies of infant feeding methods and milk protein consumption have shown correlations between ingestion of cow's milk protein and the risk of immune-mediated diabetes in humans.[33, 122, 239] Antibodies to bovine serum albumin may[112] or may not[11] be higher in newly diabetic patients than in controls. Homology between BSA (ABBOS peptide) and a 69-kDa protein of islet cells[180] could explain a triggering role of cow's milk in the autoimmune process, albeit the homology is slight. Thus, studies to evaluate the effects of avoidance of feeding cow's milk for the first 6 months of life have been designed.[110, 203] However, based on the available evidence to date, avoidance of cow's milk should not yet be recommended.[204]

BACILLE CALMETTE-GUÉRIN

One nonrandomized controlled pilot study reported that BCG administration was associated with remission of diabetes.[213] However, the control group in this study had an unusually low remission rate. A double-blind randomized placebo-controlled study is currently under way in Denver. To date, the follow-up of the whole cohort has not been encouraging.[215]

OTHER STUDIES

Diazoxide, a K channel opener that inhibits the release of insulin, has been tried in new-onset immune-mediated diabetes patients, on the hypothesis that target cell rest is likely to reduce the intensity of an autoimmune destructive process. The ten patients who were given diazoxide displayed higher basal and stimulated C-peptide level than the 10 control patients. However, metabolic control and insulin dose did not differ between groups.[26]

A preliminary study using an IL-2 receptor-targeted fusion toxin (DAB_{486}-IL-2) for 7 days in patients with immune-mediated diabetes of new onset reported reduced insulin requirements and stable C-peptide levels in 50% of cases.[170]

IN THE NEAR FUTURE

Antigen-specific tolerance has been successfully induced in NOD mice using several beta-cell autoantigen peptides, and this allows considering several possibilities in humans. Of the approaches proven in rodents models, we find that of B-chain or 8–23 B-chain peptide immunization the most promising.

Insulin B-chain appears to be the dominant epitope of insulin molecule against which T lymphocyte reactivity develops, and the critical part of insulin molecule inducing tolerance in NOD mice. Whether or not this will be applicable to humans remains to be determined. The fact that it could bind a site outside the peptide-binding-groove of the MHC II molecule in mice, acting as a superantigen, could overcome the HLA-class II presentation restriction and could allow its efficient use in humans with various HLA-class II molecules.[230] A trial of a B-chain peptide-based vaccine could be initiated in patients with diabetes of new onset, which would allow determining whether beta-cell function can be preserved, Th2 cells be induced, and Th1 cells be suppressed. If so, a trial in relatives at risk could be undertaken.

Several beta-cell antigens are targeted by the autoimmune process in humans, whereas specific epitopes of these antigens are largely unknown. Otherwise, additional beta-cell autoantigens and specific epitopes will be identified. Because the antigenic determinant spreading cascade could be heterogeneous in the human disease, therapy in the future might employ a number of autoantigens to target the polyclonal population of autoreactive T lymphocytes, thereby increasing the likelihood of successful treatment.

Moreover, the knowledge of specific epitopes would allow the use of T-lymphocyte receptor antagonists and partial agonists for manipulating the T-lymphocyte response, first in animal studies, then in humans.[106] Alternatively, the use of DNA vaccines could be interesting, because they are transcribed and translated, and

the protein they encode produced endogenously and presented to the immune system in the context of self-MHC.[156, 232]

By now, prevention trials are ongoing. If they are safe and successful, prediction of the disease in the general population would be necessary, and prevention therapies would allow eradicating the disease. Many approaches can successfully prevent diabetes in NOD mice. We contend that diabetes may be just as readily prevented in humans.

References

1. Aanstoot HJ, Kang SM, Kim J, et al. Identification and characterization of Glima 38, a glycosylated islet cell membrane antigen, which together with GAD_{65} and IA2 marks the early phases of autoimmune response in type I diabetes. J Clin Invest 1996; 97:2772–2783.
2. Aanstoot HJ, Sigurdsson E, Jaffe M, et al. Value of antibodies to GAD_{65} combined with islet cell cytoplasmic antibodies for predicting IDDM in a childhood population. Diabetologia 1994; 37:917–924.
3. Akhtar I, Gold JP, Pan LY, et al. CD4+ b cell-reactive T cell clones that suppress autoimmune diabetes in Nonobese diabetic mice. J Exp Med 1995; 182:87–97.
4. Andersen HU, Jorgensen KH, Egeberg J, et al. Nicotinamide prevents interleukin-1 effects on accumulated insulin release and nitric oxide production in rats islets of Langerhans. Diabetes 1994; 43:770–777.
5. Arden SD, Roep B, Neophytou PI, et al. Imogen 38: A novel 38-kD islet mitochondrial autoantigen recognized by T cells from a newly diagnosed type I diabetic patient. J Clin Invest 1996; 97:551–561.
6. Assan R, Feutren G, Debray-Sachs M, et al. Metabolic and immunological effects of cyclosporine in recently diagnosed type I diabetes mellitus. Lancet 1985; 1:67–71.
7. Atkinson MA, Maclaren MK. The pathogenesis of insulin-dependent diabetes. N Engl J Med 1994; 331:1428–1436.
8. Atkinson MA, Bowman MA, Campbell L, et al. Cellular immunity to a determinant common to glutamate decarboxylase, coxsackie virus in insulin-dependent diabetes. J Clin Invest 1994; 94:2125–2129.
9. Atkinson MA, Maclaren NK, Luchetta R. Insulitis and diabetes in NOD mice reduced by prophylactic insulin therapy. Diabetes 1990; 39:933–937.
10. Atkinson MA, Winter WE, Skordis N, et al. Dietary protein restriction reduces the frequency and delays the onset of insulin dependent diabetes in BB rats. Autoimmunity 1988; 2:11–20.
11. Atkinson MA, Bowman MA, Kao KJ, et al. Lack of immune responsiveness to bovine serum albumin in insulin-dependent diabetes. N Engl J Med 1993; 329:1853–1858.
12. Atkinson MA, Maclaren NK, Scharp DW, et al. 64,000 Mr autoantibodies are predictive of insulin-dependent diabetes. Lancet 1990; 335:1357–1360.
13. Atkinson MA, Kaufman DL, Newman D, et al. Islet cell cytoplasmic autoantibody reactivity to glutamate decarboxylase in insulin-dependent diabetes. J Clin Invest 1993; 91:350–356.
14. Atkinson MA, Kaufman DL, Campbell L, et al. Response of peripheral blood mononuclear cells to glutamate decarboxylase in insulin-dependent diabetes. Lancet 1992; 339:458–459.

15. Bach JF. Insulin-dependent diabetes mellitus as an autoimmune disease. Endocrinol Rev 1994; 15:516–542.

16. Baeder WL, Sredy J, Sehgal SN, et al. Rapamycin prevents the onset of insulin-dependent diabetes mellitus (IDDM) in NOD mice. Clin Exp Immunol 1992; 89:174–178.

17. Baekkeskov S, Aanstoot HJ, Christgau S, et al. Identification of the 64 K autoantigen in insulin-dependent diabetes is the GABA-synthesizing enzyme glutamic acid decarboxylase. Nature 1990; 347:151–156.

18. Baisch JM, Weeks T, Giles R, et al. Analysis of HLA-DQ genotypes and susceptibility in insulin-dependent diabetes mellitus. N Engl J Med 1990; 322:1836–1841.

19. Bharnett AH, Eff C, Leslie RD, et al. Diabetes in identical twins: A study of 200 pairs. Diabetologia 1981; 20:87–93.

20. Bennett ST, Lucassen AM, Gough SCL, et al. Susceptibility to human type I diabetes at IDDM2 is determined by tandem repeat variation at the insulin gene minisatellite locus. Nat Genet 1995; 9:284–292.

21. Bergerot I, Fabien N, Maguer V, et al. Oral administration of human insulin to NOD mice generates CD4 + T cells that suppress adoptive transfer of diabetes. J Autoimmun 1994; 7:655–663.

22. Bingley PJ, Colman P, Eisenbarth GS, et al. Standardization of IVGTT to predict IDDM. Diabetes Care 1992; 15:1313–1316.

23. Bingley PJ, Christie MR, Bonifacio E, et al. Combined analysis of autoantibodies improves prediction of IDDM in islet cell antibody-positive relatives. Diabetes 1994; 43:1304–1310.

24. Bingley PJ, Bonifacio E, Gale EAM. Can we really predict IDDM? Diabetes 1993; 42:213–220.

25. Bingley PJ, Bonifacio E, Williams AJK, et al. Prediction of IDDM in t   eral population. Strategies based on combinati   of autoantibody markers. Diabetes 1997; 46:1701–1710.

26. Bjork E, Kampe BO, Oskarsson WP, et al. Diazoxide treatment at onset preserves residual insulin secretion in adults with autoimmune diabetes. Diabetes 1996; 45:1427–1430.

27. Banas E, Carbone FR, Allison J, et al. Induction of autoimmune diabetes by oral administration of autoantigen. Science 1996; 274:1707–1709.

28. Behm BO, Manfras B, Seibler J, et al. Epidemiology and immunogenic background of islet cell antibody-positive nondiabetic schoolchildren. Diabetes 1991; 40:1435–1439.

29. Bohmer KH, Keilacker H, Kuglin B, et al. Proinsulin autoantibodies are more closely associated with type I (insulin-dependent) diabetes mellitus than insulin autoantibodies. Diabetologia 1991; 34:830–834.

30. Boitard C, Yasunami R, Dardenne M, et al. T cell-mediated inhibition of the transfer of autoimmune diabetes in NOD mice. J Exp Med 1989; 169:1669–1680.

31. Boitard C, Bendelac A, Richard MF, et al. Prevention of diabetes in nonobese diabetic mice by anti-I-A monoclonal antibodies: transfer of protection by splenic T cells. Proc Natl Acad Sci USA 1988; 85:9749–9723.

32. Borch-Johnson K, Joner G, Mandrup-poulsen T, et al. Relation between breast-feeding, incidence rates of insulin-dependent diabetes mellitus. Lancet 1984; 2:1083–1086.

33. Borsch-Johnsen K, Mandrup-Poulsen T, Zachau-Christiansen B, et al. Relation between breast-feeding and incidence of IDDM. Lancet 1984; 2:1083–1086.

34. Bottazzo GF, Florin-Christensen A, Doniach D. Islet-cell antibodies in diabetes mellitus with autoimmune polyendocrine deficiencies. Lancet 1974; 2:1279–1283.

35. Bougneres PF, Carel JC, Castagno L, et al. Factors associated with early remission of type I diabetes in children treated with cyclosporin. N Engl J Med 1988; 318:663–670.

36. Bowman MA, Campbell L, Darrow BL, et al. Immunological and metabolic effects of prophylactic insulin therapy in the NOD-scid/scid adoptive transfer model of IDDM. Diabetes 1996; 45:205–208.

37. Bruining GJ, Molenaar JL, Grobbee DE, et al. Ten-year follow-up study of islet-cell antibodies and childhood diabetes mellitus. Lancet 1989; 1:1100–1103.

38. Caillat-Zucman S, Garchon HJ, Timsit J, Assan R, Boitard C, Djilali-Saiah I, Bougneres P, Bach JF. Age-dependent HLA genetic heterogeneity of type I insulin-dependent diabetes mellitus. J Clin Invest 1992; 90:2242–2250.

39. Campbell IL, Kay TW, Oxbrow L, et al. Essential role for interferon-gamma and interleukin-6 in autoimmune insulin-dependent diabetes in NOD/Wehi mice. J Clin Invest 1991; 87:739–742.

40. Canadian-European randomized control trial group. Cyclosporin-induced remission of IDDM after early intervention: Association of 1 year of cyclosporin treatment with enhanced insulin secretion. Diabetes 1988; 37:1574–1582.

41. Cantor AB, Krisher JP, Cuthebertson DD, et al. Age and family relationship accentuate the risk of insulin-dependent diabetes mellitus (IDDM) in relatives of patients with IDDM. J Clin Endocrinol Metab 1995; 80:3739–3743.

42. Carel JC, Boitard C, Bougneres P. Decreased insulin response to glucose in islet cell antibody-negative siblings of type I diabetic children. J Clin Invest 1993; 92:509–513.

43. Carel JC, Boitard C, Eisenbarth G, et al. Cyclosporine delays but does not prevent clinical onset in glucose intolerant pre-type 1 diabetic children. J Autoimmun 1996; 9:739–745.

44. Carel JC, Bougneres PF, European Prediabetes Study Group. Treatment of prediabetic patients with insulin: Experience and future. Horm Res 1996; 45(suppl 1):44–47.

45. Castano L, Russo E, Zhou L, et al. Identification and cloning of a granule autoantigen (carboxypeptidase-H) associated with type I diabetes. J Clin Endocrinol Metab 1991; 73:1197–1201.

46. Cetkovic-Cvrlje M, Gerling IC, Muir A, et al. Retardation or acceleration of diabetes in NOD/Lt mice mediated by intrathymic administration of candidate β-cell antigens. Diabetes 1997; 46:1975–1982.

47. Chang JCC, Linarelli LG, Laxer JA, et al. Insulin-secretory-granule specific T-cell clones in human IDDM. J Autoimmun 1995; 8:221–234.

48. Chase HP, Butler-Simon N, Garg S, et al. A trial of nicotinamide in newly diagnosed patients with type I (insulin-dependent) diabetes mellitus. Diabetologia 1990; 33:444–446.

49. Chase HP, Voss MA. Diagnosis of pre type I diabetes. J Pediatr 1987; 111:807–812.

50. Chatenoud L, Thervet E, Primo J, et al. Anti CD3 antibody induces long-term remission of overt autoimmunity in non-obese diabetic mice. Proc Natl Acad Sci USA 1993; 91:123–127.

51. Chern MM, Anderson VE, Barbosa J. Empirical risk for insulin-dependent diabetes (IDD) in sibs: Further definition of genetic heterogeneity. Diabetes 1982; 31:1115–1118.

52. Christie MR, Vohra G, Champagne P, et al. Distinct antibody specificities to a 64-kD islet cell antigen in type I diabetes as revealed by trypsin treatment. J Exp Med 1990; 172:789–795.

53. Coleman DL, Kuzava JE, Leiter EH. Effect of diet on incidence of diabetes in nonobese diabetic mice. Diabetes 1990; 39:432–436.

54. Colman PJ, Nayak RC, Campbell IL, et al. Binding of cytoplasmic islet cell antibodies is blocked by human pancreatic glycolipid extracts. Diabetes 1989; 37:645–652.

55. Conrad B, Weissmahr RN, Boni Jurg, et al. A human endogenous retroviral superantigen as candidate autoimmune gene in type I diabetes. Cell 1997; 90:303–313.

56. Copeman JB, Cucca F, Hearne CM, et al. Linkage disequilibrium mapping of a type I diabetes susceptibility gene (IDDM7) to chromosome 2q31–33. Nature Genet 1995; 9:80–85.

57. Corbett JA, Mikhael A, Shimizu J, et al. Nitric oxide production in islets from nonobese diabetic mice: Aminoguanidine-sensitive and -resistant stages in the immunological diabetic process. Proc Natl Acad Sci USA 1993; 90:8992–8995.

58. Daniel D, Wegmann DR. Protection of NOD mice from diabetes by intranasal or subcutaneous administration of insulin peptide B:9–23. Proc Natl Acad Sci USA 1996; 93:956–960.

59. Davies LD, Cucca F, Goy JV, et al. Saturation multipoint linkage mapping of chromosome 6q in type I diabetes. Hum Mol Genet 1996; 5:1071–1074.

60. Davies JL, Kawaguchi Y, Bennett ST, et al. A genome wide search for human type I diabetes susceptibility genes. Nature 1994; 371:130–136.

61. De Fillipo G, Carel JC, Boitard C, et al. Long-term results of early cyclosporin therapy in juvenile IDDM. Diabetes 1996; 45:101–104.

62. Delepine M, Pociot F, Habita C, et al. Evidence for a non-MHC susceptibility locus in type I diabetes linked to HLA on chromosome 6. Am J Hum Genet 1997; 60:174–187.

63. Dotta F, Gianani R, Previti M, et al. Autoimmunity to the GM2-1 islet ganglioside before, and at the onset of type I diabetes. Diabetes 1996; 45:1193–1196.

64. DPT-1 Study Group. The diabetes prevention trial-type I diabetes (DPT-1): Enrollment report. Diabetes 1997; 46(suppl 1):163A.

65. Eisenbarth GS, Verge CF, Allen H, et al. The design of trials for prevention of IDDM. Diabetes 1993; 42:941–947.

66. Elias D, Markovits D, Reshef T, et al. Induction and therapy of autoimmune diabetes in the non-obese diabetic (NOD/Lt) mouse by a 65-kDa heat shock protein. Proc Natl Acad Sci USA 1990; 87:1576–1580.

67. Elias D, Reshef T, Birk OS, et al. Vaccination against autoimmune mouse diabetes with a T-cell epitope of the human 65-kDa heat shock protein. Proc Natl Acad Sci USA 1991; 88:3088–3091.

68. Elliott RB, Chase HP. Prevention or delay of type I (insulin-dependent) diabetes mellitus in children using nicotinamide. Diabetologia 1991; 34:362–365.

69. Elliott RB, Martin JM. Dietary protein: A trigger of insulin dependent diabetes in the BB rat? Diabetologia 1984; 26:297–299.

70. Elliott JF, Qin HY, Bhatti S, et al. Immunization with the larger isoform of mouse glutamic acid decarboxylase (GAD$_{67}$) prevents autoimmune diabetes in NOD mice. Diabetes 1994; 43:1494–1499.

71. Elliott RB, Pilcher CC, Fergusson DM, et al. A popula-tion based strategy to prevent insulin-dependent diabetes using nicotinamide. J Pediatr Endocrinol Metab 1996; 9:501–509.

72. Ellis T, Schatz D, Lan M, et al. Relationship between humoral and cellular immunity to IA-2 in IDD. Diabetes 1997; 46(suppl 1):195A.

73. Endl J, Otto H, Jung G, et al. Identification of naturally processed T cell epitopes from glutamic acid decarboxylase presented in the context of HLA-DR alleles by T lymphocytes of recent onset IDDM patients. J Clin Invest 1997; 99:2405–2415.

74. Feutren G, Papoz L, Assan R, et al. Cyclosporine increases the rate and length of remissions in insulin-dependent diabetes of recent onset. Lancet 1986; 2:119–124.

75. Field LL, Tobias R, Magnus T. A locus on chromosome 15q26 (IDDM3) produces susceptibility to insulin-dependent diabetes mellitus. Nature Genet 1995; 8:189–194.

76. Field LL, Tobias R, Thomson G, et al. Susceptibility to insulin-dependent diabetes mellitus maps to a locus (IDDM11) on human chromosome 14q24.3–q31. Genomics 1996; 33:1–8.

77. Formby B, Jacobs C, Dubuc P, et al. Exogenous administration of IL-1 alpha inhibits active and adoptive transfer of autoimmune diabetes in NOD mice. Autoimmunity 1992; 12:21–27.

78. Forsgren S, Andersson A, Hillorn V, et al. Immunoglobulin-mediated prevention of autoimmune diabetes in the non-obese diabetic (NOD) mouse. Scand J Immunol 1991; 34:445–451.

79. Foulis AK, Liddle CN, Farquharson MA, et al. The histopathology of the pancreas in type-1 (insulin-dependent) diabetes mellitus: A 25-year review of deaths in patients under 20 years of age in the United Kingdom. Diabetologia 1986; 29:267–274.

80. Fox HS. Androgen treatment prevents diabetes in nonobese diabetic mice. J Exp Med 1992; 175:1409–1412.

81. French MB, Allison A, Crem DS, et al. Transgenic expression of mouse proinsulin II prevents diabetes in nonobese diabetic mice. Diabetes 1997; 46:34–39.

82. Fukaura H, Kent SC, Pietrusewicz MJ, et al. Induction of circulating myelin basic protein and proteolipid protein-specific transforming growth factor-beta 1-secreting Th3 T cells by oral administration of myelin in multiple sclerosis patients. J Clin Invest 1996; 98:70–77.

83. Gepts W, De Mey J. Islet cell survival determined by morphology: An immunocytochemical study of the islets of Langerhans in juvenile diabetes mellitus. Diabetes 1978; 27(suppl 1):251–261.

84. Gerling IC, Serreze DV, Christianson SW, et al. Intrathymic islet cell transplantation reduces beta-cell autoimmunity and prevents diabetes in NOD/Lt mice. Diabetes 1992; 41:1672–1676.

85. Gianani R, Rabin DU, Verge CF, et al. ICA 512 autoantibody radioassay. Diabetes 1995; 44:1340–1344.

86. Gleichman H, Bottazzo GF. Progress toward standardization of cytoplasmic islet cell-antibody assay. Diabetes 1987; 36:578–584.

87. Greenbaum CJ, Kahn SE, Palmer JP. Nicotinamide's effects on glucose metabolism in subjects at risk for IDDM. Diabetes 1996; 45:1631–1634.

88. Grewal IS, Grewal KD, Wong FS, et al. Local expression of transgene encoded TNFa in islets prevents autoimmune diabetes in nonobese diabetic (NOD) mice by preventing the development of autoreactive islet-specific T cells. J Exp Med 1996; 184:1963–1974.

89. Gross DJ, Sidi H, Weiss L, et al. Prevention of diabetes mellitus in non-obese diabetic mice by linomide, a novel immunomodulating drug. Diabetologia 1994; 37:1195–1201.

90. Hagopian WA, Michelsen B, Karlsen AE, et al. Auto-antibodies in IDDM primarily recognize the 65,000-Mr rather than the 67,000-Mr isoform glutamic acid decarboxylase. Diabetes 1993; 42:631–636.

91. Hagopian WA, Sanjeevi CB, Kockum I, et al. Glutamate decarboxylase-, insulin-, and islet cell-antibodies and HLA typing to detect diabetes in a general population-based study of Swedish children. J Clin Invest 1995; 95:1505–1511.

92. Hancock WW, Polanski M, Zhang J, et al. Suppression of insulitis in non-obese diabetic (NOD) mice by oral insulin administration is associated with selective expression of interleukin-4 and -10, transforming growth factor-β, and prostaglandin-E. Am J Pathol 1995; 147:1193–1199.

93. Harrison LC, Dempsey-Collier M, Kramer DR, et al. Aerosol insulin induces regulatory CD8 γδ T cells that prevent murine insulin-dependent diabetes. J Exp Med 1996; 184:2167–2174.

94. Harrison LC, De Aizpurua H, Loudovaris T, et al. Reactivity to human islets and fetal pig proislets by peripheral blood mononuclear cells from subjects with preclinical and clinical insulin-dependent diabetes. Diabetes 1991; 40:1128–1133.

95. Harrison LC, Honeyman MC, DeAizpurua HJ, et al. Inverse relation between humoral and cellular immunity to glutamic acid decarboxylase in subjects at risk of insulin-dependent diabetes. Lancet 1993; 341:1365–1369.

96. Hasegawa Y, Yokono K, Taki T, et al. Prevention of autoimmune insulin-dependent diabetes in non-obese diabetic mice by anti LFA-1 and anti ICAM-1 mAb. Int Immunol 1994; 6:831–838.

97. Hashimoto L, Habita C, Beressi JP, et al. Genetic mapping of a susceptibility locus for insulin-dependent diabetes mellitus on chromosome 11q. Nature 1994; 371:161–164.

98. Haskins K, Wegman D. Diabetogenic T-cell clones. Diabetes 1996; 45:1299–1305.

99. Haskins K, McDuffie M. Acceleration of diabetes in young NOD mice by CD4+ islet specific T cell clone. Science 1990; 249:1433–1436.

100. Herskowitz RD, Jackson RA, Soeldner JS, et al. Pilot trial to prevent type I diabetes: Progression to overt IDDM despite oral nicotinamide. J Autoimmun 1989; 2:733–737.

101. Hiemstra HS, Duinkerken G, Benckhuijsen WE, et al. The identification of CD4+ T cell epitopes with dedicated synthetic peptide libraries. Proc Natl Acad Sci USA 1997; 94:10313–10318.

102. Higgins PJ, Weiner HL. Suppression of experimental autoimmune encephalomyelitis by the oral administration of myelin basic protein and its fragments. J Immunol 1988; 140:440–445.

103. Hurtenbach U, Lier E, Adorini L, et al. Prevention of autoimmune diabetes in non-obese diabetic mice by treatment with a class II major histocompatibility complex-blocking peptide. J Exp Med 1993; 177:1499–1504.

104. Hutchings PR, Simpson E, O'Reilly LA, et al. The involvement of Ly2+ T cells in beta cell destruction. J Autoimmun 1990; 3(suppl 1):101–109.

105. Jacob CO, Aiso S, Michie SA, et al. Prevention of diabetes in nonobese diabetic mice by tumor necrosis factor (TNF): Similarities between TNF-alpha and interleukin 1. Proc Natl Acad Sci USA 1990; 87:968–972.

106. Jameson SC, Bevan MJ. T cell receptor antagonists and partial agonists. Immunity 1995; 2:1–11.

107. Johnson TH, Crider BP, McCorkle K, et al. Inhibition of glucose transporter into rat islet cells by immunoglobulins from patients with new-onset insulin-dependent diabetes mellitus. N Engl J Med 1990; 322:653–659.

108. Julier C, Hyer RN, Davies J, et al. Insulin-IGF2 region on chromosome 11p encodes a gene implicated in HLA-DR4-dependent diabetes susceptibility. Nature 1991; 354:155–159.

109. Kagi D, Odermatt B, Seiler P, et al. Reduced incidence and delayed onset of diabetes in perforin-deficient nonobese diabetic mice. J Exp Med 1997; 186:989–997.

110. Karges W, Hammond-McKibben D, Cheung RK, et al. Immunological aspects of nutritional diabetes prevention in NOD mice: A pilot study for the cow's milk-based IDDM prevention trial. Diabetes 1997; 46:557–564.

111. Karjalainen J, Samala P, Ilonen J, et al. A comparison of childhood and adult type I diabetes mellitus. N Engl J Med 1989; 320:881–886.

112. Karjalainen J, Martin JM, Knip M, et al. A bovine albumin peptide as a possible trigger of insulin-dependent diabetes mellitus. N Engl J Med 1992; 327:302–307.

113. Karjalainen JK. Islet cell antibodies as predictive markers for IDDM in children with high background incidence of disease. Diabetes 1990; 39:1144–1150.

114. Karounos DG, Thomas JW. Recognition of common islet antigen by autoantibodies from NOD mice and humans with IDDM. Diabetes 1990; 39:1085–1090.

115. Karvonen M, Tuomilehto J, Libman I, et al. A review of the recent epidemiological data on the worldwide incidence of type I (insulin-dependent) diabetes. Diabetologia 1993; 36:883–892.

116. Kaufman DL, Clare-Salzer M, Tian J, et al. Spontaneous loss of T-cell tolerance to glutamic acid decarboxylase in murine insulin-dependent diabetes. Nature 1993; 366:69–72.

117. Kaufman DL, Erlander MG, Clare-Salzler M, et al. Autoimmunity to two forms of glutamate decarboxylase in insulin-dependent diabetes mellitus. J Clin Invest 1992; 89:283–292.

118. Keller RJ, Eisenbarth GS, Jackson RA. Insulin prophylaxis in individuals at high risk of type I diabetes. Lancet 1993; 341:927–928.

119. Kelley VE, Gaulton GN, Hattori M, et al. Anti-interleukin 2 receptor antibody suppresses murine diabetic insulitis and lupus nephritis. J Immunol 1988; 140:59–61.

120. Kennedy GC, German MS, Rutter WJ. The minisatellite in the diabetes susceptibility locus IDDM2 regulates insulin transcription. Nat Genet 1995; 9:293.

121. Koike T, Itoh Y, Ishii T, et al. Preventive effect of monoclonal anti L3T4 antibody on development of diabetes in NOD mice. Diabetes 1987; 36:539–541.

122. Kostraba JN, Cruickhanks KJ, Lawler-Heavner J, et al. Early exposure to cow's milk and solid foods in infancy, genetic predisposition, risk of IDDM. Diabetes 1993; 42:288–295.

123. Krischer JP, Schatz D, Riley WJ, et al. Insulin and islet-cell autoantibodies as time dependent covariates in the development of insulin-dependent diabetes: A prospective study in relatives. J Clin Endocrinol Metab 1993; 77:743–749.

124. Kyvik KO, Green A, Beck-Nielsen H. Concordance rates of insulin dependent diabetes mellitus: A population based study of young Danish twins. BMJ 1995; 311:913–917.

125. Lan MS, Lu J, Goto Y, Notkins AL. Molecular cloning and identification of a receptor-type protein tyrosine phosphatase IA-2, from human insulinoma. DNA Cell Biol 1994; 13:505–514.

126. Lan MS, Wasserfall C, Maclaren NK, et al. IA-2, a transmembrane protein of the tyrosine phosphatase family, is a major autoantigen in insulin-dependent diabetes mellitus. Proc Natl Acad Sci USA 1996; 93:6367–6370.

127. Landin-Olsson M, Karlsson A, Dahlquist G, et al. Islet cell and other organ-specific autoantibodies in all children developing type I (insulin-dependent) diabetes mellitus in Sweden during one year and in matched control children. Diabetologia 1989; 32:387–395.

128. Landin-Olsson M, Palmer JP, Lernmark A, et al. Predictive value of islet cell and insulin autoantibodies for type I diabetes mellitus in a population based study of newly diagnosed diabetic and matched control children. Diabetologia 1992; 35:1068–1073.

129. Larger E, Becourt, Bach JF, et al. Pancreatic islet b cells drive T cell-immune responses in the nonobese diabetic mouse model. J Exp Med 1995; 181:1635–1642.

130. Lefkowith J, Schreiner G, Cormier J, et al. Prevention of diabetes in the BB rat by essential fatty acid deficiency: Relationship between physiological and biochemical changes. J Exp Med 1990; 171:729–743.

131. Leiter EH, Serreze DV. Autoimmune diabetes in the non obese diabetic mouse: Suppression of immune defects by bone marrow transplantation and implications for therapy. Clin Immunol Immunopathol 1991; 59:323–334.

132. Lenschow DJ, Ho SC, Sattar H, et al. Differential effects of anti B7-1 and anti B7-2 monoclonal antibody treatment on the development of diabetes in the nonobese diabetic mouse. J Exp Med 1995; 181:1145–1155.

133. Lesage C, Boitard C, Carel JC, et al. Results of 3 years of screening for preclinical phase of juvenile insulin-dependent diabetes mellitus. Arch Fr Pediatr 1990; 47:709–713.

134. Levy-Marchal C, Dubois F, Noel M, et al. Immunogenetic determinants and prediction of IDDM in French schoolchildren. Diabetes 1995; 44:1029–1032.

135. Lewis CM, Canafax DM, Sprafka JM, et al. Double blind randomized trial of nicotinamide on early-onset diabetes. Diabetes Care 1992; 15:121–123.

136. Li Q, Borovitskaya AE, deSilva MG, et al. Autoantigens in insulin-dependent diabetes mellitus: Molecular cloning and characterization of human IA-2β. Proc Assoc Am Phys 1997; 109:429–439.

137. Lohman T, Leslie RDG, Hawa M, et al. Immunodominant epitopes of glutamic acid decarboxylase 65 and 67 in insulin-dependent diabetes mellitus. Lancet 1994; 343:1607–1608.

138. Lu J, Li Q, Xie H, et al. Identification of a second transmembrane protein tyrosine phosphatase, IA-2b, as an autoantigen in insulin-dependent diabetes mellitus: Precursor of the 37-kDa tryptic fragment. Proc Natl Acad Sci USA 1996; 93:2307–2311.

139. Lucassen AM, Julier C, Beressi JP, et al. Susceptibility to insulin dependent diabetes mellitus maps to a 4.1 kb segment of DNA spanning the insulin gene and associated VNTR. Nat Genet 1993; 4:305–310.

140. Lucassen AM, Screaton GR, Julier C, et al. Regulation of insulin gene expression by the IDDM associated insulin locus haplotype. Hum Mol Genet 1995; 4:501–506.

141. Lund T, O'Reilly L, Hutchings P, et al. Prevention of insulin-dependent diabetes mellitus in non-obese diabetic mice by transgenes encoding modified I-A beta-chain or normal I-E alpha-chain. Nature 1990; 345:727–729.

142. Luo DF, Buzzetti R, Rotter JI, et al. Confirmation of three susceptibility genes to insulin-dependent diabetes mellitus: IDDM4, IDDM5, and IDDM8. Hum Mol Genet 1996; 5:693–698.

143. Maki T, Ichikawa T, Blamnco R, et al. Long-term abrogation of autoimmune diabetes in nonobese diabetic mice by immunotherapy with anti-lymphocyte serum. Proc Natl Acad Sci USA 1992; 89:3434–3438.

144. Makino S, Kunimoto K, Muraoka Y, et al. Breeding of a nonobese, diabetic strain of mice. Exp Anim 1980; 29:1–13.

145. Marron MP, Raffel LJ, Garchon HJ, et al. Insulin-dependent diabetes mellitus (IDDM) is associated with CTLA4 polymorphisms in multiple ethnic groups. Hum Mol Genet 1997; 6:1275–1285.

146. Mathieu C, Laureys J, Sobis H, et al. 1,25-dihydroxyvitamin D3 prevents insulitis in NOD mice. Diabetes 1992; 41:1491–1495.

147. McCullough DK, Klaff LJ, Kahn SE, et al. Nonprogression of subclinical b-cell dysfunction among first degree relatives of IDDM patients: 5-yr follow-up of the Seattle family study. Diabetes 1990; 39:549–556.

148. Mendola G, Casamitjana R, Gomis R. Efect of nicotinamide therapy upon B-cell function in newly diagnosed type I (insulin-dependent) diabetic patients. Diabetologia 1989; 32:160–162.

149. Merriman T, Twells R, Merriman M, et al. Evidence by allelic association-dependent methods for a type I diabetes polygene (IDDM6) on chromosome 18q21. Hum Mol Genet 1997; 6:1003–1010.

150. Miller A, Lider O, Weiner HL. Antigen-driven bystander suppression after oral administration of antigens. J Exp Med 1991; 174:791–798.

151. Mirouze J, Selam JL, Pham TC, et al. Sustained insulin-induced remissions of juvenile diabetes by means of an external artificial pancreas. Diabetologia 1978; 14:223–227.

152. Miyagawa J, Yamamoto K, Hanafusa T, et al. Preventive effect of a new immunosuppressant FK-506 on insulitis and diabetes in non-obese diabetic mice. Diabetologia 1990; 33:503–505.

153. Moghaddam PH, Zwinderman AH, de Knijff P, et al. TNFa microsatellite polymorphism modulates the risk of IDDM in caucasians with the high-risk genotype HLA DQA1 0501-DQB1 0201/DQA1 0301-DQB1 0302. Diabetes 1997; 46:1514–1515.

154. Moharan G, Huang D, Tait BD, et al. Markers on distal chromosome 2q linked to insulin-dependent diabetes mellitus. Science 1996; 272:1811–1813.

155. Mollenhauer U. Insulin treatment of nondiabetic islet cell antibody positive first degree relatives: a randomized controlled trial. J Autoimmun 1993; 15(suppl):63.

156. Mor G, Yamshchikov G, Sedegah M, et al. Induction of neonatal tolerance by plasmid DNA vaccination of mice. J Clin Invest 1997; 98:2700–2705.

157. Mori Y, Suko M, Okudaira H, et al. Preventive effects of cyclosporin on diabetes in NOD mice. Diabetologia 1986; 29:244–247.

158. Mueller R, Krahl T, Sarvetnick N. Pancreatic expression of interleukin-4 abrogates insulitis and autoimmune diabetes in nonobese diabetic (NOD) mice. J Exp Med 1996; 184:1093–1099.

159. Muir A, Peck A, Clare-Salzer M, et al. Insulin immunization of nonobese diabetic mice induces a protective insulitis characterized by diminished interferon-g transcription. J Clin Invest 1995; 95:628–634.

48 Section I DIABETES MELLITUS OVERVIEW

160. Myers MA, Rabin DU, Rowley MJ. Pancreatic islet cell cytoplasmic antibody in diabetes is represented by antibodies to islet cell antigen 512 and glutamic acid decarboxylase. Diabetes 1995; 44:1290–1295.
161. Nakhooda AF, Like AA, Chappel CI, et al. The spontaneous diabetic Wistar rat: Metabolic and morphologic studies. Diabetes 1977; 26:100–112.
162. Naquet P, Ellis J, Tibensky D, et al. T cell autoreactivity to insulin in diabetic and related non-diabetic individuals. J Immunol 1988; 140:2569–2578.
163. Nepom GT. A unified hypothesis for the complex genetics of HLA association with IDDM. Diabetes 1990; 39:1153–1157.
164. Nepom BS, Schwarz D, Palmer JP, et al. Transcomplementation of HLA genes in IDDM. HLA-DQ alpha- and beta-chains produce hybrid molecules in DR3/4 heterozygotes. Diabetes 1987; 36:114–117.
165. Nistico L, Buzzetti R, Pritchard LE, et al. The CTLA4 gene region of chromosome 2q33 is linked to, and associated with, type I diabetes. Hum Mol Genet 1996; 5:1075–1080.
166. Nussenblatt RB, Caspi RR, Mahdi R, et al. Inhibition of S-antigen induced experimental autoimmune uveoretinis by oral induction of tolerance with S-antigen. J Immunol 1990; 144:1689–1695.
167. Ogawa M, Maruyama T, Hasegawa T, et al. The inhibitory effect of neonatal thymectomy on the incidence of insulitis in non-obese-diabetic (NOD) mice. Biomed Res 1985; 6:103–105.
168. Oldstone MB. Viruses as therapeutic agents. I. Treatment of nonobese insulin-dependent diabetes mellitus while maintaining general immune competence. J Exp Med 1990; 171:2077–2089.
169. Owerbach D, Lernmark A, Platz P, et al. HLA-D region beta-chain DNA endonuclease fragments differ between HLA-DR identical healthy and insulin-dependent diabetic individuals. Nature 1983; 303:815–817.
170. Pacheco-Silva A, Bastos MG, Muggia RA, et al. Interleukin 2 receptor targeted fusion toxin (DAB486-IL-2) treatment blocks diabetogenic autoimmunity in non-obese diabetic mice. Eur J Immunol 1992; 22:697–702.
171. Palmer JP, Asplin CM, Clemons P, et al. Insulin antibodies in insulin-dependent diabetics before insulin treatment. Science 1983; 22:1337–1339.
172. Panina-Bordignon P, Lang R, van Endert PM. Cytotoxic T cells specific for glutamic acid decarboxylase in autoimmune diabetes. J Exp Med 1995; 181:1923–1927.
173. Patel SD, Cope AP, Congia M, et al. Identification of immunodominant T cell epitopes of human glutamic acid decarboxylase 65 by using HLA-DR (α1 0101, β1 0401) transgenic mice. Proc Natl Acad Sci USA 1997; 94:8082–8087.
174. Patterson K, Chandra RS, Jenson AB. Congenital rubella, insulitis, and diabetes mellitus in an infant. Lancet 1981; 1:1048–1049.
175. Paxson JA, Weber JG, Kulczycki Jr A. Cow's milk-free diet does not prevent diabetes in NOD mice. Diabetes 1997; 46:1711–1717.
176. Payton MA, Hawkes CJ, Christie MR. Relationship of the 37,000–, 40,000-Mr tryptic fragments of islet antigens in insulin-dependent diabetes to the protein tyrosine phosphatase-like molecule IA-2 (ICA 512). J Clin Invest 1995; 96:1506–1511.
177. Pennline KJ, Roque-Gaffney E, Monahan M. Recombinant human IL-10 prevents the onset of diabetes in the nonobese diabetic mouse. Clin Immunol Immunopathol 1994; 71:169–175.
178. Petersen JS, Karlsen AE, Markholst H, et al. Neonatal tolerization with glutamic acid decarboxylase but not with bovine serum albumin delays the onset of diabetes in NOD mice. Diabetes 1994; 43:1478–1484.
179. Petley A, Macklin B, Renwick AG, et al. The pharmacokinetics of nicotinamide in humans and rodents. Diabetes 1995; 44:152–155.
180. Pietropaolo M, Castano L, Babu S, et al. Islet cell autoantigen 69 kD (ICA 69):molecular cloning and characterization of a novel diabetes-associated autoantigen. J Clin Invest 1993; 92:359–371.
181. Pozzilli P, Browne PD, Kolb H. Meta-analysis of nicotinamide treatment in patients with recent-onset IDDM: The nicotinamide trialists. Diabetes Care 1996; 19:1357–1363.
182. Pozzilli P, Visalli N, Boccuni ML, et al. Randomized trial comparing nicotinamide and nicotinamide plus cyclosporin in recent onset insulin-dependent diabetes (IMDIAB 1): The IMDIAB study group. Diabet Med 1994; 11:98–104.
183. Pozzilli P, Visalli N, Signore A, et al. Double blind trial of nicotinamide in recent-onset IDDM (the IMDIAB III study). Diabetologia 1995; 38:848–852.
184. Pozzilli P, Visalli N, Boccuni ML, et al. Combination of nicotinamide and steroid versus nicotinamide in recent-onset IDDM: The IMDIAB II study. Diabetes Care 1994; 17:897–900.
185. Pugliese A, Zeller M, Fernandez Jr A, et al. The insulin gene is transcribed in the human thymus and transcription levels correlate with allelic variation at the INS VNTR-IDDM2 susceptibility locus for type I diabetes. Nat Genet 1997; 15:293–297.
186. Rabin DU, Pleasic SM, Shapiro JA, et al. Islet cell antigen 512 is a diabetes-specific islet autoantigen related to protein tyrosine phosphatases. J Immunol 1994; 152:3183–3187.
187. Rabinovitch A. Immunoregulatory and cytokine imbalances in the pathogenesis of IDDM: therapeutic intervention by immunostimulation? Diabetes 1994; 43:613–621.
188. Ramiya VK, Lan MS, Wasserfall CH, et al. Immunization therapies in the prevention of diabetes. J Autoimmun 1997; 10:287–292.
189. Rappoport MJ, Jaramillo A, Zipris D, et al. Interleukin 4 reverses T cell proliferative unresponsiveness and prevents the onset of diabetes in nonobese diabetic mice. J Exp Med 1993; 178:87–99.
190. Reddy S, Bibby NJ, Elliott RB. Ontogeny of islet cell antibodies, insulin autoantibodies and insulitis in the non-obese diabetic mouse. Diabetologia 1988; 31:322–328.
191. Reed P, Cucca F, Jenkins S, et al. Evidence for a type I diabetes susceptibility locus (IDDM10) on human chromosome 10p11-q11. Hum Mol Genet 1997; 6:1011–1016.
192. Rewers M, Bugawan TL, Norris JM, et al. Newborn screening for HLA markers associated with IDDM: Diabetes autoimmunity study in the young (DAISY). Diabetologia 1996; 39:807–812.
193. Richter W, Shi Y, Baekkeskov S. Autoreactive epitopes defined by diabetes-associated human monoclonal antibodies are localized in the middle and C-terminal domains of the smaller form of glutamate decarboxylase. Proc Natl Acad Sci USA 1993; 90:2832–2836.
194. Riley WJ, Maclaren NK, Krisher J, et al. A prospective study of the development of diabetes in relatives of patients with insulin-dependent diabetes. N Engl J Med 1990; 323:1167–1172.
195. Roep B, Arden SD, de Vries RR, et al. T-cell clones

from a type-1 diabetes patient respond to insulin secretory granule protein in patients with recent onset type I diabetes. Nature 1990; 345:632–634.

196. Roep BO, Duinkerken G, Schreuder GMT, et al. HLA-associated inverse correlation between T-cell and antibody responsiveness to islet autoantigen in recent-onset insulin dependent diabetes mellitus. Eur J Immunol 1996; 26:1285–1289.

197. Roep BO. T-cell responses to autoantigens in IDDM: The search for the Holy Grail. Diabetes 1996; 45:1147–1156.

198. Roll U, Christie MR, Fuchtenbusch M, et al. Perinatal autoimmunity in offspring of diabetic parent: The German multi-center BABY-DIAB study: detection of humoral immune responses to islet antigens in early childhood. Diabetes 1996; 45:967–973.

199. Rowe R, Leech N, Nepom G, et al. High genetic risk for IDDM in the Pacific Northwest—first report from the Washington state diabetes prediction study. Diabetes 1994; 43:87–94.

200. Rubin RJ, Altman WM, Mendelson DN. Health care expenditures for people with diabetes mellitus, 1992. J Clin Endocrinol Metab 1994; 78:809A–809F.

201. Rudy G, Stone N, Harrison LC, et al. Similar peptides from two beta cell autoantigens, proinsulin and glutamic acid decarboxylase, stimulate T cells of individuals at risk for insulin-dependent diabetes. Mol Med 1995; 1:625–633.

202. Sadelain MW, Qin HY, Lauzon J, et al. Prevention of type I diabetes in NOD mice by adjuvant immunotherapy. Diabetes 1990; 39:583–589.

203. Schatz DA, Rogers DG, Brouhard BH. Prevention of insulin-dependent diabetes mellitus: an overview of three trials. Cleve Clin J Med 1996; 63:270–274.

204. Schatz DA, Maclaren NK. Cow's milk and insulin-dependent diabetes mellitus: Innocent until proven guilty. JAMA 1996; 276:647–648.

205. Schatz D, Krisher J, Horne G, et al. Islet cell antibodies predict insulin-dependent diabetes in United States school age children as powerfully as in unaffected relatives. J Clin Invest 1994; 93:2403–2407.

206. Schmidli RS, Colman PG, Bonifacio E. Participating laboratories: Disease sensitivity, specificity of 52 assays for glutamic acid decarboxylase antibodies. The second international GADAb workshop. Diabetes 1995; 44:636–640.

207. Schnell O, Eisfelder B, Standl E, et al. High-dose intravenous insulin infusion versus intensive insulin treatment in newly diagnosed IDDM. Diabetes 1997; 46:1607–1611.

208. Sempe P, Bedossa P, Richard MF, et al. Anti alpha/beta T cell receptor monoclonal antibody provides an efficient therapy for autoimmune diabetes in non-obese diabetic (NOD) mice. Eur J Immunol 1991; 21:1163–1169.

209. Serreze DV, Hamaguchi K, Leiter EH. Immunostimulation circumvents diabetes in NOD/Lt mice. J Autoimmun 1989; 2:759–776.

210. Shah SC, Malone JI, Simpson NE. A randomized trial of intensive insulin therapy in newly diagnosed insulin-dependent diabetes mellitus. N Engl J Med 1989; 320:550–554.

211. She JX. Susceptibility to type I diabetes: HLA-DQ and DR revisited. Immunol Today 1996; 17:323–329.

212. Sheehy MJ. HLA and insulin-dependent diabetes: A protective perspective. Diabetes 1992; 41:123–129.

213. Shehadeh N, Calcinaro F, Bradley BJ, et al. Effect of adjuvant therapy on development of diabetes in mouse and man. Lancet 1994; 343:706–707.

214. Silverstein J, Maclaren NK, Riley W, et al. Immunosuppression with azathioprine and prednisone in recent-onset insulin-dependent diabetes mellitus. N Engl J Med 1988; 319:599–604.

215. Slover RH, Eisenbarth GS. Prevention of type I diabetes and recurrent b-cell destruction of transplanted islets. Endocrin Rev 1997; 18:241–258.

216. Solimena M, Folli F, Aparisi R, et al. Autoantibodies to GABA-ergic neurons and pancreatic beta cells in stiff-man syndrome. N Engl J Med 1990; 322:1555–1560.

217. Srikanta S, Ganda OP, Soeldner JS, et al. First degree relatives of patients with type I diabetes mellitus:islet cell antibodies and abnormal insulin secretion. N Engl J Med 1985; 313:461–464.

218. Stiller CR, Dupre J, Gent M, et al. Effects of cyclosporine immunosuppression in insulin-dependent diabetes mellitus of recent onset. Science 1984; 223:1362–1367.

219. Taki T, Nagata M, Ogawa W, et al. Prevention of cyclophosphamide-induced and spontaneous diabetes in NOD/Shi/Kbe mice by anti-MHC class I Kd monoclonal antibody. Diabetes 1991; 40:1203–1209.

220. Tarn AC, Smith CP, Spencer KM, et al. Type I (insulin dependent) diabetes: A disease of slow clinical onset? BMJ 1987; 294:342–345.

221. Tarn AC, Thomas JM, Dean BM, et al. Predicting insulin-dependent diabetes. Lancet 1988; 1:845–850.

222. Thivolet C, Beaufrere B, Geburher L, et al. Autoantibodies and genetic factors associated with the development of type I (insulin-dependent) diabetes mellitus in first degree relatives of diabetic patients. Diabetologia 1991; 34:186–191.

223. Thomson G, Robinson WP, Kuhner MK, et al. Genetic heterogeneity, modes of inheritance, and risk estimates for a joint study of caucasians with insulin-dependent diabetes mellitus. Am J Hum Genet 1988; 43:799–816.

224. Thurau SR, Diedrichs-Mohring M, Fricke H, et al. Molecular mimicry as a therapeutic approach for an autoimmune disease: Oral treatment of uveitis-patients with an MHC-peptide crossreactive with autoantigen. First results. Immunol Lett 1997; 57:193–201.

225. Tian J, Clare-Salzer M, Herschenfeld A, et al. Modulating autoimmune responses to GAD inhibits disease progression and prolongs islet graft survival in diabetes-prone mice. Nature Med 1996; 2:1348–1353.

226. Tian J, Atkinson MA, Clare-Salzer M, et al. Nasal administration of glutamate decarboxylase (GAD 65) peptides induces Th2 responses and prevents murine insulin-dependent diabetes. J Exp Med 1996; 183:1561–1567.

227. Tisch R, Yang XD, Singer SM, et al. Immune response to glutamic acid decarboxylase correlates with insulitis in non-obese diabetic mice. Nature 1993; 366:72–75.

228. Tisch R, McDevitt H. Insulin-dependent diabetes mellitus. Cell 1996; 85:291–297.

229. Todd JA, Bell JI, McDevitt HO. HLA-DQ beta gene contributes to susceptibility and resistance to insulin-dependent diabetes mellitus. Nature 1987; 329:599–604.

230. Tompkins SM, Moore JC, Jensen PE. An insulin peptide that binds an alternative site in class II major histocompatibility complex. J Exp Med 1996; 183:857–866.

231. Trentham DE, Dynesius-Trentham RA, Orav EJ, et al. Effects of oral administration of type II collagen on rheumatoid arthritis. Science 1993; 261:1727–1730.

232. Ulmer JB, Donnely JJ, Parker SE, et al. Heterologous protection against influenza by injection of DNA encoding a viral protein. Science 1993; 259:1745–1749.

233. Vafiadis P, Bennett ST, Todd JA, et al. Insulin expression in human thymus is modulated by INS VNTR alleles at the IDDM2 locus. Nat Genet 1997; 15:289–292.

234. Vague P, Picq R, Bernal M, et al. Effect of nicotinamide treatment on the residual insulin secretion in type I (insulin-dependent) diabetic patients. Diabetologia 1989; 32:316–321.

235. Vardi P, Crisa L, Jackson RA, et al. Predictive value of intravenous glucose tolerance test insulin secretion less than or greater than the first percentile in islet cell antibody positive relatives of type I (insulin-dependent) diabetic patients. Diabetologia 1991; 34:93–102.

236. Vardi P, Ziegler AG, Mathews JH, et al. Concentration of insulin autoantibodies at onset of type I diabetes: Inverse log-linear correlation with age. Diabetes Care 1988; 11:736–739.

237. Vaysburd M, Lock C, McDevitt H. Prevention of insulin-dependent diabetes mellitus in non obese diabetic mice by immunogenic but not by tolerated peptides. J Exp Med 1995; 182:897–902.

238. Verge CF, Gianani R, Kawasaki E, et al. Prediction of type I diabetes in first degree relatives using a combination of insulin, GAD, and ICA512bdc/IA-2 autoantibodies. Diabetes 1996; 45:926–933.

239. Virtanen SM, Rasanen L, Ylonen K, et al. Early introduction of dairy products associated with increased risk of IDDM in Finnish children. Diabetes 1993; 42:1786–1790.

240. Vlahos WD, Seemayer TA, Yale JF. Diabetes prevention in BB rats by inhibition of endogenous insulin secretion. Metabolism 1991; 40:825–829.

241. Wagener DK, Sacks JM, LaPorte RE, et al. The Pittsburgh study of insulin-dependent diabetes mellitus: Risk for diabetes among relatives of IDDM. Diabetes 1982; 31:136–144.

242. Warram JH, Krolewski AS, Gottlieb MS, et al. Differences in risk of insulin-dependent diabetes in offspring of diabetic mothers and diabetic fathers. N Engl J Med 1984; 311:149–152.

243. Weiner HL. Oral tolerance: Immune mechanisms and treatment of autoimmune diseases. Immunol Today 1997; 19:335–342.

244. Weiner HL, Friedman A, Miller A, et al. Oral tolerance: Immunologic mechanisms and treatment of animal and human organ-specific autoimmune diseases by oral administration of autoantigens. Ann Rev Immunol 1994; 12:809–837.

245. Weiner HL, Mackin GA, Matsui M, et al. Double blind pilot trial of oral tolerization with myelin antigens in multiple sclerosis. Science 1993; 259:1321–1324.

246. Weiner HL. Oral tolerance for the treatment of autoimmune diseases. Annu Rev Med 1997; 48:341–351.

247. Wicker LS, Chen SL, Nepom GT, et al. Naturally processed T cell epitopes from human glutamic acid decarboxylase identified using mice transgenic for the type I diabetes-associated human MHC class II allele, DRB1 0401. J Clin Invest 1996; 98:2597–2603.

248. Wilberz S, Herberg L, Renold AE. Gangliosides in vivo reduce diabetes incidence in non-obese diabetic mice. Diabetologia 1988; 31:855–857.

249. Wogensen L, Lee MS, Sarvetnick N. Production of interleukin 10 by islet cells accelerates immune-mediated destruction of b cells in nonobese diabetic mice. J Exp Med 1994; 179:1379–1384.

250. Xie H, Notkins AL, Lan MS. IA-2, a transmembrane protein tyrosine phosphatase, is expressed in human lung cancer cell lines with neuroendocrine phenotype. Cancer Res 1996; 56:2742–2744.

251. Xie H, Zhang B, Matsumoto Y, et al. Autoantibodies to IA-2 and IA-2β in insulin-dependent diabetes mellitus recognize conformational epitopes. J Immunol 1997; 159:3662–3667.

252. Yamada K, Nonaka K, Hanafusa T, et al. Preventive and therapeutic effects of large-dose nicotinamide injections on diabetes associated with insulitis: An observation in the non-obese-diabetic (NOD) mice. Diabetes 1982; 31:749–753.

253. Yang XD, Nathan K, Tisch R, et al. Inhibition of insulitis and prevention of diabetes in nonobese diabetic mice by blocking L-selectin and very late antigen 4 adhesion receptors. Proc Natl Acad Sci USA 1993; 90:10494–10498.

254. Yang XD, Tisch R, Singer SM, et al. Effect of tumor necrosis factor A on insulin-dependent diabetes mellitus in NOD mice. I. The early development of autoimmunity and the diabetogenic process. J Exp Med 1994; 180:995–1004.

255. Zhang ZJ, Lee CSY, Lider O, et al. Suppression of adjuvant arthritis in Lewis rats by oral administration of type II collagen. J Immunol 1990; 145:2489–2493.

256. Zhang ZJ, Davidson L, Eisenbarth G, et al. Suppression of diabetes in nonobese diabetic mice by oral administration of porcine insulin. Proc Natl Acad Sci USA 1991; 88:10252–10256.

257. Zhang ZJ. Insulitis is suppressed in NOD mice by oral administration of insulin peptides and glucagon. FASEB J 1992; 6:1693.

258. Zhang B, Lan MS, Notkins AL. Autoantibodies to IA-2 in IDDM: Location of major antigenic determinants. Diabetes 1997; 46:40–43.

259. Ziegler A, Bachmann W, Rabl W. Prophylactic insulin treatment in relatives at high risk for type I diabetes. Diab Metab Rev 1993; 9:289–293.

260. Ziegler AG, Hillebrand B, Rabl W, et al. On the appearance of islet associated autoimmunity in offspring of diabetic mothers: A prospective study from birth. Diabetologia 1993; 36:402–408.

261. Ziegler AG, Dumont Herskowitz R, Jackson RA, et al. Predicting type I diabetes. Diabetes Care 1990; 13:762–775.

Chapter 3

Primary Prevention of Type 2 Diabetes Mellitus

Frank Vinicor

During the past decade, the health and economic societal burden of diabetes mellitus (DM) has become apparent.[31] Providers, purchasers, consumers, policy makers, and patients are increasingly aware that diabetes is common, serious, and costly. Further, the problems of diabetes occur particularly and disproportionately in certain segments of society, such as minority communities, elderly populations, and economically disadvantaged persons.[62] Because of these factors, and in association with a perspective that diabetes is a clinical and a public health problem,[77] efforts to reduce the devastation of this chronic disease are receiving increasing attention.

For diabetes, three levels of programmatic activities are possible: primary, secondary, and tertiary prevention strategies (Table 3.1).[78] For secondary and tertiary approaches, there is general agreement within the diabetes community and general health care system that activities do work and should be widely, broadly, and effectively applied.[20–22] The issue is no longer *if* secondary and tertiary strategies are efficacious, but *how* to make them effective at an acceptable cost.[6]

What is the status of primary prevention, especially for type 2 DM in reducing the burden of diabetes? What do we know? Is our understanding sufficient to allow us to say that proof exists to justify national policies on pri-

TABLE 3.1   PREVENTION STRATEGIES

Level of Prevention	Concept	Example
Primary	Decrease or delay onset of disease	Physical activity
Secondary	Early diagnosis and metabolic control	Glucose regulation
Tertiary	Complication detection and treatment	Retinopathy screening and treatment

mary prevention of type 2 diabetes? If not, what additional studies or information would allow us to achieve consensus about proof?

How does a person decide that he or she knows that a particular prevention or treatment strategy for any health condition will work? In other words, in medicine and health, what is proof? Approaches to this question were systematized initially by Sir Bradford Hill,[33] with subsequent reflection and amplification.[9, 12, 54] As indicated in Table 3.2, several different but interrelated criteria may need to be considered. Further, within the experimental category, a sequence of study design generally is viewed as providing increasing strength of evidence that A causes B (Table 3.3).[30] It is important to note that even if efficacy is established through careful and rigorous scientific study, other risk factors need to be considered in establishing broad-based national interventional and prevention policies.[19]

PRIMARY PREVENTION OF TYPE 2 DIABETES MELLITUS

Several factors are known to be associated with a greater likelihood of having or developing type 2 DM. Among these, age, race/ethnicity, family history, and genetic predisposition[80] cannot presently be modified or attenuated, despite exciting and important research regarding how each of these elements might be related to type 2 diabetes.

Simultaneously, several potentially modifi-

able risk factors should be considered as potential targets for primary prevention of type 2 DM.[37] (Within each of these factors, the elements listed in Tables 3.2 and 3.3 should be considered.)

Obesity

Clinically, the association between obesity and type 2 DM is striking.[58] Practitioners know that (1) type 2 DM develops most often in overweight individuals and (2) weight control or weight loss in an individual with hyperglycemia is frequently associated with partial or complete amelioration of elevated blood glucose.[74] Epidemiologic data documenting weight gain during the past two to three generations have established a clear linkage between type 2 diabetes and obesity in the population as a whole[43] and in particularly selected minority groups[10] in association with an increasing prevalence of DM in the United States.[73] More recently, interest in insulin resistance syndrome,[60] selective obesity (e.g., abdominal),[11] and possible relationships among leptin, obesity, and type 2 DM[8] all further the conviction that obesity is somehow related to type 2 DM, and that if only obesity could be ameliorated or prevented, the worldwide epidemic of DM might be avoided.[35]

Recalling the design of research studies and relationship to scientific proof (see Table 3.3), certainly levels 1 through 6 have been used and studied, and results have been published

TABLE 3.2   COMPONENTS OF "PROOF"

Category	Concept
Strength of association	Exposure to A increases B by 4/8/12 times
Temporality	Exposure to A occurs before B happens
Dose-response	The more of A, the more likely, or more of, B
Analogy	Other substances like A cause conditions like B
Consistency	Under different circumstances; in different labs; in both in vivo and in vitro, etc., A causes B
Biologic plausibility	Mechanisms exist to explain how A could cause B
Specificity	Only A causes B
Experimental	Under controlled conditions, only those exposed to A develop B

Source: Morabia A. On the origin of Hill's causal criteria. Epidemiology 1991; 2:367–369; Susser M. What is a cause and how do we know one? A grammar for pragmatic epidemiology. Am J Epidemiol 1991; 133:635–648.

(see references 40 and 46 for summary reviews). A variety of basic, clinical, and epidemiologic investigations are strongly suggestive of the impact of the interrelationships and the impact of obesity on the increased prevalence of type 2 DM. Further, some small randomized controlled trials have been completed, further suggesting the benefits of weight control.[24, 57] Presently, in the United States, a large, rigorous randomized controlled trial regarding potential primary prevention strategies, including weight control (among other behavioral approaches), has been initiated.[56] It is anticipated that this and other studies will soon provide additional scientific information regarding whether primary prevention is efficacious and what the extent of the impact will be in persons with impaired glucose tolerance at high risk for progression to type 2 DM.

Nutrients

In addition to weight gain and obesity as possible etiologic factors in type 2 DM (how *many* calories are ingested over time), attention has also focused on what *type* of calories or other specific elements are eaten, that is, the specific nutrients that are consumed.[40, 46] Fat consumption, especially unsaturated fats, has been reported to be associated with a greater likelihood of type 2 DM, particularly in special populations.[13, 52] Similarly, a recent study in a large cohort of women nurses indicated that diminished ingestion of dietary fiber and increased usage of carbohydrates (with a so-called high glycemic index) are associated with a greater incidence of type 2 DM.[65] Deficiencies in trace metals, such as chromium,[1, 17] or vitamins, such as vitamin E,[66] might be associated with insulin deficiency or resistance, with subsequent development of type 2 DM. In general, however, compared with the number and quality of studies regarding weight (see previous section) and physical activity (see subsequent section), investigations concerning specific nutrients and the development of type 2 DM require considerable validation.

Physical Activity

Several commonly noted demographic and clinical observations as well as prospective or case control studies suggest that there is a close relationship between physical inactivity and the development of type 2 diabetes mellitus.[38, 42] (Certainly, improved physical fitness is associated with improvements in glucose regulation in persons with established DM.[67]) It has been suggested that among the several possible preventive behaviors that could reduce the incidence of type 2 DM, activity is the best documented and perhaps most worthy of public health discussion and practice.[75]

It is often difficult to separate the special effects of weight control versus physical activity in the pathogenesis of type 2 DM.[40, 46] Several important large and long-term longitudinal studies have provided increasing levels of support for the value of physical activity,[32, 45, 47, 48] suggesting that physical activity is at least associated with a meaningful decrease in the incidence of type 2 DM. In male college alumni,[32] U.S. women,[47] male physicians,[48] and middle-aged Finnish men,[45] persistent physical activity performed for several years apparently resulted in a statistical and clinical meaningful reduction in the development of type 2 DM. Three factors are of interest in these investigations. (1) It appears that there may be a threshold effect regarding the intensity of physical activity and reduction in the incidence of type 2 DM.[32, 45, 47, 48] (2) The level of physical activity necessary to achieve this reduction in incidence is moderate, for example, 5.5 or more metabolic units, with a duration of activity of 40 minutes per week.[32, 45] (3) Those at greatest risk for developing future type 2 DM experienced greatest benefit from physical activity, even at levels somewhat below the so-called moderate level.[32, 45]

Some smaller randomized studies indicate that physical activity will reduce the likelihood of developing type 2 DM.[44, 57] The recent Surgeon General's Report on Physical Activity summarizes the evidence in support of the diabetes preventive benefits of physical activity.[75] These recommendations will be further scientifically explored in the Diabetes Prevention Program II.[56]

Cigarettes

The relationship between cigarette smoking and the development of type 2 DM has re-

TABLE 3.3 INCREASING STRENGTH OF STUDY DESIGN

Case report
Case series
Ecological
Cross-sectional
Case-control
Longitudinal, prospective
Randomized controlled trials

ceived recent attention. Although the benefits of never having smoked or smoking cessation are clearly justified without even considering type 2 DM,[28] studies in U.S. female nurses[63] and Dutch men[27] indicate a relatively small but meaningful impact of smoking on an increased incidence of type 2 DM, even when adjustments are made for other possible etiologic factors. The relationships between cigarettes and established DM are interesting, because of the surprisingly high frequency of smoking among persons with DM[16] and the possible synergistic interactions between cigarettes and diabetes in the genesis of diabetes complications.[71] The specific biologic mechanisms of how cigarettes could cause type 2 DM are not fully known, but recent studies suggest that cigarettes may be associated with various components of the insulin resistance syndrome,[60] including insulin resistance, hyperinsulinemia, and lipid disorders.[2, 3, 23, 29] Randomized controlled trials of cigarette usage have not and, of course, will not be carried out!

In Utero Environment

Recent important observations indicate that the in utero environment may play a major role in the subsequent development of type 2 DM. It has been recognized for many years that the presence of gestational diabetes mellitus (GDM) is associated with health risks to the newborn[15]; there is a great likelihood of the subsequent development of type 2 DM, not only in women with GDM[39] but in their offspring.[68] Parity may also be associated with a greater incidence of subsequent development of DM,[49] but these observations are not consistently supported.[50] There has been important and increasing interest in the Barker-Hale hypothesis,[4] that is, that improper fetal nutrition may be associated decades later with the development of insulin resistance syndrome,[76] including type 2 DM.[59] Particularly for GDM, glycemic control during pregnancy[25] as well as possible behavioral interventions after pregnancy[7] may be associated with a decreased likelihood of subsequent type 2 DM.[14] Further, it is possible that with improved and more appropriate fetal nutrition during the pregnancy, there will be a decreased likelihood of developing type 2 DM in offspring.[69] In both situations, additional interventional studies are necessary to confirm these exciting possibilities.

DO WE HAVE PROOF THAT PRIMARY PREVENTION WORKS FOR TYPE 2 DIABETES MELLITUS?

This simple question is, in reality, very challenging, with many approaches and answers. It is probably the aggregate of information (see Table 3.2) and the increasing strength of study design (see Table 3.3), especially the existence of rigorous randomized controlled studies,[5] that should be considered in responding to this question.[6, 33, 54, 61, 72] The answer must not be lightly arrived at, not only because of the social and economic policy implications of such decisions,[18] but also because as a general rule, for persons who are asymptomatic (without clinical manifestations that would bring the individual into contact with the health care system), ethical requirements of health promotion require a higher level of proof of efficacy and effectiveness when the health care system seeks out those with no or with unrecognized disease.[53, 70] Weight control, proper nutrition, physical activity, and not smoking are certainly good things to do for important disease conditions, such as coronary artery disease, hypertension, cancer, and chronic lung disease,[34] and it is unlikely that such behaviors will result in significant adverse health effects. However, there are legitimate concerns about launching broad-based national policies and programs before adequate understanding and proof.

In Figure 3.1, three levels of activity are delineated—investigation, demonstration, and public policy. The more information and knowledge that exists, the further to the right regarding the legitimacy, breadth, and intensity of a particular strategy, with fiscal and person-

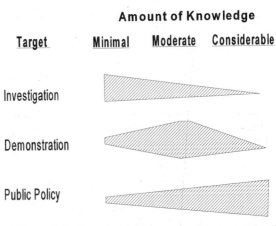

■ **Figure 3.1** Target of resources versus level of knowledge.

nel resources being directed to this level of activity.

In my judgment, additional information is certainly required before broad-based public policy and national programs in primary prevention of type 2 DM are launched, particularly in an era of economic considerations.[79] This information should include (1) results of randomized control trials, such as the Diabetes Prevention Program II[56]; (2) studies to understand how best to establish and maintain those healthy behaviors possibly associated with the prevention of type 2 DM[64]; (3) investigation to document effect size, that is, the likely benefit to individuals and populations regarding risk reduction–will it be 10%? 75%?[41]; and (4) understanding how the investment in primary prevention would impact on resource allocation in secondary or tertiary prevention programs that also can reduce the burden of diabetes.[51]

At basic, clinical, and public health levels, we have come far in understanding if and how certain risk factors for the development of type 2 DM could be manipulated to stop the onset of this increasingly frequent condition in the world.[36] In certain high-risk communities where type 2 DM appears to be exploding,[81] thoughtful, multicomponent, and evaluable demonstration projects could be implemented to begin to attenuate type 2 DM as well as increase our understanding of how to accomplish community-based interventions.[26] Further, in persons at very high risk for any of several chronic conditions that might be mitigated by primary prevention behaviors, it seems reasonable and appropriate to provide guidance and advice to that individual. However, given the impact and consequences of broad-based policy in any area of health, society must have greater information about not only *if* a primary prevention program works, but *how* and *how much*. For prevention of type 2 DM, we must be persistent, patient, and perhaps frustrated for a few more years while awaiting this critical information.

References

1. Anderson R, Cheng N, Bryden N, et al. Beneficial effects of chromium for people with Type 2 diabetes. Diabetes 1996; 45(S2):124A.
2. Attvall S, Fowelin J, Lager I, et al. Smoking induces insulin resistance: A potential link with the insulin resistance syndrome. J Intern Med 1993; 233:327–332.
3. Axeksebm M, Eliasson B, Joheim T, et al. Lipid intolerance in smokers. J Intern Med 1995; 237:449–455.
4. Barker D. Outcome of low birth weight. Horm Res 1994; 42:223–230.
5. Berlin J, Ness R. Randomized clinical trials in the presence of diagnostic uncertainty: Implications for measures of efficacy and sample size. Control Clin Trials 1996; 17:191–200.
6. Brown E, Viscoli C, Horwitz R. Preventive health strategies and the policy-makers paradox. Ann Intern Med 1992; 116:593–597.
7. Buchanan T, Catalano P. The pathogenesis of GDM: Implications for diabetes after pregnancy. Diabetes Rev 1995; 3:584–601.
8. Caro J, Sinha M, Kolaczynski J, et al. Leptin: The tale of an obesity gene. Diabetes 1996; 45:1455–1462.
9. Fletcher R, Fletcher S, Wagner E. Cause. *In* Fletcher R, Fletcher S, Wagner E (eds): Clinical Epidemiology: The Essentials. Baltimore, Williams & Wilkins, 1998, pp 208–225.
10. CDC. Update: Prevalence of overweight among children, adolescents, and adults—United States, 1988–1994. MMWR 1997; 46:199–202.
11. Chan J, Rimm E, Colditz G, et al. Obesity, fat distribution, and weight gain as risk factors for clinical diabetes in men. Diabetes Care 1994; 17:961–969.
12. Charlton B. Attribution of causation in epidemiology: Chain or mosaic? J Clin Epidemiol 1996; 49:105–107.
13. Clandinin M, Cheema S, Field C, et al. Dietary lipids influence insulin action. Ann N Y Acad Sci 1993; 683:164–171.
14. Clark C, Qui C, Amerman B, et al. Gestational diabetes: Should it be added to the syndrome of insulin resistance? Diabetes Care 1997; 20:867–871.
15. Coustan D. Diagnosis of gestational diabetes. Diabetes Rev 1995; 3:614–620.
16. Cowie C, Harris M. Physical and metabolic characteristics of persons with diabetes. *In* National Diabetes Data Group (eds): Diabetes in America, ed 2. Bethesda, Md, National Institutes of Health, National Institute of Diabetes and Digestive and Kidney Diseases, NIH Publication no. 95-1468, 1995, pp 117–164.
17. Critchfield T, Burris A. Chromium supplements: What's the story? Diabetes Forecast 1996; 49:24–26.
18. Culyer A, Harris J. The rationing debate: Maximising the health of the whole community—the case for and against. BMJ 1997; 314:667–672.
19. Detsky A, Naglie I. A clinician's guide to cost-effectiveness analysis. Ann Intern Med 1990; 113:147–154.
20. Diabetes Control and Complications Trial Research Group. The effects of intensive treatment of diabetes on the development and progression of long-term complications in insulin-dependent diabetes mellitus. N Engl J Med 1993; 329:977–986.
21. Eastman R, Javitt J, Herman W, et al. Prevention strategies for non–insulin-dependent diabetes mellitus: An economic perspective. *In* LeRoith D, Taylor S, Olefsky J (eds): Diabetes Mellitus. Philadelphia, Lippincott-Raven, 1996, pp 621–630.
22. Eastman R, Javitt J, Herman W, et al. Model of complications of NIDDM: II. Analysis of the health benefits and cost-effectiveness of treating NIDDM with the goal of normoglycemia. Diabetes Care 1997; 20:735–744.
23. Eliasson B, Tasken M-R, Smith U. Long-term use of nicotine gum is associated with hyperinsulinemia and insulin resistance. Circulation 1996; 94:878–881.
24. Eriksson K, Lindgurde F. Prevention of type 2 (non–insulin-dependent) diabetes mellitus by diet and physical exercise: The 6 year Malmo feasibility study. Diabetologia 1991; 34:891–898.
25. Eriksson U, Borg L, Forsberg H, et al. Can fetal loss be

prevented? The biochemical basis of diabetic embryopathy. Diabetes Rev 1996; 4:49–69.

26. Feinleib M. New directions for community intervention studies. Am J Public Health 1996; 86:1696–1698.

27. Feskens E, Kromhout D. Cardiovascular risk factors and the 25-year incidence of diabetes mellitus in middle-aged men: The Zutphen study. Am J Epidemiol 1989; 130:1101–1108.

28. Final Conference Report and Recommendations from American's Health Community. Tobacco Use: An American Crisis. Atlanta, U.S. Department of Health and Human Services, Public Health Service, Centers for Disease Control and Prevention, Office of Smoking and Health, 1993.

29. Frati A, Iniestra F, Ariza RC. Acute effects of cigarette smoking on glucose tolerance and other cardiovascular risk factors. Diabetes Care 1996; 19:112–118.

30. Goldberg R, Dalen J. Enhancing peer review of scientific manuscripts. Arch Intern Med 1997; 157:380–382.

31. Harris M. NIDDM: Epidemiology and scope of the problem. Diabetes Spectrum 1996; 9:26–29.

32. Helmrich S, Raglund D, Leung R, et al. Physical activity and reduced occurrence of non–insulin-dependent diabetes mellitus. N Engl J Med 1991; 325:147–152.

33. Hill BH. The environment and disease: Association or causation? Proc R Soc Med 1965; 58:295–300.

34. Jakicic J, Leermakers E. Commit to get fit: Exercise for life. Diabetes Spectrum 1996; 9:202–204.

35. Jung R, Lean M. The "wrong trousers" but the right approach to obesity. Diabetic Med 1997; 14:273–274.

36. Kenny S, Aubert R, Geiss L. Prevalence and incidence of non–insulin-dependent diabetes. In National Diabetes Data Group (eds): Diabetes in America, ed 2. Bethesda, MD, National Institutes of Health, National Institute of Diabetes and Digestive and Kidney Diseases, NIH Publication no. 95-1468, 1995, pp 47–68.

37. King H, Dowd J. Primary prevention of type 2 (NID) diabetes mellitus. Diabetologia 1990; 33:3–8.

38. King H, Kriska A. Prevention of type 2 diabetes by physical training: Epidemiology considerations and study methods. Diabetes Care 1992; 15:1794–1799.

39. Kjos S, Peters R, Xiang A, et al. Predicting future diabetes in Latino women with gestational diabetes: Utility of early postpartum glucose tolerance testing. Diabetes 1995; 44:586–591.

40. Knowler W, Narayan K, Hanson R, et al. Preventing non–insulin-dependent diabetes. Diabetes 1995; 44:483–488.

41. Kok G, Borne B, Mullen P. Effectiveness of health education and health promotion: Meta-analyses of effect studies and determinants of effectiveness. Patient Ed Counsel 1997; 30:19–27.

42. Kriska A, Blair S, Pereira M. The potential role of physical activity in the prevention of noninsulin-dependent diabetes mellitus: The epidemiological evidence. Exerc Sport Sci Rev 1994; 22:121–143.

43. Kuczmarski R. Increasing prevalence of overweight among U.S. adults: National Health and Nutrition Examination Survey 1960–1994. JAMA 1994; 272:205–211.

44. Larson J, Dela F, Kjaer M, et al. The effect of moderate exercise on postprandial glucose homeostasis in NIDDM patients. Diabetologia 1997; 40:447–453.

45. Lynch J, Helmrich S, Lakka T, et al. Moderately intense physical activities and high levels of cardiorespiratory fitness reduce the risk of non–insulin-dependent diabetes mellitus in middle-aged men. Arch Intern Med 1996; 156:1307–1314.

46. Manson J, Spelsberg A. Primary prevention of non-insulin-dependent diabetes mellitus. Am J Prev Med 1994; 10:172–184.

47. Manson J, Rimm E, Stampfer M, et al. Physical activity and incidence of non-insulin-dependent diabetes mellitus in women. Lancet 1991; 338:774–778.

48. Manson J, Nathan D, Krolewski A, et al. A prospective study of exercise and incidence of diabetes among US male physicians. JAMA 1992; 268:63–67.

49. Manson J, Rimm E, Colditz G, et al. A prospective study of parity and the subsequent development of non–insulin-dependent diabetes mellitus. Am J Med 1992; 93:13–18.

50. Manson J, Rimm E, Colditz G, et al. Parity and incidence of non–insulin-dependent diabetes mellitus. Am J Med 1992; 93:13–18.

51. Mariner W. Rationing health care and the need for credible scarcity: Why Americans can't say no. Am J Public Health 1995; 85:1439–1445.

52. Marshall J, Hoag S, Shetterly S, et al. Dietary fat predicts conversion from impaired glucose tolerance to NIDDM. Diabetes Care 1994; 17:50–56.

53. McCormick J. Health promotion: The ethical dimension. Lancet 1994; 344:390–391.

54. Morabia A. On the origin of Hill's causal criteria. Epidemiology 1991; 2:367–369.

55. Murray C, Lopez A. Alternative projections of mortality and disability by cause 1990–2020: Global burden of disease study. Lancet 1997; 349:1498–1504.

56. National Institutes of Health. Non-insulin dependent diabetes primary prevention trial. NIH Guide Grants Contracts 1993; 22:1–20.

57. Pan X, Li G, Hu Y, et al. Effects of diet and exercise in preventing NIDDM in people with impaired glucose tolerance. Diabetes Care 1997; 20:537–544.

58. Pi-Sunyer X. Health implications of obesity. Am J Clin Nutr 1991; 53:1595S–1603S.

59. Purdy L, Metzger B. Influences of the intrauterine metabolic environment on adult disease: What may we infer from size at birth? Diabetologia 1996; 39:1126–1130.

60. Reaven G. Role of insulin resistance in human disease. Diabetes 1988; 37:1595–1607.

61. Renton A. Epidemiology and causation: A realist view. J Epidemiol Commmunity Health 1994; 48:79–85.

62. Rewers M, Hamman R. Risk factors for non–insulin-dependent diabetes. In National Diabetes Data Group (eds): Diabetes in America. Bethesda, Md, Department of Health and Human Services, National Institutes of Health, National Institute of Diabetes, Digestive and Kidney Disease; 1996, pp 179–220.

63. Rimm E, Manson J, Stampfer M, et al. A prospective study of cigarette smoking and the risk of diabetes in women. Am J Public Health 1993; 83:211–214.

64. Ruggiero L, Prochaska J. Readiness for change: Application of the transtheoretical model to diabetes. Diabetes Spectrum 1993; 6:21–24.

65. Salmeron J, Manson J, Stampfer M, et al. Dietary fiber, glycemic load, and risk of non–insulin-dependent diabetes mellitus in women. JAMA 1997; 277:472–477.

66. Salonen J, Nyyssonen K, Tuomainen T-P, et al. Increased risk of non–insulin dependent diabetes mellitus at low plasma vitamin E concentrations: A four year follow up study in men. Br Med J 1995; 311:1124–1127.

67. Schafer R, Bohannon B, Franz M, et al. Translation of the diabetes nutrition recommendations for health care institutions. Diabetes Care 1997; 20:96–105.

68. Silverman B, Rizzo T, Green O, et al. Long-term prospective evaluation of offspring of diabetic mothers. Diabetes 1991; 40(S2):121–125.

69. Silverman B, Purdy L, Metzger B. The intrauterine

environment: Implications for the offspring of diabetic mothers. Diabetes Rev 1996; 4:21–35.

70. Skrabanek P. Why is preventive medicine exempted from ethical constraints? J Med Ethics 1990; 16:187–190.

71. Stamler J, Vaccaro O, Neaton J, et al. Diabetes, other risk factors, and 12-yr cardiovascular mortality of men screened in the Multiple Risk Factor Intervention Trial. Diabetes Care 1993; 16:434–444.

72. Susser M. What is a cause and how do we know one? A grammar for pragmatic epidemiology. Am J Epidemiol 1991; 133:635–648.

73. The Expert Committee on the Diagnosis and Classification of Diabetes Mellitus. Report of the expert committee on the diagnosis and classification of diabetes mellitus. Diabetes Care 1997; 20:1183–1197.

74. Therapies for obesity: Are we making progress? Diabetes Spectrum 1995; 8:333–335.

75. U.S. Department of Health and Human Services. Physical Activity and Health: A Report of the Surgeon General. Atlanta, U.S. Department of Health and Human Services, Centers for Disease Control and Prevention, National Center for Chronic Disease Prevention and Health Promotion, 1996.

76. Valdez R, Athens M, Thompson G, et al. Birth weight and adult health outcomes in a biethnic population in the USA. Diabetologia 1994; 37:624–631.

77. Vinicor F. Is diabetes a public-health disorder? Diabetes Care 1994; 17(S1):22–27.

78. Vinicor F. Challenges to the translation of the DCCT. Diabetes Rev 1994; 2:371–383.

79. Wynia M. Economic analyses, the medical commons, and patients' dilemmas: What is the physician's role? J Invest Med 1997; 45:35–43.

80. Zimmet P. The pathogenesis and prevention of diabetes in adults. Genes, autoimmunity, and demography. Diabetes Care 1995; 18:1050–1065.

81. Epidemiology and Statistics Branch, Division of Diabetes Translation, National Center for Chronic Disease Prevention and Health Promotion. CDC trends in the prevalence and incidence of self-reported diabetes mellitus, United States 1980–1994. MMWR Morb Mort Wkly Rep 1997; 46:1014–1018.

Chapter **4**

Diabetic Retinopathy

John M. Pach

INTRODUCTION

Diabetic retinopathy is a leading cause of blindness in adults. It is classified into background and proliferative types. In background diabetic retinopathy, abnormalities of retinal vascular perfusion and permeability lead to the formation of microaneurysms, intraretinal hemorrhages, and macular edema. Diabetic macular edema is the leading cause of decreased vision among diabetics. Laser photocoagulation for the treatment of macular edema is indicated when retinal thickening includes or approaches the center of fixation. Retinal ischemia can lead to the formation of neovascularization along the surface of the retina. Scatter laser photocoagulation may be done to cause regression of neovascularization and prevent complications such as vitreous hemorrhage and traction retinal detachment. Indications for intraocular surgery include nonclearing vitreous hemorrhage and traction retinal detachment involving the macula. Risk factors in the progression of diabetic retinopathy include duration, poor glycemic control, and pregnancy.

Diabetes mellitus affects about 7 million people in the United States, and it is the leading cause of new blindness in adults aged 20 to 74 years. The annual prevalence of diabetes from 1980 to 1987 increased from 25.4 to 27.6 per 1000, with African-Americans and females more commonly affected. Nearly 40,000 new cases of blindness occur each year among diabetics, and most cases are caused by diabetic retinopathy.[31]

The 10-year incidence of blindness (20/200 or less in the better eye) has been reported to be 4.8% in an older-onset non–insulin-dependent group, 4% in an older-onset insulin-dependent group, and 1.8% in a younger onset group.[28] The 10-year incidence of visual impairment (visual acuity of 20/40 or less in the better eye) was 23.9% in the older-onset non–insulin-dependent group, 37.2% in the older-onset insulin-dependent group, and 9.4% in the younger onset group.

Screening eye examinations have been shown to be cost effective. In 1991, it was estimated that at a 60% screening and treatment implementation level of type I diabetics, more than $100 million and 47,000 person-years-sight would be saved.[22] With all patients receiving appropriate eye care, savings would exceed $167 million and 79,000 person-years-sight. This assumes the cost of blindness per patient at $15,205 per year (age younger than 65 years), with $484 per year (age older than 64 years) going to the U.S. government.

BACKGROUND DIABETIC RETINOPATHY

Diabetic retinopathy is classified into background (nonproliferative) and proliferative types. Background retinopathy refers to the retinal microvascular changes that typically occur before the onset of proliferative disease. Abnormalities of retinal vascular perfusion and permeability lead to the fundus changes seen in background diabetic retinopathy. The characteristic microvascular abnormality is the formation of retinal capillary microaneurysms. The retinal capillaries are composed of two types of cells: endothelial cells and pericytes. In the normal state, there are approximately equal numbers of cells, and the pericyte to endothelial cell ratio is 1:1. In diabetics, there is a selective loss of pericytes, and the ratio of pericytes to endothelial cells is less than 1:1.[36] Preferential loss of capillary pericytes leads to microaneurysms, which are saccular dilatations of the capillary wall. The capillary basement membrane thickens as a result of various biochemical processes.[3]

Capillary dilation, abnormalities of permeability, and shunt formation may follow. Capillary closure and retinal nonperfusion result in hypoxia. The presence of intraretinal microvascular abnormality (IRMA) indicates retinal ischemia, which is often a precursor to the development of retinal neovascularization. The term *IRMA* describes a small dilated vessel that most likely represents an arteriolar venular shunt. Other indicators of retinal hypoxia are venous beading, which is an irregular dilatation of the veins, and cotton-wool spots, which represent infarcts of the nerve fiber layer of the retina and focal interruption of axoplasmic flow.

Intraretinal hemorrhages may occur from breakdown of fragile capillaries and microaneurysms. Hemorrhages in the nerve fiber layer of the inner retina are called splinter, or flame-shaped, hemorrhages. Dot-and-blot hemorrhages lie in the deeper layers of the retina. Arteriolar occlusion may lead to hemorrhagic infarcts, resulting in the formation of many larger intraretinal hemorrhages.

Mild background diabetic retinopathy is characterized by the presence of cotton-wool spots, hard exudates, and retinal hemorrhages. The presence of IRMA or numerous dot-and-blot hemorrhages is consistent with moderate background changes. With the occurrence of venous beading and more numerous hemorrhages, microaneurysms, and IRMA throughout the retina, the background changes are considered severe or preproliferative.[16]

DIABETIC MACULAR EDEMA

Abnormal permeability of the blood retinal barrier can be detected by fluorescein angiography or vitreous fluorophotometry before ophthalmoscopy.[19] Retinal edema occurs as fluid leaks from microaneurysms, IRMA, and retinal capillaries. Edema within the macula may lead to significant visual impairment in diabetics. Macular edema appears as visible thickening of the retina. Edema within the center of the macula may take the form of cysts and is referred to as cystoid macular edema (CME). Cystoid macular edema is not specific to diabetic retinopathy, but it may occur in other retinal vascular disorders, such as venous occlusive disease, and after cataract surgery. Macular edema may be present and require treatment despite normal vision. Screening for edema must include assessment of visual acuity as well as a dilated fundus examination. Hard exudates are often seen with macular edema and represent intraretinal accumulations of lipoproteins. The presence of hard exudates should alert the clinician to the presence of macular edema, which may be difficult to detect without slit lamp examination (Fig. 4.1). Examination at the slit lamp aided with the

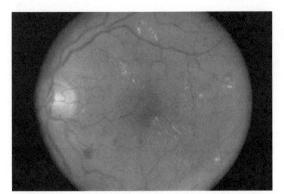

■ **Figure 4.1** Background diabetic retinopathy with scattered microaneurysms and intraretinal hemorrhages. Exudates suggest the presence of retinal thickening.

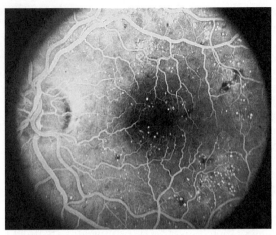

■ **Figure 4.2** Fluorescein angiogram demonstrates scattered microaneurysms throughout the macula.

use of a contact lens is needed to detect the more subtle forms of macular edema. Macular edema is a clinical diagnosis that is considered significant if retinal thickening is detected within 500 μm of the center of fixation or if there is an area of retinal thickening greater than one disc area in size within one disc area from the center of fixation.[12]

Diabetic macular edema is a leading cause of decreased vision among diabetics. The incidence of macular edema during a 10-year period in a population-based study was 20% in younger-onset diabetics and 25% in older-onset insulin-dependent types, and 14% in older-onset non–insulin-dependent types.[26] Risk factors for the development of macular edema include increased duration of diabetes in the younger-onset type, increase in diastolic blood pressure in the older-onset type, and higher glycosylated hemoglobin in both groups. The incidence of macular edema increases as the overall severity of the retinopathy worsens. The presence of proteinuria may also be a risk factor in the development of macular edema. In type I diabetics, the cumulative risk of macular edema is zero until seven years duration of diabetes. The cumulative risk increases linearly for each year of duration between 10 and 20 years, with the average annual increase of approximately 7%.[35]

Macular edema may also be classified as focal or diffuse.[4] Focal edema is characterized by clusters of microaneurysms with areas of localized retinal edema. Microaneurysms are the major source of leakage (Figs. 4.2 and 4.3). Hard exudate rings may surround areas of leakage, producing a circinate pattern (Fig. 4.4). Diffuse macular edema results from a generalized breakdown of the inner blood retinal bar-

rier in which not only the microaneurysms but also capillaries and arterioles leak (Figs. 4.5 to 4.7).[4]

TREATMENT OF DIABETIC MACULAR EDEMA

The Early Treatment Diabetic Retinopathy Study (ETDRS) assessed the effect of focal laser photocoagulation on the course of diabetic macular edema.[12, 13] The ETDRS, supported by the National Eye Institute, was a multicenter, randomized clinical trial designed to evaluate, in part, the effectiveness of photocoagulation in the treatment of diabetic macular edema. Eyes with clinically significant macular edema were assigned to immediate focal laser photocoagulation or to deferral of treatment. At 3

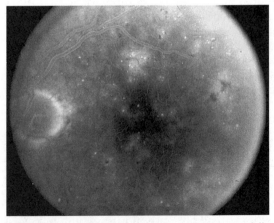

■ **Figure 4.3** Late frames of the angiogram of the patient in Figure 4–2. Several areas of dye leakage from clusters of microaneurysms are shown.

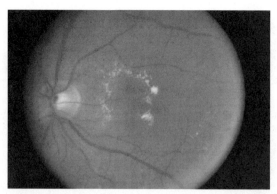

■ **Figure 4.4** Background diabetic retinopathy with exudates demarcating the area of retinal thickening. This is considered clinically significant diabetic macular edema because the exudates are within 500 μm from the center of fixation.

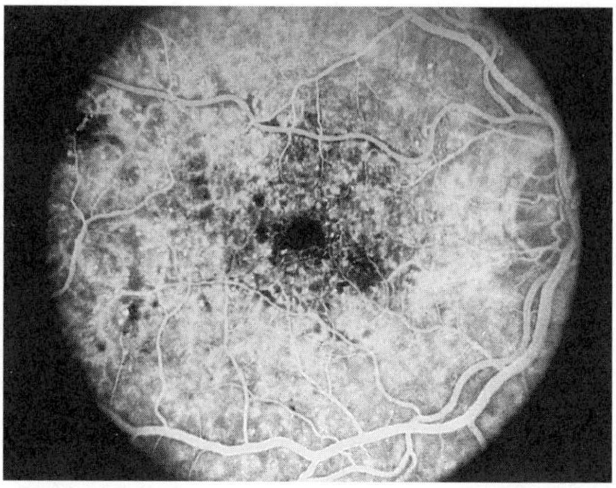

■ **Figure 4.6** Fluorescein angiogram showing effuse dilatation of the capillary bed.

years of follow-up, eyes assigned to immediate treatment were approximately one-half as likely to lose significant vision as compared with eyes assigned to deferral of treatment (12% versus 24%).

Fluorescein angiography aids in the treatment of macular edema. In cases of focal edema, microaneurysms are readily apparent and easily localized. The object of treatment is to photocoagulate the microaneurysms with 50 to 100 μm size burns. Several attempts may be needed to achieve the end point, which is a whitening around the microaneurysms and darkening of the microaneurysm itself (Fig. 4.8). It may be difficult to darken a small microaneurysm (less than 40 μm), in which case whitening of the retina around it may only be achieved. In diffuse macular edema, a grid pattern of photocoagulation burns sparing the center of the macula is used. Prompt treatment

for macular edema is recommended in eyes with retinal thickening involving the center of the macula associated with a drop in vision.[13] Thirty-five percent to 45% of untreated eyes with vision of 20/30 to 20/60 experience significant visual loss without treatment after 3 years. Treatment is less urgent when the center of the macula is not involved but the edema is within 500 μm of it and the vision is not reduced. It is acceptable to delay photocoagulation in eyes in which the fovea is not threatened. Macular edema usually progresses slowly, and treatment is more effective in preventing visual loss rather than restoring vision already lost.

Visual decline may occur after focal laser photocoagulation for diabetic macular edema from inadvertent photocoagulation of the fovea, expansion of laser scars, choroidal neovas-

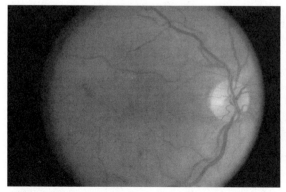

■ **Figure 4.5** Background diabetic retinopathy. Diffuse macular edema is present, with loss of the foveal reflex.

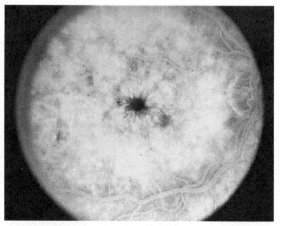

■ **Figure 4.7** Late frames of the angiogram reveal the diffuse nature of dye leakage.

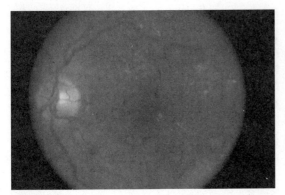

■ **Figure 4.8** Photo taken after treatment of diabetic macular edema with focal laser photocoagulation. Laser burns are light and directed at specific microaneurysms.

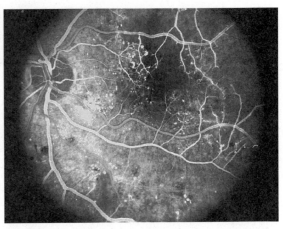

■ **Figure 4.10** Fluorescein angiogram reveals areas of capillary nonperfusion involving an area superior to the fovea. A single perifoveal capillary remains superiorly.

cularization, and submacular fibrosis.[20, 21, 33] The risk is greater when photocoagulation must be placed close to the foveal avascular zone.

Visual loss in background retinopathy may also occur from macular ischemia. Occlusion of the capillaries supplying the center of the macula or fovea leads to irreversible visual loss (Figs. 4.9 and 4.10). Macular ischemia often coexists with edema and may be the limiting factor in visual recovery.

PROLIFERATIVE DIABETIC RETINOPATHY AND VITREOUS HEMORRHAGE

In the setting of background diabetic retinopathy, occlusion of the retinal capillaries typically occurs in the retinal periphery. Retinal ischemia leads to retinal neovascularization. Ischemic retina may be the source of an angiogenic factor or factors that leads to endothelial cell pro-

liferation and new blood vessel formation on the retina or iris. The angiogenic factor in the production of neovascularization may be vascular endothelial growth factor (VEGF) or vascular permeability factor.[1, 2] The concentration of vascular endothelial growth factor was measured from vitreous samples removed during intraocular surgery. Concentrations of VEGF were higher in patients with active proliferative diabetic retinopathy than in patients with nonproliferative diabetic retinopathy, quiescent proliferative diabetic retinopathy, and nondiabetic patients. This suggests VEGF plays a role in new blood vessel formation caused by retinal ischemia.

Neovascularization that characteristically occurs on the optic disc is called neovascularization of the disc (NVD).[18] Neovascularization also is found in the retinal midperiphery and is referred to as neovascularization elsewhere (NVE) (Fig. 4.11). Angiogenic factors may diffuse anteriorly and stimulate neovascularization on the iris. Neovascularization of the iris (NVI) most often occurs on the pupillary border. It may also be found in the trabecular meshwork, which can lead to synechiae formation. This results in obstruction of aqueous humor outflow and elevated intraocular pressure, often to very high levels. This type of glaucoma, neovascular glaucoma, is difficult to treat and leads to devastating visual loss.

Retinal neovascularization proliferates on the surface of the retina or optic nerve and extends along their surfaces and into the vitreous cavity.[7] Neovascular proliferation proceeds at a variable rate. In some patients, neovascular

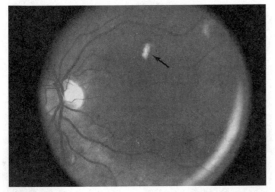

■ **Figure 4.9** Background diabetic retinopathy. *Arrow* indicates cotton-wool spot suggestive of ischemia.

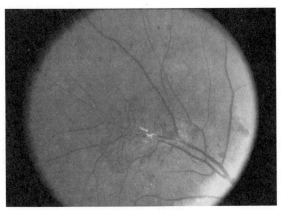

■ **Figure 4.11** Frond of neovascularization elsewhere (NVE) along the superotemporal arcade.

fronds may show little change over weeks or months and eventually become fibrotic. In other cases, the new blood vessels can increase over several weeks. In time, the new blood vessels partially regress and are replaced with fibrous tissue. During this cycle, patients are often asymptomatic. As the posterior vitreous detaches from the retina, traction on these newly formed blood vessels may lead to a vitreous hemorrhage (Fig. 4.12). When this occurs, patients report a decrease in acuity and floaters in the shape of lines, specks, or cobwebs obscuring the vision. This phase of vitreous contraction occurs in a stepwise fashion. As the vitreous detaches it may pull on the new blood vessels, often leading to recurrent vitreous hemorrhages. Hemorrhages may also occur as a result of coughing or vomiting, but more often occur during sleep.

Further contraction of the vitreous and the fibrovascular proliferation can lead to traction on the retina. The retina may then become

elevated or tented, which is termed a traction detachment. At times, the contraction can lead to hole formation in the retina, which can then create a rhegmatogenous component to the retinal detachment. Localized traction detachments may occur outside the macula and therefore do not lead to visual loss. If the traction detachment includes the macula, however, there may be profound visual loss.

TREATMENT OF PROLIFERATIVE DIABETIC RETINOPATHY

The Diabetic Retinopathy Study (DRS) evaluated the effect of panretinal photocoagulation in the treatment of proliferative diabetic retinopathy.[10, 11] The DRS was a randomized controlled clinical trial in which proliferative diabetic retinopathy was treated with scatter photocoagulation; that is, laser was directed outside the posterior pole and macula to the peripheral retina. It is placed in a random grid pattern to ablate ischemic retina (Fig. 4.13). In some cases, neovascularization can be directly treated. About 1200 to 1600 burns were placed in multiple sessions. Scatter photocoagulation reversed new blood vessel formation and reduced the rate of severe visual loss. The DRS determined that laser was effective in the treatment of proliferative diabetic retinopathy with high-risk characteristics. High-risk characteristics included disc neovascularization covering approximately one third of the disc area and vitreous hemorrhage associated with any disc neovascularization or NVE of one-half disc area in size or more. In those patients in the high-risk category, panretinal photocoagula-

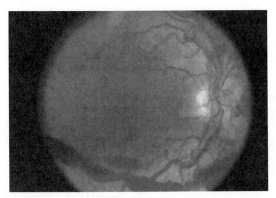

■ **Figure 4.12** Extensive frond of neovascularization of the disc (NVD) and preretinal hemorrhage.

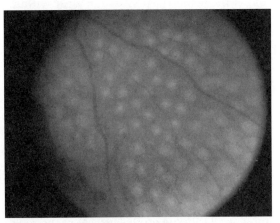

■ **Figure 4.13** Scattered laser photocoagulation burns in the retinal periphery adjacent to an area of preretinal hemorrhage.

tion reduced the rate of severe visual loss (acuity of 5/200 or worse) from 26% in the control group to 11% in the treated group at 2 years.[7] Twenty-five percent of patients treated with scatter photocoagulation required additional treatment. Indications for supplemental panretinal photocoagulation include lack of regression of neovascularization, additional neovascularization, or vitreous hemorrhage.

In eyes with early proliferative retinopathy, treatment is delayed until the high-risk category is reached. The 5-year rate of severe visual loss is low whether scatter photocoagulation is done early (3.7%) or delayed until the high-risk characteristics develop (2.6%).[15] Macular edema may occur after scatter treatment and lead to moderate visual loss (doubling of the visual angle, i.e., from 20/30 to 20/60 or 20/50 to 20/100). Therefore, in eyes with severe nonproliferative or early proliferative retinopathy, visual loss may be avoided by delaying treatment. As eyes approach the high-risk stage, scatter photocoagulation should be considered but not delayed once the criteria are met. In eyes with coexisting clinically significant macular edema and proliferative disease, focal treatment of the macular edema should be considered immediately, whereas scatter treatment should be delayed because it has an adverse effect on macular edema and visual acuity. In those eyes where scatter is necessary, focal treatment may be done simultaneously.

The presence of a vitreous hemorrhage may prevent panretinal laser photocoagulation. In those cases in which the retina is attached, treatment may be delayed until the vitreous hemorrhage clears. It may take several months for the blood to clear from the vitreous cavity to allow adequate laser photocoagulation. As a rule, if the hemorrhage does not clear within 6 months, vitreous surgery can be considered. During this time, close monitoring is essential. If the retina detaches, surgery is necessary. Often ultrasonography is needed to determine the status of the retina if vitreous hemorrhage prevents adequate visualization.

Nonclearing vitreous hemorrhage and traction macular detachments are indications for vitreous surgery. In a vitrectomy, the vitreous gel and blood are removed with needlelike instruments that cut tissue with a repetitive guillotine action and remove it with active suction. Direct tissue manipulation can also be done in which the posterior vitreous and the fibrovascular tissue on the surface of the retina can be dissected and removed through the use of intraocular scissors, picks, and forceps. Laser

photocoagulation may also be applied at the time of surgery with an intraocular probe or with an indirect ophthalmoscopic delivery system. Retinal holes and detachments require the use of various intraocular gases or air that tamponade the retina. Intraocular gas may last from days to weeks, and for treatment to be effective, the patient is usually positioned face down so the bubble can tamponade a specific area of the retina.

FACTORS IN THE PROGRESSION OF DIABETIC RETINOPATHY

Duration of diabetes is a strong risk factor in the development and progression of diabetic retinopathy.[25] In young-onset diabetics, retinopathy is not typically present at the time of diagnosis. The blood retinal barrier as determined by vitreous fluorophotometry remains intact until puberty. The prevalence of retinopathy is low in the years immediately after puberty (6% at 4 years) and increases with time (30% between 4 and 8 years).[17] Retinopathy is often present at the time of diagnosis in the older-onset type and may be severe.

The overall 10-year incidence of any retinopathy has been estimated to be 74%.[25] The rate of progression is 64%, with 17% progressing to proliferative disease during a 10-year period. Of diabetics without retinopathy, 89% of young onset (less than age 30 years) developed retinopathy during a 10-year period, as compared with 79% of older-onset insulin-dependent diabetics and 67% of older-onset insulin-independent diabetics. In addition, during a 10-year period, 30% of younger-onset diabetics developed proliferative retinopathy, compared with 24% of older-onset insulin-dependent diabetics and 10% of older-onset insulin-independent diabetics.

Glycemic control is another strong risk factor in the development of diabetic retinopathy. The Diabetes Control and Complications Trial (DCCT) studied the effect of intensive insulin treatment, with near normalization of blood glucose level, and conventional insulin therapy on the vascular and neurologic complications of insulin dependent DM.[8, 9] Intensive treatment with multiple daily injections of insulin or with an insulin pump and frequent blood glucose monitoring reduced the risk of development and progression of retinopathy when compared with conventional treatment. This effect was seen in patients with no retinopathy at baseline and duration of diabetes of 1 to 5 years (primary prevention cohort) and in those with very mild to moderate background retinopathy at baseline and duration of 1 to 15 years (secondary intervention cohort). There was an early worsening effect in the intensive treatment group within the first year that was often followed by an increasing beneficial effect over time. This substantial effect was apparent in all grades of retinopathy and increased with time.

The risk of progression was at least five times lower with intensive treatment compared with conventional treatment after 3.5 years of follow-up. There was little difference in progression of retinopathy between the two forms of treatment within the first 2 years of follow up. This may be explained by the initial adverse effect of intensive treatment and a possible inherent "momentum" of the retinopathy. Recovery after progression of retinopathy was greater with intensive treatment. In the primary prevention cohort, the rate of recovery after sustained progression was twice as great with intensive treatment compared with conventional treatment. In the secondary intervention cohort, the rate of recovery was about three times greater in the intensive group compared with the conventional group. This effect was present through the severe forms of retinopathy at baseline.

The more severe forms of retinopathy were not included in the DCCT. Initiating intensive treatment in these groups may have a significant clinical adverse effect. Close monitoring of these patients is recommended, with initiation of prompt photocoagulation if necessary.

The use of aspirin is not contraindicated in diabetics with retinopathy. Aspirin does not alter the course of retinopathy, nor does it prevent the development of high-risk proliferative retinopathy.[14] It also does not reduce the risk of visual loss or alter the occurrence, severity, and duration of vitreous hemorrhages.[6]

Increased systolic and diastolic blood pressure have been associated with a higher occurrence of retinopathy.[5, 23, 29] Proteinuria as measured by a reagent strip has also been shown to be a risk factor for development of proliferative retinopathy in younger-onset patients.[24]

Normoglycemia after successful combined pancreas and renal transplantation does not reverse or halt the progression of diabetic retinopathy.[30, 32]

Pregnant diabetics are at risk of rapid progression of retinopathy.[27, 34] If no retinopathy is present at the beginning of the pregnancy, there is little risk for vision threatening progression. Likewise, patients with quiescent retinopathy after scatter photocoagulation are at little risk of complications. Those patients with severe background or early proliferative disease are at the greatest risk of rapid progression and should be very closely observed during their pregnancies. Photocoagulation should be promptly initiated and completed in those with high-risk characteristics. The threshold for treatment may be lowered in those patients with rapid progression. In general, diabetics should be examined early in their pregnancies and closely monitored. Toxemia of pregnancy with renal involvement and elevated blood pressure may lead to macular edema, which may be severe. The edema may regress with normalization of blood pressure and diuresis.

References

1. Adamis AP, Miller JW, Bernal M, et al. Increased vascular endothelial growth factor levels in the vitreous of eyes with proliferative diabetic retinopathy. Am J Ophthalmol 1994; 118:445–450.
2. Aiello LP, Avery RL, Arrigg PG, et al. Vascular endothelial growth factor in ocular fluid of patients with diabetic retinopathy and other retinal disorders. N Engl J Med 1994; 331:1480–1487.
3. Albert DM, Jakobiec FA. Principles and Practice of Ophthalmology. Philadelphia, WB Saunders, 1994, pp 2239–2280.
4. Bresnick GH. Diabetic macular edema. Ophthalmology 1986; 93:989–997.
5. Chase HP, Garg SK, Jackson WE, et al. Blood pressure and retinopathy in Type I diabetes. Ophthalmology 1990; 97:155–159.
6. Chew EY, Klein ML, Murphy RP, et al. Effects of aspirin on vitreous/preretinal hemorrhage in patients with diabetes mellitus. Arch Ophthalmol 1995; 113:52–55.
7. Davis M. Proliferative diabetic retinopathy. Retina 1994; 1319–1359.
8. Diabetes Control and Complications Trial Research Group. The effect of intensive treatment of diabetes on the development and progression of long-term complications in insulin-dependent diabetes mellitus. N Engl J Med 1993; 329:977–986.
9. Diabetes Control and Complications Trial Research Group. The effect of intensive diabetes treatment on the progression of diabetic retinopathy in insulin-dependent diabetes mellitus. Arch Ophthalmol 1995; 113:36–51.
10. Diabetic Retinopathy Study Research Group. Preliminary report on effects of photocoagulation therapy. Am J Ophthalmol 1976; 81:383–395.
11. Diabetic Retinopathy Study Research Group. Photocoagulation treatment of proliferative diabetic retinopathy: The second report of diabetic retinopathy study findings. Ophthalmology 1978; 85:82–104.
12. Early Treatment Diabetic Retinopathy Study Research Group. Photocoagulation for diabetic macular edema. ETDRS report number 1. Arch Ophthalmol 1985; 103:1796–1806.
13. Early Treatment Diabetic Retinopathy Study Research Group. Treatment techniques and clinical guidelines for photocoagulation of diabetic macular edema. Ophthalmology 1987; 94:761–774.

14. Early Treatment Diabetic Retinopathy Study Research Group. Effects of aspirin treatment on diabetic retinopathy. ETDRS report number 8. Ophthalmology 1991; 98:757–765.

15. Early Treatment Diabetic Retinopathy Study Research Group. Early photocoagulation for diabetic retinopathy. ETDRS report number 9. Ophthalmology 1991; 98:766–785.

16. Early Treatment Diabetic Retinopathy Study Research Group. Fundus photographic risk factors for progression of diabetic retinopathy. ETDRS report number 12. Ophthalmology 1991; 98:823–833.

17. Faria de Abreu JR, Silva R, Cunha-Vaz JG. The blood-retinal barrier in diabetes during puberty. Arch Ophthalmol 1994; 112:1334–1338.

18. Four Risk Factors for Severe Visual Loss in Diabetic Retinopathy. The Third Report From the Diabetic Retinopathy Study. Arch Ophthalmol 1979; 97:654–655.

19. Frank RN. The mechanism of blood-retinal barrier breakdown in diabetes. Arch Ophthalmol 1985; 103:1303–1304.

20. Guyer DR, D'Amico DJ, Smith CW. Subretinal fibrosis after laser photo-coagulation for diabetic macular edema. Am J Ophthalmol 1992; 113:652–656.

21. Han DP, Mieler WF, Burton TC. Submacular fibrosis after photocoagulation for diabetic macular edema. Ophthalmology 1992; 113:513–521.

22. Javitt JC, Aiello LP, Bassi LJ, et al. Detecting and treating retinopathy in patients with type I diabetes mellitus. Ophthalmology 1991; 98:1565–1574.

23. Klein BEK, Klein R, Moss SE, et al. A cohort study of the relationship of diabetic retinopathy to blood pressure. Arch Ophthalmol 1995; 113:601–606.

24. Klein R, Moss SE, Klein BEK. Is gross proteinuria a risk factor for the incidence of proliferative diabetic retinopathy? Ophthalmology 1993; 100:1140–1146.

25. Klein R, Klein BEK, Moss SE, et al. The Wisconsin Epidemiologic Study of Diabetic Retinopathy. Ten-year incidence and progression of diabetic retinopathy. Arch Ophthalmol 1994; 112:1217–1228.

26. Klein R, Klein BEK, Moss SE, et al. The Wisconsin Epidemiologic Study of Diabetic Retinopathy XV. The long-term incidence of macular edema. Ophthalmology 1995; 102:7–16.

27. Moloney JBM, Drury MI. The effect of pregnancy on the natural course of diabetic retinopathy. Am J Ophthalmol 1982; 93:745–756.

28. Moss SE, Klein R, Klein BEK. Ten-year incidence of visual loss in a diabetic population. Ophthalmology 1994; 100:1062–1070.

29. Perkovich BT, Meyers SM. Systemic factors affecting diabetic macular edema. Am J Ophthalmol 1988; 105:211–212.

30. Petersen MR, Vine AK. Progression of diabetic retinopathy after pancreas transplantation. Ophthalmology 1990; 97:496–502.

31. Prevalence, incidence of diabetes mellitus—United States, 1980–1987. JAMA 1990; 264:3126.

32. Ramsay RC, Goetz FC, Sutherland DER, et al. Progression of diabetic retinopathy after pancreas transplantation for insulin-dependent diabetes mellitus. N Engl J Med 1988; 318:208–214.

33. Schatz H, Madeira D, McDonald R, et al. Progressive enlargement of laser scars following grid laser photocoagulation for diffuse diabetic macular edema. Arch Ophthalmol 1991; 109:1549–1551.

34. Sunness JS. The pregnant woman's eye. Surv Ophthalmol 1988; 32:219–238.

35. Vitale S, Maguire MG, Murphy RP, et al. Clinically significant macular edema in type I diabetes: Incidence and risk factors. Ophthalmology 1995;102:1170–1176.

36. Yanoff M, Fine BS. Pathology of the retina and vitreous. *In* Yanoff M, Fine BS (eds): Ocular Pathology. Philadelphia, Harper & Row, 1982, p 720.

Chapter **5**

Diabetic Nephropathy

David M. Wilson

DEFINITION AND EPIDEMIOLOGY

Diabetic nephropathy is a clinical syndrome characterized by persistent albuminuria, a relentless decline in glomerular filtration rate (GFR), elevated blood pressure, and increased relative mortality for cardiovascular disease. Diabetes is now the most prevalent cause of end-stage renal disease (ESRD) for patients entering dialysis transplant programs in the United States.[67]

An increasing incidence of diabetic nephropathy, despite aggressive hypertension control, raises the question of whether hypertension treatment will alter the long-term outcome. In 1993, data from the United States Renal Data System (USRDS) showed that the number of diabetic patients entering end-stage treatment programs was increasing at an annual rate of 15%.[84] Of these patients, about 50% had type 1 diabetes mellitus (DM) (juvenile-onset insulin-dependent diabetes mellitus), and 50% had type 2 DM (adult-onset non–insulin-dependent diabetes mellitus) patients. The USRDS 1996 data showed 56,600 new renal failure patients. Of these, 19,013 were diabetic, which is not as large an increase as previously and may indicate a possible leveling off of the increase in diabetic nephropathy.[85] Development of persistent proteinuria in type 1 DM presages onset of renal failure an average of 7 years later, although this is highly variable, and probability of survival has increased from 48 to 87% since the introduction of antihypertensive treatments.

About 40% of patients with type 1 DM will develop diabetic nephropathy, defined as albumin excretion greater than 300 mg/24 hours. Although the high cardiovascular mortality in diabetes is multifactorial, excess mortality in type 1 diabetes is almost entirely confined to patients with diabetic nephropathy. Cost management of patients with end-stage renal disease from diabetes exceeded $11.1 billion in 1994 in the United States. Given this huge outlay, it has been estimated that reducing the progression to ESRD from 20 to 18% of diabetics would pay for itself in decreased medical costs. Consequently, efforts for surveillance and aggressive approaches to prevent diabetic nephropathy have been increased.

Type 2 DM was initially thought to have a low incidence of renal involvement. More recently, however, a high frequency of renal involvement has been established. Nephropathy has been most clearly observed in Pima Indian patients with type 2 DM, up to 52% of whom develop nephropathy.[15, 74] Black and other nonwhite patients with type 2 DM also have a higher incidence of nephropathy.[11, 80]

PATHOLOGY

Diabetic nephropathy in humans is a specific pathologic constellation of structural abnormalities associated with characteristic immunohistochemical alterations. These glomerular, tubular, vascular, and interstitial changes are unique to diabetes (Figs. 5.1 and 5.2). Glomerular structural abnormalities show a striking correlation with renal functional changes in type 1 DM, suggesting mesangial expansion is

a critical lesion. Abnormalities occur in two patterns, the so-called nodular form (Kimmelstiel-Wilson syndrome) and, more commonly, a diffuse form. Expansion is caused by accumulation of mesangial matrix material and, to a lesser extent, expansion of the cellular compartment of the mesangium, presumably resulting in a loss of filtration surface.[26, 41, 65]

Global sclerosis of glomeruli also correlates with decreased GFR and proteinuria. Harris and colleagues postulated that the sclerosis is the result of mesangial expansion, which may result in capillary closure, or arteriolar hyalinosis, which correlates with the percent of globally sclerosed glomeruli and suggests an ischemic pathogenesis.[33] A thickened or reduplicated basement membrane of microvessels throughout the body, including the glomerulus, is a hallmark of diabetes mellitus. It is unlikely, however, that this change accounts for the decrease in GFR. In addition, expansion of the interstitial volume is increased in patients with long-standing type 1 DM regardless of whether they have developed functional abnormalities. In the study by Lane and associates, the interstitial volume changes did not correlate as well with changes in GFR as reported in other forms of renal disease.[41]

The early lesion of type 2 DM has been established in several studies. Gambara and colleagues described 52 patients with type 2 DM and overt clinical nephropathy who were biopsied for evaluation by light microscopy, immunofluorescence, and electron microscopy.[28] Nineteen patients had typical changes of diabetic nephropathy with glomerulosclerosis, glomerular hypertrophy, and arteriolar hyali-

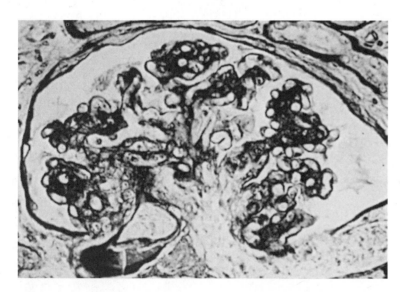

■ **Figure 5.1** Diabetic glomerulosclerosis, nodular type. (H&E, × 400.) (From Wagoner RD, Holley KE. Parenchymal renal disease: clinical and pathologic features. *In* Know FG (ed): Textbook of Renal Pathophysiology. Hagerstown, MD, Harper & Row, 1978, pp 226–253.)

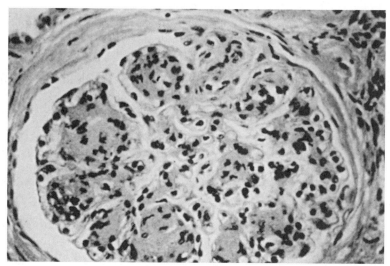

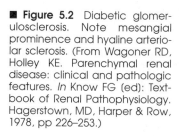 ■ **Figure 5.2** Diabetic glomerulosclerosis. Note mesangial prominence and hyaline arteriolar sclerosis. (From Wagoner RD, Holley KE. Parenchymal renal disease: clinical and pathologic features. *In* Know FG (ed): Textbook of Renal Pathophysiology. Hagerstown, MD, Harper & Row, 1978, pp 226–253.)

nosis. Sixteen patients had chronic and nonspecific changes, less glomerulosclerosis, and less hyalinosis but more ischemic glomerular disease and arteriosclerosis. Seventeen patients showed glomerular diseases superimposed on diabetic glomerulosclerosis indicating quite a heterogeneous group.

The diabetic glomerular lesions in type 2 DM are indistinguishable from those in type 1 DM when they occur. On the other hand, patients with type 2 DM and kidney disease have a much larger chance of having nondiabetic kidney disease. Parving and associates demonstrated that in the absence of retinopathy, there is a 50-50 chance that the morphological lesion will not be of a diabetic nature.[66] No prospective studies of the long-term outcome of these different pathologic groups have been undertaken. Keller and coworkers described a group of 92 consecutive type 2 DM patients in whom 13% were seen to have microalbuminuria within a year of diabetes onset.[36]

In summary, mesangial expansion, arteriolar hyalinosis, global glomerular sclerosis, and interstitial expansion are interrelated lesions in diabetic nephropathy.

PATHOGENESIS

The pathogenesis of diabetic nephropathy is multifactorial because of metabolic abnormalities, hemodynamic alterations, and various growth and genetic factors. Hyperfiltration of glomeruli is often present early in diabetes mellitus, and it has been postulated to contribute to the development of diabetic nephropathy. Hyperfiltration is thought to result from

increased glomerular hydrostatic pressure, which may be linked to the pathogenesis or progression of the nephropathy. Glomerular hyperfiltration itself, however, is unlikely to cause diabetic nephropathy because such changes do not develop in patients who have long-standing glomerular hyperfiltration from other causes, for example, after unilateral nephrectomy.

Several other hypotheses have been proposed to explain the development of diabetic nephropathy.[64] Because albuminuria is the hallmark of this disease, lesions that promote albuminuria are considered important in its pathogenesis. Such factors as integrity of the basement membrane material, size of the pores, or biochemical alteration in the incorporation of advanced glycosylation end products (AGE) could interfere with the degree of cross-linking of the membrane (see Biochemical Abnormalities).

MICROALBUMINURIA

Because therapeutic interventions only temper, but do not halt, disease progression once patients develop overt proteinuria (>300 mg/24 h or 0.30 g/d), investigators began a search for indicators of diabetic nephropathy at an earlier stage. One result was a sensitive radioimmunoassay to detect urinary albumin at ranges lower than those identified by current dipstick technology. After a series of studies evaluating urinary albumin excretion, a new normal limit was defined for excretion levels above the normal limit but below that for clinical nephropathy (30–300 mg/24 h or 20–200 µg/min or

0.46–4.6 mmol/d). These quantities were classified as *microalbuminuria*, a term which is unfortunate because the albumin excreted is normal in structure. Multiple studies regarding this level of protein excretion showed it to be somewhat variable and often a response to physiologic or hemodynamic events other than diabetes, such as exercise, position, fever, cystitis, and heart failure. Therefore, to allow for these variables, microalbuminuria must be demonstrated on two of three consecutive samples to ensure an abnormal finding.

Studies have shown that patients with this small amount of proteinuria progressed much more rapidly to diabetic nephropathy (29% within 5 years), whereas fewer than 1% of patients with normal urinary albumin excretion progressed to nephropathy. Mathiesen and colleagues studied more than 200 patients before the onset of microalbuminuria and followed them through to the development of overt proteinuria.[49] After 10 years, 29 patients had developed microalbuminuria (15%). Eight of these 29 progressed to diabetic nephropathy, and 1 died with nephropathy. Once microalbuminuria appeared, the percentage of patients receiving antihypertensive therapy increased from 10 to 45% by 4 years after the onset of microalbuminuria.

In another study, Bell and associates described a group of diabetics in whom 32% developed microalbuminuria. Of this group, 39% had retinopathy; 51%, neuropathy; 35%, hypertension; 17%, proliferative vascular disease; and 15%, ischemic heart disease.[7]

Microalbuminuria may reflect an early morphological renal lesion rather than a hemodynamic change, although Steffes and coworkers[82] have shown (in biopsies from patients with early diabetes and microalbuminuria) that the amount of microalbuminuria is independent of the presence of structural abnormalities.[64]

Subsequent studies have used albuminuria as a surrogate marker for diabetic nephropathy. These studies were carried out to assess factors leading to the onset of microalbuminuria and factors responsible for progression from microalbuminuria to the onset of albuminuria. Recently described factors necessary in studies predicting the development of microalbuminuria in type 1 diabetic patients include initial blood pressure levels, absence of a nocturnal blood pressure fall (on ambulatory blood pressure monitoring), smoking, and family history of arterial hypertension. Reduced insulin sensitivity, insertion or deletion of polymorphism

for the angiotensin-converting enzyme (ACE) gene, elevated levels of plasma renin activity, and elevated levels of plasma prorenin are also factors that predict development of microalbuminuria (Table 5.1).[77] Urinary albumin excretion (UAE) levels are found elevated in 13 to 25% of type 2 DM patients, including those with newly diagnosed and established diabetes. In type 2 DM patients, the microalbuminuria may have a different pathogenesis in that it usually follows the onset of insulin resistance and hypertension.[62] The factors listed in Table 5.1 have been documented to promote microalbuminuria in type 2 DM patients as well.

The presence of microalbuminuria is associated with cardiovascular mortality independent of diabetes. Damsgaard and colleagues found a fourfold mortality rise in a group of nondiabetics in whom the median urinary albumin excretion rate was increased from 2.5 to 7.2 µg/min (.038–.11 mmol/min).[18]

In a group of 76 type 2 DM patients studied for 9 years, 17 patients with albumin excretion rates of 30–140 µg/mL (.46–3.2 mmol/mL) developed overt proteinuria; moreover, the mortality was 148% higher than in the nonproteinuric group even in the absence of overt proteinuria. Mogensen concluded that microalbuminuria in type 2 DM patients predicted not only clinical proteinuria but increased cardiovascular mortality.[52] Although treatment trials suggest that microalbuminuria is a susceptibility factor for proteinuria and nephropathy, it is not yet clear whether treating microalbuminuria will decrease cardiovascular morbidity or mortality.

The reason for the association between albuminuria and cardiovascular risk in diabetics is not entirely clear. It is possible that increased cardiovascular risk is the result of a frequent coexistence with traditional cardiovascular risk factors, such as hyperlipidemia, coagulation abnormalities, and hypertension. Microalbuminuria may represent generalized endothelial

TABLE 5.1 FACTORS PREDICTING DEVELOPMENT OF MICROALBUMINURIA IN TYPE 1 DIABETES MELLITUS

Initial blood pressure levels
Absence of nocturnal blood pressure fall on ambulatory monitoring
Smoking
Family history of arterial hypertension
Reduced insulin sensitivity
Insertion/deletion polymorphism of angiotensin-converting enzyme gene

dysfunction, which could account for the increased cardiovascular risk.[20] Other recent studies suggest that the cardiovascular risk correlates with the levels of sialic acid. A high level of sialic acid is a strong predictor of cardiovascular morbidity and mortality in the general population and may contribute to increased risk in diabetes.[16] A correlation also exists with early autonomic dysfunction that may contribute to increased risks for early cardiac death.[55] In addition, it has been postulated that the decreased concentration of heparin sulfate in the extracellular matrix of patients with type 1 DM is an explanation for increased albuminuria and premature atherosclerosis.[19]

RISK FACTORS FOR DEVELOPMENT OR PROGRESSION OF NEPHROPATHY

Multiple risk factors for the development or progression of diabetic nephropathy are outlined in Table 5.2. A discussion of several of these factors should be instructive in understanding the pathogenesis of the nephropathy in diabetes.

Hypertension

One major risk factor for progression of diabetic nephropathy is hypertension. A higher mean arterial blood pressure at baseline is associated with increased risk of progressive renal insufficiency. A relatively small increase in mean arterial pressure (5 mm Hg) is associated with a significant increase in the risk of dou-

bling of serum creatinine. Mean arterial pressure (MAP) in a group who had doubling of creatinine was 109 mm Hg, whereas those who did not progress had a MAP of 102 mm Hg. The effect of blood pressure is more difficult to appreciate from casual office blood pressure measurements. Twenty-four-hour blood pressure recordings have been much more clearly associated with altered renal function and progression to diabetic nephropathy. Furthermore, an abnormal diurnal rhythm seems particularly predictive of a hypertension effect. There may be a closer association of progression with nighttime blood pressures than with daytime pressures. These factors have led some to suggest that the indication for starting antihypertensive treatment in diabetes is the presence of microalbuminuria as evidence of endothelial or organ damage rather than elevation of blood pressure.[54]

Normally, systemic blood pressure is not directly transmitted to the glomerulus. However, studies suggest that systemic pressure is more readily transmitted to the glomerulus in disease states such as diabetes, thus increasing the GFR. For example, in patients with essential hypertension (or in normal persons), urinary albumin excretion is not related to hypertension as directly as it is in diabetics, although elevated pressure increases albumin excretion even in normal individuals. Impaired myogenic response of the afferent arteriole in diabetic rats has been described.[33a] The response is mediated by an alteration in the eicosanoid metabolism and blunted renin angiotensin system. These data are consistent with the idea

---

TABLE 5.2   STUDIES OF RISK FACTORS FOR PROGRESSION OF NEPHROPATHY

Type 1 Diabetes Mellitus	
Hypertension	Lurbe et al.[45]; Powrie et al.[70]; Collaborative Study Group of the U.K.[50]
Microalbuminuria	Mogensen[53]
Gene polymorphisms	Doria et al.[23]
Genetic factors	Fioretto et al.[27]; Seaquist et al.[78]; Barzilay et al.[6]
Family history of hypertension	
↑ Renin activity	Anderson et al.[2]
↑ Glomerular filtration rate	Rudberg et al.[76]
↑ Duration of diabetes	Orchard et al.[63]
Nonwhite race	Smith et al.[80]
Black race	Brancati et al.[11]
Type 2 Diabetes Mellitus	
Smoking	Olivarius et al.[62]
Elevated triglycerides	Klein et al.[38]
↑ Cholesterol (males)	Klein et al.[38]
Glucosuria	Klein et al.[38]
Alcohol excess	Klein et al.[38]
Insulin resistance	Groop et al.[32]; Nosadini et al.[61]; Niskanen and Laakso[60]

that systemic pressure is directly transmitted to the glomerulus, increasing GFR.

Some studies have suggested that high blood pressure in nondiabetic parents may be a marker of susceptibility to diabetic nephropathy in their type 1 DM offspring,[86] although other studies have failed to confirm this observation. Barzilay and associates and Krolewski and colleagues recorded a higher prevalence of hypertension in the parents of type 1 DM patients with nephropathy compared with parents of normal albuminuric type 1 DM patients.[6, 39]

Cross-sectional studies of type 1 and 2 DM patients with microalbuminuria show elevated blood pressures compared with normoalbuminuric patients. In this type of study, the question of whether the blood pressure elevation is secondary to the diabetes or primary to the development of nephropathy has not been clearly established. Although these data seem quite strong, most studies have not ruled out microalbuminuria at baseline to firmly establish whether blood pressure elevation precedes the development of nephropathy. Parving and coworkers, in reviewing these studies, concluded that the contribution of elevated blood pressure plays only a minor role in development of diabetic nephropathy.[67] There is no question, however, that diabetic patients with microalbuminuria or albuminuria have more rapidly progressive diabetic nephropathy and ESRD than do normotensive diabetic patients.[35]

Studies now indicate that the level of blood pressure is associated with the future decline of the GFR in type 2 DM patients as well.[59, 73]

The level to which blood pressure must be controlled is different for different diabetic groups. The prevention of microalbuminuria in type 1 DM probably requires a limited decrease of mean blood pressure of about 5 mm Hg, whereas a greater fall in blood pressure may be advantageous in type 1 DM with overt diabetic nephropathy to a systolic pressure of 135 mm Hg. A modest increase of blood pressure is usually seen in type 2 DM patients; in this group, blood pressure should be reduced to less than 140/80 mm Hg in patients 40 to 50 years of age or 150/85 mm Hg in somewhat older patients.[59, 73]

The type of antihypertensive therapy may well be important. Lowering systemic blood pressure decreases afferent arteriolar pressure, but this decrease increases counterregulatory mechanisms that may increase efferent arteriolar pressure maintaining increased intraglomerular pressure. Medications that inhibit ACE appear to selectively inhibit efferent arteriolar constriction while lowering glomerular pressure and, presumably, decreasing transglomerular pressure and trafficking of proteins. Although ACE inhibition is a well-established treatment for preservation of renal function, there is no evidence of increased salutary effect for prevention of other diabetic complications. Early studies showed that some calcium channel blockers decrease proteinuria (nondihydropyridine group), and they may have effects similar to ACE inhibitors for reducing GFR change in type 2 DM patients.[5]

Although blood pressure control slows progression of nephropathy, therapies directed toward increased body weight, impaired glucose tolerance, hypertriglyceridemia, low high-density lipoproteins, high serum insulin, or insulin resistance may be necessary to alter cardiovascular morbidity or mortality.

In summary, hypertension may be causal for onset, although this is not well established. Hypertension, however, is certainly important in progression of diabetic renal disease. Antihypertensive therapy, particularly with ACE inhibitors and calcium channel blockers that reduce proteinuria, is useful in modulating the progression of nephropathy in patients with overt proteinuria and diabetes. Antihypertensive therapy in patients with microalbuminuria has stabilized proteinuria and renal function for several years.

Genetic Factors

One major observation in terms of understanding the pathogenesis of nephropathy may be that fewer than 50% of patients who have type 1 DM develop diabetic nephropathy. Genetic factors may be risk markers in such development. Several studies have documented familial clustering of diabetic nephropathy in type 1 DM.[9, 58, 78] As previously mentioned, presence of nephropathy in either or both parents markedly increases the likelihood of nephropathy in offspring. One identified genetic factor that may account for this is a predisposition to hypertension, in which diabetics with nephropathy have higher percentage of parents with hypertension.[6] A second factor is the ACE gene polymorphism, where an insertion-deletion in the ACE gene has been associated with increased nephropathy.[47] Clustering of an abnormal sodium/lithium transport also occurs in hypertensive parents and patients with progressive nephropathy.[23, 25, 27]

Genes involved in the regulation of blood

pressure and cardiovascular risk factors are considered candidate genes for diabetic nephropathy. Several DNA studies dealing with the ACE/insertion-deletion (I/D) polymorphism in type 2 DM patients with nephropathy have been undertaken. About 20% of these studies have shown an association between a deletion and development of diabetic nephropathy. However, a meta-analysis showed that the ACE D/D polymorphism seemed to predict increased progression of kidney disease, but most studies show that it does not predict the development of nephropathy.[83] The 2 allele is associated with increased GFR but is present in type 1 DM patients who do not progress to nephropathy.[51] An elevated plasma ACE concentration has also been found in type 1 DM patients with incipient and overt diabetic nephropathy.[47] The I/D polymorphism in the ACE enzyme gene predicts the response to ACE inhibition for progression of diabetic nephropathy in type 1 diabetic patients.[34, 56]

Two other steps in the activation of the renin-angiotensin-aldosterone system (RAS) have potential for promoting nephropathy. An altered cleavage of angiotensinogen by renin has been seen in essential hypertension as well as a polymorphism for the type 1 (angiotensin I) receptor gene. This has been demonstrated in nondiabetic patients but not in patients with diabetic microangiopathy. These data suggest a genetic predisposition for accelerated loss of kidney function in diabetic and nondiabetic glomerulopathies. One might consider more aggressive ACE inhibition or better angiotensin 2 receptor blockade in patients homozygous for the large D allele of the ACE polymorphism.

Glomerular Filtration Rate

Increased GFR early in diabetes is a risk factor for progression of nephropathy. Rudberg and colleagues studied a cohort of type 1 DM adolescents with a diabetes' duration of 8 years.[76] Patients were studied for an additional 8 years to determine the predictive value of GFR for future nephropathy. Five of 64 patients developed overt nephropathy. All had an initial GFR greater than 125 mL/min/1.73 m². The positive predictive value for incipient and overt nephropathy of an initial GFR greater than 125 mL/min was 53%. The negative predictive value of a GFR below 125 mL/min was 95%. Although initial enthusiasm for the idea that hyperfiltration is the major cause for diabetic nephropathy has waned, there is no doubt that

increased glomerular pressure enhances trafficking of glucose, lipoproteins, and other proteins through the glomerulus. Hyperfiltration likely plays some pathogenic role in the progression of nephropathy. In addition, a blunted renin angiotensin system (RAS) in the kidneys of diabetic patients leads to glomerular hypertrophy. As mentioned earlier, increased blood pressure is normally modulated at the glomerulus by several factors, including eicosanoids and the RAS, which normally dampens glomerular pressures by relaxing efferent arteriolar constriction. Failure of this system leads to an increase in glomerular pressure and links the RAS, glomerular hyperfiltration, and systemic hypertension to the progression of diabetic nephropathy.

Increases in GFR may also come from increased protein intake, which is also modulated by the RAS. Increases in the GFR from protein intake are prevented by blockade of the RAS.

Glucose Control

There is a relationship between progression of nephropathy and the level of hemoglobin A_{1C} (HbA_{1C}). A threshold for progression of about 8.1% has been established, and a rapidly increasing prevalence of nephropathy is present above 10.1%.[40] Dahl-Jorgensen and colleagues studied 45 type 1 DM patients for 7 years. Eight of 10 patients with HbA_{1C} values below 8.5% improved their albumin excretion rate, whereas patients with a mean HbA_{1C} greater than 10% had an increased albumin excretion rate from 26 to 91 mg/24 h (.39–1.4 mmol/d) ($P <.02$). Blood pressure increased significantly regardless of the HbA_{1C} levels.[17]

Race

The USRDS shows that there is an increased incidence of diabetic ESRD among African-Americans, Native Americans, and Hispanics. Brancati and associates examined the incidence of diabetic ESRD among black patients and showed a relative risk (RR) for ESRD of 3.4 (confidence interval [CI], 2.8–4.1) compared with white patients. Analysis of this risk factor showed that it was confined to type 2 DM, and blacks were not at higher risk for renal failure caused by type 1 DM.[11]

BIOCHEMICAL ABNORMALITIES

Several biochemical and immunologic abnormalities present in diabetes may promote ne-

TABLE 5.3 BIOCHEMICAL AND IMMUNOLOGIC ABNORMALITIES

Elevated sialic acid, advanced glycosylation end products, and polyol formation[13, 30, 46, 75]
Protein kinase C[21]
Increased renin-angiotensin-aldosterone system activity[56]
Increased transforming growth factor beta (rats)[90]
Increased juxtaglomerular T lymphocytes[68]

phropathy (Table 5.3). One factor in increasing extracellular matrix is transforming growth factor beta (TGF-β); it is elevated in human and experimental diabetic nephropathy. Yamamoto and associates showed a slow, progressive increase in the expression of messenger RNA for TGF-β in rats treated with streptozotozin.[90] Anderson and colleagues showed that several parts of the RAS are increased in the kidney tissues of diabetic rats, potentially explaining the prominent response to pharmacologic blockade of angiotensin II.[2]

Advanced glycation end products (AGE), which occur in diabetes and aging, result from spontaneous modification of proteins by glucose (Fig. 5.3).[3] Several studies have addressed AGEs in the pathogenesis of nephropathy. Vlassara and coworkers infused enough AGE-modified albumin in rats to elevate AGE levels to the range seen in diabetes with and without the AGE inhibitor aminoguanidine. After 5 months, the AGE content of renal tissue rose to 50% above controls, and this resulted in a 50% increase in glomerular volume and increased glomerulosclerosis. Cotreatment with aminoguanidine limited structural and functional defects. Antibodies to AGEs prevent nephropathy in mice.[87] In addition, AGEs increase mRNA expression of several growth

factors in mice[12, 14, 46, 75, 81 87 91] and increase GFR in experimental animals.[1]

Protein kinase C (PKC) is activated in rat renal glomerulus within a week of the induction of experimental diabetes. Hyperglycemia, per se, mediates protein kinase C activation. Higher levels of protein kinase C increase permeability of endothelial cells to albumin, stimulate matrix protein synthesis in mesangial cells, and are thought to be related to alterations of the glomerulus in diabetes. Protein kinase C also suppresses nitric oxide–induced cyclic guanosine monophosphate in glomeruli, thereby amplifying matrix protein synthesis in response to hyperglycemia.[21]

Myo-inositol supplementation may alter nerve conduction by changing phosphoinositide metabolism in cell regulation and the sodium potassium ATPase. Aldose reductase inhibitors link defects in myo-inositol metabolism to activation of the polyol pathway in diabetes. This metabolic defect is important in the kidney as well as in the lens and the peripheral nerves. Thus, aldolase reductase inhibitors may be effective in prevention of diabetic nephropathy.[30]

Magnesium depletion is very common in patients with type 1 and 2 DM. It correlates with elevated glycosylated hemoglobin and may play an important role in promoting diabetic nephropathy and microvascular complications. Magnesium depletion may be linked to these complications by a reduction in the rate of inositol transport and subsequent intracellular inositol depletion[29] or by reduction in the bioactivity of inositols, further impairing their function.[4] Magnesium depletion also impairs insulin sensitivity.[57]

Microvascular Changes

Pathogenesis of microvascular complications in diabetics with nephropathy is also a likely multifactorial. Atherosclerosis is thought to be associated with plasma lipoprotein profiles that are abnormal in diabetics, including an elevation in the apoprotein B component of very-low-density lipoprotein (VLDL) and low-density lipoprotein (LDL). Bucala and associates showed that advanced glycated peptides significantly impair LDL receptor-mediated clearance mechanisms and may contribute to elevated LDL levels in patients with diabetes and renal insufficiency.[13] Increases in cholesterol (20 to 25%) and in fibrinogen (20%), however, do not fully account for the tenfold higher cardiovascular mortality in diabetic patients. The

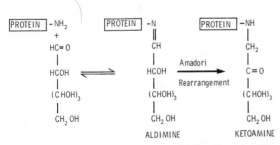

■ **Figure 5.3** The glycation of proteins in which the initial and reversible Schiff base adduct between glucose and protein amino groups (aldimine) leads via an Amadori rearrangement to the irreversible formation of a ketoamine. (From Ashby JP, Frier BM. Is serum fructosamine a clinically useful test? Diabetic Med 1988;1:118.)

Steno hypothesis suggests simultaneous development of a structural defect within the extracellular matrix of the glomeruli and of the large vessel walls.[20] The coincidence of albuminuria, as a sign of endothelial dysfunction and simultaneous development of generalized vascular hyperpermeability, supports the hypothesis.

Several potentially pathogenetic issues exist in addition to nonenzymatic glycation of the components of the extracellular matrix. Decreased concentration or sulfation of heparin sulfate appears to be present, which normally contributes to the structural stability and negative charge of the extracellular matrix. In addition, increased risk for cardiovascular disease has been associated with increased serum sialic acid concentrations, which are elevated in type 1 DM patients with microalbuminuria and clinical proteinuria and are thought to play a role as a cardiovascular risk factor or disease marker.[16] Coronary disease in type 1 diabetics increases after the onset of proteinuria, with an eightfold rise in this group compared with a group without proteinuria (40% compared with 5%).[35]

Additional risk factors for progression of nephropathy are summarized in Table 5.2. Some unique factors are associated with progression in type 2 DM that may also relate to progression of cardiovascular disease. The relationship between the following risk factors and progressive renal insufficiency is still controversial: smoking, sex, insulin levels, body mass index,[70] angiotensin and converting enzyme polymorphism DD.[24] In one study of type 2 DM, diastolic blood pressure was not proved to be a risk factor.

CLINICAL TRIALS OF TREATMENT AND PREVENTION

Several clinical trials have been undertaken to assess whether modulation of these risks would be effective in prevention.

The effect of intensive treatment of diabetes glucose control was explored in the Diabetes Control and Complications Trial. This study looked at retinopathy as evidence of microvascular disease, with observations as to the development and progression of clinical nephropathy. A total of 1441 patients were studied; 726 had no retinopathy at baseline (primary prevention) and 715 had mild retinopathy (secondary intervention cohort). Both groups were followed for 6.5 years and assessed regularly. Retinopathy was reduced 76% by intensive glucose therapy in the prevention

group, and progression was slowed in 54% of the intervention group. In these two cohorts, intensive therapy reduced the occurrence of microalbuminuria (<40 mg/24 h [.58 mmol/24h]) by 39% and reduced the occurrence of overt albuminuria (>300 mg/24 h [4.6 mmol/24h]) by 54%. This therapy was associated with a threefold increase in severe hypoglycemic episodes.[22] Wang and coworkers reviewed 16 studies concerning intensive blood glucose control.[89] This meta-analysis also showed a reduced risk of diabetic retinopathy and progression of nephropathy. The investigators, however, noted that long-term continuous subcutaneous insulin infusion was associated with increased incidence of diabetic ketoacidosis as well as with severe hypoglycemic reactions.

Several studies have assessed the prognosis of diabetic nephropathy during long-term antihypertensive treatment. Parving and associates showed that median survival with antihypertensive therapy exceeded 16 years compared with 5 and 7 years in untreated patients in the past.[66] Lewis and colleagues studied ACE inhibition in patients with overt nephropathy.[44] A randomized control trial comparing captopril with placebo in patients with greater than 500 mg of protein per day and a serum creatinine below 2.5 mg/dL (221 μmol/L) was undertaken. Of 207 patients and 202 controls, serum creatinine concentration doubled in 25 patients in the captopril group, as compared with 43 patients in the placebo group ($P < .01$) (Fig. 5.4A and B). The captopril group also showed a marked reduction in progression to ESRD requiring dialysis.

Captopril was also evaluated in patients with microalbuminuria in a randomized, double-blind placebo-controlled trial of 2 years' duration in 92 patients with no hypertension. Twelve patients receiving placebo and four receiving captopril progressed to clinical proteinuria. The geometric mean for albumin excretion rose from 52 to 76 μg/min (8–12 × 10⁻⁴ μmol/min) in the placebo group but fell from 52 to 41 μg/min (8–6.3 × 10⁻⁴ μmol/min) in the captopril group. It was concluded that captopril significantly impeded progression to clinical proteinuria and prevented an increase in the albumin excretion rate.[48]

Enalapril has also been evaluated in patients with hypertensive type 2 DM in a 5-year prospective, double-blind placebo-controlled trial showing that the drug preserved GFR better in the patients with subclinical proteinuria at baseline than other antihypertensive treatments.[71] Only 7% of enalapril-treated groups

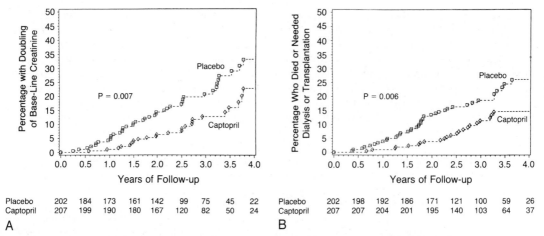

A B

■ **Figure 5.4** Cumulative incidence of events in patients with diabetic nephropathy in the captopril and placebo groups. A, The cumulative percentage of patients with the primary end point: a doubling of the base-line serum creatinine concentration to at least 2.0 mg/dL. B, The cumulative percentage of patients who died or required dialysis or renal transplantation. The numbers at the bottom of the figures are the numbers of patients in each group at risk for the event at base line and after each 6-month period. (From Lewis EJ, Hunsicker LG, Bain RP, et al. The effect of angiotensin–converting–enzyme inhibition on diabetic nephropathy. The Collaborative Study Group. N Engl J Med 1993; 329:1456–1462. Published erratum appears in N Engl J Med 1993; 330:152.)

progressed to clinical albuminuria, compared with 20% of the subjects treated with other drugs.[42, 72]

High protein intake increases GFR and is thought to accelerate progression of renal insufficiency. Moreover, in some studies, reduced protein intake has slowed progression of renal insufficiency in diabetics. In this analysis by Pedrini and associates,[69] 1413 patients were included in five studies of nondiabetic renal disease, and 108 patients were included in five studies of type 1 DM. The risk for progression of renal disease in patients on a low-protein diet was calculated using a random effects model. In the nondiabetic group, the low-protein diet significantly reduced the risk for renal failure (RR, 0.67; 95% CI, 0.5–0.89). In the five studies of type 1 DM, the low-protein diet significantly slowed the increase of urinary albumin level or the decline in GFR. Relative risk was .56 (CI = 0.4–0.77). No differences were demonstrated in blood pressure or glycosylated hemoglobin levels between low-protein and high-protein groups in the diabetics.

The one large double-blind controlled trial of protein restriction in nondiabetics with nephropathy, however, was unable to show preservation of GFR.[37] A subanalysis of this study showed the initial 4-month reduction in GFR was rapid after protein restriction. The rate of decline in GFR slowed in the treated group thereafter. It was thought that the initial de-

cline in GFR was a hemodynamic change and that, subsequently, the progression of renal disease slowed as measured by the number of functional nephrons. Investigators believed it would take 3 additional years past the conclusion of the study to detect a clear-cut difference between the diet groups. The study did show that the beneficial effect was proportional to the initial rate of decline of GFR, which may indicate that an initial fall in GFR would be predictive of long-term help by protein restriction. This large study leaves some uncertainty as to the efficacy of protein restriction in preservation of GFR in diabetes.[43]

ACUTE RENAL FAILURE

Certain situations lead to acute renal failure more frequently in diabetic than other in populations.[31] Furthermore, the high prevalence of chronic renal disease makes diabetic patients particularly susceptible to the development of acute renal failure. Several forms of acute renal failure are particularly common in diabetic patients (Table 5.4).

Radiocontrast-induced acute renal failure may account for 10% of hospital-acquired acute renal failure. Diabetic patients, in particular, are likely to have angiographic investigation because of their high prevalence of vascular disease. Although the rate of acute renal failure may have been improved somewhat with the

TABLE 5.4 FORMS OF ACUTE RENAL FAILURE

Radiocontrast media
Renal papillary necrosis
Drugs
Severe hyperglycemia
Hyperosmolar coma
Diabetic ketoacidosis
Septicemia

Data from Grenfell A. Acute renal failure in diabetics. *In* Mogensen CE (ed): The Kidney and Hypertension in Diabetes Mellitus. Boston, Kluwer Academic Publishers, 1994, pp 407–419.

introduction of low osmolality contrast agents, it has not disappeared with the use of these agents. The incidence of contrast-induced acute renal failure ranges from 9 to 16% in high-risk patients, including those with preexisting renal impairment, congestive heart failure, dehydration, poorly controlled diabetes, or associated myeloma. The incidence is about 2 to 5% in patients with these risk factors. The mechanism is uncertain but may involve direct tubular toxicity, ischemia caused by renal vasoconstriction, endothelial damage, or intratubular obstruction.

Prevention involves screening patients, avoiding unnecessary investigations, decreasing the dose of contrast, and avoiding dehydration. Preprocedure saline and mannitol with or without furosemide have been shown to reduce the incidence of contrast nephropathy.

Renal papillary necrosis occurs in patients with diabetes, chronic analgesic use, nonsteroidal anti-inflammatory drugs, pyelonephritis, urinary tract obstruction, and sickle cell anemia. Necrosis is probably present in as many as 30% of diabetics and may present as acute renal failure. Hyperglycemic hyperosmolar nonketotic coma is often associated with severe dehydration and possibly rhabdomyolysis with acute renal failure. Prevention depends on early initiation of treatment and hydration as well as careful attention to fluid and insulin therapy.

Acute renal failure is also a rare complication of diabetic ketoacidosis, occasionally associated with rhabdomyolysis. Prevention lies in prompt initiation of treatment and adequate fluid replacement. In this setting, acute renal failure should prompt early dialysis, because hyperglycemia, hyperkalemia, and acidosis are difficult to manage in oliguric patients. Septicemia causes acute renal failure in many situations. Diabetic patients are particularly prone to septicemia, especially in association with urinary tract infections.

Several drugs are important causes of acute renal failure. Three main groups are particularly important. Nonsteroidal anti-inflammatory drugs are thought to cause at least one third of all drug-induced cases of acute renal failure. Angiotensin-converting enzyme inhibitors are currently being used extensively in diabetes. Acute renal failure may occur with use of ACE inhibitors in the presence of bilateral renal artery stenosis, particularly in the presence of volume depletion, cardiac failure, and chronic renal insufficiency. This is especially true when the conditions occur in combination with nonsteroidal anti-inflammatory drugs. Diabetes does not seem to increase the risk for untoward renal effects from antibiotics, even though they are used more often because of the propensity toward sepsis in diabetic patients.

Principles for management of acute renal failure are similar to those used in other types of renal failure. Hyperkalemia is a more vexing problem in diabetics because of the fluxes resulting from ketoacidosis and hyperosmolar states, in addition to the poor excretion of potassium by the kidney.

Overall mortality from acute renal failure in patients with diabetes may be as high as 50%. Prevention is important, because acute renal failure adds considerably to the morbidity and mortality of other diabetic complications.

SCREENING AND MANAGEMENT OF MICROALBUMINURIA

Screening for and management of microalbuminuria in patients with diabetes mellitus have been codified by the Scientific Advisory Board of the National Kidney Foundation following recommendations made by an ad hoc committee of the Council on Diabetes Mellitus of the National Kidney Foundation (Figs. 5.5 and 5.6).[8] Current recommendations are outlined in Figure 5.5. Screening for microalbuminuria should be undertaken in all diabetic patients older than age 12 years on at least a yearly basis. In patients with type 2 DM, the cost-benefit ratio has not been as firmly established as it has been in type 1 DM. However, it is currently recommended that all individuals with type 2 DM younger than age 70 years with no overt renal disease be screened in a similar manner. Several factors other than diabetes can alter microalbuminuria; for example, heavy exercise, urinary tract infection, acute

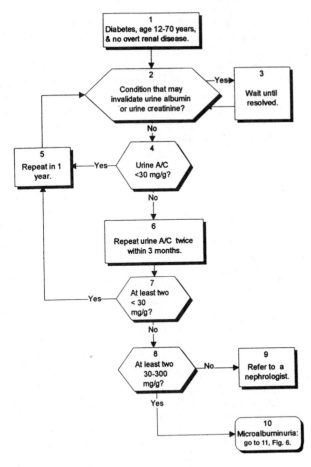

■ **Figure 5.5** Microalbuminuria screening. A/C, albumin:creatinine ratio. (From Bennett PH, Haffner S, Kasiske BL, et al. Screening and management of microalbuminuria in patients with diabetes mellitus: Recommendations to the Scientific Advisory Board of the National Kidney Foundation from an ad hoc committee of the Council on Diabetes Mellitus of the National Kidney Foundation. Am J Kidney Dis 1995; 25:107–112.)

febrile illnesses, and heart failure. Any screening should be postponed until those situations are stabilized. Similarly, drugs that alter urinary protein excretion, such as nonsteroidal anti-inflammatory drugs or ACE inhibitors, should be stopped during screening procedures.

Although timed urinary albumin excretion rates (either 24-hour or 10-hour overnight collections) are considered the most sensitive, urinary albumin-creatinine ratios are more practical and are recommended for screening purposes. The recommendation of the committee is to use a first morning specimen for the albumin-creatinine ratio, although a random specimen may be used. As outlined earlier, a ratio of greater than 30 mg/g (3×10^{-4} mmol Alb/mole creat) and less than 300 mg/g (3×10^{-4} mmol Alb/mole creat) of creatinine has been identified as the level associated with an increase in the risk for diabetic nephropathy and its complications. If urinary albumin-creatinine ratios are elevated, the abnormality should be confirmed in at least 2 of 3 samples.

If the screening albumin-creatinine ratio is in the normal range, it should be repeated on a yearly basis. If microalbuminuria is established, several management principles are recommended (see Fig. 5.6):

1. Blood glucose should be controlled to delay progression to persistent proteinuria. This can be done with dietary and intensified insulin treatment. In individuals with type 2 DM, no clear data address whether intensive insulin therapy is beneficial. However, current recommendations are that the best glycemic control possible should be the goal for patients with type 2 DM as well as those with type 1 DM.
2. If glycemic control is adequate and the increased albumin-creatinine ratio persists, ACE-inhibitor therapy should be initiated. This is appropriate in normotensive and hypertensive diabetic patients. Studies have been done with captopril and enalapril, with doses up to 50 mg, twice a day, of

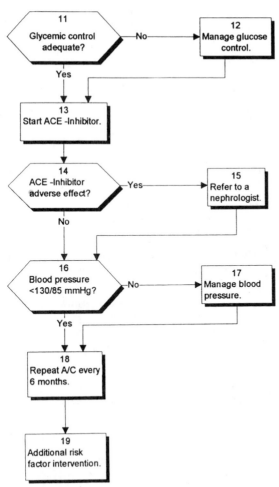

■ **Figure 5.6** Microalbuminuria management. A/C, albumin:creatinine ratio. (From Bennett PH, Haffner S, Kasiske BL, et al. Screening and management of microalbuminuria in patients with diabetes mellitus: Recommendations to the Scientific Advisory Board of the National Kidney Foundation from an ad hoc committee of the Council on Diabetes Mellitus of the National Kidney Foundation. Am J Kidney Dis 1995; 25:107–112.)

should be reduced to 130/85 mm Hg or lower in those with microalbuminuria. If this is not achieved with an ACE inhibitor alone, a low-dose diuretic agent is recommended.

5. Treatment of other risk factor interventions associated with diabetes has not been rigorously tested. Dyslipidemia is clearly an independent risk factor for progression of renal disease, but there are no intervention studies in this regard. However, because reduction in cardiovascular disease among diabetics enrolled in large lipid-lowering trials is similar to that observed for nondiabetics, it would seem appropriate to consider nonpharmacologic or pharmacologic lipid-lowering interventions. Such interventions include dietary restriction of cholesterol, weight reduction, and improvement of metabolic control. Cigarette smoking is associated with development and progression of microalbuminuria as well as with cardiovascular disease and should be vigorously discouraged in patients with diabetes.

Cost-benefit analyses for management of patients with type 1 DM and microalbuminuria using this algorithm have been undertaken.[10, 79] In these studies, considerable projected cost benefits were realized by early intervention for microalbuminuria in type 1 DM patients. Similar analyses for type 2 DM have not been performed, but it is expected that savings would be achieved in this patient population as well.

References

1. Amore A, Cirina P, Mitola S, et al. Nonenzymatically glycated albumin (Amadori adducts) enhances nitric oxide synthase activity and gene expression in endothelial cells. Kidney Int 1997; 51:27–35.
2. Anderson S, Jung FF, Ingelfinger JR. Renal renin-angiotensin system in diabetes: Functional, immunohistochemical, and molecular biological correlations. Am J Physiol 1993; 265:F477–F486.
3. Ashby JP, Frier BM. Is serum fructosamine a clinically useful test? Diabetic Med 1988; 1:118.
4. Asplin I, Galasko G, Larner J. Chiro-inositol deficiency and insulin resistance: A comparison of the chiro-inositol- and the myo-inositol-containing insulin mediators isolated from urine, hemodialysate, and muscle of control and type II diabetic subjects. Proc Natl Acad Sci USA 1993; 90:5924–5928.
5. Bakris GL, Copley JB, Vicknair N, et al. Calcium channel blockers versus other antihypertensive therapies on progression of NIDDM associated nephropathy. Kidney Int 1996; 50:1641–1650.
6. Barzilay J, Warram JH, Bak M, et al. Predisposition to hypertension: Risk factor for nephropathy and hypertension in IDDM. Kidney Int 1992; 41:723–730.

captopril and 5 to 20 mg, twice a day, of enalapril. Insufficient studies exist concerning other ACE inhibitors or calcium channel blockers to warrant inclusion in the official recommendations. The goal should be to stabilize or to decrease the albumin-creatinine ratio.

3. Because of the potential adverse effect of ACE inhibitors in diabetic patients, it is recommended that serum creatinine and potassium be monitored 1 week after beginning therapy, and consultation with nephrology personnel should be undertaken if problems are perceived.

4. If patients are hypertensive, blood pressure

7. Bell DS, Ketchum CH, Robinson CA, et al. Microalbuminuria associated with diabetic neuropathy. Diabetes Care 1992; 15:528–531.
8. Bennett PH, Haffner S, Kasiske BL, et al. Screening and management of microalbuminuria in patients with diabetes mellitus: Recommendations to the Scientific Advisory Board of the National Kidney Foundation from an ad hoc committee of the Council on Diabetes Mellitus of the National Kidney Foundation. Am J Kidney Dis 1995; 25:107–112.
9. Borch-Johnsen K, Norgaard K, Hommel E, et al. Is diabetic nephropathy an inherited complication? Kidney Int 1992; 41:719–722.
10. Borch-Johnsen K, Wenzel H, Viberti GC, et al. Is screening and intervention for microalbuminuria worthwhile in patients with insulin-dependent diabetes? BMJ 1993; 306:1722–1725.
11. Brancati FL, Whittle JC, Whelton PK, et al. The excess incidence of diabetic end-stage renal disease among blacks: A population-based study of potential explanatory factors (see comments). JAMA 1992; 268:3079–3084.
12. Brownlee M. Glycation products and the pathogenesis of diabetic complications (review). Diabetes Care 1992; 15:1835–1843.
13. Bucala R, Makita Z, Vega G, et al. Modification of low density lipoprotein by advanced glycation end products contributes to the dyslipidemia of diabetes and renal insufficiency. Proc Natl Acad Sci USA 1994; 91:9441–9445.
14. Cohen MP, Hud E, Wu VY. Amelioration of diabetic nephropathy by treatment with monoclonal antibodies against glycated albumin. Kidney Int 1994; 45:1673–1679.
15. Cowrie CC, Port FK, Wolfe RA, et al. Disparities in incidence of diabetic end-stage renal disease according to race and type of diabetes. N Engl J Med 1989; 321:1074–1079.
16. Crook MA, Earle K, Morocutti A, et al. Serum sialic acid, a risk factor for cardiovascular disease, is increased in IDDM patients with microalbuminuria and clinical proteinuria. Diabetes Care 1994; 17:305–310.
17. Dahl-Jorgensen K, Bjoro T, Kierulf P, et al. Long-term glycemic control and kidney function in insulin-dependent diabetes mellitus. Kidney Int 1992; 41:920–923.
18. Damsgaard EM, Frøland A, Jørgensen OD, et al. Microalbuminuria as predictor of increased mortality in elderly people. BMJ 1990; 300:297–300.
19. Deckert T. Nephropathy and coronary death: The fatal twins in diabetes mellitus (editorial)(review). Nephrol Dial Transplant 1994;9: 1069–1071.
20. Deckert T, Feldt-Rasmussen B, Borch-Johnsen K, et al. Albuminuria reflects widespread vascular damage. The Steno hypothesis (see comments)(review). Diabetologia 1989; 32:219–226.
21. Derubertis FR, Craven PA. Activation of protein kinase C in glomerular cells in diabetes: Mechanisms and potential links to the pathogenesis of diabetic glomerulopathy (review). Diabetes 1994; 43:1–8.
22. Diabetes Control and Complications Trial Research Group. The effect of intensive treatment of diabetes on the development and progression of long-term complications in insulin-dependent diabetes mellitus. N Engl J Med 1993; 329:977–986.
23. Doria A, Warram JH, Krolewski AS. Genetic predisposition to diabetic nephropathy: Evidence for a role of the angiotensin I—converting enzyme gene. Diabetes 1994; 43:690–695.
24. Dudley CR, Keavney B, Stratton IM, et al. U.K. Prospective Diabetes Study XV: Relationship of renin-angiotensin system gene polymorphisms with microalbuminuria in NIDDM. Kidney Int 1995; 48:1907–1911.
25. Earle K, Viberti GC. Familial, hemodynamic and metabolic factors in the predisposition to diabetic kidney disease (review). Kidney Int 1994; 45:434–437.
26. Ellis EN, Steffes MW, Goetz FC, et al. Glomerular filtration surface in type I diabetes mellitus. Kidney Int 1986; 29:889–894.
27. Fioretto P, Steffes MW, Mauer SM. Hypertension and diabetic renal disease (review). Clin Invest Med 1991; 14:630–635.
28. Gambara V, Mecca G, Remuzzi G, et al. Heterogeneous nature of renal lesions in type II diabetes. J Am Soc Nephrol 1993; 3:1458–1466.
29. Grafton G, Bunce CM, Sheppard MC, et al. Effect of Mg2+ on Na(+)-dependent inositol transport: Role of Mg2+ in etiology of diabetic complications. Diabetes 1992; 41:35–39.
30. Greene DA, Lattimer SA, Sima AA. Sorbitol, phosphoinositides, and sodium-potassium-ATPase in the pathogenesis of diabetic complications (review). N Engl J Med 1987; 316:599–606.
31. Grenfell A. Acute renal failure in diabetics. In Mogensen CE (ed): The Kidney and Hypertension in Diabetes Mellitus. Boston, Kluwer Academic Publishers, 1994, pp 407–419.
32. Groop L, Ekstrand A, Forsblom C, et al. Insulin resistance, hypertension and microalbuminuria in patients with type 2 (non–insulin-dependent) diabetes mellitus. Diabetologia 1993; 36:642–647.
33. Harris RD, Steffes MW, Bilous RW, et al. Global glomerular sclerosis and glomerular arteriolar hyalinosis in insulin dependent diabetes. Kidney Int 1991; 40:107–114.
33a. Hayashi K, Epstein M, Loutzenhiser R, Forster H. Impaired myogenic responsiveness of the afferent arteriole in streptozotocin-induced diabetic rats: role of eicosanoid derangements. J Am Soc Nephrol 1992; 2:1578–1586.
34. Jacobsen P, Tarnow L, Rossing P, et al. The insertion/deletion (I/D) polymorphism in the angiotensin-I-converting enzyme (ACE) gene predicts the progression of diabetic nephropathy during ACE inhibition (ACEI) in insulin-dependent diabetic (IDDM) patients (abstract). J Am Soc Nephrol 1995; 6:450A.
35. Jensen T, Borch-Johnsen K, Kofoed-Enevoldsen A, et al. Coronary heart disease in young type 1 (insulin-dependent) diabetic patients with and without diabetic nephropathy: Incidence and risk factors. Diabetologia 1987; 30:144–148.
36. Keller CK, Bergis KH, Fliser D, et al. Renal findings in patients with short-term type 2 diabetes. J Am Soc Nephrol 1996; 7:2627–2635.
37. Klahr S, Levey AS, Beck GJ, et al. The effects of dietary protein restriction and blood-pressure control on the progression of chronic renal disease. N Engl J Med 1994; 330:877–884.
38. Klein R, Klein BE, Moss SE. Prevalence of microalbuminuria in older-onset diabetes. Diabetes Care 1993; 16:1325–1330.
39. Krolewski AS, Canessa M, Warram JH, et al. Predisposition to hypertension and susceptibility to renal disease in insulin-dependent diabetes mellitus. N Engl J Med 1988; 318:140–145.
40. Krolewski AS, Laffel LM, Krolewski M, et al. Glycosylated hemoglobin and the risk of microalbuminuria in patients with insulin-dependent diabetes mellitus (see comments). N Engl J Med 1995; 332:1251–1255.

41. Lane PH, Steffes MW, Fioretto P, et al. Renal interstitial expansion in insulin-dependent diabetes mellitus. Kidney Int 1993; 43:661–667.

42. Lebovitz HE, Wiegmann TB, Caan A, et al. Renal protective effects of enalapril in hypertensive NIDDM: Role of baseline albuminuria. Kidney Int Suppl 1994; 45:S150–S155.

43. Levey AS, Adler S, Caggiula AW, et al. Effects of dietary protein restriction on the progression of moderate renal disease in the modification of diet in renal disease study. J Am Soc Nephrol 1996; 7:2616–2626.

44. Lewis EJ, Hunsicker LG, Bain RP, et al. The effect of angiotensin-converting-enzyme inhibition on diabetic nephropathy: The Collaborative Study Group (see comments) N Engl J Med 1993;329:1456–1462. Published erratum appears in N Engl J Med 1993; Jan 13; 330:(2)152.

45. Lurbe A, Redon J, Pascual JM, et al. Altered blood pressure during sleep in normotensive subjects with type I diabetes. Hypertension 1993; 21:227–235.

46. Makita Z, Radoff S, Rayfield EJ, et al. Advanced glycosylation end products in patients with diabetic nephropathy (see comments). N Engl J Med 1991; 325:836–842.

47. Marre M, Bernadet P, Gallois Y, et al. Relationships between angiotensin I converting enzyme gene polymorphism, plasma levels, and diabetic retinal and renal complications. Diabetes 1994; 43:384–388.

48. Mathiesen ER, Hommel E, Giese J, et al. Efficacy of captopril in postponing nephropathy in normotensive insulin dependent diabetic patients with microalbuminuria. BMJ 1991; 303:81–87.

49. Mathiesen ER, Ronn B, Storm B, et al. The natural course of microalbuminuria in insulin-dependent diabetes: A 10-year prospective study. Diabetic Med 1995; 12:482–487.

50. Microalbuminuria Collaborative Study Group United Kingdom. Risk factors for development of microalbuminuria in insulin dependent diabetic patients: A cohort study. BMJ 1993; 306:1235–1239.

51. Miller JA, Scholey JW, Thai K, et al. Angiotensin converting enzyme gene polymorphism and renal hemodynamic function in early diabetes. Kidney Int 1997; 51:119–124.

52. Mogensen CE. Microalbuminuria predicts clinical proteinuria and early mortality in maturity-onset diabetes. N Engl J Med 1984; 310:356–360.

53. Mogensen CE. Systemic blood pressure and glomerular leakage with particular reference to diabetes and hypertension (review). J Int Med 1994; 235:297–316.

54. Mogensen CE, Hansen KW, Osterby R, et al. Blood pressure elevated versus abnormal albuminuria in the genesis and prediction of renal disease in diabetes. Diabetes Care 1992; 15:1192–1204.

55. Molgaard H, Christensen PD, Hermansen K, et al. Early recognition of autonomic dysfunction in microalbuminuria: Significance for cardiovascular mortality in diabetes mellitus? Diabetologia 1994; 37:788–796.

56. Moriyama T, Kitamura H, Ochi S, et al. Association of angiotensin I-converting enzyme gene polymorphism with susceptibility to antiproteinuric effect of angiotensin I-converting enzyme inhibitors in patients with proteinuria. J Am Soc Nephrol 1995; 6:1674–1678.

57. Nadler JL, Buchanan T, Natarajan R. Magnesium deficiency produces insulin resistance and increased thromboxane synthesis. Hypertension 1993; 21:1024–1029.

58. Nelson RG, Pettitt DJ, de Courten MP, et al. Parental hypertension and proteinuria in Pima Indians with NIDDM. Diabetologia 1996; 39:433–438.

59. Nielsen S, Schmitz A, Rehling M, et al. Systolic blood pressure relates to the rate of decline of glomerular filtration rate in type II diabetes. Diabetes Care 1993; 16:1427–1432.

60. Niskanen L, Laakso M. Insulin resistance is related to albuminuria in patients with type II (non–insulin-dependent) diabetes mellitus. Metabolism 1993; 42:1541–1545.

61. Nosadini R, Solini A, Velussi M, et al. Impaired insulin-induced glucose uptake by extrahepatic tissue is hallmark of NIDDM patients who have or will develop hypertension and microalbuminuria. Diabetes 1994; 43:491–499.

62. Olivarius N, Andreasen AH, Keiding N, et al. Epidemiology of renal involvement in newly-diagnosed middle-aged and elderly diabetic patients: Cross-sectional data from the population-based study "Diabetes Care in General Practice," Denmark. Diabetologia 1993; 36:1007–1016.

63. Orchard TJ, Dorman JS, Maser RE, et al. Prevalence of complications in IDDM by sex and duration: Pittsburgh Epidemiology of Diabetes Complications Study 2. Diabetes 1990; 39:1116–1124.

64. Osterby R. Microalbuminuria in diabetes mellitus: Is there a structural basis? (editorial)(review). Nephrol Dial Transplant 1995; 10:12–14.

65. Osterby R, Parving H-H, Nyberg G, et al. A strong correlation between glomerular filtration rate and filtration surface in diabetic nephropathy. Diabetologia 1988; 31:265–270.

66. Parving H-H, Jacobsen P, Rossing K, et al. Benefits of long-term antihypertensive treatment on prognosis in diabetic nephropathy. Kidney Int 1996; 49:1778–1782.

67. Parving H-H, Tarnow L, Rossing P. Genetics of diabetic nephropathy. J Am Soc Nephrol 1996; 7:2509–2517.

68. Paulsen EP, Burke BA, Vernier RL, et al. Juxtaglomerular body abnormalities in youth-onset diabetic subjects. Kidney Int 1994; 45:1132–1139.

69. Pedrini MT, Levey AS, Lau J, et al. The effect of dietary protein restriction on the progression of diabetic and nondiabetic renal diseases: A meta-analysis. Ann Intern Med 1996; 124:627–632.

70. Powrie JK, Watts GF, Ingham JN, et al. Role of glycaemic control in development of microalbuminuria in patients with insulin dependent diabetes. BMJ 1994; 309:1608–1612.

71. Ravid M, Lang R, Rachmani R, et al. Long-term renoprotective effect of angiotensin-converting enzyme inhibition in non-insulin-dependent diabetes mellitus. Arch Intern Med 1996; 3:286–289.

72. Ravid M, Savin H, Jutrin I, et al. Long-term stabilizing effect of antiogensin-converting enzyme inhibition on plasma creatinine and on proteinuria in normotensive Type II diabetic patients. Ann Intern Med 1993; 118:577–581.

73. Ravid M, Savin H, Lang R, et al. Proteinuria, renal impairment, metabolic control, and blood pressure in type 2 diabetes mellitus. A 14-year follow-up report on 195 patients. Arch Intern Med 1992; 152:1225–1229.

74. Ritz E, Nowack R, Fliser D, et al. Type II diabetes: Is the renal risk adequately appreciated? (editorial). Nephrol Dial Transplant 1991; 6:679–682.

75. Rodby RA, Schwartz MM. Proteinuria, hematuria, hypertension, and decreased renal function in a patient with diabetes for 9 years (clinical conference). Am J Kidney Dis 1992; 20:658–667.

76. Rudberg S, Persson B, Dahlquist G. Increased glomerular filtration rate as a predictor of diabetic nephropathy: An 8-year prospective study. Kidney Int 1992; 41:822–828.

77. Ruilope LM, Rodicio JL. Microalbuminuria in clinical practice. Kidney 1995; 4:211–216.

78. Seaquist ER, Goetz FC, Rich S, et al. Familial clustering of diabetic kidney disease: Evidence for genetic susceptibility to diabetic nephropathy (see comments). N Engl J Med 1989; 320:1161–1165.

79. Siegel JE, Krolewski AS, Warram JH, et al. Cost-effectiveness of screening and early treatment of nephropathy in patients with insulin-dependent diabetes mellitus. J Am Soc Nephrol 1992; 3:S111–S119.

80. Smith SR, Svetkey LP, Dennis VW. Racial differences in the incidence and progression of renal diseases (editorial). Kidney Int 1991; 40:815–822.

81. Soulis-Liparota T, Cooper M, Papazoglou D, et al. Retardation by aminoguanidine of development of albuminuria, mesangial expansion, and tissue fluorescence in streptozocin-induced diabetic rat. Diabetes 1991; 40:1328–1334.

82. Steffes MW, Bilous RW, Sutherland DE, et al. Cell and matrix components of the glomerular mesangium in type I diabetes. Diabetes 1992; 41:679–684.

83. Tarnow L, Cambien F, Rossing P, et al. Lack of relationship between an insertion/deletion polymorphism in the angiotensin-I-converting enzyme gene and diabetic nephropathy and proliferative retinopathy in IDDM patients. Diabetes 1995; 44:489–494.

84. U.S. Renal Data System. USRDS 1993 Annual Data Report. Bethesda, National Institutes of Health, National Institute of Diabetes and Digestive and Kidney Diseases, 1993.

85. U.S. Renal Data System. USRDS 1996 Annual Data Report. Bethesda, National Institutes of Health, National Institute of Diabetes and Digestive and Kidney Diseases, 1996.

86. Viberti GC, Keen H, Wiseman MJ. Raised arterial pressure in parents of proteinuric insulin-dependent diabetics. BMJ 1987; 295:515–517.

87. Vlassara H, Striker LJ, Teichberg S, et al. Advanced glycation end products induce glomerular sclerosis and albuminuria in normal rats. Proc Natl Acad Sci USA 1994; 91:11704–11708.

88. Wagoner RD, Holley KE. Parenchymal renal disease: Clinical and pathologic features. *In* Knox FG (ed): Textbook of Renal Pathophysiology. Hagerstown, MD, Harper & Row, 1978, pp 226–253.

89. Wang PH, Lau J, Chalmers TC. Meta-analysis of effects of intensive blood-glucose control on late complications of type I diabetes (see comments). Lancet 1993; 341:1306–1309.

90. Yamamoto T, Nakamura T, Noble NA, et al. Expression of transforming growth factor beta is elevated in human and experimental diabetic nephropathy. Proc Natl Acad Sci USA 1993; 90:1814–1818.

91. Yang CW, Vlassara H, Peten EP, et al. Advanced glycation end products up-regulate gene expression found in diabetic glomerular disease. Proc Natl Acad Sci USA 1994; 91:9436-9440.

Chapter 6

Cardiovascular Disease and Diabetes

Peter C. Spittell • Robert D. Brown, Jr.

INTRODUCTION

As many as 3 to 10% of adults in the United States older than age 45 have diabetes mellitus, primarily type 2 diabetes mellitus (DM).[110, 114, 180] Of the estimated 15.7 million persons in the United States with DM, approximately one third of cases are undiagnosed.[55] Cardiovascular disease associated with DM is prevalent, occurring in a specific form (microangiopathic or endothelial proliferative changes of arterioles), usually combined with a nonspecific form (atherosclerosis and arteriosclerosis). Microangiopathic (small vessel) disease in association with diabetes is localized to small vessels and occurs in patients of all ages, whereas the nonspecific form of vascular disease (atherosclerosis) primarily involves the large arteries of the heart, brain, and lower extremities of older patients. The atherosclerotic process in diabetics is accelerated, as a result of the chronic hyperglycemia and an increased prevalence of traditional cardiovascular risk factors. Myocardial infarction, cerebrovascular disease, and occlusive peripheral arterial disease all occur with increased incidence in diabetic patients. Overall mortality from coronary artery disease (CAD) in diabetic patients is three times that of nondiabetics.[96, 172, 225]

CARDIOVASCULAR DISEASE
Pathogenesis

Patients with diabetes exhibit derangements in the metabolism of glucose, fat, and proteins, resulting in increased concentrations in the blood of glucose and atherogenic metabolites. The insulin resistance and hyperinsulinemia characteristic of type 2 DM exert a deleterious effect on the vascular endothelium, the coagulation and fibrinolytic systems, and blood lipids. Hyperglycemia adversely affects endothelial cell function by decreasing endothelium-mediated vascular reactivity, activating protein kinase C, and increasing production of vasoconstrictors, including endothelin.[216] In addition, hyperglycemia often leads to glycosylation of proteins through nonenzymatic linkage of glucose to proteins (glycation) and production of advanced glycation end products that have deleterious effects on the vascular endothelium.[41] Advanced glycosylation end products are thought to contribute to the various stage-by-stage mechanisms for atherosclerotic plaque progression.[68, 123, 185, 201] Glycation of apolipoprotein B exacerbates atherogenesis by stimulating foam cell formation and augmenting platelet aggregation.[144] Advanced glycosylation end products that accumulate in vascular tissue further promote atherogenesis by enhancing chemotaxis of monocytes; increasing production of growth factors and cytokines; stimulating vascular smooth muscle cell proliferation; and increasing binding and deposition of nonglycated low-density lipoprotein (LDL) in the arterial wall.[41, 224] Furthermore, hyperglycemia stimulates endothelial cell production of collagen IV and fibronectin, enhancing mural fibrosis.[45]

As noted, two forms of vascular disease can occur in diabetic patients: a specific form of microvascular disease (endothelial proliferative changes of arterioles), and a nonspecific macrovascular disease (atherosclerosis and arteriosclerosis). Microvascular disease, the dominant form of angiopathy in type 1 DM, is localized to small vessels and may be seen in patients of all ages. This specific microangiopathy causes thickening of the basement membrane of capillaries in the retina, conjunctiva, glomerulus, brain, pancreas, and myocardium and is clinically manifest as retinopathy, nephropathy, neuropathy, and cardiomyopathy.[82] In some cases there is also proliferation of the epithelial cells, leading to occlusion of small arterioles similar to that observed in immune arteritis. Microvascular disease is related to the severity and duration of the metabolic abnormalities associated with diabetes.[70] Importantly, at the time of initial diagnosis of diabetes, 10 to 20% of individuals already have evidence of microvascular disease.[162]

Macrovascular disease (arteriosclerosis and atherosclerosis) in persons with DM is notable for its extensive nature and rapid progression in multiple organ systems. Determinants of macrovascular disease in DM are multifactorial, reflecting in part the adverse influence of covariate cardiac risk factors such as hypertension and hyperlipidemia.[195] Hypertension, hyperlipidemia, and obesity often coexist with type 2 DM and further accelerate the atherosclerotic process.[68] At the time of initial diagnosis of diabetes, the prevalence of macrovascular disease is almost equal to that of patients with previously diagnosed diabetes.[111]

Coronary Artery Disease

Diabetes mellitus is a major risk factor for atherosclerotic CAD.[211, 238] Coronary artery disease in diabetic patients is notable for its increased prevalence (especially among female patients), premature onset, rapid rate of progression, and severity. Autopsy studies have shown the prevalence of CAD among diabetic persons to range from 18 to 75%.[87, 102, 104] Frequently associated hypertension, hyperlipidemia, obesity, and hyperglycemia combine to result in a higher incidence of heart disease in patients with diabetes. The prevalence of cardiovascular morbidity and mortality is fourfold to sixfold higher in diabetic patients compared with age- and gender-matched nondiabetic patients.[220] Furthermore, the complications of myocardial infarction (e.g., acute and chronic congestive heart failure, cardiogenic shock, and cardiac arrhythmias) are more common in patients with DM.[115, 238]

Because peripheral neuropathy, both somatic and autonomic, is commonly associated with DM, the symptoms of acute myocardial infarction (AMI) are more variable. Myocardial infarction may actually occur without pain in diabetic patients, possibly because of the loss of nerve fibers in the ischemic area.[33, 167] Not only can MI occur without symptoms, but chronic silent ischemia is not uncommon in diabetics, especially in those with peripheral diabetic autonomic nervous system abnormalities.[79, 187] Further, cardiac autonomic dysfunction in diabetic patients can result in an increase in the anginal threshold.[14, 190, 199, 246] Occasionally, silent ischemia may be present before clinical symptoms of generalized autonomic neuropathy are demonstrable.

Diabetics who do develop angina tend to have more extensive CAD than do nondiabetic patients. They are also more likely to have hypertension, cardiomegaly, diffuse hypokinesis, and previous MI.

Diabetic neuropathy involving the sympathetic or the parasympathetic nervous system (or both) may become so severe that it leads to total cardiac denervation. The changes in adrenergic nervous system function can result in tachycardia with a regular rate that shows a minimal response to physiologic stimuli (such as the Valsalva maneuver, carotid sinus pressure, or tilting) or drugs.[227] Rarely do diabetic patients with denervated hearts develop more serious arrhythmias.

Diabetic patients with AMI, regardless of the control of their diabetes before hospital admission, exhibit significantly higher mortality and morbidity than do nondiabetics.[3, 115, 211] In a large community-based study of 5322 patients with AMI and no previous history of ischemic heart disease, 333 men (9%) and 224 women (13%) had a history of diabetes.[63] The age-adjusted 28-day case fatality for women with diabetes (25%) was significantly higher than for women without diabetes (16%). The difference for men was also significant (25% with diabetes and 20% without diabetes). The increased risk for death in the diabetic patients remained after accounting for their poorer risk factor profiles. Furthermore, diabetic patients with an increased glycosylated hemoglobin level had a worse prognosis with AMI than did those with a normal level.[173] Even if they reached the hospital alive, diabetic patients were also less likely to survive than nondiabetic patients. Recurrrent infarction, heart failure, and dysrhythmias all contribute to this higher death rate.[3, 115, 200, 211, 238]

Several factors are thought to contribute to the increased mortality of diabetic patients with AMI. The size of the infarct tends to be greater in diabetic patients; diabetic patients have a greater frequency of both congestive heart failure and shock than do nondiabetics; and the diabetic patient is often in a precarious metabolic status compounded by the difficulty of adjusting insulin therapy to prevent ketoacidosis while not precipitating hypoglycemia.[3, 200, 211] The effect of AMI on carbohydrate and fat metabolism leads to stimulation of the sympathetic nervous system and increased catecholamine concentration.[57] This results in increases in circulating free fatty acid levels and reductions in glucose tolerance. The net result is that carbohydrate intolerance is common after MI, even in nondiabetics. Furthermore, the high concentrations of free fatty acid in the acute phases of MI may lead to ventricular arrhythmias.[88]

In view of the considerably higher morbidity and mortality rates for diabetic patients with AMI, initial therapy needs to be aggressive.[4] The initial emergency management of suspected AMI should include a careful cardiac history and cardiovascular examination as well as an electrocardiogram (ECG) in less than 10 minutes. Supplemental oxygen is administered and an intravenous access line and continuous ECG monitoring are established. Sublingual nitroglycerin is promptly administered (unless systolic blood pressure is less than 90 mm Hg or heart rate is less than 50 or more than 100 beats per minute). Aspirin (160 to 325 mg) is given orally and adequate analgesia with either morphine sulfate or meperidine hydrochloride is achieved. Measurements of a hematology group, serum electrolytes, glucose, magnesium, and cardiac enzyme levels are made. If the clinical presentation and ECG findings support a diagnosis of AMI, intravenous heparin is usually administered and consideration of intravenous thrombolytic therapy or possibly percutaneous transluminal coronary angioplasty (PTCA) is appropriate.

Thrombolytic agents unquestionably lower the mortality of patients with an AMI, even among patients with DM.[142, 204] Although thrombolysis has substantially improved survival of patients with MI, DM remains an independent predictor for a poor prognosis. Large randomized trials of thrombolytic therapy in AMI (Gruppo Italiano per lo Studio della Streptockinasi nell'Infarto miocardico [GISSI-2]) have demonstrated that patients with diabetes have a higher mortality at 30 days and 1 year, especially among those treated with insulin.[21, 106, 146, 248] The odds ratio for 30-day mortality for patients with diabetes is 1.77 that of patients without diabetes.[146] It appears that accelerated tissue-type plasminogen activator (t-PA) offers improved survival in diabetic patients with AMI compared with other thrombolytic agents.[146] The rates for reinfarction are similar among the different thrombolytic regimens. Diabetic retinopathy should not be considered a contraindication to thrombolytic therapy in patients with an AMI because intraocular hemorrhage is extremely uncommon (incidence of approximately 0.05%).[145] To improve outcome after AMI and thrombolytic therapy in diabetic patients, newer strategies such as peri-infarction metabolic control and primary angioplasty are areas of active investigation.[149, 210]

Administration of β-blockers to diabetics with AMI appears to reduce overall mortality, at least in the immediate post-AMI period, similar to what has been reported in nondiabetics.[107] Furthermore, in patients undergoing noncardiac and vascular surgery, aggressive perioperative β-blocker therapy may reduce cardiac events.[151] Treatment with β-adrenergic antagonists has been shown to be associated with an increased risk for impaired glucose tolerance or diabetes; this has been attributed to the worsening of insulin resistance and the deterioration of lipoprotein metabolism caused by these agents.[140] Furthermore, β-adrenergic blockers may mask the symptoms associated with hypoglycemia (except sweating) and may also prolong hypoglycemia by inhibiting glycolysis. All this has made physicians reluctant to prescribe β-adrenergic blockers for diabetic patients, although cardioselective β-adrenergic blockers have reduced mortality associated with cardiovascular causes in secondary prevention trials.[148] Fortunately, β₁-adrenergic antagonists have been shown to not prolong hypoglycemia and glucose recovery or interfere with glucagon and epinephrine response after the insulin test.

The accelerated and rapidly progressive nature of atherosclerosis in type 2 diabetes also results in higher than usual rates of re-stenosis and mortality after PTCA, development of atherosclerosis in bypass conduits after coronary artery bypass grafting (CABG), and mortality exceeding that in nondiabetic patients.[19, 26, 44] The Bypass Angioplasty Revascularization Investigation (BARI) was a clinical trial designed to test the hypothesis that an initial revascularization strategy of PTCA would compare favorably with CABG over 5 years in patients with multivessel CAD and severe angina or ischemia.[44] The one subgroup that did better with CABG was comprised of diabetic patients. In-hospital mortality was similar for CABG (1.2%) and angioplasty (0.6%), but diabetics had significantly lower 5-year all-cause survival than did nondiabetics (73% versus 91%). Among diabetics, the 5-year survival rate was 80.6% with CABG and 65.5% with PTCA ($P = 0.003$), a difference explained by a higher cardiac mortality after PTCA than after CABG (21% versus 6%).[44] Within the surgical group, 5-year cardiac mortality was only 3% when at least one internal mammary artery was used versus 18% when only saphenous vein graft conduits were used.[97] Furthermore, subsequent revascularization was often required for diabetic patients who underwent PTCA.[44] An interesting finding in the long-term angiographic follow-up of PTCA in patients with diabetes is the increased

risk of disease progression in the artery that was instrumented during balloon angioplasty.[191] This finding may explain the high adverse-event rates observed in diabetic patients in the angioplasty arm of the BARI study, most of whom had angioplasty in at least two arteries. Diabetic patients are also proposed to have a high rate of re-stenosis after PTCA because of their greater tendency to develop intimal hyperplasia. In addition, diabetic patients have a higher re-stenosis rate than do nondiabetics after coronary atherectomy (59.7% versus 47.4%, respectively).[137] Fortunately, the use of intracoronary stents in combination with PTCA has been shown to result in a lower re-stenosis rate than conventional PTCA alone in patients with diabetes.[222] Re-stenosis rates in diabetic patients treated with intracoronary stent placement are similar to nondiabetic patients (25% and 27%, respectively) 6 months after the procedure.[222] It is important to remember that CABG is strongly associated with improved survival in diabetic patients with low ejection fractions and significant CAD and should be considered as primary therapy in patients with ischemic cardiomyopathy and evidence of viable myocardium.[11]

Congestive Heart Failure

Diabetes mellitus appears to increase the risk for the development of congestive heart failure (CHF) from all causes.[3, 129] It is also an independent predictor of mortality in patients with CHF from ischemic and nonischemic etiologies.[15, 25] Even when patients with previous coronary or rheumatic heart disease are excluded, diabetic subjects have a fourfold to fivefold increased risk of CHF. This increased risk remains even after age, blood pressure, weight, and cholesterol values as well as CAD are taken into account. The increased incidence of CHF in patients with diabetes is likely caused by multiple factors, including a microangiopathy that is common and specific to diabetes, metabolic-induced changes of myocardial cell function, and the chronic sequela of CAD. Glycemic control and male gender, rather than mode of therapy (insulin versus oral hypoglycemic agent), are closely related to myocardial blood flow and myocardial flow reserve as assessed by positron emission tomography.[240] Maximal myocardial vasodilatory capacity has been reported to be reduced in angiographically normal coronary arteries, especially in patients with DM. Wall thickening and lumen narrowing of the intramural coronary microvasculature in patients with DM can result in a significant impairment in coronary flow reserve, despite angiographically normal coronary arteries.[86, 161, 168] This microvascular dysfunction has been proposed in patients with angina pectoris, normal coronary arteries, and diminished coronary flow reserve.[40] Interestingly, diabetic retinopathy, especially advanced retinopathy, is associated with and serves to identify patients with a marked restriction of coronary flow reserve.[10] Insulin-dependent diabetics with CAD appear to have "stiffer" ventricles, with greater elevation of left ventricular end-diastolic pressure, than do matched nondiabetic controls.[91] The severity of this dysfunction is related to the degree of metabolic control, and there is no clinical evidence of cardiovascular or microvascular disease.[113]

Diabetic Cardiomyopathy

There is a significant increase in the coincidence of DM and cardiomyopathy. The cardiomyopathy occurs in the absence of significant epicardial CAD or abnormalities in myocardial capillary basal lamina documented by endomyocardial biopsy.[108, 184, 214, 247] The most common histologic pattern described in diabetic cardiomyopathy is interstitial fibrosis and arteriolar hyalinization. The accumulation of periodic acid–Schiff (PAS)-positive material between muscle fibers and collections of collagen and glycoprotein extending into T tubules are specific findings.[184] Furthermore, small vessel disease is rare among patients with cardiomyopathy who are not diabetic. Systolic and diastolic dysfunction has been observed.

Management of Cardiovascular Risk Factors

Type 2 DM, which accounts for 90 to 95% of all diagnosed diabetes, is associated with risk factors that are modifiable (e.g., obesity, hyperlipidemia, hypertension) and nonmodifiable (e.g., genetic factors, older age, race/ethnicity, and positive family history). The increasing prevalence and incidence of diabetes mentioned earlier underscore the urgent need for effective intervention strategies to prevent diabetes and its complications. The high prevalence and rapid progression of atherosclerosis in type 2 diabetes is closely related to the presence of traditional cardiovascular risk factors. Although adults with type 2 diabetes have an increased incidence of hypertension and hypercholesterolemia, DM clearly confers an inde-

pendent cardiovascular risk and should be considered as a separate risk factor for atherosclerotic cardiovascular disease.[130, 211, 238] Traditional cardiovascular risk factors for CAD (cigarette smoking, hypertension, hyperlipidemia) exert an independent and additive influence. Because each risk factor for vascular disease is thought to add independently (although not equally) to the likelihood for the development of ischemic disease, the diabetic should be considered a high-risk patient in whom all correctable risk factors should be managed aggressively.[3, 115] The major focus of management in diabetic patients must be to prevent and retard the progression of atherosclerosis. Modifiable cardiovascular risk factors such as hypertension, hyperlipidemia, and tobacco use must be aggressively treated. Maintenance of euglycemia (achieving a hemoglobin A_{1c} level below 7%) is an essential element of treatment.

Diabetes

Intensive insulin therapy appears to significantly improve the prognosis for diabetic patients with AMI.[147] In a randomized trial involving 620 diabetics with AMI (about 80% of whom had type 2 DM), patients were given either standard treatment without insulin unless clinically indicated or standard treatment plus an insulin and glucose infusion followed by four daily insulin injections for at least 3 months.[147] Patients were followed for a mean of 3.4 years. By the end of follow-up, mortality was significantly lower in the intervention group (33% versus 44%). The relative reduction in mortality was 28% and the absolute risk reduction was 11%; this means that one life was saved for every nine treated patients. The effect was most pronounced in the subgroup with low cardiovascular risk and no previous insulin therapy. The major difference between the two groups, aside from mortality, was better diabetic control in the intervention group. We hope that the new guidelines, which lower the current fasting diagnostic criteria for diabetes from greater than or equal to 140 mg/dL (7.8 mmol/L) of plasma glucose to greater than or equal to 126 mg/dL (6.0 mmol/L), will allow earlier diagnosis and improved treatment and outcomes.[81]

Hyperlipidemia

Lipoprotein abnormalities, as previously mentioned, are common in patients with type 2 diabetes and likely contribute significantly to the rapidly progressive nature of atherosclerosis in these patients. Therapy of hyperlipidemia in diabetic patients should primarily be directed at treatment of the underlying metabolic abnormalities associated with diabetes. Improved metabolic control will decrease concentrations of very-low-density lipoprotein (VLDL), intermediate-density lipoprotein (IDL), and LDL cholesterol as well as increase high-density lipoprotein (HDL) cholesterol in blood.[119] Control of blood glucose by dietary measures, oral glucose-lowering agents, and/or insulin will often correct the underlying lipid abnormalities.[74, 89] Weight reduction in obese diabetic patients and exercise therapy in sedentary patients are essential and often result in significant improvements in lipoprotein abnormalities.

The goals of therapy for hyperlipidemia in patients with diabetes should adhere to the guidelines from the National Cholesterol Education Program (NCEP) Expert Panel.[164] Using these guidelines, the target LDL cholesterol value (assuming occult or overt coronary disease is present) is below 100 mg/dL (2.59 mmol/L). The target for triglycerides should be below 200 mg/dL (2.26 mmol/L).

Multiple pharmacologic agents are available to treat hyperlipidemia in diabetic patients. The most commonly used agents are gemfibrozil and 3-hydroxy-3-methylglutaryl coenzyme A (HMG CoA) reductase inhibitors. Gemfibrozil, a fibric acid derivative, has been demonstrated to lower triglycerides more than 25% in diabetic patients, with a corresponding increase in HDL cholesterol of more than 10% after 12 weeks of therapy.[223] The percent reduction in triglycerides and percent increase in HDL cholesterol are less in diabetic subjects than in nondiabetic subjects, but the incremental risk reduction for the complications of coronary heart disease (death and myocardial infarction) is greater in patients with type 2 DM.[92, 132]

The HMG CoA reductase inhibitors primarily reduce LDL cholesterol concentrations; they reduce serum triglyceride and increase HDL cholesterol levels to a lesser extent. The Scandinavian Simvastatin Survival Study (4S) demonstrated a 32% reduction in major cardiac events and a 35% reduction in LDL cholesterol over 5 years with simvastatin in patients with known coronary heart disease.[202] Based on these results, aggressive therapy of hyperlipidemia in patients with DM with either an HMG CoA reductase inhibitor or gemfibrozil will be particularly beneficial. Atorvastatin (the most recent HMG CoA reductase inhibitor approved by the Food and Drug Administration for use in clinical practice) and simvastatin are the only HMG CoA reductase inhibitors approved for treating hypertriglyceridemia, making these agents advantageous in patients with diabetes who frequently have a combined hyperlipidemia. Although HMG CoA reductase inhibitors are generally well tolerated, they may cause elevation of hepatic transaminase levels, necessitating periodic assessment of liver enzymes in patients taking these medications. In patients taking an HMG CoA reductase inhibitor in conjunction with gemfibrozil, careful follow-up for the development of myositis should be undertaken.

Hypertension

Diabetes and hypertension often coexist; in fact, at least half of all diabetic adults have hypertension, and those who are not hypertensive have an increased risk of becoming so. Compared with the general population, diabetic patients have an approximately twofold increased risk of developing hypertension and are more susceptible to the vascular consequences of high blood pressure.[176, 239] An estimated 35 to 75% of cardiovascular and renal complications in diabetic patients can be attributed to hypertension.[206] Hypertension may be essential (primary) or secondary to impaired compliance of large vessels, abnormalities of the renin-angiotensin system, diabetic nephropathy, or renal artery stenosis.[192] The renal circulation is affected in several ways, including atherosclerosis of the larger arteries and endothelial proliferation involving small arteries. The capillary basement membrane is thickened, and nodular glomerulosclerosis, a characteristic lesion of diabetes, is found. Renal complications are a significant source of morbidity and mortality in patients with DM; therefore, hypertension should be aggressively treated in the diabetic patient with the goal of normotension (blood pressure less than 140/85) throughout the day.

Aggressive treatment of hypertension in diabetic patients decreases the risk for stroke and cardiac death and attenuates the progression of nephropathy.[165] Analysis of the diabetic subset of the Systolic Hypertension in the Elderly trial (SHEP) population, which used diuretics (chlorthalidone, 12.5 to 25.0 mg/d) as the initial treatment, found a significant absolute risk reduction of major cardiovascular disease events (nonfatal plus fatal stroke, nonfatal MI, major CHD events) in elderly diabetic patients with isolated systolic hypertension.[66] The use of other classes of antihypertensive agents must take into account potential side effects as well as associated cardiovascular disease (prior myocardial infarction, reduced left ventricular systolic function, etc). Thiazide diuretics may exacerbate hyperglycemia and exert adverse effects on blood lipids. β-Adrenergic blocking agents may exacerbate elevations of LDL cholesterol and lower levels of HDL cholesterol. Central sympatholytics, direct-acting vasodilators, and α-adrenergic blocking agents may exacerbate orthostatic hypotension caused by neuropathy.

Angiotensin-converting enzyme (ACE) inhibitors are currently the drug of choice for treating hypertension in patients with diabetes because of the advantages both in terms of glucose control and in retarding the deterioration of renal function, especially in patients with microalbuminuria.[77, 117, 233, 244] Captopril has been shown to result in a 50% reduction in the combined end point of death, dialysis, or renal transplantation in patients with type 1 diabetes.[171] Long-acting ACE inhibitors offer a theoretical advantage over short-acting agents because of the likelihood of improved control of blood pressure throughout the day. In addition, ACE inhibitors slow the progression of renal disease in diabetic patients without hypertension and with or without microalbuminuria.[77] Furthermore, ACE inhibitors are beneficial in diabetic patients with dilated cardiomyopathy or previous MI resulting in reduced left ventricular function (ejection fraction less than 40%). Careful monitoring of serum creatinine is important because progressive renal insufficiency can occur in patients with bilateral renal artery stenosis. Newer agents such as carvedilol, a multiple action antihypertensive drug with nonselective (β-adrenergic receptor) and selective (α-adrenergic receptor) blocking activity, may offer advantages in patients with diabetes and hypertension, by improving glucose and lipid metabolism and reducing lipid peroxidation.[101]

Peripheral Arterial Disease

Atherosclerosis of the lower extremity arteries producing intermittent claudication or more severe ischemic symptoms is a frequent and significant manifestation of DM. In patients with type 2 DM, 8% have peripheral arterial occlusive disease (PAD) at the time of diagnosis, 15% after 10 years, and 45% after 20

years.[28, 155, 159] Furthermore, PAD in diabetics is associated with high morbidity and mortality largely because of associated cardiac and cerebrovascular disease. Diabetic patients are five times more likely to develop critical limb ischemia (ischemic rest pain, ulceration, or gangrene) than are nondiabetic patients.[155, 230] More than 60,000 lower extremity amputations performed each year result from DM complicated by ischemia and/or infection.[163] This represents 50% of all nontraumatic amputations performed in the United States annually. Diabetes itself is a major risk factor for lower extremity amputation in patients with PAD, resulting in a sevenfold increased risk of major amputation over the next 5 years.[120, 125, 155] A recent population-based study found the cumulative risk of major amputation over 25 years was 11% in both type 1 and type 2 DM.[121] When compared with lower extremity amputation rates in nondiabetics, patients with type 2 diabetes were 400 times more likely to undergo a transphalangeal amputation and 12 times more likely to require a below-knee amputation over the same time period.[121] Additional major risk factors for lower extremity amputation in diabetic patients include the development of critical limb ischemia (e.g., ischemic rest pain, ischemic ulceration, and/or gangrene).[155] Tobacco use is an important risk factor in patients with PAD. Tobacco use is associated with an elevenfold increase in risk for major amputation over 5 years in patients with DM and intermittent claudication.[155] Other risk factors reported to increase the risk of amputation in diabetic patients with PAD are duration of disease, elevated glycosylated hemoglobin, elevated diastolic blood pressure, and retinopathy. Overall, the increased amputation rate is most often due to the triad of peripheral arterial occlusive disease, peripheral neuropathy, and/or infection.

Patients with DM, particularly type 2 DM, have a distinct pattern and distribution of atherosclerosis in the lower extremity arteries. Compared with nondiabetics, there is less involvement of the aortoiliac segment, equal occurrence in the femoropopliteal segments, and more extensive disease in the infrapopliteal segments (tibial and peroneal arteries).

Clinically, patients with diabetes and PAD are younger and have more rapid onset and progression of symptoms; they usually have bilateral disease involving the tibial and peroneal arteries and small vessel disease. The majority of diabetic patients with PAD present with intermittent claudication, a characteristic

TABLE 6.1 INTERMITTENT CLAUDICATION: DIFFERENTIAL DIAGNOSIS

	Claudication	Pseudoclaudication
Onset	Walking	Standing and walking
Character	Cramp, pain	"Paresthetic"
Bilateral symptoms	Yes or no	Yes
Walking distance	Fairly constant	More variable
Relief	Standing still	Sitting down, leaning forward
Cause	Atherosclerosis	Lumbar spinal stenosis

muscular discomfort that occurs with walking and is relieved with rest and standing still. Other disorders may be confused with intermittent claudication, but a careful clinical examination will usually allow for an accurate clinical diagnosis (Table 6.1). With advanced PAD, ischemic rest pain, ischemic ulceration, and/or gangrene may occur (Fig. 6.1).

Noninvasive tests are important in the diagnosis and management of diabetic patients with PAD. Ankle-brachial index (ABI) measurement is an accurate, cost-effective, and frequently used method. Measurement of an ABI can readily be performed using a handheld continuous wave Doppler instrument and standard blood pressure cuff to determine the supine ankle systolic pressure (posterior tibial and dorsalis pedis arteries) and brachial systolic pressure. A ratio of the ankle systolic pressure to the brachial systolic pressure (ABI) provides a measurement of disease severity in patients with PAD: normal, 1.0 to 1.2; mild disease, 0.8 to 0.9, moderate disease, 0.5 to 0.8; severe disease, less than 0.5. Unfortunately,

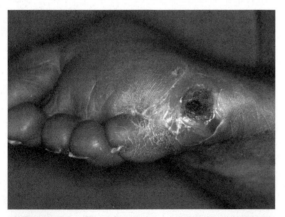

■ **Figure 6.1** Combined neurotrophic and ischemic ulceration beneath the fifth metatarsal head in a patient with diabetes mellitus and peripheral neuropathy. Note the overlying eschar consistent with an ischemic component and the surrounding callus and location over a pressure point of the foot characteristic of a neurotrophic ulcer.

patients with DM often have medial calcification (Mönckeberg's medial sclerosis) involving the infrapopliteal arterial segments, rendering these arteries noncompressible (ankle systolic pressure greater than 300 mm Hg or more than 50 mm Hg higher than brachial systolic pressure).[242] Measurement of an ABI in these patients is unreliable because of the artifactually high ankle systolic pressures. Development of medial calcification is related to the duration of diabetes, presence of hypertension, and hyperlipidemia.[152] Furthermore, medial calcification bears no relationship to the atherosclerosis that frequently involves the same arterial segments.[138] In addition, the pressures in large vessels do not necessarily reflect the adequacy of blood flow to ischemic tissue. In diabetic patients with PAD and noncompressible arteries, measurement of toe systolic pressures and segmental pressures can supply valuable additional information about large artery occlusive disease and small vessel disease.[53] Toe pressure reflects the overall obstruction in the arterial tree proximal to the digits and does not appear to be affected by the arterial noncompressibility.[52, 175] Further noninvasive assessment of PAD severity may also be accomplished by Duplex ultrasonography (combined two-dimensional ultrasound and pulsed-wave Doppler [spectral and color-flow Doppler]) or magnetic resonance angiography (MRA).[27, 51, 124, 174, 212] Duplex ultrasound and MRA both have the ability to noninvasively determine the site and severity of arterial stenosis and are accurate in diagnosing PAD when compared formally with angiography.

Transcutaneous oxygen pressure (tcPO$_2$) measurement is an adjunctive noninvasive method of measuring oxygen tension at the skin surface produced by heat-induced hyperemia. Measurement of tcPO$_2$ has been reported to predict the level at which lower extremity amputations will heal, the survival of skin grafts, and wound healing after peripheral angioplasty[6, 43, 69, 90, 109, 153, 205] Unfortunately, tcPO$_2$ is affected by many variables, including oxygen concentra-

TABLE 6.2 MEDICAL THERAPY FOR INTERMITTENT CLAUDICATION

Aggressive modification of cardiovascular risk factors
Treatment of associated coronary and carotid disease
Discontinue tobacco
Foot care and protection
Reduce weight (if obese)
Walking program
Aspirin
Pentoxifylline

tion in inspired air, lung function, hemoglobin saturation, cardiac output, and local factors such as skin thickness, edema, presence of inflammation and infection, capillary formation and skin oxygen consumption. Despite these limitations, $tcPO_2$ has recently been shown to be more useful than ABI measurements in predicting wound healing in patients undergoing peripheral angioplasty.[109]

Medical management of PAD in diabetic patients is effective and is basic to a good outcome (Table 6.2). Aggressive modification of major cardiovascular risk factors is essential. Discontinuation of tobacco use and aggressive treatment of hypertension, hyperlipidemia, and diabetes are essential components of medical therapy (see previous section). Aspirin (325 mg on alternate days) given to apparently healthy men has been shown to reduce the need for peripheral arterial surgery.[103] Whether aspirin therapy is as effective in diabetic patients with intermittent claudication requires further investigation. Our current practice is to prescribe aspirin therapy to diabetic patients with PAD, unless contraindications to its use exist. Pentoxifylline is the only oral hemorrheologic agent approved by the U.S. Food and Drug Administration for the treatment of patients with intermittent claudication.[47] Pentoxifylline has multiple effects, including reduced red blood cell rigidity and blood viscosity, inhibition of platelet aggregation, and reduced neutrophil granulocyte activation.[150, 186, 203] The most beneficial effect of pentoxifylline on walking distance in patients with intermittent claudication is seen in patients who have had stable intermittent claudication for at least 1 year and an ABI less than 0.8.[139] A regular walking program for patients with intermittent claudication is very effective.[97] The distances walked to onset of pain and to near-maximal pain increase after a program of exercise rehabilitation (walking longer than 30 minutes per session, 3 or more times per week, for greater than 6 months).[97] Foot care and protection are of para-

mount importance in diabetic patients with PAD. The combination of peripheral neuropathy, small vessel disease, and/or PAD in diabetic patients makes foot trauma more likely to be associated with a nonhealing wound or ulcer (Fig. 6.2).

In diabetic patients with intermittent claudication, angiography followed by endovascular or surgical revascularization is generally indicated because the risk of limb loss without restoration of pulsatile flow is increased and revascularization may permit a lower level of amputation.

Percutaneous transluminal angioplasty (PTA) and stenting are well documented as beneficial techniques in the treatment of iliac, femoral, and popliteal PAD.[116, 221] Percutaneous transluminal angioplasty of infrapopliteal PAD has been reported to open the majority of occluded tibioperoneal arteries (65%) and salvage the majority of limbs in diabetic patients who would otherwise have undergone amputation.[72, 109]

Peripheral arterial bypass surgery using autologous saphenous vein grafts (in situ and reversed) is effective in diabetic patients with infrapopliteal PAD. Surgical bypasses to the infrapopliteal arteries with autologous vein are commonly used for limb salvage in diabetic patients with critical limb ischemia (ischemic rest pain, ulceration, gangrene).[5, 228] The overall 5-year patency rate for autologous vein grafts (in situ and reversed) to tibial arteries is approaching 70%, with rates of limb salvage exceeding 75% at 3 years.[34, 215, 229] Over time, the distal limits of revascularization have been extended to include the pedal arteries below the ankle joint.[5, 16] Primary graft patency rates for bypasses below the ankle joint at 1 and 2 years

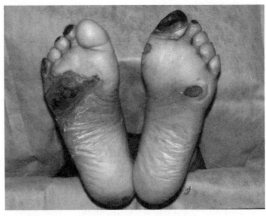

■ **Figure 6.2** Multiple areas of gangrene developed in this patient with diabetes mellitus after wearing a new pair of cowboy boots for one day.

TABLE 6.3 MAJOR CATEGORIES OF CAUSES FOR ISCHEMIC CEREBROVASCULAR DISEASE

Ischemia Source	Entity
Cardiac	Venous source with right-to-left shunt Intracardiac thrombus: atrial fibrillation, recent myocardial infarction, dilated cardiomyopathy Cardiac mass lesions: atrial myxoma Valve disease: prosthetic valve, infective endocarditis, rheumatic heart disease, calcified mitral annulus, nonbacterial thrombotic endocarditis, calcific aortic stenosis
Large vessel disease Aortic arch, carotid arteries, vertebral arteries, basilar artery, major intracranial branches	Atherosclerosis Dissection, fibromuscular dysplasia Infection Inflammatory: Takayasu's disease Other: homocystinuria, moyamoya disease, Fabry's disease
Small vessel disease	Atherosclerosis, hypertension Infections Noninfectious arteritis: connective tissue disorders, isolated central nervous system angiitis, illicit drug Migraine, hypertensive encephalopathy Other: neoplastic, MELAS (mitochondrial myopathy, encephalopathy, lactic acidosis, stroke-like episodes)
Hematologic	Major blood cell constituents: polycythemia, thrombocytosis, leukemia Thrombotic thrombocytopenic purpura, sickle cell disease and other hemoglobinopathies, disseminated intravascular coagulation Coagulation factor abnormalities Phospholipid antibody syndromes: lupus anticoagulant positivity, anticardiolipin antibodies Paraproteinemias, cryoglobulinemia
Other	Embolic syndromes: air emboli, fat emboli Cortical vein thrombosis Global hypoperfusion

are approximately 70%, with the limb salvage rates approaching 80% at 2 years.[5, 16] These techniques offer an obvious advantage to a major amputation.

Conclusion

Cardiovascular disease in the diabetic patient is prevalent and is associated with accelerated atherosclerotic disease in multiple large arteries throughout the body (cerebral, cardiac, peripheral arterial). Morbidity and mortality from cardiovascular disease is increased in patients with DM. A successful patient outcome requires a comprehensive approach and aggressive management of arterial occlusive disease that occurs in multiple organ systems and the extremities.

CEREBROVASCULAR DISEASE

Secondary complications of diabetes are important causes of morbidity and mortality.[29, 62]

In addition to microvascular complications (such as retinopathy and nephropathy) and cardiovascular disorders (such as CAD and peripheral vascular disease), cerebrovascular complications can also occur with increased occurrence among patients with types 1 and 2 DM. In addition to increased frequency, presence of diabetes also impacts on the morbidity or mortality of these disorders and the safety and efficacy of potential treatments.

Pathology

The cerebrovascular complications of diabetes are typically considered to be macrovascular in nature. The pathology of stroke, including cerebral infarction and intracranial hemorrhage, is not different in diabetic patients compared to those without diabetes.[12, 20, 30] Autopsy studies demonstrate the increased occurrence of cerebral infarction and the lower frequency of intracerebral hemorrhage.

Pathogenesis

The mechanisms causing ischemic cerebrovascular disease among diabetics are similar to those for all patients with cerebrovascular ischemia (Table 6.3) from most proximal to distal in the vascular system. The first category of disorders causing cerebrovascular infarction, transient ischemic attack (TIA), global anoxia, or syncope is cardiac disorders. Heart disease may produce cerebral ischemic symptoms by numerous mechanisms, including pump failure, causing generalized cerebral ischemia or infarction; or thromboembolism, causing focal cerebral ischemic events such as TIA and cerebral infarction.

In general, embolic events of cardiac origin are caused either from shunting of systemic venous thrombi into the arterial circulation (paradoxical embolism); intracardiac thrombi caused by dysfunction of either the ventricle, atrium, or presence of a mass lesion; or valvular heart disease. Because recent MI is a proved cardiac risk factor (Table 6.4), the increased incidence of MI in diabetics contributes to the increased occurrence of stroke. It is also important to note that silent MI may also be an important contributor to the occurrence of stroke.[100] Other cardiac lesions associated with an increased cardiac risk for cerebrovascular ischemia include dilated cardiomyopathy, which predisposes to production of intracardiac thrombi from local stagnation and also can produce arrhythmias.[243]

Global hypoperfusion may cause "border zone" ischemic infarctions, typically between the anterior and middle posterior cerebral arteries. In addition to hypotension, typically ip-silateral or bilateral arterial stenotic lesions are also present.[217] Other proven cardiac risk factors for stroke include atrial fibrillation,[38, 56, 134, 177, 213] mechanical valve,[208] and intracardiac mass. Less well-proven cardiac risks that also must be considered include sick sinus syndrome,[83] patent foramen ovale,[126, 135, 226] atherosclerotic debris in the thoracic aorta,[13, 179] hypokinetic or akinetic left ventricular segment,[71] and calcification of the mitral annulus.[32] Because of the increased occurrence of atherosclerosis in diabetics, atherosclerotic debris in the thoracic aorta may be of increased occurrence in diabetics.

Valvular lesions causing cerebral emboli include rheumatic heart disease, calcific aortic stenosis, and mitral annulus calcification. Prosthetic heart valves are also associated with an increased occurrence. Cardiac operation of all types is associated with an increased risk of cerebral ischemia, a particularly important consideration given the increased occurrence of CAD in diabetics. Infective endocarditis or nonbacterial thrombotic endocarditis are also associated with cerebral ischemic events.

The next most distal site causative for cerebral ischemic disease includes large-vessel inclusive disease. Because of the increased occurrence of atherosclerosis in diabetics, this is the most important cause of cerebral infarction in diabetics. Atherosclerosis may cause the symptoms through hemodynamic or thromboembolic mechanism. The hemodynamic compromise typically occurs when collateral circulation distal to a hemodynamically significant (>75% luminal area) becomes insufficient.

Thromboembolism is another mechanism in which atherosclerosis causes cerebral ischemic symptoms. The atherothrombotic material may be the source of emboli or cause similar hemodynamic factors because of stenosis or occlusion of the lumen. In diabetic individuals, the large-vessel occlusive disease occurs at a younger age of the population. There is little evidence that diabetes has a markedly different involvement when comparing intracranial and extracranial occlusive disease. Although this difference has been noted in African-Americans and Asians, with more intracranial occlusive disease noted, the increased incidence of diabetes in these ethnic groups did not explain the distribution.[105] Other large-vessel occlusive diseases such as fibromuscular dysplasia and carotid artery dissection may be noted but are not of markedly increased occurrence in diabetics.

Small-vessel occlusive disease is the next le-

TABLE 6.4 CARDIAC RISK FACTORS FOR CEREBRAL ISCHEMIA

Proven risk factors
  Atrial fibrillation
  Mechanical valve
  Dilated cardiomyopathy
  Recent myocardial infarction
  Intracardiac thrombus
  Intracardiac mass
Putative risk factors
  Sick sinus syndrome
  Patent foramen ovale
  Thoracic aorta atherosclerosis debris
  Spontaneous echo contrast
  Previous myocardial infarction, 2 to 6 months after
    event
  Hypokinetic/akinetic left ventricular segment
  Mitral annulus calcification

sion encountered as one progresses from proximal to distal through the arterial system. Hypertension is the most important risk factor for small-vessel arterial occlusive disease.[61] Because hypertension is markedly more common in diabetic patients, this significantly contributes to an increased frequency and severity of small-vessel occlusive disease in diabetics. Diabetes in the absence of hypertension also contributes to the increased occurrence of small-vessel occlusive disease, but the risk is lower. The typical arterial occlusive lesions (including fibrinoid necrosis, lipohyalinosis, and microaneurysms) are found typically in small arteries in the basal ganglia, thalamus, pons, cerebellum, and cortical regions. Because the perforating arteries have poor collateral circulation, blood flow obstruction leads to infarction in the limited distribution of the perforating arteries, leading to a lacunar infarct. These small (<1.5 cm in greatest diameter) infarcts cause 10 to 15% of all ischemic strokes. Higher systolic blood pressure is noted in diabetic patients compared to other age-matched patients.[18, 24, 76, 94] However, diabetes may also be an independent risk factor for lacunar infarction syndromes,[59, 241] although this has not been noted in some studies.[36, 194]

Other causes of small-vessel disease include infectious arteritis and noninfectious arteritis, but they do not have increased occurrence in diabetics.

Hematologic abnormalities of numerous types may contribute increased cerebral infarction occurrence in diabetics. Abnormalities in blood cell factors and other factors may be important. Diabetics may have higher hematocrits than do nondiabetic patients.[141] Hyperviscosity of the blood, with elevated fibrinogen, factor V, and factor VII, has also been noted.[23, 156] Increased platelet aggregation, altered red blood cell deformability, and reduced fibrinolysis in diabetics may contribute to the increased stroke risk.[23, 156]

Epidemiology

Although it is not the most important risk factor for stroke, diabetes is clearly an important independent ischemic stroke risk factor.[1, 37, 39, 42, 93, 127, 128, 131, 133, 181, 183, 189, 193, 207, 219, 245] The overall impact of diabetes as a cause of stroke is somewhat controversial and may be dependent on age and gender.[29] In one large study of males of Japanese ancestry, diabetes was noted to be an independent stroke risk factor, with a relative risk of ischemic stroke of 2.0.[1] In the same study, the risk of stroke was markedly increased for those with glucosuria compared with those without, and for those with a serum glucose value at the 80th percentile compared with the 20th percentile. In a Danish study, it was noted that the risk of stroke in diabetes was highest in the younger age groups, diminishing with age, which indicates a strong interaction of diabetes with age.[39] It is apparent that diabetes is an important risk factor for cerebral ischemia in both men and woman, although the Framingham Study[131] indicates that it may be a more important risk factor for stroke in women. In addition to the direct effect of diabetes in acceleration of atherosclerosis, diabetic autonomic neuropathy as an independent predictor of stroke has also been reported.[218]

It is apparent that hypertension is a striking risk factor for cerebral infarction. It has been debated whether diabetes is an independent risk factor apart from hypertension. In a Rochester, Minnesota, study of stroke risk factors, diabetes was an independent risk factor for first ischemic stroke after adjustment for hypertension.[67] Similar findings were noted in an Eastern Finland study, which identified diabetes as an independent risk factor.[181, 197] Cohort studies have also demonstrated that diabetes is an independent risk factor for ischemic stroke.[24, 181]

There are no data that define an increased risk of hemorrhagic stroke in diabetes.[1, 8, 42] In the Copenhagen Stroke Study, intracerebral hemorrhage was less frequent among diabetic patients.[127] The Cooperative Aneurysm Study demonstrated an inverse correlation of diabetes with subarachnoid.[8]

In addition to diabetes, one must also consider other important lifestyle factors that contribute to increased occurrence of cerebral infarction. Cigarette smoking and its effect on cerebral infarction has been demonstrated in numerous case-control and cohort studies.[2, 99, 236] Cigarette smoking also increases the risk of intracerebral hemorrhage. Alcohol use is more complicated; low to moderate use slightly decreases the risk of stroke compared with no alcohol use, but high levels of alcohol use markedly increase the risk of stroke.[46]

Hyperlipidemia is also an important issue in diabetes because the risk is elevated in diabetics. Levels of cholesterol have been more problematic in defining their potential as a risk factor for stroke. Although cholesterol is a risk factor, it appears to play a lesser role in women than in men.[122] Low levels of cholesterol were associated with a higher occurrence of subarachnoid and intracerebral hemorrhage.[122] This peculiar association was only noted in hypertensive males. In other studies, only very high levels of total cholesterol were associated with an increased risk of cerebral infarction.[39]

Stroke Severity and Mortality

In addition to increased stroke occurrence, hyperglycemia may also increase cerebral infarction size[35] and worsen the outcome. Studies have demonstrated that among diabetic patients, in-hospital and overall mortality[127, 128, 183, 207, 219] is increased after cerebral infarction.[141] However, in another study evaluating the use of naloxone in acute cerebral ischemia, the volume of infarction as seen on computed tomogram and outcome were related to neurologic deficit at admission but were not related to a history of diabetes or hyperglycemia.[7, 20, 35] Others have demonstrated that the outcome of cerebral infarction may be worse among patients with glucose values greater than 118.8 mg/dL (6.6 mmol/L).[181]

Although glucose levels at high levels increase anaerobic metabolism, which leads to cellular acidosis by raising lactic acid production, factors such as worsening cerebral edema also lead to poorer outcome after stroke.[35]

Reactive hyperglycemia after cerebral infarction may also portend a poorer prognosis.[48, 158] This stress response may be due to elevated catecholamine output.[85] The most important impact of this reactive hyperglycemia appears to be in nondiabetics.[48, 158] Another study showed that hyperglycemia combined with normal glycosylated hemoglobin may predict poorer prognosis after stroke.[65]

Clinical Syndromes

ASYMPTOMATIC CAROTID OCCLUSIVE DISEASE

The prevalence of asymptomatic carotid bruit is approximately 13% on a population basis and does increase with age.[198] In the Framingham Study, the occurrence of carotid bruit was 3.5% among those 44 to 54 years, compared with 7.0% in the 65- to 79-year-old group. The frequency of bruit detection was higher among diabetics and in those with hypertension.[234] Others have also demonstrated an increased occurrence with age and diabetics.[232] Although a bruit may indicate an underlying stenosis, a carotid bruit is merely a reflection of turbulence in the artery and is not an excellent predictor of underlying carotid stenosis in asymptomatic patients. Patients with asymptomatic carotid bruits are at greater risk than the general population for experiencing cerebral ischemic events[231, 234] and have a higher mortality.[234]

Carotid bruit is an important marker for widespread vascular occlusive disease, and it is particularly important as a predictor for the presence of CAD. In addition, the stroke rate is dependent on the degree of stenosis, with one study demonstrating a 1.3% per year risk of TIA and stroke if the carotid artery stenosis is less or equal to 75% compared with 10.5% for those with stenosis greater than 75%.[58, 169] Still others have shown that individuals with a hemodynamically significant stenosis as reflected by an abnormal oculoplethysmography (OPG) have an annual stroke rate over 3 years of 3.4% compared with 1.5% in those with normal OPG and 0.5% in normal age- and sex-matched population.[157]

The most appropriate management for patients with asymptomatic carotid artery occlusive disease is somewhat controversial. The Asymptomatic Carotid Atherosclerosis Study compared carotid endarterectomy medical management (aspirin and reduction of risk factors) in relatively healthy individuals. During 5 years after entry into the study, the risk of any stroke or death within 30 days postoperatively or any ipsilateral stroke or death after 30 days was 5.1% for surgical patients and 11% for medically treated patients.[80] The important issue was that the absolute risk reduction was very low; furthermore, the resultant 66% relative risk reduction in men was statistically significant, but the reduction of 17% was not statistically significant in women.

Even among asymptomatic patients, one must consider potential predictors of stroke in major surgical procedures. For CABG, diabetic patients appear to be at increased risk. Diabetes has been demonstrated to be an independent risk factor for stroke after CABG.[182] Another study showed that aortic calcification, mural thrombi, and diabetes predicted postoperative permanent neurologic deficits.[143] The etiology for the stroke events after CABG is multifactorial. The increased likelihood of large-vessel atherosclerosis in diabetic patients contributes to the occurrence of stroke, with higher occurrence of embolic aortic debris of carotid occlusive disease leading to watershed-type cerebral infarcts.

TRANSIENT ISCHEMIC ATTACKS/CEREBRAL INFARCTION

A TIA is defined as an episode of focal loss and brain function attributed to cerebral ischemia lasting less than 24 hours, localized to a limited region of the brain.[166] In general, only 40% of thrombotic strokes are preceded by a TIA. Although TIAs occur more frequently than expected in patients with diabetes,[178] diabetics more commonly have cerebral infarction without a preceding TIA compared with nondiabetics.[73] Among patients with TIA not dying for another reason within the 5 years after a TIA, 33% will have a stroke, with 20% occurring within the first month and 50% within the first year after TIA.[118]

Patients with diabetes have reduced survival after TIA. In one analysis of 451 patients with TIA, diabetes was an independent predictor of reduced survival. Other independent predictors included increasing age, cigarette smoking, previous contralateral cerebral infarction, carotid distribution symptoms, and presence of ischemic heart disease.[118] The reasons for this reduced survival is consistent with the diffuse nature of atherosclerotic occlusive disease. Supporting this are data indicating that TIA is associated with an increased occurrence of morbidity and mortality from ischemic heart disease.[54, 160]

When a patient is seen with a TIA or cerebral infarction, it is useful to decide whether the cerebral event is related to cardiac, large vessel, small vessel, or hematologic disease. In a given patient, it may be difficult to ascertain whether an ischemic event is because of embolus or thrombosis, although there may be some clinical features which would favor embolus: homonymous hemianopsia without motor or sensory dysfunction, inferior middle cerebral artery division ischemia, rapidly resolving severe deficit of abrupt onset, top of the basilar syndrome, posterior inferior cerebellar artery events, and spontaneous hemorrhagic transformation. One must also consider the potential for an infarction in a smaller vessel distribution leading to a lacunar infarct. In general, these events present with certain stroke syndromes, including pure motor stroke, pure sensory stroke, clumsy-hand dysarthria syndrome, sensorimotor stroke, and ataxic-hemiparesis. Because the risk of lacunar infarction is likely to be higher in patients without diabetes, it is particularly important to be aware of these clinical syndromes.[95]

In essentially all patients with cerebral vascular disease (such as TIA or cerebral infarction), the initial evaluation includes a computed tomographic (CT) examination of the head performed without contrast. This provides a noninvasive method of differentiating nonhemorrhagic and hemorrhagic cerebral vascular disease. In addition, patients with symptoms clinically suggestive of TIA often demonstrate cerebral infarction on CT imaging.[160] Other baseline studies should be performed, including a complete blood count, prothrombin time, activated partial thromboplastin, serum chemistry group, erythrocyte sedimentation rate, and comprehensive lipid analysis. In most patients, urinalysis, chest radiography, and electrocardiogram are also required.

Although magnetic resonance imaging (MRI) is better than CT scanning in defining early infarction and in evaluating the posterior fossa, MRI has some difficulty in defining early hemorrhage.

The additional evaluation is based on the symptoms at the presentation. In patients with clinical symptoms suggesting ischemia of the anterior (carotid) circulation (Table 6.5), the first step is aggressive evaluation of the extracranial carotid system, particularly in light of the increased occurrence of extracranial atherosclerosis in patients with diabetes.

Carotid ultrasonography is a very sensitive means for estimating the degree of extracranial carotid stenosis, with an overall accuracy of greater than 90%.[209] Oculoplethysmography is also accurate in predicting the presence of a hemodynamically significant stenosis. Magnetic resonance angiography can noninvasively visualize the extracranial and intracranial arterial and venous circulations.[188] Advantages over standard arteriography include imaging without administration of contrast medium and elimination of the risks associated with arterial puncture. However, some problems

TABLE 6.5 CLINICAL SYMPTOMS WITH ISCHEMIA OF ANTERIOR (CAROTID) CIRCULATION

Motor dysfunction of contralateral extremities and/or face
  Clumsiness
  Weakness
  Paralysis
  Slurred speech
Visual loss in ipsilateral eye
Contralateral homonymous hemianopia or quadrantanopia
Dominant hemisphere: Language deficit, may include problem with expressive speech, comprehension, calculation, reading, naming, or writing
Nondominant hemisphere: Visuospatial deficit, inattention, denial of deficit, or hemineglect
Sensory deficit of contralateral extremities and/or face
  Numbness or loss of sensation
  Paresthesias

with the technique include difficulty in distinguishing between high-grade vessel stenosis and occlusion and low sensitivity for detecting intimal irregularities; it may overestimate the degree of stenosis.

In most cases, if the presence of a high-grade carotid stenosis in a vessel appropriate for the distribution of the TIA or stroke is detected, then a patient's surgical candidacy must be considered. The need for cerebral arteriography before surgery is controversial. Because cerebral angiography is associated with a risk of stroke of approximately 1%,[84] the surgeon may consider operating based on the ultrasound or MRA. However, the largest surgical trials addressing a potential efficacy of carotid endarterectomy for symptomatic carotid occlusive disease evaluated levels of atherosclerosis using angiographic determinant.[78, 154, 170]

Carotid endarterectomy has been determined to be an efficacious treatment for patients with TIA or minor cerebral infarction when associated with an extracranial internal carotid stenosis of greater than 70%.[170] In patients who are not surgical candidates, anticoagulation with warfarin is typically considered in those with a high-grade extracranial internal carotid artery stenosis.[49]

If noninvasive arterial evaluation fails to demonstrate a significant stenosis or other cause in the extracranial site, transesophageal echocardiogram is performed to evaluate for a more proximal source. This is particularly true in light of increasing evidence indicating the association of aortic arch atherosclerotic debris and cerebral infarction.[13, 179] Likewise, if the transesophageal is also negative, evaluation of the distal intracranial circulation with MRA or transcranial Doppler[50] is used. If all of these studies fail to demonstrate a clear cause in patients with a single event, treatment with aspirin is usually used.

Although the most appropriate dose of aspirin is unclear, 325 mg of aspirin is typically used.[17, 75] Ticlopidine hydrochloride, an antiplatelet agent acting in a pharmacologically dissimilar fashion from aspirin, is used in individuals who are aspirin intolerant or allergic, those with recurrent spells on aspirin therapy who do not have an event more appropriately treated with warfarin, or those with gastric ulcer disease precluding aspirin use. There is some evidence that ticlopidine may be more efficacious in women and in those with vertebral basilar distribution ischemia.[14, 98, 112] In patients on ticlopidine, monitoring of blood

TABLE 6.6 CLINICAL SYMPTOMS WITH ISCHEMIA OF POSTERIOR (VERTEBROBASILAR) CIRCULATION

Motor dysfunction of any combination of extremities and/or face (bilateral or alternating symptoms suggest the posterior circulation; other brain stem symptoms* are often associated).
  Clumsiness
  Paralysis
  Ataxia
Loss of vision of one or both homonymous visual fields. Bilateral visual field deficit suggests posterior circulation involvement.
Sensory deficit of extremities and/or face (bilateral or alternating symptoms suggest the posterior circulation; other brain stem symptoms* are often associated).
  Numbness or loss of sensation
  Paresthesias

*The following typically occur but are not diagnostic if occurring in isolation: ataxic gait, ataxic extremities, vertigo, diplopia, dysphagia, dysarthria.

counts biweekly for the first 3 months is needed because of the risk of neutropenia.

Patients with posterior circulation distribution ischemia (Table 6.6) are usually evaluated with MRA[188] or transcranial Doppler.[50] Transcranial Doppler is about 75% sensitive for detecting hemodynamically significant stenosis in the distal intracranial segments of the vertebral arteries or in the basilar artery. If transcranial Doppler or MRA suggests the presence of a stenosis, therapeutic options include empiric uses of warfarin; arteriography is considered in selected patients. Although warfarin use for symptomatic intracranial arterial stenosis is somewhat controversial, warfarin is usually used in this setting.[49, 60] The duration of warfarin used in this circumstance is poorly defined. However, at least short-term anticoagulation is used if a stenosis is detected in the vertebral or basilar artery. Further cardiac imaging with transesophageal echocardiography is typically used if the MRA is negative. Treatment is then based on the transesophageal echocardiogram findings. Again, if the transesophageal echocardiogram is negative, one may consider initial therapy with aspirin or with ticlopidine.

In all subgroups of patients with TIA and cerebral ischemia, if the noninvasive evaluation is negative, then other studies may be needed, including Holter monitoring.[64] Particularly in younger patients, evaluation for hypercoagulable state with comprehensive hematologic studies is required. In selected patients, even if the noninvasive studies and transesophageal echocardiogram are negative, further evaluation with arteriography to define the presence of intracranial atherosclerosis or very proximal extracranial stenosis may also be needed. This is also important in light of the increased occurrence of atherosclerosis in patients with diabetes.

Surgical Management of Cerebrovascular Disease

In selected patients with symptomatic carotid stenosis, carotid endarterectomy is considered. The North American Symptomatic Carotid Endarterectomy trial (NASCET) demonstrated that surgery was efficacious compared to medical management with aspirin in patients with high-grade (>70% defined on arteriogram) symptomatic carotid stenosis.[170] There is some evidence that the risk of early complications after carotid endarterectomy is higher in diabetics.[196]

In addition to appropriate medical or surgical management, aggressive management of atherosclerosis risk factors is imperative. This includes treatment of high blood pressure if present, hyperlipidemia, diabetes, and cigarette smoking cessation.[9, 136, 235] In addition, appropriate levels of exercise and weight reduction in obese patients are important.

Conclusion

Diabetes in an important and independent risk factor for cerebral vascular occlusive disease. Although other important risk factors such as hypertension may be more powerful predictors, diabetes leads to premature and more rapidly progressive atherosclerosis. In addition, the mortality after cerebral infarction is higher in diabetic patients. It is important for the clinician to aggressively manage diabetes[237] to potentially reduce the risk of stroke and to reduce the size of cerebral infarction. Diabetes also has implications on the safety and efficacy of some treatments and interventions such as carotid endarterectomy. Future studies will continue to evaluate the usefulness of aggressive diabetes therapy for reducing the risk of stroke, of importance to diabetics in the setting of acute stroke.

References

1. Abbott RD, Dunahue RP, MacMahon SW, et al. Diabetes and the risk of stroke. The Honolulu Heart Program. JAMA 1987; 257:949–952.
2. Abbott RD, Yn Y, Reed DM, et al. Risk of stroke in male cigarette smokers. N Engl J Med 1986; 315:717–720.
3. Abbott RD, Donahue RP, Kannel WB, et al. The impact of diabetes on survival following myocardial infarction in men vs women: The Framingham Study. JAMA 1988; 260:3456.
4. ACC/AHA Guidelines for the Management of Patients With Acute Myocardial Infarction: A report of the American College of Cardiology/American Heart Association Task Force on Practice Guidelines. J Am Coll Cardiol 1996; 28:1328.
5. Acer E, Veith FJ, Gupta SK. Bypasses to plantar arteries and other tibial branches: An extended approach to limb salvage. J Vasc Surg 1988; 8:1434.
6. Achaver BM, Kirby SB, Litke DL. Transcutaneous PO2 in flaps: A new method of survival prediction. Plast Reconstr Surg 1980; 65:738–741.
7. Adams H, Olinger C, Marler J, et al. Comparison of admission serum glucose concentration with neurologic outcome in acute cerebral infarction. Stroke 1988; 19:455–458.
8. Adams JP Jr, Putnam SF Kassel NF, et al. Prevalence of diabetes mellitus among patients with subarachnoid hemorrhage. Arch Neurol 1987; 41:1033–1035.
9. Agewall S, Wikstrand J, Samuelsson O, et al. The efficacy of multiple risk factor intervention in treated hypertensive men during long-term follow-up. J Intern Med 1994; 236:651–659.
10. Akasaka T, Yoshida K, Hozumi T, et al. Retinopathy identifies marked restriction of coronary flow reserve in patients with diabetes mellitus. J Am Coll Cardiol 1997; 935–941.
11. Alderman EL, Fisher LD, Litwin P, et al. Results of coronary artery surgery in patients with poor left ventricular function (CASS). Circulation 1983; 68:785–795.
12. Alex M, Baron E, Goldbert S, et al. An autopsy study of cerebrovascular accidents in diabetes mellitus. Circulation 1962; 25:663–673.
13. Amarenco P, Duyckaerts C, Tzourio C, et al. The prevalence of ulcerated plaques in the aortic arch in patients with stroke. N Engl J Med 1992; 326:221–225.
14. Ambepityia G, Lopelman PG, Omgra D. Exertional myocardial ischemia in diabetes: A quantitative analysis of anginal perceptual threshold and the influence of autonomic function. J Am Coll Cardiol 1990; 15:72.
15. Andersson B, Waagstein F. Spectrum and outcome of congestive heart failure in a hospitalized population. Am Heart J 1993; 126:632–640.
16. Andros G, Harris RW, Salles-Cunha SX, et al. Bypass grafts to the ankle and foot. J Vasc Surg 1988; 7:785.
17. Antiplatelet Trialists' Collaboration. Collaborative overview of randomised trials of antiplatelet therapy. I. Prevention of death, myocardial infarction, and stroke by prolonged antiplately therapy in various categories of patients. BMJ 1994; 308:81–106.
18. Arauz-Pacheco C, Raskin P. Hypertension in diabetes mellitus. Endocrinol Metab Clin North Am 1996; 25:401–423.
19. Aronson D, Bloomgarden Z, Rayfield EJ. Potential mechanisms promoting restenosis in diabetic patients. J Am Coll Cardiol 1996; 27:528–535.
20. Asplund K, Hagg F, Helmers C, et al. The natural history of stroke in diabetic patients. Acta Med Scand 1980; 207:417–424.
21. Barbash GI, White HD, Modan M, et al, and the Investigators of the International Tissue Plasminogen/Streptokinase Mortality Trial: Significance of diabetes mellitus in patients with acute myocardial in-

farction receiving thrombolytic agents. J Am Coll Cardiol 1993; 22:707–713.

22. BARI Investigators. Influence of diabetes on 5-year mortality and morbidity in a randomized trial comparing CABG and PTCA in patients with multivessel disease. Circulation 1997; 96:1761–1769.

23. Barnes AJ, Locke P, Scudder PR, et al. Is hyperviscosity a treatable component of diabetic microcirculatory disease? Lancet 1977; 2:789–791.

24. Barrett-Connor E, Khaw KT. Diabetes mellitus: An independent risk factor for stroke? Am J Epidemiol 1988:128:116–123.

25. Bart BA, Shaw LK, McCants CB Jr, et al. Clinical determinants of mortality in patients with angiographically diagnosed ischemic or nonischemic cardiomyopathy. J Am Coll Cardiol 1997; 30:1002–1008.

26. Barzilay JI, Krommal RA, Bittner V, et al. Coronary artery disease and coronary artery bypass grafting in diabetic subjects aged >65 years (report from the Coronary Artery Surgery Study [CASS] registry). Am J Cardiol 1994; 74:334–339.

27. Baum RA, Rutter CM, Sunshine JH, et al. Multicenter trial to evaluate vascular magnetic resonance angiography of the lower extremity. JAMA 1995; 274:875–880.

28. Beach KW, Brunzell JD, Conquest LL, et al. The correlation of arteriosclerosis obliterans with lipoproteins in insulin-dependent and noninsulin-dependent diabetes. Diabetes 1979; 28:836–840.

29. Bell D. Stroke in the diabetic patient. Diabetes Care 1994; 17:213–219.

30. Bell ET. A postmortem study of vascular disease in diabetics. Arch Pathol 1952; 53:444–455.

31. Bellavance A for the Ticlopidine Aspirin Stroke Study Group. Efficacy of Ticlopidine and aspirin for prevention of reversible cerebrovascular ischemic events: The Ticlopidine Aspirin Stroke Study. Stroke 1993; 24:1452–457.

32. Benjamin EJ, Plehn JF, D'Agostino RB, et al. Mitral annular calcification and the risk of stroke in an elderly cohort. N Engl J Med 1992; 327:374–379.

33. Bennet T, Hosking DJ, Hampton JR. Cardiovascular control in diabetes mellitus. Br Med J 1975; 2:585.

34. Bergamini TM, Towne JB, Bandyk DF, et al. Experience with in situ saphenous vein bypasses during 1981 to 1989: Determinant factors of long-term patency. J Vasc Surg 1991; 13:137.

35. Berger L, Hakim AM. The association of hyperglycemia with cerebral edema in stroke. Stroke 1986; 17:865–871.

36. Bogousslavsky J, Castillo V, Kumral E, et al. Stroke subtypes and hypertension: Primary hemorrhage vs infarction, large- vs small-artery disease. Arch Neurol 1996; 53:265–269.

37. Bornstein NM, Aronovich BD, Karepov VG, et al. The Tel Aviv Stroke Registry: 3600 consecutive patients. Stroke 1996; 27:1770–1773.

38. Boston Area Anticoagulation Trial for Atrial Fibrillation Investigators. The effect of low-dose warfarin on the risk of stroke in patients with non-rheumatic atrial fibrillation. N Engl J Med 1990; 323:1505–1511.

39. Boysen G, Nyboe J, Appleyard M, et al. Stroke incidence and risk factors for stroke in Copenhagen, Denmark. Stroke 1988; 19:1345–1353.

40. Bradley AJ, Alpert JS. Coronary flow reserve. Am Heart J 1991; 122:1116–1128.

41. Brownlee M. Glycation and diabetic complications. Diabetes 1994; 43:836–841.

42. Burchfiel CM, Curb JD, Rodriguez BL, et al. Glucose intolerance and 22-year stroke incidence: The Honolulu Heart Program. Stroke 1994; 25:951–957.

43. Burgess EM, Masten FA, Wyss CR, et al. Segmental transcutaneous measurements of PO2 in patients requiring below-the-knee amputation for peripheral vascular insufficiency. J Bone Joint Surg 1982; 64:378–382.

44. Bypass Angioplasty Revascularization Investigation (BARI) Investigators: Comparison of coronary bypass surgery with angioplasty in patients with multivessel disease. N Engl J Med 1996; 335:217–225.

45. Cagliero R, Roth T, Roy S, et al. Characteristics and mechanisms of high-glucose-induced over-expression of basement membrane components in cultured human endothelial cells. Diabetes 1991; 40:102–110.

46. Camargo CA Jr. Moderate alcohol consumption and stroke: The epidemiologic evidence. Stroke 1989; 20:1611–1626.

47. Cameron H, Walker P, Ramsay L. Drug treatment of intermittent claudication: A critical analysis of the methods and findings of published clinical trials, 1965–1985. Br J Clin Pharmacol 1988; 26:569.

48. Candelise L, Landi G, Orazio EN, et al. Prognostic significance of hyperglycemia in acute stroke. Arch Neurol 1985; 42:661–663.

49. Caplan LR. Anticoagulation for cerebral ischemia. Clin Neuropharmacol 1986; 9:399–414.

50. Caplan LR, Brass LM, DeWitt LD, et al. Transcranial Doppler ultrasound: Present status. Neurology 1990; 40:696–700.

51. Caputa MR, Masui T, Gooding GA, et al. Popliteal and tibioperoneal arteries: Feasibility of two-dimensional time-of-flight MR angiography and phase velocity mapping. Radiology 1992; 182:387–392.

52. Carter SA, Lezack JD. Digital systolic pressures in the lower limb in arterial disease. Circulation 1971; 43:905–914.

53. Carter SA, Tate RB. Value of toe pulse waves in addition to systolic pressures in the assessment of the severity of peripheral arterial disease and critical limb ischemia. J Vasc Surg 1996; 24:258–265.

54. Cartlidge NEF, Whisnant JP, Elveback LR. Carotid and vertebral-basilar transient cerebral ischemic attacks: A community study, Rochester, Minnesota. Mayo Clin Proc 1977; 52:117–120.

55. Centers for Disease Control. National Diabetes Fact Sheet: National Estimates and General Information on Diabetes in the United States. Atlanta, U.S. Department of Health and Human Services, 1997.

56. Cerebral Embolism Task Force. Cardiogenic brain embolism. Arch Neurol 1986; 43:71–84.

57. Ceremuzynski L. Hormonal and metabolic reactions evoked by acute myocardial infarction. Circ Res 1981; 48:767.

58. Chambers BR, Norris JW. Outcome in patients with asymptomatic neck bruits. N Engl J Med 1986; 315:860–865.

59. Chamorro A, Sacco RL, Mohr JP, et al. Clinical-computed tomographic correlations of lacunar infarction in the stroke data bank. Stroke 1991; 22:175–181.

60. Chimowitz MI, Kokkinos J, Strong J, et al. The warfarin-aspirin symptomatic intracranial disease study. Neurology 1995; 45:1488–1493.

61. Christlieb AR. The hypertension of diabetes. Diabetes Care 1982; 5:50–58.

62. Chukwuma C, Tuomilehto J. Diabetes and the risk of stroke. J Diabetes Complications 1993; 4:250–262.

63. Chun BY, Dobson AJ, Heller RF. The impact of diabetes on survival among patients with first myocardial infarction. Diabetes Care 1997; 20:704–708.

64. Come PC, Riley MF, Bivas NK. Roles of echocardiography and arrhythmia monitoring in evaluation of patients with suspected systemic embolism. Ann Neurol 1983; 13:527–531.

65. Cox NH, Lorains JW. The prognostic value of blood glucose and glycosylated haemoglobin estimation in patients with stroke. Postgrad Med J 1986; 62:7–10.

66. Curb JD, Pressel SL, Cutler JA, et al. Diuretics reduced cardiovascular disease events in diabetic and nondiabetic patients. JAMA 1996; 276:1886–1892.

67. Davis PH, Dambrosia JM, Schoenberg BS, et al. Risk factors for ischemic stroke: A prospective study in Rochester, Minnesota. Ann Neurol 1987; 22:319–327.

68. DeFronzo RA. Insulin resistance, hyperinsulinemia, and coronary artery disease: A complex metabolic web. Coron Artery Dis 1992; 3:11–25.

69. Devehat LE, Khodabandehlou T. Transcutaneous oxygen pressure and hemorheology in diabetes mellitus. Int Angiol 1990; 9:259–262.

70. Diabetes Control and Complications Trial Research Group. The effect of intensive treatment of diabetes on the development and progression of long-term complications in insulin-dependent diabetes mellitus. N Engl J Med 1993; 329:977–986.

71. DiPasquale G, Andreoli A, Grazi P, et al. Cardioembolic stroke from atrial septal aneurysm. Stroke 1988; 19:640–643.

72. Dorros G, Lewin RF, Jamnadas P, et al. Below the knee angioplasty: Tibioperoneal vessels, the acute outcome. Cathet Cardiovasc Diagn 1990; 19:170–178.

73. Drielsma RF, Burnett JR, Gray-Weale AC, et al. Carotid artery disease: The influence of diabetes mellitus. J Cardiovasc Surg 1988; 29:692–696.

74. Dunn FL. Treatment of lipid disorders in diabetes mellitus. Med Clin North Am 1988; 72:1379.

75. Easton JD. Antiplatelet therapy for prevention of ischemic stroke. Cerebrovasc Dis 1992; 2(suppl):6–13.

76. Epstein M, Sowers JR. Diabetes mellitus and hypertension. Hypertension 1992; 19:403–418.

77. EUCLID Study Group. Randomized placebo-controlled trial of lisinopril in normotensive patients with insulin-dependent diabetes and normoalbuminuria or microalbuminuria. Lancet 1997; 349:1787–1792.

78. European Carotid Surgery Trialists Collaborative Group. MRC European Carotid Surgery Trial: Interim results for symptomatic patients with severe (70–99%) or with mild (0–29%) carotid stenosis. Lancet 1991; 337:1235–1243.

79. Ewing DJ, Campbell IW, Clarke BF. Assessment of cardiovascular effects in diabetic autonomic neuropathy and prognostic implications. Ann Intern Med 1980; 92:308.

80. Executive Committee for the Asymptomatic Carotid Atherosclerosis Study: Endarterectomy for asymptomatic carotid artery stenosis. JAMA 1995; 273:1421–1428.

81. Expert Committee on the Diagnosis and Classification of Diabetes Mellitus. Report of the Expert Committee on the Diagnosis and Classification of Diabetes Mellitus. Diabetes Care 1997.

82. Factor SM, Okun EM, Minase T. Capillary microaneurysms in the human heart. N Engl J Med 1980; 302:384.

83. Fairfax AJ, Lambert CD, Leatham A. Systemic embolism in chronic sinoatrial disorder. N Engl J Med 1976; 295:190–192.

84. Faught E, Trader SD, Hanna GR. Cerebral complications of angiography for transient ischemia and stroke: Prediction of risk. Neurology 1979; 29:4–15.

85. Feibel JH, Hardy PM, Campbell RG, et al. Prognostic value of the stress response following stroke. JAMA 1977; 238:1374–1376.

86. Fein FS, Zonnenblich EH. Diabetic cardiomyopathy. Prog Cardiovasc Dis 1985; 27:255–270.

87. Feldman M, Feldman M Jr: The association of coronary occlusion and infarction with diabetes mellitus: A necropsy study. Am J Med Sci 1954; 228:53–56.

88. Flink EB, Brick JE, Shane SR. Alterations of long-chain free fatty acid and magnesium concentrations in acute myocardial infarction. Arch Intern Med 1981; 141:441.

89. Frantz MJ, et al. Nutrition principles for the management of diabetes and related conditions (review). Diabetes Care 1994; 17:490.

90. Franzeck UK, Talke P, Bernestein EF, et al. Transcutaneous PO2 measurements in health and peripheral occlusive disease. Surgery 1982; 91:156–163.

91. Frater RWM, Oka Y, Kadish A, et al. Diabetes and coronary artery surgery. Mt Sinai J Med 1982; 49:237.

92. Frick MH, et al. Helsinki Heart Study: Primary Prevention Trial with gemfibrozil in middle aged men with dyslipidemia. N Engl J Med 1987; 317:1237.

93. Fujishima M, Kiyohara Y, Kato I, et al. Diabetes and cardiovascular disease in a prospective population survey in Japan: The Hisayama Study. Diabetes 1996; 45:S14–S16.

94. Fuller JF. Hypertension and diabetes: Epidemiologic aspects as a guide to management. J Cardiovasc Pharmacol 1993; 21:S63–S66.

95. Gandolfo C, Caponnetto C, Del Sette M, et al. Risk factors in lacunar syndromes: A case control study. Acta Neurol Scand 1988; 77:22–26.

96. Garcia MJ, McNamara PM, Gordon T, et al. Morbidity and mortality of diabetics in the Framingham population: Sixteen year follow-up study. Diabetes 1974; 23:105–111.

97. Gardner AW, Poehlman ET. Exercise rehabilitation programs for the treatment of claudication pain: A meta-analysis. JAMA 1995; 274:975–980.

98. Gent M, Blakely JA, Easton JD, et al. The Canadian American Ticlopidine Study (CATS) in thromboembolic stroke. Lancet 1989; 1:1215–220.

99. Gill JS, Shipley MJ, Tsementzis SA, et al. Cigarette smoking: A risk factor for hemorrhagic and nonhemorrhage stroke. Arch Intern Med 1989; 149:2053–2057.

100. Ginsberg HN. Relationship of diabetes mellitus and coronary artery disease. Clin Diabetes 1988; 6:78–81.

101. Giugliano D, Acampora R, Marfella R, et al. Metabolic and cardiovascular effects of carvedilol and atenolol in non–insulin-dependent diabetes mellitus and hypertension: A randomized, controlled trial. Ann Intern Med 1997; 126:955–959.

102. Goldenberg S, Alex M, Blumenthal HT: Sequelae of arteriosclerosis of the aorta and coronary arteries: a statistical study in diabetes mellitus. Diabetes 1958; 7:98–108.

103. Goldhaber S, Manson J, Hennekens C, et al. Low-dose aspirin and subsequent peripheral arterial surgery in the Physician's Health Study. Lancet 1992; 340:143.

104. Goodale F, Daoud AS, Florentin R, et al. Chemicoanatomic studies of arteriosclerosis and thrombosis in diabetics. I. Coronary arterial wall thickness, thrombosis, and myocardial infarcts in autopsied North Americans. Exp Mol Pathol 1962; 1:353–363.

105. Gorelick PB, Caplan LR, Hier DB, et al. Racial differences in the distribution of anterior circulation occlusive disease. Neurology 1984; 34:54–59.

106. Granger CB, Califf RM, Young S, et al. Outcome of patients with diabetes mellitus and acute myocardial

infarction treated with thrombolytic agents. J Am Coll Cardiol 1993; 21:920–925.

107. Gunderson T, Kjekshus J. Timolol treatment after myocardial infarction in diabetic patients. Diabetes Care 1983; 6:285.

108. Hamby RI, Soneraich S, Sherman L. Diabetic cardiomyopathy. JAMA 1974; 229:1749.

109. Hanna GP, Fujise K, Kjellgren O, et al. Infrapopliteal transcatheter interventions for limb salvage in diabetic patients: Importance of aggressive interventional approach and role of transcutaneous oximetry. J Am Coll Cardiol 1997; 30:664–669.

110. Harris M: Summary. *In* Harris MI, Cowie CC, Stern MP, et al, eds. Diabetes in America, ed 2. Washington, DC, National Institutes of Health, 1995. NIH publication no. 95-1468.

111. Harris MI. Undiagnosed NIDDM: Clinical and public health issues. Diabetes Care 1993; 16:642.

112. Hass WK, Easton JD, Adams HP, et al for the Ticlopidine Aspirin Stroke Study Group. A randomized trial comparing ticlopidine hydrochloride with aspirin for the prevention of stroke in high-risk patients. N Engl J Med 1989; 321:501–507.

113. Hausdorf G, Rieger U, Koepp P. Cardiomyopathy in childhood diabetes mellitus: Incidence, time of onset, and relation to metabolic control. Int J Cardiol 1988; 19:225.

114. Helms RB. Implications of population growth on prevalence of diabetes: A look at the future. Diabetes Care 1992; 15(suppl 1):6–9.

115. Herlitz J, Malmberg K, Karlson BW, et al. Mortality and morbidity during a five-year follow-up of diabetics with myocardial infarction. Acta Med Scand 1988; 224:31.

116. Hewes RC, White RI, Murray RR. Long term results of superficial femoral artery angioplasty. Am J Roentgenol 1986; 146:1025–1029.

117. Houston MC. Treatment of hypertension in diabetes mellitus. Am Heart J 1989; 118:819.

118. Howard G, Toole J, Frye-Pierson J, et al. Factors influencing the survival of 451 transient ischemic attack patients. Stroke 1987; 18:552–557.

119. Hughes TA, Clements RS, Rairclough PK. Effects of insulin therapy on lipoproteins in non-insulin dependent diabetes mellitus (NIDDM). Atherosclerosis 1987; 67:105–114.

120. Hughson WG, Mann JI, Tibbs DJ, et al. Intermittent claudication: Factors determining outcome. Br Med J 1978; 1:1377–1379.

121. Humphrey LL, et al. The contribution of non-insulin-dependent diabetes to lower-extremity amputation in the community. Arch Intern Med 1994; 154:885.

122. Iso H, Jacobs DR Jr, Wentworth D, et al. Serum cholesterol levels and six-year mortality from stroke in 350 977 men screened for the Multiple Risk Factor Intervention Trial. N Engl J Med 1989; 320:904–910.

123. Jacoby RM, Nesto RW. Acute myocardial infarction in the diabetic patient: Pathophysiology, clinical course and prognosis. J Am Coll Cardiol 1992; 20:736–744.

124. Jager KA, Phillips DJ Martin RL, et al. Noninvasive mapping of lower limb arterial lesions. Ultrasound Med Biol 1985; 11:515–521.

125. Jonason T, Ringqvist I. Diabetes mellitus and intermittent claudication: Relation between peripheral vascular complications and location of the occlusive atherosclerosis in the legs. Acta Med Scand 1985; 218: 217–221.

126. Jones HR, Caplan LR, Come PC, et al. Cerebral emboli of paradoxical origin. Ann Neurol 1983; 13:314–319.

127. Jorgensen HS, Nakayama H, Raaschou HO, et al. Stroke in patients with diabetes: The Copenhagen Stroke Study. Stroke 1994; 25:1977–1984.

128. Jorgensen HS, Nakayama H, Raaschou HO, et al. Effect of blood pressure and diabetes on stroke in progression. Lancet 1994; 344:156–159.

129. Kannel W, Hjortland M, Castelli W. Role of diabetes in congestive heart failure: The Framingham Study. Am J Cardiol 1974; 29:34.

130. Kannel WB, D'Agostino RB, Wilson PW, et al. Diabetes, fibrinogen, and risk of cardiovascular disease: The Framingham experience. Am Heart J 1990; 120:672–676.

131. Kannel WB, McGee DL. Diabetes and cardiovascular disease: The Framingham Study. JAMA 1979; 241:2035–2038.

132. Koskinen P, et al. Coronary heart disease incidence in NIDDM patients in the Helsinki Heart Study. Diabetes Care 1992; 15:820.

133. Kuusisto J, Mykkanen L, Pyorala K, et al. Non-insulin-dependent diabetes and its metabolic control are important predictors of stroke in elderly subjects. Stroke 1994; 25:1157–1164.

134. Laupacis A, Albers G, Dunn M, et al. Antithrombotic therapy in atrial fibrillation. Chest 1992; 102(suppl): 426S–433S.

135. Lechat P, Mas JL, Lascault G, et al. Prevalence of patent foramen ovale in patients with stroke. N Engl J Med 1988; 318:1148–1152.

136. Leonberg S, Elliott F. Prevention of recurrent stroke. Stroke 1981; 12:731–735.

137. Levine GN, Jacobs AK, Keeler GP, et al. Impact of diabetes mellitus on percutaneous revascularization (CAVEAT-I). Am J Cardiol 1997; 79:748–755.

138. Lindbom A. Arteriosclerosis and arterial thrombosis in the lower limb: A roentgenological study. Acta Radiol 1950; 1:80.

139. Lindgarde F, Jelnes R, Bjorkman H, et al. Conservative drug treatment in patients with moderately severe chronic occlusive peripheral arterial disease. Circulation 1989; 80:1549–1556.

140. Lithell HO. Effect of antihypertensive drugs on insulin, glucose, and lipid metabolism. Diabetes Care 1991; 14:203–209.

141. Lithner F, Asplund K, Eriksson S, et al. Clinical characteristics in diabetic stroke patients. Diabete Metab 1988; 14:15–19.

142. Lynch M, Gammage MD, Lamb P, et al. Acute myocardial infarction in diabetic patients in the thrombolytic era. Diabete Med 1994; 11:162–165.

143. Lynn GM, Stefanko K, Reed JF, et al. Risk factors for stroke after coronary artery bypass. J Thorac Cardiovasc Surg 1992; 104:1518–1523.

144. Lyons TJ, Lopes-Virella MF, Baystle JW. Glycation, oxidation, and glyoxidation in the pathogenesis of atherosclerosis in diabetes. Mod Med 1993; 61(suppl 2): 4–8.

145. Mahaffey KW, Granger CB, Toth CA, et al. Diabetic retinopathy should not be a contraindication to thrombolytic therapy for acute myocardial infarction: Review of ocular hemorrhage incidence and location in the GUSTO-I trial. J Am Coll Cardiol 1997; 30:1606–1610.

146. Mak KH, Moliterno DJ, Granger CB, et al. Influence of diabetes mellitus on clinical outcome in the thrombolytic era of acute myocardial infarction. J Am Coll Cardiol 1997; 30:171–179.

147. Malmberg K for the DIGAMI (Diabetes Mellitus Insulin Glucose Infusion in Acute Myocardial Infarction)

Study Group. Prospective randomised study of intensive insulin treatment on long term survival after acute myocardial infarction in patients with diabetes mellitus. BMJ 1997; 314:1512–1515.

148. Malmberg K, Herlitz J, Hjalmarson A, et al. Effects of metoprolol on mortality and late infarction in diabetics with suspected acute myocardial infarction: Retrospective data from two large studies. Eur Heart J 1989; 10:423–428.

149. Malmberg K, Ryden L, Efendic S, et al. Randomized trial of insulin-glucose infusion followed by subcutaneous insulin treatment in diabetic patients with acute myocardial infarction (DIGAMI study): Effects on mortality at 1 year. J Am Coll Cardiol 1995; 26:57–65.

150. Mandell GL, Novick WJ. Pentoxifylline and Leukocyte Function. Somerville, NJ, Hoechst-Roussel Pharmaceuticals, 1988.

151. Mangano DT, Layug EL, Wallace A, et al for the Multicenter Study of Perioperative Ischemia Research Group. Effect of atenolol on mortality and cardiovascular morbidity after noncardiac surgery. N Engl J Med 1996; 335:1713–1720.

152. Maser RE, et al. Cardiovascular disease and arterial calcification in insulin-dependent diabetes mellitus: Interrelation and risk factor profiles. Arterioscler Thromb 1991; 11:958.

153. Matsen FA, Wyss CR, Pedegana CR. Transcutaneous oxygen tension measurement in peripheral vascular disease. Surg Gynecol Obstet 1980; 150:525–528.

154. Mayberg MR, Wilson SE, Yatsu F, et al. Carotid endarterectomy and prevention of cerebral ischemia in symptomatic carotid stenosis. JAMA 1991; 266:3289–3294.

155. McDaniel MD, Cronenwett JL. Basic data related to the natural history of intermittent claudication. Ann Vasc Surg 1989; 3:273–277.

156. McMillan DE. Blood flow, diabetes, and atherogenesis. In Plum F, Pulsinelli W (eds): Cerebrovascular Diseases. New York, Raven Press, 1985, pp 97–103.

157. Meissner I, Wiebers DO, Whisnant JP, et al. The natural history of asymptomatic carotid artery occlusive lesions. JAMA 1987; 258:2704–2710.

158. Melamed E. Reactive hyperglycemia in patients with acute stroke. J Neurol Sci 1976; 29:267–275.

159. Melton LJ III, et al. Incidence and prevalence of clinical peripheral vascular disease in a population-based cohort of diabetic patients. Diabetes Care 1980; 3:650.

160. Murros K, Evans G, Toole J, et al. Cerebral infarction in patients with transient ischemic attacks. J Neurol 1989; 236:182–184.

161. Nahser PJ, Brown RE, Oskarsson H, et al. Maximal coronary flow reserve and metabolic coronary vasodilation in patients with diabetes mellitus. Circulation 1995; 91:635–640.

162. Nathan DM. Long-term complications of diabetes mellitus. N Engl J Med 1993; 328, 1676.

163. National Diabetes Advisory Board: The national long-range plan to combat diabetes. Bethesda, Md, U.S. Department of Health and Human Services, Public Health Service, National Institutes of Health, 1987, p 87. NIH publication no. 88–1587.

164. National Cholesterol Education Program (NCEP) Expert Panel: Summary of second report of the National Cholesterol Education Program (NCEP) Expert Panel on detection, evaluation, and treatment of high blood cholesterol in adults (adult treatment panel II). JAMA 1993; 269:3015–3023.

165. National High Blood Pressure Education Program Working Group. National High Blood Pressure Education Program Working Group Report on Hypertension in Diabetes. Hypertension 1994; 23:145–158.

166. National Institute of Neurological Disorders and Stroke Ad Hoc Committee. Classification of cerebrovascular diseases III. Stroke 1991; 21(4):637–680.

167. Nesto RW, Phillips RT, Kett KG, et al. Angina and exertional myocardial ischemia in diabetic and nondiabetic patients: Assessment by exercise thallium scintigraphy. Ann Intern Med 1988; 108:170.

168. Nitenberg A, Valensi P, Sachs R, et al. Impairment of coronary vascular reserve and Ach-induced coronary vasodilatation in diabetic patients with angiographically normal coronary arteries and normal left ventricular systolic function. Diabetes 1993; 32:1017–1023.

169. Norris JW, Zhu CZ, Bornstein NM, et al. Vascular risks of symptomatic carotid stenosis. Stroke 1991; 22:1485–1490.

170. North American Symptomatic Carotid Endarterectomy Trial Collaborators. Beneficial effect of carotid endarterectomy in symptomatic patients with high-grade carotid stenosis. N Engl J Med 1992; 325:445–453.

171. Orth S, Nowicki M, Wiecek A, et al. Nephroprotective effect of ACE inhibitors. Drugs 1993; 46(suppl 2):189–196.

172. Ostrander LD Jr, Epstein FH. Diabetes, hyperglycemia and atherosclerosis: New research directions. In Fajans SS (ed): Diabetes Mellitus. Washington, DC, Department of Health, Education, and Welfare, 1976. DHEW Publication no. NIH 76-854.

173. Oswald GA, Corcoran S, Yudkin JS. Prevalence and risks of hyperglycaemia and undiagnosed diabetes in patients with acute myocardial infarction. Lancet 1984; 1:1264–1267.

174. Owen RS, Carpenter JP, Baum RA, et al. Magnetic resonance imaging of angiographically occult runoff vessels in peripheral arterial occlusive disease. N Engl J Med 1992; 326:1577–1581.

175. Paaske WP, Tonnesen KH. Prognostic significance of distal blood pressure measurements in patients with severe ischaemia. Scand J Thorac Cardiovasc Surg 14:105–108.

176. Pell S, D'Alonzo A. Some aspects of hypertension in diabetes mellitus. JAMA 1967; 202:104.

177. Petersen P, Boysen G, Godtfredsen J, et al. Placebo-controlled, randomized trial of warfarin and aspirin for prevention of thromboembolic complications in chronic atrial fibrillation: The Copenhagen AFASAK study. Lancet 1989; 1:175–179.

178. Polumbo PJ, Elveback LR, Whisnant JP. Neurologic complications of diabetes mellitus: Transient ischemic attacks as opposed to strokes. Eur J Vasc Surg 1987; 1:259–262.

179. Pop G, Sutherland GR, Koudstaal PJ, et al. Transesophageal echocardiography in the detection of intracardiac embolic sources in patients with transient ischemic attacks. Stroke 1990; 21:560–565.

180. Porte D. B-cells in type II diabetes. Diabetes 1991; 40:166–180.

181. Pulsinelli EA, Levy DE, Sigsbee B, et al. Increased damage after ischemic stroke in patients with hyperglycemia with or without established diabetes mellitus. Am J Med 1983; 74:540–544.

182. Rao V, Christakis G, Weisel R, et al. Risk factors for stroke following coronary bypass surgery. J Cardiac Surg 1995; 10:468–474.

183. Rastenyte D, Tuomilehto J, Domarkiene S, et al. Risk factors for death from stroke in middle-aged lithuanian men. Stroke 1996; 27:672–676.

184. Regan FJ, Lyons MM, Ahmed SS, et al. Evidence of cardiomyopathy in familial diabetes mellitus. J Clin Invest 1977; 60:885.

185. Reichard P, Nilsson BY, Rosenqvist U. The effect of long-term intensified insulin treatment on the development of microvascular complications of diabetes mellitus. N Engl J Med 1993; 329:304–309.

186. Reid HL, Dormandy JA, Bernes AJ, et al. Impaired red cell deformability in peripheral vascular disease. Lancet 1976; 1:666.

187. Resnekov L. Silent myocardial ischemia: Therapeutic implications. Am J Med 1985; 79:3A30.

188. Riles TS, Eidelman EM, Litt AW, et al. Comparison of magnetic resonance angiography, conventional angiography and duplex scanning. Stroke 1992; 23:341–346.

189. Rohr J, Kittner S, Feeser B, et al. Traditional risk factors and ischemic stroke in young adults: The Baltimore-Washington cooperative young stroke study. Arch Neurol 1996; 53:603–607.

190. Roy TM, Peterson HR, Snider HL, et al. Autonomic influence on cardiac performance in diabetic subjects. Am J Med 1989; 87:382.

191. Rozenman Y, Sapoznikov D, Mosseri M, et al. Long-term angiographic follow-up of coronary balloon angioplasty in patients with diabetes mellitus: A clue to the results of the BARI study. J Am Coll Cardiol 1997; 30:1420–1425.

192. Rubler S. Cardiac manifestations of diabetes mellitus. Cardiovasc Med 1977; 2:823.

193. Sacco RL. Risk factors and outcomes for ischemic stroke. Neurology 1995; 45:S10–S14.

194. Sacco SE, Whisnant JP, Broderick JP, et al. Epidemiological characteristics of lacunar infarcts in a population. Stroke 1991; 22:1236–1241.

195. Sachneider DJ, Sobel BE. Determinants of coronary vascular disease in patients with type II diabetes mellitus and their therapeutic implications. Clin Cardiol 1997; 20:433–440.

196. Salenius JP, Harju E, Riekkinen H. Early cerebral complications in carotid endarterectomy: Risk factors. J Cardiovasc Surg 1990; 31:162–167.

197. Salonen JT, Puska P, Tuomilehto J, et al. Relation of blood pressure, serum lipids, and smoking to the risk of cerebral stroke: A longitudinal study in Eastern Finland. Stroke 1982; 13:327–333.

198. Sandok BA, Whisnant JP, Furlan AJ, et al. Carotid artery bruits: Prevalence survey and differential diagnosis. Mayo Clin Proc 1982; 57:227–230.

199. Sato N, Hachimoto H, Takiguchi Y, et al. Altered responsiveness to sympathetic nerve stimulation and agonist of isolated left atria of diabetic rat: No evidence for involvement of hypothyroidism. J Pharmacol Exp 1989; 87:382.

200. Savage MP, Krolewski AS, Kenien GG, et al. Acute myocardial infarction in diabetes mellitus and significance of congestive heart failure as a prognostic factor. Am J Cardiol 1988; 48:767.

201. Savage PJ, Soad MF. Insulin and atherosclerosis: Villain, accomplice, or innocent bystander? (editorial). Br Heart J 1993; 69:473–475.

202. Scandinavian Simvastatin Survival Study: Randomized trial of cholesterol lowering in 4444 patients with coronary heart disease: The Scandinavian Simvastatin Survival Study (4S). Lancet 1994; 344:1383–1389.

203. Schroer R. Antithrombotic potential of pentoxifylline, a hemorheologically active drug. Angiology 1985; 36:387.

204. Second International Study on Infarct Survival Collaborative Group. Randomised trial of intravenous streptokinase, oral aspirin, both, or neither among 17,187 cases of suspected acute myocardial infarction: ISIS-2. Lancet 1988; 2:535–40.

205. Shoemaker WC, Vidyasagar D. Physiological and clinical significance of PtcO2 measurements. Crit Care Med 1981; 9:689–690.

206. Sowers JR, Epstein M. Diabetes mellitus and associated hypertension, vascular disease, and nephropathy: An update. Hypertension 1995; 26(6 pt 1):869–879.

207. Stegmayr B, Asplund K. Diabetes as a risk factor for stroke. A population perspective. Diabetologia 1995; 38:1061–1068.

208. Stein PD, Kantrowitz A. Antithrombotic therapy in mechanical and biological prosthetic heart valves and saphenous vein bypass grafts. Chest 1989; 95(suppl): 107S–117S.

209. Steinke W, Hennerici M, Rautenberg W, et al. Symptomatic and asymptomatic high-grade carotid stenoses in Doppler color-flow imaging. Neurology 1992; 42:131–138.

210. Stone GW, Grines CL, Browne KF, et al. Does primary angioplasty improve prognosis of patients with diabetes and acute myocardial infarction? (abstract). J Am Coll Cardiol 1995; 25(suppl):401A.

211. Stone PH, Muller JE, Hartwell T, et al. The effect of diabetes mellitus on prognosis and serial left ventricular function after acute myocardial infarction: Contribution of both coronary disease and diastolic left ventricular dysfunction to the adverse prognosis. J Am Coll Cardiol 1989; 14:49.

212. Strandness DE Jr. Duplex scanning for diagnosis of peripheral arterial disease. Herz 1988; 13:372–378.

213. Stroke Prevention in Atrial Fibrillation Investigators. The stroke prevention in atrial fibrillation study: Final results. Circulation 1991; 84:527–539.

214. Sutherland CGG, Fisher BM, Frier BM, et al. Endomyocardial biopsy pathology in insulin-dependent diabetic patients with abnormal ventricular function. Histopathology 1989; 14:593.

215. Taylor LM, Edwards JM, Porter JM. Present status of reversed vein bypass grafting: Five-year results of a modern series. J Vasc Surg 1990; 11:193.

216. Tesfamariam B, Brown ML, Cohen RA. Elevated glucose impairs endothelium-dependent relaxation by activating protein kinase C. J Clin Invest 1991; 87:1643–1648.

217. Torvik A. The pathogenesis of watershed infarctions in the brain. Stroke 1984; 15:221–223.

218. Toyry JP, Niskanen LK, Lansimies EA, et al. Autonomic neuropathy predicts the development of stroke in patients with non-insulin-dependent diabetes mellitus. Stroke 1996; 27:1316–1318.

219. Tuomilehto J, Rastenyte D, Jousilahti P, et al. Diabetes mellitus as a risk factor for death from stroke. Stroke 1996; 27:210–215.

220. Ursitupa MI, Niskanen LK, Siitonen O, et al. 5-year incidence of atherosclerotic vascular disease in relation to general risk factors, insulin level, and abnormalities in lipoprotein composition in non-insulin-dependent diabetic and nondiabetic subjects. Circulation 1990; 82:27–36.

221. van Andel GJ, van Erp WFM, Krepel VM, et al. Percutaneous transluminal dilatation of the iliac artery: Long term results. Radiology 1985; 156:321–323.

222. Van Belle E, Banters C, Hubert E, et al. Restenosis rates in diabetic patients: A comparison of coronary stenting and balloon angioplasty in native coronary vessels. Circulation 1997; 96:1454–1460.

223. Vinik A, Colwell JA and the Hyperlipidemia in Diabetes Investigators: Effects of gemfibrozil on triglyceride levels in patients with NIDDM. Diabetes Care 1993; 16:37.

224. Vlassara H. Recent progress on the biologic and clinical significance of advanced glycosylated end products. J Lab Clin Med 1994; 124:19–30.

225. Waller BF, Palumbo PJ, Lie JT, et al. Status of the coronary arteries at necropsy in diabetes mellitus with onset after age 30 years: Analysis of 229 diabetic patients with and without clinical evidence of coronary heart diseae and comparison of 183 control subjects. Am J Med 1980; 69:498.

226. Webster MWI, Smith HJ, Sharpe DN, et al. Patent foramen ovale in young stroke patients. Lancet 1988; 2:11–12.

227. Weise F, Heydenreich F, Gehrig W, et al. Heart rate variability in diabetic patients during orthostatic load: A spectral analytic approach. Klin Wochenschr 1990; 68:26.

228. Wengerter KR, Yang PM, Veith FJ, et al. A twelve-year experience with the popliteal-to-distal artery bypass: The significance and management of proximal disease. J Vasc Surg 1992; 15:143.

229. Wengerter KR, Veith FJ, Gupta SK, et al. Prospective randomized multicenter comparison of in situ and reversed vein infrapopliteal bypasses. J Vasc Surg 1991; 13:189.

230. West KW. Epidemiology of diabetes and its vascular complications: Report to U.S. National Commission of Diabetes. Scope and Impact of Diabetes 1975; 3:56–60.

231. Wiebers DO, Whisnant JP, Sandok BA, et al. Prospective comparison of a cohort with asymptomatic carotid bruit and a population-based cohort without carotid bruit. Stroke 1990; 21:984–988.

232. Willeit J, Kiechl S. Prevalence and risk factors of asymptomatic extracranial carotid artery atherosclerosis: A population-based study. Arteriosclerosis Thrombosis 1993; 13:661–668.

233. Williams GH. Converting enzyme inhibitors in the treatment of hypertension. N Engl J Med 1988; 319:1517.

234. Wolf P, Kannel W, Sorlie P, et al. Asymptomatic carotid bruit and risk of stroke. JAMA 1981; 245:1442–1445.

235. Wolf PA, Belanger AJ, D'Agostino RB. Management of risk factors. Neurol Clin 1992; 10:177–191.

236. Wolf PA, D'Agostino RB, Kannel WB, et al. Cigarette smoking as a risk factor for stroke: The Framingham Study. JAMA 1988; 259: 1025–1029.

237. Wolffenbuttel BHR, van Haeften TW. Prevention of complications in non-insulin-dependent diabetes mellitus (NIDDM). Drugs 1995; 50:263–288.

238. Woods KL, Samanta A, Burden AC. Diabetes mellitus as a risk factor for acute myocardial infarction in Asians and Europeans. Br Heart J 1989; 62:118.

239. Working Group on Hypertension in Diabetes. Statement on hypertension in diabetes mellitus: Final report. Arch Intern Med 1987; 147:830.

240. Yokoyama I, Momomura SI, Ohtake T, et al. Reduced myocardial flow reserve in non-insulin-dependent diabetes mellitus. J Am Coll Cardiol 1997; 30:1472–1477.

241. You R, McNeil JJ, O'Malley HM, et al. Risk factors for lacunar infarction syndromes. Neurology 1995; 45:1483–1487.

242. Young MJ, et al. Medial arterial calcification in the feet of diabetic patients and matched non-diabetic control subjects. Diabetologia 1993; 36:615.

243. Zarich SW, Nesto RW. Diabetic cardiomyopathy. Am Heart J 1989; 118:1000–1012.

244. Zatz R, Dunn BR, Meyer TW, et al. Prevention of diabetic glomerulopathy by pharmacological amelioration of glomerular capillary hypertension. J Clin Invest 1986; 77:1925.

245. Zeiler K, Siostrzonek P, Lang W, et al. Different risk factor profiles in young and elderly stroke patients with special reference to cardiac disorders. J Clin Epidemiol 1992; 45:1383–1389.

246. Zola B, Kahn JK, Juni JE, et al. Abnormal cardiac function in diabetic patients with autonomic neuropathy in the absence of ischemic heart disease. J Clin Endocrinol Metab 1986; 63:208.

247. Zoneraich S. Diabetes and the heart. Springfield, Ill, Charles C Thomas, 1978, p 303.

248. Zuanetti G, Latini R, Maggioni AP, et al on behalf of GISSI-2 Investigators. Influence of diabetes on mortality in acute myocardial infarction: Data from the GISSI-2 study. J Am Coll Cardiol 1993; 22:1788–1794.

Chapter **7**

Peripheral Vascular Disease

Matthew J. Young • *Andrew J. M. Boulton*

INTRODUCTION

Diabetic peripheral vascular disease has a number of clinical associations. However, few of these have been proved amenable to improvement by control of hyperglycemia or specific therapy. The onset of vascular disease seems to influence the development of peripheral neuropathy, resulting in neuroischemic limbs that are a particular clinical problem to diabetic foot care teams. The development of improved radiologic and surgical limb salvage techniques has proved to be of benefit in reducing amputation rates. Postamputation care can also be effective in improving quality of life by preventing second amputations. Despite these powerful arguments in favor and the apparent drive to achieve the St. Vincent targets, few centers have adopted these techniques in full, and the amputation rates in diabetic patients remain disappointingly high.

Joslin first reported that gangrene was a menace to diabetic patients in 1934.[76] More than 60 years later, despite the development of sophisticated surgical reconstruction and interventional radiologic techniques, the rate of lower limb amputation is still 15 times higher in diabetic patients compared with nondiabetic patients,[113] and foot problems remain one of the commonest reasons for hospital admission among diabetic patients. In addition, more than 50% of diabetic amputees need an amputation in the contralateral limb during the first 4 years after the loss of the first leg.[35] Although

105

amputations are still performed in diabetic patients with neuropathic lesions, which might otherwise have been prevented had they received care in a multidisciplinary diabetic foot clinic,[37, 155] the majority of amputations are performed on dysvascular limbs. It is the stated aim of the World Health Organization (WHO) and International Diabetes Federation (IDF) in Europe, as part of the St. Vincent Declaration, to achieve a 50% reduction in the numbers of amputations performed for diabetic gangrene.[166] Most of the St. Vincent's targets can be achieved by the development of multidisciplinary foot care teams,[37, 155] but the remainder will require fundamental changes in the approach to vascular disease in diabetes.

The mechanisms underlying the development of peripheral vascular disease in diabetes are only partly understood, and primary prevention strategies are difficult to employ because of the natural history of the disease. More than 10% of type 2 (non–insulin dependent) diabetic patients have peripheral vascular disease at diagnosis.[156] Macrovascular disease is the largest single cause of mortality in diabetic patients, and it is the cause of death in more than 50% of type 2 diabetes patients, on average within 5 years after diagnosis.[151] Therefore, screening and secondary prevention methods may prove to be the best hope of saving limbs in diabetic patients.

PATHOGENESIS

The mechanisms underlying the development of peripheral vascular disease in diabetes are drawn from observations of cardiovascular and cerebrovascular disease that have been studied in greater detail.[124] An additional confounding factor is that individual studies often use varying criteria, ranging from palpation of pulses to Doppler pressures and arteriography, to describe peripheral vascular disease, and surveys of peripheral vascular disease do not always record diabetes and may misclassify patients. Such differences in methodology can often make conclusions difficult to compare across papers.

Any proposed mechanisms have to explain why vascular disease develops earlier and more aggressively in diabetic patients, particularly type 2 patients, and why females lose their premenopausal protection, whereas, conversely, unless they develop proteinuria, type 1 (insulin dependent) diabetic patients have only a marginally higher lifetime risk of developing macrovascular disease when compared

with nondiabetic subjects. New research into cellular adhesion molecules and vascular permeability factor is adding to the understanding of the basic cellular mechanisms underlying atherogenesis[32] but, at a clinical level, most pathogenetic factors have been proposed on the basis of cross-sectional surveys, with few, if any, true prospective studies of risk factor profiles and nearly no studies of intervention strategies. Despite this, a number of factors appear to be associated with the development of peripheral vascular disease in diabetic patients.

Hyperglycemia

In cross-sectional epidemiologic surveys, including the Framingham study,[55] the Multiple Risk Factor Intervention Trial (MRFIT),[149] and WHO survey,[28] diabetic patients have between two and four times the prevalence of peripheral vascular disease as that found in nondiabetic patients. A number of studies have also suggested that the prevalence of macrovascular disease may be related to the level of hyperglycemia, although one study found that this relationship was only found in men,[8, 44, 51] and a further study has found no relationship.[11] This excess of macrovascular disease is not only found in diabetic patients but also in those with impaired glucose tolerance and, indeed, formed the basis of the diagnosis of impaired glucose tolerance in the Whitehall study. Once other factors have been corrected, more than 75% of the excess mortality from cardiovascular disease, and therefore by extrapolation peripheral vascular morbidity, was attributable to the presence of diabetes.[51]

The mechanism by which hyperglycemia promotes the development of vascular disease remains unproved, but it is reasonable to postulate that glucose might damage endothelial cells by an as yet undetermined mechanism, thus increasing permeability of the endothelium to plasma proteins and lipids.[91] In addition, endothelial cell damage reduces prostacyclin production and increases platelet adhesion to the endothelium (see Rheological and Fibrinolytic Changes). Thus, an increase in the constituents and processes involved in the development of atheroma plaques appears to be promoted by hyperglycemia, and this may explain part of the increase in peripheral vascular disease in diabetic patients.

In addition to the proposed direct effects of hyperglycemia on atheroma development, glycation of the extracellular matrix is known to increase collagen cross-links and thus decrease arterial compliance by reducing the elasticity of the media. Increased arterial stiffness is a common finding in diabetic patients and a factor associated with the development of vascular disease. Stiff arteries lead to systolic hypertension, which in turn results in direct endothelial damage and increased endothelial shear stress. Both are likely to promote the development of atheroma plaques in an individual.

Glycated collagen also appears to be chemotactic to monocytes and has increased affinity for binding low-density lipoprotein (LDL) molecules, further constituents of the atheroma plaque, and therefore is likely to promote atherogenesis.[13]

In addition to the lack of clear evidence that prevailing glycemia, as measured either as fasting blood glucose or glycated hemoglobin, is directly related to the incidence of peripheral vascular disease, no study has as yet demonstrated that reducing hyperglycemia modulates risk. Most studies of glycemic control, including the Diabetes Control and Complications Trial (DCCT),[25] have examined the effects of improved glycemic control on microvascular disease. The United Kingdom Prospective Diabetes Study (UKPDS)[156] has been designed to examine the role of glycemic control on the development of macrovascular disease in type 2 diabetic patients. There have been no final results as to whether this can be achieved, and the results of the UKPDS are likely to provoke considerable debate about the treatment of type 2 diabetes.

Rheological and Fibrinolytic Changes

Diabetes is associated with a number of procoagulant effects that are more prominent in patients with complications and a defect in fibrinolysis. However, the small size of some studies,[167] the failure to define adequately the patient groups with a mix of different complications and levels of complications, and the failure to control for smoking have further confused this question.

Increased levels of von Willebrand factor[30] and fibrinogen[6, 53, 95] have been reported in diabetes and are thought to increase the risk of macrovascular disease, particularly in patients with type 2 diabetes.[110, 111]

The balance of platelet aggregation dissociation is also regulated by the balance of thromboxane (TXA$_2$, although this is usually measured as the stable compound TXB$_2$ in most studies), which promotes platelet aggregation, and the prostanoids, prostaglandin E$_1$, and prostacyclin,[108] which reduce it. There is evidence in experimental diabetes that the balance of thromboxane and prostacyclins is disturbed, with an excess of thromboxane synthesis,[56, 80] and this has also been reported in humans.[67] Prostacyclin synthesis has also been reported to be reduced in animals with experimental diabetes[163] and in diabetic patients.[74, 145, 169] This results in a relative excess of thromboxane, which, when taken together with evidence of increased thromboxane receptors on platelets in patients with type 1 diabetes,[107] may partially explain the abnormal platelet function and the significantly increased platelet aggregation reported in diabetic patients.[22, 24, 118, 119] This increase in platelet aggregability may in turn lead to increased atheroma production or an increased tendency to in situ thrombosis once an atheroma plaque fissures.

Overall, the fibrinolytic system is believed to be impaired in patients with diabetes,[147] and this may be more abnormal in patients with poor diabetes control. The main activators of the fibrinolytic system are tissue plasminogen activator (t-PA) and urokinase-like plasminogen activator (u-PA). Circulating t-PA is produced by the vascular endothelium; u-PA is produced by the liver and a number of other cell lines. There are two plasminogen activator inhibitors, PAI-1 and PAI-2. Plasminogen activator inhibitor 1 is found in plasma, hepatocytes, endothelial cells, and platelets.[61] It has been suggested that high insulin levels, either because of resistance or pharmacologic treatment, are associated with increased PAI-1 levels.[78, 79] However, a number of euglycemic clamp and related studies of patients who are not insulin resistant have failed to show such a relationship. It has therefore been suggested that obesity and hypertension may be the main correlates of PAI-1 activity[6, 60, 86, 129] and that impaired fibrinolysis may explain some or all of the increased risk of atherosclerosis associated with these conditions.[8, 157]

In type 1 diabetes, studies measuring the activity of each fibrinolytic parameter have shown lower t-PA or t-PA/PAI-1 activity ratios in type 1 diabetes compared with controls.[6, 48, 167] Wieczorek and colleagues also demonstrated that there was an attenuated fibrinolytic response after venous occlusion or insulin induced hypoglycemia in type 1 diabetes.[167] They suggested that this abnormality in fibrinolysis might be caused by an underlying endothelial defect. In type 2 diabetes, there is a consensus that fibrinolytic activity is reduced.[52, 54, 61, 143, 162] Overall, the pattern of procoagulant state and reduced fibrinolysis appears to be consistent in diabetic patients with macrovascular disease.[104]

Smoking

Smoking is strongly associated with the risk of macrovascular disease in cross-sectional prevalence studies, and this association may be stronger in diabetic patients than nondiabetic patients. The increased prevalence of macrovascular disease associated with smoking appears to be modulated by direct effects causing endothelial damage; increased concentrations of von Willebrand factor, possibly as a consequence of endothelial damage; and by further impairing fibrinolysis. Interestingly, despite this association with peripheral vascular disease, the lifetime quantity smoked was only predictive of amputation in diabetes patients diagnosed before the age of 30 in the Wisconsin study,[112] but not among older-onset diabetic patients. Reiber and associates found no difference in lifetime smoking history between diabetic veterans undergoing amputation and diabetic control subjects.[135] Selby and Zhang also found no clear association between smoking and lower limb amputations.[144] Thus, smoking does not appear to contribute substantially to the excess risk for amputation among type 2 diabetic patients. This is despite its clear association with peripheral vascular disease and remains to be explained. A vigorous antismoking education program is nevertheless to be encouraged, especially in young type 1 patients, because of other associated risk factors.

The quoted smoking rate in most diabetes clinics is usually lower than the 33% often quoted in the general population of the United Kingdom. However, studies that examine objective markers of smoking, such as urinary cotinine levels or carbon monoxide (CO) concentrations, suggest true smoking prevalence rates are actually higher. In turn, these studies provide evidence that all our efforts to reduce smoking in the diabetic population are to little effect, despite recognition of the health dangers of smoking in the diabetic population.[100]

Hypertension

Hypertension is a major correlate for the development and progression of peripheral vascular disease in all the epidemiologic surveys of peripheral vascular disease.[55, 122] Hypertension is present in about 50% of type 2 diabetic patients at diagnosis.[156] There is evidence that if hypertension is inadequately treated in diabetic patients, then the rate of progression of peripheral vascular disease is greater than in those patients with good blood pressure control.[122]

The effects of hypertension are difficult to view in isolation. Type 2 diabetes is commonly found in association with the insulin resistance/hyperlipidemia syndrome. Type 1 diabetes is usually associated with hypertension, which is usually found in association with microalbuminuria and proteinuria, which are in turn are associated with lipid abnormalities, fibrinolytic disturbance, and increased macrovascular risk.

Dyslipidemia

Diabetic patients have an excess of lipid abnormalities when compared with the general population, but this is not particularly marked in patients with peripheral vascular disease. This is also true in diabetic patients, particularly type 2 patients, in whom triglyceride concentrations may be a significant risk marker for peripheral vascular disease.[11, 84] However, despite this association, no therapeutic trial has yet demonstrated a reduction in the development of peripheral vascular disease with lipid altering therapy. In addition, although a small plaque regression study has shown changes in coronary angiographic appearance,[43] no sizable study has examined the role of secondary prevention with lipid-lowering therapy to determine the effects on the progression of peripheral vascular disease and amputation rate. Such data may emerge from subgroup analyses of major cardiovascular secondary prevention trials recently completed and currently being undertaken in diabetic patients, but until then, such treatment, in the absence of myocardial infarction,[134] remains speculative.

Insulin Resistance and Hyperinsulinemia

The metabolic syndrome, *syndrome X*, and its constituents, hyperinsulinemia, hyperlipidemia, hypertension, and central abdominal obesity, are associated with decreased fibrinolysis and are, individually, as described above, significant risk factors for peripheral vascular disease. In particular, hyperinsulinemia has emerged as one of the strongest independent risk factors in a number of epidemiologic surveys.[31, 49, 165] It is unclear whether this is a specific effect of insulin or whether this is mediated through the association of hyperinsulinemia with obesity and impaired fibrinolysis.

Proteinuria

The development of microalbuminuria and subsequent dipstick-positive proteinuria marks a significant stage in the risk-factor profile for the development of peripheral vascular disease. In type 1 diabetic patients, the development of proteinuria increases the prevalence of vascular disease by more than 34 times that of nonproteinuric type 1 diabetic patients.[72] In type 2 diabetic patients, proteinuria is a marker of increased cardiovascular disease risk, but the association with peripheral vascular disease is not as strong as in type 1 diabetes, possibly because the risk of peripheral vascular disease is already increased in type 2 diabetic patients.[101]

The increased prevalence of peripheral vascular disease in diabetic patients with proteinuria is probably modulated through the association of nephropathy and an increased prevalence of hypertension, increased Lp(a) lipoprotein concentrations, and greater degrees of dyslipidemia in diabetic patients. In particular, proteinuria is associated with an increased serum total cholesterol concentration, increased LDL levels, increased triglyceride concentrations, and variable effects on high-density lipoprotein (HDL) (HDL concentrations are usually reported to be lower), which create a significantly more adverse and atherogenic risk profile in proteinuric patients.

Proteinuria is also associated with an increase in Lp(a) concentrations. Lipoprotein(a) is probably no higher in type 2 diabetic patients than the general population,[65] but in type 1 diabetic patients, and in particular those with macroproteinuria, there is probably an increase in Lp(a) concentrations with an attendant rise in atherosclerotic risk.[66]

Vascular Permeability Factor

It has been suggested that much of the increase in the prevalence of macrovascular disease in diabetic patients can be explained by the effects of diabetes on vascular permeability factor (VPF).[32] Vascular permeability factor is a short heparin-binding glycopeptide produced in the subendothelial smooth muscle cells and pericytes of the vascular tree. It is believed to modulate the entry of macromolecules such as lipoproteins through endothelial pores. In experimental studies, VPF is also chemotactic to monocytes.

The production of VPF from endothelial smooth muscle cells can be modulated in vitro by altering the prevailing glucose concentration in the experimental model, by simulating the effects of pulsatile blood pressure changes on the deformity of vascular smooth muscle, and by altering levels of hypoxia. If these experimental results are confirmed, then this may supply a unifying hypothesis for the final common pathway for many of the associated risk factors for peripheral vascular disease.

EPIDEMIOLOGY

The definition of peripheral vascular disease varies in different epidemiologic surveys. Cofactors such as peripheral neuropathy may reduce the pain of intermittent claudication or even ischemic rest pain. Although such symptoms are usually a reliable indicator of peripheral vascular insufficiency, painful peripheral neuropathy may sometimes be difficult to distinguish from ischemic pain. In addition, medial arterial calcification, more prevalent in diabetic patients and especially in those with peripheral neuropathy, can falsely elevate ankle systolic pressure levels, thus rendering normal values inaccurate in excluding occlusive peripheral vascular disease.[23, 29, 42, 171] Nevertheless, the presence of an abnormally low value (ankle-brachial systolic pressure ratio <0.9) or the nature of the Doppler signal is still useful indicators of disease. However, for screening most asymptomatic patients, the most useful measure is still the peripheral pulses. The absence of two or more foot pulses is diagnostic of peripheral vascular disease, and the palpation of pulses remains the cornerstone of foot screening in the annual review of diabetic patients.

Using the absence of two or more peripheral pulses as a diagnostic criterion, the UKPDS reported that 11% of type 2 diabetic patients had peripheral vascular disease at diagnosis.[156] Other surveys have put the point prevalence of peripheral vascular disease in type 2 diabetes at up to 34%, depending on the criteria used.[160] The detection of excess peripheral vascular disease in type 2 patients at diagnosis is indicative of prolonged hyperglycemia before diagnosis and supports the role of impaired glucose tolerance and hypertension in the pathogenesis of peripheral vascular disease. Similar surveys in type 1 diabetic patients have put the prevalence of peripheral vascular disease at around 9%. These prevalence rates are around two to four times those seen in the nondiabetic population.[12]

Diabetic patients may develop atheroma and occlusive vascular disease at any site in the vascular tree, but it is often stated that the majority of diabetic peripheral vascular disease is distal to the popliteal trifurcation. This is not the case. There does not appear to be a significant difference between the prevalence of proximal vascular disease (aortoiliac and femoral segments) between diabetic and nondiabetic patients. Distal vascular disease (peroneal and tibial arteries) is probably more prevalent in diabetic patients, but not in all studies.[77, 89, 105, 106, 153] Even in the presence of tibioperoneal disease there may be patent vessels in the foot (the crural vessels). The implications for treatment are outlined in the therapy section.

Overall, amputation rates in diabetic patients are about 15 times higher than in nondiabetic patients.[113] The prevalence of major amputation in diabetic patients in hospital and community surveys in the United Kingdom has been measured at around 2%.[94, 114] These prevalence rates are relatively low, and this is probably because the median survival after amputation is so short in diabetic patients. Patients survived for a median of 22 months after amputation in a study done in Newcastle upon Tyne.[27] In a Northwest England regional survey, 24% of diabetic patients who had major amputation and survived to attend a limb-fitting center died within 18 months of amputation, compared with only 15% of nondiabetic peripheral vascular disease patients.[1] In both groups the main cause of death after amputation is the progression of other macrovascular problems, resulting in cardiac death or stroke.

NEUROPATHY AS A MANIFESTATION OF VASCULAR DISEASE

Although minor neurophysiologic abnormalities can be found in the majority of diabetic patients, using careful clinical criteria, diabetic peripheral neuropathy is usually found in less than one third of all patients,[172] and it is therefore likely that other factors play a role. Although other pathogenic mechanisms, including immunologic mechanisms[131] and those relating to disturbances in the balance of nerve growth factors,[87] have been proposed in the pathogenesis of diabetic peripheral neuropathy, opinion is generally divided between the role of metabolic abnormalities,[10, 20] including those of the polyol pathway,[63] and the role of microvascular disease[32, 93] as the principal cause of diabetic peripheral neuropathy. Within an individual, however, both mechanisms are likely to be at work, and indeed, the two may be related,[10, 93] probably through oxidative stress, free radical damage, and vasoconstriction caused by reduced nitric oxide formation.

Clinical surveys of ulceration and amputation in diabetic patients clearly demonstrate that neuropathy and peripheral vascular disease coexist in more than 50% of attendees at diabetic foot clinics.[38, 155] Therefore, in addition to the microvascular mechanisms proposed in the development of peripheral neuropathy, there is a clear indication that neuropathy and peripheral vascular disease are associated. This assumption is further supported by considerable evidence from experimental and clinical studies that demonstrate that lower limb vascular disease and peripheral ischemia can adversely affect nerve function. The loss of nerve function after interruption of the blood supply is termed *ischemic conduction failure*.[93] This is usually tested in humans by applying a sphygmomanometer cuff around the limb to be tested and inflating above systolic blood pressure and measuring nerve function at timed intervals. Measuring the reduction in vibration perception using this technique, Steiness[150] reported that diabetic patients with peripheral neuropathy demonstrated resistance to ischemic conduction failure and suggested that endoneurial hypoxia might be responsible for this phenomenon. This *resistance to ischemic conduction failure* is a feature of diabetic neuropathy and is thought to point to a role for endoneurial hypoxia in the pathogenesis of diabetic neuropathy.[93] Direct measurement of endoneurial oxygen tension has demonstrated that this is reduced in chronically hyperglycemic rats, and oxygen supplementation in hyperbaric chambers can ameliorate the fall in nerve conduction velocities that usually occurs.[93] Nondiabetic rats kept in a low oxygen environment have also been shown to develop a peripheral neuropathy.[92] Experimental assessments of nerve blood flow have confirmed that this is also reduced in diabetic rats,[15] and more recent research has demonstrated that a surgically created proximal arteriovenous shunt can significantly reduce nerve function in the rat hind limb by reducing distal blood flow.[146] Studies by Cameron and associates and others have shown that experimental neuropathy can be prevented in streptozocin-diabetic rats by treatment with vasodilators from the induction of diabetes.[16] Repeated muscle stimulation with electric shocks has been shown to improve angiogenesis and ameliorate the decline in nerve conduction seen in experimental animals.[14] Angiotensin-converting enzyme (ACE) inhibitors may also be able to prevent the development of conduction velocity slowing in experimental diabetes.[15]

In humans, direct measurement of endoneurial oxygen tension has also shown that the diabetic sural nerve is hypoxic compared with nondiabetic controls and that the sural oxygen tension was lower than that of the overlying vein.[115] It could be reasoned that if diabetic peripheral neuropathy is the result of reduced endoneurial blood flow or hypoxia, then a direct reduction in blood flow or impaired tissue oxygenation in nondiabetic patients should result in peripheral nerve dysfunction and the same histologic features as those found in diabetes. Malik and coworkers reported that microangiopathy and myelinated fiber loss can also be found in nerve biopsies from nondiabetic hypoxic chronic obstructive airways disease patients,[96] up to 20% of whom may develop a mild but clinically detectable peripheral neuropathy.[117] These patients also show the same electrophysiologic features as diabetic patients, including resistance to ischemic conduction failure.[99] As in animal models, the creation of arteriovenous shunts for hemodialysis has been demonstrated to lead to a distal neuropathy in a number of case reports.[82, 139, 168] Epidemiologically, peripheral neuropathy has been found to be associated with peripheral vascular disease,[98] and clinical assessments of peripheral vascular disease have been shown to correlate with peripheral nerve function with a greater degree of neuropathy in the more ischemic limb.[132] Similarly, peripheral nerve function is directly proportional to transcutaneous oxygen tension in diabetic patients, although this might be an effect of shunting and not a causal factor in the development of the neuropathy.[170] In addition, a reduction in motor conduction velocity[70] and morphological abnormalities, including a reduction in myelinated fiber density, have been reported in patients with peripheral vascular disease.[141]

Reversal studies have as yet given mixed results. Small-scale studies of vasodilators have resulted in small increases in nerve conduction velocity in experimental diabetes.[17] Such improvement has not yet been shown in double-blind, controlled studies in humans, although the improvement in peripheral neuropathy reported in trials with γ-linolenic acid (Scotia Pharmaceuticals, Guildford, Surrey, U.K.) has in part been attributed to improved microvascular blood flow,[81] and an open-label study of the use of the ACE inhibitor lisinopril (Zeneca Pharmaceuticals, Macclesfield, U.K.) in humans has also shown improvements in nerve conduction.[137] Arterial reconstructive surgery in small numbers of nondiabetic and short-duration type 2 diabetic patients with single femoral artery occlusion and no peripheral gangrene has been reported to result in an increase in peripheral transcutaneous oxygen tension and short-term improvements in conduction velocity.[170, 173] Larger, longer studies of mixed diabetic and nondiabetic groups,[70] or mixed type 1 and type 2 patients,[161] both of which included patients with peripheral gangrene undergoing limb salvage operations, have failed to demonstrate significant reversal of neurological deficit. In the latter studies, the likelihood of irreversible diabetic or ischemic damage may have limited the potential for reversal. Therefore, therapeutic modalities aimed at early intervention in endoneurial ischemia may still provide the best hope for the prevention and treatment of diabetic peripheral neuropathy.

DETECTION AND ASSESSMENT OF PERIPHERAL VASCULAR DISEASE
History and Examination

Peripheral vascular disease in diabetic patients usually has the same clinical presentation as that seen in nondiabetic patients. Patients usually complain of intermittent (exercise induced) claudication, which progresses with severity of disease to rest pain, ulceration, and gangrene.[88] However, the symptoms of peripheral ischemia may be masked by coexisting peripheral neuropathy, and diabetic patients may not complain of pain even in the presence of tissue necrosis. There does not appear to be good evidence for so-called neuropathic pseudoclaudication in carefully studied, well-defined groups of diabetic patients.[127]

As outlined previously, in the absence of symptomatic ischemia, the foot pulses are the best guide to the presence of peripheral vascular disease in diabetic patients, and two or more absent foot pulses is a commonly adopted standard. Foot pulses may be absent even when the popliteal pulses are present because of tibioperoneal disease; therefore, the presence of a popliteal pulse should not preclude further investigations where indicated.

Although areas of cyanosis or peripheral necrosis also indicate arterial insufficiency, it is more common to detect hair loss, cool feet, and thinning of the skin. The presence of dependency rubor, where the foot is red and flushed when below heart level, and elevation pallor, where the skin of the foot blanches and becomes pale on elevation above the arterial inflow pressure, is a simple clinical test to establish the presence of reduced arterial inflow to the feet.

Medial arterial calcification is another common finding in diabetic patients and can be recognized on radiographs by its pipe-stem appearance.[37] Medial arterial calcification is reported to be associated with diabetic peripheral somatosensory and autonomic neuropathy[46, 58] and is more prevalent with increasing age, duration of diabetes, and serum creatinine. Medial arterial calcification is significantly associated with an increased prevalence of cardiovascular mortality,[71, 85, 116] although this may also be related to the increase in medial arterial calcification associated with diabetic nephropathy, which is an independent marker of increased mortality in diabetes.[72] Medial arterial calcification, when present, is known to alter the pulse waveform, resulting in a uniphasic, high-pitched, fast-velocity waveform, and falsely elevated ankle pressures in diabetic patients even in the presence of occlusive peripheral vascular disease diagnosed by other methods.[23, 29, 42] However, although it is not thought to adversely affect tissue oxygenation in the foot, it is known that diabetic patients undergoing major amputation have higher ankle pressures than nondiabetic amputees with peripheral vascular disease, and this is believed to be caused by the effect of medial arterial calcification on ankle systolic pressures. A recent semiquantitative survey of medial arterial calcification in the diabetic foot has demonstrated that medial arterial calcification is present in diabetic patients with ankle systolic pressures as low as 50 mm Hg.[171] It also demonstrated that medial arterial calcification is more prevalent in the ankle region than in the forefoot. For this reason, toe systolic pressure measurements might be less prone to interference from medial arterial calcification than ankle pressure measurements. A recent study that demonstrated that toe systolic pressures are reduced in diabetic patients with peripheral neuropathy, despite normal or increased ankle systolic pressures, would support this view.[152] However, toe pressures are considerably more difficult and time-consuming to measure than ankle pressures and the equipment required, a

laser Doppler or impedance plethysmograph, is not available in most centers. For these reasons, they are not in routine use.

Despite these problems, if used appropriately, ankle pressures still have a place in the diagnosis of peripheral vascular disease. The ankle/brachial pressure index is usually around 1 to 1.2. A level of less than 0.9 is usually taken to be indicative of occlusive arterial disease. A level of less than 0.3 or an ankle systolic pressure of less than 50 mm Hg is indicative of critical ischemia in the presence of tissue damage or rest pain. The equivalent toe pressure systolic is 30 mm Hg or less.[133] All cases where the ankle systolic pressure is low can be accepted as indicative of occlusive vascular disease. If the ankle systolic pressure is more than 75 mm Hg above the brachial systolic pressure, then this is highly indicative of medial arterial calcification, and the ankle pressure cannot be used to indicate lower extremity arterial disease.[120] In all other cases, and particularly in elderly and neuropathic diabetic patients, an ankle systolic pressure or ankle/brachial pressure index that is normal or elevated should be interpreted with caution.

Segmental Pressures and Doppler Waveform Analysis

More sophisticated methods of Doppler ultrasound screening for peripheral vascular disease include segmental Doppler pressures and Doppler waveform analysis. By measuring systolic pressures above and below the knee as well as in the foot it is possible to estimate the site of an arterial occlusion, but this is no substitute for angiography in determining the suitability of a patient for surgery. Doppler waveform analysis and duplex scanning adds significant information by measuring flow velocity and direction in addition to systolic pressures. Localized fast turbulent flow (>160 cm/s) indicates the site of a stenosis of more than 70% of luminal area.[109] Unidirectional or attenuated flow suggests failure of perfusion. High-pitched unidirectional flow is, however, also often found in association with medial arterial calcification. By comparing flow velocity and cross-sectional area at a number of sites, Doppler waveform analysis and duplex scanning can give functional information about the site and degree of stenosis, and they are commonly used in the carotid arteries to estimate carotid stenoses before surgery. At present, it is as accurate as angiography for locating single stenoses above the popliteal segment, but it is less reliable at locating multiple stenoses and stenoses below the popliteal segment. Therefore, it is only used as an alternative to diagnostic angiography in a small number of centers. Both techniques are, however, routinely used in graft surveillance programs to monitor the patency of bypass grafts.

Transcutaneous Oxygen Tension

Transcutaneous oxygen ($tcPO_2$) measurements are increasingly being used to determine tissue viability in patients with ulceration and incipient gangrene. Perilesional measurements can be used in isolation or as a chest/foot ratio to allow for systemic hypoxia in patients with chronic obstructive airway disease and other chest problems. Unlike ankle pressure measurements, transcutaneous oxygen tensions do not seem to be influenced by medial arterial calcification.[18] A value of less than 50 mm Hg would be suggestive of ischemia. Peri-ulcer transcutaneous oxygen levels of less than 30 mm Hg (4 kPa) are indicative of tissue that is 39 times less likely to heal without revascularization than peri-ulcer areas with higher $tcPO_2$. In practice, this measurement has been used to determine the need for revascularization or amputation, and indeed the level of amputation, in diabetic patients.[125]

Plain Radiography

Standard x-ray films can be used to demonstrate the extent of medial arterial calcification and thus to determine the usefulness of Doppler pressure measurements.

Magnetic Resonance Angiography

The techniques of magnetic resonance angiography (MRA) have been used in cerebral circulatory and cardiac assessment. Rapid reversal sequence imaging using high resolution coils delineates moving blood flow while suppressing background static tissue. At present, MRA tends to overestimate the presence of stenoses if turbulent flow creates slow moving eddies and therefore apparent filling defects in the column of blood. For this reason, the reliability of MRA in diabetic patients and smaller lower limb arteries remains to be clarified, especially in routine clinical use.[103]

Arteriography

Despite advances in ultrasound, angioscopy, and magnetic resonance imaging, arteriography is widely regarded as the gold standard of techniques for the diagnosis of occlusive vascular disease. This is principally because it provides structural information for surgical reconstruction or angioplasty by clearly delineating the site of arterial occlusion or stenosis anatomically. Angiography does not provide any functional information and should always be interpreted in the context of the clinical condition of each patient.

Good quality angiographic images are difficult to obtain in many patients and, because of the potential adverse renal effects of intravenous contrast, arterial puncture angiography should only be performed in centers with adequate facilities and sufficient numbers of patients to ensure adequate experience in the technique. This is particularly true of angioplasty. Although it is recognized that many diabetic patients have tibioperoneal occlusions, distal runoff vessels may reform at the ankle or dorsal arch. Therefore, all angiograms in diabetic patients should examine the vascular tree to the toes.

Intra-arterial puncture and angioplasty may release showers of debris from disrupted atheromatous plaques, causing distal embolization. The likelihood of distal embolization may be minimized by listening for bruits at the femoral puncture site, visualizing the puncture site with ultrasound, or using intravenous rather than intra-arterial contrast injections. Intravenous contrast is, however, less desirable because of the superior images obtained with intra-arterial digital subtraction arteriography, which also usually requires lower doses of contrast. Despite this and the use of nonionic contrast media, there is still a significant risk of contrast nephropathy, which can occur in up to 40% of angiograms in diabetic patients with proteinuria and renal impairment.[59] For this reason, all angiograms in diabetic patients should be performed with the patient well hydrated, and an intravenous infusion should be running before and after the procedure.[68]

THERAPY FOR PERIPHERAL VASCULAR DISEASE

Nonpharmacologic Therapy

The best advice for any stable patient with claudication and no evidence of tissue loss is to stop smoking and keep walking. There is considerable evidence that to be effective, the patient should walk to the point of claudicating and even some distance with claudication.

It is believed that this may encourage the proliferation of collateral circulation.[68]

Although the long-term benefit is a disputed area among vascular surgeons, reconstructive surgery for diabetic patients with claudication should be considered if walking distance reduces and before the onset of tissue loss. A recent survey has clearly demonstrated an improved quality of life for such patients.[126] Reducing claudication distance is a sign of impending critical ischemia in diabetic patients who have a greater tendency to early and more aggressive progression of arterial disease. Diabetic patients also have a higher amputation rate for similar initial grades of arterial disease than nondiabetic patients.[102] There is such clear evidence that tissue loss has a significantly adverse effect on limb prognosis that surgery before the onset of critical ischemia has its advocates in many centers.

In common with all patients with at-risk diabetic feet, those patients with peripheral vascular disease should be educated about general foot care and appropriate shoes. This education should preferably be performed in small groups or as individual one-to-one education and be repeated regularly.[40] Routine chiropody should be arranged, particularly if the patient is partially sighted or lives alone without a spouse to care for the feet.

Some authorities also recommend weight loss, which will at least make vascular access or postamputation mobilization easier if surgery is required; a low-fat diet; modest alcohol consumption; reduced salt diet, perhaps to aid blood pressure control; and vitamins A, C, and E to reduce the risk of atheroma plaque fissuring and thrombotic arterial occlusion.[3] Little clinical evidence supports the effectiveness of these recommendations.

Pharmacologic Therapy

Antihypertensive Therapy. As outlined above, uncontrolled hypertension is one of the principal predictors of progression of peripheral vascular disease. No study has shown a direct reduction in amputation rate from blood pressure control but, particularly in view of the association between proteinuria and vascular disease in diabetic patients, blood pressure control is likely to be a priority. The treatment of blood pressure in diabetic patients with peripheral disease is more complicated than in nondiabetic patients. Therapy with ACE inhibitors needs careful monitoring as significant renal artery disease may be found in up to 50% of diabetic patients with peripheral vascular disease. Beta-blockers are not wholly contraindicated in peripheral vascular disease but should be reviewed regularly after prescription.[148]

Lipid Lowering Therapy. The scant evidence comparing diabetic and nondiabetic subjects suggests that there is no difference, in terms of correction of dyslipidemia, between the response of diabetic and nondiabetic patients to lipid lowering therapy. However, although the role of lipid lowering therapy is clear in patients after myocardial infarction, there is as yet no "4S" (Scandinavian Simvastatin Survival Study) equivalent in evaluating the effectiveness of lipid lowering therapy in patients with peripheral vascular disease.[134]

Aspirin. In a similar situation to that outlined for lipid-lowering therapy, although there is good evidence for the effectiveness of aspirin in the treatment of unstable angina, myocardial infarction, and transient ischemic attacks, it has yet to be proved that aspirin saves legs or improves claudication distance.[5] Despite this lack of formal scientific evidence, aspirin is now commonly prescribed in hope and on theoretical grounds. In addition, because of the widespread nature of diabetic vascular disease, there may be tangible benefits in protecting the cardiac and cerebral circulation.

Formal Anticoagulation. Administration of warfarin is the usual practice after synthetic grafting, but it probably has little to offer in routine clinical use for diabetic patients with peripheral vascular disease.[3]

Oxpentifylline. Case reports still emerge with one or two patients in whom oxpentifylline is considered to be of benefit. These are probably exceptions, and controlled trials continually suggest that there is little or no worthwhile additional benefit from its use.[83] If oxpentifylline is tried, then there is probably a delay of at least 6 to 8 weeks before any benefit can be expected.

Vasodilators. The main determinant of blood flow in end arteries is the degree of proximal stenosis. In critical and exercise induced ischemia, distal hypoxia is likely to be a stimulus to maximal dilatation of distal vessels. In addition, at least theoretically, vasodilatation beyond a fixed stenosis is likely to worsen blood flow across the stenosis, as seen with aortic stenosis and ACE inhibitor therapy. For these reasons, vasodilators, including calcium channel antagonists, would appear to have little to offer in the management of intermittent claudication on first principles, and this seems to be borne out in clinical trials.[21, 148]

Naftidrofuryl. The efficacy of naftidrofuryl is yet to be proved beyond doubt.

CRITICAL ISCHEMIA

The definition of critical ischemia causes particular problems when applied to diabetic patients. Rest pain is a hallmark of critical ischemia and yet may be absent in diabetic patients with concomitant peripheral neuropathy.[154] The ankle pressure may be falsely elevated and therefore remain above the usual cutoff of an ankle pressure of less than 50 mm Hg or an ankle-brachial systolic ratio of less than 0.3. As described previously, a toe systolic pressure of less than 30 mm Hg can be used, but this is not available in routine practice in most centers. Similarly a perilesional tcPO$_2$ of less than 30 mm Hg (4 kPa) is not a routine measurement in most centers. Significant occlusive vascular disease, particularly proximal disease, can be present in diabetic patients with clinical signs of vascular disease even when there are palpable pulses.[4, 140] Even areas of tissue necrosis can be misleading, because digital infarction can occur in infected toes even when the arterial supply is adequate.[39] However, most digital necrosis and areas of tissue necrosis elsewhere on the foot are likely to be indicators of inadequate arterial inflow.

Clinicians must keep a high index of suspicion for the presence of critical ischemia in diabetic patients because all the standard tests might be misleading. Therefore, in the absence of adequate, reliable simple clinical measures, it has been advocated that a diabetic foot ulcer showing no signs of healing after 6 weeks of optimal medical management is an indication for an urgent referral to vascular surgery.

Initial Management of Critical Ischemia

Despite the increasing trend for successful outpatient management of diabetic foot disease, patients with critical ischemia require admission to hospital. All such patients should be treated as though the ulcer is infected, because clinical signs may be modified by the ischemia and diabetes. Control of infection in such cases

means the use of broad-spectrum antibiotics, with emphasis on antistreptococcal and staphylococcal cover. Combination therapy for initial blind treatment of deep infection might be ampicillin, flucloxacillin and metronidazole, or ciprofloxacin and metronidazole, or ciprofloxacin and clindamycin, although this is often based on personal choice rather than hard scientific evidence.[158] Similarly, diabetes control should be optimized if possible, because there is evidence to suggest that healing is impaired with poor blood glucose control, although this does not necessarily mean a need for insulin in a patient who does not take insulin.

Heparinization. A small-scale study of low-molecular-weight heparin has demonstrated additional benefit in critical ischemia and ulcer healing time in diabetic patients.[75] It is a common clinical practice to give heparin to patients with critical ischemia, but again this seems to be based on anecdote and clinical experience, not truly evidence-based trials.

Prostacyclin. Prostacyclin is often prescribed on theoretical grounds in critical ischemia and has a limited degree of success in Buerger's disease.[47] To date, prostacyclin infusions have not been proved to prevent amputations, although they may prove to be a possible adjuvant in minimizing tissue loss and reducing ischemic rest pain in patients not suitable for reconstructive surgery. However, many of these patients are frail and elderly, and the side effects of prostacyclin infusions may be poorly tolerated, particularly if higher doses are used.[62] In addition, for state-funded health care systems, the cost of such infusions may be prohibitive.

Thrombolysis. Intra-arterial thrombolysis may achieve recanalization of acute arterial thromboses in 60% of cases if the limb is still viable when therapy commences, that is, still sensate, motor function present, and capillary return present.[34] Unfortunately, such a situation is rare in clinical practice, and thrombolysis tends to be performed in centers of interest rather than being generally adopted as first-line therapy for critical ischemia.[130]

Sympathectomy. Chemical sympathectomy is often used by surgeons when they do not wish to perform reconstructive surgery. Neuropathic and neuroischemic diabetic patients usually have an associated peripheral autonomic neuropathy, and, therefore, have had an "autosympathectomy," which makes such an approach superfluous.[142, 174] The role of sympathectomy in pure ischemia is difficult to determine because of the lack of effective controlled trials.

Reconstructive Surgery and Limb Salvage in the Diabetic Patient

Despite the cost of interventional radiology, reconstructive surgery, and reoperating or redoing angioplasty for recurrent disease, it is always less expensive to try to save a limb than to remove a limb if the patient has a reasonable life expectancy. Rehabilitation and social costs mean that each amputation can cost in excess of £25,000 ($18,000).[164] Thus, it is financially as well as clinically important to try to reduce amputations.

INTERVENTIONAL RADIOLOGY IN THE ISCHEMIC DIABETIC LIMB

Angioplasty. The technique of percutaneous transluminal angioplasty using an inflatable balloon was first described in 1976.[64] Positioned at the site of an atheromatous narrowing within an artery, the balloon stretches the vessel, thus splitting the plaque and restoring luminal area. Re-endothelialization then has to occur over the fissured plaque, and it is usual to use intravenous heparin to prevent thrombotic occlusion in the first 24 hours after angioplasty. In general, the success rate for recanalization of an arterial occlusion by angioplasty is proportionate to the length of stenosis or thrombosis. Recanalization can usually be achieved in more than 90% of short stenoses in appropriately skilled hands.[97] Even a good technical result with total recanalization of an occluded vessel does not always lead to clinical improvement in the limb if the distal runoff is poor, and this may require further treatment to the distal vessels. Angioplasty has been performed at the level of the tibial and peroneal arteries since 1982 and may be the first-line therapy in patients with other medical conditions or in whom vein is not available for distal bypass.[26]

Arterial tears and early thrombotic occlusion are the main adverse events associated with angioplasty. Fortunately, the incidence of these problems is low. However, there remains a problem with long-term reocclusion. Even in technically successful angioplasties with good runoff, intimal hyperplasia or recurrence of native disease leads to reocclusion rates that approach 50% overall, depending on the duration of follow-up. However, these rates are similar in diabetic and nondiabetic patients. Re-angioplasty may be possible, and, even if a vessel does restenose or occlude, there may have been sufficient duration of improved circulation to facilitate healing or to allow a plane of tissue viability to establish or lead to the closure of the lesion. Once a lesion is closed, the blood supply requirements may be lower than those for an ulcerated limb, and limb salvage rates are usually higher than patency rates in most series.

There is evidence that in iliac vessels or situations where restenosis is likely, stenting the artery wall can prevent re-occlusion.[73, 121] Iliac angioplasty with or without stenting can also be used to increase arterial inflow to the limb and improve the chances of a lower bypass remaining patent.

Atherectomy. It is rare to achieve a successful angioplasty result in arterial stenoses and occlusions of more than 10 cm in length.[97] For this reason, atherectomy has been attempted in such cases to remove the plaque. Atherectomy can lead to distal embolization of atheroma material. Although the 1-year patency rate achieved in most series is less than 50%, for the reasons outlined in the previous section, this may enable tissue closure and limb salvage. It is probably best reserved for centers with experience in this technique at present.[34]

SURGICAL MANAGEMENT OF ISCHEMIC DIABETIC LIMBS

Indications for Revascularization. Many surgeons talk of an aggressive limb salvage approach in the management of the ischemic diabetic limb.[57] Such an approach is often, and probably should always be, based on appropriate patient selection. The patient should be expected to have a reasonable life expectancy. It should be remembered that concomitant cardiac and cerebrovascular disease are likely to result in death in more than 50% of amputees within 5 years. It is the practice of many American surgeons to attend to these vascular beds at the same time as or before revascularization of the lower limbs.[45] To follow such a policy requires greater resources than are likely to be available in most state-funded health care systems. In general, the patient must be able to undergo what is usually a lengthy operation, particularly for distal bypass, and pre-existing lung or cardiac pathology may limit the ability of the patient to withstand the operation or limit its effectiveness. If the patient has a low functional capacity with poor potential for rehabilitation beyond a wheelchair, then such an approach is not tenable. Similarly, if the patient is not motivated to walk or to stop smoking, the graft patency will be jeopardized.

If surgery to vessels below the knee is required, then this has to be performed with a vein as the conduit. Synthetic grafts, even with vein cuffs, have such low patency rates as to render attempts at below-knee reconstructive surgery using such materials pointless.[19, 90] If the leg veins are varicosed or have been harvested for coronary artery grafting, then arm vein can be used but this adds to the technical aspects and duration of the operation. If a short length of vein can be found, popliteal artery to foot bypass may be almost as successful as femoral artery to distal bypass.[128] Similarly, the patient must have suitable anatomy with adequate inflow and a patent foot vessel on which to graft. If the nature and extent of infection and necrosis is such that it encroaches on the potential graft site, then again the likelihood is that the graft will fail, once again highlighting the need for control of infection.

Any center that wishes to perform reconstructive surgery, particularly distal surgery, needs a graft surveillance program to assess the clinical progress of patients and to audit results. In the follow-up period, the other vascular trees, coronary and carotid arteries, and the other limb may need attention to reduce the coexisting morbidity and mortality and to improve patient outcomes.

The nature of diabetes as a systemic disorder usually implies that in those patients requiring reconstructive surgery, there are other associated complications. Intensive care time is often longer in diabetic patients, and the perioperative management of diabetes control, cardiac and renal impairment, and radiologic investigation require a team approach to the management of surgery in such patients.[69]

Proximal Arterial Reconstruction. These operations are divided into inflow procedures, usually aortoiliac surgery, where synthetic graft materials are usually used, and where, because of high flow rates, the graft patency is excellent. For aortobifemoral grafts, the 5-year patency rate is commonly more than 85%. The patency of aortobifemoral grafts is the same in the diabetic and nondiabetic patient, but, because of associated cardiovascular disease,

overall patient survival rates are lower in diabetic patients.

Reconstructive surgery below the inguinal ligament is usually referred to as an outflow procedure. The usual operation is the femoropopliteal bypass graft around a superficial femoral occlusion. Synthetic graft materials can be used for these operations, but vein grafts have better secondary patency rates. Regardless of the conduit used, the long-term patency depends on the flow rate through the graft, which in turn is influenced by the runoff vessels. In most series, the 5-year patency averages 70%, although reoperation and redo-angioplasty rates are higher in diabetic patients in some series.[9] Despite the predilection for vascular disease to be multilevel and to affect the infrapopliteal vessels in diabetes, there appears to be no significant difference in patency rates between diabetic and nondiabetic patients. This may be because of patient selection, but there also is some evidence that femoral disease and distal disease do not always coexist in diabetic patients. In addition, because of high coexisting mortality, graft patency may exceed the life expectancy of the patient.[9]

Distal Reconstructive Operations. These operations are all outflow procedures performed to vessels below the popliteal artery. As outlined above, autologous vein is the only suitable conduit for these procedures, which can limit the suitability of many patients for surgery. In general, these operations are performed for limb salvage. If a tibial or pedal vessel is present on intra-arterial digital subtraction angiography, then it is a cost-effective alternative to primary amputation in suitable patients.[123] The flow rate may mean that in many cases the graft may have failed by 1 year, but the limb can be saved if the lesion has closed and, in selected centers, 5-year limb salvage rates approach 85% despite a graft patency of only 68%.[128]

Amputations. Despite the increased availability of distal reconstructive surgery and interventional radiologic techniques, not all amputations are avoidable. However, as a counsel of perfection, every diabetic patient with actual or suspected peripheral vascular disease should be reviewed by a vascular surgeon before an amputation is contemplated.[138] In many cases, reconstructive surgery may limit the extent of the amputation or the level of amputation that can be accurately assessed. It is rarely necessary for amputations to be performed as an emergency procedure, and the operation should be planned and performed, or at least supervised, by a senior surgeon.

In simple terms, a better quality stump leads to better quality rehabilitation and increases the likelihood of successful walking after amputation.[159] At present, the overall picture is disappointing. It is unclear how many diabetic patients who have amputations die shortly after operation, or because of comorbidity, are never referred to limb centers. The patients who are referred are generally believed to be younger and fitter than those who are not referred. However, even in this group of selected patients, the mortality rate is high and ambulation low. A study from Northwest England has highlighted that 18 months after amputation, 24% of amputees referred to the Disablement Services Centre for limb fitting had died, and of the survivors only 50% were walking using their artificial limbs.[27] The reasons for low limb-walking rates include cardiac disease, stump volume changes (particularly in nephropathic patients), stump injuries (resulting from associated neuropathy), and problems fitting the limb because of associated poor vision or cheiroarthropathy.[159]

Once an amputation has been performed, the contralateral limb requires particular care. Up to 66% of remaining limbs may develop ulceration or gangrene in the first year after amputation, and the rate of bilateral amputation approaches 50% after 3 years.[136] A coordinated approach to the podiatric, diabetic and other medical needs of diabetic amputees, sadly lacking in most centers, can significantly improve the fate of the remaining limb[2, 50] and should be recommended to all centers providing diabetic foot care and amputee rehabilitation.

References

1. Abbott CA, Vileikyte L, Carrington A, et al. Mobility and mortality in diabetic and peripheral vascular disease unilateral lower limb amputees. Diabetic Med 1995; 12(suppl 2):S36
2. Abbott CA, Carrington AL, Boulton AJM. Reduced bilateral amputation rate in diabetic patients: Effect of a foot care clinic. Diabetic Med 1996; 13(suppl 7):S45.
3. Allen BT, Anderson CB, Walker WB, et al. Vascular surgery. In Levin ME, O'Neal LW (ed): The Diabetic Foot. St Louis, Mosby–Year Book, 1988, pp 385–422.
4. Andros G, Harris RW, Dulawa LB, et al. The need for arteriography in diabetic patients with gangrene and palpable pulses. Arch Surg 1984; 119:1260.
5. Antiplatelet Trialists' Collaboration. Collaborative overview of randomised trials of antiplatelet therapy. I: Prevention of death, myocardial infarction and stroke by prolonged antiplatelet therapy in various categories of patients. Br Med J 1994; 308:81–106.
6. Auwerx J, Bouillon R, Collen D, et al. Tissue-type plasminogen activator antigen and plasminogen activator inhibitor in diabetes mellitus. Arteriosclerosis 1988; 8:68–72.
7. Barrett-Connor E, Witzam JL, Holdbrook M. Plasma lipids and diabetes mellitus in an adult community. Am J Epidemiol 1983; 117:186–192.
8. Barrett-Connor E, Wingard DL, Criqui MH, et al. Is borderline hyperglycaemia a risk factor for cardiovascular disease? J Chronic Dis 1984; 37:773–779.
9. Bartlett FF, Gibbons GW, Wheelock FC. Aortic reconstruction for occlusive disease: Comparable results in diabetics. Arch Surg 1986; 121:1150–1153.
10. Bays HE, Pfeifer MA. Peripheral diabetic neuropathy. Med Clin North Am 1988; 72:1439–1464.
11. Beach KW, Strandness DE. Arteriosclerosis obliterans and associated risk factors in insulin dependent and non-insulin dependent diabetes. Diabetes 1980; 29:882–888.
12. Brand PN, Abbott RD, Kannel WB. Diabetes, intermittent claudication and risk of cardiovascular events: The Framingham study. Diabetes 1989; 38:504–509.
13. Brownlee M, Cerami A, Vlassara H. Advanced glycation end products in tissue and the biochemical basis of diabetic complications. N Engl J Med 1988; 318:1315–1321.
14. Cameron NE, Cotter MA, Robertson S. Chronic low frequency electrical activation for one week corrects nerve conduction velocity deficits in rats with diabetes of three months duration. Diabetologia 1989; 32:759–761.
15. Cameron NE, Cotter MA, Low PA. Nerve blood flow in early experimental diabetes in rats: Relation to conduction deficits. Am J Physiol 1992; 261:E1–E8.
16. Cameron NE, Cotter MA, Robertson S. Angiotensin converting enzyme inhibition prevents development of muscle and nerve dysfunction and stimulates angiogenesis in streptozotocin-diabetic rats. Diabetologia 1992; 35:12–18.
17. Cameron NE, Cotter MA. Potential therapeutic approaches to the treatment or prevention of diabetic peripheral neuropathy: Evidence from experimental studies. Diabetic Med 1993; 10:593–605.
18. Chanteleau E, Ma XY, Herrnberger S, et al. Effect of medial arterial calcification on O_2 supply to exercising diabetic feet. Diabetes 1990; 39:513–516.
19. Cheshire NJW, Wolfe JHN, Noone MA, et al. The economics of femorocrural reconstruction for critical leg ischaemia with and without autologous vein. J Vasc Surg 1992; 15:167–175.
20. Clements RS, Bell DSH. Diagnostic, pathogenetic and therapeutic aspects of diabetic neuropathy. Special Topics Endocrinol Metab 1982; 2:1–42.
21. Coffman JD. Vasodilator drugs in peripheral vascular disease. N Engl J Med 1979; 300:713–717.
22. Colwell JA, Halushka PV, Sarji KE, et al. Platelet function and diabetes mellitus. Med Clin North Am 1978; 62:753–766.
23. Cutajar CL, Marston A, Newcombe JF. Value of cuff occlusion pressures in assessment of peripheral vascular disease. BMJ 1973; 2:392–395.
24. Dallinger KJC, Jennings PE, Toop MJ, et al. Platelet aggregation and coagulation in insulin dependent diabetics with and without microangiopathy. Diabetic Med 1987; 4:44–48.
25. DCCT Research Group. The effect of intensive treatment of diabetes on the development and progression

of long term complications in insulin dependent diabetes mellitus. N Engl J Med 1993; 329:977–986.

26. Dean MRE. Percutaneous transluminal angioplasty of the popliteal and posterior tibial arteries. *In* Vecht RJ (ed): Angioplasty. London, Pitman, 1984, pp 34–47.

27. Deerochanawong C, Home PD, Alberti KGMM. A survey of lower limb amputation in diabetic patients. Diabetic Med 1992; 9:942–946.

28. Diabetes Drafting Group. Prevalence of small vessel and large vessel disease in diabetic patients from 14 centres. The WHO multinational study of vascular disease in diabetics. Diabetologia 1985; 28:615–640.

29. Dormandy J (ed). European Consensus Document on Critical Limb Ischaemia. Berlin, Springer Verlag, 1989.

30. Dornan TL, Rhymes IL, Cederholm-Williams SA, et al. Plasma hemostatic factors and diabetic retinopathy. Eur J Clin Invest 1983; 13:231–235.

31. Ducimetiere P, Eschwage E, Papoz L, et al. Relationship of plasma insulin levels to the incidence of myocardial infarction and coronary heart disease mortality in a middle-aged population. Diabetologia 1980; 19:205–210.

32. Dvorak HF, Brown LF, Detmar M, et al. Vascular permeability factor/vascular endothelial growth factor, microvascular hyperpermeability, and angiogenesis. Am J Pathol 1995; 146:1029–1039.

33. Dyck PJ. Hypoxic neuropathy: Does hypoxia play a role in diabetic neuropathy? Neurology 1989; 39:111–118.

34. Dyet JF. High speed rotational angioplasty in occluded peripheral arteries. J Intervent Radiol 1992; 172:725–730.

35. Earnshaw JJ, Westby JC, Gregson RHS. Local thrombolytic therapy of acute peripheral ischaemia with tissue plasminogen activator: A dose ranging study. Br J Surg 1988; 75:1196–1200.

36. Ebskov B, Josephsen P: Incidence of reamputation and death after gangrene of the lower extremity. Prosthet Orthot Int 1980; 4:77–80.

37. Edmonds ME, Morrison N, Laws JW, et al. Medial arterial calcification and diabetic neuropathy. BMJ 1982; 284:928–930.

38. Edmonds ME, Blundell MP, Morris ME, et al. Improved survival of the diabetic foot: The role of the specialist foot clinic. QJ Med 1986; 232:763–771.

39. Edmonds M, Foster A, Greenhill M, et al. Acute septic vasculitis not diabetic microangiopathy leads to digital necrosis in the neuropathic foot. Diabetic Med 1992; 9(suppl 1):P85.

40. Edmonds ME, van Acker K, Foster AVM. Education and the diabetic foot. Diabetic Med 1996; 13(suppl 1):S61–S64.

41. Eisenberg RC, Bank WO, Hedgecock MW. Renal failure after major arteriography. AJR 1981; 136:859–862.

42. Emanuele MA, Buchanan BJ, Abraira C. Elevated leg systolic pressures and arterial calcification in diabetic occlusive vascular disease. Diabetes Care 1981; 4:289–292.

43. Ericsson CG, Hamsten A, Nilsson J, et al. Angiographic assessment of the effects of bezafibrate on progression of coronary artery disease in young male post-infarction patients. Lancet 1996; 347:849–853.

44. Eschwage E, Ducimetiere P, Papoz L, et al. Blood glucose and coronary heart disease. Lancet 1980; 2:472–473.

45. Estes JM, Pomposelli FB. Lower extremity arterial reconstruction in patients with diabetes mellitus. Diabetic Med 1996; 13(suppl 1):S43–S57.

46. Everhart JE, Pettitt DJ, Knowler WC, et al. Medial arterial calcification and its association with mortality and complications of diabetes. Diabetologia 1988; 31:16–23.

47. Fiessinger JN, Schafer M. Trial of iloprost versus aspirin treatment for critical limb ischaemia thromboangiitis obliterans. Lancet 1990; 335:555–557.

48. Fisher BM, Quin JD, Rumley A, et al. Effects of acute insulin-induced hypoglycaemia on hemostasis, fibrinolysis and hemorheology in insulin-dependent diabetic patients and control subjects. Clin Sci 1991; 80:525–531.

49. Fontbonne AM, et al. Insulin and cardiovascular disease: A Paris prospective study. Diabetes Care 1991; 6:461–469.

50. Foster A, Fraser S, Walters H, et al. Improving the outlook of diabetic amputees. Diabetic Med 1995; 12(suppl 2):S36

51. Fuller JH, Shipley MJ, Rose G, et al. Mortality from coronary heart disease and stroke in relation to degree of glycaemia: The Whitehall Study. J Chronic Dis 1979; 32:721–728.

52. Fuller JH, Keen H, Jarrett RJ, et al. Haemostatic variables associated with diabetes and its complications. BMJ 1979; 2:964–966.

53. Ganda OP, Arkin CF. Hyperfibrinogenemia: An important risk factor for vascular complications in diabetes. Diabetes Care 1992; 15:1245–1250.

54. Garcia Frade LJ, de la Calle H, Torade MC, et al. Hypofibrinolysis associated with vasculopathy in non-insulin dependent diabetes mellitus. Thromb Res 1990; 59:51–59.

55. Garcia ML, McNamara PM, Gordon T, et al. Morbidity and mortality in diabetics in Framingham population: Sixteen year follow up study. Diabetes 1974; 23:105–111.

56. Gerrard JM, Stuart MJ, Rao GHR. Alteration in the balance of prostaglandin and thromboxane synthesis in diabetic rats. J Lab Clin Med 1980; 95:950–958.

57. Gibbons GW. Vascular surgery: Its role in foot salvage. *In* Boulton AJM, Connor H, Cavanagh PR (eds): The Foot in Diabetes. Chichester, U.K., John Wiley and Sons, 1994, pp 177–190.

58. Goebel F-D, Fuessi HS. Mönckeberg's sclerosis after sympathetic denervation in diabetic and non-diabetic subjects. Diabetologia 1983; 24:348–350.

59. Gomes AS, Low JF, Baker JD, et al. Acute renal dysfunction in high risk patients after angiographic comparison of ionic and non-ionic contrast media. Radiology 1989; 170:65–68.

60. Grant PJ, Medcalf RL. Hormonal regulation of hemostasis and the molecular biology of the fibrinolytic system. Clin Sci 1990; 78:3–11.

61. Grant PJ. Disorders of the fibrinolytic system in diabetes mellitus. Treating Diabetes 1991; 34:8–11.

62. Grant SM, Goa KL. Iloprost: A review of its pharmacodynamic and pharmacokinetic properties. Drugs 1992; 43:889–924.

63. Greene DA, Lattimer SA, Sima AAF. Are disturbances of sorbitol, phosphoinositide, and Na^+-K^+-ATPase regulation involved in pathogenesis of diabetic neuropathy? Diabetes 1988; 37:688–693.

64. Gruntzig A. Die perkutane Rekanalization chronischer arterieller Veschlusse (Dotter Princip) mit einem neuen Dilationskatheter. ROFO 1976; 124:80.

65. Haffner SM, Morales PA, Stern MP, et al. Lp(a) concentrations in NIDDM. Diabetes 1992; 41:1267–1272.

66. Haffner SM. Lipoprotein(a) and diabetes. Diabetes Care 1993; 16:835–840.

67. Halushka PV, Rogers RC, Loadholt CB, et al. In-

creased platelet thromboxane synthesis in diabetes mellitus. J Lab Clin Med 1981; 97:87–96.

68. Hiatt WR, Regensteiner JG, Hargaten ME, et al. Benefit of exercise conditioning for patients with peripheral arterial disease. Circulation 1990; 81:602–609.

69. Hirsch IB, White PF. Medical management of surgical patients with diabetes. In Levin ME, O'Neal LW (eds): The Diabetic Foot. St Louis, Mosby–Year Book, 1988, pp 423–432.

70. Hunter GC, Song GW, Nayak NN, et al. Peripheral nerve conduction abnormalities in lower extremity ischemia: The effects of revascularisation. J Surg Res 1988; 45:96–103

71. Janka HU, Stadl E, Mehnert H. Peripheral vascular disease in diabetes mellitus and its relation to cardiovascular risk factors: Screening with Doppler ultrasonic technique. Diabetes Care 1980; 3:207–213.

72. Jensen T, Borch-Johnsen K, Kofoed-Enevoldsen A, et al. Coronary heart disease in young type 1 (insulin-dependent) diabetic patients with and without diabetic nephropathy: Incidence and risk factors. Diabetologia 1987; 30:144–148.

73. Joffre F, Rousseau H, Puel J. Arterial stenting. J Intervent Radiol 1989; 4:155–159.

74. Johnson M, Harrison HE, Raftery AT, et al. Vascular prostacyclin may be reduced in diabetes in man. Lancet 1979; 1:325–326

75. Jorneskog G, Brismar K, Fagrel B. Low molecular weight heparin seems to improve local capillary circulation and healing of chronic foot ulcers in diabetic patients. Vasa 1993; 22:137–142.

76. Joslin EP: The menace of diabetic gangrene. N Engl J Med 1934; 211:16–20.

77. Jude E, Shaw J, Chalmers N, et al. Peripheral vascular disease (PVD) in diabetic and non-diabetic patients: A comparison. Diabetic Med 1996; 13(suppl 7):P71.

78. Juhan-Vague I, Roul C, Alessi MC, et al. Increased plasminogen activator inhibitor activity in insulin dependent diabetic patients: Relationship with plasma insulin and the acute phase response. Thromb Haemostas 1989; 61:370–373.

79. Juhan-Vague I, Alessi MC, Vague P. Increased plasma plasminogen activator inhibitor 1 levels. A possible link between insulin resistance and atherothrombosis. Diabetologia 1991; 34:457–462.

80. Karpen CW, Pritchard KA, Merola AJ, et al. Alterations of the prostacyclin-thromboxane ratio in streptozotocin-induced diabetic rats. Prostaglandins Leukot Med 1982; 8:93–103.

81. Keen H, the Gamma-Linolenic Acid Multicentre Trial Group. Treatment of diabetic neuropathy with gamma-linolenic acid. Diabetes Care 1993; 16:8–15

82. Knezevic W, Mastalgia FL. Neuropathy associated with Brescia-Cimino arteriovenous fistulas. Arch Neurol 1984; 41:1184–1192.

83. Kokesh J, Kazmers A, Zierler RE. Pentoxifylline in the nonoperative management of intermittent claudication. Ann Vasc Surg 1991; 5:66–70.

84. Laakso M, Pyorala K. Lipid and lipoprotein abnormalities in diabetic patients with peripheral vascular disease. Atherosclerosis 1988; 74:55–63.

85. Lachman AS, Spray TL, Kerwin DM, et al. Medial calcinosis of Mönckeberg: A review of the problem and a description of a patient with involvement of peripheral, visceral and coronary arteries. Am J Med 1977; 63:615–622.

86. Landin K, Tengborn L, Chmielewska J, et al. The acute effect of insulin on tissue plasminogen activator and plasminogen activator inhibitor in man. Thromb Haemost 1991; 65:130–133.

87. Levi-Montalcini R. The nerve growth factor 35 years later. Science 1987; 237:1154–1162.

88. Levin ME. The diabetic foot: Pathophysiology, evaluation and treatment. In Levin ME, O'Neal LW (eds): The Diabetic Foot. St Louis, Mosby–Year Book, 1988, pp 1–50.

89. LoGerfo FW, Coffman JD: Vascular and microvascular disease of the foot in diabetes. N Engl J Med 1984; 311:1615–1619.

90. LoGerfo FW, Gibbons GW. Ischaemia in the diabetic foot: Modern concepts and management. Clin Diabetes 1989; 7:72–75.

91. Lorenzi M, Cagliero E, Toledo S. Glucose toxicity for human endothelial cells in culture. Delayed replication, disturbed cell cycle and accelerated death. Diabetes 1985; 34:621–627.

92. Low PA, Schmelzer JD, Ward KK, et al. Experimental chronic hypoxic neuropathy: Relevance to diabetic neuropathy. Am J Physiol 1986; 250:E94–99.

93. Low PA. Recent advances in the pathogenesis of diabetic neuropathy. Muscle Nerve 1987; 10:121–128.

94. Macleod AF, Williams DRR, Sonksen PH, et al. Risk factors for foot ulcers in diabetic patients attending a hospital clinic. Diabetologia 1991; 34(suppl):A39.

95. MacRury SM, Lennie SE, McColl P, et al. Increased red cell aggregation in diabetes mellitus: Association with cardiovascular risk factors. Diabetic Med 1993; 10:13–20.

96. Malik RA, Masson EA, Sharma AK, et al. Hypoxic neuropathy: Relevance to human diabetic neuropathy. Diabetologia 1990; 33:311–318.

97. Mansell PI, Gregson R, Allison SP. An audit of lower limb angioplasty in diabetic patients. Diabetic Med 1992; 9:84–90.

98. Maser RE, Steenkiste AR, Dorman JS, et al. Epidemiological correlates of diabetic neuropathy: Report from Pittsburgh Epidemiology of Diabetes Complications study. Diabetes 1989; 38:1456–1461.

99. Masson EA, Church SE, Woodcock AA, et al. Is resistance to ischemic conduction failure induced by hypoxia? Diabetologia 1988; 31:762–765.

100. Masson EA, MacFarlane IA, Priestley CJ, et al. Failure to prevent nicotine addiction in young people with diabetes. Arch Dis Childhood 1992; 67:100–102.

101. Mattock MB, Keen H, Viberti GC, et al. Coronary heart disease and albumin excretion rate in type 2 (non-insulin dependent) diabetic patients. Diabetologia 1988; 31:82–87.

102. McAllister FF. The fate of patients with intermittent claudication managed conservatively. Am J Surg 1976; 132:593–595.

103. McCaulay TR, Monib A, Dickey KW, et al. Peripheral vascular occlusive disease: Accuracy and reliability of time of flight MR angiography. Radiology 1994; 192:351–357.

104. Meade TW, Chakrabarti R, Haines AP, et al. Haemostatic function and cardiovascular death: Early results of a prospective study. Lancet 1980; 1:1050–1053.

105. Melton LJ, Macken KM, Palumbo PJ, et al. Incidence and prevalence of clinical peripheral vascular disease in a population based cohort of diabetic patients. Diabetes Care 1980; 3:650–654.

106. Menzoian JO, LaMorte WW, Paniszyn CC, et al. Symptomatology and anatomic patterns of peripheral vascular disease: Differing impact of smoking and diabetes. Ann Vasc Surg 1989; 3:224–228.

107. Modesti PA, Abbate R, Gensini GF, et al. Platelet thromboxane A2 receptors in type 1 diabetes. Clin Sci 1991; 80:101–105.

108. Moncada S, Vane JR. Pharmacology and endogenous roles of prostaglandins, endoperoxides, thromboxane A1 and prostacyclin. Pharmacol Rev 1979; 30:293–315.
109. Moneta GL, Yeager RA, Lee RW, et al. Non-invasive localisation of arterial occlusive disease: A comparison of segmental Doppler pressures and arterial duplex mapping. J Vasc Surg 1993; 17:578–582.
110. Morrish NJ, Stevens LK, Fuller JH, et al. Incidence of macrovascular disease in diabetes mellitus: The London cohort of the WHO Multinational Study of Vascular Disease in Diabetics. Diabetologia 1991; 34:584–589.
111. Morrish NJ, Stevens LK, Fuller JH, et al. Risk factors for macrovascular disease in diabetes mellitus: The London follow-up to the WHO Multinational Study of Vascular Disease in Diabetics. Diabetologia 1991; 34:590–594.
112. Moss SE, Klein R, Klein BEK. The prevalence and incidence of lower extremity amputation in a diabetic population. Arch Intern Med 1992; 152:610–661.
113. Most RS, Sinnock P. The epidemiology of lower extremity amputations in diabetic individuals. Diabetes Care 1983; 6:87–91.
114. Neil HAW, Thompson AV, Thorogood M, et al. Diabetes in the elderly: The Oxford community diabetes study. Diabetic Med 1989; 6:608–613.
115. Newrick PG, Wilson AJ, Jakubowski J, et al. Sural nerve oxygen tension in diabetes. BMJ 1986; 293:1053–1054.
116. Nillson SE, Lindholm H, Bülow S, et al. The Kristianstad survey 63–64 (calcifications in arteries of lower limbs). Acta Med Scand 1967; 428(suppl):1–46.
117. Nowak D, Bruch M, Arnaud F, et al. Peripheral neuropathies in patients with chronic obstructive pulmonary disease: A multicenter prevalence study. Lung 1990; 168:43–51.
118. O'Donnell MJ, Le Guen CA, Lawson N, et al. Platelet behaviour and haemostatic variables in type 1 (insulin dependent) diabetic patients with and without albuminuria. Diabetic Med 1991; 8:624–628.
119. O'Malley BC, Timperley WR, Ward JD, et al. Platelet abnormalities in diabetic peripheral neuropathy. Lancet 1975; 2:1274–1280.
120. Orchard TJ, Strandness DE. Assessment of peripheral vascular disease in diabetes. Diabetes Care 1993; 16:1199–1209.
121. Palmaz JC, Laborde JC, Rivera FJ. Stenting of the iliac arteries with the Palmaz stent: Experience from a multicentre trial. Cardiovasc Intervent Radiol 1992; 15:291–297.
122. Palumbo PJ, O'Fallon WM, Osmundson PJ, et al. Progression of peripheral occlusive vascular disease: What factors are predictive? Arch Intern Med 1991; 151:717–721.
123. Panayiotopoulos YP, Tyrrell MR, Arnold FJL, et al. Results and cost analysis for distal (tibial/pedal) arterial reconstruction for limb salvage in diabetic and non-diabetic patients. Diabetic Med 1997; 14:214–220.
124. Papoz L, Costagliola D, Massan V. Epidemiology of the micro- and macrovascular complications of diabetes. In Tchobroutsky G, Slama G, Assan R, et al (eds): Vascular Complications of Diabetes. Paris, Editions Pradel, 1994, pp 63–69.
125. Pecoraro RE, Ahroni JH, Boyko EJ, et al. Chronology and determinants of tissue repair in diabetic lower-extremity ulcers. Diabetes 1991; 40:1305–1313.
126. Pell JP, Lee AJ, on behalf of the Scottish Vascular Audit Group. Impact of angioplasty and arterial reconstructive surgery on the quality of life of claudicants. Scott Med J 1997; 42:47–48.
127. Pickstock PG, Voight A, Singh BM. Claudication without macrovascular disease: Does diabetic neuropathic pseudoclaudication exist? Diabetic Med 1997; 14 (suppl 1):S55.
128. Pomposelli JB, Jepson SJ, Gibbons GW, et al. A flexible approach to infra popliteal vein grafts in patients with diabetes mellitus. Arch Surg 1991; 126:724–729.
129. Potter van Loon BJ, De Bart ACW, Radder JK, et al. Acute exogenous hyperinsulinaemia does not result in elevation of plasma plasminogen activator inhibitor-1 (PAI-1) in humans. Fibrinolysis 1990; 4(suppl 2):93–94.
130. Priollot P. Arterial disease in the diabetic. In Tchobroutsky G, Slama G, Assan R, et al (eds): Vascular Complications of Diabetes. Paris, Editions Pradel, 1994, pp 145–150.
131. Rabinowe SL, Brown FM, Watts M, et al. Anti-sympathetic ganglia antibodies and postural blood pressure in IDDM subjects of varying duration and patients at high risk of developing IDDM. Diabetes Care 1989; 12:1–6.
132. Ram Z, Sadeh M, Walden R, et al. Vascular insufficiency quantitatively aggravates diabetic neuropathy. Arch Neurol 1991; 48:1239–1242
133. Ramsey DE, Manke DA, Sumner DS. Toe blood pressure: A valuable adjunct to ankle pressure measurement for assessing peripheral arterial disease. J Cardiovasc Surgery 1983; 24:43–46.
134. Randomised trial of cholesterol lowering in 4444 patients with coronary heart disease. The Scandinavian Simvastatin Survival Study (4S). Lancet 1994; 344:1383–1389.
135. Reiber GE, Pecoraro RE, Koepsell TD. Risk factor for amputation in patients with diabetes mellitus. Ann Intern Med 1992; 117:97–105.
136. Reiber GE. The epidemiology of diabetic foot problems. Diabetic Med 1996; 13(suppl 1):S6–S11.
137. Reja A, Tesfaye S, Harris N, et al. Improvement in nerve conduction and quantitative sensory tests following treatment with lisinopril. Diabetic Med 1993; 10:S18.
138. Report of the diabetic foot amputation and amputation group. Diabetic Med 1996; 13(suppl 4):S27–S42
139. Riggs JE, Moss AH, Labosky DA, et al. Upper extremity ischemic monomelic neuropathy: A complication of vascular access procedures in uremic diabetic patients. Neurology 1989; 39:997–998.
140. Rivers SP, Scher L, Veith FJ. Indications for distal reconstruction in the presence of palpable pedal pulses. J Vasc Surg 1990; 12:552–557.
141. Rodriguez-Sanchez C, Sanchez MM, Malik RA, et al. Morphological abnormalities in the sural nerve from patients with peripheral vascular disease. Histol Histopathol 1991; 6:63–71.
142. Ryder REJ, Marshall R, Johnson K, et al. Acetylcholine sweat spot test for autonomic denervation. Lancet 1988; 1:1303–1305.
143. Schneider SH, Kein HC, Khachdurian AK, et al. Impaired fibrinolytic response to exercise in type II diabetes: Effects of exercise and physical training. Metabolism 1988; 37:924–929.
144. Selby JV, Zhang D. Risk factors for lower extremity amputation in persons with diabetes. Diabetes Care 1995; 18(4):509–516.
145. Silberkane NO, Silberbauer K, Schernthauer G, et al. Decreased vascular prostacyclin in juvenile-onset diabetes. N Engl J Med 1979; 300:366–367.
146. Sladky JT, Tschoepe RL, Greenberg JH, et al. Peripheral neuropathy after chronic endoneurial ischemia. Ann Neurol 1991; 29:272–278.

147. Small M, Lowe GDO, MacCuish AC, et al. Thrombin and plasmin activity in diabetes mellitus and their association with glycemic control. J Med 1987; 65:1025–1031.

148. Solomon SA, Ramsay LE, Yeo WW, et al. B blockade and intermittent claudication: Placebo controlled trial of atenolol and nifedipine and their combination. BMJ 1991; 303:1100–1104.

149. Stamler J, Vaccaro O, Neaton JD, et al. Diabetes, other risk factors and 12-yr cardiovascular mortality in men screened in the Multiple Risk Factor Intervention Trial. Diabetes Care 1993; 16:434–444.

150. Steiness IB. Vibratory perception in diabetics during arrested blood flow to the limb. Acta Med Scand 1959; 163:195–205.

151. Stengard JH, Juomiluto J, Pekkanen J, et al. Changes in glucose tolerance and mortality during a five year follow up: The Finnish cohorts of the Seven Countries Study. Diabetologia 1992; 35:760–765.

152. Stevens MJ, Goss DE, Foster AVM, et al. Abnormal digital pressure measurements in diabetic neuropathic foot ulceration. Diabetic Med 1993; 10:909–915.

153. Strandness DE Jr, Priest RE, Gibbons GE, et al. Combined clinical and pathologic study of diabetic and non diabetic peripheral arterial disease. Diabetes 1964; 13:366–372.

154. Thomas JH, Sterrs JL, Keisjerian SM, et al. A comparison of diabetics and nondiabetics with threatened limb loss. Am J Surg 1988; 156:481–483.

155. Thomson FJ, Veves A, Ashe H, et al. A team approach to diabetic foot care: The Manchester experience. Foot 1991; 2:75–82.

156. UK Prospective Diabetes Study Group. UK Prospective Diabetes Study XII. Differences between Asian, Afro-Carribean and White Caucasian type 2 diabetic patients at diagnosis of diabetes. Diabetic Med 1994; 11:670–677.

157. Vague J. The degree of masculine differentiation of obesities: A factor determining predisposition to diabetes, atherosclerosis, gout and uric acid calculous disease. Am J Clin Nutr 1956; 4:20–28.

158. van der Meer JWM, Koopmans PP, Lutterman JA. Antibiotic therapy in diabetic foot infection. Diabetic Med 1996; 13(suppl 1):S48–S51.

159. Van Ross E. Rehabilitation of the diabetic amputee: Its role in foot salvage. In Boulton AJM, Connor H, Cavanagh PR (eds): The Foot in Diabetes. Chichester, U.K., John Wiley and Sons, 1994, pp 229–239.

160. Veves A, Uccioli L, Manes C, et al. Comparison of risk factors for foot ulceration in diabetic patients attending teaching hospital outpatient clinics in four different European states. Diabetic Med 1994; 11:709–711.

161. Veves A, Donaghue VM, Sarnow MR, et al. The impact of reversal of hypoxia by revascularisation on the peripheral nerve function of diabetic patients. Diabetologia 1996; 39:344–345.

162. Walmsley D, Hampton KK, Grant PJ. Contrasting fibrinolytic responses in type 1 (insulin-dependent) and type 2 (non-insulin-dependent) diabetes. Diabetic Med 1991; 8:954–959.

163. Ward KK, Low PA, Schmelzer JD, et al. Prostacyclin and noradrenaline in peripheral nerve of chronic experimental diabetes. Brain 1989; 112:197–208.

164. Waugh NR. Amputations in diabetic patients: A review of rates, relative risks and resource use. Community Med 1988; 10:279–288.

165. Welborne TA, Wearne K. Coronary heart disease and cardiovascular mortality in Busselton with reference to glucose and insulin concentrations. Diabetes Care 1979; 2:154–160.

166. WHO/IDF. Diabetes care and research in Europe: The St Vincent Declaration. Diabetic Med 1990; 7:360.

167. Wieczorek I, Pell ACH, McIver B, et al. Coagulation and fibrinolytic systems in type 1 diabetes: Effects of venous occlusion and insulin-induced hypoglycaemia. Clin Sci 1993; 84:79–86.

168. Wilbourn AJ, Furlan AJ, Hulley W, et al. Ischemic monomelic neuropathy. Neurology 1983; 33:447–451.

169. Ylikorkala O, Kaila J, Viinikka L. Prostacyclin and thromboxane in diabetes. BMJ 1981; 283:1148–1150.

170. Young MJ, Veves A, Walker MG, et al. Correlations between nerve function and tissue oxygenation in diabetic patients: Further clues to the aetiology of diabetic neuropathy? Diabetologia 1992; 35:1146–1150.

171. Young MJ, Adams JE, Anderson GF, et al. Medial arterial calcification in the feet of diabetic patients and matched non-diabetic control subjects. Diabetologia 1993; 36:615–621.

172. Young MJ, Boulton AJM, Macleod AF, et al. A multicentre study of the prevalence of diabetic peripheral neuropathy in the United Kingdom hospital clinic population. Diabetologia 1993; 36:150–154.

173. Young MJ, Veves A, Smith JV, et al: Restoring limb blood flow improves nerve function in diabetic patients. Diabetologia 1995; 38:1051–1054.

174. Young RJ, Zhou YQ, Rodriguez E, et al. Variable relationship between peripheral somatic and autonomic neuropathy in patients with different syndromes of diabetic polyneuropathy. Diabetes 1986; 35:192–197.

Neuropathic Assessment

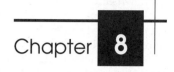

Chapter 8

Neuropathy Tests and Normative Results

Ian A. Grant • Peter O'Brien • Peter James Dyck

INTRODUCTION

There is consensus that symptoms, neurologic abnormalities (impairments), nerve conduction (NC) abnormalities, quantitative sensory test (QST) abnormalities, and quantitative autonomic test (QAT) abnormalities are useful for the detection, characterization, and quantitation of diabetic neuropathies. Symptom scores that tally and assess severity and change are useful for evaluation of symptoms, but interpretation must be performed by trained physicians to provide reliable results.

Decreased or absent ankle reflexes, increased vibration threshold (especially when quantitated with an adequate system such as computer assisted sensory evaluator [CASE IV]), and inability to walk on the heels are important clinical assessments to detect worsening. The Neuropathy Impairment Score of lower limbs (NIS[LL]) is a useful scored measure, but trained physicians to administer this test are needed.

We have developed several standard calibrated tests, administered rigorously and using percentile reference values corrected for anatomical site, age, sex, and physical characteristics based on study of appropriate large randomly selected cohorts in which neurologic disease has been excluded. Using percentile abnormalities of test results corrected for age, sex, and physical characteristics allows the investigator to follow the changes caused by diabetic neuropathy. The choice of the level of the percentile value chosen as abnormal and the choice of minimal criteria have a strong influence on frequency of diabetic patients declared to have diabetic polyneuropathy (DPN). The most sensitive criteria are those based on abnormalities of NC; NIS and vibration threshold are less sensitive criteria, and cold and heat-pain sensation are even less sensitive.

Two approaches have been found useful in quantitating the severity of DPN: (1) staging and (2) using a composite score such as NIS(LL)+7 tests. The latter has been shown to demonstrate a monotone* worsening over time. In controlled clinical trials of therapy of diabetic neuropathy, assuming that worsening can be prevented but improvement will not occur, longitudinal data from the Rochester Diabetic Neuropathy Study (RDNS) indicate that a meaningful difference could be found in 3 years with persons in each arm of the trial.

This chapter is concerned with evaluative procedures, tests, and reference values that make it possible to detect DPN sensitively (recognition of peripheral neuropathy given that it is present), accurately (ability to assess severity as it is), and reproducibly (obtaining the same result in repeated measurement). We also discuss the drawbacks of using simple, unvalidated approaches.

THE USE OF NEUROPATHY TESTS IN MEDICAL PRACTICE AND RESEARCH

It would be desirable to detect and comprehensively characterize diabetic neuropathies simply, accurately, and reproducibly, but unfortunately this does not appear possible without using sophisticated tests, adequate reference values, and composite scores. In this respect, it is not unlike many other diseases, such as atherosclerosis, in that the underlying condition is not readily detected or quantitated before the occurrence of the catastrophic event (the heart attack or stroke). To detect, characterize, and quantitate atherosclerosis before the adverse event strikes is not a simple matter.

Similarly, in diabetic neuropathies (for example, polyneuropathy or DPN), it would be desirable to detect, characterize, and quantitate DPN periodically to anticipate the development of sensory, autonomic, or motor symptoms (such as unsteadiness, pain, postural hypotension, gastroparesis, impotence, sweating disturbances, or weakness) or adverse outcomes (such as Charcot's joints, plantar ulcers, foot amputation, or impaired functions of daily living).

Is it worthwhile to detect, characterize, and quantitate DPN for use in medical practice? For the most part, it appears that general physicians and diabetologists are not doing it, suggesting that they do not believe it is worthwhile, they do not know how to do it, or they do not have adequate approaches to do so. There are three reasons why we believe it is increasingly important to monitor for DPN: (1) information, (2) prevention, and (3) intervention. Patients and physicians would like to know if DPN is present and how severe it is for reassurance or for an indication that intervention is necessary. Reasons 2 and 3 can be combined. If physicians and patients were aware of the severity of neuropathic impairment of the patients' feet, it might spur them to use preventive or therapeutic measures. For example, based on present thinking, it might spur them to insist on more rigorous glycemic control, improved foot care, or remedial pharmacologic intervention (as such agents become available for use).

The need for adequate and appropriate detection, characterization, and quantitation of DPN for use in epidemiologic studies and controlled clinical trials has been emphasized by our recent longitudinal assessment of DPN in the RDNS cohort. A prevalence cohort of approximately 200 diabetic patients was followed for 2 to 10 years. We assessed a variety of symptoms, clinical signs, and tests for their ability to recognize statistically significant and monotone worsening and the magnitude of that worsening. In such an analysis, one assumes that, as a group, diabetic patients worsen over time—an assumption that is reasonable based on available epidemiologic studies. We found that the choice of evaluation procedures, how they are performed and analyzed, their standardization, and the adequacy of reference values are critically important to the design and successful conduct of epidemiologic studies and controlled clinical trials. Appropriate end points and adequate reference values are needed to minimize the number of

---

*Monotone in this sense refers to change in a measured variable that is in the same direction in repeated measurements over time. The direction of the change, not the magnitude, is considered. For example, yearly nerve conductions in a diabetic patient may demonstrate a progressive decrease in the amplitude of the sural sensory nerve action potential (SNAP) with each measurement. The degree to which the sural SNAP consistently shows worsening, during worsening of DPN, is the degree of monotonicity of the test. If, on the other hand, the sural SNAP did not consistently show worsening, it would not be as consistent or monotone a test.

patients and the duration of trials to manageable levels.

WHY CHARACTERIZE AND QUANTITATE NEUROPATHY SYMPTOMS, IMPAIRMENTS, TEST ABNORMALITIES, OVERALL SEVERITY, AND OUTCOME?

Simply detecting whether one or more of the diabetic neuropathies are present or absent is of little importance unless they cause (or will cause in the future) symptoms, interfere with life's activities, or act as risk factors for poor health outcomes. Such a judgment (whether the patient has one of the neuropathies discussed previously) is of even less value if the diagnosis is based on uncontrolled flimsy evidence or criteria. Even if the diagnosis of neuropathy is based on high-quality tests and evaluations, if the neuropathy is not now or later accompanied by symptoms, impaired health, or resultant complications, the recognition of these surrogate measures is of little importance. It is, therefore, necessary to begin to candidly look at the various neuropathy tests and try and understand whether and how they help in diagnosis, characterization, and predicting outcome.

In DPN, early and reliable detection, characterization, and quantitation may be of help for information (patient and physician), especially if it will lead to intervention that will ameliorate or arrest the process so that bad health or life outcomes will be avoided. Because there now is clear evidence that chronic total hyperglycemic exposure is deleterious for DPN (and also for retinopathy and nephropathy), real efforts can be made to limit this risk factor and prevent a degree of worsening. In this chapter, we discuss the strengths and limits of clinical tests to recognize a clinically meaningful change in DPN. To predict symptoms or poor health outcomes, it is reasonable to ask what degree of alteration exists in NC, heart beat variation with deep breathing, or muscle stretch reflex. It is now clear that only a small percentage of patients with test abnormalities will develop symptomatic stages of clinical impairment or any real degree of health problems.

In diabetic lumbosacral radiculoplexus neuropathy or diabetic thoracolumbar radiculoneuropathy, concern about nonmeaningful test results is perhaps of less concern because physicians are not assessing for asymptomatic impairment. Generally, therefore, these patients have problematic degrees of symptoms that often necessitate extensive medical evaluation, intervention, pain management, and cessation of gainful employment.

In upper limb mononeuropathies, carpal tunnel syndrome and cubital tunnel syndrome are associated with problematic degrees of symptoms that often necessitate extensive medical evaluation and intervention, pain management, and cessation of gainful employment.

In DPN, carpal tunnel syndrome, and cubital tunnel syndrome, there may be characteristic electrophysiologic findings. These abnormalities help in characterization and in diagnosis, but whether the lesions are symptomatic and whether and how they should be treated have to be decided by other approaches and criteria.

NEUROPATHIC SYMPTOMS

Volunteered Symptoms. Use of the problem-based approach commonly used by physicians makes it likely that only symptoms of concern to the patient, generally those with some degree of magnitude or persistence, are recorded. Generally, complainers are more apt to report symptoms than noncomplainers. Use of only volunteered symptoms makes it likely that unevenness will occur among symptoms, among patients, among physicians, and even among cohorts. This approach, therefore, is generally not used for epidemiologic or controlled clinical trials because of this variability and because investigators want to inquire into whether certain specific symptoms occur and to determine their magnitude and persistence.

Tally of Symptoms From Checklists. Use of a checklist to ask patients about symptoms encountered in DPN is a useful approach. The approach has the advantage of systematically ascertaining which symptoms are (or are not) experienced by the patient. If one simply tallies symptoms from previously obtained medical records and a symptom has not been documented, one may not know whether the symptom was not experienced or was not asked about or recorded. The major symptoms encountered in DPN are listed in the neuropathy symptoms score (NSS) (Table 8.1). This relatively simple survey requires only a few minutes to take. To be useful, however, the physician must take whatever time is needed to ensure that the symptoms relate to the neuropathy studied, for example, DPN. A tally of these symptoms provides some information

TABLE 8.1 THE NEUROLOGICAL SYMPTOM SCORE

Score 1 point for the presence of each symptom:	Score
I. Symptoms of muscle weakness	
A. Bulbar	
1. Extraocular	____
2. Facial	____
3. Tongue	____
4. Throat	____
B. Limbs	
5. Shoulder girdle and upper arm	____
6. Hand	____
7. Hip girdle and thigh	____
8. Leg	____
II. Sensory disturbance	
A. Negative symptoms	
9. Difficulty identifying objects in mouth	____
10. Difficulty identifying objects in hands	____
11. Loss of feeling in feet or unsteadiness (touch, heat, pain)	____
B. Positive symptoms	
12. Numbness, asleep feeling, like Novocain, prickling at any site	____
13. Pain—burning, deep aching, tenderness at any site	____
III. Autonomic symptoms	
14. Postural fainting	____
15. Impotence	____
16. Loss of urinary control	____
17. Night diarrhea	____
18. Gastroparesis	____
Total	____

about the symptoms in DPN and, in cohort studies, shows worsening over time. The NSS considers only the presence or absence of symptoms and does not consider severity.

There are more robust measures of worsening of symptoms over time. The neuropathy symptom profile (NSP) is a patient-completed questionnaire—32 major detailed, true-and-false questions—scored by optical character recognition technology, regarding symptoms encountered in neuropathy.[9] It has the following important features: (1) it is a standard test; (2) the profile of score abnormalities has been shown to differ among neuropathies of various causes; and (3) percentile responses for age, gender, and physical features have been estimated for the various parts of the test. However, in longitudinal evaluation of a diabetic cohort, the NSP score was not shown to detect worsening over time—patients actually showed improvement. Because physician-evaluated symptoms (e.g., NSS and neuropathy symptoms and change [NSC], see subsequent section), neurologic impairment, and other tests showed serial worsening, we do not believe that the NSP can be used for sensitive and accurate assessment of change in DPN with time.

Assessment of Severity and Change of Neuropathic Symptoms. A variety of testing instruments have been developed to assess severity of symptoms at one point in time and to follow change serially.

Visual Analog Scales of Pain. In many studies, patients are asked to place a mark, representing the magnitude of a symptom (such as pain), on a horizontal line of standard length with the understanding that one end of the line represents no pain and the other end represents the most severe pain imaginable. This procedure can also be done on a video screen. The distance along the line to the marked point is then measured. This visual analog scaling has been used especially for measurement of pain.

Graphic Rating Scales. A graphic rating scale is essentially a visual analog scale, modified so that descriptive terms are placed at intervals along the line. The patient is required to place a mark representing symptom severity at any point on the line, as with the visual analog scale. This approach might be useful in increasing patient understanding. However, Scott and Huskisson have compared the responses of groups of patients with various painful conditions using several types of graphic rating scales and found that, with some configurations, responses tend to cluster around the sites of the descriptive terms.[27] They concluded that this may decrease the sensitivity of the scale, reducing its ability to detect small differences in symptom severity.

Total Symptom Score. Ziegler and colleagues developed a physician-administered symptom scale used in the longitudinal assessment of patients with diabetic neuropathy in a therapeutic trial.[30] In the total symptom score (TSS), patients are asked to rate four symptoms (pain, burning, paresthesias, and numbness) according to the two variables of intensity and frequency; intensity is graded as absent, slight, moderate, or severe; and frequency is graded as occasional, frequent, or continuous. Increasing symptom severity with respect to each variable is assigned a numeric value that increases in equidistant steps (Table 8.2). A total score is thus derived, ranging from 0 (asymptomatic) to 14.64 (all four symptoms are present, severe, and continuous).

If this test is used, it would be advisable to clarify the terms, because words such as *pain* and *burning* are overlapping and ambiguous.

TABLE 8.2 SCORING APPROACH FOR THE NEUROPATHIC SYMPTOMS INCLUDED IN THE TOTAL SYMPTOM SCORE (PAIN, BURNING, PARESTHESIA, NUMBNESS)

Symptom Frequency	Symptom Intensity			
	Absent	*Slight*	*Moderate*	*Severe*
Occasional	0	1.00	2.00	3.00
Frequent	0	1.33	2.33	3.33
(Almost) continuous	0	1.66	2.66	3.66

From Ziegler D, Hanefeld M, Ruhnau KJ, et al. Treatment of symptomatic diabetic peripheral neuropathy with the anti-oxidant alpha-lipoic acid: A 3-week multicenter randomized controlled trial (ALADIN Study). Diabetologia 1995; 38:1425.

Prickling (pins and needles) should perhaps be used for paresthesia. Another word for *numbness* should be used, because its meaning is not precisely understood; it could mean loss of feeling, asleep numbness, dead, or other.

Neuropathy Symptoms and Change (NSC). We recommend this assessment because it is comprehensive and standard, has been validated in healthy subjects and in a variety of neuropathies, and depends on the judgment of a physician (for example, a neurologist). It provides three measures of symptoms: number (and kind), severity, and change (as compared with a specific previous date). Questions are grouped by function into motor, sensory, and autonomic symptoms. Test results for these three functions can be considered as a global score, as three separate scores, or as additional subscores. Table 8.3 contains examples of some of the most useful motor, sensory, and autonomic questions. The physician administering the test is required to make certain judgments; if questions are answered positively, sympathetic cross examination is used to determine whether the symptom is present beyond what is encountered in health and whether it is caused by the condition being evaluated, for example, DPN.

To illustrate, if one is assessing for DPN, symptoms attributable to a previous Bell's palsy or a coexisting carpal tunnel syndrome are not included. A neurologist can usually make such judgments and decrease the noise from symptoms not caused by DPN.

The NSC has been tested in serial evaluation of patients with chronic inflammatory demyelinating polyneuropathy (CIDP), multifocal motor neuropathy with persistent conduction block, and diabetic neuropathy. Patients' symptoms may vary considerably from one evaluation to the next, either spontaneously or with treatment (for example, plasma exchange or intravenous immunoglobulin [IVIg] infusion).

This variability can be monitored using the three scales of NSC or other instruments such as the Neuropathy Impairment Score (NIS) (see next section); electrophysiologic variables such as summated compound muscle action potential amplitudes of the ulnar, peroneal, and tibial nerves; summated sensory nerve action potential amplitudes of the ulnar and sural nerves; and vibratory detection threshold on the toe using CASE IV. When there is a large or intermediate degree of change, all these measures move in the same direction (improving or worsening). By contrast, when the change is small, discrepancies among tests are anticipated. How well do these scales of NSC reflect objective worsening or improvement as measured by neuropathic impairment? The analysis is not complete, but it would appear that NSC severity and NSC change are better measures of improvement or worsening than is a simple tally of number of symptoms. It is unclear what is the minimum degree of change in severity of DPN detectable by the NSC. Questions of this kind are under study in our laboratory at this time.

NEUROPATHIC IMPAIRMENTS

Neurologic examination and quantitation of deficit is another important approach in making judgments about occurrence, characterization, and severity of DPN. In certain diabetic studies (such as the Diabetes Control and Complications Trial [DCCT][3]), neurologists made a judgment as to whether patients had clinically evident DPN, questionable DPN, or did not have DPN. Although criteria for this judgment were suggested in the DCCT, it is unclear what severity of DPN constitutes clinically evident DPN; different neurologists may use different minimal criteria. One might find absent bilateral ankle reflexes compelling evidence, another might insist on decreased clinical vibration loss, and a third might use all the above

TABLE 8.3 EXAMPLE QUESTIONS FROM THE NEUROPATHY SYMPTOMS AND CHANGE QUESTIONNAIRE
(fill in 1 circle per symptom; if yes [under symptom], fill in 1 circle for severity and 1 circle for change)

Symptoms of Weakness

Upper Limbs

Symptom	Yes	No	Severity +	++	+++	Same	Better +	++	+++	Worse −	−−	−−−
						Are symptoms the same, better or worse than (specify date)?						
Weakness of hands, e.g., to zipper, button, handle coins, manipulate a key, or other	○	○	○	○	○	○	○	○	○	○	○	○
Weakness when straightening fingers												

Lower Limbs

Symptom	Yes	No	Severity +	++	+++	Same	Better +	++	+++	Worse −	−−	−−−
Weakness of legs so that you slap your feet in walking or cannot carry your weight on your heels	○	○	○	○	○	○	○	○	○	○	○	○
Weakness of legs so that you cannot walk on your toes or forefoot	○	○	○	○	○	○	○	○	○	○	○	○

Sensory Symptoms

Symptom	Yes	No	Severity +	++	+++	Same	Better +	++	+++	Worse −	−−	−−−
Decrease (or inability) to feel the surface features, size, shape or texture of what you touch	○	○	○	○	○	○	○	○	○	○	○	○

If yes, choose only one:

In legs only (feet are included) ○
In arms only (hands are included) ○
In legs and arms ○
In mouth, face, or head only ○
Other than any of the above ○

Symptom	Yes	No	Severity +	++	+++	Same	Better +	++	+++	Worse −	−−	−−−
Decrease (or inability) to recognize hot from cold Etc., as above	○	○	○	○	○	○	○	○	○	○	○	○

Autonomic Symptoms

Symptom	Yes	No	Severity +	++	+++	Same	Better +	++	+++	Worse −	−−	−−−
Feel faint or actually faint, only upon sitting or standing, not explained by use of blood pressure medication or psychologic stress	○	○	○	○	○	○	○	○	○	○	○	○
Loss of bladder control, not caused by gynecologic problems in women or prostate problems in men	○	○	○	○	○	○	○	○	○	○	○	○

plus appropriate symptoms. There are four major problems with this approach: (1) the neurologic examination is not sufficiently standardized; (2) the grading of abnormalities is not standardized or continuous; (3) the minimal criteria for abnormality are not given as one number; and (4) overall severity is not expressed numerically.

The Medical Research Council (MRC) grading scale of muscle strength is a very useful approach for quantifying muscle weakness, but it was designed to quantitate recovery of paralyzed muscles after nerve injury. For assessment of generalized neuropathic impairment, it is not ideal because (1) it measures only muscle strength and does not include abnormalities of sensation or muscle stretch reflexes; (2) severe degrees of muscle weakness are emphasized; (3) it is not a linear measure of muscle weakness; and (4) it does not provide an indication of which muscles should be tested or which muscles should be included for an overall score.

Neuropathy Impairment Score (NIS). This instrument was originally called the Neurologic Disability Score and was developed to express overall neurologic impairment from peripheral neuropathy as a single numeric value. The test items were chosen to provide an overall measure of severity of muscle weakness, decrease or loss of muscle stretch reflexes, and sensory loss. The intention was to provide a clinically relevant balance among these three types of deficit. The score was developed for use in controlled trials and epidemiologic studies of patients with chronic inflammatory demyelinating neuropathy, neuropathy associated with monoclonal gammopathy of uncertain significance (MGUS), DPN, and other varieties of neuropathy. The grading approach used is based on elements of the Mayo Clinic examination approach and the MRC. What makes NIS unique are the following:

- The choice of examination items included
- De-emphasis of the contribution of reflexes and sensation
- Use of standard sites of sensory examination on toe and finger
- Expression of results as points for percentile abnormality considering site, age, sex, applicable physical variables, and physical fitness
- Use of a single summated number to express overall impairment

Thought was given to use of gradations in

function that might be recognized by a neurologist. Muscle strength was graded from 0 to 4 as follows: normal (grade 0), 25% weak (grade 1), 50% weak (grade 2), 75% weak (grade 3), and paralyzed (grade 4). Between grades 3 and 4 are several subdivisions: flicker of muscle without moving joint (grade 3.75), movement of joint with gravity eliminated (grade 3.5), and joint movement against gravity (grade 3.25). Reflexes were graded as normal (grade 0), decreased (grade 1), or absent (grade 2). Touch pressure, vibration, joint position and motion, and pinprick were assessed in the terminal phalanx of index finger and great toe and were graded as normal (grade 0), decreased (grade 1), or absent (grade 2). The NIS is shown in Table 8.4. A computerized version has been developed for automatic entry of individual and group evaluation into a computer database.

For DPN, the NIS of the lower limbs (NIS[LL]) is preferable. This is because neuropathic deficits are confined to the lower extremities in most patients with DPN; consideration only of the lower limbs therefore eliminates the dilutional effect of the (usually) neurologically normal upper limbs. A composite score that includes NIS(LL) and seven electrophysiologic, quantitative sensory, and autonomic tests for which percentile abnormalities of tests are transformed to points (to be equivalent to NIS points) is also available (NIS[LL]+7). Other composite scores combining NIS(LL) and tests for small fiber function or large fiber function are also available.

The NIS by itself has been shown to provide a good measure of cross-sectional and longitudinal change in such conditions as inherited neuropathy, CIDP, MGUS neuropathy, and other neurologic disorders. It has been shown to improve with treatment (for example, prednisone versus placebo, plasma exchange [PE] versus sham PE, and PE versus IVIg in CIDP; PE versus sham PE in MGUS neuropathy). It has also been shown to worsen over time in diabetic neuropathy and in inherited neuropathy.

We have used the NIS extensively in our medical practice simply to monitor worsening or improvement. We have tested its reproducibility in individual observers and among different observers. A high degree of reproducibility was found for trained observers.

Functional Scales. The previous approaches assess specific neurologic functions individually and then derive an overall measure of

TABLE 8.4 NEUROPATHY IMPAIRMENT SCORE

Name _____ Accession # _____
Age _____ Sex _____ Date _____

Objective: To provide a single score of neuropathic deficit and subset score (cranial nerve, muscle weakness, reflexes, and sensation) abnormalities, abstracted from a neurologic examination in which all of the assessments are made.

Scoring: The examiner scores deficits by what he or she considers to be normal considering test, anatomical site, age, gender, height, weight, and physical fitness. **Muscle weakness is scored:** normal = 0; 25% weak = 1; 50% weak = 2; 75% weak = 3; and paralyzed = 4. Additional scoring of weakness: just able to move limb against gravity = 3.25; just able to move limb when gravity eliminated = 3.5; and flicker of muscle without movement = 3.75. Patients to age 75 years should be able to walk on toes and heels. Inability to arise from kneeled position is not scored as abnormal after the age of 60 years. **Reflexes and sensation are scored:** normal = 0, decreased = 1, and absent = 2. For patients 50–69 years old, ankle reflexes that are decreased are graded 0, and when absent are graded 1. For patients ≥70 years, absent ankle reflexes are graded 0. **Touch-pressure, pinprick, and vibration** are assessed on the dorsal surface of the terminal phalanx of index finger and great toe. Joint motion is tested by moving the terminal phalanx of the index finger and great toe.

			Right	Left	Sum
Cranial Nerves	1	3rd nerve			
	2	6th nerve			
	3	Facial weakness			
	4	Palate weakness			
	5	Tongue weakness			
Muscle Weakness	6	Respiratory			
	7	Neck flexion			
	8	Shoulder abduction (deltoid)			
	9	Elbow flexion (biceps brachii)			
	10	Brachioradialis			
	11	Elbow extension (triceps brachii)			
	12	Wrist flexion			
	13	Wrist extension			
	14	Finger flexion			
	15	Finger spread (interossei)			
	16	Thumb abduction (thenar)			
	17	Hip flexion (iliopsoas)			
	18	Hip extension (gluteus max.)			
	19	Knee flexion (biceps femoris)			
	20	Knee extension (quadriceps)			
	21	Ankle dorsiflexors (tibialis ant. +)			
	22	Ankle plantar flexors (gastroc. soleus)			
	23	Toe extensors			
	24	Toe flexors			
Reflexes	25	Biceps brachii			
	26	Triceps brachii			
	27	Brachioradialis			
	28	Quadriceps femoris			
	29	Triceps surae/gastroc. soleus			

Table continued on opposite page

TABLE 8.4 NEUROPATHY IMPAIRMENT SCORE *Continued*

			Right	Left	Sum
Sensation Index finger: (terminal phalanx)	30	Touch pressure			
	31	Pinprick			
	32	Vibration			
	33	Joint position			
Great toe: (terminal phalanx)	34	Touch pressure			
	35	Pinprick			
	36	Vibration			
	37	Joint position			
				TOTAL _____	

From Dyck PJ, Litchy WJ, Lehman KA, et al. Variables influencing neuropathic end points: The Rochester Diabetic Neuropathy Study of Healthy Subjects (RDNS-HS). Neurology 1995; 45:1115.

neurologic status from the composite of those functions. An alternative (and often complementary) approach is to assess the patient's ability to perform certain defined functional tasks such as specific activities of daily living, that is, to measure disability. At the most complex level, one can assess the patient's overall ability to function independently, that is, to measure handicap.

Hughes and colleagues[14] developed a functional scale for assessment of treatment in Guillain-Barré syndrome. This scale categorized patients according to ability to walk with or without support, need for assisted ventilation, and mortality. These parameters have little value for patients with DPN because they were designed to evaluate the severe and generalized weakness typical of Guillain-Barré syndrome but rare in DPN.

Overall independence is measured by the Rankin scale[25] and modified Rankin scale[28] (Table 8.5). These scales were developed for use in prognostic studies of cerebrovascular disease, but have subsequently been used more widely, including in therapeutic trials for peripheral neuropathies.[21]

NERVE CONDUCTION AND NEEDLE ELECTROMYOGRAPHY

This is discussed in detail in Chapter 16. Here we simply wish to show how attributes of NC may be added to the NIS(LL) to provide a broader or composite score of DPN. Abnormality of attributes of NC may be expressed as a value below or above a certain cutoff value (see Procedure for Setting Normal Values), or

preferably as a defined percentile value as obtained by comparison with a healthy subject cohort. Abnormal conduction velocities and amplitudes are in the lower percentiles (for example, <1st or <2.5th), whereas abnormal latencies are in the upper percentiles (for example, >99th or >97.5th). As we describe in a subsequent section, using special computer programs it is possible to calculate the specific percentile value of an NC attribute of a patient by considering age, sex, and applicable physical characteristics if an adequate normative study has been done, and the influence of the variables on measured attributes of NC have been estimated.

When such information is available, it is possible to transform an NC abnormality to a point score. For example, values at the ≥95–

TABLE 8.5 MODIFIED RANKIN SCALE

Grade 0	No symptoms
Grade 1	No significant disability despite symptoms; able to carry out all usual duties and activities
Grade 2	Slight disability; unable to carry out all previous activities, but able to look after own affairs without assistance
Grade 3	Moderate disability; requiring some help, but able to walk without assistance
Grade 4	Moderately severe disability; unable to walk without assistance and unable to tend to own bodily needs without assistance
Grade 5	Severe disability; bedridden, incontinent, and requiring constant nursing care and attention

From Rankin J. Cerebral vascular accidents in patients over the age of 60. 2: Prognosis. Scott Med J 1957; 2:200.

99th percentile = 1 point, ≥99th–99.9th percentile = 2 points, and ≥99.9th percentile = 3 points if the abnormality is in the high tail of the distribution. This point score can be added to the NIS(LL) to provide composite scores. In the NIS(LL)+7 tests, the average of NC values with responses is used rather than a simple summation of transformed points.

QUANTITATIVE SENSORY TESTS

The subject is covered in Chapter 10. Here we discuss only how a percentile abnormality of a QST can be transformed and used in composite scores.

Assuming that the percentile value of a given sensory test abnormality can be calculated, it is possible to convert this value to a point abnormality by the same rules listed earlier: <95th percentile = 0; ≥95th–99th percentile = 1; ≥99th–99.9th percentile = 2; and ≥99.9th percentile = 3. This point value can subsequently be used in the generation of composite scores. For example, in the NIS(LL)+7 score, we add lower limb QST scores and autonomic scores to the NIS(LL).

QUANTITATIVE AUTONOMIC TESTS

A variety of laboratory tests are available for the evaluation of autonomic function. Most are noninvasive and quantitative. Autonomic testing can be used to establish the presence of autonomic dysfunction; determine the population (classes) of autonomic neurons or fibers affected; determine the distribution of deficits; quantitate severity; follow the course of autonomic involvement over time; and evaluate response to treatment.

The specific tests used will vary among laboratories, but it is reasonable to include, where possible, studies that evaluate vagal, adrenergic, and sympathetic sudomotor function. Available tests have been reviewed in detail by Low.[17] The Autonomic Laboratory at the Mayo Clinic has developed an autonomic reflex screen (ARS) consisting of quantitative sudomotor axon reflex test (Q-SART) recordings from the forearm and three lower limb sites, heart rate response to deep breathing and Valsalva maneuver, and blood pressure response to Valsalva maneuver, deep breathing, and tilt.[18]

Quantitative data regarding autonomic function should be interpreted in light of age. Cardiovascular reflexes, as measured by both heart rate response to deep breathing and by Valsalva ratio, decrease progressively with age.[19, 22, 24] In contrast, there appears to be relatively little if any decrease in Q-SART responses with age.[22]

Autonomic dysfunction as measured by the above tests can be expressed as a global score. This approach has the same advantages as do global scores of somatic neuropathy. Low has developed a Composite Autonomic Scoring Scale (CASS) to express abnormalities measured with the ARS as a single numeric value between 0 and 10.[16] A score of 1 to 3 is assigned for each of the sudomotor and cardiovascular components of the test, and a score of 1 to 4 is assigned for the adrenergic component of the test, with each score normalized for age and sex; these are added to give a composite score of between 0 and 10 (Table 8.6). Patients with a score of 0 to 3 are considered to have mild autonomic failure; those with a score of 4 to 6, moderate failure; and those with a score of 7 or more, severe failure. This score has been validated in groups of patients with and without symptomatic autonomic failure; a score of 7 was found to differentiate between the two groups, with a sensitivity of 94% and a specificity of 100%.

MORPHOMETRY OF SURAL NERVE

Although routine assessment of nerve biopsy specimens in most medical centers is principally qualitative, quantitation (or morphometry) of specific types of pathologic findings can be performed. A quantitative approach is useful in the diagnosis of a variety of conditions in individual patients in daily practice. More importantly, in clinical studies in which pathologic end points are used as measures of disease presence or severity or efficacy of treatment, morphometric approaches are necessary in reliably measuring such end points and detecting changes over time. Morphometry has several advantages over subjective assessment of nerve pathology: (1) it is quantitative and allows statistical analysis; (2) it facilitates assessment of a large data set; (3) it reduces observer bias; and (4) it is readily adapted to computerization for both image processing and analysis.[31] The pathologic alterations in sural nerve that occur in diabetes are discussed in Chapter 19.

Morphometric techniques can be used to assess myelinated fibers, unmyelinated fibers, or interstitial structures such as blood vessels. Myelinated fibers are most commonly studied. In general, studies are performed on either

TABLE 8.6 ORDER OF PHYSICAL VARIABLES SIGNIFICANTLY ASSOCIATED IN STEPWISE MULTIPLE LINEAR REGRESSION ANALYSIS WITH MOTOR NERVE CONDUCTION VALUES AND THEIR MODEL COEFFICIENTS*†

End Points	First	Second	Third
Motor Nerve Conduction‡			
Ul Amp	Age, −0.041		
Ul CV	Age, −0.118	Sex, 3.981	
Ul DL	Age, 0.005	Ht, 0.011	
Ul F-Wave L	Ht, 0.157	Age, 0.056	Sex, −1.592
Med Amp	Age, −0.061		
Med CV	Age, −0.109	Sex, 1.853	
Med DL	Sex, −0.179	Age, 0.008	BSA, 0.417
Med F-Wave L	Sex, −1.437	Ht, 0.143	Age, 0.060
Per Amp	Age, −0.042		
Per CV	Age, −0.121	Ht, −0.214	
Per DL	Ht, 0.020		
Per F-Wave L	Ht, 0.405	Age, 0.108	
Tib Amp	Age, −0.114	BSA, −4.796	
Tib CV	Age, −0.114	Ht, −0.248	
Tib DL	Age, 0.009	Ht, 0.016§	
Tib F-Wave L	Ht, 0.138	Age, 0.422	

*The physical variables assessed were age, gender (sex), height, weight, body mass index, and surface area.
†All variables listed in the table are $P<.001$.
‡Abbreviations: Ul, ulnar; Med, median; Per, peroneal; Tib, tibial; Amp, amplitude; CV, conduction velocity; DL, distal latency; L, latency; Ht, height; BSA, body surface area.
§$P=.001<P<.01$.
From Dyck PJ, Litchy WJ, Lehman KA, et al. Variables influencing neuropathic end points: The Rochester Diabetic Neuropathy Study of Healthy Subjects (RDNS-HS). Neurology 1995; 45:1115.

semi-thin or thin transverse sections or teased nerve fiber preparations. Characteristics of fibers that can be assessed in transverse sections are number, density (number per unit area), distribution, size (diameter or area), shape, relationship of axon to myelin sheath thickness, and pathologic condition. The diameter distribution of myelinated fibers or their axons can be determined and expressed as a histogram; alterations from normal can be observed as a change in the size or position of one or both peaks, which represent large and small myelinated fiber populations (see Table 8.1).

Techniques are also available for assessing the distribution of myelinated fibers within or among fascicles at a given level of nerve or among different levels. Alterations from the normal distribution are useful in demonstrating focal or multifocal pathologic processes, including fiber loss and fiber regeneration.

Normative data were obtained by Dyck and colleagues using nerve tissue obtained from healthy subjects of various ages.[7] Material from several levels between dorsal and ventral spinal roots and distal sural nerve was studied. In the sural nerve, there is considerable variability in myelinated fiber number and density among individuals, and this variability increases with age. In contrast, fiber size distribution is relatively constant among normal subjects and shows less variability with age. In either case, this variability is not so great as to preclude differentiation of normal and diseased nerves where the disease in question affects histologic parameters. This differentiation may be aided by the use of a percentile approach if an adequate number of samples from healthy subjects is available.

Evaluation of teased nerve fibers may also provide useful quantitative data. Dyck and associates[8] have introduced a system of classification of teased fiber conditions. Nine conditions are recognized, as summarized here:

A. Normal
B. Excessive myelin irregularity
C. Segmental or paranodal demyelination
D. As in condition C, with thinly myelinated internodes indicating remyelination
E. Axonal degeneration
F. Thinly myelinated internodes indicating remyelination, without demyelination
G. Focal myelin thickening
H. Normally myelinated internodes with superimposed myelin ovoids, indicating fiber regeneration
I. Several normal proximal internodes adjacent to a row of myelin ovoids, indicating wallerian degeneration

Observer judgment may introduce a certain

degree of variability; this is usually minimal except where fixation or staining are suboptimal or where surgical artifact is present.

Several studies have used morphometric measures of sural nerves as the primary end point, especially to assess for efficacy of aldose reductase inhibitors. Assessed were numbers of myelinated fiber (MF)/mm^2, MF diameter histogram, and teased fiber conditions. A consensus group of the Peripheral Nerve Society expressed some reservation about the use of morphometric end points as efficacy measures because (1) degenerating profiles (a myelin ovoid) may be mistaken for an MF; (2) an MF profile may be nonfunctional; and (3) the potential benefits may not be outweighed by the morbidity and high cost of the procedure.[4]

Nerve Endings in Punch Skin Biopsies

Bolton and associates[1, 5] showed that morphometric assessment of skin nerve endings (for example, the Meissner corpuscle) may provide a marker of the severity of sensory neuropathy. Various authors (Yasuda and colleagues,[29] Kennedy and coworkers,[15] McCarthy and associates[20]) have reintroduced the use of punch biopsies so that the density of nerve endings might be used as a quantitative indicator of peripheral neuropathy. These approaches might be considered for use in controlled clinical trials in DPN. We think there are three limitations of the procedure for this purpose: (1) there is still insufficient information of how well present methods actually detect all nerve fibers; (2) the counted nerve fiber may not be functional; and (3) it is unclear what degree of change (in number of nerve endings) over time should be considered meaningful of clinical change.

PROCEDURES FOR SETTING NORMAL VALUES

As we state in a paper on this issue, "The judgment regarding the presence or absence of disease and the need to perform further testing or to treat may depend importantly on whether measured patient characteristics are within 'normal limits.'"[20] Too frequently, reference values are far from ideal, mainly because of unrepresentative selection of healthy subjects, inadequate sample size, lack of medical evaluation of subjects, failure to measure variables that influence the attribute studied, and failure to use appropriate statistical analysis. Developing better normal values might result in

more sensitive (detecting disease when it is present) and specific (not detecting disease when it is absent) identification of disease. If tests are expressed as a percentile for age, sex, and applicable physical characteristics, it may be possible to follow the disease progression, as measured by the characteristic, free of other influences than the disease itself.

It is not possible to set normal limits for all the tests previously described. One cannot set normal limits for disease scores such as the NSC and NIS because they are designed to measure severity of disease, not variability in healthy subjects. The neurologist uses previous experience and judgment to decide whether a finding is abnormal or not. By contrast, attributes of NC, modalities of QST, and different QAT percentile responses can be set.

Selection of the Reference Cohort. Considerable care needs to be used to select the reference cohort so that it will adequately serve as the norm or standard. Ideally, one begins by randomly selecting persons from the general population. These persons should be representative of the population by age, gender, ethnic origin, and perhaps physical characteristics. Next, one should exclude certain persons from this list. Those patients who have diseases that the test will be used to diagnose should be excluded. For neuropathy tests, we generally have excluded patients with neuropathy, neurologic diseases, or diseases predisposing to neuropathy (e.g., untreated hypothyroidism, malnutrition, alcoholism, and malignancy). Patients with static mononeuropathy need not be excluded, but of course the affected nerve is not used as a control.

Sometimes a reference value departs so far from the norm that it needs to be excluded simply as an outlier. Consider the case of a patient selected for NC reference values whose conduction velocities are in the range of 20 to 30 m/s—unequivocally outside of the normal range. From previous experience, this patient, although asymptomatic, probably has inherited neuropathy and should be excluded from the reference population. However, caution must be exercised in using results of the test for which normal values are being derived as an exclusion criteria for that test, because circularity can easily develop and an erroneously narrow range of normal values can be obtained. This practice should be limited to cases where the test result clearly indicates disease and should ideally be correlated clinically.

Even after a representative cohort has been

selected from census lists, this representation may be lost because of uneven agreement to participate. How might one detect the imbalance that has been introduced? It may be possible to ascertain whether an agreement-to-participate bias has been introduced by comparing available data of participating and nonparticipating groups. Such factors as age, sex, ethnic origin, occupation, and physical characteristics might be used for this purpose.

Use of Friends, Laboratory Personnel, and Hospital Workers as the Reference Cohort. This approach is sometimes used, but it is not good practice. It is not that such persons should not be asked to participate, but they may not be representative of the community for which they will provide normal values.

More Than Age Should Be Taken Into Account. Usually, age is an important variable influencing normal values. It is convenient, therefore, to display and understand a graph in which one displays the normal value and age and defines a normal limit. But other physical characteristics and ethnic origin may relate importantly to normal values. To illustrate, we found that vibratory detection threshold relates importantly to anatomical site, age, gender, body surface area, and body mass index. Assuming that the appropriate statistical analyses have been done and with the general availability of personal computers, it is then possible to derive the percentile value of a test using applicable variables. That it is complex is no longer an adequate reason not to use it.

Cost Effectiveness of Prospectively Assessing Large Healthy Subject Cohorts. The cost of selecting, evaluating, and analyzing data from a healthy subject cohort can be considerable. Some thought must therefore be given to whether the improved estimate of abnormality and reliable detection of disease that results is worthwhile. The use of generalized and accurate reference values are perhaps more easily justified for epidemiologic or research studies. In diabetes, a serial decrease in the value of NC velocity (m/s) or increase in vibratory detection threshold (ln μm of displacement) may not reflect a true worsening of neuropathy. It may reflect a combination of worsening polyneuropathy, age, and increasing weight. To isolate the change to neuropathy, it would therefore be better to follow the percentile response that has been corrected for the factors other than DPN.

Use of Referred Patients Without Neuromuscular Disease as the Reference Cohort. This practice is not recommended. Patients who are referred to an electromyography laboratory and are not found to have electrophysiologic evidence of neuromuscular disease are not ideal controls. Because they were referred for symptoms, they may suffer from undiagnosed disease. It is unclear that they are representative of the general population. It is flawed reasoning to use subjects who passed a test to serve as controls for the same test.

Statistical Methods for Computing Normal Values. It is essential that appropriate statistical methods be used in computing normal percentiles. An algorithm that will accommodate most situations encountered in clinical practice is described in the next section.[23]*

A Single Dependent Variable

In considering the statistical techniques that are useful in obtaining normal values, we start with the simplest situation: only one characteristic (or, in statistical language, one dependent variable) for which reference values are desired, and no explanatory variables (independent variables) such as age or gender are to be considered. In the past, interest has centered on the 2.5th and 97.5th percentiles, commonly referred to as a normal range. However, in view of the wide availability of computers, there is no need to restrict attention to the resulting dichotomy of normal/abnormal. It will be more informative to indicate the actual percentile attained by an individual patient, and computing each of the percentiles (from 1 through 99) is easily done with a computer.

Notationally, we will refer to the Pth percentile for a variable Y as Y(P), for P = 1,...,99.

Notice that Y(P) is defined as the value such that P% of values in the reference population is less than Y(P). To estimate Y(P) from a study population, one simply selects the corresponding percentile in the set of study values. This method is simple and universally valid, requiring no esoteric mathematical assumptions. Notice, however, that it will require large sample sizes to estimate very large or very small percentiles. This is not unreasonable. For example, common sense would indicate that, if we are to estimate the 99th percentile (that value below which 99% of persons fall), we would need at least 99 subjects in our study. Conversely, it

*This text from O'Brien IA, Dyck PJ. Procedures for setting normal values. Neurology 1995; 45:17–23, with permission.

should be apparent that a sample of 15 subjects, for example, would not suffice.

Unfortunately, there is a common misconception that statistical wizardry can obviate this need for large sample sizes in setting normal values. This misconception is based on the erroneous belief that 95% of values in any population can be expected to lie within the mean ± 2 standard deviations. This assertion is sometimes qualified to be true only if the mean and standard deviation are computed from large sample sizes, and is based on the assumption that values in a population must follow what statisticians refer to as a Gaussian, or normal, distribution. The use of the label "normal distribution" is unfortunate, since there is no basis for assuming that values in any population must follow such a distribution.

The lack of any rational basis for assuming values in a population to follow a Gaussian distribution was pointed out eloquently by Elveback and coworkers.[11-13] We will only add here that, if the hypothesis were true, it would necessarily imply the possibility of negative values in the population, a circumstance that is often impossible. On the other hand, if one accepts that a Gaussian distribution is not a mathematical necessity but might only hold approximately, one must be concerned with the accuracy of the approximation (strictly speaking, one might argue that any statement is true "approximately"). In this case, however, one must acknowledge that judging the accuracy of a normal distribution in estimating normal percentiles in any specific instance would require knowledge of the true percentiles. Simply having a bell shaped curve is not sufficient to ensure close agreement of percentiles.

The observation that the "normal law of errors" lacks both a mathematical and an empirical basis was also pointed out eloquently by Poincaré[12]: "Everyone believes in the normal law of error, the physicists because they think that the mathematicians have proved it to be a mathematical necessity, the mathematicians because they believe that physicists have established it by laboratory demonstration."

In order to illustrate the issues raised thus far, we consider a population of serum urea values obtained from consecutive patients at the Mayo Clinic. The population consisted of 5,594 values that were stored on a computer. We then generated a true random sample from this population (Table 8.7). Note that the 95th percentile may be estimated by the value 82, the 95th largest value. In fact, any number

TABLE 8.7 DISTRIBUTION OF SERUM UREA VALUES IN A SAMPLE (n = 100) RANDOMLY DRAWN FROM A POPULATION (n = 5594)*

Value (mg/dl)	Frequency and Percentile (P)	Value (mg/dl)	Frequency and Percentile (P)
173	1	36	2
103	1	35	6
95	1	34	2
88	1	33	3
82	1 (P_{95})	32	9 (P_{50})
68	1	31	4
66	1	30	6
52	2	29	6
50	1 (P_{90})	28	2
46	1	27	2 (P_{25})
45	2	26	2
44	1	25	4
42	5	24	6
41	3	23	3 (P_{10})
40	5 (P_{75})	22	2
39	2	20	5 (P_8)
38	1	19	1
37	3	18	1
		16	1

*Means of sample is 36.56; SD is 20.27.
From O'Brien PC, Shampo MA. Statistics for clinicians: 10. Normal values. Mayo Clin Proc 1981; 56:639–640. By permission of Mayo Foundation.

between 69 and 82 will exceed 95% of values in the sample, and thus any of these could be used to estimate the 95th percentile. Rather than choosing the largest, one usually chooses an intermediate value, and various strategies are available for making the choice. Note also that the mean minus 2 standard deviations yields a negative number.

In order to illustrate the need for large sample sizes in estimating percentiles, we generated 9 additional samples of size 100 from this population (Table 8.8). Notice that estimates of the mean and median are quite stable, indicating that n = 100 is a large sample size for estimating a typical value. (Note also that medians are more appropriate than means when the distribution of values is skewed, as in the present instance, with the largest values in the population more spread out than the smallest values.) However, the upper percentiles vary markedly from one sample to the next. In general, we recommend that a sample size of 100 should be considered a minimum for reliably estimating normal values.

A Single Independent Variable

Next, suppose that values of Y vary with age. In this case, one would wish to estimate percentiles taking into account the ages of persons

TABLE 8.8 MEAN AND SELECTED PERCENTILES OF SERUM UREA VALUES IN 10 SAMPLES
(n = 100 FOR EACH)

Sample	Mean (mg/dl)	Values for Selected Percentiles			
		P_{50}	P_{00}	P_{05}	P_{99}
1*	36.56	32	50	82	173
2	33.92	31	50	57	103
3	34.24	31	50	62	123
4	33.00	31	43	52	86
5	33.47	31	46	60	220
6	36.67	32	48	56	172
7	35.15	30	52	61	123
8	38.93	32	50	69	388
9	32.31	30	48	56	93
10	86.57	32	46	55	174
SD†	2.07	0.8	2.7	8.8	89.3
Population values‡	35.33	31	48	60	124

*From Table 8.7.
†SDs of the 10 values listed directly above.
‡From population of 5594 values.
From O'Brien PC, Shampo MA. Statistics for clinicians: 10. Normal values. Mayo Clin Proc 1991; 56:639–640. By permission of Mayo Foundation.

in the population. The methodology for doing so is described below.

Step 1: Visually inspect a scatterplot of the data for outliers. If present, these values are to be deleted from the regression analyses that follow, but not from the estimation of percentiles at the end (Steps 6 and 7).

Step 2: Visually inspect for skewness, possibly indicating the need to transform the data (taking logarithms of original values, for example).

Step 3: Evaluate whether the average value of Y changes with age. This may be performed by constructing a regression equation relating Y to age, having the form: $\hat{Y} = b_0 + b_1$ age. The decision whether or not to adjust for age at this point would depend on several factors. Is the association statistically significant? Is the association with age of sufficient magnitude to warrant considering an adjustment? In assessing this, one might compare the standard deviation of the Y values to the standard deviation of the differences between the Y values actually observed and the corresponding estimates obtained from the regression equation. (These differences are referred to as the residuals from regression.) Alternatively, one might compare the squared values of these quantities, which statisticians refer to as the variance. The percent reduction in variance of Y is given by a statistic called R-squared. If the association is found to depend on age, one might then wish to consider adding higher order terms (age squared, for example) to the estimation equa-

tion. If no adjustment is made for age at this point, $\hat{Y}$ is set equal to the mean.

Step 4: It is equally important to consider whether the variability in Y values changes with age. This is commonly the case, since the aging process can be expected to progress at different rates, and in different forms, in individual subjects in the population. For percentiles above the 50th, one may estimate the effect of age on variability by regressing the positive residuals (R) against age, obtaining an equation of the form: $\hat{R} = C_0 = C_1$ age. The need to adjust for an association with age at this point is judged in a manner analogous to the method described in step 2. If no adjustment is made, $\hat{R}$ is set equal to 1.

Step 5: For each subject (including the outliers excluded from the regression analyses), compute an age adjusted Z score: $Z = (Y - \hat{Y})/\hat{R}$.

Step 6: Compute the percentiles for Z, using the methodology described in the section on a single dependent variable, obtaining Z(P) for P = 1,...,99. (We have explicitly described the algorithm for the upper percentiles. The lower percentiles are obtained in the same manner, but using the absolute value of the negative residuals in step 3).

Step 7: To obtain percentiles for Y as a function of age, one computes $Y(P) = \hat{R} Z(P) + \hat{Y}$.

Multiple Explanatory Variables

In practice, one may have a variety of characteristics that may influence the measurement of interest, such as age, gender, weight, height, occupation. The methodology for incorporating such variables is easily accomplished, using the basic principles described in the preceding section. However, in developing the analogous regression equations for $\hat{Y}$ and $\hat{R}$ (accounting for factors that influence average values and variability, respectively), we recommend using a step-wise regression approach. Thus, in the regression equation for $\hat{Y}$, for example, one first identifies the variable that best predicts Y. After including this variable in the prediction equation, one then identifies which of the remaining variables adds the most information (provides the best prediction of Y) beyond the information already available from the first variable to enter. One continues in this way until none of the remaining variables provide a statistically significant improvement in the prediction of Y. This process yields a prediction equation of the form: $\hat{Y} = b_0 + b_1$ *age* $+ b_2$ *weight* $+ \dots$.

One obtains an equation for $\hat{R}$ in similar fashion, computes Z scores as described previously, ultimately obtaining percentiles for Y. Although the computations become more complicated than in the case of a single explanatory variable, they are easily carried out using step-wise regression algorithms that are standard with most statistical software packages. Once the equations for obtaining percentiles have been developed, one simply enters the selected explanatory variables to obtain the corresponding percentiles.

In some instances, it may be desirable to have percentiles available in tabular or graphical form, rather than (or in addition to) computerized printout of percentiles. Approximate tabulations may be obtained by defining strata by dividing the explanatory variables into intervals. One may then compute a selected percentile of interest (such as the 95th) for the midpoint of each interval, then tabling these percentiles. Graphical displays may be calculated by retaining one variable (such as age) as a quantitative variable. For each of the strata defined by the remaining explanatory variables, one may graph $\hat{Y}$ against the single quantitative variable (age), including both data points and the estimated percentile line. Such graphical displays will be helpful in verifying that the algorithm performed appropriately.

Multiple Independent Variables and Multiple Dependent Variables

One is sometimes confronted with a battery of test results. Recognizing that healthy patients may often have one or two unusual values, one may desire to identify patients with a pattern of values that require further medical attention. Building on the analysis described in the preceding section, one may evaluate the possibility of unusual patterns by focusing on the Z scores obtained in the study of each dependent variable. Specifically, for each subject in the reference population, one computes the distance between the multivariate array of Z scores from the mean of the Z scores. The statistical measure of distance used is called Mahalanobis' distance, and the computations required are easily performed on most statistical software packages. Letting D represent the distance computed for each subject, one may set percentiles for these D values using the algorithm in the preceding section.

REFERENCE VALUES FOR NEUROPATHY END POINTS

We have not developed reference values for such symptom scores as NSS and NSC because we consider them to be disease scores. To illustrate, the physician evaluating the patient does not score paresthesia as present and caused by peripheral polyneuropathy unless he or she judges it to be in the appropriate anatomical region and beyond physiologic norms in duration and severity. By contrast, the scales of the NSP and percentile scores have been derived.

Likewise, most scores for neuropathic impairment are disease scores. In NIS (see Table 8.4), muscle weakness is graded as a percent of normal considering age, gender, and physical fitness and attributes, that is, it is considered to be an abnormality. Likewise, muscle stretch reflexes and sensation are to be graded as disease scores and only when they are unequivocally abnormal.

Reference values for attributes of NC have been published by various investigators. One of the larger series of subjects is the one now in use in the Mayo electromyography laboratory, developed by E. H. Lambert and colleagues. The subjects were not randomly selected from the population; rather, several hundred persons were recruited from several sources. Nerve conduction values were plotted against age and a lower limit was set by eye—approximately at the first percentile. In an important paper in which 104 healthy subjects had NC studies, Rivner and colleagues[26] found that height had a strong inverse relationship with sural, peroneal, and tibial conduction velocity. Height was also significantly correlated with distal latency for many nerves. Other authors generally agreed that height or limb length played a role in influencing attributes of NC.[2] We showed that a variety of variables influenced NC attributes.[7] The healthy subject cohort (HS-RDNS) was selected at random from the Rochester, Minn., population so as to obtain 15 men and 15 women for each hemidecade for persons 18 to 74 years without neuropathy, neurologic disease, or diseases predisposing to neuropathy. We used the approaches of O'Brien and colleagues[22] to determine the covariates for the major attributes of NC.[10] The three covariates that were found to influence NC attributes often were age, height, and sex—and occasionally body surface area or body mass index. As shown in Tables 8.6, 8.9, and 8.10, the order was not the same for

all attributes. Age or height was often the most important covariate. We concluded that with the general availability of personal computers and percentile responses for age and these physical characteristics, it was now possible and desirable to estimate percentile responses specific for age, height, sex, and applicable variables. We noted that "continued use of normal limits tables, which are corrected only for age, provides quite inadequate reference values, especially for some attributes of NC and especially for the extremes of height and weight."[10]

Quantitative Sensory Tests. We have developed reference values for vibratory detection threshold (VDT), cooling detection threshold (CDT), and heat-pain threshold (HP 0.5) and

TABLE 8.9 THE ORDER OF PHYSICAL VARIABLES SIGNIFICANTLY ASSOCIATED IN STEPWISE MULTIPLE REGRESSION ANALYSIS WITH SENSORY NERVE CONDUCTION VALUES AND THEIR MODEL COEFFICIENTS*†

End Points	First	Second	Third
Sensory Nerve Conduction‡			
Su Amp	Age, -0.199	BSA, -10.134	
Su CV	Ht, -0.364	Age, -0.134	
Su DL	Ht, 0.016	Age, 0.007	
Wrist-Index Med Amp	Age, -0.825	Sex, 14.297	BSA, -16.063
Wrist-Index Med CV	Age, -0.167	Ht, -0.138	
Wrist-Index Med DL	Age, 0.006	BSA, 0.298	
Palm-Wrist Left Ul Amp‖	BSA, -49.920	Age, -0.618	Sex, 12.909
Palm-Wrist Left Ul DL	Age, 0.003	Ht, 0.005	
Palm-Wrist Left Med Amp	BSA, -89.616	Age, -1.988	Sex, 33.703
Palm-Wrist Left Med DL	BSA, 0.372	Age, 0.005	
Palm-Wrist Right Ul Amp	Sex, 15.034	Age, -0.657	Wt, -0.272
Palm-Wrist Right Ul DL	Age, 0.004	Ht, 0.005	
Palm-Wrist Right Med Amp	BSA, -90.341	Age, -2.069	Sex, 30.035
Palm-Wrist Right Med DL	Age, 0.007	Wt, 0.005	
Wrist-Fifth Ul Amp	Age, -0.608	Sex, 20.218	
Wrist-Fifth Ul CV	Age, -0.133	Sex, 3.408	
Wrist-Fifth Ul DL	Age, 0.005	Ht, 0.008	
Palm-Wrist Left Ul CV	Age, -0.133	Sex, 4.463	
Palm-Wrist Left Med CV	Age, -0.181	Ht, -0.117	Sex, 1.970§
Palm-Wrist Right Ul CV	Age, -0.149	Sex, 3.819	
Palm-Wrist Right Med CV	Age, -0.162	Sex, 3.533	
Summated CMAP (Ul, Per, Tib)	Age, -0.195	Wt, -0.073	
Summated SNAP	BSA, -47.128	Age, -0.873	Sex, 7.460§
Autonomic			
Heart period Valsalva	Age, -0.010		
Heart period deep breathing	Age, -0.245		
CASS	Age, 0.008		

*The physical variables assessed were: age, gender (sex), height, weight, body mass index, and surface area.
†All variables listed in the table are $P<.001$, unless they were identified by a section mark when their P value is $.001<P<.01$.
‡Abbreviations: Su Amp, sural amplitude; Su DL, sural distal latency; Med Amp, median amplitude; Med CV, median conduction velocity; Med DL, median distal latency; Ul AMP, ulnar amplitude; Ul DL, ulnar distal latency; Ul CV, ulnar conduction velocity; CASS, composite autonomic scoring scale; Ht, height; BSA, body surface area; Wt, weight; CMAP, compound muscle action potential; SNAP, sensory nerve action potential; Ul, ulnar; Per, peroneal; Tib, tibial.
§$P=.001<P<.01$.
‖Height was also significant by association with this attribute (coefficient of 0.521; $P<0.01$).
From Dyck PJ, Litchy WJ, Lehman KA, et al. Variables influencing neuropathic end points: The Rochester Diabetic Neuropathy Study of Healthy Subjects (RDNS-HS). Neurology 1995; 45:1115.

TABLE 8.10 INFLUENCE OF AGE, HEIGHT, AND WEIGHT ON 1st OR 99th PERCENTILE: NORMAL LIMITS OF SOME ATTRIBUTES OF NERVE CONDUCTION

		CMAP 1st Percentile (mV)				MNCV 1st Percentile (m/s)				DL 99th Percentile (ms)			
		Peroneal		Tibial		Peroneal		Tibial				Peroneal	
Ht	Wt	30 y	70 y	30 y	70 y	30 y	70 y	30 y	70 y	30 y	70 y	30 y	70 y
6'6	250	1.59	0	1.51	0	36.7	31.9	35.5	30.9	6.90	6.90	5.49	5.86
6'6	170	1.59	0	4.24	0	36.7	31.9	35.5	30.9	6.90	6.90	5.49	5.86
6'0	250	1.59	0	3.14	0	39.9	35.1	39.3	34.7	6.59	6.59	5.24	5.61
6'0	150	1.59	0	5.30	.73	39.9	35.1	39.3	34.7	6.59	6.59	5.24	5.61
5'6	200	1.59	0	4.77	.20	43.2	38.4	43.1	38.5	6.28	6.28	5.00	5.37
5'6	125	1.59	0	6.49	1.93	43.2	38.4	43.1	38.5	6.28	6.28	5.00	5.37

CMAP, compound muscle action potential; MNCV, motor nerve conduction velocity; DL, distal latency; Ht, height; Wt, weight.
From Dyck PJ, Litchy WJ, Lehman KA, et al. Variables influencing neuropathic end points: The Rochester Diabetic Neuropathy Study of Healthy Subjects (RDNS-HS). Neurology 1995; 45:1115.

an intermediate pain response (HP 5.0) using the more than 300 persons in the HS-RDNS cohort. As shown in Table 8.6, the covariates for VDT are site, age, body surface area, and body mass index. For CDT, they are site, age, and body mass index. Our studies of HP 0.5 and 5.0 have not been completed.

Quantitative Autonomic Tests. As shown in Table 8.10, only age was a covariate for heart period variation with Valsalva, deep breathing, and CASS in our healthy subject studies.

References

1. Bolton CF, Winkelmann RK, Dyck PJ. A quantitative study of Meissner's corpuscles in man. Neurology 1966; 16:1–9.
2. Campbell WW Jr, Ward LC, Swift TR. Nerve conduction velocity varies inversely with height. Muscle Nerve 1981; 4:520.
3. DCCT Research Group: The Diabetes Control and Complications Trial (DCCT): Design and methodologic considerations for the feasibility phase. Diabetes 1986; 35:530.
4. Diabetic polyneuropathy in controlled clinical trials: Consensus Report of the Peripheral Nerve Society. Ann Neurol 1995; 38:478.
5. Dyck PJ, Winkelmann RK, Bolton CF. Quantitation of Meissner's corpuscles in hereditary neurologic disorders. Neurology 1966; 16:10–17.
6. Dyck PJ, Davies JL, Litchy WJ, et al. Longitudinal assessment of diabetic polyneuropathy using a composite score in the Rochester Diabetic Neuropathy Study Cohort. Neurology 1997; 49:229–239.
7. Dyck PJ, Giannini C, Lais A. Pathologic alterations of nerves. In Dyck PJ, Thomas PK, Low PA, et al (eds): Peripheral Neuropathy. Philadelphia, WB Saunders, 1993, p 514.
8. Dyck PJ, Johnson WJ, Lambert EH, et al. Segmental demyelination secondary to axonal degeneration in uremic neuropathy. Mayo Clin Proc 1971; 46:400.
9. Dyck PJ, Karnes J, O'Brien PC, et al. Neuropathy symptom profile in health, motor neuron disease, diabetic neuropathy, and amyloidosis. Neurology 1986; 36:1300.
10. Dyck PJ, Litchy WJ, Lehman KA, et al. Variables influencing neuropathic end points: The Rochester Diabetic Neuropathy Study of Healthy Subjects (RDNS-HS). Neurology 1995; 45:1115.
11. Elveback LR, Taylor WF. Statistical methods of estimating percentiles. Ann N Y Acad Sci 1969; 161:538–548.
12. Elveback LR, Guillier CL, Keating FR Jr. Health, normality, and the ghost of Gauss. JAMA 1970; 211:69–75.
13. Elveback LR. A discussion of some estimation problems encountered in establishing "normal values." In Gabrieli ER (ed): Clinically Oriented Documentation of Laboratory Data. New York, Academic Press, 1972, pp 117–137.
14. Hughes RAC, Newsom-Davis JM, Perkin GD, et al. Controlled trial of prednisolone in acute polyneuropathy. Lancet 1978; 2:750.
15. Kennedy WR, Wendelschafer-Crabb G, Johnson T. Quantitation of epidermal nerves in diabetic neuropathy. Neurology 1996; 47:1042.
16. Low PA. Composite autonomic scoring scale for laboratory quantification of generalized autonomic failure. Mayo Clin Proc 1993; 68:748.
17. Low PA. Clinical Autonomic Disorders: Evaluation and Management. Boston, Little, Brown, 1993.
18. Low PA. Autonomic nervous system function. J Clin Neurophysiol 1993; 10(1):14.
19. Low PA, Opfer-Gehrking TL, Proper CJ, et al. The effect of aging on cardiac autonomic and postganglionic sudomotor functions. Muscle Nerve 1990; 13:152.
20. McCarthy BG, Hsieh ST, Stocks A, et al. Cutaneous innervation in sensory neuropathies: Evaluation by skin biopsy. Neurology 1995; 45:1848.
21. Notermans NC, Lokhorst HM, Franssen H, et al. Intermittent cyclophosphamide and prednisone treatment of polyneuropathy associated with monoclonal gammopathy of undetermined significance. Neurology 1996; 47:1227.
22. O'Brien IA, O'Hare P, Corrall RJ. Heart rate variability in healthy subjects: Effect of age and the derivation of normal ranges for tests of autonomic function. Br Heart J 1986; 55:348.
23. O'Brien PC, Dyck PJ. Procedures for setting normal values. Neurology 1995; 45:17.
24. Persson A, Solders G. RR variations: A test of autonomic function. Acta Neurol Scand 1983; 67:285.
25. Rankin J. Cerebral vascular accidents in patients over the age of 60. 2: Prognosis. Scott Med J 1957; 2:200.
26. Rivner MH, Swift TR, Crout RO, et al. Toward more

rational nerve conduction interpretations: The effect of height. Muscle Nerve 1990; 13:232–239.

27. Scott J, Huskisson EC. Graphic representation of pain. Pain 1976; 2:175.

28. UK-TIA Study Group. The UK-TIA aspirin trial: Interim results. Br Med J 1988; 296:316.

29. Yasuda H, Kikkawa R, Hatanaka I, et al. Skin biopsy as a beneficial procedure for morphological evaluation of diabetic neuropathy. Acta Pathol Jpn 1985; 35:1.

30. Ziegler D, Hanefeld M, Ruhnau KJ, et al. Treatment of symptomatic diabetic peripheral neuropathy with the anti-oxidant alpha-lipoic acid: A 3-week multicenter randomized controlled trial (ALADIN Study). Diabetologia 1995; 38:1425.

31. Zimmerman IR, Karnes JL, O'Brien PC, et al. Imaging system for nerve and fiber tract morphometry: Components, approaches, performance, and results. J Neuropathol Exp Neurol 1980; 39:409.

Quantitative Motor Assessment

K. R. Mills

INTRODUCTION

Failure of muscle to generate sufficient force leads to motor impairment and often produces disability. The etiology, distribution, and severity of muscle weakness are important diagnostic features in many conditions. Although clinical examination remains the prime method of assessing muscle weakness, in many situations, such as the trial of therapeutic agents, it is preferable—some would say mandatory—to have some quantitative method of measuring the force of muscle contraction.

TYPES OF MUSCLE CONTRACTION

The function of muscle is to transform energy, stored as high energy phosphate, into force and heat. Muscle force may be exerted without a change in muscle length, in which case the muscle contraction is described as *isometric.* Force is measured in newtons (N), 1 N being the force that, if applied to a mass of 1 kg, gives it an acceleration of 1 meter per second squared ($m \cdot s^{-2}$). An example of an isometric contraction is the key grip, in which the opponens pollicis and first dorsal interosseous muscles produce sufficient force to hold the key between the thumb and index finger; the muscles exert this force without changing length. More commonly, muscle force is translated into movement; force is directed through tendons to bones that act as levers acting around the fulcrum at joints. The product of the force and the lever length is termed *torque* and is measured in newton-meters (Nm). Muscle contractions in which the muscle shortens in length are termed *concentric contractions*. Conversely, contraction may be associated with a lengthening of muscle, in which case the contraction is termed *eccentric*. Muscle contractions in which the velocity of shortening or lengthening is constant are termed *isokinetic*. In a simple exercise in which a subject moves on and off a step, the quadriceps muscle of one leg shortens as it raises the body up, that is, it is working concentrically. As the subject steps down, the other quadriceps muscle contracts yet lengthens to lower the body weight to the ground, that is, it is working eccentrically. Interestingly, although concentric contractions use about five times as much energy as do eccentric contractions, eccentric contractions have a much greater propensity to cause muscle damage and pain.[30] Muscle power, strictly speaking, is defined as the rate of force production over time. Thus, a 50% maximal muscle contraction maintained for 10 seconds has the same power as a 100% maximal contraction maintained for 5 seconds. The range of forces generated by different human muscles varies enormously; high jumpers generate sufficient force in their calf muscles to propel their body weight 7 feet off the ground; eye muscles, in contrast, work on a constant load (the globe) and are able to produce minute deviations of the visual axis. The harnessing of such a wide range of force-generating capability is the province of the central nervous system.

PHYSIOLOGY

A voluntary motor act presumably begins in frontal premotor cortex, which is where the action is planned. Psychologists distinguish cued voluntary acts, such as "press the button when you hear the bell," from self-initiated motor acts. In either case, the "motor program" for the desired movement is assembled and routed to the primary motor cortex. The appropriate command signals are transmitted over the corticospinal tract to the spinal motoneurons. Other descending tracts undoubtedly also influence the motoneurons, which integrate the command signals and discharge over the motor axons to the fine nerve terminals in the muscle. The nerve impulses are transmitted across the neuromuscular junctions and set up action potentials in the muscle fiber membrane. A single spinal motoneuron may innervate between 2 and 3000 single muscle fibers. The motoneuron, its axon, and the muscle fibers it controls form a *motor unit*. The size of motor units (the number of muscle fibers per motoneuron) is related to the muscle function; postural muscles have large motor units, whereas eye muscles have very small motor units. Human muscle fibers are basically of two types, which differ in their physiologic, metabolic, and staining characteristics. Type I fibers are characterized by pale staining for ATPase at pH 9.4, slow twitches, and predominantly oxidative metabolism. Type II fibers have dark staining, fast twitches, and glycolytic metabolism. All human muscles contain both fiber types in varying proportions. The type of a fiber is governed by the size and firing characteristics of the spinal motoneuron by which it is innervated. Thus, small motoneurons, with slow intrinsic firing rates, tend to be connected to thin axons and type I fibers. Large motoneurons have higher natural firing rates and thicker peripheral axons and innervate type II fibers. There is no mixing of fiber types within a motor unit. Muscle fiber excitation is translated into contraction by a complex sequence of reactions, in which calcium is intimately involved, that ultimately results in actin and myosin filaments forming cross bridges that slide over one another. Execution of the movement itself is monitored by receptors in muscle, skin, and joints that feed back the information to the central nervous system, allowing error correction and movement modification to be achieved.

The strength of a muscle contraction therefore depends on many factors, some local to the muscle itself (such as the number of fibers), some related to the spinal cord mechanisms (such as the rate of firing of spinal motoneurons), and some in the brain (such as the voluntary "effort" exerted). Muscle weakness is defined as a failure of a muscle to generate the expected force. Patients may complain of weakness, but they are more commonly describing some disability that results from a loss of force. Thus, patients may have difficulty rising from a chair or may drop objects. A loss of overall strength must be distinguished from muscle fatigue. Fatigue in the clinical setting is often used loosely to describe tiredness, loss of concentration, or malaise, but it is used in this chapter in a more restricted sense to describe an inability to maintain the expected force of contraction, that is, fatigue is time dependent.

Dysfunction of any of the systems in the chain of command from cortex to muscle can lead to muscle weakness. Stroke, motoneuron disease, peripheral neuropathy, and myopathy all lead to muscle weakness. Clinical and investigative methods can be used to determine the cause of muscle weakness. For instance, the characteristic features of upper motoneuron weakness and its common association with hyperreflexia and hypertonia are well known to clinicians. Similarly, weakness resulting from a lesion in the lower motoneuron pathway (from the perikaryon of the spinal motoneuron distally) often has a characteristic distribution and is associated with muscle wasting.

Techniques are available for measuring the function of all elements of the system. The motor cortex can be stimulated and the responses of muscles measured to allow an assessment of conduction in the corticospinal tracts.[16, 17, 24, 28] Percutaneous magnetic brain stimulation of appropriate intensity can evoke responses in many voluntary muscles; the response is much larger if the muscle is simultaneously voluntarily activated.[17] The central motor conduction time, representing cortical activation and conduction down the corticospinal tract to the spinal motoneurons, can be measured by subtracting from the total conduction time from cortex to muscle the peripheral conduction time.[16] Motor roots or nerves may be stimulated to measure conduction in peripheral nerve segments.[25] The neuromuscular junction can be assessed by measuring the muscle responses to repetitive nerve stimulation or the more sensitive technique of single fiber electromyography (EMG).[36] Motor unit and muscle fiber function can to some extent be quantified by EMG. The assessment of muscle force, however, has the advantage of being a measurement directly related to the patient's disability.

METHODS FOR ASSESSING MUSCLE STRENGTH

Clinical Examination

The examiner assesses the strength of individual muscle groups by applying a counter force to the limb to overcome the patient's voluntary force. Accurate diagnosis requires an assessment of the severity and distribution of weakness and can be achieved rapidly by the experienced examiner. The Medical Research Council (MRC) scale[1] (Table 9.1) has stood the test of time as being a robust and clinically useful

TABLE 9.1 THE MRC SCALE FOR ASSESSING MUSCLE STRENGTH

0: No contraction
1: Flicker or trace of contraction
2: Active movement, with gravity eliminated
3: Active movement against gravity
4: Active movement against gravity and resistance
5: Normal strength

method for quantifying muscle strength in patients. The scale, however, is nonlinear and ordinal. This means that a change of scale from say 4 to 3 does not imply the same loss of strength as from 3 to 2.[2, 23] In addition, the scale uses gravity as a benchmark against which strength is tested; clearly, the weight of the limb and the length of the lever system over which the muscle operates are important. Weakness of gastrocnemius, for instance, is difficult to assess unless it is very weak because it acts over a short lever system at the ankle. Furthermore, MRC grade 2 weakness, such as active movement with gravity eliminated, will clearly be different for the quadriceps muscle raising the leg than for a small muscle of the hand raising a finger. The effect of gravity is often ignored in routine clinical examination and in classifying patterns of weakness. Hip flexion is usually tested with the patient supine, that is, gravity is included in the estimate. In contrast, hip extension is usually tested with gravity eliminated. Pyramidal weakness, said to affect shoulder abduction more than adduction, finger and elbow extension more than flexion, hip flexion more than extension, and dorsiflexion more than plantar flexion, may in fact be an artifact of the assessment procedures because of differences in strength between agonists and antagonists and the effects of gravity.[8, 9]

Clinical examination of strength is also important in the detection of "hesitancy" or "submaximal effort." Fluctuations in the strength of a voluntary contraction are easily appreciated; pain from joints or muscle may also contribute to this hesitancy. In addition, co-contraction of agonists and antagonists such as occurs in dystonia may be detectable, as will the gradually increasing force encountered in extrapyramidal disorders. An estimate of the voluntary effort being exerted during a contraction can be obtained with the twitch superposition technique.[33] The rationale behind this is that if all muscle fibers are active during a contraction, then supramaximal stimulation of the periph-

Force (% max)

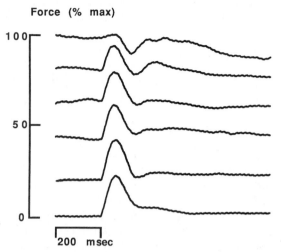

■ **Figure 9.1** Force of voluntary isometric index finger abduction was measured with a strain gauge placed next to the proximal interphalangeal joint. The subject was required to exert fixed fractions of his maximal force while a supramaximal electrical stimulus to the ulnar nerve at the wrist was given 200 msec into the sweep. The twitch superimposed on the voluntary force plateau is easily seen. When the subject exerts his maximum, the stimulus produces no extra force. The small reduction in force is caused by electrical silencing of the muscle that results from collision of antidromic stimulus-induced action potentials with orthodromic voluntary activity. Note also that maximal force can only be sustained for a short time before fatigue begins.

eral nerve should not result in any further force being generated. Figure 9.1 shows a force record from a normal subject performing voluntary contractions of various strengths. A supramaximal nerve shock applied during the contraction results in a twitch that is superimposed on the voluntary force. When the contraction is submaximal, additional force is produced by the shock; when the force is maximal, no additional force is produced. The technique is most easily applied to intrinsic hand muscles, where the peripheral nerve is accessible to stimulation, but it has been applied to other muscles such as the quadriceps, where intramuscular nerve terminals can be activated by large pad electrodes. The technique has been used to document submaximal muscle activation in chronic fatigue syndrome,[37] but it could also be useful in distinguishing upper motoneuron lesions, where the central drive is reduced but the force-generating capacity of the muscle is intact.

Dynamometry

The use of a device to measure the force of a muscle quantitatively has the advantage over

clinical assessment in having a continuous scale for which normal values can be determined.[4, 42] The scale will also be equally accurate and sensitive over its entire range. A wide range of devices have been used, such as spring balances,[32] cable tensiometers, and dynamometers.[40] The most useful devices measure force at a constant muscle length (isometric force) or at a constant velocity of movement (isokinetic force). The simplest device is a hand-held dynamometer, usually connected to an electronic recording device, with which the examiner assesses the force required to "break" the best effort of the patient.[43] Clearly, the positioning of the instrument on the limb needs to be standardized.[39] Often, the first trial must be discarded because the patient failed to appreciate exactly what was required. Usually, three or four trials are then collected, and either the highest value or the average of the three highest values that are within about 10% of each other are taken as representing the maximum force. The patient must be positioned so as to isolate the muscle group under test, when possible, eliminating gravity. Vigorous verbal encouragement may be needed to ensure the subject is producing his or her maximum. It should also be remembered that a subject can only produce his or her maximum force for a few seconds before fatigue begins (see Fig. 9.1).

A hand-held dynamometer has been used to measure the muscle strength in a wide range of muscle groups,[38, 41, 44, 45] with standardized positions of the device on the limb. Normal ranges have been determined (Table 9.2), and the technique has been validated for clinical use. For instance, the intertrial variability and interrater variability both have coefficients of variation of about 10%.[14, 15, 43] It is useful to be able to examine a trace of the force output on some recording device or computer screen. Patients who are pain-free produce a clear plateau of force, and hesitancy of effort is easily detected as a fluctuating force trace.

Several factors have been found to influence muscle strength, and these must be taken into account when assessing patients. Cross-sectional studies, for instance, indicate that isometric strength reaches its maximum in the second and third decades; from the fifth decade onward, it declines by about 15% per decade.[18, 46] Muscle strength, at least in proximal muscles, is higher in males than in females (see Table 9.2). Strength also varies throughout the menstrual cycle in women, reaching a peak at midcycle, possibly because of the increase in estrogen that occurs at that time.[34] In certain

TABLE 9.2 NORMAL VALUES FOR MYOMETRY

| | Muscle Strength (Newtons) | | | |
| | Males | | Females | |
	Mean	SD	Mean	SD
Neck flexion (supine)	139	37	68	13
Neck flexion (sitting)	176	39	95	19
Shoulder abduction	232	39	151	28
Elbow flexion	254	27	184	31
Elbow extension	161	30	117	20
Grip	405	66	236	34
Pinch grip	86	14	58	15
First dorsal interosseous	45	8	35	6
Abductor pollicis brevis	27	9	34	7
Abductor digiti minimi	23	5	22	5
Hip flexion	263	40	172	35
Hip abduction	263	37	218	31
Knee extension (R)	443	119	292	82
Knee extension (L)	421	122	287	81

SD, standard deviation.
From Wiles C, Karni Y, Nicklin J. Laboratory testing of muscle function in the management of neuromuscular disease. J Neurol Neurosurg Psychiatry 1990; 53:384.

conditions, it may also be relevant at which time of day assessments are made; in rheumatoid arthritis, grip strength is less early in the morning.[13]

The technique has successfully been applied to children[35] and has been used in a variety of neurologic conditions, including amyotrophic lateral sclerosis,[3, 14] Guillain-Barré syndrome,[21] and inflammatory muscle disease.[38] It has also proved useful in the serial study of patients undergoing treatment and can act as an early warning of deterioration.[44]

Electromyography and Compound Muscle Action Potential Amplitude as Indirect Measures of Muscle Force

The electrical activity associated with a muscle contraction can be recorded either with surface electrodes or with intramuscular needles. The former method records activity from a large volume and is therefore a representative average of the whole muscle activity. Needle electrodes are selective and record from only a small volume of tissue. Conventional electromyography (EMG) electrodes "see" a volume of muscle of radius about 1 mm. In relation to the assessment of overall strength, therefore, surface electrodes are preferable. The EMG signal must be processed in some way to give a measure of the overall electrical activity. This can be done by integrating the signal over a specified time or by measuring the root mean square value. What is the relationship between EMG and force? In a simple system where a single muscle produces the force under study such as abduction of the index finger by the first dorsal interosseous muscle, the relationship between force and EMG is linear (Fig. 9.2). A problem arises where the movement is not achieved by a single muscle; for instance, in elbow flexion, EMG may be recorded from the biceps muscle, but force of elbow flexion is generated by the biceps, brachioradialis, and brachialis muscles. In this situation, the relationship between EMG and force is nonlinear. Attempts have been made to quantify the relationship in patients to give an estimate of the "efficiency" of muscle contraction, that is, the force per unit EMG activity, but this has not proved to be a clinically useful measure.

Another estimate of the volume of active tissue in a muscle, particularly small muscles of the hand, is provided by the amplitude or area of the compound muscle action potential (CMAP) produced by supramaximal stimulation of the peripheral nerve. The amplitude, usually measured from the initial negative component, is closely correlated with the area of the CMAP, and there seems little point in using the latter measure. The CMAP increases with increasing strength of stimulation and then reaches a maximum when it is assumed that all motor axons are being activated. Each axon activates the fibers in its motor unit and

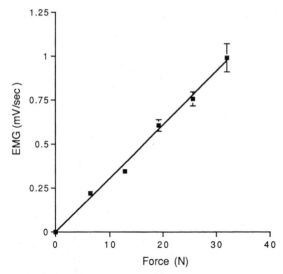

■ **Figure 9.2** Electrical activity (EMG) was recorded with surface electrodes over the first dorsal interosseous muscle. The force of index finger abduction was recorded with a strain gauge. Electrical activity was rectified and integrated over 1 sec while the subject held forces of 20, 40, 60, 80, and 100% maximum. The mean and standard deviation (SD) of 5 trials at each force level are shown. The relation between force and EMG is linear for this muscle, allowing a prediction of force to be made from EMG. In other muscles, the relationship is nonlinear.

produces a single fiber action potential. These summate to produce the CMAP. In a normal population, CMAP amplitudes of the abductor pollicis brevis muscle, for example, are not normally distributed but skewed to the left. There is also much variation between individuals depending on occupation, handedness, and other variables. Nevertheless, the absolute amplitude of the CMAP in intrinsic hand and foot muscles is usually above 5 mV, and this is a useful index clinically. Furthermore, the CMAP amplitude or area can be measured from different stimulation points on the nerve, allowing motor conduction velocity to be measured and the detection of conduction block.[22, 31] This important cause of muscle weakness is due to focal demyelination of peripheral nerve; conduction block leading to muscle weakness may be present in the absence of muscle wasting. It is detected by measuring the size of the CMAP evoked by nerve stimulation below and above the block. A decrease in amplitude of more than 50% is usually taken as secure evidence of conduction block. The CMAP amplitude has a nonlinear relationship to the MRC scale (Fig. 9.3) but correlates linearly with an arbitrary estimate (nil, mild, moderate, or severe) of the degree of wasting.[23]

MUSCLE FATIGUE

Just as the absolute force generating capacity of muscle may be compromised by dysfunction of one component of the pathway from motor cortex to muscle, so the ability of muscle to maintain a force may be similarly disturbed. When a healthy subject attempts to maintain a continuous maximal muscle contraction, force very quickly begins to fall.[20] The mechanical response of the muscle to nerve stimulation slows in speed, and adaptive changes in the spinal outflow occur. The firing rate of motoneurons is modulated downward to optimize the force production.[5, 6] As the maximal contraction proceeds, the muscle's energy-providing mechanisms and the neuromuscular junctions begin to fail, but in healthy subjects, no single cause of force decline has been identified. In patients, fatigue can occur from failure of central and peripheral mechanisms. Thus, muscle fatigue can arise centrally in multiple sclerosis[7] or peripherally either at the neuromuscular junction, as in myasthenia gravis, or in the muscle fiber itself, such as in myotonic dystrophy.[10] Several techniques are available to study muscle fatigue in patients.

By recording the electrical and mechanical response of a muscle to repetitive peripheral nerve stimulation, information can be obtained

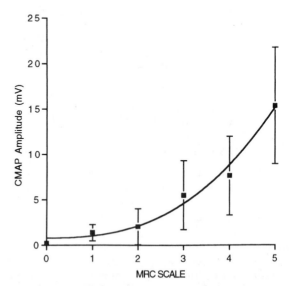

■ **Figure 9.3** The compound muscle action potential (CMAP) amplitude in the first dorsal interosseous muscle was measured in 50 patients with amyotrophic lateral sclerosis who were seen at 3-month intervals. The Medical Research Council (MRC) score in the muscle was also recorded. There is a nonlinear relation between them. Mean and standard deviation (SD) of CMAP amplitude are shown.

about the site of fatigue.[20] If the electrical response of the muscle and the CMAP remain the same size and yet the twitch produced by the muscle falls in size, then the abnormality is in the muscle itself. If the CMAP also falls in size, then an abnormality of the neuromuscular junction is likely. In healthy subjects, repetitive peripheral nerve stimulation at frequencies up to about 10 Hz causes no change in CMAP amplitude, and the twitch produced is of constant size. The twitch duration is approximately 100 ms; when the frequency of stimulation exceeds 10 Hz, the mechanical effects begin to summate and produce an unfused tetanus that becomes fused when the frequency reaches 30 Hz. The electrical response of normal muscle begins to decline at frequencies in excess of 70 Hz, indicating failure of the neuromuscular junction. In conditions where neuromuscular transmission is compromised, junctions may begin to fail at much lower stimulation frequencies because the safety factor of transmission is reduced.

The relationship between the frequency of stimulation and the force output of the muscle may be useful in analyzing certain types of fatigue.[12] The characteristic frequency-force curve can be obtained by stimulation of peripheral nerve trunks or by stimulation of intramuscular nerves with large pad electrodes. Essentially similar curves have been obtained from adductor pollicis,[12] biceps,[19] sternomastoid,[27] diaphragm,[26] and quadriceps[12] muscles. In this context, another form of contractile fatigue is recognized. After a period of heavy exercise, the frequency-force curve becomes shifted to the right. Whereas in the fresh state, 20 Hz stimulation would be expected to generate about 70% maximum force, in the fatigued state, the same stimulation generates only 30% maximum force.[11] This so-called "low frequency fatigue" occurs in the face of a maintained CMAP, that is, the abnormality lies distal to the neuromuscular junction. It probably results from impaired calcium release or transfer from the sarcoplasmic reticulum. Low frequency fatigue has been documented to occur in many human muscles, including small hand muscles, sternomastoid, and the diaphragm. It occurs after a prolonged period of intense activity or if the muscle is made ischemic by more moderate exercise. Eccentric contractions of muscle are more potent in causing low-frequency fatigue than concentric contractions.[30] This type of contractile fatigue can last many hours, and the time course of recovery differs from the return to normal of other indicators

of fatigue, such as muscle pH and phosphocreatine. Additionally, the contractile fatigue does not correlate with the rise in creatine phosphokinase or the muscular pain that follows prolonged muscular exercise.[29] Although low-frequency fatigue has been shown to occur in the diaphragm,[26] its role as a cause of chronic respiratory insufficiency remains to be fully determined.

References

1. Aids to the Examination of the Peripheral Nervous System. London, Ballière Tindall (on behalf of the Guarantors of Brain), 1986.
2. Aitkens S, Lord J, Bernauer E. Relationship of manual muscle testing to objective strength measurements. Muscle Nerve 1989; 12:173.
3. Andre P, Hedlund W, Finison L. Quantitative motor assessment in amyotrophic lateral sclerosis. Neurology 1986; 36:937.
4. Beasley W. Quantitative muscle testing: Principles and applications to research and clinical services. Arch Phys Med Rehabil 1961; 42:398.
5. Bigland-Ritchie B, Johansson R, Lippold O. Changes in motoneuron firing rates during sustained maximal voluntary contractions. J Physiol 1983; 340:355.
6. Bigland-Ritchie B, Johansson R, Lippold O. Contractile speed and EMG changes during fatigue of sustained maximal voluntary contractions. J Neurophysiol 1983; 50:313.
7. Boniface SJ, Mills KR, Schubert M. Responses of single spinal motoneurons to magnetic brain stimulation in healthy subjects and patients with multiple sclerosis. Brain 1991; 114:643.
8. Colebatch J, Gandevia S. The distribution of muscular weakness in upper motor neuron lesions affecting the arm. Brain 1989; 112:749.
9. Colebatch J, Gandevia S, Spira P. Voluntary muscle strength tests in hemiparesis: Distribution of weakness at the elbow. J Neurol Neurosurg Psychiatry 1986; 49:1019.
10. Cooper R, Stokes M, Edwards R. Physiological characterisation of the "warm up" effect of activity in patients with myotonic dystrophy. J Neurol Neurosurg Psychiatry 1988; 51:1134.
11. Edwards R, Hill D, Jones D, et al. Fatigue of long duration in human skeletal muscle after exercise. J Physiol 1977; 272:769.
12. Edwards R, Young A, Hosking G, et al. Human skeletal muscle function: Description of tests and normal values. Clin Sci Mol Med 1977; 52:283.
13. Ferraz M, Ciconelli R, Araujo P, et al. The effect of elbow flexion and time of assessment on the measurement of grip strength in rheumatoid arthritis. J Hand Surg [Am] 1992; 17:1099.
14. Goonetilleke A, Modarres-Sadeghi H, Guiloff R. Accuracy, reproducibility, and variability of hand held dynamometry in motor neuron disease. J Neurol Neurosurg Psychiatry 1994; 57:326.
15. Heinonen A, Sievanen H, Viitasalo J, et al. Reproducibility of computer measurement of maximal isometric strength and electromyography in sedentary middle-aged women. Eur J Appl Physiol 1994; 68:310.
16. Hess CW, Mills KR, Murray NM, et al. Magnetic brain stimulation: Central motor conduction studies in multiple sclerosis. Ann Neurol 1987; 22:744.

17. Hess CW, Mills KR, Murray NMF. Responses in small hand muscles from magnetic stimulation of the human brain. J Physiol 1987; 388:397.

18. Hurley B: Age, gender and muscular strength. J Gerontol A Biol Sci Med Sci 1995; 50:41.

19. Ismail H, Ranatunga K. Isometric tension development in a human skeletal muscle in relation to the working range of movement: The length:tension relationship of biceps brachii muscle. Exp Neurol 1978; 62:595.

20. Jones D: Muscle fatigue due to changes beyond the neuromuscular junction. *In* Human Muscle Fatigue: Physiological Mechanisms. Ciba Foundation Symposium 82. London, Pitman, 1981, vol 82, p 178.

21. Karni Y, Archdeacon L, Mills KR, et al. Clinical assessment and physiotherapy in Guillain-Barré syndrome. Physiotherapy 1984; 70:282.

22. Lewis R, Sumner A. The electrodiagnostic distinctions between chronic familial and acquired demyelinative neuropathies. Neurology 1982; 32:592.

23. Mills K. Wasting, weakness and the MRC scale in the first dorsal interosseous muscle. J Neurol Neurosurg Psychiatry 1997; 62:541.

24. Mills KR. Magnetic brain stimulation: A tool to explore the action of the motor cortex on single human spinal motoneurons. Trends Neurosci 1991; 14:401.

25. Mills KR, Murray NMF. Electrical stimulation over the human vertebral column: Which neural elements are excited? Electroencephalogr Clin Neurophysiol 1986; 63:582.

26. Moxham J, Morris A, Spiro S: Contractile properties and fatigue of the diaphragm in man. Thorax 1981; 36:164.

27. Moxham J, Wiles C, Newham D, et al. Sternomastoid muscle function and fatigue in man. Clin Sci 1980; 59:463.

28. Murray NM: Magnetic stimulation of cortex: Clinical applications. J Clin Neurophysiol 1991; 8:66.

29. Newham D, Jones D, Edwards RHT. Large and delayed plasma creatine kinase changes after stepping exercise. Muscle Nerve 1983; 6:36.

30. Newham D, Mills K, Quigley B, et al. Pain and fatigue after concentric and eccentric muscle contractions. Clin Sci 1983; 64:55.

31. Olney R, Miller R. Conduction block in compression neuropathy: Recognition and quantification. Muscle Nerve 1984; 7:662.

32. Ritchie Russell W, Fischer-Williams M. Recovery of muscular strength after poliomyelitis. Lancet 1954; 1:330.

33. Rutherford O, Jones D, Newham D. Clinical and experimental application of the twitch superimposition technique for the study of human muscle activation. J Neurol Neurosurg Psychiatry 1986; 49:1288.

34. Sarwar R, Beltran Niclos B, Rutherford O. Changes in muscle strength, relaxation rate and fatiguability during the human menstrual cycle. J Physiol 1996; 493:267.

35. Scott O, Hyde S, Goddard C, et al. Quantitation of muscle function in children: A prospective study in Duchenne muscular dystrophy. Muscle Nerve 1982; 5:291.

36. Stålberg E, Trontelj J. Single fibre electromyography. *In* Studies in Healthy and Diseased Muscle, ed 2. New York, Raven Press, 1994.

37. Stokes M, Cooper R, Edwards R. Normal muscle strength and fatiguability in patients with effort syndromes. BMJ 1988; 297:1014.

38. Stoll T, Bruhlman P, Stucki G, et al. Muscle strength assessment in polymyositis and dermatomyositis: Evaluation of the reliability and clinical use of a new, quantitative, easily applicable method. J Rheumatol 1995; 22:473.

39. Su C, Lin J, Chien T, et al. Grip strength in different positions of the elbow and shoulder. Arch Phys Med Rehabil 1994; 75:812.

40. Tornvall G. Assessment of physical capabilities with special reference to the evaluation of maximal voluntary isometric muscle strength and maximal working capacity. Acta Physiol Scand 1963; 58(suppl 201):1.

41. van der Ploeg R, Fidler G, Oosterhuis H. Hand-held myometry: Reference values. J Neurol Neurosurg Psychiatry 1991; 54:244.

42. van der Ploeg R, Oosterhuis H, Reuvencamp J. Measuring muscle strength. J Neurol 1984; 231.

43. Wiles C, Karni Y. The measurement of muscle strength in patients with peripheral neuromuscular disorders. J Neurol Neurosurg Psychiatry 1983; 46:1006.

44. Wiles C, Karni Y, Nicklin J. Laboratory testing of muscle function in the management of neuromuscular disease. J Neurol Neurosurg Psychiatry 1990; 53:384.

45. Ylinen J, Ruuska J. Clinical use of neck isometric strength measurement in rehabilitation. Arch Phys Med Rehabil 1994; 75:465.

46. Young A, Stokes M, Crowe M. The size and strength of the quadriceps muscles in old and young men. Clin Physiol 1985; 5:145.

Chapter **10**

Quantitative Sensory Assessment

Guillermo A. Suarez • Peter James Dyck

INTRODUCTION

Clinical assessment of sensation, the approach most commonly used by physicians, provides information about sensory abnormalities. However, it has several limitations including (1) the characteristics of the stimuli are undefined and variable; (2) the sequential steps of testing are not standardized; (3) the test performed varies among physicians; (4) results are not compared with normal results considering age, sex, site, and other variables; and 5) provides limited information on hypersensitive phenomena. Therefore, bedside approaches can detect only gross sensory loss and perhaps altered sensation among regions.

Sensitive and reliable approaches are necessary to detect and characterize the symptoms and deficits of diabetic neuropathy. For the reliable assessment of sensory thresholds for specific modalities of sensation at a given site, for the evaluation of hypersensitivity, and for epidemiologic and controlled clinical trials, quantitative sensory testing is needed.

The focus of this chapter is on microprocessor-controlled quantitative sensory examination to evaluate sensation using physical stimuli that activate mechanoreceptors, cool receptors, and nociceptors. Most of our results will be based on use of Computer Assisted Sensory Examination, system 4 (CASE IV), because it is the system we developed and with which we have seen results. Several other systems have become available since the introduction of CASE IV.[26, 27, 33, 34, 46] Direct electrical stimulation of the skin might also be considered.

ANATOMY AND PHYSIOLOGY OF SENSORY SYSTEMS

The somatic sensory system processes different kinds of stimuli that subjectively are experienced as different modalities of sensation. Thus, spatial, temporal, directional, and rate deformation of the skin and superficial tissues may be experienced as superficial touch, deep touch (pressure), rumbling, vibration, crawling, object recognition, and others. Interplay of various classes of receptors may induce stickiness, wetness, sharpness, lancinating pain, deep aching pain, and so on.

The anatomical elements of the somatic sensory system include receptors (also known as cutaneous sensory units), the dorsal root ganglion neuron (primary afferent neuron) with a peripheral afferent fiber, cell body, and centrally projected fiber synapsing with second order neurons in the spinal cord or brain stem. Somatic sensory information is relayed next to the thalamus and then to the cerebral cortex by two major ascending pathways, the dorsal column-medial lemniscus system conveying touch and proprioception and the anterolateral system mediating pain and temperature.

Receptors are distributed diffusely over the surface of the body, and there is substantial variability in receptor density with site and age. In healthy individuals, there is a dramatic reduction in receptor density with age (Fig. 10.1). Receptors may be classified according to their response properties. The receptors that respond to innocuous mechanical stimuli are called *mechanoreceptors*. A second class of receptors excited by small changes in temperature is known as *thermoreceptors*. The third group is consistently activated by noxious (tissue-damaging) stimuli of various types and is called *nociceptors* (Latin "nocere," to injure). *Nociceptors* can be further subdivided on the basis of the stimulus.

1. *Mechanical nociceptors* are activated by strong mechanical stimulation, for example, sharp objects.
2. *Thermal nociceptors* are activated selectively by cold or heat. In humans, heat nociceptors respond when the temperature of their receptive area is above 45°C; cold nociceptors are stimulated by noxious cold stimuli.

3. *Polymodal nociceptors* respond to different types of noxious stimuli.

Receptors are located in the superficial skin and deeply in the dermis and subcutaneous tissues. The classes of receptors found in glabrous (hairless) skin are Meissner's corpuscles, Merkel's receptors (also known as slowly adapting type I receptors), both located in the dermal papillae, and bare or "free" nerve endings. The receptors of the hairy skin are hair receptors (different types), bare nerve terminals, and Merkel's receptors with a slightly different organization compared to those found in the glabrous skin. Subcutaneous receptors include the pacinian corpuscle, a rapidly adapting receptor, and Ruffini's corpuscle, also known as slowly adapting type II receptor, both found beneath glabrous and hairy skin. Figure 10.2 illustrates the location of various types of receptors.

Mechanoreceptors and their sensory fibers provide information about direction, timing, shape, and spatial characteristics of the stimuli. Some receptors, such as the pacinian corpuscle, respond selectively to vibratory stimuli. Mechanoreceptors may be classified according to their pattern of response to a constant stimuli. Rapidly adapting receptors respond at the beginning and at the end but not during the duration of the stimulus, whereas slowly adapting receptors respond continuously to a steady stimulus.

Examples of two rapidly adapting receptors are Meissner's corpuscle located in the superficial skin and the pacinian corpuscle in the subcutaneous tissue. Merkel's corpuscle (superficial skin) and Ruffini's corpuscle (subcutaneous) are examples of slowly adapting receptors. Mechanoreceptors can also be classified depending on their threshold (high or low), by the size of their receptive field (large or small), and by whether their borders are sharp or sloping. The physiologic characteristics of mechanoreceptors found in experimental animal and human skin have been studied in detail.[3, 32, 36]

The main types of mechanoreceptors found in the superficial glabrous skin are a rapidly adapting receptor, the Meissner's corpuscle, and a slowly adapting receptor, the Merkel's receptor. These two receptors have small receptive fields, on average 2 to 4 mm. The size of the receptive field of a group of receptors determines the capacity to resolve spatial differences of objects. Deeply distributed receptors such as the rapidly adapting pacinian corpuscle and Ruffini receptor have large

MEISSNER'S CORPUSCLES PLANTAR SURFACE GREAT TOE WITH AGE-SPECIFIC CHE

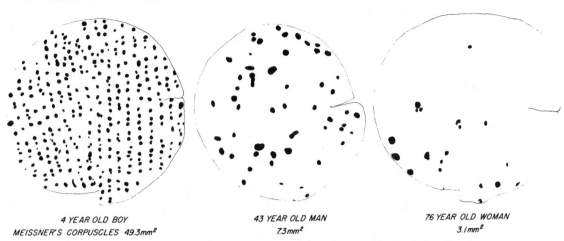

4 YEAR OLD BOY
MEISSNER'S CORPUSCLES 49.3mm²

43 YEAR OLD MAN
7.3mm²

76 YEAR OLD WOMAN
3.1mm²

■ **Figure 10.1** Appearance and distribution of Meissner's corpuscles in horizontal sections of 3-mm punch biopsy specimens of skin from the plantar surface of great toes in normal subjects (by method of superimposition of horizontal sections). The concentrations of Meissner's corpuscles are as follows: 4-year-old boy, 49.3/mm²; 43-year-old man, 7.3/mm²; and 76-year-old woman, 3.1/mm². (From Bolton CF, Winkelman RK, Dyck PJ. A quantitative study of Meissner's corpuscles in man. Neurology 1996; 16:1.)

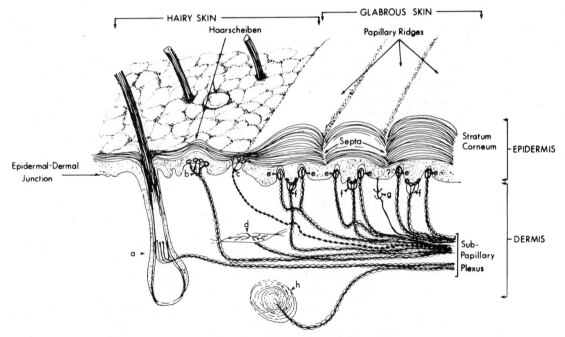

■ **Figure 10.2** Schematic drawing showing the location of various receptors in hairy and glabrous skin of primate. *a*, Hair follicle with "palisade" endings (G₁-, G₂-hair); *b*, Haarscheiben ("touch dome") neurite complex terminating on Merkel's cell (type I); *c*, "free" nerve ending (actually coated by Schwann cell) penetrating basal lamina and terminating among keratinocytes (myelinated nociceptor; cooling receptor?); *d*, Ruffini's ending (type II; SA II); *e*, Meissner's corpuscle found in dermal papillae (RA glabrous skin receptor; field receptor); *f*, Merkel's cell–neurite complex found on intermediate ridge of dermal papillae (SA I); *g*, "free" nerve ending stemming from unmyelinated axon (C polymodal? cooling? warming?); *h*, pacinian corpuscle (pacinian corpuscle receptor). (From Light AR, Perl ER. Peripheral sensory systems. *In* Dyck PJ, et al. (eds). Peripheral Neuropathy, ed 2. Philadelphia, WB Saunders, 1984, p 216.)

receptive fields. Receptors with small receptive areas can resolve fine spatial differences, whereas receptors with large receptive fields can only detect coarse spatial differences. The sensitivities of the rapidly adapting receptors can be separated according to their response to a sinusoidal mechanical stimuli. A low-frequency sinusoidal mechanical stimuli most consistently excites the Meissner's corpuscle located in the superficial skin. Pacinian corpuscles are most responsive to high-frequency stimuli. The stimulation of Meissner's receptors evokes a well-localized sensation, consistent with the small size of the receptive field, and feels like a fluttering in the skin. Conversely, stimulation of pacinian corpuscle evokes a response poorly localized because of the large receptive field and feels like a diffuse vibration or humming sensation. Natural complex stimuli, the ones most frequently encountered in everyday life, are different than the relatively pure sensory responses described above and often are perceived with multiple qualities. The study of textures may be considered an example of complex stimuli that activates several types of mechanoreceptors. Johnson and Lamb[31] studied texture discrimination by analyzing the patterns of response of different mechanoreceptors of the glabrous skin in the hands of monkeys. Their observations suggest that different components of the stimulus information are processed by both rapidly and slowly adapting receptors. It appears that rapidly adapting receptors provide speed of information, whereas the spatial characteristics of the stimuli are conveyed through slowly adapting receptors. In addition to the mechanoreceptors described above, there are other receptors that transduce thermal sensations of cold and warmth and pain.[3]

There are separate spots on the skin of humans where thermal stimulation evokes a warm or cold sensation. The threshold for activation of these spots is lower than in other areas of the skin. Warm and cold spots are innervated by thermoreceptors. There are two types of thermoreceptors, warmth and cold receptors. Warmth or warm receptors are selectively activated with skin warming above the neutral level (30 to 34°C), and their response rate increases with progressively warmer stimuli. When the temperature reaches approximately 45°C, warmth is not perceived, and the subject experiences heat-pain. In this range of painful thermal stimuli (>45°C), the discharge frequency of warm receptors is, in fact, reduced. Therefore, thermal receptors convey warmth sensation, whereas heat pain is mediated by nociceptors. Cold or cooling receptors are the second type of thermoreceptors and discharge at skin surface temperatures ranging between 25 and 30°C. The frequency of firing is proportional to the magnitude and rate at which temperature is lowered. These sensory units are able to respond to small changes in skin temperature (0.1°C), and at the lower end of their temperature range (<20°C), they often discharge in bursts. The duration and frequency of these burst discharges may play a role in temperature regulation.[25] In addition, cold receptors exhibit an interesting phenomenon called *paradoxical cold*. When a noxious heat stimulus of 45°C or more is applied to a single cold spot on the skin, it is perceived by the subject as cold, not hot. This paradoxical response has been related to the sensation of cold from brief contact with hot objects.[8]

Sensory information is transmitted to the central nervous system (CNS) via fibers that conduct action potentials at different rates. The velocity of the impulse is related to the diameter of the fiber. The faster a fiber transmits the information to the CNS the sooner the CNS can process and act on the information. Afferent fiber groups are classified based on conduction velocity and fiber size. When the human sural nerve is stimulated in vitro with shocks of increasing intensity, one successively elicits Aα, (also called A$\alpha\beta$), Aδ, and C potentials. A numerical nomenclature is generally used for muscle afferents: I (large myelinated); II (small myelinated); III (smaller myelinated); and IV (unmyelinated). Table 10.1 shows the relationship between receptor types and afferent fiber groups.

There is selective loss of modalities of sensation and degeneration of certain classes of sensory fibers in different disorders. In Friedreich's ataxia, for example, there is abnormally elevated sensory thresholds to vibration and touch-pressure. This correlates well with the known selective involvement of the Aα peak in the compound action potential and loss of large myelinated fibers in this disorder. In diabetic neuropathy, selective involvement of fibers has been reported. Several investigators[2, 4, 41] have described loss of small myelinated and unmyelinated fibers in some cases of painful distal diabetic neuropathy. Dyck and colleagues,[16] in a morphometric study of sural nerve biopsies from 32 patients with diabetic neuropathy, found no evidence of selective fiber involvement, suggesting that these types represent extremes of the normal distribu-

TABLE 10.1 CUTANEOUS SENSORY RECEPTORS

Modality	Receptor	Primary Afferent
Vibration	Pacinian corpuscle	Aαβ (myelinated)
Touch-pressure	Meissner's corpuscle (RA)	Aαβ (myelinated)
	Merkel's cell–neurite complex (SA I)	
	Ruffini's ending (SA II)	
Warm		C (unmyelinated)
Cold	Unmyelinated neurite complex	Aδ (myelinated)
Heat-pain	?	C (unmyelinated)
Cold-pain	Unmyelinated neurite–Schwann cell	Aδ (myelinated)
	Complex in basal epidermis	
	?	C (unmyelinated)

RA, rapidly adapting receptor; SA I, slowly adapting type I receptor; SA II, slowly adapting type II receptor.
From Gruener G, Dyck PJ. Quantitative sensory testing: methodology applications and future directions. J Clin Neurophysiol 1994; 11(6):568–583.

tion and not a different disorder. Recently, Llewelyn[35] reported similar findings, that is, no polar distribution of fiber involvement, confirming the prior observation.

In this chapter, we have reviewed a variety of distinct somatic sensory receptors with different physiologic characteristics. Three implications can be derived from these observations.

1. To infer the class of sensory fibers (systems) that are affected in disease, the investigator may need to evaluate several modalities of sensation.
2. In the assessment of sensory thresholds, anatomical variability (for example, site and age) needs to be recognized.
3. Because of the complexity and multiple qualities of somatic sensation, its assessment requires modality-specific evaluation, which can be performed with automated systems such as quantitative sensory testing (QST).

Quantitative sensory testing is based on psychophysics and attempts to evaluate the subject's response to standardized, quantified, and modality-specific stimuli (vibration, warm, cold, heat-pain). It is also useful to assess and characterize hypersensitive phenomena such as hyperalgesia and allodynia. We will now review sensory thresholds and QST in diabetes, and in the next sections we will discuss the equipment and testing methodology used in QST.

SENSORY THRESHOLDS IN DIABETES

Quantitative sensory testing is used to evaluate sensory thresholds in health and disease. Detection thresholds are increasingly being used to detect, characterize, and quantitate the degree and pattern of sensory loss in different

neurologic diseases, especially neuropathy. The assessment of sensory thresholds in diabetic patients is useful for the following reasons.

1. To determine whether sensation is normal or abnormal, taking into account modality, site, age, and sex.
2. To correlate thresholds with the clinical sensory examination.
3. To characterize sensory abnormalities in different types of diabetes (types 1 and 2).
4. To relate sensory thresholds to measured attributes of nerve conduction studies and to morphometric abnormality.
5. To infer the class of fibers that are affected in different types of diabetic neuropathy.
6. To follow the course of the sensory abnormality in a patient.
7. To assess changes in thresholds used as primary end points in epidemiologic and controlled clinical trials.
8. To allow for comparison of results among different medical centers.

The validation and methodological approaches of QST were reviewed in a consensus report from the Peripheral Neuropathy Association.[9] The evaluation of thresholds provides a standardized test that directly assesses distal sensory loss—a common neurologic symptom in diabetic neuropathy. Dyck and colleagues provided information on sensitivity, specificity, and reproducibility of detection thresholds in a cohort of diabetic patients with and without neuropathy.[15]

Although initially debated,[5–7, 37] there is now considerable evidence to support the concept that elevated thresholds are the correlate of clinical sensory loss. The following observations indicate that elevated thresholds are useful as indices of neuropathy.

1. Steiness[42] found that elevated sensory thresholds at the foot were associated with areflexia at the ankles in a group of patients with diabetic neuropathy.
2. Several reports describe an association between abnormal sensory thresholds and reduced conduction velocity on nerve conduction studies.[29, 30, 38]
3. Altered sensory thresholds are associated with neuropathologic abnormalities.[11, 13, 39, 40, 44]

Further evidence confirming that sensory thresholds are an expression of neuropathy have been provided by studies demonstrating a statistical association between the two. Dyck and colleagues,[11] in a study of 180 diabetic patients, found that there was a high degree of concordance among raised sensory thresholds and neuropathy assessed by neuropathic symptoms, deficits, and attributes of nerve conduction studies. In a subsequent prospective epidemiologic study—the Rochester Diabetic Neuropathy Study (RDNS)[15]—380 diabetic patients were evaluated. In this study, abnormal sensory thresholds were statistically associated with different tests used to evaluate and adequately characterize diabetic polyneuropathy. Neuropathy symptoms were assessed by the use of the Neuropathy Symptom Profile (NSP)[12] and the Neuropathy Symptom Score (NSS).[21] Neurologic deficits were evaluated by use of the Neuropathy Impairment Score (formerly known as the Neuropathy Disability Score[21]). Several attributes of nerve conduction studies as well as quantitative autonomic examination were performed to diagnose and stage severity of diabetic polyneuropathy. The high degree of concordance between test abnormalities reflects a common condition—diabetic neuropathy.[15]

INSTRUMENTS TO EVALUATE SENSATION

Here we shall review computer system approaches to assess sensation. A comprehensive review of hand-held devices and other instruments to assess sensation is beyond the scope of this chapter, and readers are referred to recent reviews on this subject.[17] We will focus our discussion on a system, CASE III and IV, that we developed. Lindblom and Tegner introduced similar instruments to evaluate sensation.[34] Verdugo and Ochoa reported a method to assess small-fiber function, the quantitative somatosensory thermotest, and validated its usefulness in healthy subjects and large series

of patients.[46] However, our emphasis will be on the CASE systems because our experience relates to their use.

In 1975, Dyck and colleagues introduced automated systems to quantitative sensory testing.[24] These microprocessor-controlled systems deliver appropriate and quantitated stimulus to reproduce the sensations tested over a broad range of intensities using algorithms of testing and finding thresholds. These systems are cost effective because they can be operated by technicians as well as physicians. Computerized systems have several advantages over hand-held devices in patient evaluation. With automated systems, the stimulus, algorithm of testing, and finding threshold are specifically controlled, lending themselves especially useful for reliable evaluation of sensory threshold and for epidemiological and controlled clinical trials.

The CASE IV system was designed to evaluate vibratory (VDT), cooling (CDT), and warming (WDT) detection thresholds as well as heat-pain via a numerical visual analog scale (1 to 10) of pain (HPVAS). This battery of tests allows noninvasive, standardized, sensitive, and specific assessment of large-fiber (VDT) and small-fiber sensory function (CDT, WDT, HPVAS). The earlier version of the system (CASE III) measured touch-pressure at discrete grid points over the surface of the skin; however, this required long testing periods, possibly raising threshold inappropriately because of inattention or drowsiness.

Computer-Assisted Sensory Examination System IV (CASE IV)

The CASE IV system* consists of the following components.

1. A personal computer, with video screen and keyboard for entry of biographic data and for display of operator instructions and menu
2. A printer to print the results
3. Base unit or electronic controller, containing power supplies and electronic circuits
4. A visual cueing device, displaying a yellow light (get ready) and a green light (test in progress)
5. A patient response key, to indicate the appearance and or disappearance of stimuli (real or null) depending on the algorithm used and the choice of one or two in the forced-choice method

---

*Manufactured by W. R. Medical Electronics, Stillwater, MN.

6. A vibration and thermal stimulator
7. A vibration and thermal calibration system

The software was written in the C language and can be programmed to have different testing routines.

TESTING CONDITIONS AND PATIENT PREPARATION

The testing environment should allow the patient or subject to concentrate and be attentive to testing events. Ideally, the test should be performed in an isolated or dedicated room to minimize disturbing sounds or interruptions. The room should be comfortable, with enough light and air circulation. The patient must be alert and cooperative. Patients with mental retardation or dementia cannot reliably be tested, and children younger than 8 years of age are unable to be attentive for the duration of the test to provide reliable results. The area (for example, foot or hand) to be tested should have an intact skin without skin lesions, dermatitis, or infected or necrotic skin. Vibration testing sites usually include the base of the great toenail and the base of the nail of the index finger. Thermal testing sites include the dorsal surface of the foot and hand. Other sites could also be used.

A sensory technician describes the testing procedure and responses needed, having the subject follow along using large cue cards displayed before the patient. We recommend administering a pretest trial with a detectable sample stimulus to help the patient recognize the stimulus and to determine whether the patient knows how to respond. The patient is then instructed to provide the "best" answer at detection of just-detectable stimuli. When the testing is completed, a report is generated that includes patient's name, sex, site, clinic number, date, and other variables such as weight and height. The test results are presented and compared with normative data or percentiles. A cutoff value for abnormality is determined (for example, >99th percentile). A physician interprets the results and provides a written commentary.

STIMULI

For the assessment of sensation, it is important that the stimulus be appropriate to the modality tested. It should induce the sensation to be tested, for example, vibration, cooling, warming, or heat-pain. For the detection of vibratory thresholds, the physical stimuli consists of a sinusoidal waveform at right angles to the surface of the skin at a given frequency. The stimulus to elicit touch-pressure sensation needs to induce a punctuate sheer force perpendicular to the site tested.[28] The assessment of cold, warm, and heat-nociception sensation requires ramps (linear or another defined ramp) or pulses of temperature change to be delivered to specific areas.[45] In each modality tested, the waveform must be precisely described and should remain constant throughout the full range of stimulus intensities or magnitudes. The stimuli also need to be quantifiable in units of force or displacement (touch-pressure), displacement (vibration), or differences in temperature (Δ C) and cover a broad range of intensities to allow the study of sensitive and insensitive sites in patients and control subjects. Background conditions during stimulus administration, such as temperature of the transducer during temperature testing and the load of the transducer during vibratory testing, should remain constant.

The system should be periodically calibrated to ascertain that it will provide identical stimuli at different times and at different medical institutions.

TESTING METHODOLOGY

To obtain sensitive, specific, and reproducible QST results it is important to critically describe the methods of programmed testing (algorithms). In general, there are two types of testing algorithms and finding thresholds: the stimulus (that is, the waveform, intensity, and presentation of the stimuli) and the subject's response or response paradigm.

Two modes of stimulus presentation are used: the method of limits and the tracking method. The method of limits uses gradual changes of stimulus intensity. Different approaches may be used, such as gradually increasing the intensity of stimulation to the point of detection ("appearance" threshold); gradually decreasing the intensity of stimulation to the point of disappearance ("disappearance" threshold); or a combination of the above, also known as the Békésy method. In the tracking method, the subject's response determines the stimulus intensities used. For example, when the subject correctly identifies the stimulus (appearance threshold), the next stimulus given is of lower intensity, with continuous reduction of the intensity until the stimulus is no longer felt (disappearance threshold).

At this point (turnaround point) the next stimulus would be of a higher magnitude. This sequence is performed several times to obtain mean values of appearance and disappearance thresholds. This response paradigm is known as following "a simple up-down rule." The degree of stimulus change can consist of gradual changes in intensity, stepwise changes of known magnitudes or based on studies using the just noticeable differences (JND) in intensities.[24] The response paradigm is the second component of the testing algorithm. Three patterns are generally described. The first one is referred to as the *two-interval forced choice*.[14] A stimulus is delivered as paired stimulus events, one actual and the other a null event. This is indicated to the subject by the serial display of the numbers 1 and 2. Chance determines whether the stimulus is in the first or second interval. The subject, by depressing a response key, indicates the interval that he or she judges contains the actual stimulus. Depending on whether the individual is successful at identifying the real stimulus, subsequent stimuli are given at greater or lesser stimulus intensities. The subject's threshold is generally defined as the ability to correctly identify 75% of the time the interval having the stimulus. A typical sequence is shown in Figure 10.3.

The second variety uses a *yes-no paradigm*, which presents an actual stimulus or a null stimulus during each stimulus event. The ability of the subject or patient to correctly identify the stimulus event half of the time is consid-

ered the threshold. The third method is a variation of the yes-no paradigm. In this sequence, the subject grades its intensity along a scale. A commonly used scale is the visual analog scale (VAS) or a numerical (1 to 10) scale, which can be graded 0 (no sensation) or from 1 to 10 (minimal to maximal sensation for the sensory modality being scaled). This method is frequently used for the estimation of heat-pain detection threshold (HPDT). It has the additional advantage of allowing the detection of suprathreshold, defined as a sensation of a specific intensity or grade.

As we have discussed, both the stimulus and response paradigm need to be carefully described. Regardless of the method used (limits, tracking), there are other variables that can influence the test performance. The actual threshold can be influenced by the time between stimuli, the ramp rate of stimulus magnitude, the number of stimuli presented, the number of turnarounds, the use of null stimuli, and how responses are evaluated to determine threshold.[14] These events should be described, and the testing parameters of the algorithm should be validated using computer simulations and tests on healthy control subjects and patients. Sensitivity and specificity should be provided by comparing the complete testing algorithm with a comparative gold standard or, if one is not available, by using a comparative test that measures nerve function. The establishment of normative data is necessary so that the responses can be expressed in percentiles. As we reviewed earlier, normal values should be obtained in healthy subjects for sensory modality, site, age, sex, and physical covarieties. Because of the variation in receptor density, receptor location, and skin thickness, control data should be available for each site tested.

We shall now turn our attention to the description of the methods used to evaluate VDTs, CDTs, and WDTs as well as heat-pain responses using the CASE systems.

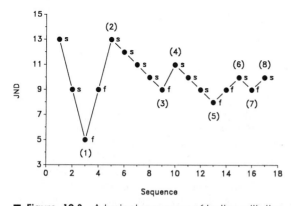

■ **Figure 10.3** A typical sequence of testing with the forced-choice algorithm. The abbreviated rules by which the stimulus increases or decreases and the method of calculating the threshold are given in the text. *JND*, just noticeable difference; *s*, success; *f*, failure. The numbers in parentheses indicate the turnarounds. (From Dyck PJ, et al: Comparison of algorithms of testing for use in automated evaluation of sensation. Neurology 1990; 40:1607.)

VIBRATORY DETECTION THRESHOLD USING CASE IV

Vibratory Transducer

The stimulator probe is a flat disc, 9 mm in diameter, coated with Teflon (to minimize heat loss). It is mounted by a shaft to an optical scanning motor whose vertical displacement is directly proportional to current (Fig. 10.4). The transducer is affixed to the front part of a bal-

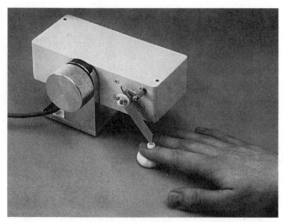

■ **Figure 10.4** The stimulator probe and vibratory stimulus transducer used in computer-assisted sensory examination (CASE IV).

ance arm, allowing the probe to rest on the part to be tested with sufficient mass (30 g) so as not to respond to rapid displacement but to move up or down with the movement of the anatomical part being tested. A sinusoidal 125-Hz waveform is used; to avoid sudden onset and offset, the stimulus interval is increased and decreased exponentially. The waveform has the characteristics of a charging and discharging capacitor (Fig. 10.5). Twenty-five discrete levels of stimulation are used, ranging from 0.01 to 577 μm of displacement. These magnitudes of different levels of stimulus intensities are distributed based on estimates of JND. The displacement of the stimulating

probe is periodically calibrated using a laser beam.

Vibratory Threshold Determination With CASE IV

Several modifications took place during the development of testing procedures of the CASE systems. When the algorithms and different ramps were compared to forced-choice testing, it was noted that slow linear ramps were impractical, because they were excessively time consuming to detect threshold in insensitive subjects or sites. Fast ramps had the problem of overestimating threshold. Fortunately, other methods have been developed and tested as more efficient ways of detecting threshold.[19]

A two-interval forced-choice method and a 4, 2, and 1 stepping algorithm are the preferred methods to assess vibratory threshold. In both, the vibratory stimulus consists of 125 Hz-sinusoidal oscillations with 25 discrete levels of magnitude of vibratory stimulus available. The forced-choice method has been previously discussed. The 4, 2, and 1 stepping algorithm uses a combination of features from the method of limits, other features of a tracking paradigm, and null stimuli. Testing begins at an intermediate level (level 13) and increases or decreases the magnitude by 4 steps, 2 steps, and 1 step, according to whether the subject felt or did not feel the stimulus. For instance, the stimulus would be decreased (if perceived by the subject) or increased (if not felt) by 4 steps to the

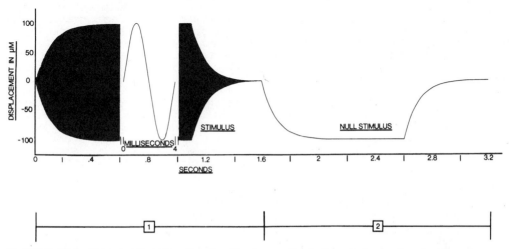

■ **Figure 10.5** The waveform for vibration. The line on the bottom indicates the duration of stimulus events of a forced-choice pair. The duration of each is 1.6833 seconds. (Modified from Dyck PJ, et al. Introduction of automated systems to evaluate touch-pressure, vibration, and thermal cutaneous sensation in man. Ann Neurol 1978; 4:502–510.)

point of turnaround. Turnaround is when the stimulus is perceived at the higher level when was not felt at lower levels or the opposite, when it was not felt at the lower level but had been perceived at the higher level. Following the first turnaround, stepping was in steps of 2 and then in steps of 1. A total of 20 stimulus events are used, with 5 of them being randomly assigned null stimuli, but no more than two can occur consecutively. An affirmative response (felt the stimulus) to more than one null stimulus terminates the program. The patient is instructed again and the test re-run. If the subject identifies the null stimulus as a true stimulus three times after the test is re-run twice, this indicates that the algorithm is not suited for this individual. A supersensitive site is defined as the individual correctly identifying three stimuli at level 1 (lowest intensity). Along the same lines, an insensitive site is defined when the subject fails to identify three consecutive times at maximum intensity (level 25). To estimate threshold, only the turnaround values arrived by single stepping are analyzed, and threshold is defined as the mean of the turnaround levels observed. The average time required for this algorithm is approximately 3 minutes, an important reduction in time when compared with the time needed for the forced-choice testing, approximately 13 minutes. Figure 10.6 illustrates the waveforms used in different algorithms of vibratory testing.

CASE SYSTEMS FOR TESTING TOUCH-PRESSURE THRESHOLDS

We previously reviewed touch-pressure or tactile sensation, which is mediated by receptors with small receptive fields and sharp edges. Because of this receptor configuration, it is appropriate to evaluate touch-pressure detection thresholds (T-PDT) using punctuate stimuli at grid points. The CASE III system assesses T-PDT at 9 points, 1 mm apart, using a 3 × 3 grid. Each patient is tested separately by using the tip of a stylus (a sphere 0.64 mm in diameter and coated with Teflon). The stylus is mounted to a galvanometer motor that controls the intensity of the stimulus (Fig. 10.7), and the entire system is affixed to an electromechanical translator. To avoid the abruptness of onset and offset, the stimulus waveform has the characteristics of a charging and discharging capacitor with a time constant of 0.02 sec. The sensation produced feels like a tap or a touch. Twenty-one levels of stimulus intensities are used, ranging from a total load of 2.9 to 1200

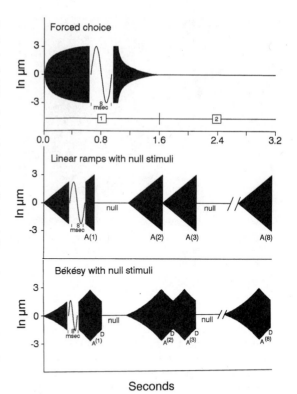

■ Figure 10.6 Shown here are the waveforms used in forced-choice testing (*top*), linear ramps with null stimulus (*middle*), and Békésy with null stimuli (*bottom*). Although sinusoidal waveforms at 125 Hz are used for all three algorithms, the rate and shape of the increase of intensity and the method of testing differ. In alternative forced-choice testing, the observer is asked to choose the interval, associated with the display of the numbers 1 and then 2, that had a vibratory stimulus. The rules of testing and finding threshold are described in the text. In linear ramp testing with null stimuli (*middle*), the intensity of vibratory stimuli increases to the point at which the response key is depressed. After the initial stimulus, seven stimuli and four null stimuli are presented as described in the text. A(1), A(2), A(3), and A(8) indicate the first, second, third, and eighth appearance thresholds in a typical sequence. Null stimuli are shown as ``null.'' In Békésy testing with null stimuli (*bottom*), the rate of increase of the vibratory stimulus follows an exponential function based on our previous study of just noticeable difference. The $A^{(1)D}$, $A^{(2)D}$, $A^{(3)D}$, and $A^{(8)D}$ refer to the first, second, third, and eighth ``appearance'' and ``disappearance'' thresholds. Null stimuli are indicated by the word ``null.'' (From Dyck PJ, et al: Comparison of algorithms of testing for use in automated evaluation of sensation. Neurology 1990; 40:1607.)

mg. A tracking method[24] and a forced-choice algorithm are used to detect T-PDT.

Touch-pressure detection threshold is currently performed in selected patients or upon specific request. We have substituted T-PDT for VDT as a measure of large-fiber mechanorecep-

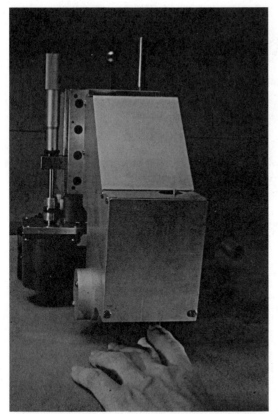

■ Figure 10.7 Touch-pressure stimulator assembly is shown attached to the mechanical translator as touch-pressure of the index finger is being tested. The finger is cradled in clay and the stimulator stylus rests on the skin just proximal to the base of the nail. (From Dyck PJ, Zimmerman IR, O'Brien PC, et al. Introduction of automated systems to evaluate touch-pressure, vibration, and thermal cutaneous sensation in man. Ann Neurol 1978; 4:502.)

tor sensory function, because VDT can be performed more rapidly and has been shown to provide comparable information.[17]

COOL, WARM, AND HEAT-PAIN SENSATION

As we have reviewed earlier in the section on anatomy and physiology of sensory systems, cold, warm, and heat-pain sensation are conveyed by small myelinated fibers (Aδ) and unmyelinated fibers (C fibers). The majority of unmyelinated C fibers are thought to be nociceptors, and many are polymodal nociceptors responding to intense mechanical and heat and cold stimulation. When a subject is stimulated with ramps of increasing temperature up to 40°C, the evoked response is usually a warm or hot sensation. As the temperature increases

above 40°C, the subjects report burning, pricking-heat, or pain. Temperatures in the heat-nociceptive range, 42 to 45°C or above, produce frank pain. In elderly healthy individuals, at some anatomical sites (feet and legs) no warm sensation is felt, but pain is not experienced. As the temperature of the thermode is increased to the heat-nociceptive range the subject may not experience a warm feeling, but reports only burning pain. In these subjects, one has to infer that specific thermal receptors were either not present or stimulated under the thermode and only polymodal nociceptors had been activated. This appears to be related to the low and variable distribution of warm receptors. This low density of warm receptors was observed by earlier investigators and confirmed later by others.[22] With cold stimulation, as the thermode temperature is reduced from skin temperature, the subject experiences a cool sensation before reporting a painfully cold sensation. The implications from these observations is that to test CDT and WDT, one should not test in the nociceptive range. Alternatively, if one detects thresholds within the range of temperatures in the nociceptive range, these results should be reported as heat nociception or cold nociception.

COLD, WARM, AND HEAT-PAIN DETECTION THRESHOLDS USING CASE IV

The components of the CASE system have been reviewed in previous sections. The thermal stimulus is delivered via a thermode with a 10-cm² surface area (a smaller surface area is also available). The thermode can provide small or large ramps or pulses of cooling or heating at the thermode testing surface. The thermode consists of two thermoelectric units (TEU), separated by an aluminum block, and a water chamber through which water circulates to dissipate heat. The TEU 1 rests on the skin area to be tested, and the TEU 2 keeps the aluminum block at a constant skin temperature. The TEU 1 delivers ramps of heating or cooling to the skin using a Peltier effect. When a current is applied, the temperature at the ends of the thermode charge in the opposite direction. For instance, a desired wave of cooling is given by applying a variable current to TEU 1. By reversing the direction of the current to TEU 1, a warming stimulus is then obtained. Temperature ramps or pulses in the form of pyramids or trapezoid shapes can be delivered

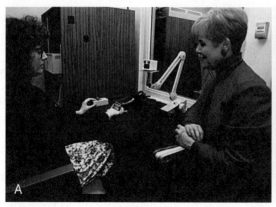
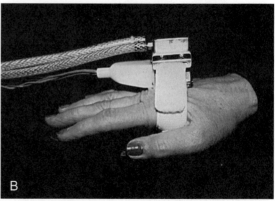

■ **Figure 10.8** Use of CASE IV to assess cool, warm, or heat-pain detection thresholds on the dorsal surface of the hand. *A,* The subject is sitting on a dental chair, which can be positioned so that the hand (or foot) rests comfortably on the testing table. The thermode assembly is firmly strapped in place; the right hand of the subject activates the number 1 or 2 response key to indicate whether the sensation studied—for example, a cooling pulse—occurs during the display of ''1'' or ''2'' on the visual cueing device. The visual cueing device is mounted on a multijointed mechanical arm so that it can be positioned for comfort at eye level. In this test, the examining technician has previously entered the biographic and testing information and simply monitors the test to ensure that further instruction is not needed; that drowsiness, should it occur, is detected; and whether any malfunction occurs. The electronic controller, computer, and keyboard are rack-mounted just beyond the testing table. *B,* A close-up view of the thermode assembly. The umbilical cord to the thermode has two components: electrical cords (lower) and circulating fluid hoses. (From Dyck PJ, et al: Cool, warm, and heat-pain detection thresholds: Testing methods and inferences about anatomic distribution of receptors. Neurology 1993; 43:1500–1508.)

at predefined rates and levels using available computer software.

TESTING METHODS

The skin temperature is recorded with an infrared thermometer, and TEU 2 adjusts the temperature of the aluminum block to this temperature. True skin temperature is considered the baseline temperature. To adjust the thermode to skin temperature a special subroutine is used. The TEU 1 current is turned off, and the current to TEU 2 is continuously adjusted so that there is no difference in temperature between the thermocouples near the skin and in the aluminum block. In practice, this appears to provide a baseline temperature that does not feel cold or warm. Afterward, the aluminum block is maintained at a steady-state baseline temperature (skin) by providing current to TEU 2 in the appropriate direction as required. Current flow to TEU 1 is delivered by computer instructions to create the stimulus waveform desired. Thermodes are calibrated periodically using a high-quality mercury thermometer in a water bath and a special subroutine to ensure that in the range of 10 to 50°C the temperature does not change more than 0.5°C.[22] The CDT and WDT can be estimated specifying

different baselines and maximal temperatures, different pulses or ramps of change of temperature, and different algorithms of testing. Ascending or descending linear ramps of temperature change are used in the different algorithms of testing (Fig. 10.9). Ramp rates may be modified between 0 and 4°C/s. It is the initial change in temperature in either direction (cooling or warming) from skin temperature (baseline) that is the effective stimulus felt as cold or warm, and not the return to baseline. Twenty-five discrete steps of stimulus intensities over a broad range of magnitudes are available, and range from 1 (smallest) to step 25 (largest). The maximum temperatures are 49°C held for 10 seconds for HPVAS, 45°C for 10 seconds for WDT, and 9°C for 10 seconds for CDT. Different algorithms of testing have been evaluated for estimation of CDT, WDT, and HPDT.[22] Multiple linear or exponential ramps of temperature change with null stimuli, Békésy algorithm, the two-alternative forced-choice algorithm, and the 4, 2, and 1 stepping algorithm with null stimuli were analyzed in patients with neuropathy and healthy controls. The approach to find threshold with these methods is similar to the one described earlier for detecting vibratory threshold. As previously observed for VDT, in CDT and WDT

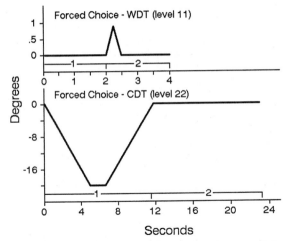

■ **Figure 10.9** Shown are thermal pulses used in forced choice; 4, 2, and 1 stepping; and operator-chosen stepping algorithms of testing described in text. In the upper frame, we show a pyramidal thermal pulse with initial warming and then cooling at 4°C/s. We refer to this as a "warming" stimulus because it is the initial direction of temperature change from skin temperature (shown as 0), which is the effective stimulus. Note that the apex of the pulse is positioned at the midpoint of the second testing interval. In forced-choice testing, two stimulus intervals are used (shown here), but in other algorithms, single-stimulus intervals are used. In assessing cool detection threshold (CDT) or warm detection threshold (WDT) by forced choice (or another algorithm of testing), 25 magnitudes of stimulus intensities (levels) are available for testing. In the lower frame, we show a cooling flat-topped pyramidal stimulus at level 22 in stimulus period 1. (From Dyck PJ, Zimmerman IR, O'Brien PC, et al. Introduction of automated systems to evaluate touch-pressure, vibration, and thermal cutaneous sensation in man. Ann Neurol 1978; 4:502.)

the use of linear or exponential ramps of temperature to the point of threshold consistently overestimated threshold. Slow thermal ramps gave acceptable results but were impractical because of the excessive time required to test insensitive sites or subjects. Algorithms that used defined levels of stimulus magnitudes distributed in steps, such as the forced-choice and the 4, 2, and 1 stepping method, performed well. The first choice among the algorithms tested is the forced-choice method, because it has the minimum of subject and observer bias and has been extensively validated. It has two disadvantages: (1) it is time-consuming and (2) it is not the method of choice to test heat-pain because repeated testing is not well tolerated in the heat-pain zone and may alter threshold with repetitive testing. For CDT, a 4, 2, and 1 stepping algorithm with a yes-no response paradigm was found to be an efficient method of assessing cold thresh-

olds. A similar method is used for determining warm thresholds. However, as we have reviewed earlier, because of the low density of warm receptors at some sites (such as the foot), estimation of WDT may not be as useful as estimating other modalities in the evaluation of neuropathy. For this reason, we preferentially assess CDT in the evaluation of patients with diabetic and other neuropathies.

HEAT-PAIN THRESHOLDS

A standard method to assess heat-pain thresholds using CASE IV has been recently reviewed.[23] Briefly, the site to be tested should be inspected to avoid diseased or infected skin. Skin temperature is taken with an infrared thermometer, and if it is below 32°C, the limb is warmed. The thermode is applied and set at 34°C, allowing the skin temperature to adapt. Subsequently, the sensory technician reads a set of instructions to the patient or subject. These instructions are also displayed on a card placed in front of the patient. Pulses of warming heat of different intensities are given, and the patient is instructed to provide responses according to the stimulus felt using a modified yes-no paradigm with a numerical scale from 1 (least) to 10 (most). If the patient feels nothing or warm or hot but without discomfort the response should be 0. If there is some degree of discomfort or pain the patient should grade its severity from 1 to 10. Number 1 would correspond to the lowest level of discomfort or pain and number 10 to the most severe pain. Stimuli are given in steps of two of increasing magnitudes, and generally a heat-pain sensation is first reported at stimulus steps 19–21. Thereafter, single steps are used until a VAS of 5 or greater is first reached or a level 25 has been tested. The largest stimuli produce erythema without causing skin damage or blistering. Two stimulus waveforms are generally used: (1) pyramidal-shaped stimuli with a maximal temperature to 55 to 60°C and (2) pyramidal- and trapezoid-shaped stimuli to 49°C. We prefer the second approach because the margin of safety is higher at lower temperatures, and testing for a prolonged period of time in the 55°C temperature range induces pain and tissue damage. The HPDT is defined as the halfway point between a nonpainful (0 = 0) and painful stimulus (1 = 1) and referred to as HP:0.5. Then, an intermediate heat-pain response (5 = 5) is chosen and referred to as HP:5.0. This serves to terminate further increments in stimulus intensities that are not well tolerated, and perception and grading may then be altered.[47] In some insensitive sites, HP:5.0 cannot be estimated; in such cases the next highest level is estimated (for example, HP:4.0, 3.0, or 1.0). The difference in steps between HP:5.0 and HP:0.5 is HP:5 to 0.5. The algorithm of testing that appears to perform well is the nonrepeating ascending algorithm with null stimuli (NRA-NS), which begins testing at a level below threshold (step 13) and increases by steps of two until step 21 or pain is perceived (≥1), and then increases by single steps until greater than HP:5.0 is reached or step 25 has been tested (whichever is first). This algorithm has been extensively tested and is generally completed in 8 to 15 minutes.[23] We demonstrate the use of the HP test in the following examples. Figure 10.10 shows the lowered HP:0.5 and HP:5.0 after injection of intradermal nerve growth factor (NGF), providing evidence that NGF lowers HP thresholds in humans.[20] Figure 10.11 illustrates the use of the heat-pain test in three diabetic patients. It shows a normal response, an elevated threshold that may be seen in diabetic polyneuropathy, and representative cases of hyperalgesia (steeper-than-normal stimulus-response line) and hypoalgesia (a less steep line). The reproducibility of the test is within 1 or more stimulus steps 76% of the time for HP:0.5 and 88% for HP:5.0. The standardized approach to test heat-pain reviewed here allows us to estimate detection thresholds and the stimulus necessary to elicit an intermediate heat-pain response. These results can be compared with normal values obtained from healthy controls. It is now possible to estimate normal limits on healthy individuals considering age, anatomical site, gender, and other physical variables. Normal percentiles specific for age, site, gender, weight, and other physical variables are preferred over normal limits tables.[18]

DETECTION THRESHOLDS IN HEALTH

It is well accepted that normative values are necessary in order to recognize abnormality in disease. Therefore, detection thresholds for vibration, touch-pressure, and cooling were evaluated in more than 300 healthy subjects between ages of 8 and 80 years, without neuropathy or diseases known to predispose to neuropathy. For touch-pressure and vibratory sensations, the sites tested include the dorsal surface of the terminal phalanx at the base of the nail for the great toe and index finger, the lateral leg, volar forearm, anterior thigh, lateral

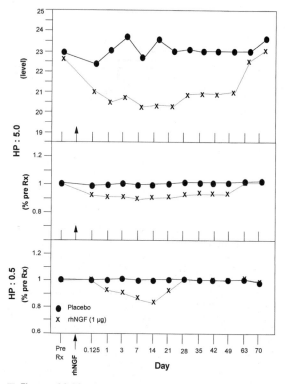

■ **Figure 10.10** Sequential heat-pain (HP) responses from a healthy subject (male, 66 years) who received 1 μm of recombinant human nerve growth factor (rhNGF) intradermally into the volar forearm on one side and a similar volume of saline into the other. In the upper panel, we show serial values of the HP:5.0 (by stimulus steps needed to induce this degree of pain). Notice the similarity of threshold prior to NGF injection at onset, the normal variability of the HP:5.0 of the saline-injected side over the duration of the experiment, and the dramatic lowering of the HP:5.0 on the rhNGF injected side that persisted for many weeks. In the middle panel, we show these results plotted as a percent of baseline values. In the lower panel, we show the HP:0.5 changes with time plotted as a percent of baseline. The outcome of this study has been confirmed in a study of 16 healthy subjects using dosages of 1 and 3 μg of rhNGF.[20] In addition to showing how stable threshold measures of heat-pain can be over long time periods, it provides evidence that NGF can lower heat-pain thresholds in humans, a result anticipated from tests in the rat model using the tail-flick test. Rx, treatment. (From Dyck PJ, et al: A standard test of heat-pain responses using CASE IV. J Neurol Sci 1996; 136:54–63.)

shoulder, and maxillary region. For cooling, the areas tested include the same sites listed above. There is considerable variability among subjects for anatomical sites and age. Detection thresholds for all modalities increased with age with the exception of the face. For touch-pressure threshold of the toe, a sex difference was noted, with higher values in men, especially

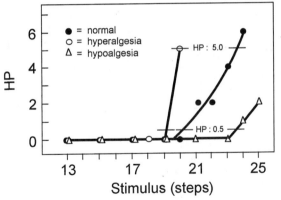

■ **Figure 10.11** A superimposition of the plotted values of three diabetic patients illustrating a normal response, one with hyperalgesia and one with hypoalgesia. Note that it is possible to estimate the HP:0.5 and the HP:5.0 for the first two but only the HP:0.5 for the third. In the third case, it is possible (and useful for percentile estimation) to estimate the HP:2. HP, heat-pain. (From Dyck PJ, et al: A standard test of heat-pain responses using CASE IV. J Neurol Sci 1996; 136:54–63.)

after the age of 50 years. Figures 10.12 and 10.13 show the mean values of vibratory threshold at the finger and at the toe using CASE III. None of these subjects had insensitive points at the finger. The opposite occurred at the toe, with frequent insensitive points in individuals older than 50 years. Because insensitive points are commonly encountered in disease, both the threshold of sensitive points and the number of insensitive points are taken into account for vibratory threshold of the toe. This explains the less steep regression line against age at the toe, because points with unknown

threshold were excluded. For this reason, it is impossible to compare the slope of the regression line of the threshold for the toe with that for the finger. Nevertheless, it is clear that thresholds are elevated with age. In Figure 10.14, we show the VDTs using CASE IV in healthy subjects. The solid lines represent the 98th percentile and the broken lines the 95th percentile, illustrating the normal values. Thresholds increase with age, and there is a significant difference between sexes. Threshold differences by modality of sensation by site and age are shown in Figure 10.15. For touch-pressure sensation expressed as displacement, the finger is the most sensitive, followed by the toe (in women and young men) and then the face. For vibration sensation, the most sensitive site is the finger, followed by the toe and face in young subjects. In old individuals, the toe is the least sensitive. For cooling sensation, the face is most sensitive, followed by the hand and then the foot.

Dyck and colleagues reported variables influencing neuropathic end points in the healthy subject component of the RDNS.[18] This included the evaluation of more than 330 randomly selected healthy subjects, with at least 15 men and women without neuropathy, for each hemidecade between 18 and 74 years of age. This study demonstrated that other physical variables in addition to age influence the setting of abnormal limits for QST. The main variables that influenced vibratory and cooling thresholds were age, followed by body surface area and body mass index. The novel observation of increased threshold with increasing sur-

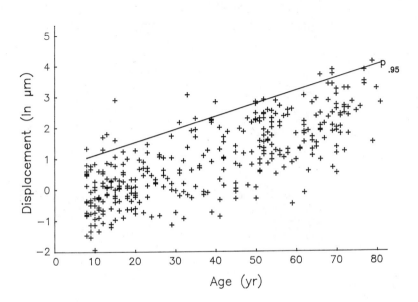

■ **Figure 10.12** Average values of vibratory thresholds of sensitive grid points at the finger in natural logarithm (ln) μm of displacement against age in 328 (151 male and 177 female) healthy subjects. (From Dyck PJ, Karnes JL, O'Brien PC, et al. Detection thresholds of cutaneous sensation in humans. In Dyck PJ, Thomas PK, Griffin J, et al (eds): Peripheral Neuropathy, ed 3. Philadelphia, WB Saunders, 1993, pp 706–728.)

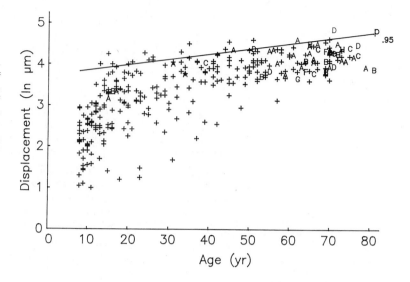

■ **Figure 10.13** Average values of vibration thresholds of sensitive grid points at the toe in natural logarithm (ln) μm of displacement against age in 305 (151 male and 154 female) healthy subjects. (From Dyck PJ, Karnes JL, O'Brien PC, et al. Detection thresholds of cutaneous sensation in humans. In Dyck PJ, Thomas PK, Griffin J, et al (eds): Peripheral Neuropathy, ed 3. Philadelphia, WB Saunders, 1993, pp 706–728.)

face area correlates well with the topographic distribution of sensory receptors. Percentile values for site, age, gender, and other physical variables of healthy subjects are stored in the memory of the CASE computer to be available for comparison to patient values. The choice of a specific percentile used (for example, 90th or 99th) as an abnormal value depends on the goal of the study. For screening purposes, sensitivity is preferred over specificity. Thus, the 90th percentile would be the value of choice.

When specificity is the main goal, the 99th percentile may be used to define the normal limits.

CUTANEOUS SENSORY THRESHOLDS IN DIABETIC NEUROPATHY

The use of QST in various neuropathic conditions has been reviewed elsewhere.[17] In this section, we will provide an overview of QST in diabetic polyneuropathy. This was the area

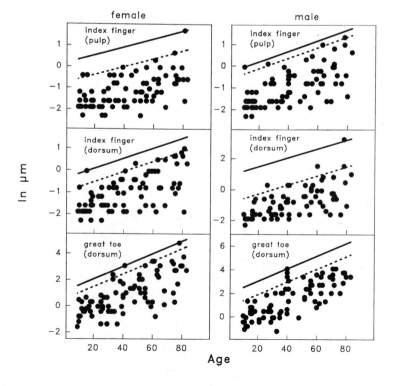

■ **Figure 10.14** The vibratory detection threshold using CASE IV in healthy subjects. The broken line represents the estimated 95th percentile; the solid line the 95th+ percentile line. (From Dyck PJ, Karnes JL, O'Brien PC, et al. Detection thresholds of cutaneous sensation in humans. In Dyck PJ, Thomas PK, Griffin J, et al (eds): Peripheral Neuropathy, ed 3. Philadelphia, WB Saunders, 1993, pp 706–728.)

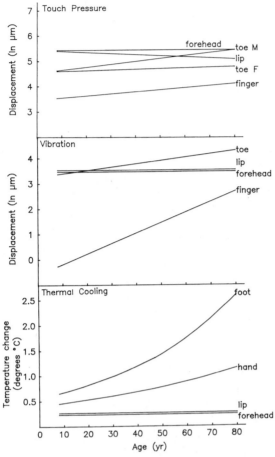

■ **Figure 10.15** Threshold regression lines in health against age and modality of sensation and site, as described in text. In, natural logarithm. (From Dyck PJ, Karnes JL, O'Brien PC, et al. Detection threshold of cutaneous sensation in humans. *In* Dyck PJ, Thomas PK, Griffin J, et al. Peripheral Neuropathy, ed 3. Philadelphia, WB Saunders, 1993, pp 706–728.)

in which QST underwent one of its first systematic applications, helping to detect and characterize peripheral nerve involvement and staging for severity in diabetic neuropathy.

Steiness[42, 43] performed detailed biothesiometric measurements of the vibratory perception threshold (VPT) in 100 normal subjects and 63 patients with diabetes mellitus and analyzed the results statistically. He provided evidence that in healthy controls, VPT is similar on both sides of the body, increases with age, and is higher in the great toe than for other anatomical sites tested. For patients with diabetic neuropathy, Steiness demonstrated the following.

1. The VPT of both upper and lower limbs is significantly increased in diabetic patients.
2. Higher VPTs at the great toe were associated with longer duration of diabetes.

3. VPT values were not associated with hyperglycemic control.
4. VPT values were not associated with neuropathic symptoms, but a positive correlation was observed with sensory loss and areflexia.

Other studies[11, 13] based on the evaluation of 180 patients with diabetes mellitus had shown that abnormal thresholds as determined by CASE were evidence of peripheral nerve involvement and were statistically associated with scored neuropathic symptoms and deficits, nerve conduction abnormalities, and pathologic abnormalities of sural nerve. More recent studies[15] based on the evaluation of 380 diabetic patients from the RDNS have confirmed previous observations. These studies have used standardized, prospectively performed, reproducible, and validated neuropathy tests and compared the results with large and matched control values obtained by the same approaches as done in patients. Neuropathic symptoms and deficits were comprehensively evaluated using the NSS, NSP, and NDS, now called the NIS. Attributes of motor and sensory nerve conduction studies and quantitative autonomical studies were also performed in this cohort. The QST included the evaluation of vibratory and cooling thresholds using CASE. Abnormality of vibratory and cooling threshold was defined as 99th or greater percentile as judged by comparison with previously performed studies. In this cohort, statistically significant associations were found between abnormality of one evaluation or test and abnormality of any other evaluation or test. Vibratory and cooling thresholds were strongly associated with clinical deficits as measured by the NDS and attributes of nerve conduction studies ($P = 0.001$). Vibratory and cooling thresholds were also useful in setting minimal criteria for the diagnosis of polyneuropathy. Using a stepwise discriminant analysis, nerve conduction studies were the most important test in predicting polyneuropathy, followed by Valsalva ratio and then vibratory and cooling thresholds. The QST correlated with increasingly severe stages of diabetic polyneuropathy. These correlations were statistically significant for vibratory and cooling thresholds for asymptomatic neuropathy with ability to walk on heels (N1a) and for more severe symptomatic neuropathy with inability to walk on heels (N2b). These results indicate that sensory abnormalities as measured by CASE provide a reliable, reproducible, and sensitive index of diabetic neuropathy.

USE OF QUANTITATIVE SENSORY TESTING TO EVALUATE THERAPY

The results of QST may be used as primary or secondary end points in controlled clinical trials in diabetic and other neuropathies.[10] In diabetic neuropathy, QST provides meaningful information regarding distal sensory loss. Vibratory and touch-pressure thresholds are ideally suited to assess large-fiber sensory function. Cooling and heat-pain thresholds are appropriate measures for evaluation of small-fiber sensory function.

The value of QST with standardized techniques to measure cooling and heat-pain thresholds will be discussed in relation to experimental diabetic trial data on NGF. Nerve growth factor may play a role in prevention or treatment of human diabetic polyneuropathy,[1] and phase III clinical trials are under way to further elucidate its role. The usefulness of a standard heat-pain threshold using CASE IV was demonstrated in a study of intradermal recombinant human NGF in humans. Dyck and coworkers studied 16 healthy subjects and tested whether intradermal NGF as compared to saline induces hyperalgesia (lowered heat-pain threshold or a steeper-than-normal stimulus-response curve) or alters cutaneous sensation.[20] They found a significantly lowered heat-pain threshold (HP:0.5) and intermediate level of pain (HP:5.0) at 1, 3, and 7 days after NGF injection. An example is provided in Figure 10.9. No abnormality of vibratory or cooling detection thresholds was observed. Quantitative sensory testing will be used in other controlled clinical trials in diabetic polyneuropathy.

Summary

Somatic sensory receptors are morphologically distinct with different physiologic characteristics.

Quantitative sensory testing provides a reliable and standardized evaluation of cutaneous sensory thresholds and helps to characterize hypersensitive phenomena such as hyperalgesia.

Sensory thresholds vary with site, age, sex, and other physical variables in healthy individuals.

Quantitative sensory testing is especially suited for epidemiologic and controlled clinical trials in diabetic and other neuropathies because (1) it uses a defined stimulus that is appropriate for the modality tested, such as VDT, WDT, CDT, or HNDT; (2) the stimulus waveforms are precisely described, quanti-

tated, and of a wide range of magnitudes; (3) the testing algorithms have been validated in patients and control subjects; and (4) there is information on sensitivity, specificity, accuracy, and reproducibility.

Vibratory detection threshold of the toe is significantly elevated in patients with diabetic polyneuropathy.

In diabetic neuropathy, elevated sensory thresholds are statistically associated with neuropathic symptoms, deficits, and neuropathologic abnormalities of sural nerve. Both VDT and CDT correlated with increasingly severe stages of diabetic polyneuropathy.

The measurement of small-nerve fiber function with CDT and HNDT using CASE is useful for the evaluation of potential new therapeutic agents such as NGF in prevention or treatment of diabetic polyneuropathy.

Sensory abnormalities as measured by CASE provide a reliable, reproducible, and sensitive index of diabetic neuropathy.

References

1. Apfel SC, Arezzo JC, Brownlee M, et al. Nerve growth factor administration protects against experimental diabetic sensory neuropathy. Brain Res 1994; 634:7.
2. Archer AG, Watkins PJ, Thomas PK. The natural history of acute painful neuropathy in diabetes mellitus. J Neurol Neurosurg Psychiatry 1983; 46:491.
3. Birder LA, Perl ER. Cutaneous sensory receptors (review). J Clin Neurophysiol 1994; 11:534.
4. Brown MJ, Martin JR, Asbury AK. Painful diabetic neuropathy: A morphometric study. Arch Neurol 1976; 33:164.
5. Chochinow RH, Ullyot LE, Moorhouse JA. Sensory perception thresholds in patients with juvenile diabetes and their close relatives. N Engl J Med 1972; 286:1233.
6. Collins WS, Zilinsky JD, Boas LC. Impaired vibratory sense in diabetes. Am J Med 1946; 1:638.
7. Conomy JP, Barnes KL, Conomy JM. Cutaneous sensory function in diabetes mellitus. J Neurol Neurosurg Psychiatry 1979; 42:656.
8. Dodt E, Zotterman Y. The discharge of specific cold fibers at high temperatures. Acta Physiol Scand 1952; 26:358.
9. Dyck PJ. Quantitative sensory testing: A consensus report from the Peripheral Neuropathy Association. Neurology 1993; 43:1050.
10. Dyck PJ. Diabetic polyneuropathy in controlled clinical trials: Consensus report of the Peripheral Nerve Society. Ann Neurol 1995 38:478.
11. Dyck PJ, Bushek W, Spring EM, et al. Vibratory and cooling detection thresholds compared with other tests in diagnosing and staging diabetic neuropathy. Diabetes Care 1987; 10:432.
12. Dyck PJ, Karnes J, O'Brien PC, et al. Neuropathy symptom profile in health, motor neuron disease, diabetic neuropathy, and amyloidosis. Neurology 1986; 36:1300.
13. Dyck PJ, Karnes JL, Daube J, et al. Clinical and neuropathological criteria for the diagnosis and staging of diabetic neuropathy. Brain 1985; 108:861.
14. Dyck PJ, Karnes JL, Gillen DA, et al. Comparison of

algorithms of testing for use in automated evaluation of sensation. Neurology 1990; 40:1607.

15. Dyck PJ, Karnes JL, O'Brien PC, et al. The Rochester Diabetic Neuropathy Study: Reassessment of tests and criteria for diagnosis and staged severity. Neurology 1992; 42:1164.

16. Dyck PJ, Karnes JL, O'Brien PC, et al. The spatial distribution of fiber loss in diabetic polyneuropathy suggests ischemia. Ann Neurol 1986; 19:440.

17. Dyck PJ, Karnes JL, O'Brien PC, et al. Detection thresholds of cutaneous sensation in humans. *In* Dyck PJ, Thomas PK, Griffin J, et al (eds): Peripheral Neuropathy. Philadelphia, WB Saunders, 1993, p 706.

18. Dyck PJ, Litchy WJ, Lehman KA, et al. Variables influencing neuropathic endpoints: The Rochester Diabetic Neuropathy Study of Healthy Subjects (RDNS-HS). Neurology 1995; 45:1115.

19. Dyck PJ, O'Brien PC, Kosanke JL, et al. A 4, 2, and 1 stepping algorithm for quick and accurate estimation of cutaneous sensation threshold. Neurology 1993; 43:1508.

20. Dyck PJ, Peroutka S, Rask C, et al. Intradermal recombinant human nerve growth factor induces pressure allodynia and lowered heat-pain threshold in humans. Neurology 1997; 48:501.

21. Dyck PJ, Sherman WR, Hallcher LM, et al. Human diabetic endoneurial sorbital, fructose, and myo-inositol related to sural nerve morphometry. Ann Neurol 1980; 8:590.

22. Dyck PJ, Zimmerman IR, Gillen DA, et al. Cool, warm, and heat-pain detection thresholds: Testing methods and inferences about anatomic distribution of receptors. Neurology 1993; 43:1500.

23. Dyck PJ, Zimmerman IR, Johnson DM, et al. A standard test of heat-pain responses using CASE IV. J Neurol Sci 1996; 136:54.

24. Dyck PJ, Zimmerman IR, O'Brien PC, et al. Introduction of automated systems to evaluate touch-pressure, vibration, and thermal cutaneous sensation in man. Ann Neurol 1978; 4:502.

25. Dykes RW. Coding of steady and transient temperatures by cutaneous "cold" fibers serving the hand of monkeys. Brain Res 1975; 98:485.

26. Fruhstorfer H, Lindlom U, Schmidt WG. Method for quantitative estimation of thermal thresholds in patients. J Neurol Neurosurg Psychiatry 1976; 39:1071.

27. Goldberg JM, Lindblom U. Standardized method of determining vibratory perception thresholds for diagnosis and screening in neurological investigation. J Neurol Neurosurg Psychiatry 1979; 42:793.

28. Greenspan JD, McGillis SLB. Stimulus features relevant to the perception of sharpness and mechanically evoked cutaneous pain. Somatosens Mot Res 1991; 8:131.

29. Gregersen G. Vibratory perception threshold and motor conduction velocity in diabetics and non-diabetics. Acta Med Scand 1968; 183:61.

30. Halar EM, Milutinoviv J, Brozovich FV, et al. Uremic neuropathy: Correlation of nerve conduction velocity and clinical findings. Arch Phys Med Rehabil 1978; 59:564.

31. Johnson KO, Lamb GD. Neural mechanisms of spatial tactile discrimination: Neural patterns evoked by Braille-like dot patterns in the monkey. J Physiol (Lond) 1981; 310:117.

32. Light AR, Perl ER. Peripheral sensory systems. *In* Dyck PJ, Thomas PK, Griffin JW, et al (eds): Peripheral Neuropathy. Philadelphia, WB Saunders, 1993, p 149.

33. Lindblom U. Touch perception threshold in human glabrous skin in terms of displacement amplitude on stimulation with single mechanical pulses. Brain Res 1974; 82:205.

34. Lindblom U, Tegner R. Quantification of sensibility in mononeuropathy, polyneuropathy, and central lesions. *In* Munsat TL (ed): Quantification of Neurologic Deficit. Boston, Butterworths, 1989, p 171.

35. Llewelyn JG, Gilbey SG, Thomas PK, et al. Sural nerve morphometry in diabetic autonomic and painful sensory neuropathy: A clinicopathological study. Brain 1991; 114:867.

36. Martin JH, Jessell TM. Modality coding in the somatic sensory system. *In* Kandel ER, Schwartz JH, Jessell TM (eds): Principles of Neural Science. New York, Elsevier, 1991, p 341.

37. Mirsky IA, Futterman P, Broh-Kahn RH. The quantitative measure of vibration perception in subjects with and without diabetes mellitus. J Lab Clin Med 1953; 41:221.

38. Nielsen VK. The peripheral nerve function in chronic renal failure. Acta Med Scand 1972; 191:287.

39. Nielsen VK, Lund FS. Diabetic polyneuropathy: Corneal sensitivity, vibratory perception and Achilles tendon reflex in diabetics. Acta Neurol Scand 1979; 59:15.

40. Russell JW, Karnes JL, Dyck PJ. Sural nerve myelinated fiber density differences associated with meaningful changes in clinical and electrophysiologic measurements. J Neurol Sci 1996; 135:114.

41. Said G, Slama G, Salva J. Progressive centripetal degeneration of axons in small fibre diabetic polyneuropathy. Brain 1983; 106:791.

42. Steiness IB. Vibratory perception in normal subjects: A biothesiometric study. Acta Med Scand 1957; 158:315.

43. Steiness IB. Vibratory perception in diabetics: A biothesiometric study. Acta Med Scand 1957; 158:327.

44. Steiness IB. Influence of diabetic status on vibratory perception during ischemia. Acta Med Scand 1961; 170:319.

45. Stevens JC, Marks LE. Spatial summation and the dynamics of warmth sensation. Percept Psychophys 1971; 9:391.

46. Verdugo R, Ochoa JL. Quantitative somatosensory thermotest: A key method for functional evaluation of small caliber afferent channels. Brain 1992; 115:893.

47. Yarnitsky D, Simone DA, Dotson RM, et al. Single C nociceptor responses and psychophysical parameters of evoked pain: Effect of rate of rise of heat stimuli in humans. J Neurophysiol 1992; 450:581.

Cardiovascular Assessment

Michael Pfeifer

INTRODUCTION

Cardiovascular autonomic neuropathy has been less well studied in diabetes than sensorimotor neuropathy. This is because the symptoms of autonomic neuropathy may be subtle and occur late in the course of diabetes and because reproducible, clinically applicable techniques for the assessment of cardiovascular autonomic nervous system (ANS) integrity are relatively new. However, studies of cardiovascular ANS activities are warranted because neuropathy of this system is frequently present in diabetic patients,[36, 38, 84, 89] is an important cause of diabetic morbidity,[21, 42, 70, 80] and in fact may carry a higher risk of mortality than sensorimotor neuropathy.[21] Both the absence of pain during myocardial infarction and the occurrence of sudden death have been attributed to autonomic neuropathy in diabetic parents.[21, 42, 70] In addition, one study reported a 50% mortality within 3 years of the clinical diagnosis of various kinds of autonomic neuropathy in a group of diabetic patients.[21, 36, 38] The authors concluded that cardiovascular ANS neuropathy played a major role in the increased mortality. There are several excellent reviews that have detailed the morbidity and mortality of diabetic autonomic neuropathy,[21, 22, 38] including cardiovascular autonomic neuropathy.

Until recently, diabetic autonomic neuropathy was thought to be a late complication of diabetes. However, this impression was traceable to the fact that frank clinical manifestations of autonomic neuropathy could be detected only after damage had progressed beyond the body's ability to compensate. As techniques were developed, it became clear that results of assessments of the cardiovascular ANS[84, 89] and other portions of the ANS[13, 32, 43, 73, 83, 89, 102] may be abnormal early in the course of diabetes, before the appearance of overt signs and symptoms. Further, these newer techniques have documented the frequent coexistence and often simultaneous progression of sensorimotor and cardiovascular ANS neuropathies.[88, 104]

IMPORTANCE OF ASSESSMENT OF THE CARDIOVASCULAR AUTONOMIC NERVOUS SYSTEM

In discussing the importance of the assessment of the cardiovascular ANS, we have elected to address research and clinical applications separately. Assessment of cardiovascular autonomic function is very important in diabetic research. Inclusion of such assessment in research protocols will lead to a better understanding of the natural history of cardiovascular autonomic neuropathy, its relationship to morbidity and mortality, and the possible effectiveness of glucose control and other treatment modalities in altering nerve function. Furthermore, some of the available techniques are quantitative and can be directly related to physiologic and pathophysiologic responses (e.g., exercise intolerance and postural hypotension).

At present, assessment of the cardiovascular ANS may afford some clinical insight in the management of selected patients. For example, this assessment may assist the physician in making clinical judgment as to whether the patient should be placed on an exercise regimen. In the future, if any treatment modality is proved to alter the course of diabetic neuropathies, then a means for the early identification of patients at high risk for developing symptomatic neuropathy will be of great importance in clinical practice. In one retrospective study of 67 asymptomatic adult diabetic patients, the usefulness of several neural tests in predicting the later development of neuropathic symptoms was evaluated.[110] Measures that were evaluated included dark-adapted pupil size after parasympathetic nervous system (PNS) blockade, pupillary latency time, heart rate, RR variation before and after sympathetic nervous system (SNS) blockade, the Valsalva ratio, and nerve conduction velocities of the peroneal,

median motor, and median sensory nerves. Presence and absence of SNS and ANS symptoms were determined by a single examiner who used the scoring method described by Dyck et al.[28] Results were analyzed by linear logistic regression models, which took into account the possible effects of the patient's age, sex, adiposity, and glycemic control as well as the duration and type of diabetes. RR variation, one of the specific measures of cardiovascular autonomic function described later in this chapter, and the duration of diabetes were important in all three models: the model for sensorimotor neuropathy, the model for autonomic neuropathy, and the model for either sensorimotor or autonomic neuropathy. In a small (n = 9) prospective study, the RR variation correctly predicted whether symptoms would occur in eight of nine patients ($P <$ 0.05).[110] Thus, it appears that the development of a predictive index for all forms of diabetic neuropathy is feasible and that a measure of cardiovascular ANS function, such as RR variation, may be an important component of this index. Prospective clinical trials to evaluate these linear logistic regression models are now in progress.

SYNDROMES OF CARDIOVASCULAR AUTONOMIC NEUROPATHY

The syndromes of cardiovascular autonomic neuropathy can most easily be discussed by considering the early and late manifestations of the efferent, afferent, and reflex pathways.

Efferent Abnormalities

Early abnormalities of the efferent pathway may lead to denervation supersensitivity. Increased response of systolic blood pressure to infusions of norepinephrine in diabetic patients with cardiovascular autonomic neuropathy have been demonstrated by Scobie and colleagues.[96] Hilsted and coworkers[60] found exaggerated responses of heart rate and greater drop of mean arterial pressure in diabetic patients with cardiovascular autonomic neuropathy than in diabetic patients without cardiovascular autonomic neuropathy or in nondiabetic persons. This denervation supersensitivity may account for the increased cardiovascular lability seen in some diabetic patients.

During anesthesia after long duration of diabetes mellitus, the denervation supersensitivity may lead to denervation atrophy and account, in part, for the greater incidence of heart failure seen in diabetic patients without coronary disease. In fact, one study demonstrated a relationship between diastolic dysfunction and the degree of autonomic dysfunction.

Afferent Abnormalities

Decreased sensation of the heart may help to explain the greater incidence of painless myocardial ischemia in diabetic patients compared to nondiabetic patients.

Abnormal Reflex Arcs

EXERCISE INTOLERANCE

In normal persons, the ANS is important in the cardiovascular response to exercise. During the early stages of exercise there is a decrease in cardiac PNS activity[46] followed by an increase in vascular SNS activity.[20, 94] At maximal levels of exercise (near-exhaustion), there is a release of epinephrine.[35, 82] These responses increase cardiac output, ejection fraction, blood pressure, and heart rate and thus supply increased amounts of oxygen and nutrients needed by the brain and skeletal muscles.

Cardiac performance has been evaluated in nondiabetic cardiac-denervated humans and dogs. In humans, the studies were performed in heart transplant recipients who presumably had total cardiac denervation.[50] Cardiac output was below normal in these subjects at rest and increased (although remaining abnormal) late in exercise as a result of the effects of increased circulating catecholamines on the heart. Similar results have been reported in acutely denervated healthy dogs.[27] In still other studies, the effects of β-adrenergic blockade have been evaluated in normal humans. During exercise, heart rate, systolic blood pressure, left ventricular ejection fraction, and cardiac output were decreased in these patients.[90, 101] In dogs, the effects of an atropine-induced decreased cardiac PNS resulted in an increase in heart rate but a decrease in stroke volume and left ventricular pressure.[1] Therefore, an abnormal decrease in PNS, a decrease in SNS, or both appear to have functional effects that diminish cardiac performance during exercise.

In diabetic patients evaluated by graded exercise, it was found that the worse the cardiovascular autonomic neuropathy, the more abnormal the cardiovascular performance, systemic peripheral resistance, and change in heart rate.[55, 57, 86] The increase in plasma norepinephrine during exercise was smaller in the patients with postural hypotension. Thus, cardiovascular ANS neuropathy appears to contribute to the poor exercise tolerance observed in many diabetic patients.

POSTURAL HYPOTENSION

The syndrome of postural hypotension is characterized by posture-related weakness, dizziness, visual impairment, and presyncope. A detailed discussion of the causes of postural hypotension is included in an excellent review by Thomas and associates.[107] Although the definition of postural hypotension varies among investigators, it is generally accepted that a decrease, upon standing, of 10 mm Hg in diastolic blood pressure or 30 mm Hg in systolic blood pressure is sufficient to establish the diagnosis. When a normal person changes from a recumbent to an upright position, a baroreceptor-mediated reflex produces increased SNS tone in the heart and blood vessels in order to prevent venous pooling, decreased venous return, and decreased cardiac output with resulting hypotension. Diastolic blood pressure rarely falls and may increase slightly, and systolic blood pressure often transiently decreases. But these changes in normal persons are much smaller than those used to define hypotension. The increase in sympathetic tone to the peripheral vasculature results in an increase in the neurotransmitter norepinephrine within the cleft at the neuroeffector junction, thus increasing the plasma norepinephrine level.[17, 24, 25, 115] In patients with nondiabetic autonomic neuropathy (e.g., Shy-Drager syndrome) the inability to increase SNS tone of the blood vessels is reflected by a lack of rise in plasma norepinephrine concentration upon standing.[115]

In diabetic patients with postural hypotension, the response of plasma norepinephrine concentration to standing is variable. Like patients with Shy-Drager syndrome, some orthostatic, diabetic patients have no increase in plasma norepinephrine upon standing,[17, 25, 59] a finding consistent with vascular sympathetic neuropathy. Other diabetic patients with orthostatic hypotension show an increase in plasma norepinephrine upon standing that is similar in magnitude to that seen in normal subjects. However, since this increase is less than expected for the degree of hypotension, these patients are also considered to have vascular autonomic neuropathy. Still other diabetic patients have a supernormal (greater than 2 SD above the mean for normal subjects[25]) increase in their plasma norepinephrine concentration upon standing. This supernormal response has been found to occur in patients with intravascular volume contraction, specifically, a reduction in red blood cell mass.[108] Unlike the first two types of diabetic patients, these patients may not have vascular autonomic neuropathy. Other causes for orthostatic hypotension have been suggested. It has been postulated that an inadequate increase in heart rate is a cause of orthostatic hypotension in some diabetics.[103] Vasovagal syncope as well as the effects of medications (such as nitroglycerin[62] and even insulin[51, 71, 79, 81]) should be considered in the differential diagnosis of orthostatic hypotension in diabetic patients. It also is important to bear in mind that the symptoms of hypoglycemia and vestibular dysfunction may be similar to and be confused with the symptoms of orthostatic hypotension. Figure 11.1 is an algorithm that may be helpful in establishing the cause of postural dizziness in diabetic patients. Management of orthostatic hypotension in diabetic patients includes volume repletion and control of glycosuria, use of elastic stockings[16] and military antigravity suits, high salt intake,[107] mineralocorticoids,[16] vasoconstrictors,[3, 9, 44, 95] β-blockers,[12, 72] and atrial pacing.[76] Long duration vasoconstrictors usually produce supine hypertension, but nasal phenylephrine (Neo-Synephrine; 10% ophthalmic solution, one to three drops every 4 hours while upright) avoids this problem and may be efficacious.

CARDIAC DENERVATION SYNDROME

A fixed pulse rate of 80 to 90 beats per minute that is unresponsive to mild exercise, stresses, or sleep indicates nearly complete cardiac denervation.[22, 61, 70] By this definition, cardiac denervation has been documented in some diabetic patients.[70] Cardiac denervation has been offered as an explanation for the increased incidence of painless myocardial infarction in diabetic patients.[11, 22, 38, 42, 61, 80] Some authors have also suggested that some cases of sudden death in diabetic patients are caused by adrenergic supersensitivity from cardiac denervation (cardiac denervation supersensitivity).[22, 36, 38]

The presence of cardiac denervation supersensitivity in diabetic patients has been suggested by two studies. In one study, diabetic patients with autonomic neuropathy who were challenged by hypoglycemia had the same increase in plasma epinephrine but a greater increase in heart rate compared with normal subjects.[58] In the other study, long-term diabetic patients showed an increased sensitivity to intravenous infusions of catecholamines compared with normal controls.[17] Increased numbers or sensitivity of end-organ adrenergic receptors has been suggested as an explanation for denervation supersensitivity.[114] An alternative explanation would be impairment of ANS counterregulation. For example, an exaggerated response to epinephrine could be due to a lack of cardiac counterregulation by the PNS (i.e., PNS neuropathy). Whatever the explana-

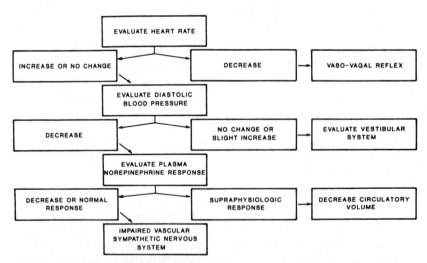

■ **Figure 11.1** Flow chart of the evaluation of postural dizziness. Several distinct etiologies can result in postural dizziness in diabetic patients. Provided that a drug-induced cause has been eliminated and hypoglycemia has been excluded, this flow chart indicates which of the four major etiologies is the probable cause.

tion, cardiac denervation supersensitivity does appear to occur in some diabetic patients. Whether this supersensitivity is actually the cause of sudden death is still open to question.

Since myocardial ischemia may not cause typical anginal chest pain in diabetic patients,[11] severe coronary artery disease may be clinically occult. Therefore, vague thoracic or epigastric symptoms in a diabetic patient may represent myocardial ischemia and should be regarded with a high index of suspicion. Thus, liberal use of nuclear medicine cardiovascular exercise stress tests or comparable studies in such patients is warranted, especially if cardiovascular autonomic neuropathy has been diagnosed previously.[42] Furthermore, diabetic patients who are likely to have cardiovascular autonomic neuropathy should be strongly advised to have cardiac stress testing before undertaking an exercise program.

DIFFICULTIES IN ASSESSING THE CARDIOVASCULAR AUTONOMIC NERVOUS SYSTEM

Unlike the peripheral, sensorimotor nervous system in which individual nerves can be tested directly, the ANS usually studied by observation of end-organ function. Such studies involve the application of a standardized stimulus to the afferent limb of a complex reflex arc involving a sensory, afferent nerve, central processing elements, efferent nerve, neuroeffector junctions, and end-organ response. An abnormality at any point in the reflex arc can alter end-organ function. To make matters more complicated, most organ systems are dually innervated with parasympathetic and sympathetic nerves that often work in opposition. For example, SNS stimulation of the heart tends to increase the heart rate, whereas PNS stimulation of the heart tends to decrease it. Thus, a fast heart rate could result from either decreased PNS activity (autonomic neuropathy) or increased sympathetic nervous system activity (stress). Furthermore, the cardiac SNS has both chronotropic and inotropic properties. On the other hand, vascular tone is believed to be regulated by the SNS without direct opposition of the PNS. Thus, even though the neuroanatomy of the cardiovascular system is reasonably well understood, interpretations of cardiovascular ANS tests must take into account the complexity of the involved reflex arcs.

SPECIFIC METHODS FOR ASSESSMENT OF THE CARDIOVASCULAR AUTONOMIC NERVOUS SYSTEM

Many techniques have been used to assess the cardiovascular ANS (Table 11.1). Although most are simple to perform, relatively noninvasive, and quantitative, only three will be discussed in detail. These three were selected for discussion because they have been cited frequently in the literature, are sufficiently reproducible (after proper patient preparation) to be clinically useful, and involve reflex arcs that are reasonably well understood.

RR Variation

It has long been known that the heart rate increases with inspiration and decreases with expiration. In electrocardiographic terms, the RR interval shortens during inspiration and lengthens during expiration. Figure 11.2 illustrates these changes in a normal and a diabetic subject. This sinus arrhythmia (or beat-to-beat variation in RR interval) during quiet respiration has been used as an index of cardiac PNS activity since 1973 because of a study that showed that atropine (a PNS antagonist), but not propranolol (a beta-adrenergic antagonist), alters RR variation in normal subjects.[112] However, a subsequent study showed that isoproterenol (a β-adrenergic agonist) decreases the RR variation.[84] Therefore, RR variation is not always an exact reflection of PNS activity because increased cardiac SNS activity is capable of affecting RR variation.

There are several ways of measuring (quantifying) RR variation. In a review that compared five ways of describing RR variation, the investigators concluded that the standard deviation of the mean RR interval during a period of quiet breathing was one of two methods that best differentiated between diabetic patients with and without autonomic damage.[35] The other method was the difference between the maximum and minimum heart rates recorded over a period of time during deep breathing at six breaths per minute. However, RR variation determined by either the standard deviation of the mean RR interval or the "max-minus-min" method does have some inherent problems. A gradual trend over time that results in a global change (increase or decrease) in the mean RR interval (heart rate) may result in a false elevation in RR variation measured by either of these methods. A fast basal heart rate will pro-

TABLE 11.1 METHODS TO EVALUATE CARDIOVASCULAR AUTONOMIC NERVOUS SYSTEM ACTIVITY

Test	Description	References
Face into cold water	Immersion of face into cold water; measure change in heart rate	4, 6, 52
Cold pressor	Measure changes in blood pressure after immersing arm in cold water	46, 50
Skin temperature	Measure skin temperature (related to vascular flow) in ambient room temperature	71
Finger wrinkling	Observe presence or absence of finger wrinkling after hand immersion in water (vascular flow)	14
Startle	Measure change in heart rate after a sudden loud noise	44
Mental stress	Measure change in heart rate during mental arithmetic	6, 63, 64, 98
Lower body negative pressure	Measure heart rate changes during a decrease in pressure	30
Carotid massage	Measure change in heart rate during carotid massage	63, 64
Neck suction	Measure change in heart rate during negative carotid pressure	29
Phenylephrine	Measure change in heart rate during increased blood pressure and baroreceptor stimulation	4, 6, 63, 64
Amyl nitrite	Measure change in heart rate during a decrease in blood pressure by amyl nitrite administration	63, 64
Handgrip	Measure change in heart rate and blood pressure during half maximal handgrip	33, 35, 39, 104
Exercise	Measure change in heart rate during exercise	28, 53–55, 79
Heart rate	Observe resting heart rate or heart rate trends over 24 hours	8, 33, 35, 36, 40
Plasma catecholamines	Measure plasma catecholamines during resting and stimulated states	16
Postural testing	Measure plasma catecholamines, heart rate, and blood pressure before and after assuming the upright posture	4, 6, 24, 28, 33, 35, 63, 64, 95, 100, 104
RR variation	Measurement of the degree of sinus arrhythmia during deep respiration	4, 6, 28, 33, 35, 77
Valsalva	Measure heart rate and blood pressure during Valsalva maneuver	4, 6, 7, 28, 33, 35, 63, 64

duce smaller RR intervals and, for statistical reasons, one would expect a smaller standard deviation and a smaller difference between the maximum and minimum RR intervals. In order to eliminate these problems, a new method of describing RR variation has been developed.[109] It has been termed the *circular mean resultant*. This method, which is based on vector analysis, eliminates the effects of trends in heart rate over time and greatly attenuates the effect of basal heart rate and ectopic beats on the calculated variability of heart rate. Normative values are found in Table 11.2. Furthermore, recent studies have shown that this calculation of RR variation is the most reproducible.

Several specific protocols for the measurement of RR variation have been described.[4, 5, 35, 84, 109] In general, these protocols involve continuous electrocardiographic measurements of heart rate over a defined period of time. Patients are required to breathe at a standardized respiratory rate (usually five or six times per minute) since respiratory rate has been found to alter RR variation.[84] Patient position affects RR variation[5] and, therefore, current protocols require a standardized patient position, although there is not yet a consensus as to the preferred position. However, we prefer

the supine position since RR variation was not altered in normal subjects studied in the recumbent position after modest acute volume depletion.[89] In contrast, volume changes during upright posture may result in a marked increase in cardiovascular SNS tone that may in turn alter RR variation.[108]

Other factors may potentially alter RR variation. Vascular SNS activity is altered by a variety of factors such as eating,[97] obesity,[97] drinking coffee,[91, 93] and smoking.[48] Therefore, it seems prudent to have subjects avoid as many of these factors as possible when RR variation is evaluated. Furthermore, medicines often taken by diabetic patients may alter the ANS. Insulin is known to increase plasma norepinephrine and heart rate and may decrease arterial blood pressure in patients with neuropathy,[17, 51, 71, 79, 81] Over-the-counter medications may also alter ANS activity. Sodium salicylate has been known to potentiate plasma norepinephrine and epinephrine responses to hypoglycemia in normal humans.[75] In our preliminary studies, sodium salicylate augments RR variation. Since salicylates have also been reported to augment cholinergic responses in several species,[26] it is possible that over-the-counter products such as aspirin (acetylsali-

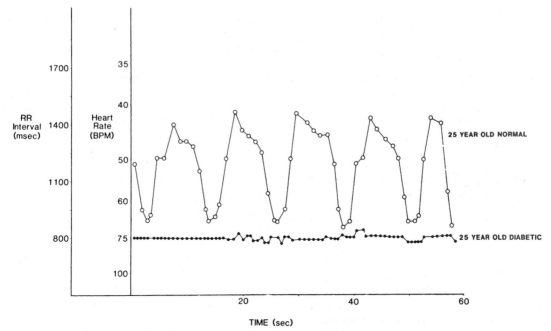

■ **Figure 11.2** Changes in heart rate during deep breathing in a normal and a diabetic subject. The variation in heart rate (sinus arrhythmia) during breathing is termed RR variation. Its magnitude is clearly less in this 25-year-old diabetic patient with severe autonomic neuropathy than in the normal subject. Both patients were breathing at a fixed rate of 5 breaths per minute. (From Pfeifer MA, and Greene DA: Current Concepts. The Upjohn Company, 1985.)

cylic acid) may also alter ANS tests. For this reason, medicines such as aspirin, antihistamines, and nasal sprays should be avoided prior to testing. Other factors such as aging[85] can affect RR variation. Recent studies have shown that myocardial ischemia and end-stage cardiac failure can also result in abnormal RR variation. The Diabetes Control and Complication Trial demonstrated that intensive glucose management can both prevent the onset of abnormal RR variation and slow the deterioration of RR variation over time. In order to avoid many of these and other potential confounding factors in the measurement of RR variation, we prefer to do measurement of RR variation under the following conditions:

1. In a quiet, relaxed atmosphere, preferably in the morning
2. After an overnight (8-hour) fast
3. With patient using a device to help guide the timing of breathing
4. After the patient has practiced the procedure several times
5. After the patient has had at least 15 minutes of supine rest
6. In patients who have avoided tobacco products (8 hours), ethanol (24 hours), and over-the-counter medicines (8 hours)
7. After patients have avoided prescription medicine known to alter ANS activities (including insulin) for at least 8 hours (unless the patient is on an insulin pump,

TABLE 11.2 NORMATIVE VALUES FOR RR VARIATION AND VALSALVA RATIO STRATIFIED BY AGE

Age	n	Value*	95% Normative Values
RR variation			
11–20	52	62.0 ± 26.4	31.9–117.0
21–30	162	57.6 ± 21.6	23.0–95.8
31–40	144	51.1 ± 21.5	21.5–90.3
41–50	77	39.9 ± 16.6	16.9–71.0
51–60	20	34.0 ± 20.0	7.2–63.4
61–70	23	29.1 ± 14.5	5.0–60.0
>70	11	16.8 ± 8.2	0.0–27.0
Valsalva			
11–20	40	2.37 ± 0.37	1.83–3.01
21–30	128	2.02 ± 0.45	1.37–2.88
31–40	111	1.89 ± 0.42	1.36–2.76
41–50	55	1.73 ± 0.29	1.24–2.30
51–60	9	1.77 ± 0.31	1.20–2.15
61–70	8	1.63 ± 0.19	1.18–1.88
>70	3	1.78 ± 0.23	†

*Values expressed as ± SD.
†95% normative values not determined given small n.

in which case the basal infusion rate of insulin should be maintained before and during the study)

8. In patients who have not experienced vigorous exercise or severe emotional upset in the past 24 hours
9. In patients who have not had a hypoglycemic episode in the last 8 hours or an acute illness (e.g., acute viral upper respiratory tract infection) in the past 48 hours
10. In patients who are not otherwise stressed (e.g., acute myocardial infarction)

In addition, β-blockade (propranolol) can be used to help further prevent SNS alterations of RR variation.[84, 85, 89] Normal values and reproducibility for measurements of RR variation vary depending on the protocol and descriptive measure (standard deviation of the mean, "max-minus-min," circular mean resultant) used. Therefore, each center should establish its own range of normal values.

In one study in which two groups of normal subjects had both RR variation and the Valsalva ratio determined before and after graded doses of atropine (PNS blockade), RR variation became less than saline at a lower dose (0.7 mg) of atropine than did the Valsalva ratio (2.0 mg).[87] Thus, less PNS blockage was needed before a change in RR variation could be detected. However, at very high levels of atropine, the RR variation could not decrease further (i.e., there was no difference in 2.0 mg and 4.0 mg of atropine), whereas the Valsalva ratio could decrease further at these high doses. Thus, RR variation appears to be more sensitive to ANS blockade (impairment), but the Valsalva ratio may be more useful in severe impairment. In a separate study, three groups of age- and sex-comparable subjects were compared.[87] RR variation was diminished in diabetic subjects who had no neuropathic symptoms and even further reduced in diabetic subjects with symptoms of autonomic neuropathy. The Valsalva ratio was less only in patients who had autonomic neuropathy. Thus, RR variation may be more sensitive than the Valsalva ratio, but the Valsalva ratio may be more useful in the more severely neuropathic patients in longitudinal studies. Furthermore, Figure 11.3 shows that in a group of type 1 and a group of type 2 diabetic subjects, whose known duration of disease was less than 24 months, there was (as a group) abnormal RR variation.[89] Thus, RR variation is sensitive enough to pick up these abnormalities early after the diagnosis of diabetes mellitus has been made.

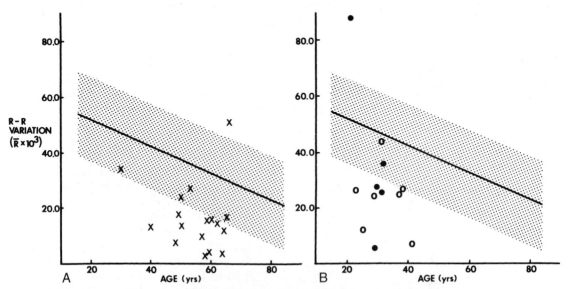

■ **Figure 11.3** RR variation in a patient with a recent (less than 24 months) diagnosis of diabetes mellitus. RR variation after beta-adrenergic blockade[77] was determined by the vector analysis technique.[101] The bold lines represent the regression lines and the shaded areas the 70% confidence band for normal subjects.[78] After age adjustment, the group of non–insulin-dependent diabetic patients *(left panel)* and insulin-dependent diabetics *(right panel)* had significantly smaller RR variation. (From Pfeifer MA, et al: Autonomic neural dysfunction in recently diagnosed diabetic subjects. Diabetes Care, 7:477, 1984.)

Valsalva Maneuver

The Valsalva maneuver consists of forced expiration against a standardized resistance for a specified period of time. Although test conditions should be rigidly standardized for each laboratory, reported protocols have used pressures ranging from 30 to 40 mm Hg (usually 40 mm Hg) and an open loop system that precludes maintenance of measured expiratory pressure by the use of cheek musculature. The most commonly used time periods vary from 10 to 20 seconds.

The physiology of the changes associated with the Valsalva maneuver were well described by Sharpey-Schafer in 1965.[99] When a subject begins the Valsalva maneuver, blood pressure falls, peripheral vascular resistance rises, and tachycardia occurs. These changes appear to be secondary to decreased venous return to the heart, which leads to decreased cardiac output, resulting in a baroreflex-mediated increase in vascular and cardiac SNS activity and tachycardia. Toward the end of the Valsalva maneuver, the subject's blood pressure returns from a hypotensive level toward the subject's baseline blood pressure. Immediately after the Valsalva maneuver (post-Valsalva), venous return to the heart increases due to a release of mechanical resistance to venous flow, and cardiac output increases despite continued constriction of the vascular bed. This increase in cardiac output results in transient hypertension, which leads to bradycardia from an increase in cardiac PNS activity. It has been found that the post-Valsalva bradycardia can be totally abolished with atropine.[67] The transient, post-Valsalva hypertension can be prevented by SNS blockade.[34]

Initially, measurement of the responses of the Valsalva maneuver was assessed by relating the increase in diastolic blood pressure after the maneuver to the decrease in pulse pressure during the maneuver.[98] A more recent method has been to relate a decrease in heart rate after the Valsalva maneuver to the resting heart rate.[4] However, the former method is probably less reliable than the currently used methods,[34] and the latter method is closely related to the more commonly used index, the Valsalva ratio.[36] The Valsalva ratio is the maximum heart rate during the Valsalva maneuver divided by the slowest heart rate after the Valsalva maneuver. Classically, a Valsalva ratio of greater than 1.50 is normal.[68] Table 11.2 gives normative values by age. Although this is a simple and reproducible index,[2] a low Valsalva

ratio can be due to a decrease in cardiac PNS activity, cardiac SNS activity, vascular SNS activity, or a decrease in baroreceptor sensitivity. Thus, it seems that it serves as a general cardiovascular ANS test rather than a specific PNS or SNS evaluator. The Diabetes Control and Complication Trial demonstrated that the deterioration of the Valsalva ratio over time could be slowed by tight glucose control. Since this involves complex reflex arcs of both PNS and SNS pathways, a variety of factors could theoretically affect the Valsalva ratio (see earlier discussion). Therefore, avoidance of possible confounding factors would seem prudent. As stated previously, the Valsalva ratio is not as sensitive as the RR variation, but may reflect the presence of clinically evident diabetic autonomic neuropathy (see section on RR variation). An example of a normal and an abnormal response to the Valsalva maneuver is shown in Figure 11.4.

Plasma Catecholamines

Norepinephrine is released from the adrenal medulla and postganglionic sympathetic neurons.[23, 65] Plasma norepinephrine remains normal after adrenalectomy.[23] Therefore, plasma norepinephrine arises primarily from spillover from postganglionic sympathetic neuroeffector junctions. It has been found that the wider the junctions, the greater the spillover of norepinephrine into the plasma.[65] Since the sympathetic neuromuscular junctions are wide and in close proximity to the blood stream, these junctions appear to be the most important source of plasma norepinephrine.[23] A study in dogs suggests that sympathetic neuromuscular junctions in the heart do not make an important contribution to plasma norepinephrine.[53] In humans, norepinephrine increases with either mild or severe stress. Thus, plasma norepinephrine appears to be an index of vascular SNS activity.

In one study, it was found that basal plasma norepinephrine was not elevated in diabetic patients.[25] However, in two studies of patients who had a very long duration of diabetes, it was found that plasma norepinephrine concentration[18] and the arterial content of norepinephrine[77] were decreased. These two activities are decreased in long-term diabetics. In poorly controlled diabetic patients, norepinephrine responses to exercise are exaggerated.[19, 105] However, as has been previously shown, exaggerated norepinephrine responses may be due to volume contraction.[108] In contrast, patients

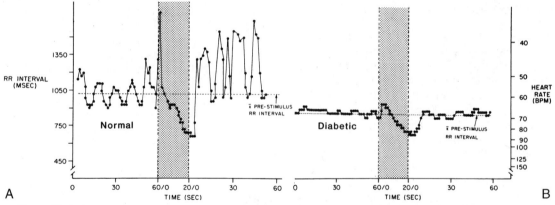

■ **Figure 11.4** Heart rate responses to the Valsalva maneuver. The shaded areas represent a Valsalva maneuver of 40 mm Hg for 20 seconds. The *left panel* illustrates a typical response of a normal subject. Before and after the Valsalva maneuver sinus arrhythmia (RR variation) to breathing is evident. During the Valsalva period there is a gradual increase in heart rate (shorter RR intervals). After the Valsalva period a baroreflex-mediated bradycardia is observed. The diabetic subject with clinical evidence of autonomic neuropathy *(right panel)* has no evidence of RR variation, and the reflex bradycardia after the Valsalva period is lacking.

with orthostatic hypotension have a smaller rise in norepinephrine during exercise.[57] Thus, if factors (such as volume status) are properly controlled, patients with SNS vascular neuropathy have decreased norepinephrine responses to mild (see section on the postural hypotension syndrome) and severe (exercise) cardiovascular stress. In addition to volume, factors such as obesity,[97] eating,[97] coffee drinking[91, 93] and smoking[48] may be associated with increased plasma norepinephrine. Therefore, although plasma norepinephrine is a good index of vascular SNS activity, studies in which plasma norepinephrine is used should be carefully standardized.

Plasma norepinephrine and epinephrine can be determined by radioenzymatic assay.[23, 33, 82] This single-isotope method involves use of catechol-O-methyl transferase plus [³H]-S-adenosyl-L-methionine. The labeled metanephrine and normetanephrine formed by this enzyme reaction are separated by thin-layer chromatography, extracted, and then counted.

Postural Testing

The syndrome of postural hypotension has been described earlier. It has recently been suggested that heart rate responses to postural change (supine to upright) may be used as an index of ANS activity.[34, 39, 103] Although potentially useful, these tests are relatively new and await further validation by multiple centers.

SUMMARY

At our present stage of understanding, it appears that cardiovascular autonomic neuropathy can occur early in the course of diabetes, may be present before the appearance of overt signs and symptoms, carries a risk of morbidity and mortality when associated with clinical signs and symptoms, and is often present (at least subclinically) in conjunction with both sensorimotor and the ANS neuropathies.

It is now possible to quantitatively assess neuroreflex arcs of the cardiovascular system. Currently, these tests have a role in diabetes related research and potentially a role in screening tests in clinical medicine. However, proper assessment of these complicated pathways requires rigid standardization and avoidance of factors that may interfere with the test results.

ACKNOWLEDGMENTS

The authors thank Sheila Green for her secretarial assistance.

References

1. Atkins JM, Horwitz LD. Cardiac autonomic blockade in exercising dogs. J Appl Physiol 1977; 42:878.
2. Baldwa VS, Ewing DJ. Heart rate response to the Valsalva maneuver: Reproducibility in normals and relation to variation in resting heart rate in diabetics. Br Heart J 1977; 39:641.
3. Bannister R. Chronic autonomic failure with postural hypotension. Lancet 1979; 2:404.

4. Bennett T, Farquhar IK, Hosking DJ, et al. Assessment of methods for estimating autonomic nervous control of the heart in patients with diabetes mellitus. Diabetes 1978; 27:1167.

5. Bennett T, Fentem PH, Fitton D, et al. Assessment of vagal control of the heart in diabetes: Measures of RR interval variation under different conditions. Br Heart J 1977; 39:25.

6. Bennett T, Hosking DJ, Hampton JR. Cardiovascular control in diabetes mellitus. Br Med J 1975; 2:585.

7. Bennett T, Hosking DJ, Hampton JR. Vasomotor responses to the Valsalva maneuver in normal subjects and in patients with diabetes mellitus. Br Heart J 1979; 42:422.

8. Bennett T, Riggott PA, Hosking DJ, et al. Twenty-four hour monitoring of heart rate and activity in patients with diabetes mellitus: A comparison with clinic investigators. Br Med J 1976; 1:1250.

9. Benowitz NL, Byrd R, Schambelan M, et al. Dihydroergotamine treatment for orthostatic hypotension from Vacor rodenticide. Ann Intern Med 1989; 92:387.

10. Bevan JA. Some functional consequences of variation in adrenergic synaptic cleft width and in nerve density and distribution. Fed Proc 1977; 36:2439.

11. Bradley RF, Schonfeld A. Diminished pain in diabetic patients with acute myocardial infarction. Geriatrics 1962; 17:322.

12. Brevetti G, Chiariello M, Lavecchia G, et al. Effects of propranolol in a case of orthostatic hypotension. Br Heart J 1979; 41:245.

13. Buck AC, McRae CU, Reed PI, et al. Abnormal detrusor function in asymptomatic diabetes. Br J Surg 1973; 60:310.

14. Bull C, Henry JA. Finger wrinkling as a test of autonomic function. Br Med J 1977; 1:551.

15. Burgos L, Ebert T, Assidao C, et al. Increased intraoperative cardiovascular morbidity in diabetics with autonomic neuropathy. Diabetes Spectrum 1990; 3:28.

16. Chobanian AV, Volicet I, Tifft CP, et al. Mineralocorticoid-induced hypertension in patients with orthostatic hypotension. N Engl J Med 1979; 301:68.

17. Christensen NJ. Catecholamines and diabetes mellitus. Diabetologia 1979; 16:211.

18. Christensen JJ. Plasma catecholamines in long-term diabetics with and without neuropathy and in hypophysectomized patients. J Clin Invest 1972; 51:779.

19. Christensen JJ. Plasma norepinephrine and epinephrine in untreated diabetics, during fasting, and after insulin administration. Diabetes 1974; 23:1.

20. Christensen JJ, Brandshorg O. The relationship between plasma catecholamine concentration and pulse rate during exercise and standing. Eur J Clin Invest 1977; 3:299.

21. Clarke BF, Campbell IW, Ewing FJ. Prognosis in diabetic autonomic neuropathy. Horm Metab Res 1980; 9(suppl):101.

22. Clarke BF, Ewing DJ, Campbell IW. Diabetic autonomic neuropathy. Diabetologia 1979; 17:196.

23. Cryer PE. Isotope derivative measurement of plasma norepinephrine and epinephrine in man. Diabetes 1976; 25:1071.

24. Cryer PE. Physiology and pathophysiology of the human sympathoadrenal neuroendocrine system. N Engl J Med 1980; 303:436.

25. Cryer PE, Silverberg AB, Santiago JV, et al. Hypoadrenergic and hyperadrenergic postural hypotension. Am J Med 1978; 64:407.

26. Delbarre B, Aron E, Dumas G, et al. Action de l'acide acctylsalicylique suz le systeme nerveux vegetalif. Experientia 1971; 27:920.

27. Donald DE, Shepard JT. Response to exercise in dogs with cardiac denervation. Am J Physiol 1963; 205:393.

28. Dyck PJ, Sherman WR, Hallcher LM, et al. Human diabetic endoneurial sorbitol, fructose, and myo-inositol related to sural nerve morphometry. Ann Neurol 1980; 8:590.

29. Dysberg T, Benn J, Sandahl-Christiansen J, et al. Prevalence of diabetic autonomic neuropathy measured by simple bedside tests. Diabetologia 1981; 20:190.

30. Eckberg DL, Cavanaugh MS, Mark AL, et al. A simplified neck suction device for activation of carotid baroreceptors. J Lab Clin Med 1975; 85:167.

31. Eckberg DL, Orshan CR. Respiratory and baroreceptor reflex interactions in man. J Clin Invest 1977; 59:780.

32. Ellenberg M, Weber H. The incipient asymptomatic diabetic bladder. Diabetes 1967; 16:331.

33. Evans MI, Halter JB, Porte D Jr. Comparison of double and single-isotope enzymatic derivative methods for measuring catecholamine in human plasma. Clin Chem 1978; 24:567.

34. Ewing DJ. Cardiovascular reflexes and autonomic neuropathy. Clin Sci Molec Med 1978; 55:321.

35. Ewing DJ, Borsey DQ, Bellavere F, et al. Cardiac autonomic neuropathy in diabetes: Comparison of measures of RR interval variation. Diabetologia 1981; 21:18.

36. Ewing DJ, Campbell IW, Clarke BF. Assessment of cardiovascular effects in diabetic autonomic neuropathy and prognostic implications. Ann Intern Med 1980; 92(part 22):308.

37. Ewing DJ, Campbell IW, Clarke BF. Heart rate changes in diabetes mellitus. Lancet 1981; 1:183.

38. Ewing DJ, Campbell IW, Clarke BF. The natural history of diabetic autonomic neuropathy. QJ Med 1980; 49:95.

39. Ewing DJ, Campbell IW, Murray A, et al. Immediate heart rate response to standing: Simple test for autonomic neuropathy in diabetes. Br Med J 1978; 1:145.

40. Ewing DJ, Irving JB, Ken F, et al. Cardiovascular responses to sustained handgrip in normal subjects and in patients with diabetes mellitus: A test of autonomic function. Clin Sci Molec Med 1974; 46:295.

41. Ewing DJ, Neilson JMM, Travis P. New method for assessing cardiac parasympathetic activity using 24-hour electrocardiogram. Br Heart J 1984; 52:396.

42. Faerman I, Faccio E, Meleti J, et al. Autonomic neuropathy and painless myocardial infarction in diabetic patients: Histologic evidence of their relationship. Diabetes 1977; 26:1147.

43. Faerman I, Maler M, Jadzinsky M, et al. Asymptomatic neurogenic bladder in juvenile diabetes. Diabetologia 1971; 7:168.

44. Fouad FM, Tarazi RC, Bravo EL. Dihydroergotamine in idiopathic orthostatic hypotension: Short-term intramuscular and long-term oral therapy. Clin Pharmacol Ther 1981; 30:782.

45. Frank J II, Frewin DB, Robinson SM, et al. Cardiovascular responses in diabetic dysautonomia. Aust NZ J Med 1972; 1:1.

46. Freyschuss U. Cardiovascular adjustment to somatomotor activation. Acta Physiol Scand 1970; 324(suppl):1.

47. Friedman HS, Sacerdote A, Bandu I, et al. Abnormalities of the cardiovascular response to cold presser test in Type 1 diabetes: Correlation with blood glucose control. Arch Intern Med 1984; 144:43.

48. Gash A, Karliner JS, Janowsky D, et al. Effects of smoking marijuana on left ventricular performance and plasma norepinephrine: Studies in normal men. Ann Intern Med 1978; 89:448.

49. Gelber D, Pfeifer MA, Schumer M, et al. Reliability and comparison of methods to calculate heart rate variability. Diabetes 1995; 44:66A.

50. Griepp RB, Stinson EB, Dong E Jr, et al. Hemodynamic performance of the transplanted human heart. Surgery 1971; 70:88.

51. Gundersen HJG, Christensen NJ. Intravenous insulin causing loss of intravascular water and albumin and increased adrenergic nervous activity in diabetics. Diabetes 1977; 26:551.

52. Hague R, Scarpello J, Sladen G, et al. Autonomic function tests in diabetes mellitus. Diabetes Metab 1978; 4:227.

53. Halter JB, Kelley KO, Gould KL. Effects of adrenergic stimulation of cardiac handling of catecholamines in vivo. Clin Res 1981; 29:83.

54. Helstad DD, Abbound FM, Eckstein JW. Vasoconstrictor response to stimulated diving in man. J Appl Physiol 1968; 25:542.

55. Hilsted J. Pathophysiology in diabetic autonomic neuropathy: Cardiovascular, hormonal, and metabolic studies. Diabetes 1982; 31:730.

56. Hilsted J, Galbo H, Christensen NJ. Impaired cardiovascular responses to graded exercise in diabetic autonomic neuropathy. Diabetes 1979; 28:313.

57. Hilsted J, Galbo H, Christensen NJ. Impaired cardiovascular responses of catecholamines, growth hormone, and cortisol to graded exercise in diabetic autonomic neuropathy. Diabetes 1980; 29:257.

58. Hilsted J, Madsbad S, Krarup T, et al. Hormonal, metabolic, and cardiovascular responses to hypoglycemia in diabetic autonomic neuropathy. Diabetes 1981; 30:626.

59. Hilsted J, Parving HH, Christensen NJ, et al. Hemodynamics in diabetic orthostatic hypotension. J Clin Invest 1981; 68:1427.

60. Hilsted J, Richter E, Madsbad S, et al. Metabolic and cardiovascular responses to epinephrine in diabetic autonomic neuropathy. N Engl J Med 1987; 317:421.

61. Hosking DJ, Bennett T, Hampton JR. Diabetic autonomic neuropathy. Diabetes 1978; 27:1043.

62. Hume L, Ewing DJ, Campbell IW, et al. Provocation of postural hypotension by nitroglycerin in diabetic autonomic neuropathy. Diabetes Care 1980; 3:27.

63. Kahn JK, Zola B, Juni JE, et al. Radionuclide assessment of left ventricular diastolic filling in diabetes mellitus with and without cardiac autonomic neuropathy. J Am Coll Cardiol 1986; 7(6):1303.

64. Kannel WB, Levy D, Cupples LA. Left ventricular hypertrophy and risk of cardiac failure: Insights from the Framingham study. J Cardiovasc Pharmacol 1987; 6:S135.

65. Kipin IJ. Plasma levels of norepinephrine. Ann Intern Med 1978; 88:671.

66. Langer A, Freeman RM, Josse R, et al. Detection of silent myocardial ischemia in diabetes mellitus. Am J Cardiol 1991; 67:1073.

67. Leon DF, Shaver JA, Leonard JJ. Reflex heart rate control in man. Am Heart J 1970; 80:729.

68. Levin AB. A simple test of cardiac function based upon the heart rate changes induced by the Valsalva maneuver. Am J Cardiol 1966; 18:90.

69. Lloyd-Mostyn RN, Watkins PJ. Defective innervation of heart and diabetic autonomic neuropathy. Br Med J 1975; 3:15.

70. Lloyd-Mostyn RN, Watkins PJ. Total cardiac denervation in diabetic autonomic neuropathy. Diabetes 1976; 25:748.

71. Mackey JD, Hayakawa H, Watkins PJ. Cardiovascular effects of insulin: Plasma volume changes in diabetics. Diabetologia 1978; 15:453.

72. Man in 'T Veld AJ, Schalekamp MADH. Pindolol acts as beta-adrenoceptor agonist in orthostatic hypotension: Therapeutic implications. Br Med J 1981; 282:929.

73. Mandelstam P, Siegel CI, Lieber A, et al. The swallowing disorder in patients with diabetic neuropathy gastroenteropathy. Gastroenterology 1969; 56:1.

74. Margolis JR, Kannel WS, Feinleib M, et al. Clinical features of unrecognized myocardial infarction-silent and symptomatic. Am J Cardiol 1973; 32(1):1.

75. Metz S, Halter J, Robertson RP. Sodium salicylate potentiates neurohumoral responses to insulin-induced hypoglycemia. J Clin Endocrinol Metab 1980; 51:93.

76. Moss AJ, Glaser W, Topol E. Atrial tachypacing in the treatment of a patient with primary orthostatic hypotension. N Engl J Med 1980; 302:1456.

77. Neubauer B, Christensen JJ. Norepinephrine, epinephrine, and dopamine contents of the cardiovascular system in long-term diabetics. Diabetes 1976; 25:6.

78. Odel HM, Roth GM, Keating FR Jr. Autonomic neuropathy stimulating the effects of sympathectomy as a complication of diabetes mellitus. Diabetes 1955; 4:92.

79. Page MMcB, Smith RBW, Watkins PJ. Cardiovascular effects of insulin. Br Med J 1976; 1:430.

80. Page MMcB, Watkins PJ. Cardiorespiratory arrest and diabetic autonomic neuropathy. Lancet 1978; 1:14.

81. Page MMcB, Watkins PJ. Provocation of postural hypotension by insulin in diabetic autonomic neuropathy. Diabetes 1976; 25:90.

82. Passon PG, Peuler JD. A simplified radiometric assay for plasma norepinephrine and epinephrine. Anal Biochem 1973; 51:618.

83. Pfeifer MA, Cook D, Brodsky J, et al. Quantitative evaluation of sympathetic and parasympathetic control of iris function. Diabetes Care 1982; 5:518.

84. Pfeifer MA, Cook D, Brodsky J, et al. Quantitative evaluation of cardiac parasympathetic activity in normal and diabetic man. Diabetes 1982; 31:339.

85. Pfeifer MA, Halter JB, Weinberg CR, et al. Differential changes of autonomic nervous system function with age in man. Am J Med 1983; 75:249.

86. Pfeifer MA, Peterson H, Snider H, et al. Relationship of diabetic autonomic neuropathy to cardiac performance. Clin Res 1985; 33:851.

87. Pfeifer MA, Weinberg CR, Cook D, et al. Sensitivity of RR variation and the Valsalva ratio in the assessment of diabetic autonomic neuropathy. Clin Res 1983; 31:394.

88. Pfiefer MA, Weinberg CR, Cook DL, et al. Correlations among autonomic, sensory, and motor neural function tests in untreated noninsulin dependent diabetics. Diabetes Care 1985; 8:576.

89. Pfeifer MA, Weinberg CR, Cook DL, et al. Autonomic neural dysfunction in recently diagnosed diabetic subjects. Diabetes Care 1984; 7:447.

90. Port S, Cobb FR, Jones RH. Effects of propranolol on left ventricular function in normal men. Circulation 1963; 61:358.

91. Robertson D, Johnson GA, Robertson RM, et al. Comparative assessment of stimuli that release neuronal and adrenomedullary catecholamines in man. Circulation 1979; 59:637.

92. Robertson D, Wade D. Management of severe idiopathic orthostatic hypotension with phenylephrine nasal spray. Clin Res 1979; 27:237.

93. Robertson D, Wade D, Workman R, et al. Tolerance to the humoral and hemodynamic effects of caffeine in man. J Clin Invest 1981; 67:1111.

94. Robinson BF, Epstein SE, Beiser GD, et al. Control of heart rate by the autonomic nervous system. Circ Res 1966; 19:400.

95. Schirger A, Sheps SG, Thomas JE, et al. Midodrine: A new agent in the management of idiopathic orthostatic hypotension and Shy-Drager syndrome. Mayo Clin Proc 1981; 56:429.

96. Scobie IN, Rogers PT, Brown PM, et al. Supersensitivity to both tyramine and noradrenaline in diabetic autonomic neuropathy. J Neurol Neurosurg Psychiatry 1987; 50(3):275.

97. Schwartz RS, Halter J, Bieman EL. The relationship of abnormal dietary-induced thermogenesis in obesity to plasma triiodothyronine and norepinephrine. Clin Res 1980; 28:405.

98. Sharpey-Schafer EP. Effects of Valsalva's maneuver on the normal and failing circulation. Br Med J 1955; 1:693.

99. Sharpey-Schafer EP. *In* Handbook of Physiology. Washington, DC, American Physiological Society, 1965, pp 1875.

100. Sheps SG. Use of an elastic garment in the treatment of orthostatic hypotension. Cardiology 1976; 61(suppl 1):271.

101. Sorensen SG, Ritchie JL, Caldwell JH, et al. Serial exercise radionuclide angiography: Validation of count derived changes in cardiac output and quantitation of maximal exercise ventricular volume change after nitroglycerin and propranolol in normal men. Circulation 1980; 61:600.

102. Stewart IM, Hosking DJ, Preston BJ, et al. Oesophageal motor changes in diabetes mellitus. Thorax 1976; 31:278.

103. Sundkvist G, Lilja B, Almer LO. Abnormal diastolic blood pressure and heart rate reactions in tilting in diabetes mellitus. Diabetologia 1980; 19:433.

104. Tackman W, Kaeser HE, Berger W, et al. Autonomic disturbances in relation to sensorimotor peripheral neuropathy in diabetes mellitus. J Neurol 1981; 224:273.

105. Tamberlane WV, Sherwin RS, Koivisto V, et al. Normalization of the growth hormone and catecholamine response to exercise in juvenile onset diabetic subjects treated with a portable insulin infusion pump. Diabetes 1979; 28:785.

106. Taylor SH, Meeran MK. Different effects of adrenergic beta-receptor blockade on heart rate response to mental stress, catecholamines, and exercise. Br Med J 1973; 4:256.

107. Thomas JE, Schirger A, Fealey RD, et al. Orthostatic hypotension. Mayo Clin Proc 1981; 56:117.

108. Tohmeh JF, Shah SD, Cryer PE. The pathogenesis of hyperadrenergic postural hypotension in diabetic patients. Am J Med 1979; 67:772.

109. Weinberg CR, Pfeifer MA. An improved method for measuring heart-rate variability: Assessment of cardiac autonomic function. Biometrics 1984; 40:855.

110. Weinberg CR, Pfeifer MA. Development of a predictive model for symptomatic neuropathy (SN) in diabetes. Diabetes 1983; 32:38.

111. Weiner D, Ryan T, Parson L, et al. Significance of silent myocardial ischemia during exercise testing in patients with diabetes mellitus: A report from the Coronary Artery Surgery Study (CASS) registry. Am J Cardiol 1991; 68:729.

112. Wheeler T, Watkins PJ. Cardiac denervation in diabetes. Br Med J 1973; 4:584.

113. Wieling W, Borst C, VanBrederode JFM, et al. Testing for autonomic neuropathy: Heart rate changes after orthostatic maneuvers and static muscle contractions. Clin Sci 1983; 64:581.

114. Williams LT, Lefkowitz RJ. Receptor Binding Studies in Adrenergic Pharmacology. New York, Raven Press, 1978, p 37.

115. Ziegler MG, Lake CR, Kopin IJ. The sympathetic-nervous system defect in primary orthostatic hypotension. N Engl J Med 1977; 296:293.

Chapter 12

Assessment of Pupil Function

Shirley A. Smith • Stephen E. Smith

INTRODUCTION

The pupil is frequently abnormal in diabetic patients. The most obvious abnormalities are its small size, a reduced light reflex and failure to dilate in darkness, redilatation lag, and a poor response to atropine-like mydriatic drugs. Additionally, there may be structural abnormality of the iris in the form of rubeosis, readily visible to the naked eye and made up of neovascularization, which may be sufficient to stiffen the structure of the iris and further immobilize the pupil. The extent to which abnormality of the pupil is caused by autonomic neuropathy or by rubeotic change varies among patients and may be hard to discern without laboratory investigation. Both appear to be correlated with the severity and duration of the diabetes.

METHODS OF MEASUREMENT

The resting diameter of the pupil is readily measured clinically with a ruler or the graticule in the eyepiece of an ophthalmic slit lamp. At best, however, measurement can yield a result only to the nearest 0.5 mm, and even this may be hard to achieve in darkly pigmented eyes because of the difficulty of seeing the pupil margin clearly. Furthermore, care is needed with illumination because light falling on the eye along the visual axis will elicit a light reflex, thus diminishing the diameter of the pupil that is recorded. Light directed at the eye from

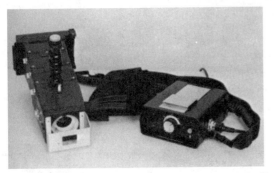

■ **Figure 12.1** Polaroid pupil camera. (From Smith SA, Dewhirst RR. A simple diagnostic test for pupillary abnormality in diabetic autonomic neuropathy. Diabet Med 1986; 3:38–41.)

the side or from below minimizes this source of error. Care is also needed to ensure that the subject is focusing on a distant object to avoid further pupil constriction from the near reflex. Inevitably, clinical measurements of this type are poorly repeatable.

The most reliable pupil measurements are obtained in darkness, either photographically or with a specialized infrared pupillometer. A simple fixed-focus Polaroid camera equipped with ring flash and an appropriate darkness hood provides highly repeatable measurements with a coefficient of variation of only 3% (Fig. 12.1).[25] Comparable measurements may be obtained with a fundal camera such as the Canon CR3–45NM using the built-in accessory + 12 diopter lens system.[24]

Extension of such static measurements to include dynamic recordings of the amplitude of the light reflex as well as its velocity of constriction and redilatation requires the use of a pupillometer such as the Applied Science Laboratories Model 1050 (Fig. 12.2) or the simpler Pupilscreen or Pupilscan instruments. In all cases, measurement of the pupil is obtained

under infrared illumination by a video or a diode system, and a visible light source is incorporated to permit initiation and recording of a light reflex. For the more complex Model 1050, this light source can be focused in the plane of the pupil, thus permitting closed-loop stimulation of the retina rather than open-loop stimulation, in which the amount of light entering the eye is limited by the size of the pupil. Such equipment is largely used for research and found in only a few specialized laboratories.

Measurement of pupillary function for testing autonomic integrity may be invalidated if the patient has severe rubeosis iridis or is receiving drug therapy affecting α-adrenergic or muscarinic receptor function (as with certain antipsychotic and antidepressive agents), or if the pupils have been dilated for fundal inspection in the preceding 48 hours.[28]

DARKNESS PUPIL DIAMETER

A small pupil is common in diabetic neuropathy.[3, 7, 9, 17, 20, 21, 29] This can be demonstrated most clearly when pupil size is measured in darkness. Pupils also become smaller in healthy subjects with advancing age, and it is therefore important to use an age-related normal range to identify miosis.[25, 26] A screening study of 359 unselected diabetic patients found that 21.7% had abnormally small pupils for age.[23]

Significant associations between small pupils and a wide range of diabetic complications have been recorded: cardiovascular autonomic dysfunction[26] (Fig. 12.3), peripheral sensory loss,[9, 29] retinopathy,[6] and nephropathy.[9] Patients are more likely to have small pupils if their hyperglycemia has been of marked severity and duration.[9, 29] Acute hyperglycemia, as in untreated diabetes, may cause miosis that reverses when normoglycemia is established.[1, 8]

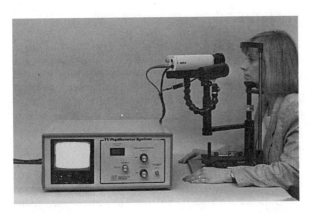

■ **Figure 12.2** Applied Science Laboratories Model 1050 Pupillometer. (Courtesy of Applied Science Laboratories, Bedford, MA.)

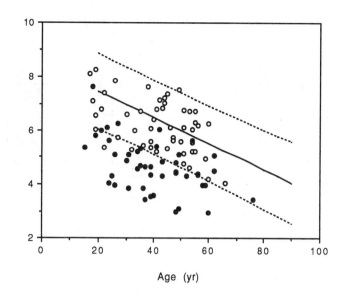

■ Figure 12.3 Darkness pupil diameters in diabetic patients with *(closed circles)* and without *(open circles)* cardiovascular autonomic neuropathy. *Interrupted lines* indicate the 95% confidence intervals of the normal range (original data).

The common occurrence of a small pupil with intact light reflexes, in contrast to the rarity of a large pupil with poor light reflexes, suggests that the sympathetic iris innervation is more susceptible to damage than the parasympathetic innervation. Histologic studies of irides removed from diabetic patients during cataract surgery have confirmed that loss of nerve terminals occurs preferentially from the dilator pupillae.[4, 12] The reason for the greater susceptibility of the sympathetic nerves is unknown but may be related to the greater length of the nerve pathway.

RESPONSE TO TOPICAL MYDRIATIC AGENTS

The mydriatic response to directly acting sympathomimetic agents is exaggerated in patients with diabetic autonomic neuropathy,[6, 26] suggesting that there is denervation supersensitivity, such as in Horner's syndrome.[14, 30] In one

study,[26] mydriatic responses were tested in 34 diabetic patients divided into four groups according to how well their pupils dilated in darkness. The groups were balanced for age, but those with small pupils had poorer glycemic control and poorer neurologic function in general (Table 12.1). Severe miosis was associated with supersensitivity to 2% phenylephrine, but normal responsiveness was associated with the indirect-acting sympathomimetic 0.5% hydroxyamphetamine (Fig. 12.4). These findings indicate that diabetic miosis is neuropathic in origin but that the postganglionic neuron remains functionally intact. It would be surprising if diabetes interrupted any specific part of the sympathetic pathway; more probably the deficit results from a composite of mildly reduced function throughout.

Instillation of tropicamide, the atropine-like anticholinergic agent, into diabetic eyes often produces less mydriasis than in healthy eyes, presumably because of the loss of effective pu-

TABLE 12.1 CLINICAL CHARACTERISTICS OF DIABETIC SUBJECTS DIVIDED INTO FOUR GROUPS ON THE BASIS OF THEIR DARKNESS PUPIL DIAMETER

Group	N	Age (y) Mean (Range)	Duration (y) Mean (Range)	HbA$_1$ (%) Mean (Range)	Mean Pupil Diameter (mm) Observed-Expected	Sinus Arrhythmia (% of normal), Mean ± SEM
1	9	35.4 (18–50)	10.6 (2–23)	10.2 (5.5–18.7)	0.18	94 ± 12
2	9	33.3 (19–50)	18.0 (6–40)	10.9 (7.8–14.6)	−1.10	100 ± 12
3	10	33.3 (19–48)	15.3 (4–26)	12.2 (9.2–18.4)	−1.80	67 ± 13*
4	6	34.2 (15–49)	23.0 (11–36)	13.5 (9.5–18.9)	−2.85	40 ± 9*

*Significantly different from normal ($=100\%$); $P < 0.05$.
From Smith SA, Smith SE: Evidence for a neuropathic aetiology in the small pupil of diabetes mellitus. Br J Ophthalmol 1983 67:89–93.

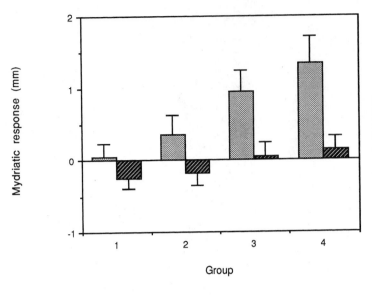

■ **Figure 12.4** Phenylephrine and hydroxyamphetamine responses in diabetic patients graded by darkness pupil diameter. The smallest pupils (group 4) have the greatest responses to the mydriatics. (Data from Smith SA, Smith SE. Reduced pupillary light reflexes in diabetic autonomic neuropathy. Diabetologia 1983; 24:330–332.)

pil dilator function discussed previously. Some observers have measured pupil size after treating the eye with a large dose of an anticholinergic to obtain evidence of dilator function and indirectly of the state of diabetic damage.[18, 20] From a practical standpoint, full mydriasis in the diabetic patient before fundoscopy requires the combined influence of tropicamide and phenylephrine.[11] Such a combination is usually as effective as in healthy eyes (Fig. 12.5), and it permits full visualization of, and access to, the peripheral retina.

LIGHT REFLEX AMPLITUDE

The amplitude of the pupillary constriction to light is reduced in diabetic autonomic neuropa-thy.[10, 27] This reduction is usually found only in pupils that are already small from sympathetic dysfunction. Thus, in severely affected patients, pupil size remains almost constant despite wide changes in illumination. Iris myopathy is not necessarily responsible because drugs are often effective in changing pupil size. Presumably, the iris in such patients is essentially denervated in both autonomic branches.

Testing for reduction of the parasympathetically mediated light constriction may be complicated by the presence of other ocular pathology that limits the effectiveness of the light stimulus. Retinopathy and optic nerve disease will give an afferent pupil defect, and these may well be present to some extent in patients

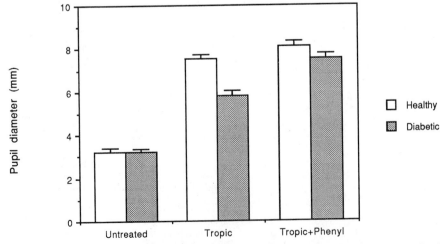

■ **Figure 12.5** Mydriatic responses to tropicamide *(Tropic)* with or without phenylephrine *(Phenyl)* in healthy subjects and diabetic patients. (Data from Huber MJE, Smith SA, Smith SE. Mydriatic drugs for diabetic patients. Br J Ophthalmol 1985; 69:425–427.)

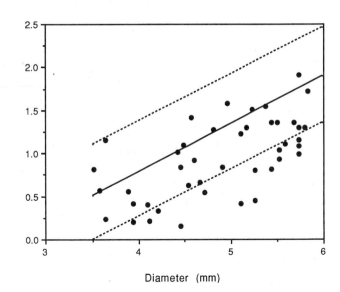

■ Figure 12.6 Reduced light reflexes in patients with diabetic autonomic neuropathy. *Interrupted lines* indicate the 95% confidence intervals of the normal range. (Data from Smith SA, Smith SE. Reduced pupillary light reflexes in diabetic autonomic neuropathy. Diabetologia 1983; 24: 330–332.)

being examined for neuropathy. This can be overcome by relating the intensity of the stimulating light to the visual perception threshold measured by a forced-choice method,[2, 27] enabling the efferent side of the reflex arc to be tested independently.

Establishing the presence of a true reduction in the reflex arc is complicated further by the limited movement range of pupils already made small by sympathetic dysfunction. The extent of this mechanical restriction has been investigated[27] by comparing responses in diabetic patients with those of elderly nondiabetic subjects with senile miosis. Reflex amplitudes were reduced in pupils made miotic by old age or diabetes, but the reduction was greater in diabetic pupils (Fig. 12.6), presumably because of added parasympathetic dysfunction. The enhanced response of the diabetic pupil to cholinomimetic agents such as pilocarpine,[6] indicating denervation supersensitivity, supports this hypothesis.

LIGHT REFLEX LATENCY, VELOCITY, AND REDILATATION TIME

More complex measures of pupil function, which can be recorded only with a dynamic pupillometer, are frequently abnormal in diabetic autonomic neuropathy. Measurement of latency has been used as an autonomic function test.[18–20] Reflexes are slow in onset and time course, giving prolonged latency times and reduced maximum velocities of constriction and redilatation.[29] These measures are, however, strongly related to reflex amplitude in neuropathic and nonneuropathic pupils, and they do not reliably distinguish one from the other. The sole exception is detectable in the shape of the redilatation curve, specifically in the delay that occurs in its second half (Fig. 12.7). This corresponds to the redilatation lag that occurs in Horner's syndrome.[30] It is most readily recorded by determining the three-quarter recovery time.

■ Figure 12.7 Pupillometer traces showing single reflex responses to flashes of bright light. Compared with the two nondiabetic subjects (*left* and *right*), the diabetic patient (*middle*) had a small darkness diameter, normal reflex amplitude, and delayed redilatation from the reflex.

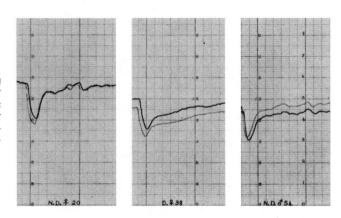

PUPIL CYCLE TIME

Pupil cycle time has been described for the detection of afferent pupil defects caused by conditions such as optic neuritis.[16] Regular oscillations of the pupil are induced by focusing a narrow beam of light on the pupil margin with a slit lamp. The period of these oscillations—the pupil cycle time—is prolonged in diabetic patients with autonomic neuropathy,[15] and the test has therefore been advocated as a diagnostic test for pupillary (efferent) dysfunction. However, the proportion of pupils that fail to oscillate, the low repeatability of the test, and the confounding influence of associated afferent sensory deficits limit the usefulness of this measure.

HIPPUS

In the light, the normal pupil diameter is never quite constant but oscillates continuously over a small range. This phenomenon, known as hippus, or pupillary unrest, is always symmetrical in the two eyes and is therefore likely to be central in origin.[13] Diabetics with neuropathy show reduced hippus,[5, 29] which suggests that central control of the pupillary autonomic innervation may be affected.

CONCLUSION

A number of pupillary autonomic function tests are available that compare favorably for repeatability with conventional cardiovascular tests. There is significant correlation with cardiovascular autonomic testing, although this is not strong and some patients are found to have abnormal pupils with normal cardiac vagal function and vice versa.[22] In diabetes, the patterns of autonomic nerve damage vary from patient to patient, so testing a variety of autonomic functions is recommended when documenting autonomic neuropathy in the individual case.

References

1. Boutros G, Insler MS. Reversible pupillary miosis during a hyperglycaemic episode: Case report. Diabetologia 1984; 27:50–51.
2. Fison PN, Garlick DJ, Smith SE. Assessment of unilateral afferent pupillary defects by pupillography. Br J Ophthalmol 1979; 63:195–199.
3. Friedman SA, Feinberg R, Podolak E, et al. Pupillary abnormalities in diabetic neuropathy: A preliminary study. Ann Intern Med 1967; 67:977–983.
4. Fujii T, Ishikawa S, Uga S. Ultrastructure of iris muscles in diabetes mellitus. Ophthalmologica 1977; 174:228–239.
5. Gundersen HJG. An abnormality of the central autonomic nervous system in long-term diabetes: Absence of hippus. Diabetologia 1974; 10:366.
6. Hayashi M, Ishikawa S. Pharmacology of pupillary responses in diabetics: Correlative study of the responses and grade of retinopathy. Jpn J Ophthalmol 1979; 23:65–72.
7. Hreidarsson AB. Pupil motility in long-term diabetes. Diabetologia 1979; 17:145–150.
8. Hreidarsson AB. Acute, reversible autonomic nervous system abnormalities in juvenile insulin-dependent diabetes: A pupillographic study. Diabetologia 1981; 20:475–481.
9. Hreidarsson AB. Pupil size in insulin-dependent diabetes: Relationship to duration, metabolic control, and long-term manifestations. Diabetes 1982; 31:442–448.
10. Hreidarsson AB, Gundersen HJG. The pupillary response to light in Type 1 (insulin dependent) diabetes. Diabetologia 1985; 28:815–821.
11. Huber MJE, Smith SA, Smith SE. Mydriatic drugs for diabetic patients. Br J Ophthalmol 1985; 69:425–427.
12. Ishikawa S, Bensaoula T, Uga S, et al. Electron microscopic study of iris nerves and muscles in diabetes. Ophthalmologica 1985; 191:172–183.
13. Lowenstein O, Loewenfeld IE. The pupil. In Davson H (ed): The Eye. New York, Academic Press, 1969, vol. 3, pp 255–337.
14. Maloney WF, Younge BR, Moyer NJ. Evaluation of the causes and accuracy of pharmacological localization in Horner's syndrome. Am J Ophthalmol 1980; 90:394–402.
15. Martyn CN, Ewing DJ. Pupil cycle time: A simple way of measuring an autonomic reflex. J Neurol Neurosurg Psychiatry 1986; 49:771–774.
16. Miller SD, Thompson HS. Pupil cycle time in optic neuritis. Am J Ophthalmol 1978; 85:635–642.
17. Namba K, Utsumi T, Kitazawa A. Diabetes mellitus and the pupil: A preliminary report. Nippon Ganka Gakkai Zasshi 1980; 84:398–405.
18. Pfeifer MA, Cook D, Brodsky J, et al. Quantitative evaluation of sympathetic and parasympathetic control of iris function. Diabetes Care 1982; 5:518–528.
19. Pfeifer MA, Weinberg CR, Cook D, et al. Differential changes of autonomic nervous system function with age in man. Am J Med 1983; 75:249–258.
20. Pfeifer MA, Weinberg CR, Cook DL, et al. Autonomic neural dysfunction in recently diagnosed diabetic subjects. Diabetes Care 1984; 7:447–453.
21. Rundles RW. Diabetic neuropathy: General review with report of 125 cases. Medicine 1945; 24:111–160.
22. Smith SA. Diagnostic value of the Valsalva ratio reduction in diabetic autonomic neuropathy: Use of an age-related normal range. Diabetic Med 1984; 1:295–297.
23. Smith SA. Horner's syndrome in diabetes mellitus. Diabetic Med 1987; 4:381.
24. Smith SA. Testing pupillary autonomic function with a retinal camera. Diabetic Med 1989; 6:175–176.
25. Smith SA, Dewhirst RR. A simple diagnostic test for pupillary abnormality in diabetic autonomic neuropathy. Diabetic Med 1986; 3:38–41.
26. Smith SA, Smith SE. Evidence for a neuropathic aetiology in the small pupil of diabetes mellitus. Br J Ophthalmol 1983; 67:89–93.
27. Smith SA, Smith SE. Reduced pupillary light reflexes in diabetic autonomic neuropathy. Diabetologia 1983; 24:330–332.
28. Smith SE: Mydriatic drugs for routine fundal inspection. Lancet 1971; 2:837–839.
29. Smith SE, Smith SA, Brown PM, et al. Pupillary signs in diabetic autonomic neuropathy. BMJ 1978; 2:924–927.
30. Thompson HS. Diagnosing Horner's syndrome. Trans Am Acad Ophthalmol Otolaryngol 1977; 83:840–842.

Chapter 13

Sudomotor Neuropathy

Phillip A. Low • Robert D. Fealey

INTRODUCTION

Quantitation of autonomic sudomotor function provides important information on peripheral autonomic failure in diabetic neuropathy. It complements the evaluation of measurements of motor and sensory deficits. This chapter will focus on some methods of evaluating distal sudomotor deficits and the use of sudomotor evaluation to assess the severity and distribution of diabetic autonomic neuropathy. We will also attempt to define the value of the thermoregulatory sweat pattern in diabetic neuropathy.

TESTS OF SUDOMOTOR FUNCTION

Thermoregulatory Sweat Test

In 1938, List and Peet reported that sweat induced by externally heating the body was a reliable and reproducible way of activating efferent sympathetic sudomotor pathways. The skin sweat distribution was demonstrated via Minor's starch and iodine technique.[16] A similar sweating test devised by Roth[27] and Brown and Adson[2] was used to depict the effects of surgical sympathectomy graphically. The thermal sweating technique, referred to as the thermoregulatory sweat test (TST), became a useful and widely used method to study sympathetic autonomic involvement in disease states, including diabetes mellitus.[1, 3, 13, 21 23 25 28] A summary of the results found when using the TST to study diabetes is shown in Table 13.1. The

TABLE 13.1 REPORTED THERMOREGULATORY
SWEAT TEST RESULTS IN DIABETIC NEUROPATHY

Author	No. Patients Studied	Percentage Abnormal
Rundles[28]	13	85
Odel et al.[25]	40	73
Barany and Cooper[1]	23	74
Martin[23]	20	100
Goodman[11]	35	83
Low et al.[21]	10	100
Fealey et al.[9]	51	94

most common abnormality found was loss of sweating, often asymmetrical, in a "stocking" distribution. Infrequently, the pattern mimicked bilateral lumbar sympathectomy,[25] and such patients had excessive sweating in the upper body. When areas of anhidrosis in the feet were further tested via direct heating, faradic stimulation, and intradermal acetylcholine, a postganglionic sympathetic lesion was suggested.[1] Although asymptomatic diabetics may have normal thermoregulatory sweating,[23] the literature is scarce on this point. Abnormalities of sweating tend to correlate with electromyographic and clinical evidence of neuropathy.[11, 14, 21, 23, 31]

In 1989, we reported TST results of 51 patients suspected of having diabetic neuropathy on the basis of clinical examination and detailed laboratory tests excluding other causes of neuropathy.[9] Each record was reviewed for details of the initial signs and symptoms, the findings on neurologic examination and electromyography (EMG), and other relevant test results.

The TSTs were done in the Mayo Thermoregulatory Laboratory using a technique modified from Guttmann's quinizarin sweat test.[8, 12] Subjects were heated in a cabinet (air temperature 44 to 50°C, humidity 40 to 50%, skin temperature 39 to 39°C), raising mean oral temperature 1.5°C in 35 to 45 minutes. Alizarin red powder was used to demonstrate sweat patterns over the whole anterior body surface. Characteristic peripheral neuropathy syndromes of diabetes such as length-dependent small fiber neuropathy or anterior truncal neuropathy were associated with equally characteristic TST abnormalities.

Figure 13.1 shows individual cases exhibiting the representative sweat distributions encountered. Pathologic loss of sweating occurred distally in 65% (case 43), segmentally in 25% (case 3), and only in isolated dermatomes

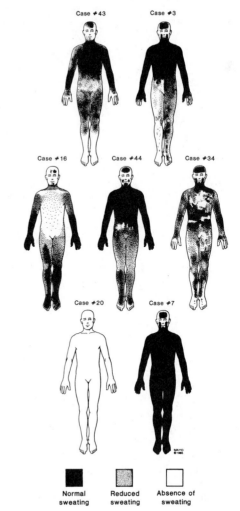

■ **Figure 13.1** Thermoregulatory sweat distributions in patients with diabetes mellitus: representative cases of the 51 subjects studied are shown.

or peripheral nerve distributions (focal or multifocal anhidrosis) in 25% (case 44); it was most common (78%) to observe a combination of two or more patterns (such as distal and focal/multifocal) in the same patient (case 34). Eight patients having global (>80% body surface anhidrosis) sweat loss (case 20) had clinically severe autonomic neuropathy; and in the entire group, the percentage of body surface anhidrosis correlated highly with the degree of clinical dysautonomia (Fig. 13.2).[9]

Three patients with normal sweating had minimal abnormalities on neurologic examinations or EMG.

Fourteen patients had focal truncal neuropathic pain or paresthesias, with 12 of the 14 having corresponding focal anhidrotic patches (Fig. 13.3). One patient had focal loss of sweat-

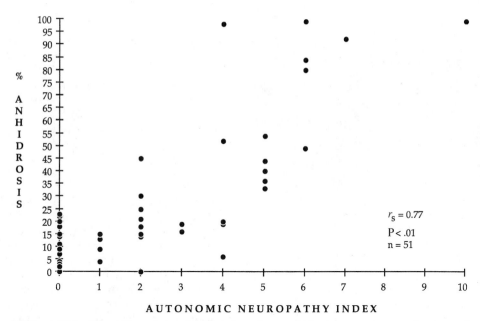

$r_s = 0.77$

$P < .01$

$n = 51$

AUTONOMIC NEUROPATHY INDEX

■ **Figure 13.2** Correlation of degree of body surface anhidrosis versus degree of autonomic neuropathy. 0 = none, 10 = severe. (From Fealey RD, Low PA, Thomas JE. Thermoregulatory sweating abnormalities in diabetes mellitus. Mayo Clin Proc 1989; 64:617.)

ing on the contralateral side, and one with coexisting autonomic neuropathy had diffuse truncal anhidrosis. Focal truncal anhidrosis is highly correlated with EMG findings of paraspinal fibrillation potentials. Patients with a previous contralateral episode of truncal neuropathy who had symptomatically recovered usually still showed an obvious zone of anhidrosis in the appropriate dermatome.

Twelve of 13 patients having distal anhidrosis of the lower extremities on the TST had abnormal quantitative sudomotor axon reflex test (QSART) responses indicative of a postganglionic axonopathy. Additional observations during the past 5 years confirm the comparable sensitivity of the TST and QSART in the diagnosis of distal diabetic and idiopathic small fiber neuropathies.[30]

Patients with normal QSART (usually in the forearm) and absent thermoregulatory sweating continue to be seen, although this is uncommon. This combination suggests a preganglionic site for the autonomic lesion, which has been described in autopsy studies.[17, 21, 26]

We have observed patients who on serial studies show a rare reversal of deficits affecting the entire forehead on one side. Anatomically, the lesion is likely to be in the superior cervical ganglion; such an observation raises the intriguing possibility that such reversible lesions represent examples of neuropathology caused by immune-mediated mechanisms (such as au-

toantibodies to cervical ganglia), reported to be very prevalent in patients with type 1 diabetes mellitus.[5]

The ability of a properly done TST to demonstrate the distribution of the often multifocal neuropathy of diabetes, the anatomically diagnostic deficits of certain clinical syndromes (such as truncal neuropathy), the quantitative correlation of percentage anhidrosis and clinical autonomic involvement, and the ability to follow patients serially (via digital photography) suggest a continuing role of the TST in the diagnosis, management, and investigation of diabetic neuropathy.

Quantitative Sudomotor Axon Reflex Test

In the QSART, one population of eccrine sweat glands is stimulated by acetylcholine (ACh) and iontophoresed through intact skin; the evoked sweat output is recorded from a second population of sweat glands.[18, 20] The multicompartmental sweat cell (attached to skin using elastic straps, attached to posts [Fig. 13.4G]) consists of a central recording compartment 1 cm in diameter (Fig. 13.4A) surrounded by an air gap 1.5 mm wide (Fig. 13.4B), separating the recording compartment from a circular stimulus moat 4 mm wide (Fig. 13.4C) that is filled with 10% ACh via a cannula (Fig. 13.4E). Any residual air is forced out through a second

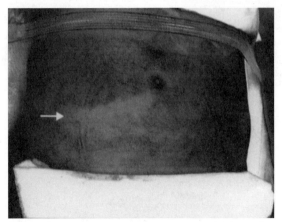

■ **Figure 13.3** Digital camera image of a diabetic patient with right abdominal wall burning pain. Normal sweating skin turns the indicator powder brownish purple, but the denervated skin fails to sweat, remaining orange in color. The curvilinear deficit *(arrow)* can be seen approximating the anterior T11 dermatome, providing evidence of a neuropathic etiology.

ropathy. The response may be (A) normal, (B) absent, (C) reduced, or (D) persistent (Fig. 13.5). Short latencies are sometimes seen with pattern D. This pattern of persistent sweat activity describes a sweat response that fails to turn off when the stimulus ceases; it is often seen in painful diabetic and other neuropathies and in some cases of florid reflex sympathetic dystrophy. A pattern of excessive QSART response is sometimes seen in the upper extremities of patients with diabetic neuropathy (Fig. 13.5).

We performed QSART recordings on 73 consecutive patients with diabetic neuropathy (based on neurologic history, examination, and nerve conduction studies) and related these findings to heart period responses (Valsalva maneuver and deep breathing) and to blood pressure recordings in the supine and standing positions.[22] QSART recordings were made in the forearm distally and the foot proximally.

An abnormal response was defined as a response that fell below the first centile when matched with controls by age and sex. Abnormal heart period responses to deep breathing or Valsalva maneuver alone each occurred in 67% of patients. Abnormal responses to both tests (a more reliable indicator of vagal abnormality than a single test) occurred in 55% of patients. A reduced or absent QSART response on the foot occurred in 58% of patients (Fig. 13.6), but sudomotor response was reduced in the forearm in only 9% of patients.

Heart period and QSART response were concordant in 64% of patients. In a typical recording, the heart period responses were impaired and the foot response was absent, whereas the forearm response was present and excessive (Fig. 13.7). In 14% of patients, postganglionic sudomotor failure occurred when

cannula. Nitrogen is passed through a gas inlet and outlet (Fig. 13.4*D*). Acetylcholine is iontophoresed using a constant current generator. Anodal current is passed via the anodal electrode (Fig. 13.4*F*) connected to the stimulus well. The cathode is a 4 × 6 cm rectangular lead strip wrapped in flannel and soaked in isotonic saline. Sweat droplets in compartment A are evaporated off by a nitrogen stream of constant flow and humidity, and the sweat output is quantitated by a sudorometer.

Under controlled conditions, the QSART provides a reproducible, sensitive, and accurate measurement of postganglionic sudomotor function, with a coefficient of variation less than 20%.[18, 20] There are now several recognized abnormal QSART patterns in peripheral neu-

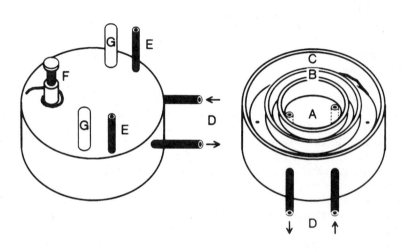

■ **Figure 13.4** The multicompartmental sweat cell for quantitative sudomotor axon reflex measurements. *A,* Central recording compartment; *B,* air gap; *C,* circular stimulus moat; *D,* gas inlet and outlet; *E,* cannula; *F* and *G,* see text for a more detailed description.

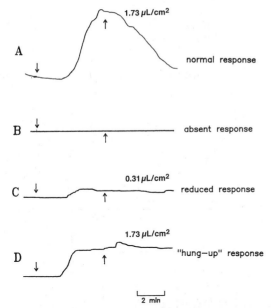

■ Figure 13.5 Quantitative sudomotor axon reflex test (QSART) sweat patterns showing (A) normal, (B) absent, (C) reduced, and (D) persistent sweat activity. Arrows indicate onset and cessation of stimulus.

heart period responses were still normal. Representative recordings are shown in Figure 13.8. In a similar percentage of patients, abnormal vagal function occurred when postganglionic sudomotor function using QSART was normal.

Twenty-six percent of the patients had orthostatic hypotension. In this subset of patients (Fig. 13.9), the frequency of heart period and QSART abnormalities was very high (89% and

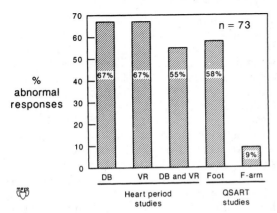

■ Figure 13.6 The frequency of patients having abnormalities detected with quantitative sudomotor axon reflex test (QSART) and heart period measurements. DB, deep breathing; VR, Valsalva response; F-arm, forearm.

83%, respectively), confirming the impression that orthostatic hypotension represents a late manifestation of widespread sympathetic failure, occurring at a time when other more sensitive indices of sympathetic and parasympathetic failure have long become abnormal. We concluded that distal sympathetic failure does not lag behind vagal failure when sensitive and quantitative recording methods are used. We used conservative criteria for distal sympathetic failure, requiring a reduced or absent sweat volume at the proximal foot level to qualify. A higher incidence of abnormalities would have been found had we accepted hypohidrosis at a more distal site or had we included abnormalities such as the "hung-up" sweat response.

Sweat Imprint Method

Drops of sweat will produce an imprint on soft impression material. Kennedy and colleagues used the Silastic impression method[14] to count and size sweat droplets on the dorsum of the foot just proximal to the medial two digits. Sweating was stimulated by iontophoresis by 1% pilocarpine (2 mA for 5 minutes); the sweat output was quantitated from the same population of sweat glands that was stimulated. They measured 81 patients with type 1 diabetes who were 20 to 72 years of age (mean, 35.3 years). Seventy of these patients had chronic renal failure or had had a kidney transplant.[14]

The results of sweat quantitation correlated well with pain perception. Patients with impairment of pinprick sensation had a reduced density of sweat droplets of reduced diameters, and the quantitative abnormalities paralleled the severity of impairment of pain perception. There was a low concordance between sweat function and conduction velocity. In tests using this method, sudomotor abnormalities occurred only in patients with severe somatic neuropathy (muscle compound action potential less than 0.5 mV) and appeared to develop later than vagal abnormalities.[14]

Skin Potential Recordings

Abnormalities in skin potential responses were found by Goadby and Downman in about a third of patients with diabetic neuropathy.[10] They noted marked variability in the responses. Shahani and associates[29] studied skin potentials in 33 patients with neuropathy, of whom 5 had diabetic neuropathy. Skin potentials were absent in all 5. They reported that

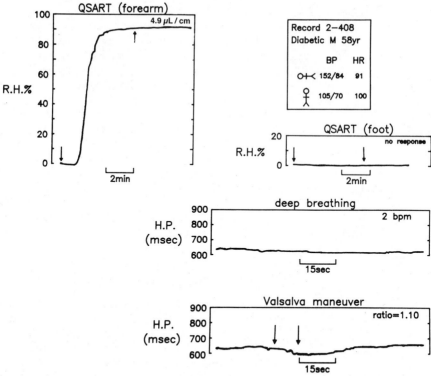

■ **Figure 13.7** Representative recordings showing absent quantitative sudomotor axon reflex test (QSART) recording on the foot and abnormal heart period (H.P.) recordings. The forearm response is excessive. R.H., relative humidity; BP, blood pressure; HR, heart rate; bpm, beats per minute.

patients with absent skin potentials tended to have an axonal or mixed type process on EMG and in single teased fiber studies; morphometry of sural nerve showed loss of myelinated and unmyelinated axons. Fagius and Jameson[7] studied the effects of an aldose reductase inhibitor on galvanic skin response of diabetic patients. They also noted marked variability of responses. Fagius[6] performed microneurographic recordings of sympathetic activity in the peroneal and median nerves of patients with diabetic neuropathy. In 64% of patients, sympathetic activity was not recordable, correlating well with impaired skin potential recordings.

The major advantage of the method is its simplicity, so that it can be used in any EMG laboratory. The disadvantages are its large variability and the tendency of the responses to habituate, although claims for a low coefficient of variation have appeared.[15] There is general agreement that a loss of skin potential is abnormal. Controversy exists as to whether a reduction of skin potential or a reduction in latency are reliable abnormalities. There is some evidence that unmyelinated fibers conduct with-

out slowing or not at all.[32] The test has been reported to correlate well with QSART,[24] but in our experience, it is often present when QSART is clearly impaired. Potentials are reported to become reduced with aging.[4]

Comparison of Methods to Measure Sudomotor Activity

Of the methods available (Table 13.2), the Kennedy Silastic method is a good and quantitative one that differs from QSART recordings in several essential respects. The two methods are complementary, the Silastic method[14] providing a sweat output histogram, whereas the QSART recording provides a dynamic quantitation of sweat output. The principles of the two methods are quite different. The Silastic method depends on the function of a directly stimulated sweat gland (the denervated gland losing its sudomotor response), whereas QSART depends on the integrity of the axon reflex rather than sweat gland function. Perhaps because of the longer pathway tested in QSART (sympathetic C → branch point → sympathetic C), this test detects sudomotor failure before the Silastic method does. The

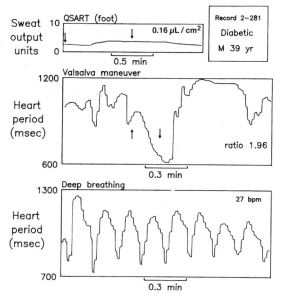

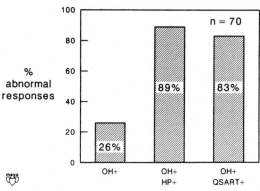

■ **Figure 13.9** Left bar shows the frequency of patients with orthostatic hypotension (OH+). Center and right bars indicate the percentage of heart period (HP) (OH+, HP+) and quantitative sudomotor axon reflex test (QSART) abnormalities (OH+, QSART+) in those patients who have orthostatic hypotension.

■ **Figure 13.8** Representative recordings showing markedly reduced quantitative sudomotor axon reflex test (QSART) foot recording and completely normal heart period recordings. bpm, beats per minute.

second major advantage is the real-time sudorometry using QSART. This property has enabled us to detect persistent sweat activity; it also permits a study of other sweating reflexes, such as somatosympathetic reflexes.

The TST is a straightforward simple test that provides important information on the distribution of sweat activity. Because of the sampling problems inherent in quantitative tests such as the Silastic and QSART recordings, which record from minute areas of skin, the TST provides important complementary information. Diabetic neuropathy appears to be

characterized by multifocal nerve involvement. The patient with, for instance, diabetic thoracic radiculopathy may have a diagnostic TST pattern but may lack distal anhidrosis (and have a normal Silastic or QSART recording). The TST and QSART in combination can be used to define the site of the lesion causing anhidrosis (preganglionic as opposed to postganglionic).

The skin potential recording is dynamic but subject to great variability because it readily habituates[17] and is a function of many factors.[17] Although it has a limited role in the EMG laboratory, it is unsuitable for clinical trials.

Composite Autonomic Scoring Scale

Because sudomotor function is affected by the confounding effects of age and sex, we sought

TABLE 13.2 COMPARISON OF QSART, SILASTIC IMPRINT, AND SKIN POTENTIAL METHODS

Parameter	QSART	Silastic Imprint	Skin Potential
Principle	Axon-reflex pathway integrity	Sweat gland response to direct stimulation	Integrity of somatosympathetic pathways
Stimulus	Acetylcholine	Pilocarpine	Various
Afferent	Sympathetic C	Nil	Groups II and III
Efferent	Sympathetic C	Nil	Sympathetic B and C
Effector	Sweat gland	Sweat gland	Sweat gland secretion and epithelium
Response			
Latency	Long (1–2 m)	Brief (seconds)	Brief (seconds)
Turn on	Rapid	Rapid	Rapid
Turn off	Relatively fast (1–2 m)	Extremely slow (> 2 h)	Fast (seconds)
Neuropathy detection	+ + +	+ +	+ +
Advantages	Sensitive, reproducible	Sensitive, reproducible	Simple
Disadvantages	Special equipment	Complex	Variable (habituation)

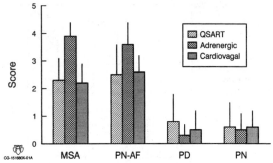

■ **Figure 13.10** Individual scores ± SD, normalized for age and sex differences, for quantitative sudomotor axon reflex test (QSART), adrenergic function, and cardiovagal function in patients with multisystem atrophy (MSA), peripheral neuropathy and autonomic failure (PN-AF), Parkinson's disease (PD), and peripheral neuropathy but no autonomic symptoms (PN). (From Low PA: Composite autonomic scoring scale for laboratory quantification of generalized autonomic failure. Mayo Clin Proc 1993; 68:748.)

to provide a composite autonomic scoring scale (CASS) that corrects for these confounding factors.[19] The CASS scores autonomic deficits in sudomotor, cardiovagal, and adrenergic function from 0 (no deficit) to 10 (maximal deficit). The sudomotor subset of CASS (CASS$_{sudo}$) is scored from 0 to 3 based on four recording sites (distal forearm, proximal leg, distal leg, proximal foot) and is graded using the normal range for age and sex for each site. Normative data are based on 357 normal subjects aged 10 to 83 years, evenly distributed by age and sex. The CASS$_{sudo}$ scores of 1, 2, and 3 represent mild, moderate, and severe postganglionic sudomotor failure, respectively.

To validate CASS, we studied autonomic function in four groups of patients. These were multiple system atrophy, N = 18; autonomic neuropathies (idiopathic, Sjögren's syndrome, diabetic, amyloid, paraneoplastic, cisplatin), N = 20; Parkinson's disease, N = 20; peripheral neuropathy (without autonomic complaints), N = 20. The CASS$_{sudo}$ scores were multiple system atrophy, 2.4 ± 0.8; autonomic neuropathy, 2.5 ± 1.1; Parkinson's disease, 0.8 ± 1.0; and peripheral neuropathy, 0.6 ± 0.9 (Fig. 13.10).

References

1. Barany FR, Cooper EH. Pilomotor and sudomotor innervation in diabetes. Clin Sci 1956; 15:533.
2. Brown GE, Adson AW. Physiologic effects of thoracic and of lumbar sympathetic ganglionectomy or section of the trunk. Arch Neurol Psychiatry 1929; 22:322.
3. Clarke BF, Ewing DJ, Campbell IW. Diabetic autonomic neuropathy (review). Diabetologia 1979; 17:195.
4. Drory VE, Korczyn AD. Sympathetic skin response: Age effect. Neurology 1993; 43:1818.
5. Ejskjaer N, Arif S, Dodds W, et al. Prevalence of autoantibodies against nervous tissue structures in a population of insulin-dependent diabetic patients (abstract). Clin Auton Res 1997; 7:104.
6. Fagius J. Microneurographic findings in diabetic polyneuropathy with special reference to sympathetic nerve activity. Diabetologia 1982; 23:415.
7. Fagius J, Jameson S. Effects of aldose reductase inhibitor treatment in diabetic polyneuropathy: A clinical and neurophysiological study. J Neurol Neurosurg Psychiatry 1981; 44:991.
8. Fealey RD. Thermoregulatory sweat test. In Daube JR (ed): Clinical Neurophysiology. Philadelphia, FA Davis, 1996, p 396.
9. Fealey RD, Low PA, Thomas JE. Thermoregulatory sweating abnormalities in diabetes mellitus. Mayo Clin Proc 1989; 64:617.
10. Goadby HK, Downman CB. Peripheral vascular and sweat-gland reflexes in diabetic neuropathy. Clin Sci Mol Med 1973; 45:281.
11. Goodman JI. Diabetic anhidrosis. Am J Med 1966; 41:831.
12. Guttmann L. Management of quinizarin sweat test (QST). Postgrad Med J 1947; 23:353.
13. Hosking DJ, Bennett T, Hampton JR. Diabetic autonomic neuropathy (review). Diabetes 1978; 27:1043.
14. Kennedy WR, Sakuta M, Sutherland D, et al. Quantitation of the sweating deficit in diabetes mellitus. Ann Neurol 1984; 15:482.
15. Levy DM, Reid G, Rowley DA, et al. Quantitative measures of sympathetic skin response in diabetes: Relation to sudomotor and neurological function. J Neurol Neurosurg Psychiatry 1992; 55:902.
16. List CF, Peet MM. Sweat secretion in man. I: Sweating responses in normal persons. Arch Neurol Psychiatry 1938; 39:1228.
17. Low PA. Quantitation of autonomic responses. In Dyck PJ, Thomas PK, Lambert EH, et al (eds): Peripheral Neuropathy. Philadelphia, WB Saunders, 1984, p 1139.
18. Low PA. Sudomotor function and dysfunction. In Asbury AK, McKhann GM, McDonald WI (eds): Diseases of the Nervous System. Philadelphia, WB Saunders, 1986, p 596.
19. Low PA. Composite autonomic scoring scale for laboratory quantification of generalized autonomic failure. Mayo Clin Proc 1993; 68:748.
20. Low PA, Caskey PE, Tuck RR, et al. Quantitative sudomotor axon reflex test in normal and neuropathic subjects. Ann Neurol 1983; 14:573.
21. Low PA, Walsh JC, Huang CY, et al. The sympathetic nervous system in diabetic neuropathy: A clinical and pathological study. Brain 1975; 98:341.
22. Low PA, Zimmerman BR, Dyck PJ. Comparison of distal sympathetic with vagal function in diabetic neuropathy. Muscle Nerve 1986; 9:592.
23. Martin MM. Involvement of autonomic nerve-fibres in diabetic neuropathy. Lancet 1953; 1:560.
24. Maselli RA, Jaspan JB, Soliven BC, et al. Comparison of sympathetic skin response with quantitative sudomotor axon reflex test in diabetic neuropathy. Muscle Nerve 1989; 12:420.
25. Odel HM, Roth GM, Keating FR Jr. Autonomic neuropathy simulating the effects of sympathectomy as a complication of diabetes mellitus. Diabetes 1955; 4:92.
26. Olsson Y, Sourander P. Changes in the sympathetic nervous system in diabetes mellitus: A preliminary report. J Neurovisc Relat 1968; 31:86.
27. Roth G. Clinical test for sweating. Mayo Clin Proc 10:383, 1935.

28. Rundles RW. Diabetic neuropathy: General review with report of 125 cases. Medicine 1945; 24:111.

29. Shahani BT, Halperin JJ, Boulu P, et al. Sympathetic skin response: A method of assessing unmyelinated axon dysfunction in peripheral neuropathies. J Neurol Neurosurg Psychiatry 1984; 47:536.

30. Stewart JD, Low PA, Fealey RD. Distal small fiber neuropathy: Results of tests of sweating and autonomic cardiovascular reflexes. Muscle Nerve 1992; 15:661.

31. Thomas PK, Eliasson SG. Diabetic neuropathy. *In* Dyck PJ, Thomas PK, Lambert EH, et al (eds): Peripheral Neuropathy. Philadelphia, WB Saunders, 1984, p 1773.

32. Tzeng SS, Wu ZA, Chu FL. The latencies of sympathetic skin responses. Eur Neurol 1993; 33:65.

Chapter **14**

Assessment of Diabetic Sexual Dysfunction and Cystopathy

Claire C. Yang • William E. Bradley

INTRODUCTION

Sexual dysfunction and cystopathy frequently occur in patients with diabetes mellitus.[15, 17] The principal evidence of sexual dysfunction in the male is erectile failure. This can be evaluated by a series of laboratory tests, which attests to the multifactorial origin of the complaint. Cystopathy requires a cystometric study for its detection. Regular follow-up is necessary to avoid further deterioration of the bladder and or renal function. Treatment is discussed in Chapter 40.

Both disabilities are caused by dysfunction of the autonomic and somatic nervous systems secondary to the disease. Although rarely life threatening, sexual dysfunction and cystopathy can have a tremendous impact on the diabetic patient's well-being.

Sexual dysfunction in the male can be evaluated using innovative laboratory methods.[6, 29, 35, 49] These methods have clearly defined the organic causes of impotence and have frequently indicated its multifactorial origin (Table 14.1). No similar methods are currently available for evaluation of female sexual dysfunction, so the prevalence and diagnosis of this problem has been difficult to appraise.[9]

Diabetic cystopathy is a result of impairment

TABLE 14.1 LABORATORY EVALUATION OF DIABETIC GENITOURINARY COMPLICATIONS

  I. Erectile function
     A. Assessment of erectile capacity: continuous nocturnal penile tumescence and rigidity monitoring
     B. Neurologic factors
        1. Nerve conduction velocity of dorsal nerve of the penis
        2. Bulbocavernosus reflex
        3. Urethroanal reflex
        4. Pudendal cortical evoked response
     C. Vascular factors
        1. Arterial
           a. Duplex sonography and color Doppler analysis
           b. Arteriography
           c. Penile/brachial blood pressure index
        2. Venous
           a. Infusion cavernosography and cavernosometry
     D. Psychologic factors
        1. Continuous nocturnal penile monitoring
        2. Minnesota Multiphasic Personality Inventory
     E. Hormonal factors
        1. Serum testosterone
        2. Serum follicle-stimulating hormone, luteinizing hormone, prolactin
 II. Bladder function
     A. Uroflow and postvoiding residual volume measurement
     B. Cystometry/videourodynamics
     C. Electrodiagnostic testing
        1. Urethro-anal reflex
        2. Pudendal studies

of the sensory component of detrusor muscle innervation. Symptoms of bladder dysfunction typically are less prominent than those of male sexual dysfunction. The patient is unaware of difficulty until late in the development of the disease. Bladder evaluation techniques are applicable to male and female patients.

ASSESSMENT OF MALE SEXUAL DYSFUNCTION

Anatomy and Physiology

The penis consists of three spongy erectile bodies: the two corpora cavernosa and the corpus spongiosum with the urethra in its center (Fig. 14.1). The two cavernous bodies are composed of a fibrous-tissue covering called the tunica albuginea, and this surrounds the spongy tissue, which is composed primarily of vascular sinusoidal tissue. Blood is supplied to the penis from the penile branches of the internal pudendal artery. Each of the paired penile arteries divides into three vessels to the penis: (1) the

deep artery of the penis, which runs through the entire corpus cavernosum; (2) the dorsal artery of the penis, which supplies the penile skin and the glans penis; and (3) the bulbourethral artery, which supplies the corpus spongiosum and urethra. The venous return is more variable. The vascular sinusoids are drained through numerous subtunical veins that then drain into a series of larger veins along the outer aspect of the tunica albuginea, called the emissary and circumflex veins. An intricate system of drainage connects these vessels to the pelvic venous plexus.

The nerve supply to the penis is derived primarily from the S2 to S4 spinal cord segments. The somatosensory innervation is primarily provided through the dorsal nerve of the penis, a terminal branch of the pudenal nerve. The perineal nerve also supplies sensation from the ventral aspect of the penis and the scrotum. The autonomic innervation of the penis is provided through the cavernous nerve, which arises from the pelvic plexus.

With afferent stimulation to the central nervous system through the dorsal nerve of the penis or through the cranial nerves, efferent impulses are delivered through the pelvic plexus to the cavernous nerve in each corpus cavernosum. Subsequent neurotransmitter release, including nitric oxide, vasoactive intestinal polypeptide (VIP), and acetylcholine, produces relaxation of the sinusoidal smooth muscle and decreases the peripheral resistance of the penis. There is a resultant increase in blood flow through the deep penile arteries. The subsequent vascular engorgement of the sinusoids creates an increase in intracorporal pressure as the tunica albuginea resists distention. This pressure compresses the subtunical

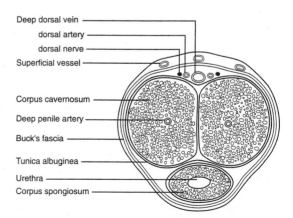

■ **Figure 14.1** Cross-sectional anatomical diagram of penis.

and emissary veins, prohibiting venous drainage from the corporal bodies, which acts to maintain the erection. Through this mechanism, penile tumescence and rigidity occur.

Ejaculation is the expulsion of seminal fluid from the urethra by contraction of the bulbocavernosus muscle and other muscles of the perineum. The motor innervation of the bulbocavernosus muscle is a branch of the pudendal nerve. Emission, which precedes ejaculation, is the deposition of seminal fluid into the posterior urethra by contraction of the smooth muscles of the male adnexa. This phenomenon is mediated through the sympathetic hypogastric nerves. With ejaculation, the bladder neck closes (also mediated by the hypogastric nerves) and allows antegrade propulsion of seminal fluid.

Diabetes is probably the single most frequent cause of impotence in the United States. The primary etiology of impotence in diabetic men is thought to be neuropathy of the somatic and autonomic innervation of the penis, with penile vasculopathy the secondary cause. Psychological and hormonal factors may also have a role in diabetic impotence. The prevalence of erectile dysfunction in the diabetic population ranges from 35 to 59%.[17, 32, 38] There does not seem to be a relationship between the occurrence of impotence and the duration of diabetes,[43] and impotence may be a presenting sign of the disease.[17] Similarly, the type of diabetic treatment does not correlate with the occurrence of impotence,[11, 32, 36] but poor glucose control is associated with a higher incidence.[2]

History and Physical Examination

Patients presenting with sexual dysfunction will complain of loss of erectile rigidity, inability to sustain an erection, and decreased genital sensation. Other complaints may include impairment of libido and diminished force or loss of ejaculatory function.[16] The symptoms typically are of insidious onset and may have occurred during a period of several years.[32] There may be concurrent symptoms of bladder dysfunction, peripheral neuropathy, neuropathic ulcers, and enteropathy. Impotence in the diabetic male has been associated with the subsequent development of other diabetic complications.[37]

Other significant points to elicit in the medical history include concurrent medical problems that are known to cause or exacerbate impotence, such as atherosclerotic vascular disease,[48] previous genital or pelvic surgery,[20] and

neurologic disease.[3] Many medications, particularly antihypertensive and psychotropic preparations are also known to contribute to erectile dysfunction.[13] Alcohol abuse may contribute to impotence.

The physical examination of the impotent patient includes examination of the phallus for structural deformities, descent and size of both testes, and genital and perineal sensation. The presence of a bulbocavernosus reflex demonstrates the integrity of the sacral reflex arc, but absence of the reflex is not necessarily pathologic. Neurologic abnormalities of the lower extremities may be suggestive of pathology in sacral nerve distributions. Stigmata of other diabetic sequelae should be noted.

Laboratory Evaluation

ASSESSMENT OF ERECTILE FUNCTION

Continuous Penile Monitoring. Overall erectile capacity can be assessed with the use of continuous nocturnal penile tumescence and rigidity monitoring during sleep.[29] Normal sleep is characterized by four or five episodes of penile rigidity and associated circumferential expansion (tumescence). Organic impotence will manifest as diminished nocturnal erectile activity. A normal nocturnal penile tumescence and rigidity monitoring study in a man complaining of erectile dysfunction is highly suggestive of psychogenic impotence,[29] and this information may prevent unnecessary endocrine, neural, and vascular evaluations.

Continuous recording of penile circumferential expansion and rigidity is performed by a portable monitor (Rigiscan Plus, Osbon Corp., Augusta, GA). The monitor consists of two major components: a penile tumescence and rigidity data recording unit and a microprocessor. The data recording unit has two loops, one of which is placed around the base and the other at the tip of the penis at the coronal sulcus. With the expansion of the penis, and consequently of the loop, the microprocessor detects circumferential changes as compared with the subject's baseline measurement, and tumescence is expressed in centimeters. The monitor also performs penile rigidity measurements by applying a predetermined force to each loop every 3 minutes. Rigidity is expressed as a function of displacement when the loop tightens around the penis. A rigidity of 100% represents no linear displacement, and for each 0.5 mm of loop shortening the rigidity measure is reduced by 2.3%. The number and

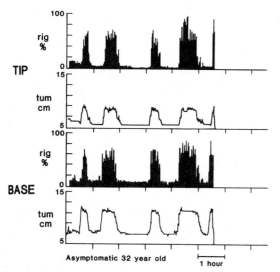

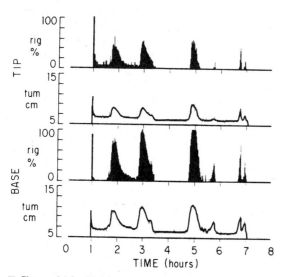

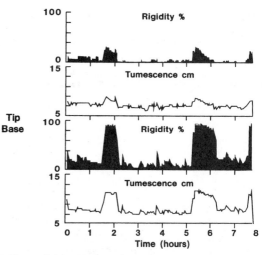

■ **Figure 14.2** Continuous penile tumescence and rigidity monitoring, with recording loops at the base of the penis and coronal sulcus. Each episode of tumescence (circumferential expansion) is accompanied by rigidity. Tumescence is measured in centimeters, and rigidity is expressed as a percentage, with 100% rigidity that of a solid cylinder. Subject is a 32-year-old man with normal sexual function.

■ **Figure 14.4** Rigi-Scan results showing dissociation of base and tip rigidity with lower maximum amplitude of tip rigidity, indicative of distal penile softening.

duration of erectile episodes are also recorded (Fig. 14.2). Penile monitoring is then performed during two or three successive nights, after which the results are evaluated. Monitoring can also be performed for real-time analysis of tumescence in the awake state. Penile erection is obtained by visualization of erotic stimuli,

■ **Figure 14.3** Rigi-Scan results of a 50-year-old man showing decreased frequency and duration of erectile episodes as well as a decrease in maximum amplitude of penile rigidity.

mechanical stimulation, or pharmacologic erection. Continuous monitoring has now replaced previous techniques for assessment of penile erections, including the stamp test and the snap-gauge band.[14]

Abnormalities of erectile function are represented by decreases in the frequency and duration of episodes of tumescence and rigidity (Fig. 14.3). In addition, there are two specific abnormalities known as dissociation and uncoupling. Dissociation is characterized by softening of the distal penile shaft concurrent with normal penile base rigidity (Fig. 14.4). This may become exaggerated to produce uncoupling, which is attainment of penile tumescence without development of any substantial rigidity. Diabetic erectile dysfunction can manifest with any of these abnormalities. Nocturnal penile tumescence studies are abnormal even in diabetic men reporting normal erectile function, perhaps a harbinger of future sexual dysfunction.[39]

After the initial evaluation of erectile function by continuous nocturnal tumescence and rigidity monitoring, the etiology of impotence in the diabetic patient can be defined through further laboratory testing. The basis for erectile dysfunction in diabetic males can be traced to one or a combination of factors, such as neurologic, vascular, psychologic, or hormonal etiologies.

Neurologic Evaluation. Sexual activity relies on the somatic and the autonomic nervous systems for normal function, and neuropathy

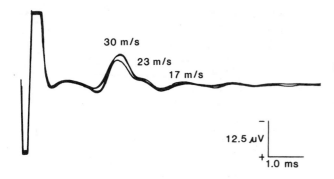

■ **Figure 14.5** Nerve conduction velocity measurement of dorsal nerve of penis in a normal patient. The three peaks with differing conduction velocities in meters per second indicate three different axonal populations.

of both systems is considered to be the predominant cause of sexual dysfunction in diabetic men.[2, 15] In the evaluation of patients with impotence, a neuropathic cause can be defined by electrophysiologic testing of reflex sexual pathways. As of this writing, electrophysiologic testing of the afferent and autonomic innervation of the corpora cavernosa is technically not possible. Histologic studies of the cavernous nerve in diabetic men,[18, 42] measurement of autonomic detrusor dysfunction,[17] and corpora cavernosa smooth muscle electromyography[46] have been used to indirectly diagnose penile autonomic neuropathy.

More amenable to laboratory evaluation is the somatic innervation of the penile shaft, consisting of the pudendal sensory axons in the peripheral as well as central nervous system pathways. These pathways and their conduction velocity can be precisely measured by electrophysiologic testing.[2, 6, 11, 23, 30, 33] The importance of the pudendal nerve in male erectile function is evident from animal and human studies,[4, 24, 25] and the neuropathic effects of diabetes on this nerve can result in impotence.

The effect of diabetic neuropathy is to slow the peripheral conduction velocity, as measured in electrophysiologic testing. This manifests in the genitourinary system as penile neuropathy. Neuropathic changes can also occur in central nervous system pathways and produce central nervous system impotence. The normal conduction velocity of the dorsal nerve of the penis (DNP), a branch of the pudendal nerve, has been measured[6] (Fig. 14.5). Stimulation and recording are performed along the length of the dorsal aspect of the penis. Penile dissections have demonstrated undulations in the DNP while the penis is flaccid.[50] These undulations are unfurled with erection or penile stretch. Thus, a more accurate measurement of the nerve conduction velocity is obtained with the penis on stretch or with a pharmacologic erection, and either maneuver should be used

when performing this test. The velocity of the potential is reduced in diabetic impotent patients, and this is the most sensitive test of penile neuropathy[30] (Fig. 14.6). This slowing correlates well with the clinical presence of peripheral neuropathy and reduction in the conduction velocity of the sural nerve, and the degree of slowing is augmented with penile stretch.[33]

The latency of the bulbocavernosus reflex has been used to define disease of the cauda equina and conus medullaris in patients with diabetes mellitus.[30] This reflex is elicited by stimulation of the dorsal nerve of the penis and recording the electromyographic response in the bulbocavernosus muscle or anal sphincter (Fig. 14.7). The normal reflex latency is 28 to 42 ms. With neuropathic change in the afferent axons occurring in diabetes, there can be slowing of conduction and increase in the reflex latency, although the sensitivity of this test has been questioned.[12, 41] A variation of this reflex, with stimulation of the vesicourethral junction (visceral afferents) rather than the dorsal nerve of the penis, has been reported to be a more sensitive indicator of diabetic neurogenic impotence.[43] Description of this technique is reported in the section on diabetic cystopathy.

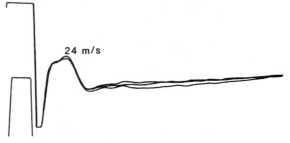

■ **Figure 14.6** Abnormal nerve conduction velocity measurement of dorsal nerve of penis. This study was performed in a patient with diabetic penile neuropathy. The nerve conduction velocity of 24 m/s is considerably below the normal mean.

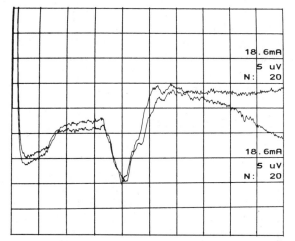

■ **Figure 14.7** Bulbocavernosus reflex latency measurement. The response is elicited by stimulation of the dorsal nerve of the penis and measured in the bulbocavernosus muscle. Normal latency is 28 to 42 ms, and this can be prolonged in diabetics with erectile dysfunction. Time base = 10 ms/div.

The latency of the cortical pudendal evoked response (Fig. 14.8) has been used to define spinal cord, brain stem, and cerebral causes of impotence. The evoked response of the dorsal nerve of the penis is measured at the cortex at the Cz' position (international 10–20 system). The latency of the normal pudendal cortical evoked response in the male ranges from 37 to 45 ms.[23] Diabetic neuropathic change in the peripheral nerves may result in prolonged latency and altered morphology of these responses.

Bemelmans and colleagues found 23 of 27 impotent diabetic patients (85%) had electrodiagnostic proof of urogenital or peripheral neuropathy, as compared with 40% of potent diabetic patients and 44% of impotent nondiabetic patients.[2] Daniels reported 23 of 24 impotent diabetic men had an abnormal bulbocavernosus reflex latency, as compared with 12 of 21 potent diabetics.[11] The prevalence of genital sensory neuropathy in impotent diabetics underscores the importance of somatosensory input for activation of the sexual reflex.

Vascular Evaluation—Arterial. Atherosclerotic disease is common in diabetic patients, and penile arterial flow can be compromised by peripheral vascular disease, with resultant erectile dysfunction. The penile arteries can be assessed noninvasively by duplex sonography and color Doppler analysis, evaluating the pulsation, diameter, and blood flow velocity of these vessels.[35] Injection of pharmacologic vasodilating agents simulates the blood flow changes that occur with spontaneous erection and is helpful in assessing the functional capability of the penile arteries.

If there is significant abnormality, arteriography can be performed by selective catheterization of the internal iliac or pudendal arteries. Generally, arteriography is reserved for patients considered for arterial revascularization of the penis. The indications for this are few, especially in the diabetic population. Another technique to evaluate the penile arteries is measurement of penile/brachial blood pressure index. An index below 0.75 is suggestive of inadequate penile arterial flow.

Vascular Evaluation—Venous. Infusion cavernosography and cavernosometry are techniques used to document abnormal arteriovenous communications and consequent venous leakage.[49] Cavernosography is performed by injection of a radiopaque contrast agent into one of the corpora, followed by a roentgenographic study (Fig. 14.9). Cavernosometry involves infusion of saline or contrast to maintain an artificial erection with simultaneous intracorporal pressure monitoring. This is performed through special cannulae placed into the corpora cavernosa. An erection may be obtained with concurrent injection of vasodilating agents. Little to no venous drainage is observed in normal persons during erection. With detumescence, there is rapid drainage of contrast and decrease of intracorporeal pressure. Impotence can be a result of venous insufficiency, which is manifested as leakage of blood from the corpora during tumescence, and a failure to generate intracorporeal pressures ad-

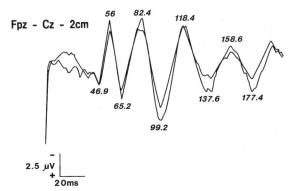

■ **Figure 14.8** Cortical evoked response elicited by stimulation of the dorsal nerve of the penis. The numbers listed at the wave peaks are the response latencies, measured from the moment of stimulation.

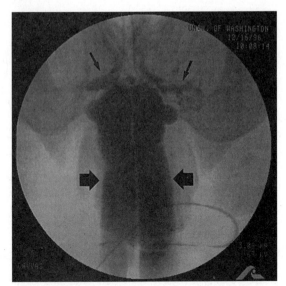

■ **Figure 14.9** Radiograph taken during cavernosography. The two corpora cavernosa seen beneath the symphysis pubis are designated by *large arrows*, and the infusion cannula is inserted into the left corpus. Abnormal venous leakage is noted by *small arrows*. Little to no venous outflow from the corpora is seen in normal persons.

equate to attain penile rigidity. This leakage is believed to be caused by incompetence of the subtunical and emmisary veins.[34] Abnormalities of these tests may also be due to patient anxiety, which can hinder an erectile response.

Psychological Evaluation. Psychological evaluation is important whether or not organicity is indicated by laboratory investigation. Use of the Minnesota Multiphasic Personality Inventory test,[27, 40] followed by an interview with a psychologist trained in treating patients who have sexual complaints, is especially helpful. Detailed reviews of the relevant psychological evaluation may be obtained from other sources.[8, 47]

Hormonal Evaluation. Prospective investigations have not determined hormonal derangements (glucose metabolism notwithstanding) to be a significant cause of impotence in diabetic men,[2, 17, 32] and our experience corroborates this. In the man with normal libido and testicular volume, a serum testosterone level is obtained as a screening measure.[28] If it is low or if clinical signs of hypogonadism are present, serum prolactin, follicle-stimulating hormone (FSH), and luteinizing hormone (LH) levels should also be determined, and a more detailed assessment is obtained as needed.

The cause of impotence in patients with diabetes mellitus is often multifactorial; the aim of laboratory testing is to define which of these causes is contributing to impairment of erectile function. Subsequently, appropriate treatment can be instituted.

EJACULATORY FUNCTION

The prevalence of ejaculatory dysfunction in diabetics is unknown. A man may have retrograde, weak, or no ejaculation at all. The most common dysfunction is retrograde ejaculation, which may occur with diabetic autonomic neuropathy.[16] Autonomic neuropathy results in a failure of the bladder neck to contract with the pelvic floor musculature, allowing semen into the bladder. Weak ejaculation or anejaculation is thought to be the sequela of peripheral neuropathy.[30] This can be assessed by pudendal electrodiagnostic testing as previously described under Neurologic Evaluation.

ASSESSMENT OF BLADDER FUNCTION AND DETECTION OF DIABETIC CYSTOPATHY

Diabetic cystopathy is an insidious and apparently progressive disease in which there is impairment of bladder sensation. It is a frequent occurrence in type 1 diabetes mellitus, and, at its end stages, it is associated with detrusor areflexia and increased residual urine volume after voiding.

Anatomy and Neurophysiology

The bladder is composed of a lattice of smooth muscle fibers that converge at the vesical outlet, or bladder neck. Visceral afferent and autonomic (parasympathetic) innervation of the detrusor is mediated through the pelvic nerve, which arises primarily from the S3–S4 spinal cord segments, although there is variability between individuals. The trigone, or bladder base, and bladder neck have an embryonic derivation separate from the detrusor, and receive their innervation from the sympathetic outflow through the hypogastric nerve. This nerve originates from T11–L2 spinal levels. The external urethral sphincter is a striated skeletal muscle under voluntary control, innervated by a branch of the pudendal nerve (S2–S4).

The normal micturition cycle involves two phases: (1) bladder filling and urine storage and (2) bladder emptying. Bladder filling requires accommodation of increasing volumes at low intravesical pressure and appropriate sensation. At normal bladder capacity (350 to 450 mL), sensations of fullness are transmitted through detrusor afferents, nerves that provide reflex excitation through the central nervous system to the motor innervation to the detrusor.[5] Cerebral inhibitory functions suppress detrusor reflex activity until it is socially acceptable to urinate. Voiding requires a detrusor contraction of adequate magnitude and duration to completely empty the bladder, with an appropriate relaxation of the sphincters. Findings from neuropathologic studies suggest that diabetic cystopathy may be initially confined to bladder afferents. It is thought that the neuropathic process affects the autonomic innervation at a late stage and rarely involves the urethral striated-muscle sphincter.

The precise incidence of urinary bladder dysfunction in patients with diabetes mellitus is unknown, with reported figures of 48 to 71%.[19, 22, 26] There is a very strong correlation between diabetic peripheral somatic neuropathy and cystopathy.[7, 22] There are no pathognomonic symptoms associated with the neuropathic change in the sensory nerves that the patient can identify, and diabetics with voiding dysfunction may not have classic diabetic cystopathy.[31] Older men may often have complaints of urinary frequency, decreased force of stream, sense of incomplete emptying, and nocturia, symptoms that are usually attributed to voiding dysfunction as a result of prostatic enlargement. Clinically, the patient gradually increases his bladder volume and voids less frequently, because of an impaired sensation to void. Women and men with advanced disease may report on detailed questioning that they void as infrequently as twice a day. Some patients with complete detrusor failure may report incontinence as a result of an overdistended bladder. The percentage of patients with end-stage diabetic cystopathy in a cohort of diabetics with voiding dysfunction is reported to be less than 10%.[31, 45]

History and Physical Examination

In addition to the patient's voiding habits, concurrent medical problems, previous pelvic or spinal surgery, and history of urinary tract infections are important to note during history taking. The physical examination includes palpation and percussion of the lower abdomen to assess for a distended bladder. In men, the physical examination is similar to that as described in the section on male sexual function. In women, genital and perineal sensation is assessed, and a bimanual examination is performed to evaluate pelvic floor muscle strength and support, genital tissue integrity, a bulbocavernosus reflex, and anal sphincter tone. Abnormalities in the genital examination may reveal concurrent problems, such as bladder prolapse and poorly estrogenized vaginal mucosa, that may be contributing to a woman's

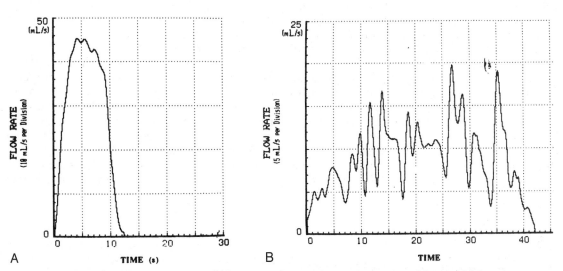

■ **Figure 14.10** Urine flow rate measurements. *A,* Normal flow curve, 34-year-old female. Peak flow rate is 48 mL/s, and voided volume is 375 mL. *B,* Urine flow of 35-year-old man with detrusor areflexia and diabetic cystopathy. The multiple peaks in the curve reflect abdominal straining, which manifests as increased urine flow. Peak flow rate is 19 mL/s, and voided volume is 423 mL.

urinary tract complaints. Other signs of diabetic sequelae, especially peripheral neuropathy, should be noted in all patients. Urinalysis and urine culture are performed as indicated.

Laboratory Evaluation

Urine Flow and Postvoiding Residual Volume Measurement. Screening measures for cystopathy can be performed in the office by obtaining a urine flow measurement and postvoiding residual volume. The latter can be obtained using a new, noninvasive ultrasound device, specifically designed for bladder volume measurements.[10] A residual volume can also be obtained through straight catheterization. A large postvoiding residual volume is a common finding with diabetic cystopathy. Urine flow rates are measured by having the patient void into a uroflometer. The uroflometer is a load-cell mounted in the well of a commode whose output is an instantaneous differential of the weight of the flow column and is therefore a measurement of urinary flow rate. The urine flow of a patient with diabetic cystopathy and an areflexic bladder has a classic "straining" appearance (Fig. 14.10).

Cystometry. If the patient demonstrates an abnormal urine flow and increased postvoiding residual urine volume, further evaluation is warranted with cystometry. Cystometry consists of filling the bladder with known volumes of fluid or gas (carbon dioxide) via a urethral catheter and measuring resulting bladder pressure changes. Sensation of bladder filling is also recorded. The most important observation of cystometry is the presence or absence of a detrusor reflex contraction evoked by this procedure, and whether it can be suppressed.[1] In the normal person, the initial sensation of bladder distention occurs within the first 200 mL of filling, and a detrusor contraction can be suppressed on command (Fig. 14.11). Early diabetic cystopathy is evident as an increase in threshold of occurrence of a detrusor reflex contraction with retained ability to voluntarily

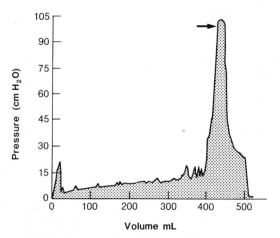

■ **Figure 14.11** Plot of normal cystometrogram. At a filling volume of 400 mL, a detrusor reflex contraction appeared and was evident as a rise in intravesical pressure, to a peak of 105 cm/H_2O pressure. At the *arrow*, the subject was asked to suppress the contraction, which resulted in a sharp decline in intravesical pressure. The subject's ability to voluntarily suppress a detrusor reflex contraction was evidence of normal urinary control.

suppress it. With voiding, the contraction may be of low magnitude and poorly sustained, thus leaving residual urine after voiding. As the disease progresses, there is greater impairment of bladder sensation with subsequent detrusor areflexia. This is caused by a combination of chronic overdistention and autonomic neuropathy, resulting in increased bladder capacity and large postvoiding residual urine volume (Fig. 14.12). When asked to void, the patient is often noted using a Valsalva's maneuver to void, generating pressure extravesically to empty the bladder contents.

Detrusor hyperrelexia, the inability to suppress a detrusor contraction, has also been found in diabetic patients.[1, 31, 45] This occurrence implies that the cortical or spinal regulatory tracts innervating the detrusor muscle have been interrupted. Detrusor hyperreflexia can occur concurrently with diminished bladder sensation and contractions of low magnitude.

Cystometry is often performed in the context

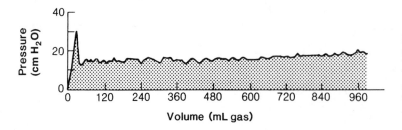

■ **Figure 14.12** Cystometrogram showing detrusor areflexia in patient with diabetic cystopathy. The bladder capacity was greatly enlarged, and no detrusor contraction was present.

of the videourodynamic study. Rather than using gas as the medium, radiopaque contrast is infused into the bladder. Fluoroscopy is used to visualize the bladder during filling for structural abnormalities, and then during voiding, to ascertain bladder outlet patency. In addition, the use of fluid allows for measurement of flow velocity and residual volume. Concurrent electromyography of the external urethral sphincter can be performed with needle or surface electrodes and can be used to detect abnormal sphincter activity such as detrusor-sphincter dyssynergia and uninhibited sphincter relaxation.[5]

Electrodiagnostic Testing. In theory, diabetic cystopathy can be detected through electrophysiologic studies of detrusor innervation, although such tests in humans are not available at this time. However, studies of adjacent nerves, such as through stimulation of the vesicourethral junction, can be used to provide analogous information on detrusor innervation.[1, 43, 44] Sensation from the vesicourethral junction is mediated through the visceral afferent fibers of the pelvic plexus, the same plexus through which detrusor sensation is carried. A urethral catheter adapted with circumferentially mounted electrodes is used for stimulation. Cortical evoked potentials are measured over the sensory cortex at Cz', and normal latencies range from 44 to 82 ms. In diabetics, these responses are more likely to be absent rather than delayed.[44] The evoked response latency measured in the pelvic skeletal musculature, recorded in the bulbocavernosus muscle in males and the anal sphincter in females, has a transit time of 50 to 70 ms in healthy subjects (Fig. 14.13).[5] The response can be measured with needle electrodes in the muscle, surface

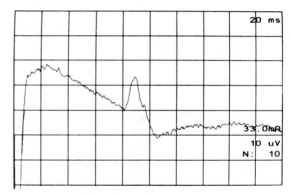

■ **Figure 14.14** Urethroanal reflex measured in 37-year-old woman with autonomic neuropathy. Latency is prolonged at 81 ms.

electrodes, or electrodes mounted on an anal plug. This reflex latency can be increased in diabetics with neuropathy of the visceral afferents (Fig. 14.14). Electrodiagnostic testing of the pudendal nerves and its branches may also be helpful in the estimation of detrusor innervation.

Diabetic cystopathy is a frequent accompaniment of type I diabetes, caused by neuropathic change in the detrusor afferent innervation. The clinical results are gradual bladder enlargement and detrusor hyporeflexia or areflexia. Increased residual urine volume and impairment in voiding occur. As a result, there may be a greater predisposition to urinary tract infection and renal deterioration. Yearly assessment with urine flow and postvoiding residual measurement should be performed on all patients with type 1 diabetes and symptomatic neuropathy, and cystometry or videourodynamic studies should be performed as a baseline and when deemed appropriate by the health care provider.

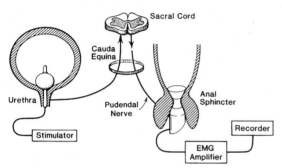

■ **Figure 14.13** Schematic diagram of urethroanal reflex measurement. Catheter-mounted electrodes stimulate the vesicourethral junction, and the evoked response in the anal sphincter is measured by an anal plug.

References

1. Andersen JT, Bradley WE. Early detection of diabetic visceral neuropathy: An electrophysiologic study of bladder and urethral intervention. Diabetes 1976; 25:1100.
2. Bemelmans BLH, Meuleman EJH, Doesburg WH, et al. Erectile dysfunction in diabetic men: The neurological factor revisited. J Urol 1994; 151:884.
3. Benet AE, Melman A. The epidemiology of erectile dysfunction. Urol Clin North Am 1995; 22:699.
4. Bors E, Comarr AE. Effect of pudendal nerve operations on the neurogenic bladder. J Urol 1954; 72:666.
5. Bradley WE. Diagnosis of urinary bladder dysfunction in diabetes mellitus. Ann Intern Med 1980; 92:323.
6. Bradley WE, Lin JT, Johnson B. Measurement of the conduction velocity of the dorsal nerve of the penis. J Urol 1984; 131:6.

7. Buck AC, Reed PI, Siddiq YK, et al. Bladder dysfunction and neuropathy in diabetes. Diabetologia 1976; 12:251.

8. Buetler LE, Scott FB, Karacan I. Psychological screening of impotent men. J Urol 1976; 116:193.

9. Campbell LV, Redelman MJ, Borkman M, et al. Factors in sexual dysfunction in diabetic female volunteer subjects. Med J Australia 1989; 151:550.

10. Cardenas DD, Egan K, Krieger JN, et al. Residual urine measurements in patients with spinal cord injury: Measurement with a portable ultrasound instrument. Arch Phys Med Rehabil 1988; 69:514.

11. Daniels JS. Abnormal nerve conduction in impotent patients with diabetes mellitus. Diabetes Care 1989; 12:449.

12. Desai KM, Dembny K, Morgan H, et al. Neurophysiological investigation of diabetic impotence: Are sacral response studies of value? Br J Urol 1988; 61:68.

13. Drugs that cause sexual dysfunction: An update. Med Lett 1992; 34:73.

14. Ek A, Bradley WE, Krane RJ. Snap gauge band: New concept in measuring penile rigidity. Urology 1983; 21:63.

15. Ellenberg M. Diabetic neurogenic vesical dysfunction. Arch Intern Med 1966; 117:348.

16. Ellenberg M. Retrograde ejaculation in diabetic neuropathy. Ann Intern Med 1966; 65:1237.

17. Ellenberg M. Impotence in diabetes: The neurologic factor. Ann Intern Med 1971: 75:213.

18. Faerman I, Glocer L, Fox D, et al. Impotence and diabetes: Histological studies of the autonomic nervous fibers of the corpora cavernosa in impotent diabetic males. Diabetes 1974; 23:971.

19. Fagerberg S-E, Kock NG, Petersen I, et al. Urinary bladder disturbances in diabetics. I: A comparative study of male diabetics and controls aged between 20 and 50 years. Scand J Urol Nephrol 1967; 1:19.

20. Finkle AL, Taylor SP. Sexual potency after radical prostatectomy. J Urol 1981; 125:350.

21. Frimodt-Møller C. Diabetic cystopathy. I: A clinical study on the frequency of bladder dysfunction in diabetics. Dan Med Bull 1976; 23:267.

22. Frimodt-Møller, C. Diabetic cystopathy. A review of the urodynamic and clinical features of neurogenic bladder dysfunction in diabetes mellitus. Dan Med Bull 1978; 25:49.

23. Haldeman S, Bradley WE, Bhatia NN, et al. Pudendal somatosensory evoked response. Arch Neurol 1982; 39:280.

24. Hart BL. Sexual reflexes in the male rat after anesthetization of the glans penis. Behav Biol 1972; 7:127.

25. Herbert J. The role of the dorsal nerves of the penis in the sexual behaviour of the male rhesus monkey. Physiol Behav 1973; 10:293.

26. Ioanid CP, Noica N, Pop T. Incidence and diagnostic aspects of the bladder disorders in diabetics. Eur Urol 1981; 7:211.

27. Jefferson TW, Glaros A, Spevack M, et al. An evaluation of the Minnesota Multiphasic Personality Inventory as a discriminator of primary organic and primary psychogenic impotence in diabetic males. Arch Sex Behav 1989; 18:117.

28. Johnson AR, Jarow JP. Is routine endocrine testing of impotent men necessary? J Urol 1992; 147:1542.

29. Kaneko S, Bradley WE. Evaluation of erectile dysfunction with continuous monitoring of penile rigidity. J Urol 1986; 136:1026.

30. Kaneko S, Bradley WE. Penile electrodiagnosis: Value of bulbocavernosus reflex latency versus nerve conduction velocity of dorsal nerve of the penis in diagnosis of diabetic impotence. J Urol 1987; 137:933.

31. Kaplan SA, Te AE, Blaivas JG. Urodynamic findings in patients with diabetic cystopathy. J Urol 1995; 153:342.

32. Kolodny RC, Kahn CB, Goldstein HH, et al. Sexual dysfunction in diabetic men. Diabetes 1974; 23:306.

33. Lin JT, Bradley WE. Penile neuropathy in insulin-dependent diabetes mellitus. J Urol 1985; 133:213.

34. Lue TF, Tanagho EA. Physiology of erection and pharmacologic management of impotence. J Urol 1987; 137:829.

35. Lue TF, Mueller SC, Jow YR, et el. Functional evaluation of penile arteries with duplex ultrasound in vasodilator-induced erection. Urol Clin North Am 1989; 16:799.

36. Maatman TJ, Montague DK, Martin LM. Erectile dysfunction in men with diabetes mellitus. Urology 1987; 29:589.

37. McCulloch DK, Young RJ, Prescott RS, et al. The natural history of impotence in diabetic men. Diabetologia 1984; 26:437.

38. McCulloch DK, Campbell IW, Wu FC, et al. The prevalence of diabetic impotence. Diabetologia 1980; 18:279.

39. Nofzinger EA, Reynolds CF, Jennings JR, et al. Results of nocturnal penile tumescence studies are abnormal in sexually functional diabetic men. Arch Intern Med 1992; 152:114.

40. Osborne D: Psychologic evaluation of impotent men. Mayo Clin Proc 1976; 51:363.

41. Parys BT, Evans CM, Parsons KF. Bulbocavernosus reflex latency in the investigation of diabetic impotence. Br J Urol 1988; 61:59.

42. Saenz de Tejada I, Goldstein I. Diabetic penile neuropathy. Urol Clin North Am 1988; 15:17.

43. Sarica Y, Karacan I: Bulbocavernosus reflex somatic and visceral nerve stimulation in normal subjects and in diabetics with erectile impotence. J Urol 1987; 138:55.

44. Sarica Y, Karatas M, Bozdemir H, et. al. Cerebral responses evoked by stimulation of the vesico-urethral junction in diabetics. Electroenceph Clin Neurophysiol 1996; 100:55.

45. Starer P, Libow L. Cystometric evaluation of bladder dysfunction in elderly diabetic patients. Arch Intern Med 1990; 150:810.

46. Stief CG, Djamilian M, Anton P, et al. Single potential analysis of cavernous electrical activity in impotent patients: A possible diagnostic method for autonomic cavernous dysfunction and cavernous smooth muscle degeneration. J Urol 1991; 146:771.

47. Teifer L, Schuetz-Mueller D. Psychological issues in diagnosis and treatment of erectile disorders. Urol Clin North Am 1995; 22:767.

48. Virag R, Bouilly P, Frydman D. Is impotence an arterial disorder? A study of arterial risk factors in 400 impotent men. Lancet 1984; 1:181.

49. Wespes E, Delcour C, Struyven J, et al. Pharmacocavernosometry-cavernosography in impotence. Br J Urol 1986; 58:429.

50. Yang CC, Bradley WE, Berger RE. Unpublished data.

Chapter **15**

Assessment of Gastrointestinal Function

Allison Malcolm • Michael Camilleri

INTRODUCTION

Diabetes mellitus can affect nearly every site in the gastrointestinal (GI) tract. It may result in symptoms such as dysphagia, heartburn, nausea and vomiting, abdominal pain, constipation, and diarrhea and fecal incontinence.

EPIDEMIOLOGY

Although GI symptoms are not generally regarded to be major causes of morbidity in diabetic patients, 76% of diabetic patients evaluated at a tertiary referral center had GI symptoms.[17] These estimates may have been biased as a result of tertiary referral; in another study, the prevalence of GI symptoms was no greater in diabetic patients than in controls from the same community in Finland.[27] In the study by Janatuinen and associates, however, the diabetic patients consumed more laxatives than the controls.[27] In a preliminary study by Maleki and colleagues in the United States, constipation was more common in the diabetic population than in community controls.[33] Because functional GI symptoms[12, 38] and abnormal psychiatric profiles[8] are prevalent in the general population, the true impact of diabetes on GI symptoms is difficult to assess.

The reported prevalence of GI symptoms in diabetes varies among studies (Table 15.1). In

TABLE 15.1 PREVALENCE OF GASTROINTESTINAL SYMPTOMS IN DIABETIC PATIENTS IN DIFFERENT STUDIES

Symptom	Frequency (%)	Reference
Dysphagia	2–27	17, 36
Nausea and vomiting	7–29	17, 36
Abdominal pain	18–34	14, 17
Diarrhea	0–22	17, 36
Constipation	2–60	17, 36
Fecal incontinence	1–20	17, 36

gastroparesis, this depends on the type of patients studied, the criteria for diagnosis of gastroparesis, and the methods used to evaluate gastric emptying. Gastroparesis, which is defined by gastric emptying abnormalities demonstrated scintigraphically, occurred in about 50% of type 1 and 2 diabetic patients seen at a university medical center in Australia.[25, 26] In other studies, nausea and vomiting occurred in 7 to 29% of patients with diabetes.[17, 36] The finding that gastroparesis was equally prevalent in type 1 and 2 diabetic patients is contrary to the popular belief that motor disorders are more common in patients with type 1 diabetes. This may reflect the increasing length of survival in patients with type 2 diabetes and the propensity to develop neurologic and other complications with increasing duration of disease.

PATHOPHYSIOLOGY

The GI tract is under intrinsic and extrinsic neural control. Extrinsic control involves parasympathetic input (excitatory to nonsphincteric muscle) and sympathetic input (excitatory to GI sphincters and inhibitory to nonsphincteric muscles). Just as diabetes can cause peripheral somatic neuropathy, it can also produce gut neuropathy, which in turn leads to GI symptoms such as vomiting, diarrhea, and fecal incontinence.

The pathogenesis of GI tract complications in diabetes is poorly understood. Although autonomic neuropathy is likely to be a major factor, other factors contribute as well (Table 15.2).

Motor Dysfunction. In tertiary referral centers, motor dysfunction is often seen in patients with type 1 and type 2 diabetes mellitus of prolonged duration, typically more than 5 years. Most patients have associated peripheral somatic neuropathy and evidence of auto-

nomic neuropathy, such as abnormal pupillary responses, anhidrosis, gustatory sweating, orthostatic hypotension, impotence, retrograde ejaculation, and urinary dysfunction.[5, 29, 31] Vagal nerve dysfunction (autovagotomy) and sympathetic nerve damage probably contribute to the motor dysfunction; the relative contributions of damage to the two extrinsic neural systems is unknown. Vagal dysfunction is probably critical in the causation of gastric stasis,[29] but it is unclear whether the rapid small bowel transit that is commonly seen in these patients is the result of vagotomy or loss of the sympathetic "brake." Several of the intestinal motor abnormalities observed in symptomatic diabetic patients are indistinguishable from those seen in patients with other syndromes associated with postganglionic sympathetic lesions.[5] Parasympathetic denervation is also thought to be important in the development of constipation.[4] Sympathetic dysfunction likely contributes to nocturnal stool incontinence caused by reduced resting anal tone.[49]

Sensory Dysfunction. Sensory dysfunction may contribute to induction or reduction of GI symptoms in diabetes. Samsom and associates showed increased sensory perception during gastric distention in diabetic patients.[47] On the other hand, diabetic patients with severe nausea and vomiting exhibit normal perceptual and electroencephalographic responses to esophageal electrical stimulation, whereas patients with mild symptoms exhibit impaired perception.[45] These findings suggest that a visceral sensory neuropathy may initially increase and later reduce the severity of gut symptoms in patients with diabetes; this is comparable to the effects of peripheral sensory neuropathy leading to paresthesias initially and numbness later.

TABLE 15.2 MECHANISMS OF GASTROINTESTINAL COMPLICATIONS IN DIABETES

Motor dysfunction
Sensory dysfunction
Abnormal mucosal fluid absorption
Deranged pancreatic function
Altered glucose control (acute and chronic)
Alterations in gastrointestinal peptides and
  neurotransmitters
Ischemia
Electrolyte disturbances
Uremia
Diabetic ketoacidosis

Impaired Mucosal Fluid Absorption. Because adrenergic nerves normally stimulate intestinal reabsorption of fluids and electrolytes, decreased adrenergic function may contribute to diabetic diarrhea. Chang and colleagues demonstrated that the enterocyte in diabetic rat models has impaired α_2-adrenergic tone.[7] They also described the therapeutic potential of an α_2-adrenergic agonist, clonidine, in the treatment of diabetic diarrhea in humans. Clonidine may correct abnormal fluid transport and motor dysfunction.

Pancreatic Exocrine Insufficiency. Decreased pancreatic enzyme and bicarbonate secretion in response to stimuli such as secretin or cholecystokinin has been well documented in diabetes.[15, 22] Progression to steatorrhea or overt pancreatic insufficiency is rare, however, because of the large functional reserve of the exocrine pancreas.[11] Possible mechanisms for the impaired exocrine function in diabetes include microangiopathy and insulin deficiency; insulin is normally trophic to acinar cells, and insulin deficiency may result in pancreatic atrophy. Abnormal secretion of hormones such as glucagon, somatostatin, and pancreatic polypeptide may affect pancreatic exocrine function. Other putative mechanisms are listed in Table 15.3.

Altered Glucose Control. It is becoming increasingly evident that altered glucose control influences GI function. In type 1 diabetes, acute hyperglycemia reduces solid gastric emptying.[21] In type 2 diabetes, the relationship between the glucose level at the time of the gastric emptying test and the impairment of gastric emptying of liquids suggests that acute hyperglycemia delays gastric emptying.[26] However, in type 2 diabetes with elevated levels of blood glucose but no evidence of autonomic neuropathy, gastric emptying of solids is normal.[19] In healthy volunteers, acute hyperglycemia slows gastric emptying, reduces gastric

phase III migrating motor complexes, and causes abnormal myoelectric activity of the stomach.[21, 28, 42] Fraser and coworkers demonstrated that acute hyperglycemia induces premature intestinal phase III migrating motor complexes but reduces intestinal fed activity and retards intestinal transit.[20] In the colon, acute hyperglycemia blunts the reflex colonic response to gastric distention with a balloon.[54] Whether the effects of acute and chronic hyperglycemia are similar is unclear. Chronic poor glycemic control is likely to be important in the development of gut autonomic neuropathy because tight metabolic control influences long-term complications of diabetes mellitus, such as neuropathy.[9]

Gastrointestinal Peptides and Neurotransmitters. Altered hormonal control is likely to influence GI function and symptoms. Vasoactive intestinal peptide, an inhibitory transmitter, is present in increased concentrations in myenteric plexus and smooth muscle in experimental animal models of diabetes. The significance of this finding is unclear; it may reflect an adaptive response to sympathetic denervation or be a cause of the inhibition of gut motor function. Neuropeptide Y, serotonin, substance P, and calcitonin gene-related peptide are reduced in concentration in submucosal neurons of rats with experimental diabetes, which is consistent with alterations in visceral sensation and peptidergic control of the peristaltic reflex. There are no available studies of enteric (intrinsic) innervation in patients with diabetes mellitus. Alterations in glucose control may also alter circulating levels of glucose counterregulatory hormones (e.g., glucagon, epinephrine, somatostatin, growth hormone, and cortisol) that may affect GI motility. However, when formally tested, exogenous administration of glucagon at concentrations that mimic postprandial circulating levels in patients with diabetes does not alter gastric emptying.[50] The effects of physiologic concentrations of other counterregulatory hormones have not been fully evaluated.

Ischemia. Atherosclerotic disease of medium and large vessels that cause acute or chronic mesenteric arterial ischemia may occur in the diabetic population. Microangiopathy may contribute to neuropathy and to the histopathologic abnormalities that have been observed in gut smooth muscle.[13]

Electrolyte Imbalance, Uremia, and Diabetic Ketoacidosis. Symptoms such as nausea,

TABLE 15.3 POSSIBLE MECHANISMS OF IMPAIRED EXOCRINE PANCREATIC FUNCTION IN DIABETES

Insulin deficiency
Diabetic microangiopathy leading to fibrosis
Suppressing effect of high glucagon levels
Other gut hormones: somatostatin, pancreatic
    polypeptide
Autoimmune destruction
Disrupted enteropancreatic cholinergic reflex

vomiting, and diffuse abdominal pain are commonly seen in diabetic ketoacidosis. Differential diagnosis may be difficult because such abdominal symptoms may mask an underlying abdominal inflammatory process (such as diverticulitis, appendicitis) that may have triggered the condition. Hyperglycemia and hypokalemia may aggravate the chronic motility disorder in patients with diabetic gastroparesis.

CLINICAL ASSESSMENT

The assessment of GI dysfunction in patients with diabetes begins with a complete history and physical examination. Abnormalities may predominate in one segment of the gut, but more often multiple levels are involved (Fig. 15.1).

Dysphagia and Heartburn

Gastroesophageal reflux disease, esophageal candidiasis, and esophageal dysmotilities may cause esophageal symptoms in patients with diabetes.[43] Motor abnormalities include abnormal (usually low) lower esophageal sphincter pressure and alterations in the amplitude, frequency, and shape of propagated contractions in the esophagus. Abnormalities of motor function are correlated with signs of peripheral somatic or autonomic neuropathy[24] but not always with symptoms.

Upper GI endoscopy should be performed in patients with dysphagia, heartburn, or odynophagia to exclude reflux disease, candidal esophagitis, or incidental malignancy. Specialized tests that assess esophageal motor function play a relatively minor role in clinical practice. Chest pain should not necessarily be attributed to esophageal motor dysfunction because of the high prevalence of coronary artery disease in the diabetic population.

Nausea and Vomiting

Gastroparesis diabeticorum was a term first used by Kassander in 1958 to describe the atony and delayed gastric emptying that is sometimes seen in diabetic patients.[29] Typical symptoms include nausea, vomiting (usually 1 to 2 hours postprandially), weight loss, bloating, and early satiety.[31] Attacks of nausea and vomiting follow a variable course, may last from days to months, and may occur in cycles. A succussion splash may be evident on clinical examination, and a large gastric residual is often present after an overnight fast.[17] The gastroparesis syndrome may result in worsening of diabetic control, malnutrition, or bleeding caused by Mallory-Weiss tears as a result of repeated retching and vomiting. Affected patients often have concomitant retinopathy, nephropathy, peripheral somatic neuropathy, and other forms of autonomic neuropathy. The differential diagnosis of nausea and vomiting in a patient with diabetes should include gastric outlet obstruction caused by chronic peptic ulcer disease, or neoplasms, metabolic derangements, effects of medications (e.g., psychotropics, antihypertensive agents), biliary disease, and psychogenic vomiting.

Studies have shown that symptoms and gastric motor abnormalities in diabetes are not always closely correlated.[25, 26, 31] Recent data

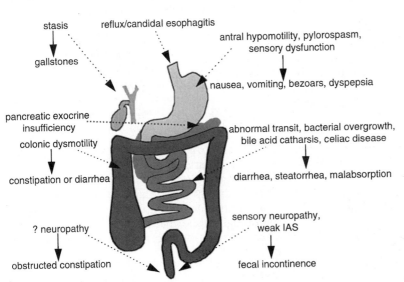

stasis
reflux/candidal esophagitis
antral hypomotility, pylorospasm, sensory dysfunction
gallstones
nausea, vomiting, bezoars, dyspepsia
pancreatic exocrine insufficiency
abnormal transit, bacterial overgrowth, bile acid catharsis, celiac disease
colonic dysmotility
constipation or diarrhea
diarrhea, steatorrhea, malabsorption
? neuropathy
sensory neuropathy, weak IAS
obstructed constipation
fecal incontinence

■ **Figure 15.1** Mechanisms of gastrointestinal symptoms in diabetic patients. IAS, internal anal sphincter.

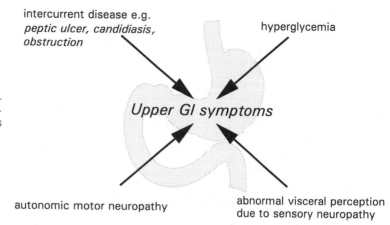

■ **Figure 15.2** Proposed mechanisms contributing to upper gastrointestinal symptoms in diabetes mellitus.

suggest that the gastric accommodation to ingestion of a meal is impaired in diabetics, and this may contribute to GI symptoms such as nausea, bloating, and early satiety. Moreover, just as a peripheral sensory neuropathy can be associated with painful dysesthesias, gastric distention induces more pain in diabetic patients than in controls.[47] Presumably, this applies until the afferent fibers lose all function. Figure 15.2 shows the possible pathophysiology of upper GI symptoms in diabetes.

The diagnosis of gastroparesis requires demonstration of a delay in gastric emptying. Barium studies and scintigraphy using labeled liquid meals are of limited value because the gastric emptying of liquids and semisolids (e.g., mashed potatoes) may be normal, even in the presence of moderately severe symptoms. Assessment of solid emptying is more sensitive, and a standardized method with a well-defined normal range is required. At the Mayo Clinic, a sequence of three scans is taken 2, 4, and 6 hours after ingestion of a standard solid and liquid meal (Fig. 15.3). A single radiolabel that tags the solid phase of the meal is used in our studies. The proportion of radioisotope retained in the stomach at 2 and 4 hours distinguishes normal function from gastroparesis with a sensitivity of 90% and a specificity of 70%.[6] In early diabetes, rapid gastric emptying has also been reported.[44]

Delayed gastric emptying also predisposes patients to gastric bezoar formation, which when found on endoscopy or barium studies is a sign of antral hypomotility. Bezoars may lead to gastric outlet obstruction and subsequent nausea, vomiting, and abdominal distention.

Gastropyloroduodenal manometry is a specialized technique used for research purposes and selected clinical situations (Fig. 15.4). Hypomotility of the gastric antrum is probably the major cause of motor dysfunction and impaired emptying in diabetes, but impaired relaxation or contraction of the fundus, pylorospasm, antropyloroduodenal incoordination, and small bowel dysmotility may also contribute to gastric stasis.[5, 40, 47] Assessment of the

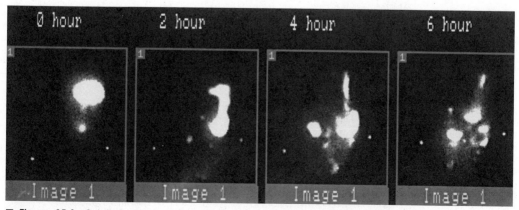

■ **Figure 15.3** Scintigraphic transit study showing delayed gastric emptying.

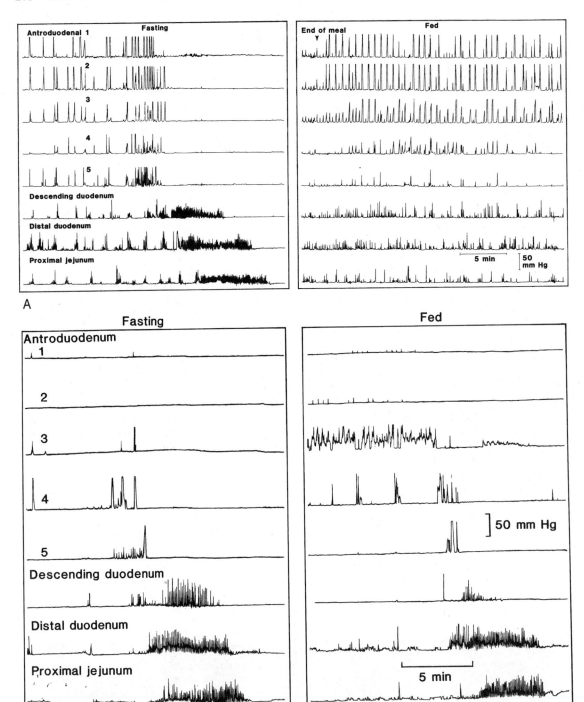

■ Figure 15.4 *A*, Normal manometric profile (fasting and postprandial). The migrating motor complex characteristic of the fasting state is demonstrated by the presence of quiescence (phase I), intermittent activity (phase II), and an activity front (phase III). Postprandial profile shows high-amplitude, irregular but persistent phasic pressure activity at all levels. (From Malegalada J-R, Camilleri M, Stanghellini V: Manometric Diagnosis of Gastrointestinal Motility Disorders. New York, Thieme Publishers, 1986.) *B*, Manometric profile in a 26-year-old female with diabetes and autonomic neuropathy, showing abnormal propagation of phase III of interdigestive motor complex and lack of a well-developed antral component in fasting tracing. Postprandially, note antral hypomotility, pylorospasm, and failure of meal to induce a feed pattern. (From Colemont LJ, Camilleri M: Chronic intestinal pseudo-obstruction: Diagnosis and treatment. Mayo Clin Proc 1989; 64:60–67.)

pressure profiles of the stomach and small bowel is necessary in some patients: those with selective abnormalities of antral function may tolerate feeding delivered directly into the small bowel, whereas those with a more generalized motility disorder may not tolerate enteral feeding.

Diarrhea and Fecal Incontinence

The prevalence of diarrhea in patients with diabetes who are seen at tertiary referral centers varies from 8 to 22%.[17, 59] Diabetic diarrhea is characterized by its chronicity, severity, and association with a long history of diabetes (at least 8 years).[30] It is often nocturnal[53] and may be associated with fecal incontinence. Bouts of diarrhea can be episodic and interspersed with periods of normal bowel movements or constipation.

Several mechanisms may result in diarrhea in these patients. Clinical features of "diabetic diarrhea" are nonspecific; the diagnosis is usually made by excluding other disorders. These include small bowel bacterial overgrowth, small bowel dysmotility caused by autonomic neuropathy, anorectal dysfunction, celiac sprue, impairment of exocrine pancreatic function, altered intestinal secretion, consumption of sorbitol-containing foods, or effects of medications (laxatives, antacids, or biguanides).

The assessment of a patient with diabetes and diarrhea starts with a detailed history, paying particular attention to diet, medication intake, and identification of features that suggest fecal incontinence or malabsorption. Sorbitol, found in many dietetic foods, chocolate, artificial sweeteners, and chewing gum is a common cause of diarrhea in diabetic individuals and may do so in amounts as little as 10 g.[1] Laxatives, antacids, or biguanides such as phenformin or metformin may cause diarrhea.[10] Patients often will not volunteer the symptom of fecal incontinence and may complain of "diarrhea" even though stool volume or consistency may be unaltered. Anorectal examination allows assessment of anal sphincter pressure (resting and squeeze) and rectal and anal sensation, all of which may be reduced. Weakness at rest reflects internal anal sphincter dysfunction (sympathetic innervation), which is most commonly abnormal in diabetes[4]; weakness during squeeze reflects external anal sphincter dysfunction.

If there are features to suggest malabsorption, such as anemia, macrocytosis, hypoalbuminemia, or steatorrhea, small bowel or pancreatic pathology needs to be considered. Steatorrhea may be confirmed with a 48- or 72-hour fecal fat study. Fecal fat in the range of 7 to 14 g/d may result from altered small bowel motor or secretory function alone.[18] Bacterial overgrowth in the small intestine is usually diagnosed by quantitative culture of jejunal aspirates, more than 10^5 aerobes or more than 10^3 anaerobes per milliliter. Alternatively, one of the breath tests could be used, in which expired H_2 or $^{14}CO_2$ is measured after oral ingestion of simple substrates, such as glucose or ^{14}C D-xylose, that are metabolized by enteric bacteria. A diagnostic trial of antibiotics could be considered, but spontaneous remissions are common in diabetic diarrhea, and a response does not necessarily prove bacterial overgrowth.

Anemia and low serum folate may suggest celiac sprue, which occurs with increased frequency in type 1 diabetes.[62] This was confirmed in a U.S. Army Medical Center study, where sprue occurred in 6.4% of diabetics[46] as compared with 0.02 to 0.1% in a U.S. community population.[57] A genetic predisposition to both diseases occurs with HLA types B8, DR3, and DQ.[16, 39, 52] The association with celiac sprue may also be partly the result of hormonal and immunologic factors.[35] Currently, small bowel biopsy is indicated for diagnosis, but antigliadin antibodies (and others such as antireticulin and antiendomysial antibodies) may be used as screening tests. When significant steatorrhea is found, exocrine pancreatic insufficiency should be considered and can be identified by direct pancreatic function testing, such as the secretin or cholecystokinin stimulation test. A trial of oral pancreatic enzymes may be considered if these tests are unavailable. Bile acid malabsorption is a more rare cause of diarrhea in these patients, but empiric treatment with cholestyramine may be considered.[48]

Intestinal motor function can be evaluated by measurement of transit measures or small bowel manometry. Abnormal patterns of motility, however, do not determine which patients have slow or fast transit. Estimation of breath hydrogen after ingestion of substrates such as lactulose are suboptimal measures of orocecal transit. Accurate, noninvasive, and relatively inexpensive scintigraphic methods can simultaneously measure gastric, small bowel, and colonic transit.[60] An algorithm for the investigation of diabetic patients with diarrhea is given in Chapter 39.

Evaluation of anorectal function should include anorectal manometry, with testing of compliance and sensation to distention of a balloon. Sphincter electromyography or pudendal nerve conduction tests are mostly used as research tools. Anorectal ultrasound may identify incidental defects in the anal sphincter or thinning of the perineal body, which may be coincident and occur commonly with multiparous women.[55] Rectoceles, intussusception, and pelvic floor dysfunction may be evaluated with a defecating proctogram. Rectoceles are clinically significant only if they preferentially fill and fail to empty during attempted defecation.

Constipation

Constipation is a common symptom in patients with diabetes mellitus,[17] yet little is known about its pathophysiology. It typically alternates with diarrhea. The hypothesis that autonomic neuropathy plays a role is supported by a study by Battle and colleagues in which the postprandial gastrocolonic response was im-

paired in patients with diabetes and peripheral neuropathy.[4] A careful rectal examination at rest and with straining should be performed to exclude mucosal lesions, rectal prolapse, rectoceles, and pelvic floor dysfunction (excess perineal descent or failure of puborectalis to relax).

The extent of evaluation in a diabetic patient with constipation depends on the severity of constipation and the associated symptoms. Digital examination, sigmoidoscopy, and barium enema or full colonoscopy should be performed to exclude malignancy, especially if weight loss or bleeding is present. A management algorithm is shown in Figure 15.5. Empirical treatment with increased dietary fiber (20 to 30 g/d) in combination with bulk or osmotic laxatives should be the first step.

Evaluation of anorectal and pelvic floor function is indicated for more resistant cases; these problems may occur as a complication of diabetes or as an unrelated problem. Such "obstructed constipation" is an important cause of constipation in the general population[54] and in

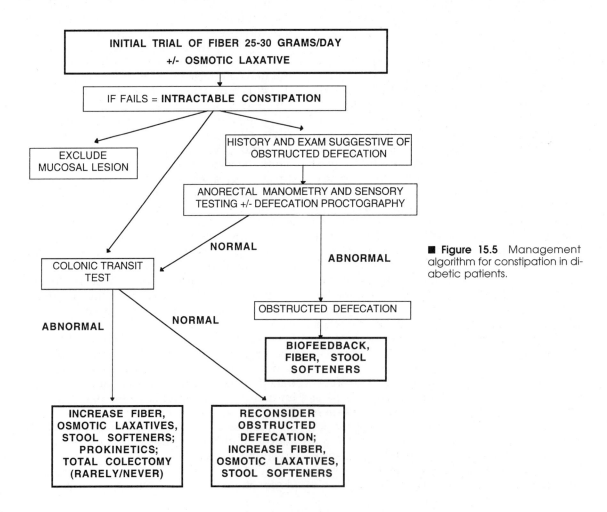

■ Figure 15.5 Management algorithm for constipation in diabetic patients.

those who are seen in tertiary centers.[32] Features from the history to suggest these disorders of the defecation process include inability to initiate defecation, digitation to facilitate defecation, assumption of contorted postures during defecation, feelings of incomplete evacuation, and rectal discomfort. Patients may report that even enemas are ineffective. Anorectal manometry with balloon expulsion and defecography best assesses these disorders. If anorectal function is normal, colonic transit time should be evaluated using noninvasive, accurate, inexpensive tests such as radiopaque markers or scintigraphy.[60]

Acute and Chronic Abdominal Pain

Several conditions may cause abdominal pain in patients with diabetes mellitus (Table 15.4). Patients may have significant abdominal pain caused by thoracolumbar radiculopathy without evidence of GI pathology.[32] A history of a chronic, remitting, burning dermatomal pain may suggest this diagnosis, and electromyography and a thermoregulatory sweat test may confirm the diagnosis. Antidepressants such as amitriptyline and desipramine may be useful to control painful neuropathy.[37] When neuropathy develops, diabetic patients may actually have less abdominal pain. Just as "silent infarcts" occur in diabetics with coronary artery disease, "silent mesenteric ischemia" has been reported.[51] This theory is supported by studies showing lack of pain from jejunal balloon distention,[63] rectal balloon distention,[61] or esophageal electrical stimulation[45] in diabetic patients compared with controls.

Diabetic patients have a predilection for gallstones as a result of altered gallbladder contractility; thus, biliary colic or cholecystitis may cause abdominal pain in diabetes.[3] Mesenteric ischemia may occur because of generalized arteriosclerosis. Small intestinal ischemia causes

diffuse postprandial midabdominal pain and later abdominal distention. Colonic ischemia may cause pain and rectal bleeding from ischemic colitis.

Diffuse abdominal pain, usually with nausea and vomiting, may be seen with diabetic ketoacidosis. Symptoms usually resolve quickly after administration of intravenous fluids, electrolytes, and insulin. Motor disorders of the GI tract may cause significant abdominal pain if associated with distention such as acute gastric dilatation or ileus.

Acute pancreatitis is twice as common in type 1 diabetics compared with the incidence in age-matched controls,[23, 34] but the incidence of clinically significant chronic pancreatitis is not increased. More commonly, diabetes results from chronic pancreatitis. The relationship between diabetes and pancreatic cancer is controversial, but in 80% of patients with pancreatic carcinoma and diabetes, diabetes is discovered within a year after the cancer has become clinically obvious, suggesting that it is the basis of the diabetes.[41]

SUMMARY AND PROSPECTS

Patients with diabetes can have a broad spectrum of GI manifestations with diverse pathophysiologies. Several tertiary referral center studies have shown that GI symptoms are frequent in diabetic patients, but population-based data regarding prevalence are rare. It is unknown how these complications affect quality of life, mortality, and glycemic control in the typical patient with diabetes.

Sensory dysfunction and motor dysfunction contribute to the symptom profile. Symptoms may be heightened early in disease or reduced in patients with more severe diabetic neuropathy. Acute hyperglycemia can affect certain aspects of GI function. These areas must be further clarified in future studies. With the results of the Diabetes Control and Complications Trial, we can also advise patients of the proved benefits of tight metabolic control on the development of long-term complications, such as neuropathy.

Documentation of the mechanisms contributing to the symptom complex may be helpful in the selection of therapy (see Chapter 39). Diagnostic modalities to appraise motor and sensory function are available. A single physician should coordinate and prioritize treatment of the diabetes itself and the various complications. Medications used to treat associated diseases, such as depression or hypertension, may

---

TABLE 15.4 CAUSES OF ABDOMINAL PAIN IN DIABETES MELLITUS

Thoracolumbar radiculopathy
Biliary colic and cholecystitis
Mesenteric ischemia
Diabetic ketoacidosis
Acute gastric dilatation
Ileus
Pancreatic disease: pancreatitis, pancreatic cancer
Incidental causes: diverticulitis, irritable bowel
  syndrome, etc.

alter motor and sensory function of the gut. As gastroenterologists become more aware of the importance of the neuromuscular apparatus of the gut in the development of GI symptoms, communication between neurologists and gastroenterologists is important to achieve better patient care.

References

1. Badiga MS, Jain NK, Casanova C, et al. Diarrhea in diabetics: The role of sorbitol. J Am Coll Nutr 1990; 9:578.
2. Barnett JL, Owang C. Serum glucose concentration as a modulator of interdigestive gastric motility. Gastroenterology 1988; 94:739.
3. Bartoli E, Ferrari E, Saporetti N, et al. Prevalence of cholelithiasis in diabetes mellitus: A cholecystosonographic study. Diagn Radiol 1987; 12:43.
4. Battle WM, Snape WJ Jr, Alava A, et al. Colonic dysfunction in diabetes mellitus. Gastroenterology 1980; 79:1217.
5. Camilleri M, Malagelada J-R. Abnormal intestinal motility in diabetics with gastroparesis syndrome. Eur J Clin Invest 1984; 14:420.
6. Camilleri M, Zinsmeister AR, Greydanus MP, et al: Towards a less costly but accurate test of gastric emptying and small bowel transit. Dig Dis Sci 1991; 36:609.
7. Chang EB, Fedorak RN, Field M. Experimental diabetic diarrhea in rats: Intestinal mucosal denervation, hyposensitivity and treatment with clonidine. Gastroenterology 1986; 91:564.
8. Clouse RE, Lustman PJ. Gastrointestinal symptoms in diabetic patients: Lack of association with neuropathy. Am J Gastroenterol 1989; 84:868.
9. Crofford OB: Diabetes control and complications. Annu Rev Med 1995; 46:267.
10. Dandona P, Fonseca V, Mier A, et al. Diarrhea and metformin in a diabetic clinic. Diabetes Care 1983; 6:472.
11. DiMagno EP, Go VL, Summerskill WH. Relations between enzyme outputs and malabsorption in severe pancreatic insufficiency. N Engl J Med 1973; 288:813.
12. Drossman DA, Li Z, Andruzzi E, et al. U.S. householder survey of functional gastrointestinal disorders: Prevalence, sociodemography, and health impact. Dig Dis Sci 1993; 38:1569.
13. Duchen LW, Anjorin A, Watkins PJ, et al. Pathology of autonomic neuropathy in diabetes mellitus. Ann Intern Med 1980; 92:301.
14. Dyck PJ, Kratz KM, Karnes JL, et al. The prevalence by staged severity of various types of diabetic neuropathy, retinopathy, and nephropathy in a population-based cohort: The Rochester Diabetic Neuropathy Study. Neurology 1993; 43:817.
15. El-Newihi J, Dooley CP, Saad C, et al. Impaired exocrine pancreatic function in diabetics with diarrhea and peripheral neuropathy. Dig Dis Sci 1988; 33:705.
16. Falchuk ZM, Rogentine GN, Strober W. Predominance of histocompatability antigen HLA-B8 in patients with gluten-sensitive enteropathy. J Clin Invest 1972; 51:1602.
17. Feldman M, Schiller LR. Disorders of gastrointestinal motility associated with diabetes mellitus. Ann Intern Med 1983; 98:378.
18. Finek KD, Fordtran JS. The effect of diarrhea on fecal fat excretion. Gastroenterology 1992; 102:1936.
19. Frank JW, Saslow SB, Camilleri M, et al. Mechanism of accelerated gastric emptying and hyperglycemia in Type II diabetes mellitus. Gastroenterology 1995; 109:755.
20. Fraser R, Russo A, Dent J, et al. Effects of hyperglycemia on small intestinal motility and transit in healthy humans. Gastroenterology 1995; A601.
21. Fraser RJ, Horowitz M, Maddox AF, et al. Hyperglycemia slows gastric emptying in type I (insulin-dependent) diabetes mellitus. Diabetologia 1990; 33:675.
22. Frier M, Saunders JHB, Wormsley KG, et al. Exocrine pancreatic function in juvenile-onset diabetes mellitus. Gut 1976; 17:685.
23. Hillemeir C, Gryboski J. Diabetes and the gastrointestinal tract in the pediatric patient. Yale J Biol Med 1983; 56:195.
24. Hollis JB, Castell DO, Braddom RL. Esophageal function in diabetes mellitus and its relation to peripheral neuropathy. Gastroenterology 1977; 73:1098.
25. Horowitz M, Harding PE, Maddox A, et al. Gastric and oesophageal emptying in insulin-dependent diabetes mellitus. J Gastroenterol Hepatol 1986; 1:97.
26. Horowitz M, Harding PE, Maddox AF, et al. Gastric and oesophageal emptying in patients with Type II (non–insulin-dependent) diabetes mellitus. Diabetologia 1989; 32:151.
27. Janatuinen E, Pikkarainen P, Laakso M, et al. Gastrointestinal symptoms in middle-aged diabetic patients. Scand J Gastroenterol 1993; 28:427.
28. Jebbink RJA, Samsom M, Bruifs J, et al. Hyperglycemia induces abnormalities of gastric myoelectrical activity in patients with type I diabetes mellitus. Gastroenterology 1994; 107:1390.
29. Kassander P. Asymptomatic gastric retention in diabetics (gastroparesis diabeticorum). Ann Intern Med 1958; 48:797.
30. Katz LA, Spiro HM. Gastrointestinal manifestations of diabetes. N Engl J Med 1966; 273:1350.
31. Kim CH, Kennedy FP, Camilleri M. Measurement of small bowel and colonic transit: Indications and methods. Mayo Clin Proc 1992; 67:1169.
32. Longstreth GF, Newcomer AD. Abdominal pain caused by diabetic radiculopathy. Ann Intern Med 1977; 86:166.
33. Maleki D, Camilleri M, Van Dyke CT, et al. Gastrointestinal symptoms in non-insulin-dependent diabetes mellitus (NIDDM) in a U.S. community: A pilot prevalence study. Gastroenterology 1996; 110:A27.
34. Malone JI. Juvenile diabetes and acute pancreatitis. J Pediatr 1975; 85:825.
35. Mann NS, Mann SK. Celiac sprue and diabetes mellitus. J Clin Gastroenterol 1993; 16:4.
36. Maser RE, Pfeifer MA, Dorman JS, et al. Diabetic autonomic neuropathy and cardiovascular risk. Arch Intern Med 1990; 150:1218.
37. Max MB, Lynch SA, Muir J, et al. Effects of desipramine, amitriptyline and fluoxetine on pain in diabetic neuropathy. N Engl J Med 1992; 326:1250.
38. Maxton DG, Whorwell PJ. Functional bowel symptoms in diabetes mellitus: The role of autonomic neuropathy. Postgrad Med J 1991; 67:991.
39. Mazzilli MC, Ferrante P, Mariani P, et al. A study of Italian pediatric celiac disease patients confirms that the primary HLA association is to the DQ (alpha 1*0501, beta 1*0201) heterodimer. Hum Immunol 1992; 33:133.
40. Mearin F, Camilleri M, Malagelada J-R. Pyloric dysfunction in diabetics with recurrent nausea and vomiting. Gastroenterology 1986; 90:1919.

41. Nix GAJJ, Schmitz PIM, Wilson JHP, et al. Carcinoma of the head of the pancreas: Therapeutic implications of endoscopic retrograde cholangiopancreatography findings. Gastroenterology 1984; 87:37.

42. Oster-Jorgensen E, Pedersen SA, Larsen ML. The influence of induced hyperglycemia on gastric emptying rate in healthy humans. Scand J Clin Lab Invest 1990; 50:831.

43. Parkman HP, Schwartz SS. Esophagitis and gastroduodenal disorders associated with diabetic gastroparesis. Arch Intern Med 1987; 147:1477.

44. Phillips WT, Schwartz JG, McMahan CA. Rapid gastric emptying of an oral glucose solution in type 2 diabetic patients. J Nucl Med 1992; 33:1496.

45. Rathmann W, Enck P, Frieling R, et al. Visceral afferent neuropathy in diabetic gastroparesis. Diabetes Care 1991; 14:1086.

46. Rensch MJ, Merenich JA, Lieberman M, et al. Gluten-sensitive enteropathy in patients with insulin dependent diabetes mellitus. Ann Intern Med 1996; 124:564.

47. Samsom M, Salet GA, Roelofs JM, et al. Compliance of the proximal stomach and dyspeptic symptoms in patients with type I diabetes mellitus. Dig Dis Sci 1995; 40:2037.

48. Scarpello JH, Hague RV, Cullen DR, et al. The 14C-glycocholate test in diabetic diarrhea. Br J Med 1976; 2:673.

49. Schiller LR, Santa Ana CA, Schmulen AC, et al. Pathogenesis of fecal incontinence in diabetes mellitus. N Engl J Med 1982; 307:1666.

50. Schjoldager B, Lawaetz O, Christiansen J. Effect of pancreatic glucagon and its I-21 fragment on gastric emptying in man. Scand J Gastroenterol 1988; 23:726.

51. Selby CD, Dennis MJS, Whincup PH. Painless mesenteric infarction in a patient with diabetes. Diabetic Care 1987; 10:259.

52. Shanahan F, McKenna R, McCarthy CF, et al. Coeliac disease and diabetes mellitus: A study of patients with HLA-typing. QJM 1982; 203:329.

53. Sheridan EP, Baily CC. Diabetic nocturnal diarrhea. JAMA 1946; 130:632.

54. Sims M, Hasler W, Chey WD, et al. Acute hyperglycemia inhibits gastrocolonic and colonic peristaltic reflexes measured by an electronic barostat in healthy humans. Gastroenterology 1994; 108:A566.

55. Sultan AH, Kamm MA, Hudson CN, et al. Anal-sphincter disruption during vaginal delivery. N Engl J Med 1993; 329:1905.

56. Surrenti E, Rath DM, Pemberton JH, et al. Audit of constipation in a tertiary referral gastroenterology practice. Am J Gastroenterol 1995; 90:1471.

57. Talley NJ, Valdovinos M, Petterson TM, et al. Epidemiology of celiac sprue: A community-based study. Am J Gastroenterol 1994; 89:843.

58. Talley NJ, Weaver AL, Zinsmeister AR, et al. Functional constipation and outlet delay: A population-based study. Gastroenterology 1993; 105:781.

59. Valdovinos MA, Camilleri M, Zimmerman BR. Chronic diarrhea in diabetes mellitus: Mechanisms and an approach to diagnosis and treatment. Mayo Clin Proc 1993; 68:691.

60. von der Ohe MR, Camilleri M. Measurement of small bowel and colonic transit: Indications and methods. Mayo Clin Proc 1992; 67:1169.

61. Wald A, Tunuguntla K. Anorectal sensorimotor dysfunction, fecal incontinence and diabetes mellitus. N Engl J Med 1984; 310:1282.

62. Walsh CH, Cooper BT, Wright D, et al. Diabetes mellitus and celiac disease. A clinical study. QJM 1978; 47:89.

63. Whalen GE, Soergel KH, Geenan JE. Diabetic diarrhea: A clinical and pathophysiological study. Gastroenterology 1969; 56:1021.

Chapter **16**

Electrophysiologic Testing in Diabetic Neuropathy

Jasper R. Daube

ROLE OF NEUROPHYSIOLOGIC TESTS

Electrophysiologic tests provide reliable and reproducible approaches to the detection and characterization of nerve, muscle, and neuromuscular junction disease.[40] Nerve conduction tests are used to localize lesions and to describe the type and severity of the pathophysiologic process, including alterations in function that are not recognized clinically. These evaluations are useful in following the course of neuropathy and in assessing response to treatments.[21] The techniques are also helpful in deciding which fibers are involved.[11] Sensory fibers are tested by recording nerve action potentials and somatosensory evoked potentials (SEPs).[28, 64] Nerve conduction recordings of compound muscle action potentials, F-wave and distal latencies, and needle electromyographic recordings provide data about the function of motor axons. Small myelinated fibers mediating autonomic function and pain cannot be tested by standard nerve conduction studies[50] (see Chapters 11 to 15). Nerve conduction studies are most valuable in assessing diabetic neuropathy when used in conjunction with clinical assessment, quantitative sensory testing, and autonomic function testing.[42]

In nerve conduction studies, two equally important measures, amplitude and conduction velocity, can be precisely quantitated[34] (Fig. 16.1). Although conduction velocity is the best known, amplitude has the most clinical significance. The amplitude is a function of the number and size of the nerve or muscle fibers, the range of conduction velocities of fibers, and technical factors. If the latter are well controlled and the range of conduction velocities

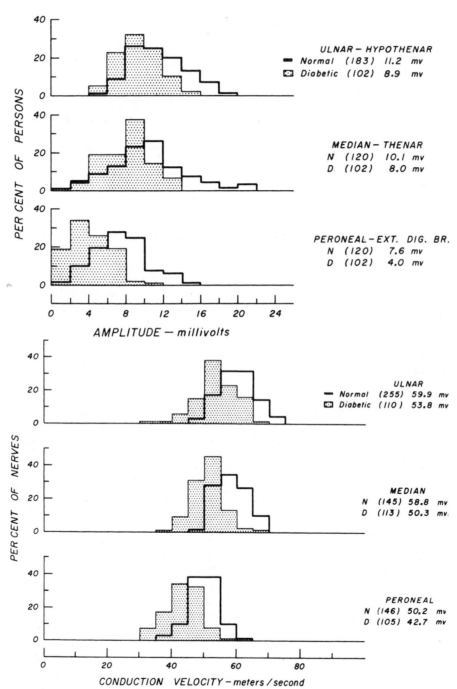

■ **Figure 16–1.** The distribution of amplitudes *(top)* and conduction velocities *(bottom)* in the upper and lower extremities in a group of unselected patients with diabetes is shown in the shaded histogram. The normal distribution is shown in the bar graph. (From Mulder DW, et al: The neuropathies associated with diabetes mellitus. Neurology, 11:275, 1961.)

is not great, the amplitude provides an indication of the number of functioning axons in a nerve, and of the amount of muscle still innervated. If the range of conduction velocities of nerve fibers is greater than normal, the action potential becomes dispersed so that the area of the potential is a better estimate of the number of functioning axons than amplitude. Recently developed methods of estimating the number of motor units in a muscle provide additional useful information. Generally, amplitude or area measures are directly related to the patient's clinical deficit in the nerve and muscle tested. For example, an absent peroneal response from the extensor digitorum brevis would be associated with severe atrophy or absent muscle on the dorsum of the foot. If the nerve damage is primarily distal, anterior tibial muscle strength might still be normal.

Changes in the amplitude of evoked responses with repetitive stimulation are used to measure both the function of the neuromuscular junction, which may be involved in some neural diseases, and the ability of nerve to discharge repetitively. An early manifestation of some axonal disorders is loss of the ability to carry repetitive impulses, particularly at higher rates. Repetitive stimulation or measures of refractory period and accommodation can identify peripheral nerve disorders when other physiologic and histologic measures are still normal.

The conduction velocity, whether measured in meters per second or as a latency in milliseconds over a fixed distance, is a function of a number of physiologic properties. Fiber size, myelination, nodal and internodal length, and external and internal axonal resistance play a role in the speed of conduction. A patient's symptoms and deficits with a neuropathy cannot be inferred from the speed of nerve conduction. A patient with a severe nerve conduction abnormality may have no, or few, symptoms or deficits, and vice versa.

Quantitation of spontaneous and voluntary potentials on needle electromyography (EMG) is more difficult and less reliable than nerve conduction studies[34]; however, EMG quantitation can provide additional information about neural dysfunction not identified from nerve conduction studies. Measures of the size of voluntary motor unit potentials can identify remodeling of the motor unit occurring in slowly progressive, chronic neural disorders. Measurement of the density of spontaneous fibrillation potentials with the muscle at rest can identify destruction of axons that is not recognized clinically or on nerve conduction studies.

A refinement of standard needle electromyography, single fiber electromyography (SFEMG)[34, 127] provides precise quantitation of muscle changes in response to peripheral nerve disease. Fiber density measurements define the number of muscle fibers that are innervated by a single motor unit. The fiber density increases with loss of peripheral axons and reinnervation of denervated muscle fibers by remaining viable axons through collateral sprouting. Jitter, an indirect but quantitative measure of end plate potential amplitude and thereby of neuromuscular transmission, is altered in disorders with ongoing collateral sprouting as well as disorders of the neuromuscular junction.

Both nerve conduction studies and EMG are useful in determining the distribution of the neuropathic abnormality. They are of help in deciding whether there is proximal and or distal involvement and in distinguishing focal from multifocal disease.[33] They may also be helpful in defining the membrane abnormality in diabetic axons.[68]

In diabetes, nerve conduction and EMG may be particularly helpful in localizing the pathology to a single nerve and to the specific segment of nerve involved. The identification of a thoracic radiculopathy in a patient with chest or abdominal pain, described in a later section, is a prime example. Localized changes in amplitude (conduction block) or velocity along the length of the nerve may be used to identify a focal lesion[34] (Fig. 16.2). Both conduction block and localized slowing can occur in diabetic neuropathy. In patients with diabetic neuropathy, determination of the distribution of involvement is not only confirmatory, but often adds new, clinically unsuspected information. Fibrillation potentials may occur in foot muscles in some diabetic patients before clinical deficit or nerve conduction changes. Nerve conduction studies and responses to repetitive stimulation are often abnormal before there is clinical evidence of impaired function. Somatosensory evoked potentials, H reflexes, and F wave latencies (Fig. 16.3) can show abnormal proximal function with no changes on distal clinical or electrical testing.[8, 99] A purely distal distribution of deficits can help identify a length-dependent neuropathy.

Neurophysiologic testing can distinguish new disease from an old, unrelated problem, such as the residuals of a radiculopathy caused by a herniated disc.[33] The presence of a superimposed problem, such as carpal tunnel syn-

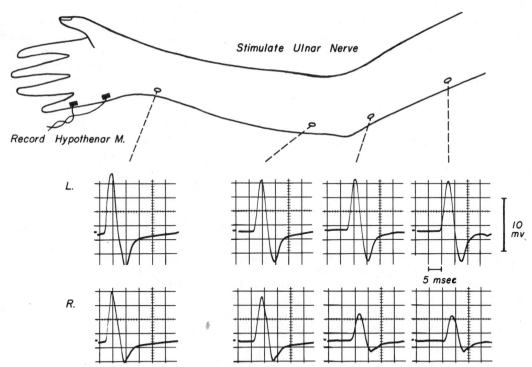

■ Figure 16–2. Conduction block at the elbow in the right ulnar nerve in a patient with an ulnar neuropathy. The amplitude of the evoked response is markedly reduced above a localized segment of the nerve. The conduction block may or may not be associated with localized slowing of conduction. (From Clinical Examination in Neurology, 5th ed. Philadelphia, W. B. Saunders Company, 1981.)

drome, with a generalized neuropathy can be precisely localized and defined. A pattern of electrophysiologic abnormalities typical of diabetic neuropathy may even suggest the presence of diabetes mellitus before it has been recognized clinically.

Electrophysiologic test results may allow inferences to be made about underlying patho-

logic alterations of nerve fibers.[11] In wallerian degeneration, there is a reduction in amplitude with little or no decrease in conduction velocity. Axonal degeneration of large, fast-conducting fibers results at most in only mild changes in conduction velocity. Fibrillation potentials and changes in motor unit potentials on EMG are the typical findings with axonal destruc-

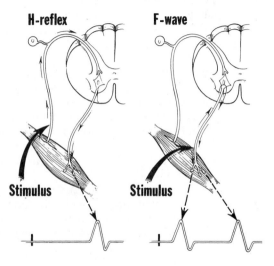

■ Figure 16–3. Schematic diagram of the origin of H reflexes and F waves. Stimulation is applied to the mixed nerve for both responses. The H reflex is elicited with lower voltage stimuli that selectively activate the sensory axons from the muscle, while the F wave is elicited with supramaximal stimuli that activate antidromic action potentials in motor axons.

tion. In contrast, changes in the diameter of axons or changes in myelination will result primarily in changes in rate of conduction, either latency or conduction velocity. Focal compressive or ischemic lesions result in an abrupt reduction in amplitude (conduction block) along the length of the nerve, which can be localized to segments as short as 1 cm.

In diabetic neuropathy, electrophysiologic testing is helpful in characterizing the evolution of the disorder and following its course.[33] Some inferences can be drawn about the acuteness of the pathologic process from a single evaluation. The presence of mild generalized conduction changes with motor unit potential changes, but no fibrillation potentials, indicates a slow, chronic process. Prominent fibrillation potentials or a localized conduction block suggests a more acute or rapidly progressive process. If the patient is tested periodically, changes in amplitude and conduction velocity can be used to follow the course of the disease or response to treatment.

CRITICAL FACTORS IN NEUROPHYSIOLOGIC TESTING AND INTERPRETATION

Nerve conduction studies are not reliable (reproducible) without good technique and control for physiologic variables.[15] Reproducibility of nerve conduction requires consistency of methods, including electrode locations, distances, and temperature. F-wave latencies are the most reproducible, with only a 2 to 3% variation; amplitudes have the lowest reproducibility (10 to 15%), and conduction velocity and distal latency are intermediate (4 to 7%).[23, 128] Other demographic factors, such as age, gender, and anthropomorphic factors, also play a part in determining the nerve conduction values in patients with diabetes.[2] The effect of these variables likely is different in diabetic neuropathy than in normal nerve.[36] Physicians engaged in electrophysiologic testing must therefore not only control for each of the critical factors, but also must know how much variability is present in their results. Reliability should be tested in both normal subjects and patients with disease by a series of tests given over short intervals with all pertinent variables controlled.

Selection of the nerve and parameter to test cannot be made solely on the basis of reliability. The sensitivity and specificity must also be considered. Sensitivity refers to the rate of detection of an abnormality that is present; specificity refers to the rate of apparent identification of an abnormality that is not present. Electrophysiologic tests are not sensitive to small-fiber damage, but they can be more sensitive than clinical or histologic studies in identifying motor axon damage. In some conditions, sensory amplitudes show earlier and more prominent changes than do motor conduction velocities. F-wave latencies are more sensitive in diffuse neuropathies, whereas latencies over short segments are more sensitive to focal abnormalities. F waves have been reported to be the most sensitive measure of diabetic neuropathies.[6] Specificity is reduced when variables such as age, temperature, and anomalous innervation are not taken into account. Because nerve conduction parameters and EMG results vary with patient age and limb temperature, temperature must be controlled and results must be compared to age-matched controls. Limb temperatures must be monitored throughout testing; if limb temperature is low, it should be corrected by warming the limb.

The techniques used in nerve conduction studies must be rigorous. Stimulating and recording electrodes must be placed in the correct and the same locations (e.g., anatomical landmarks) to provide reproducible size, shape, and latencies of potentials in the same patient, and among patients. Anomalous innervation, occurring in 20% of normal subjects, results in variations in responses that must not be mistaken for abnormalities caused by nerve disease.

Normal values for each nerve conduction parameter should be based on a large number of subjects of both genders and all ages, without either diseases of nerve or diseases predisposing to nerve disease. The data on normal subjects should be expressed as a mean, standard deviation, and range. Normal ranges should be defined by 3 SD from the mean, or for data that are not normally distributed, by ranges of normal values. Interpretations of changes in diabetic neuropathy can then be made for either single individuals or populations of patients. The results in single individuals should be considered to be clearly abnormal only if their values are outside the normal range. This will not occur in most patients until there has been a major change. In contrast, abnormalities in a population of patients may be recognized when most individual values are within the normal range, but the mean value is significantly different from that of controls. Thus, small changes in disease occurring in a

TABLE 16.1 EVOLUTION OF EMG CHANGES AFTER AXONAL DAMAGE*

	Acute <7 d	Subacute 10 d–6 w	Chronic, Progressive 6 w–3 mo	Residual
Fibrillation potentials	None	Proximal	Many	Distal, small, few
Fasciculation potentials	Rare	Rare	Rare	Occasional
Motor unit potentials	Reduced recruitment	Reduced recruitment Polyphasic Vary	Long duration High amplitude Polyphasic Vary	Long duration High amplitude (especially distal)
Complex repetitive discharges	None	None	Rare	Occasional
Compound muscle action potential amplitude	Normal	Low	Low	(Low)
Motor conduction velocity	Normal	(Slightly low)	(Slightly low)	(Slightly low)
F wave	Absent	Absent	Absent	(Prolonged)
H reflex	(Prolonged)	(Prolonged)	(Prolonged)	(Absent)

*Items in parentheses may be present.

population may not be evident in single individuals.

Correct interpretation of results depends on recognition by the electromyographer that neurophysiologic alterations are different in acute, subacute, and chronic processes (Tables 16.1 and 16.2).[33] Conduction block, loss of F waves, and reduced recruitment without motor unit potential changes suggest an acute process. Polyphasic, varying, motor unit potentials, and increased jitter provide evidence for ongoing reinnervation and attempts at recovery. Long-duration, stable motor unit potentials with low amplitude-evoked potentials are evidence of long-standing disease. In neurogenic disease, fibrillation potentials are evidence of denervation not compensated by innervation. Therefore, fibrillation potentials suggest the presence of either active disease or severe disease that precludes reinnervation. Fibrillation potentials are usually associated with low amplitude-evoked responses, but their time course of development is different. The first electrophysiologic change after acute nerve injury is poor recruitment of motor unit potentials on EMG. Three to 5 days after axonal disruption with nerve injury, the amplitudes of evoked responses on nerve conductions fall. Fibrillation potentials do not develop until 14 to 21 days after axonal loss.

Residual alterations in nerve conduction and EMG findings from a previous neuropathic disease must be recognized by the electromyographer. Complete clinical recovery from radiculopathy, carpal tunnel syndrome, or even generalized disorders will usually leave residual abnormalities. The changes are most prominent in the motor unit potentials, but conduction velocity and amplitudes can also remain abnormal. A diabetic patient will show different abnormalities when absent ankle reflexes are caused by a mild early diabetic peripheral neuropathy than when it is the residual of old sacral radiculopathies or cauda equina damage.

NERVE CONDUCTION AND ELECTROMYOGRAPHY FINDINGS IN DIABETIC PATIENTS

The neurophysiologic findings in published series of patients with diabetic neuropathy vary with the patient population tested and with the type and distribution of neuropathy. Differences in patient selection undoubtedly account for major differences between series. To illustrate, in one series only symptomatic patients were included,[11] whereas others studied consecutive patients encountered in a diabetic clinic.[92, 108]

The clinical and pathologic manifestations

TABLE 16.2 COMPOUND MUSCLE ACTION POTENTIAL AMPLITUDE AFTER FOCAL PERIPHERAL NERVE INJURY

	0–5 d	After 5 d	Recovery
Conduction block			
Proximal stimulation	Low	Low	Increases
Distal stimulation	Normal	Normal	Normal
Axonal disruption			
Proximal stimulation	Low	Low	Increases
Distal stimulation	Normal	Low	Increases

of neuropathy in diabetes vary considerably among patients. Neurophysiologic abnormalities will reflect these differences. The frequency and severity of neurophysiologic abnormality is high in patients with symptomatic neuropathy and much lower in diabetics without symptoms of neuropathy. The electrophysiologic findings vary with the distribution of the neuropathy, for example, in a symmetric sensory neuropathy versus an asymmetric process such as femoral neuropathy. Most but not all patients with mononeuropathy, monoradiculopathy, painful neuropathies and autonomic neuropathies caused by diabetes have electrophysiologic findings of a diffuse neuropathy.[108]

The clinical electromyographer should be familiar with the symptoms and signs of the variety of neuropathies that may occur in a patient with diabetes so that the appropriate tests are selected for each patient's specific problem. The variety of nerve disorders seen with diabetes precludes the use of standard sets of either nerve conduction studies or EMG. The tests must be individually selected on the basis of the clinical picture to provide the data that will help answer the questions posed by the primary physician.

The neurophysiologic changes in different types and degrees of neuropathy are summarized in this section, but it should be remembered that overlap of findings among these groups is usual.

Asymptomatic Patients

Published reports of EMG and nerve conduction findings in asymptomatic diabetic patients with no clinical signs of neuropathy often group them with patients who have minimal findings, such as slight reduction in ankle jerks or mild reduction in vibratory sensation. Although this lumping of patients increases the frequency of neurophysiologic abnormality, it precludes the need to distinguish patients who have similar findings caused by aging that are generally considered to be of little clinical consequence.

Most studies of asymptomatic diabetic patients have focused on the mean values of nerve conduction studies, which have been found to differ from normal for all nerves tested—sensory and motor, both proximal and distal in arms and legs.[39, 41, 83, 113] Some studies have shown the abnormalities to be more prominent with longer duration of diabetes,[44, 45, 48, 61] but others have not.[53, 111] The severity of nerve conduction abnormality was correlated with the severity of hyperglycemia in two reports.[44, 61] This correlation is most prominent in the peroneal conduction studies.[80] No differences have been found in patients with type 1 and type 2 diabetes mellitus.[126]

Conduction velocity changes in asymptomatic patients are of mild to moderate degree, with mean values for motor conduction 10 to 30% below the normal mean, an abnormality that reflects disease of large axons.[38] Amplitude has been significantly reduced, often to a greater degree than the conduction velocity, in the few studies that report amplitude. Sensory nerve action potential amplitude is reduced up to 60% in the legs; up to half the patients had amplitudes outside the normal range. Sensory nerve action potentials and SEP are generally more sensitive in identifying mild abnormalities than are motor conduction studies.[28, 64, 80, 95]

The amplitude and conduction changes are most prominent in the distal segments of nerves and in the legs,[45, 76] especially in the peroneal motor conduction values. Some patients may have greater slowing in proximal segments.[28, 57, 129] Large fibers are generally most affected, but slower conducting fibers may be selectively involved.[29] Population studies show a mild to moderate reduction in mean values, suggesting a mild, generalized neuropathy. But when individual, asymptomatic, diabetic patients are examined, a different perspective is obtained. As many as 20% have multiple values that are outside the normal range that indicate the presence of a subclinical peripheral neuropathy. Among these patients, the involvement of different nerves is not always generalized and symmetric. Some of the patients have abnormal values in only single nerves, especially the peroneal nerve or median nerve at the wrist. In other patients, ulnar nerve conduction across the elbow, SEP, or F-wave latencies are abnormal.[8, 64] The increased incidence of abnormalities at sites of common compression is consistent with damage occurring at potential sites of nerve entrapment or repeated occupational pressure.

Although most studies have searched for abnormalities in nerve conduction studies, asymptomatic diabetic patients clearly also have significant abnormalities on EMG.[48] There may be changes in size or configuration of motor unit potentials or fibrillation potentials in distal muscles. These changes may precede abnormality of nerve conduction.[48, 65, 80, 92] The fibrillation potentials occur most commonly in the intrinsic foot muscles (in a different distribution and to a greater extent than seen in normal individuals). Fibrillation potentials can also be found elsewhere, including in paraspinal muscles. Needle examination is therefore needed for an adequate assessment of patients with suspected diabetic neuropathy.

The abnormalities on nerve conduction studies and needle examination may be present within a month of recognition of the diabetic state in some patients. This finding suggests either of two conclusions: (1) that long periods of hyperglycemia may not be needed to develop this complication or (2) that significant hyperglycemia may have been overlooked for long periods of time.

Moderate Symmetric Peripheral Neuropathy

The electrophysiologic changes in patients with this pattern of clinical findings parallel the clinical findings. Sensory manifestations usually overshadow a mild motor abnormality.

Sensory Neuropathy. In patients with the clinical findings of a sensory neuropathy, the most common and severe abnormality is a reduction in the amplitude of sensory nerve action potentials, particularly in the legs.[20, 56] The sensory potentials often cannot be recorded with standard, surface techniques and require averaging and needle recording electrodes near the nerves. The responses are lost first in the plantar nerves, and then later in the sural and superficial peroneal nerves.[105] When responses can be recorded, they have mildly prolonged latencies and minimally reduced conduction velocities. Needle electrode recordings from sensory nerves show that some fibers are conducting much more slowly. Reduced amplitude sensory nerve action potentials are usually also found in the arms, although to a lesser degree than in the legs. The median antidromic sensory potential recorded from the digit is one of the most reliable measurements of amplitude and is reduced significantly in most patients.[20] The amplitude reduction in the median nerve may be greater than that in the ulnar nerve sensory action potential, most likely because of damage occurring in the carpal tunnel. The radial nerve usually shows the least change in the hand.

Abnormalities in sensory conduction are usually present with each type of measurements, but they may be more prominent in or limited to one of them. For example, some patients have prolongation of distal latencies, others have mainly slowing of conduction ve-

locity, and still others have prolongation of SEP recorded at the neck or lumbar spine. Although the selective abnormalities in any one of these measures could be caused by greater abnormality in the distal, middle, or proximal segments of a nerve, the SEP latency increase may result from the longer segment of nerve being tested.

Motor conduction studies may be normal in diabetic patients with sensory neuropathy, but they most commonly show mild abnormalities. Peroneal conduction velocity is usually in the 30 to 40 m/s range, with amplitudes slightly low or borderline. There is usually an associated reduction in motor unit number estimate. Some patients may also show focal slowing of conduction or, less commonly, focal conduction block, especially of the ulnar nerve at the elbow, the median nerve at the wrist, or the peroneal nerve at the knee. F-wave latencies are on the average longer, just as they are for asymptomatic diabetic patients. Both H reflexes and blink reflexes include sensorimotor components and are also usually of increased latency to a mild or moderate degree in patients with sensory neuropathies.[75, 129]

Most reports of electrophysiologic studies in diabetic patients with sensory neuropathies do not report the findings on EMG. Nearly all patients with sensory neuropathy on clinical evaluation have abnormalities on needle examination. The most common change is impaired recruitment, with an increase in the duration and amplitude of the motor unit potentials. The motor unit potential changes are mild and distal in distribution, with the most apparent changes in the peroneal distribution; however, not infrequently intrinsic hand muscles show the same abnormalities. In up to 25% of patients with sensory neuropathies, there are also fibrillation potentials present, particularly in the intrinsic foot muscles. As in asymptomatic diabetic patients, the abductor hallucis muscle is the most reliably and readily examined of these muscles. Persistent fibrillation potentials in this foot muscle provide evidence of motor axon damage that may not be evident clinically.

Mixed Motor and Sensory Neuropathy. The findings in patients with sensorimotor neuropathies, both adults and children, are similar to those for patients with sensory neuropathies, with an increased frequency and severity of abnormality.[11, 82, 95]

Sensory potentials show the greatest changes, especially in amplitude in the legs, where they are often absent with surface recording methods; arm sensory potentials are abnormally low in 30 to 50% of these patients.[20] Sensory conduction velocities show moderate slowing in the arms to mean values of 40 to 50 m/s. The slowing is due to fiber loss when amplitudes are grossly reduced.[11] Distal sensory latencies are comparably prolonged by 20 to 30%.[39] Somatosensory evoked potentials are prolonged at the spine in 75% of these patients and often cannot be recorded with leg stimulation. Scalp SEP may still be recorded with absent sensory nerve action potentials and can provide estimates of conduction velocity with severe neuropathy.[95]

The characteristic that distinguishes these patients from those with primarily sensory neuropathies is the presence in all of them of more prominent motor conduction abnormality.[48, 56, 83] Compound muscle action potentials and motor unit number estimates in the legs are reduced by an average of 50% or more, with many of the patients having no distal motor responses.[78, 92] Arm amplitudes are generally in the normal range, although with a reduction of the mean value below that of normal subjects. Motor conduction velocities may be as low as 20 m/s, and mean values can be under 30 m/s.[21, 78, 92] The extent of abnormality on nerve conduction studies is generally related to the severity of neuropathy[13, 96] and is reported to parallel the duration of diabetes or metabolic control in some studies,[60, 73, 80–82, 92, 96] especially in children,[45, 55, 117] but it does not in other studies.[53, 73, 79, 123]

Studies of the correlation of duration of diabetes and blood sugar control differ in their conclusions in part because of different patient populations and in part because of the absence of adequate control for the age of the patients and the type of diabetes, which both affect nerve conduction. (See Chapter 18 for a discussion of the relationship of hypoglycemia control in preventing and ameliorating diabetic neuropathy.)

Although the changes on nerve conduction studies are generally worse distally,[76] patients with generalized neuropathies have prolongation of proximal conduction as well, with long F-wave and blink reflex latencies.[75, 129] F-wave latencies are prolonged in proportion to the peripheral slowing of conduction and have as high a frequency of abnormality as peroneal motor conduction velocity. Estimates of the relative proximal and distal slowing can be made by comparing the distal conduction velocities with the F-wave latencies. Although the abnormalities are typically diffuse, usually the slowing is greater distally and worse in the legs in patients with diffuse neuropathies. Blink reflexes are sometimes outside the normal range, and diabetics can have mean values 20% longer than the normal population, indicating that there can be major involvement of the proximal nerves.[75]

It is common to find evidence of localized slowing, and at times of conduction block, in generalized peripheral neuropathy.[56, 95] These changes may not be accompanied by symptoms or signs of focal neuropathy. Individual patients may have focal abnormalities in one or more nerves. Most commonly, prolongation of the median motor and sensory distal latencies with low amplitude sensory nerve action potential is found. This finding is similar to the changes found in carpal tunnel syndrome and makes it more difficult to distinguish superimposed median compression neuropathy at the wrist that warrants specific treatment. No criteria have been published that define the extent of slowing that is evidence of a focal lesion that can be expected to respond to decompression. In general, a superimposed compression neuropathy should be considered in a symptomatic patient when the slowing is greater: (1) in the suspect region, e.g., the carpal tunnel, than in a more distal segment of the nerve; (2) in the suspect region than in other nerves in the same limb; (3) than in the same nerve in the opposite limb; and (4) when the latency is prolonged 1 m/s or more outside the normal range.

Needle examination is abnormal in all patients with generalized sensorimotor deficits. There are motor unit potential changes in all distal muscles of the arms and legs, worse in the legs, with fibrillation potentials in many distal muscles both below the knee and in the intrinsic hand muscles. As many as 20% of these patients have fibrillation potentials in the paraspinal muscles as well.[10]

Painful Neuropathies

Painful neuropathies with diffuse, mainly distal pain, burning, and dysesthesia may have little neurologic deficit on examination. If they do, the changes are similar to those described for moderate, generalized neuropathy.[17] In patients without clinical deficit, the changes can be quite minimal.[7] They usually resemble those in asymptomatic patients with mild reduction in sensory amplitudes and mild slowing of conduction velocity.[17] However, some patients with severe pain have normal EMG and nerve conduction studies. The clinical and electrodiagnostic findings are consistent with involvement of small fibers, which are not tested on standard electrodiagnostic studies. Reports of slow-fiber conduction studies have not included diabetic patients. Computerized estimates of the distribution of conduction velocities (DCV) from the nerve action potentials have shown loss of smaller fibers, but these estimates have not been applied in patients with painful, diabetic neuropathies. The DCV analysis would be unlikely to show abnormalities in this group, because the small pain fibers are not activated in standard nerve conduction studies. In occasional patients there may be prolongation of the F-wave latencies or SEP, indicating the presence of proximal plexus or nerve root damage that may be the source of the painful symptoms. However, it is not clear that these changes are any more prominent in subjects with painful neuropathies than in the general population of diabetic patients.

Proximal Motor Neuropathy

Diabetic amyotrophy is a clinical problem that has been described in the literature under a number of terms described in Chapter 5. It includes proximal motor weakness that may be asymmetric and generally is associated with pain. It will be discussed as a proximal motor neuropathy, because this is the usual electrodiagnostic picture.

The EMG findings are typical enough that when they occur, the pattern of findings can be used to suggest the diagnosis of diabetes.[98] Patients with this disorder have electrophysiologic evidence of a mild or moderate generalized peripheral neuropathy, usually with sensorimotor findings, as described in the earlier sections.[115, 119, 134] The amplitude reductions and slowing of conduction velocity may be mild. The proximal abnormalities are most prominent in the needle examination, but there is often evidence of proximal abnormality in nerve conduction studies as well.[26] In particular, F waves may be absent or slowed out of proportion to the peripheral conduction abnormalities.[24] Blink reflexes may also be prolonged.

The major finding is the presence of prominent fibrillation potentials in proximal muscles, usually with mild to moderate motor unit potential changes.[10, 25] The fibrillation potentials are found most prominently in muscles innervated by L2 to L4 spinal nerves. Although the

femoral-innervated thigh muscles are the most commonly reported as abnormal, iliopsoas, adductor and gracilis muscles are usually also abnormal. Other proximal hip girdle muscles may show fibrillation potentials, but to a lesser extent. The paraspinal muscles typically have extensive fibrillation potentials bilaterally at multiple, lumbar and low thoracic levels. The wide distribution of the paraspinal fibrillation potentials into thoracic levels distinguishes this disorder from lumbar disc diseases.[67] The distribution suggests multiple, lumbosacral radiculopathies, multiple segmental nerve neuropathy, or less likely, spinal cord lesions.[116] Abdominal muscles often also have fibrillation potentials.

Most authors have found the motor unit potential changes of some reduction in recruitment, with an increase in duration and amplitude, but usually of only a mild to moderate degree.[10, 25] The motor unit potential change may be limited to an increase in proportion of polyphasic motor unit potential, especially in the paraspinal muscles. The arms usually show only mild nerve conduction slowing and amplitude reduction with mild increase in motor unit potential size in distal muscles.

The clinical symptoms and signs usually slowly subside. As they do, the fibrillation potentials gradually decrease in density. However, they may remain present for many months after the clinical symptoms of pain or proximal weakness have subsided. The motor unit potential changes remain present indefinitely.

Autonomic Neuropathy

Patients who present clinically with primarily autonomic symptoms and diabetes usually have mild abnormalities on conduction studies.[47, 124] The changes are similar to those described for asymptomatic patients and those occurring with painful neuropathy. There is a high frequency of combined urodynamic and electrophysiologic abnormalities in patients without obvious neuropathy.[19] It appears that the incidence of electrophysiologic changes is greater in autonomic neuropathy than in asymptomatic diabetic subjects.[14, 118]

Although there have been reports of electrophysiologic measurement of autonomic function, none of them has been developed and standardized for routine application in an electromyographic laboratory. Measurement of the skin potential under sympathetic control is used clinically, but it has not been adequately standardized.[77, 84] The recordings from sympathetic axons with intraneural electrodes is too difficult technically for use other than for research or experimental purposes,[50] but it has shown loss of sympathetic function in diabetic patients.[51]

Hyperinsulin Neuropathies

There have been occasional reports of electrophysiologic studies of patients with atrophy associated with hypoglycemia. Most of these have been in patients with insulinomas and have suggested the presence of a neuropathy from excess insulin.[30, 70, 91] Although rare, this possibility should also be considered in a patient with electrophysiologic evidence of neuropathy and diabetes, especially if severe insulin reactions have occurred. The electrophysiologic changes are more those of an axonal neuropathy. There is a loss of compound muscle action potential amplitude, with minimal or no slowing of conduction velocity. The motor fibers are generally more involved than sensory fibers. There is a loss of motor unit potentials with fibrillation potentials prominent in both proximal and distal muscles. Recovery occurs with regeneration of damaged axons rather than collateral sprouting of intact axons.[79]

Focal Neuropathies

Mononeuropathies are common in diabetes and generally occur at the same sites as mononeuropathies in nondiabetic subjects; these occur more frequently and often are multifocal in patients with diabetes. These are not related to the severity, duration, or control of the diabetes.[54, 56] Electromyography and nerve conduction studies readily provide evidence of their presence, severity, and location. Electrophysiologic testing of a diabetic patient with focal symptoms should proceed in the same manner as for a nondiabetic patient with focal symptoms; testing should include, in particular, the common sites of damage such as the ulnar nerve at the elbow and median nerve at the wrist. However, interpretation of results must be more cautious, because the diabetic patient will almost always have some electrophysiologic evidence of a mild, diffuse neuropathy with greater slowing at common sites of compression. Therefore, the investigator cannot rely on comparisons with normal conduction values to identify a superimposed focal neuropathy. Greater slowing than that found at similar sites in diabetic patients without focal lesions must be shown.

The identification of a focal lesion on nerve conduction studies is most reliable if a measurable conduction block is present, because that does not occur in asymptomatic patients. In the absence of conduction block, focal slowing of conduction can be used to identify a focal abnormality, if the slowing is of moderate severity and greater than the slowing in other segments of the nerve and in other nerves in that patient.[20, 97] For example, in a patient with a painful hand, carpal tunnel syndrome cannot be confirmed unless the slowing of conduction in the carpal tunnel is greater than that seen in the ulnar nerve, the contralateral median nerve, and other nerves, and the actual latency value is at least 0.5 if not 1.0 m/s greater than the upper limit of normal.

Mononeuropathies in the Arm. Median neuropathy at the wrist and ulnar neuropathy at the elbow are the most common mononeuropathies in the arm in diabetic patients, just as they are in the general population.[54, 65] The associated electrophysiologic changes are localized slowing of conduction or conduction block (Fig. 16.4). Sensory conduction abnormalities occur before those on motor conduction. Needle examination abnormalities are usually late changes, but they may be seen early with an acute or severe lesion. The changes are similar but of greater severity if the patient has pain, paresthesia, weakness, or atrophy. The best predictor of success of carpal tunnel surgery in diabetic patients is finding localized nerve conduction changes in the carpal tunnel.[4]

An idiopathic brachial plexopathy can occur in patients with diabetes, possibly related to the diabetes. Studies have not compared the incidence of plexopathy in diabetic populations and the general population to determine whether they are chance associations. When brachial plexopathies do occur, they show changes primarily on needle examination with loss of motor unit potentials and prominent fibrillation potentials; occasionally reduction in evoked potential amplitudes is seen with little or no slowing in conduction velocity.

Mononeuropathies in the Leg. Peroneal neuropathy at the knee is the most common focal abnormality in the leg in diabetic patients, who may present with such an abnormality as the first sign of their diabetes.[54, 114]

A localized conduction block is usually seen

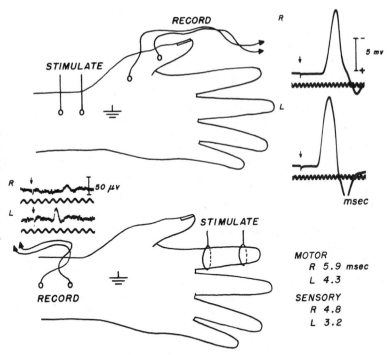

■ **Figure 16–4.** Prolonged motor and sensory distal latencies in the right hand of a patient with carpal tunnel syndrome. The sensory nerve action potential amplitude is reduced on the right as well. (From Clinical Examinations in Neurology, 5th ed. Philadelphia, W. B. Saunders Company, 1981.)

superimposed on generalized slowing of conduction and low amplitude evoked responses. Localized slowing of conduction can occur but should be at least 15 m/s slower than that in the distal segment of the nerve and than in other nerves, to be certain that the slowing is not just part of the generalized neuropathy.

Patients with diabetes sometimes develop major vessel occlusions with secondary ischemic neuropathies, especially in the legs.[32, 102] The electrical picture in these cases typically has signs of a combination of distal nerve and muscle damage. The compound muscle action potentials and sensory nerve action potentials are markedly reduced or absent in all nerves in the involved extremity. Conduction velocities, when they are obtainable, are mildly reduced. Needle examination of muscles shows prominent fibrillation potentials of increasing density in more distal muscles associated with polyphasic motor unit potentials that are mixed in size, both large and small. The muscle often is fibrotic, with a firm resistance to needle insertion.[32]

Lumbosacral plexopathies occur in diabetics with a frequency suggesting a greater incidence than in the general population. Clinically, these can resemble the entity of proximal motor neuropathy described earlier. A plexopathy can be distinguished by the absence of paraspinal fibrillation potentials and the unilateral loss of peripheral sensory nerve action potentials.

Mononeuropathies in the Trunk. The radiculopathies that occur in diabetic patients without compressive or structural lesions can be reliably identified by EMG.[74, 85, 122] In some patients, EMG provides the only explanation of severe abdominal or chest pain in a patient with painful thoracic radiculopathy caused by diabetes. Patients with this disorder usually have mild changes on nerve conduction studies similar to those of asymptomatic diabetic patients or those with a mild sensory neuropathy.[88, 122] The critical findings are prominent fibrillation potentials in a localized area in the paraspinal muscles.[85] These can be identified only by careful examination at multiple paraspinal levels bilaterally, with the patient fully relaxed. Relaxation is best obtained with the patient lying on the side, with back, hips, knees, and head fully flexed. The fibrillation potentials can also be found in the appropriate abdominal muscles or intercostal muscles, a particularly helpful finding when the patient's relaxation is incomplete and paraspinal muscle assessment is difficult. Such focal radiculopathies at the upper lumbar levels can be distinguished from proximal motor neuropathy by the localization of the fibrillation potentials to one side.

Cranial Neuropathies. The increased incidence of facial neuropathy in diabetic patients[1] is associated with a prolonged facial nerve latency.[75] In more severe cases with facial weakness, there is a loss of motor unit potentials and prominent fibrillation potentials.[87] Facial compound muscle action potentials may be markedly reduced, but the facial nerve latency usually shows only mild prolongation. Except for involvement of the fifth nerve on blink reflex testing, neuropathies of other cranial nerves cannot be confirmed on electrical testing.[75]

MONITORING TREATMENT OF DIABETES

In addition to the identification, localization, and definition of severity of neuropathy in diabetes, nerve conduction studies have been used to follow the course of neuropathy during treatment, in particular to identify beneficial effects from treatment. In some early reports of nerve conduction studies in diabetes, a relationship between the control of the diabetes and the extent of abnormality on nerve conduction studies was found.[60, 72, 80, 81] This suggested that nerve conduction studies could be used to monitor the neuropathy more reproducibly than clinical testing. Studies of alternate treatment methods such as intensive therapy,[59, 101, 105, 111] the insulin pump,[90, 100, 112, 113, 130] arterial reconstruction,[5] and drugs[9, 21, 49, 60, 63, 71] have relied heavily on nerve conduction studies to determine the value of the treatments. Each such study must be carefully reviewed to be certain that there are matched controls, that all the necessary variables have been properly controlled (including limb temperature, location of stimulating and recording electrodes, and methods of measurement of amplitude and latency), and that the parameters are measured. Quantitative measurement of amplitudes and latencies should be assessed in addition to the commonly used measurement of conduction velocity. The reproducibility of the measurements should be defined. Changes with time, in both treatment arms, are then compared statistically. When multiple measurements are taken, a change in one of a number of parameters must be shown to be more than a chance occurrence.

Most studies testing a variety of treatment modalities have shown only a small[9, 49, 59, 63, 71, 90, 101, 113, 130, 133] or no change in conduction velocity.[21, 60, 111, 112] Improvements in nerve conduction studies with therapy are sometimes in only one or two nerves that could occur by chance. The most significant changes have been seen in F-wave latency, SEP, and sensory nerve action potentials. Intensive diabetes treatment to achieve strict control of hyperglycemia has slowed the progression of abnormalities compared with controls.[94, 113] Clear improvement of the major abnormalities have been shown in conduction studies in patients undergoing pancreatic transplantation and early in the treatment of children.[3, 117, 94]

SPECIAL ELECTRICAL TESTS

A number of specialized electrical tests have been used in diabetic patients to provide information about the pathophysiology of the disease and the severity of the neuropathy and to recognize subclinical abnormalities not shown with EMG and nerve conduction studies. The DCV method (described earlier) of determining the distribution of conduction velocities is one such test.[38] A number of others are being used.

Evoked Response Testing

The abnormalities of SEP recorded from the spine and scalp have been described earlier.[28, 64] Visual-evoked potentials and auditory-evoked potentials have also been measured in diabetic subjects and show minimal or no abnormalities.[37, 52, 132] Changes, when present, may be related to longer duration of disease.

Refractory Period Testing

Normal nerve has an upper limit to the rate at which it can conduct impulses, which is defined by the refractory period. Stimulating a nerve with paired stimuli at short intervals can determine the length of the refractory period. Refractory period testing has been suggested as another method of identifying subclinical neuropathy. Refractory periods are abnormal in patients with diabetes, not only in those with clinical or electrical evidence of neuropathy but also in those with normal nerve conduction studies.[109, 125] Rapid, repetitive stimulation depends on the refractory period and is abnormal in diabetic patients with and without neuropathy; their nerves cannot conduct impulses at rates as rapid as those in normal persons.[89, 125]

Accommodation and Resistance to Ischemia

Nerve conduction in diabetic subjects, as in patients with other metabolic neuropathies, is more resistant to ischemia than in normal subjects and is correlated with control of diabetes.[62, 69, 110] Resistance to ischemia has been recommended as the most sensitive indicator of peripheral nerve dysfunction in diabetes. The phenomenon appears to be the result of lower metabolic needs for maintaining conduction in a partially depolarized nerve.[106] Recent studies tracking axonal threshold by accommodation and other tests of membrane function have provided further insight into the membrane abnormalities of metabolic and toxic neuropathies.[12] Diabetic distal latencies show a greater sensitivity to alcohol than those in normal subjects.[72]

Motor Unit Number Estimates

The reduction in number of motor units in a muscle because of peripheral nerve disease can be estimated in cooperative subjects with graded, threshold stimulation during nerve conduction studies.[18, 31] The method requires careful attention to recording methods and well-defined normal values. Moderate to severe reductions in number of motor units have been found in patients with diabetic neuropathy, even without clinical evidence of neuropathy.[18, 65]

Single-Fiber Electromyography

Quantitative measurements of the motor unit potentials with a very small electrode can measure the density of fibers innervated by a single motor unit (fiber density) and minimal abnormalities of neuromuscular transmission (jitter).[16, 120, 127] These methods show changes in fiber density or jitter in patients with diabetic neuropathy, especially with more severe abnormalities. In some patients, SFEMG may detect abnormalities before nerve conduction.[22] Reinnervation does not occur as extensively as it does in some other neuropathies, either because of less axonal destruction or limited capacity for regeneration.

Macro Electromyography

A method of recording averaged motor unit potentials in a muscle with a long recording surface on a needle electrode while triggering with a separate single-fiber electrode provides a better estimate of the size of motor units in a muscle. This method helps to distinguish slow, chronic disorders from more rapid processes, and it distinguishes disorders with a capability for reinnervation from those without.[119] Macro EMG in diabetic patients has had only limited application.

CONCLUSION

Diabetic patients with or without clinical evidence of neuropathy have prominent, diffuse, and multifocal abnormalities of nerve conduction and EMG. The multifocal nature of the neurophysiologic abnormalities must be taken into account in postulations regarding mechanisms causing a neuropathy, providing evidence of focal damage of the type that might occur with an ischemic or immune-mediated neuropathy.

References

1. Adour KK, Wingerd JW, Doty HE. Prevalence of concurrent diabetes mellitus and idiopathic facial paralysis (Bell's palsy). Diabetes 1975, 24:449.
2. Albers JW, Brown MB, Sima AA, et al. Nerve conduction measures in mild diabetic neuropathy. Neurology 1996, 46:85–91.
3. Allen RD, Al-Harbi IS, Morris JG, et al. Diabetic neuropathy after pancreas transplantation. Transplantation 1997, 63:830–838.
4. Al-Qattan MM, Manktelow RT, Bowen CV. Outcome of carpal tunnel release in diabetic patients. J Hand Surg 1994, 19:626–629.
5. Akbari CM, Gibbons GW, Habershaw, et al. The effect of arterial reconstruction on the natural history of diabetic neuropathy. Arch Surg 1997; 132:148–152.
6. Anderson H, Stalberg E, Falck B. F-wave latency: The most sensitive nerve conduction parameter in patients with diabetes mellitus. Muscle Nerve 1997; 20:1296.
7. Archer AG, Watkins PJ, Thomas PK, et al. The natural history of acute painful neuropathy in diabetes mellitus. J Neurol Neurosurg Psychiatry 1983; 46:491.
8. Argyropoulos CJ, Panayiotopoulos CP, Scarpalezos S, et al. F-wave and M-response conduction velocity in diabetes mellitus. EMG Clin Neurophysiol 1979; 19:443.
9. Bassi S, Albizzati MG, Calloni E, et al. Electromyographic study of diabetic and alcoholic polyneuropathic patients treated with gangliosides. Muscle Nerve 1982; 5:351.
10. Bastron JA, Thomas JE. Diabetic polyradiculopathy: Clinical and electromyographic findings in 105 patients. Mayo Clin Proc 1981; 56:725.
11. Behse F, Buchthal F, Carlsen F. Nerve biopsy and conduction studies in diabetic neuropathy. J Neurol Neurosurg Psychiatry 1977; 40:1072.
12. Bostock H, Cikurei K, Burke D. Threshold tracking techniques in the study of human peripheral nerve. Muscle Nerve 1998; 21:137–158.
13. Braddom RL, Hollis JB, Castell DO. Diabetic peripheral neuropathy: A correlation of nerve conduction

studies and clinical findings. Arch Phys Med Rehab 1977; 58:308.

14. Braune HJ. Early detection of diabetic neuropathy: A neurophysiologic study on 100 patients. EMG Clin Neurophys 1997; 37:399–407.

15. Bril V. Role of electrophysiological studies in diabetic neuropathy. Can J Neurol Sci 1994; 21:8–12.

16. Bromberg MB, Scott DM, Ad Hoc Committee of the AAEM Single Fiber Special Interest Group (member). Single fiber EMG reference values: Reformatted in tabular form. Muscle Nerve 1994; 17:820–821.

17. Brown MJ, Martin JR, Asbury AK. Painful diabetic neuropathy: A morphometric study. Arch Neurol 1976; 33:164.

18. Brown WF, Feasby T. Estimates of motor axon loss in diabetics. J Neurol Sci 1974; 23:275.

19. Buck AC, Reed PI, Siddiq YK, et al. Bladder dysfunction and neuropathy in diabetes. Diabetologia 1976; 12:251.

20. Casey EB, Le Quesne PM. Digital nerve action potentials in healthy subjects, and in carpal tunnel and diabetic patients. J Neurol Neurosurg Psychiatry 1972; 35:612.

21. Chakrabarti AK, Samantaray SK. Diabetic peripheral neuropathy: Nerve conduction studies before, during and after carbamazepine therapy. Aust NZ J Med 1976; 6:565.

22. Chang CW, Chuang LM. Correlation of HbA1c concentration and single fiber EMG findings in diabetic neuropathy. EMG Clin Neurophys 1996; 36:425–432.

23. Chaudry V, Corse AM, Freimer ML, et al. Inter- and intraexaminer reliability of nerve conduction measurements in patients with diabetic neuropathy. Neurology 1994; 44:1459–1462.

24. Chokroverty S. Proximal nerve dysfunction in diabetic proximal amyotrophy: Electrophysiology and electron microscopy. Arch Neurol 1982; 39:403.

25. Chokroverty S, Teyes MG, Rubino FA, et al. The syndrome of diabetic amyotrophy. Ann Neurol 1977; 2:181.

26. Chopra JS, Hurwitz LJ. Femoral nerve conduction in diabetes and chronic occlusive vascular disease. J Neurol Neurosurg Psychiatry 1968; 31:28.

27. Claus D, Mustafa C, Vogel W, et al. Assessment of diabetic neuropathy. Muscle Nerve 1993; 16:757–768.

28. Cracco J, Castells S, Mark E. Spinal somatosensory evoked potentials in juvenile diabetes. Ann Neurol 1984; 15:55.

29. Cummins KL, Dorfman LJ. Nerve conduction velocity distributions: Studies of normal and diabetic human nerves. Ann Neurol 1981; 9:67.

30. Danta G. Hypoglycemic peripheral neuropathy. Arch Neurol 1969; 21:121.

31. Daube JR. Estimating the number of motor units in a muscle. J Clin Neurophysiol 1995; 12:585–594.

32. Daube JR, Dyck PJ. Neuropathy due to peripheral vascular diseases. In Dyck PJ, et al (eds): Peripheral Neuropathy. Philadelphia, WB Saunders, 1984, p 1458.

33. Daube JR. Clinical applications of recent developments in EMG. In Struppler A, Weindl A (eds): Electromyography and Evoked Potentials. New York, Springer-Verlag, 1985, p 123.

34. Daube JR. Nerve conduction studies. In Aminoff MJ (ed): Electromyography in Clinical Practice, ed 4. Addison-Wesley, 1998.

35. Department of Neurology. Clinical Examinations in Neurology, ed 7. Philadelphia, WB Saunders, 1997.

36. Dioszeghy P, Stelberg E. Changes in motor and sensory nerve conduction parameters with temperature

in normal and diseased nerve. EEG Clin Neurophysiol 1992; 85:229–235.

37. Donald MW, Bird CE, Lawson JS, et al. Delayed auditory brainstem responses in diabetes mellitus. J Neurol Neurosurg Psychiatry 1981; 44:641.

38. Dorfman LJ, Cummins KL, Reaven GM, et al. Studies of diabetic polyneuropathy using conduction velocity distribution (DCV) analysis. Neurology 1983; 33:773.

39. Downie AW, Newell DJ. Sensory nerve conduction in patients with diabetes mellitus and controls. Neurology 1961; 11:876.

40. Dyck PJ, Davies JL, Litchy WJ, et al. Longitudinal assessment of diabetic polyneuropathy using a composite score in the Rochester Diabetic Neuropathy Study cohort. Neurology 1997; 49:229–239.

41. Dyck PJ, Karnes JL, O'Brien PC, et al. The Rochester Diabetic Neuropathy Study: Reassessment of tests and criteria for diagnosis. Neurology 1992; 42:1164–1170.

42. Dyck PJ, Melton LJ, O'Brien PC, et al. Approaches to improve epidemiological studies of diabetic neuropathy. Diabetes 1997; 46(suppl 2):S5–8.

43. Duck SC, Wei FF, Parke J, et al. Role of height and glycosylated hemoglobin in abnormal nerve conduction in pediatric patients with type 1 diabetes. Diabetes Care 1991; 14:386–392.

44. Eeg-Olofsson O, Petersen I. Childhood diabetic neuropathy: A clinical and neurophysiological study. Acta Paediatr Scand 1966; 55:163.

45. Eng GD, Hung W, August GP, et al. Nerve conduction velocity determinations in juvenile diabetics: Continuing study of 190 patients. Arch Phys Med Rehab 1976; 57:1.

46. Eriksson KF, Nilsson H, Lindgarde F, et al. Diabetes mellitus but not impaired glucose tolerance is associated with dysfunction in peripheral nerves. Diabetic Med 1994; 11:279–285.

47. Ewing DJ, Burt AA, Williams IR, et al. Peripheral motor nerve function in diabetic autonomic neuropathy. J Neurol Neurosurg Psychiatry 1976; 39:453.

48. Fagerberg SE, Petersen I, Steg G, et al. Motor disturbances in diabetes mellitus: A clinical study using electromyography and conduction velocity determination. Acta Med Scand 1963; 174:711.

49. Fagius J, Jameson S. Effects of aldose reductase inhibitor treatment in diabetic polyneuropathy—a clinical and neurophysiological study. J Neurol Neurosurg Psychiatry 1981; 44:991.

50. Fagius J, Wallin B. Sympathetic reflex latencies and conduction velocity in normal man. J Neurol Sci 1980; 47:433.

51. Fagius J, Wallin BG. Sympathetic reflex latencies and conduction velocities in patients with polyneuropathy. J Neurol Sci 1980; 47:449.

52. Fedele D, Martini A, Cardone C, et al. Impaired auditory brainstem-evoked responses in insulin-dependent diabetic subjects. Diabetes 1984; 33:1085.

53. Fedele D, Negrin P, Fardin P, et al. Motor conduction velocity (MCV) in insulin-dependent and noninsulin-dependent diabetics with and without clinical peripheral neuropathy. Diabete Metab 1980; 6:189.

54. Fraser DM, Campbell IW, Ewing DJ, et al. Mononeuropathy in diabetes mellitus. Diabetes 1979; 28:96.

55. Gamstorp I, Shelburns SA, Engelson G, et al. Peripheral neuropathy in juvenile diabetics. Diabetes 1966; 15:411.

56. Gilliatt RW, Willison RG. Peripheral nerve conduction in diabetic neuropathy. J Neurol Neurosurg Psychiatry 1962; 25:11.

57. Ginzburg M, Lee M, Ginzburg J, et al. Changes in the Erb's point-axilla conduction velocity in motor nerves in the early electrodiagnostic detection of latent diabetic neuropathy. EMG Clin Neurophysiol 1983; 23:303.
58. Graf RJ, Halter JB, Halar E, et al. Nerve conduction abnormalities in untreated maturity onset diabetes: Relationship to levels of fasting plasma glucose and glycosylated hemoglobin. Ann Intern Med 1979; 90:298.
59. Graf RJ, Halter JB, Pfeifer MA, et al. Glycemic control and nerve conduction abnormalities in non-insulin-dependent diabetic subjects. Ann Intern Med 1981; 94:307.
60. Greene DA, Brown MJ, Braunstein SN, et al. Comparison of clinical course and sequential electrophysiological tests in diabetics with symptomatic polyneuropathy and its implications for clinical trials. Diabetes 1981; 30:139.
61. Gregersen G. Diabetic neuropathy: Influence of age, sex, metabolic control, and duration of diabetes on motor conduction velocity. Neurology 1967; 17:972.
62. Gregersen G. A study of the peripheral nerves in diabetic subjects during ischaemia. J Neurol Neurosurg Psychiatry 1968; 31:75.
63. Gregersen G, Borsting H, Theil P, et al. Myoinositol and function of peripheral nerves in human diabetics. Acta Neurol Scand 1978; 58:241.
64. Gupta PR, Dorfman LJ. Spinal somatosensory conduction in diabetes. Neurology 1981; 31:841.
65. Hansen S, Ballantyne JP. Axonal dysfunction in the neuropathy of diabetes mellitus: A quantitative electrophysiological study. J Neurol Neurosurg Psychiatry 1977; 40:555.
66. Hendriksen PH, Oey PL, Wieneke GH, et al. Subclinical diabetic polyneuropathy: Early detection. J Neurol Neurosurg Psychiatry 1993; 56:509–514.
67. Hirsh LF. Diabetic polyradiculopathy simulating lumbar disc disease. Report of four cases. J Neurosurg 1984; 60:183.
68. Horn S, Quastoff S, Grafe P, et al. Abnormal axonal inward rectification in diabetic neuropathy. Muscle Nerve 1996; 19:1268–1275.
69. Horowitz SH, Ginsberg-Fellner F. Ischemia and sensory nerve conduction in diabetes mellitus. Neurology 1979; 29:695.
70. Jaspan JB, Wollman RL, Bernstein L, et al. Hypoglycemic peripheral neuropathy in association with insulinoma: Implication of glucopenia rather than hyperinsulinism. Medicine 1982; 61:33.
71. Judzewitsch RG, Jaspan JB, Polonsky KS, et al. Aldose reductase inhibition improves nerve conduction velocity in diabetic patients. N Engl J Med 1983; 308:119.
72. Juntunen J, Salmi T, Sainio K, et al. Acute effects of alcohol on the peripheral nerves in diabetic polyneuropathy: A clinical and neurophysiological study. J Neurol Neurosurg Psychiatry 1982; 45:452.
73. Kaar M-L, Saukkonen M, Pitkanen M, et al. Peripheral neuropathy in diabetic children and adolescents. A cross-sectional study. Acta Paediat Scand 1983; 72:373.
74. Kikta DG, Breuer AC, Wilbourn AJ. Thoracic root pain in diabetes: The spectrum of clinical and electromyographic findings. Ann Neurol 1982; 11:80.
75. Kimura J. An evaluation of the facial and trigeminal nerves in polyneuropathy: Electrodiagnostic study in Charcot-Marie-Tooth disease, Guillain-Barré syndrome, and diabetic neuropathy. Neurology 1971; 21:745.
76. Kimura J, Yamada T, Stevland NP. Distal slowing of motor nerve conduction velocity in diabetic polyneuropathy. J Neurol Sci 1979; 42:291.
77. Knezevic WV, Bajada S. Peripheral autonomic surface potential: A quantitative technique for recording sympathetic conduction in man. J Neurol Sci 1985; 67:239.
78. Kraft GH, Guyton JD, Huffman JD. Follow-up study of motor nerve conduction velocities in patients with diabetes mellitus. Arch Phys Med Rehab 1970; 51:207.
79. Lambert EH, Mulder DW, Bastron JA. Regeneration of peripheral nerves with hyperinsulin neuronopathy. Neurology 1960; 10:851.
80. Lamontagne A, Buchthal F. Electrophysiological studies in diabetic neuropathy. J Neurol Neurosurg Psychiatry 1970; 33:442.
81. Laor A, Bialik V, Kanter Y. Study of risk factors for nerve conduction abnormalities in diabetes. EMG Clin Neurophysiol 1985; 25:175.
82. Laor A, Kanter Y, Bialik V. Prediction of diabetic vascular complications by nerve conduction data. Israel J Med Sci 1984; 20:505.
83. Lawrence DE, Locke S. Motor nerve conduction velocity in diabetes. Arch Neurol 1961; 5:483.
84. Levy DM, Reid G, Rowley DA, et al. Quantitative measures of sympathetic skin response in diabetes. J Neurol Neurosurg Psychiatry 1992; 55:902–908.
85. Longstreth GF, Newcomer AD. Abdominal pain caused by diabetic radiculopathy. Ann Intern Med 1977; 86:166.
86. Ludvigsson J, Johannesson G, Heding L, et al. Sensory nerve conduction velocity and vibratory sensibility in juvenile diabetes. Relationship to endogenous insulin. Acta Paediatr Scand 1979; 68:739.
87. Lundgren A, et al. Facial palsy in diabetes mellitus. Adv Otorhinolaryngol 1977; 22:182.
88. Massey EW. Diabetic truncal mononeuropathy: Electromyographic evaluation. Acta Diabet Lat 1980; 17:269.
89. Miglietta O. Neuromuscular transmission defect in diabetes. Diabetes 1973; 22:719.
90. Morrell B, Meyer M, Porr O, et al. Microalbuminuria and nerve conduction velocity in type I diabetes during conventional therapy and during continuous IV insulin infusion. Acta Diabet Lat 1984; 21:303.
91. Mulder DW, Bastron JA, Lambert EH. Hyperinsulin neuronopathy. Neurology 1956; 6:627.
92. Mulder DW, Lambert EH, Bastron JA, et al. The neuropathies associated with diabetes mellitus. Neurology 1961; 11:275.
93. Multicenter Group. Effect of intensive diabetes treatment on nerve conduction. Ann Neurol 1995; 38:869–880.
94. Navarro X, Sutherland DE, Kennedy WR. Long-term effects of pancreatic transplantation on diabetic neuropathy. Ann Neurol 1997; 42:727.
95. Noel P. Sensory nerve conduction in the upper limbs at various stages of diabetic neuropathy. J Neurol Neurosurg Psychiatry 1973; 36:786.
96. Odusote K, Ohivovoriale A, Roberts O. Electrophysiologic quantification of distal neuropathy in diabetes. Neurology 1985; 35:1432.
97. Padua L, Monaco LO, Valente EM. A useful electrophysiologic parameter for diagnosis of carpal tunnel syndrome. Muscle Nerve 1996; 19:48.
98. Pascoe MK, Low PA, Windebank AJ, et al. Subacute diabetic proximal neuropathy. Mayo Clinic Proc 1997; 72:1123–1132.
99. Palma V, Serra LL, Armentano V, et al. Somatosensory evoked potentials in non-insulin dependent diabetics with neuropathy. Diabetes Res 1994; 25:91–96.

100. Pietri A, Ehle AL, Raskin P. Changes in nerve conduction velocity after six weeks of glucoregulation with portable insulin infusion pumps. Diabetes 1980; 29:668.

101. Porter D Jr, Graf RJ, Halter JB, et al. Diabetic neuropathy and plasma glucose control. Am J Med 1981; 70:195.

102. Raff MC, Asbury AK. Ischemic mononeuropathy and mononeuritis multiplex in diabetes mellitus. N Engl J Med 1968; 279:17.

103. Ratzmann KP, Raschke M, Gander I, et al. Prevalence of peripheral and autonomic neuropathy in newly diagnosed type II diabetes. J Diabetic Complications 1991; 5:1–5.

104. Redmond JM, Mckenna MJ, Feingold M, et al. Sensory testing versus nerve conduction velocity in diabetic polyneuropathy. Muscle Nerve 1992; 15:1334–1339.

105. Reeves ML, Seigler DE, Ayyar DR, et al. Medial plantar sensory response. Sensitive indicator of peripheral nerve dysfunction in patients with diabetes mellitus. Am J Med 1984; 76:842.

106. Ritchie JM. Note on the mechanism of resistance to anoxia and ischemia in pathophysiological mammalian nerve. J Neurol Neurosurg Psychiatry 1985; 48:244.

107. Robinson LR, Stolov WC, Rubner DE. Height is an independent risk factor for neuropathy in diabetic men. Diabetes Res 1992; 16:97–102.

108. Sangiorgio L, Iemmolo R, LeMoli R, et al. Diabetic neuropathy: Prevalence, concordance between clinical and electrophysiologic testing. Panminerva Med 1997; 39:1–5.

109. Schutt P, Muche H, Lehmann HJ. Refractory period impairment in sural nerves of diabetics. J Neurol 1983; 229:113.

110. Seneviratne KN, Peiris OA. Effect of ischaemia on the excitability of sensory nerves in diabetes mellitus. J Neurol Neurosurg Psychiatry 1968; 31:348.

111. Service FJ, Daube JR, O'Brien PC, et al. Effect of blood glucose control on peripheral nerve function in diabetic patients. Mayo Clin Proc 1983; 58:283.

112. Service FJ, Daube JR, O'Brien PC, et al. Effect of artificial pancreas treatment on peripheral nerve function in diabetes. Neurology 1981; 31:375.

113. Service FJ, Rizza RA, Daube JR, et al. Near normoglycemia improved nerve conduction and vibration sensation in diabetic neuropathy. Diabetologia 1985; 28:722–727.

114. Shahani B, Spalding JMK. Diabetes mellitus presenting with bilateral foot-drop. Lancet 1969; 2:930.

115. Skanse B, Gydell K. A rare type of femoral-sciatic neuropathy in diabetes mellitus. Acta Med Scand 1956; 155:463.

116. Slager UT. Diabetic myelopathy. Arch Pathol Lab Med 1978; 102:467.

117. Solders G, Thalme B, Brandt L, et al. Nerve conduction and autonomic nerve function in diabetic children: A 10-year follow-up study. Acta Paediatr 1997; 86:361–366.

118. Spitzer A, Lang E, Claus D, et al. Cardiac autonomic involvement and peripheral nerve function in patients with diabetic neuropathy. Funct Neurol 1997; 12:115–122.

119. Stalberg E, Fawcett P. Macro EMG in healthy subjects of different ages. J Neurol Neurosurg Psychiatry 1982; 45:870.

120. Stalberg E, Trontelj JV. Single Fiber Electromyography. New York, Raven Press, 1994.

121. Subramony SH, Wilbourn AJ. Diabetic proximal neuropathy; clinical and electromyographic studies. J Neurol Sci 1982; 53:293–301.

122. Sun SF, Streib EW. Diabetic thoracoabdominal neuropathy: Clinical and electrodiagnostic features. Ann Neurol 1981; 9:75.

123. Tackmann W, Kaeser HE, Berger W, et al. Sensory and motor parameters in leg nerves of diabetics: Intercorrelations and relationships to clinical symptoms. Eur Neurol 1981; 20:344.

124. Tackmann W, Kaeser HE, Berger W, et al. Autonomic disturbances in relation to sensorimotor peripheral neuropathy in diabetes mellitus. J Neurol 1981; 224:273.

125. Tackmann W, Lehmann HJ. Conduction of electrically elicited impulses in peripheral nerves of diabetic patients. Eur Neurol 1980; 19:20.

126. Tchen PH, Fu CC, Chiu HC. Motor evoked potentials in diabetes mellitus. J Form Med Assoc 1992; 91:20–23.

127. Thiele K, Stalberg E. Single fiber EMG findings in polyneuropathies of different etiology. J Neurol Neurosurg Psychiatry 1975; 38:881.

128. Tjon-A-Tsien AM, Lamkes HH, van der Kamp-Huyts AJ, et al. Large electrodes improve nerve conduction repeatability in controls as well as in patients with diabetic neuropathy. Muscle Nerve 1996; 19:689–695.

129. Troni W. Analysis of conduction velocity in H pathway. Part 2. An electrophysiological study in diabetic polyneuropathy. J Neurol Sci 1981; 51:235.

130. Troni W, Carta Q, Cantello R, et al. Peripheral nerve function and metabolic control in diabetes mellitus. Ann Neurol 1984; 16:178.

131. Tsigos C, White A, Young RJ. Discrimination between painful and painless diabetic neuropathy. Diabetes Med 1992; 9:359–365.

132. Verma A, Bisht MS, Ahuja GK. Involvement of central nervous system in diabetes mellitus. J Neurol Neurosurg Psychiatry 1984; 47:414.

133. Ward JD, Barnes CG, Fisher DJ, et al. Improvement in nerve conduction following treatment in newly diagnosed diabetics. Lancet 1971; 1:428.

134. Williams IR, Mayer RF. Subacute proximal diabetic neuropathy. Neurology 1976; 26:108.

Diabetic Polyneuropathy

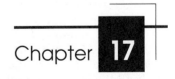

Chapter 17

Epidemiology

L. Joseph Melton III • Peter James Dyck

INTRODUCTION

Although originally developed to investigate epidemics of infectious diseases, epidemiology today has evolved to include studies of the distribution and determinants of disease in general. Epidemiologic investigators may report on descriptive studies of the frequency and impact of disease in different populations as well as analytic studies of risk factors for disease onset or progression; all are relevant to the problem of diabetic neuropathy. It is necessary to know the impact of neuropathy on persons with diabetes and on society because this establishes its priority for research support and for the instigation of control efforts. Equally important is the description of frequency and natural history of diabetic neuropathy because this provides an opportunity to generate hypotheses about etiology and facilitates the identification of high-risk populations for screening, prophylaxis, or therapy. Unfortunately, many gaps and discrepancies exist in the currently available data, which are discussed later in the chapter. In this chapter, the frequency and impact of diabetic neuropathy are covered in general terms, and some of the factors responsible for the generally poor quality of epidemiologic data on this subject are assessed. We describe what is known about the incidence, prevalence, and risk factors for diabetic polyneuropathy that have been discovered in epidemiologic investigations. Other forms of neuropathy are discussed in Chapters 30 to 39.

IMPACT OF DIABETIC NEUROPATHY

Improved estimates of the magnitude of the health problem resulting from diabetic neuropathy would permit better planning by public health agencies, medical care providers, the pharmaceutical industry, and lay health societies. Thus, it is necessary to estimate not only the frequency but the actual health burden of the condition. To illustrate, the frequency of absent ankle reflexes or decreased perception to the tuning fork provides some information about the prevalence of diabetic polyneuropathy but little meaningful information about its implications for poor health. What is needed are data on the frequency of symptoms of pain, weakness or unsteadiness, impotence, and so on, as well as measures of the overall severity of neuropathy and the impact this has on reduced quality of life, work loss resulting from disability, etc. None of these aspects have been particularly well documented. There has been real improvement in estimating the severity of diabetic polyneuropathy, but more needs to be known about morbidity, mortality and the contribution of neuropathy to plantar ulcers, Charcot's joints, and other poor outcomes and to overall social costs.

Mortality

As measured by death certificate data on the underlying cause of death, neuropathy appears to contribute little to mortality. In the United States in 1991, only 2096 deaths (from a total of almost 2.2 million) were attributed to all diseases of the peripheral nervous system combined.[36] Even among those with diabetes, deaths are rarely assigned to neuropathy. From 48,951 deaths attributed to diabetes in the United States in 1991, only 329 referred to diabetes with neurologic manifestations of any kind.[36] However, national death data are notoriously incomplete; diabetes appears on the death certificate in less than half of all deaths among diabetic patients.[16] Moreover, limitations on the number of conditions that can be listed and certain conventions in assigning the cause of death probably contribute to the underrepresentation of neuropathy on death certificates. For example, cardiovascular disease is responsible for about half of all diabetic deaths, but the possible role of autonomic neuropathy in sudden unexpected death has not been fully accounted for.

Morbidity

In contrast with the almost complete lack of information about neuropathy-related mortality, data on the morbidity associated with diabetic neuropathy exist but are difficult to interpret. For example, estimates of the proportion of diabetics having neuropathy have ranged from 5 to 100%.[52] The 1965 National Health Interview Survey found that in the month preceding interview, 26.5% of diabetic persons in the sample experienced extreme tiredness, 22.5% had leg pain, and 18.6% had sudden weakness.[1] The nature of these complaints was not further characterized and, although they may be attributable to diabetic neuropathy, such symptoms are not rare in the general population. More recently, the National Health Interview Survey questioned a large representative sample of United States adults specifically about symptoms of sensory neuropathy, defined as a positive history in the previous 3 months of numbness or loss of feeling in the hands or feet, painful sensations or tingling in the hands or feet, or decreased ability to feel hot or cold.[19] Among those with self-reported diabetes, 37.9% had one or more of these symptoms, compared with only about 10% of the population without diabetes. However, the extent to which diabetics are more likely to report such symptoms is unknown, and the testing instrument was unable to discriminate diabetic polyneuropathy from other disorders.

Data are similarly limited with respect to the impact of neuropathy on functional status, although an abundance of anecdotal information suggests that a substantial number of diabetic individuals are incapacitated by pain, weakness, chronic diarrhea, neurotropic ulcers resulting in some cases in lower extremity amputation, or orthostatic hypotension; sexual impotence in men is also a common complaint.[52] The National Nursing Home Survey found that 6.2% of all nursing home residents had "paralysis or palsy" not related to stroke, arthritis, or rheumatism,[49] but the etiology of the condition was not further specified. Although diabetes had been diagnosed in 13.3% of all residents, it is not known whether diabetic neuropathy precipitated the institutionalization of any of these individuals. It has long been held that real disability is present in 40% of diabetic neuropathy patients,[28] but this is almost certainly an overestimate resulting from referral bias (see Methodological Problems, Research Setting). It has been reported that 44% of patients with type 1 diabetes mellitus (DM) who have "definite" neuropathy have a disability, and 74% of patients with type 2 DM who have sensory neuropathy have some limitations in activity.[51] Men with type 1 DM and neuropathy have much lower levels of physical activity.[25] However, the most detailed population-based study found a much lower frequency of serious polyneuropathy.[7]

Cost

Although the complications of diabetes are said to account for more than 40% of the total economic impact of the condition,[21] limitations of the diagnostic coding system preclude the collection of detailed national data concerning medical services used in the care of diabetic neuropathy. Recent data on hospitalizations for neuropathy and related disorders, for example, are shown in Table 17.1. Diabetic polyneuropathy was listed as a discharge diagnosis on 92,000 occasions in the United States in 1991, but it was rarely the first-listed diagnosis, that is, the reason for admission.[17] Unfortunately, this figure cannot be used to assess the frequency of the condition in the population because episodes of hospitalization were counted and not individual patients. The role, if any, of diabetes in the remaining admissions for neuropathy that are enumerated in Table 17.1 is unclear. In the same year, 175,000 patients were discharged with a diagnosis of "diabetes with neurological manifestations." Only 25,000 of these hospitalizations listed diabetes with neurologic manifestations as the primary diagnosis.[17] However, even this subset of cases was associated with 153,000 days of hospital care.

This compares with more than 3 million hospital days for all first-listed discharge diagnoses for diabetes in the United States in 1991. Interestingly, this represents a substantial reduction from the 440,000 hospital days attributed to the neurologic manifestations of diabetes in 1983,[24] before the introduction of measures to reduce the frequency and duration of hospitalizations generally.

Data on outpatient care in the United States are collected by the National Ambulatory Medical Care Survey. In 1985, there were 26,000 visits to primary care providers (in this instance including endocrinologists and diabetologists as well as general internists and family practitioners) for neurologic complications of diabetes and 12,000 visits to other specialists for this problem.[18] The latter appears to be an undercount because there were 50,000 visits to neurologists by diabetic individuals. There were a total of 8.1 million diabetes-related visits to primary care physicians and 1.9 million visits to specialists. One regional survey has shown that neurologic conditions (neuropathy, autonomic insufficiency, paresthesias, and impotence) were responsible for an average of 0.3 clinic encounters per patient per year and 0.2 hospitalizations per year of follow-up among diabetic individuals.[2] By comparison, all diabetes-related conditions accounted for an average of 9.2 clinic visits and 1.3 hospitalizations per year of follow-up among the diabetic residents of that community.

Expenditures for the care of diabetic neuropathy, including inpatient and outpatient services, were estimated at $240 million in 1986.[21] The details are shown in Table 17.2. Altogether,

TABLE 17.1 DISCHARGES FROM SHORT-STAY NONFEDERAL HOSPITALS IN 1991, BY FIRST-LISTED AND ALL-LISTED DIAGNOSES

Category	First-Listed Diagnoses		All-Listed Diagnoses
	Number	*Days of Care*	*Number*
Disorders of autonomic nervous system	5,000	29,000	48,000
Peripheral autonomic neuropathy in disorders classified elsewhere	—	—	35,000
Trigeminal nerve disorders	8,000	38,000	15,000
Facial nerve disorders	—	—	23,000
Disorders of other cranial nerves	—	—	—
Nerve root and plexus disorders	7,000	23,000	16,000
Mononeuritis of upper limb and mononeuritis multiplex	21,000	34,000	56,000
Mononeuritis of lower limb	7,000	27,000	28,000
Hereditary and idiopathic peripheral neuropathy	8,000	71,000	51,000
Inflammatory and toxic neuropathy	7,000	111,000	107,000
Polyneuropathy in diabetes	—	—	92,000

From Graves EJ. Detailed diagnoses and procedures, National Hospital Discharge Survey, 1991. National Center for Health Statistics. Hyattsville, MD, DHHS Publication No. PHS 94-1776, Vital Health Stat 13(115), 1994.

TABLE 17.2 HEALTH CARE EXPENDITURES IN 1986 ATTRIBUTABLE TO TYPE 2 DIABETES MELLITUS, BY CONDITION AND TYPE OF SERVICE (IN $ MILLIONS)

	Type of Service					
Condition	Hospital	Physician	Drugs	Nursing Home	Other	Total
Diabetes mellitus*	2626	1478	593	2019	117	6833
Circulatory disorders	1692	508	177	1386	86	3849
Visual disorders	141	156	42	33	15	387
Neuropathy	218	14	5	0	3	240
Nephropathy	87	10	4	0	3	104
Skin ulcers	106	26	10	0	3	145
Total	4870	2192	831	3438	227	11,558

*Includes diabetic ketoacidosis, diabetic coma, and unspecified diabetic complications.
From Huse DM, Oster G, Killen AR, et al. The economic costs of non-insulin-dependent diabetes mellitus. JAMA 1989; 262(19):2708.

$218 million (91%) of total health care expenditures for diabetic neuropathy were attributed to hospital charges. This seems incommensurate with the frequency of diabetic neuropathy in clinic populations.[52] The role of neuropathy in foot ulcers and amputations[41, 45] also suggests that the cost of this condition has been underestimated. This notion is reinforced by the conclusion that neuropathy was responsible for only 2% of the expenditures for care of type 2 DM generally in the United States in 1986.[21] Until better data are available on the number of excess or early deaths caused by diabetic neuropathy, the number of possibly preventable hospitalizations, the amount of wages lost, or the medical and social services expended a result of neuropathy-induced disability, diabetic neuropathy will remain disadvantaged as a focus for research funding or therapeutic initiatives relative to other diabetic complications whose social impact is better documented.

FREQUENCY OF DIABETIC NEUROPATHY

Methodological Problems

Reliable information about the frequency of diabetic neuropathy in different environments and under different personal or social conditions might provide insights into the causes of this disorder and the underlying pathophysiologic mechanisms responsible. At present, however, there is a great deal of conflicting information in the literature concerning the incidence and prevalence of diabetic neuropathy, its occurrence by age and sex, and the types of neuropathy encountered in different patient groups. Although there are inherent difficulties

in studying diabetic neuropathy, much of the confusion results from methodological problems. Some of the more important of these problems are discussed below.

Research Setting. A relatively small proportion of diabetic individuals residing in the community are seen at specialized diabetes clinics or other tertiary medical centers. Consequently, it is unlikely that patients who are referred for such care are representative of those who are not. For example, the overall prevalence of microvascular complications was 26% in diabetic residents in one community. Among those who were seen in a diabetes clinic, the prevalence was 34%, and among the subset of patients who were hospitalized during the previous year, the prevalence was 40%.[34] Others have made similar observations.[47] These trends are exaggerated among diabetic patients attending tertiary referral centers so that cases reported from diabetes centers, transplant centers, dialysis units, ophthalmology clinics, or neuromuscular clinics represent highly biased patient series. In addition to overestimating the prevalence of neuropathy, this referral bias may also alter the apparent mix of neuropathy types because those needing specialized management would be disproportionately selected from among all patients in the community. In a population-based study of maturity-onset diabetic residents of Rochester, Minnesota, distal polyneuropathy accounted for 72% of the neuropathy observed.[40] A predominance of peripheral neuropathy was also found by Fry and associates,[15] who described the selection process aptly:

Two-thirds of our cases had symmetrical peripheral neuropathy, whereas Sullivan (1958), for example, reported that out of 42 patients with diabetic neuropathy admitted to a neurological ward, 31 had asymmetrical motor lesions. Similarly all our patients with amyotrophy and most of those with isolated nerve palsies were seen by a neurologist and often presented at the neurological department. This was not true, however, of patients with symmetrical peripheral neuropathy, relatively few of whom were referred for a neurological opinion.

Clinical Spectrum. It is well known that the epidemiologic patterns of microvascular complications differ from those of the macrovascular complications of diabetes. Even among the macrovascular diseases, moreover, patterns may differ for coronary heart disease, cerebrovascular disease, and peripheral vascular disease. Although information about the frequency of occurrence and the risk factors for vascular disease in general might be of some interest, real progress in unraveling the etiologic factors responsible for the various forms of vascular disease depends on precise definition of specific pathophysiologic syndromes. The same is true for neuropathy, which incorporates a variety of specific and nonspecific syndromes.[52] As discussed in Chapter 30, it seems reasonable to divide diabetic neuropathies into the following varieties: diabetic polyneuropathy, lumbosacral plexus neuropathy, truncal radiculopathy, diabetic mononeuropathies (e.g., carpal tunnel syndrome and tardy ulnar palsy), diabetic oculomotor neuropathy, and perhaps others (e.g., diabetic autonomia and hypoglycemic neuropathy). However, mixing the different types of diabetic neuropathy together results in a variable estimate of the frequency of diabetic polyneuropathy.

Definitions. Lack of consistency in the basic definition of diabetic neuropathy makes the results of the many studies done to date difficult to compare. For example, in a population-based survey in Kristianstad, Sweden, Nilsson and coworkers[38] assessed the neurologic status of patients via ankle jerk and malleolar vibratory perception and found that the prevalence of absent Achilles' jerk and absent vibratory sense increase with age and with duration of diabetes. Both deficits, however, were also seen in nondiabetic controls. Mayne[31] also found that impaired or absent ankle jerk was more common among diabetics than nondiabetic controls (impaired reflex, 30 versus 15%; absent reflex, 46 versus 12%), as was impaired or ab-

sent vibratory sense at the ankles (impaired sense, 32 versus 17%; absent sense, 23 versus 8%). However, he was impressed with the frequency of these findings in nondiabetic individuals and concluded that absent ankle jerks and diminished vibration sense at the ankles were not sufficient grounds for the diagnosis of neuropathy.[31] This approach has been taken by others, for example, by Pirart (see section on Frequency) who excluded from his neuropathy cases all patients older than 65 years who had only isolated Achilles' reflex loss or slight diminution of vibrating sense, along with patients of any age who had absent tendon reflexes without symptoms or other signs of neuropathy.[42] To confuse matters further, Ellenberg[10] found that absent ankle jerk reflexes were very uncommon in normal people and concluded that unless there was some other overt neurologic disease, absent reflexes were mostly the result of diabetic neuropathy. In fact, none of these manifestations is an adequate representation of diabetic polyneuropathy, which is the sum of the symptoms, dysfunctions, and impairments of sensory, autonomic, and motor nerve fibers. This issue is discussed extensively in Chapter 18.

Diagnostic Criteria. For any disease, diabetic neuropathy included, there is a range of possible manifestations. Generally, as the diagnostic tests that are used become more sensitive, the disease becomes more common (for example, the apparent incidence or prevalence increases as milder cases are identified) and, simultaneously, the disease becomes less severe on average. Thus, tests that measure abnormalities of nerve conduction indicate that the majority of diabetics have neuropathy but that the condition is subclinical in many.[8] However, the use of sensitive measures raises questions about the meaning of an abnormality. Thus, if one measurement is used and the 95th percentile is used to define an abnormal level, 5% of patients could be declared "abnormal" by chance alone.[39] This percentage increases to about 23% if any abnormality among five different tests is the basis for diagnosis. Conversely, evaluations based on clinical symptomatology will yield the smaller proportion of patients who have significant neuropathy but will miss some asymptomatic individuals with a substantial degree of objective impairment.[8] Moreover, it is not sufficient to equate one patient's polyneuropathy (diagnosed by one abnormal attribute of nerve conduction, for example) with another's polyneuropathy consisting of severe symptoms, neuropathic impairments, and a bad outcome. A solution to this problem is proposed in Chapter 18.

Attribution. It is not always clear the extent to which any given impairment is the result of diabetes per se. For example, a sizable number of healthy people lose ankle reflexes and vibration sensation in old age. This was shown 30 years ago in a population-based survey in Kristianstad, Sweden, where absent ankle jerk was observed in 27% of diabetic men aged 60 to 79 years compared with 21% of normal men; comparable figures for women were 24% and 25%.[38] Likewise, it has been shown that vibratory thresholds are more closely associated with age and gender than with diabetes, although thresholds did decline with duration of diabetes.[30] In the individual patient, however, it may be impossible to determine the relationship between absent reflexes and diabetes.[52] Moreover, a confounding neurologic disease occurred in 2% of type 1 and 7% of type 2 patients in the Rochester Diabetic Neuropathy Study.[7] In these patients, it was not possible to determine the extent to which the polyneuropathy was attributable to the coexisting disease. If these coexisting neurologic abnormalities had been spuriously attributed to diabetic polyneuropathy, its prevalence would have been erroneously increased by about 5%.

Population at Risk. Because the frequency of diabetic neuropathy is usually assessed relative to the size of the population of diabetic individuals generally, it is necessary to have a reliable estimate of this number. Although identification of patients with type 1 diabetes is relatively straightforward because of their need for more intensive management, it is very difficult to completely identify those with type 2 disease. Moreover, the specific diagnostic criteria for diabetes that are used can have a considerable effect on the results. Thus, only 84% of Rochester residents considered diabetic at Mayo Clinic from 1945 to 1969 met later National Diabetes Data Group criteria for diabetes.[33] This change to more stringent diagnostic criteria reduced the number of diabetic patients and would likely have increased the relative frequency of neuropathy, presuming that the risk is greatest among the most severely affected patients. Conversely, inclusion of milder degrees of glucose intolerance would have the opposite effect. In many studies, the diagnostic criteria for diabetes are not even provided.

Frequency

Incidence. In contrast to the legitimate difficulties encountered in defining diabetic neuropathy, the problems introduced by confusion between incidence and prevalence rates for the condition are needless. Incidence rates measure the likelihood of acquiring the condition. To determine the incidence of diabetic neuropathy, all new cases that occur in some circumscribed population during a specified period must be identified. An incidence rate would then be calculated as follows:

Incidence (per 1000 person-years) =

$$\frac{\text{Number of new cases of diabetic}}{\text{neuropathy diagnosed in study period}} \times 1000$$
$$\frac{}{\text{Person-years of observation among}}$$
subjects at risk during the study period

In a strict sense, incidence rates refer to the occurrence of the disease among those actually at risk. Because this information is rarely available, incidence rates are often calculated for the entire population, with the implied assumption that everyone is at risk. No estimates have been made of the incidence of diabetic neuropathy in the general population, but studies have been carried out among cohorts of diabetics. Pirart found that the incidence of neuropathy generally increased from about 3 cases per 100 diabetic patients per year to about 19 cases per 100 previously unaffected patients per year during the 25-year period of his study.[43] In the typical clinical series, some new cases are identified but the population from which the cases originated cannot be precisely described, a fact that precludes the calculation of an incidence rate.

Cumulative Incidence. Another measure of risk is the cumulative incidence rate, where the proportion of subjects who develop neuropathy over time is calculated for various durations of follow-up using life-table methods. Few have been able to follow a cohort of diabetic individuals and obtain the necessary data to calculate the cumulative incidence of neuropathy. Palumbo and associates[40] followed all 995 Rochester, Minnesota, residents who were initially diagnosed with maturity-onset diabetes in the period 1945 to 1969 and who were free of neuropathy at first diagnosis. They found that the actuarially estimated cumulative incidence of a subsequent clinical diagnosis of distal polyneuropathy was 4% by 5 years and rose to 15% by 20 years after the diagnosis of diabetes. After 20 years of follow-up, the cumulative incidence of carpal tunnel syndrome was 1.3%; mononeuropathy, 0.6%; autonomic neuropathy, 0.3%; and all other neuropathies combined, 1.1%. The median time between the diagnosis of diabetes and the first diagnosis of neuropathy was 9 years. However, the assessment of neuropathy in this cohort was based on medical record review and doubtless represents an undercount, especially of the more subtle manifestations of neuropathy. If there were no survival disadvantage for patients with diabetic neuropathy and no net migration in or out of the community, then the cumulative incidence rate should be comparable to population-based prevalence rates (see next section). Unfortunately, these conditions are rarely—if ever—fulfilled, so comparison of cumulative incidence data with prevalence data is tenuous.

Prevalence. If the incidence of diabetic neuropathy cannot be determined, it may still be possible to define its prevalence, that is, the proportion of persons in a population at some specific time who have the condition. Prevalence rates for diabetic neuropathy would be calculated as follows:

Prevalence (%) =

$$\frac{\text{Number of existing cases of diabetic neuropathy at a point in time}}{\text{Number of individuals in the population at that point in time}} \times 100$$

Prevalence data often provide the best assessment of the burden of disease in the community. However, the clinical spectrum of any disorder is better reflected by the incidence cases because they represent all known occurrences in the population. Prevalence cases represent the survivors, who may have very different characteristics. Most existing data on the frequency of neuropathy are prevalence data from specific clinical practices. Only recently have there been population-based studies of the prevalence of peripheral neuropathy, which are reviewed in subsequent sections.

Prevalence rates can be determined for the population generally but, to our knowledge, only three such studies have been reported. Savetteri and colleagues found that the prevalence of diabetic neuropathy was 0.7% among individuals 40 years or older who resided in two regions of Sicily.[48] Subjects who responded positively to a questionnaire (previous diagnosis of peripheral neuropathy or symptoms of

sensory change, paralysis or weakness of limbs, paralysis of face or drooping of mouth) or who failed tests of balance or heel-to-toe walking were examined by a neurologist. In a survey of general practitioners in two regions of Italy, the prevalence of symptomatic polyneuropathy (two or more neuropathic symptoms and two or more of bilateral impairment of strength, sensation, or deep tendon reflexes) was 3.6% and 3.3%, respectively, in Varese and San Giovanni Rotondo.[4] Forty-four percent of these patients had diabetes, so, the prevalence of symptomatic diabetic polyneuropathy might be roughly 1.5%. In a survey of the Parsi community in Bombay, the prevalence of any peripheral neuropathy was 2.4% and of diabetic peripheral neuropathy alone, 0.4%.[3] Neuropathy was ascertained by questionnaire (trouble in walking not caused by arthritis, weakness or numbness on one side of the body lasting more than 24 hours, weakness/numbness/tingling in hands or feet lasting more than 24 hours, clumsiness in use of hands for fine work) and confirmed by a neurologist (sensory or motor change or hyporeflexia).

It is much more common to assess the prevalence of neuropathy only among those with diabetes. In Rochester, Minnesota, for example, 870 residents were known to have diabetes by National Diabetes Data Group criteria on January 1, 1986, of whom 380 were enrolled in the Rochester Diabetic Neuropathy Study.[7] On the basis of medical record review, the prevalence of peripheral neuropathy was very similar among participants in this study compared with nonparticipants (12.4 versus 13.5%, respectively), despite the older average age of the nonparticipants. The volunteers then underwent an extensive evaluation for neuropathy (Neuropathy Symptom Score and Neuropathy Disability Score given by a neurologist; patient-completed Neuropathy Symptoms Profile; conduction in ulnar, peroneal, tibial, and sural nerves; vibratory detection and cooling detection thresholds in the foot; and heartbeat variation to deep breathing or Valsalva). From these assessments, 60.8% of the subjects were judged to have some form of diabetic neuropathy, and 47.6% had diabetic polyneuropathy. The proportions with polyneuropathy were similar for those with type 1 DM compared with type 2 DM, although the latter group had more severe manifestations (Table 17.3). However, the prevalence of symptomatic polyneuropathy was only 15% among the patients with type 1 DM and only 13% among those with type 2 DM.[7]

TABLE 17.3 PREVALENCE (%) OF DIABETIC POLYNEUROPATHY* BY STAGED SEVERITY IN THE ROCHESTER DIABETIC NEUROPATHY STUDY

Age	Type 1 Diabetes Mellitus†				Type 2 Diabetes Mellitus†			
	NO‡	N1	N2a	N2b	NO	N1	N2a	N2b
<20	100	0	0	0	0	0	0	0
20–39	50	42	2	6	73	18	9	0
40–59	34	38	21	7	55	30	15	0
>60	40	40	13	7	53	34	11	2
Total	46	39	9	6	55	32	12	1

*Polyneuropathy was defined as two or more abnormalities from among neuropathic symptoms as measured with neuropathy symptom score, neuropathic deficits as measured with neuropathy disability score, quantitative sensory examination (vibration detection threshold or cool detection threshold) or quantitative autonomic examination (deep breathing or Valsalva) with at least one being an abnormality of nerve conduction or an abnormality of quantitative examination.
†The separation into category of disease was based on C-peptide response to infused glucagon.
‡NO, no neuropathy; N1, subclinical neuropathy; N2a, symptomatic, mild; and N2b, symptomatic neuropathy, more severe. There were no patients with N3, disabling neuropathy.
Modified from Dyck PJ, Kratz KM, Karnes JL, et al. The prevalence by staged severity of various types of diabetic neuropathy, retinopathy, and nephropathy in a population-based cohort: The Rochester Diabetic Neuropathy study. Neurology 1993; 43(4):817.

The prevalence rate of 54% for any diabetic polyneuropathy (symptomatic or asymptomatic) among type 1 DM patients in Rochester[7] contrasts with an estimate of only 37% based on the first 400 subjects from the Pittsburgh Epidemiology of Diabetes Complications Study.[29] However, the prevalence of diabetic polyneuropathy was a comparable 58% among patients with type 1 DM 30 years or older in that study (the mean age of the patients with type 1 DM in Rochester was 41 years), despite the fact that neuropathy was assessed only on the basis of abnormalities in two or more of sensory or motor signs, symptoms consistent with neuropathy, or decreased tendon reflexes. The prevalence of neuropathy (two or more of symptoms [numbness, burning, prickling, deep aching, tenderness, and tingling]; loss of light touch; impairment of pain perception or absent ankle jerks [<70 years old] on neurologic examination; or abnormal vibration thresholds [Bioesthesiometer] of medial malleolus or great toe) among 213 residents of East Dorset, England with type 1 diabetes was 13%,[54] whereas the prevalence of sensory neuropathy (bilateral diminution of pinprick sensation in the feet) among patients with type 1 DM in rural Australia was 8%.[23] In the Piemonte region of Italy, 7% of 467 patients with type 1 DM had asymptomatic neuropathy (at least one abnormality among neurologic evaluation, vibration sensation, and heart rate response to deep breathing or blood pressure response to standing up) and 21% more had symptomatic neuropathy (abnormalities on a structured questionnaire in addition to objective evidence of neuropathy);

the prevalence of sensory abnormalities alone was 17%.[53]

Compared with the 45% prevalence of any diabetic polyneuropathy (symptomatic or asymptomatic) among patients with type 2 DM in Rochester,[7] the prevalence of distal symmetrical neuropathy among 279 individuals with type 2 DM in the San Luis Valley Diabetes Study was only 25.8%.[12] Neuropathy was discerned from a 5-minute assessment by a nurse practitioner of ankle reflexes and temperature sensation combined with a history of pain, numbness, burning or tingling at rest in both legs or feet in the previous 6 months. Neuropathy was considered to be present if two of three criteria (positive history, decreased ankle reflexes bilaterally or abnormal temperature sense bilaterally) were met. However, 97% of affected individuals were symptomatic by history, so a more appropriate comparison may be with the 13% of Rochester type 2 DM patients with symptomatic polyneuropathy.[7] The symptomatic patients in the Rochester Diabetic Neuropathy Study, however, also had to have had at least one objective abnormality of nerve conduction or autonomic function. The prevalence of neuropathy (two or more of symptoms, loss of light touch, impairment of pinprick, absent ankle reflexes, or abnormalities of vibration perception) among the 864 type 2 diabetics in East Dorset was 17%.[54] The prevalence of impaired vibration perception in a survey of diabetic residents of Oxford, England, aged 20 to 74 years was 23%; less than 2% would have been expected on the basis of normal values.[37] The prevalence of peripheral neuropathy (subjective paresthesias in feet, absent deep tendon reflexes in knees or ankles, absent position or vibratory sensation in feet, or altered pinprick sensation in a stocking distribution) in a Native American population was 12%.[44]

In other instances where the frequency of neuropathy is assessed at a specific point in time (such as at the time of diagnosis of diabetes or at the time of evaluation in a diabetes referral center), the resulting data are also prevalence rates, *not* incidence rates. Thus, Pirart[43] found that the prevalence of neuropathy rose from about 8% at the time of diagnosis to about 50% at the 25-year point in the follow-up in his cohort of 2795 diabetics seen from the onset of their disease. The prevalence after 20 years in Pirart's study was more than 40%, and this was twice the figure reported for the cumulative incidence at 20 years in the Palumbo data.[40] As a microcosm of the problem of data comparability in diabetic neuropathy research, one cannot tell if the higher Pirart figure results from the different definition of neuropathy, from more complete case ascertainment as a result of regular exams, or from the fact that the patients were not from the general community but were obtained from the practices of a diabetologist, a specialty clinic, and two university hospitals.[42] Because of variability in definitions, method of ascertainment, patient selection, and statistical error resulting from small patient numbers, the differences among estimates of neuropathy prevalence that were published in earlier years (Table 17.4) are essentially uninterpretable.[6]

Although prevalence is related to incidence (prevalence $\approx$ incidence $\times$ mean duration of disease), prevalence rates are unreliable estimators of incidence (and thus of the risk of diabetic neuropathy) because they are affected by changes in duration, selective survival, patient migration, and other factors.[32] Thus, if survival is impaired in those with neuropathy, then prevalence rates (which are calculated for the survivors remaining at some point in time) could greatly underestimate the true risk of acquiring the disorder. These and related problems have long led to calls for reliance in diabetes research on inception cohorts followed from the time of initial diagnosis onward.[22] Such calls have been unanswered, but it must be admitted that inception cohorts are difficult to define in diabetes because the actual onset of the disease often predates its clinical recognition. In the case of type 2 DM, the interval between onset and diagnosis can be decades long.[55] Thus, the complications of diabetes, including peripheral neuropathy,[14] can be present at the time of diagnosis of diabetes without necessarily indicating that the complications arose in the absence of diabetes. This was aptly demonstrated by Mincu[35] in a study of 10,000 newly discovered diabetic residents of Bucharest. Overall, 11.6% had diabetic neuropathy at the time of diagnosis, but the figures ranged from 4% of those who had had symptoms for less than 5 months before diagnosis up to 19% in patients who had been symptomatic for more than 15 months before diagnosis. The lower prevalence of diabetic neuropathy at diagnosis among patients with juvenile-onset diabetes (1.4%) compared to those with maturity-onset diabetes (14.1%) might thus be partly

TABLE 17.4 REPORTED PREVALENCE OF SYMPTOMS AND SIGNS OF NEUROPATHY IN DIABETES

Source	Measurement	Number of Patients	% Neuropathy
Cleveland, 1953	Subjective complaints	261	62
Salford, U.K., 1953	General findings	100	57
Brussels, 1965	Objective signs	1175	21
Stockholm, 1950	Objective signs	150	49
Rochester, MN, 1961	Electromyography, objective signs	103	42
Philadelphia, 1958	Impotence	198	55
New York, 1952	Skin vessel dilatation	16	44
London, 1960	Abnormal Valsalva maneuver	337	20
Toronto, 1961	Objective signs	100	52
Cincinnati, 1951	General signs	77	35
Chicago, 1966	Objective signs, motor conduction velocity	107	10
Aarhus, Denmark, 1968	Motor conduction velocity	14	100
London, 1971	Motor conduction velocity	39	100
Edinburgh, 1977	Motor conduction velocity, autonomic vascular tests	10	100

From U.S. Department of Health, Education, and Welfare. Diabetes Data. Compiled 1977. National Institutes of Health. DHEW Publication No. NIH 78-1468. Washington, DC, U.S. Government Printing Office, 1978.

because of differences in the duration of diabetes before diagnosis.[35]

RISK FACTORS FOR DIABETIC NEUROPATHY
Methodological Problems

There are also methodological problems in associating specific neuropathic syndromes with putative risk factors, including even diabetes itself, because neuropathy does occur in its absence. Consequently, there is some background level of neuropathy that would be expected to occur among diabetic individuals solely by chance, given that they are exposed to the same toxins and trauma as are other members of the population. The excess of neuropathy among diabetic men found by some but not all investigators has been attributed to this phenomenon because occupational and ethanol-related neuropathy appear to be more frequent in men.[43] Determining the characteristics of diabetic patients is relatively easy, therefore, compared with deciding whether these characteristics differ from expected. The existence of chronic diseases and abnormal physiologic states could simply result from the fact that many of the patients are relatively old. A variety of study designs are available with which to assess these relationships, and they have different strengths and weaknesses.

Experiments. The degree to which the presence of diabetes augments the risk of neuropathy in humans can be assessed through experimental or observational studies. A direct experiment, in which the investigator controls the exposure (diabetes) and assigns it randomly to various study patients, would be unethical. However, a clinical trial of withholding diabetes (tight control versus usual therapy) is ethical and would provide the best data concerning the relationship between diabetes and the risk of subsequent neuropathy. Such experiments are difficult to conduct, however, and rarely have involved a sufficient number of subjects to provide convincing data on the risk of various forms of diabetic neuropathy. Thus, Holman and colleagues[20] found a statistically significant improvement in vibration sensory threshold in the intensive control arm of a randomized clinical trial among 74 type 1 diabetics, whereas Service and associates[50] found no significant differences in glucose control or in a variety of measures of peripheral nerve function between the rigorous versus conventional

control arms in a randomized clinical trial among 33 patients with types 1 and 2 DM. Likewise, there was no change in vibration sense among 15 patients randomized to continuous subcutaneous insulin infusion compared with 15 other patients with type 1 DM who were maintained on conventional treatment.[26] However, there was a significant reduction in nerve conduction velocities among 54 patients randomly assigned to conventional therapy compared with 48 patients on more intensive treatment,[46] and comparable results were seen in a similar small study.[5] A notable exception to these limitations is the large Diabetes Control and Complications Trial (see Risk Factors) but this trial involved only type 1 DM. No comparable study has yet been undertaken among the patients with type 2 DM, who represent the great majority of diabetic individuals in the community.

Observational Studies. Investigators are usually forced to rely on observational studies: those in which the investigator neither controls nor randomly assigns the exposure of interest (diabetes). The two main types of observational studies that can be used to assess the relationship between diabetes and neuropathy are the cohort study and the case-control study. In a cohort study, a group of people with diabetes and a comparable group without diabetes are followed in an identical manner to determine the subsequent occurrence of neuropathy. The degree of increased risk of neuropathy associated with diabetes is then measured by the relative risk:

Relative risk =

$$\frac{\text{Incidence of neuropathy among those with diabetes}}{\text{Incidence of neuropathy among those without diabetes}}$$

No large cohort studies have been undertaken to evaluate the risk of neuropathy in this fashion. However, studies have been carried out within cohorts of diabetic subjects to identify more specific risk factors for the development of neuropathy. In these instances, the particular clinical characteristics become the exposures of interest. In the Pittsburgh Epidemiology of Diabetes Complications Study, for example, the risk of distal symmetrical polyneuropathy (two or more of symptoms, sensory signs, or decreased tendon reflexes) over 4 years was 13%.[27] However, the relative risk was 3.2 for the 220 type 1 patients with poor control (glycosylated hemoglobin 11% or greater) compared with the 438 subjects with fair control

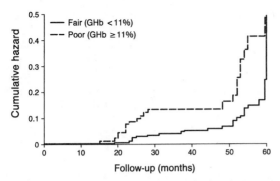

■ **Figure 17.1** Risk of distal symmetrical polyneurop-athy (life table method) by glycemic control (GHb, glycosylated hemoglobin) among Pittsburgh Epidemi-ology of Diabetes Complications Study subjects who participated in a clinical examination at baseline (1986–1988) and who were followed every 2 years. (From Lloyd CE, Becker D, Ellis D, et al. Incidence of complications in insulin-dependent diabetes mellitus: A survival analysis. Am J Epidemiol 1996; 143(5):431.)

(glycosylated hemoglobin below 11%) (Fig. 17.1). The association of neuropathy with gly-cemic control persisted (P <0.001) even after adjusting for duration of diabetes.

Case-control studies of diabetic neuropathy are more common because they are easier to conduct. In a case-control study, patients with neuropathy of a particular type are compared with those without neuropathy. The presence or absence of diabetes as well as other potential risk factors is assessed in the same manner for cases and controls. The degree of risk associ-ated with any particular factor in a case-control study (diabetes) is then estimated by the odds ratio, which is a good estimate of the relative risk (the quantity actually desired) if three con-ditions are fulfilled: (1) the cases studied are representative of all neuropathy cases in the underlying population in terms of the expo-sure of interest (diabetes); (2) the controls are representative of all individuals without neu-ropathy in the population in terms of the fre-quency of diabetes; and (3) the disease (neu-ropathy) is rare. If either the cases or the controls are unrepresentative, the odds ratio will not accurately reflect the true relative risk. Hospital or referral center cases and control subjects selected from these sources are rarely representative of the underlying general popu-lation in terms of diabetes or other potentially important risk factors. Thus, population-based case-control studies conducted in the commu-nity would be expected to provide much more reliable data. This same approach can be used within a population of diabetic subjects to identify risk factors that are associated with the

development of neuropathy over and above diabetes per se. Most of the case-control studies published to date are of this sort.

Risk Factors

Relationship With Diabetes. Several popu-lation-based studies have assessed the excess risk of neuropathy among patients with diabe-tes compared with other groups. Thus, 2392 self-reported diabetic subjects in the National Health Interview Survey[19] were asked the fol-lowing question:

During the past three months have you had: a) numbness or loss of feeling in your hands and feet other than from your hands or feet falling asleep; b) a painful sensation or tingling in your hands or feet? Do not include normal foot aches from standing or walking for long periods; c) decreased ability to feel hot or cold in things you touch?

A total of 37.9% complained of one or more symptoms of numbness (28.2%), pain or tin-gling (26.8%), or decreased ability to feel hot or cold (9.8%) in the hands or feet during the previous 3 months.[19]

The overall prevalence of one of these symp-toms was greater for the 2268 patients with type 2 DM (39.8% for women and 36.0% for men) than for the 124 with type 1 DM (30.2%). These figures were much higher than the prev-alence of any symptom among a representative sample of more than 20,000 nondiabetic sub-jects from this household survey (11.8% and 9.8% for women and men, respectively). Like-wise, the prevalence of peripheral neuropathy in the San Luis Valley Diabetes Study (two or more of positive history, decreased ankle reflexes, or abnormal temperature sense) was 27.8% among 277 subjects with type 2 DM compared with 11.2% among 89 subjects with impaired glucose tolerance and 3.5% among a group of 486 nondiabetic subjects sampled from the same communities.[12] Compared with a similar prevalence of 2.9% in nondiabetic subjects in East Dorset, the prevalence of lower limb neuropathy (two or more of symptoms, loss of light touch, impairment of pinprick, absent ankle reflexes, or abnormal vibration perception) among diabetic residents of the community was 16.3%.[54]

Other Risk Factors. The more important question is the mechanism by which diabetes exerts its adverse effects on nerve function. A number of more specific risk factors have been evaluated in population-based studies of types 1 and 2 DM. For example, the Pittsburgh Epidemiology of Diabetes Complications Study compared the characteristics of 135 type 1 DM patients with diabetic polyneuropathy as previously described and 228 unaffected subjects with type 1 DM (Table 17.5). In multivariate analyses, the independent predictors of neuropathy were increasing duration of diabetes, hyperglycemia (glycosylated hemoglobin [HbA₁]), lower high-density lipoprotein levels, cigarette smoking, and the presence of overt nephropathy or proliferative retinopathy.[29] In a feasibility study for the Diabetes Control and Complications Trial, 278 patients with type 1 DM were evaluated at 21 clinical centers, and 39% were found to have symptoms, signs, or abnormal reflexes attributed to diabetic peripheral neuropathy.[11] Those with neuropathy were older, more likely to be men and taller, and had a longer duration of disease. They were also more likely to have retinopathy, but HbA_{1c} levels were not different. However, the ability to generalize these findings is uncertain because patients were excluded who had renal impairment, hypertension, or neuropathy for which treatment was indicated. Increasing age and longer duration of diabetes were risk factors for diabetic neuropathy in the Piemonte study,[53] and height and retinopathy were independent predictors of neuropathy among patients with type 1 DM in East Dorset.[54]

A similar analysis of peripheral neuropathy among 277 patients with type 2 DM was reported from the San Luis Valley Diabetes Study.[13] Characteristics of the 77 patients with neuropathy as previously described were compared with 200 type 2 DM patients without neuropathy (Table 17.6). The independent predictors of neuropathy in a multivariate analysis were increasing age, greater duration of diabetes, hyperglycemia (increased glycohemoglobin), and insulin use. These investigators could not confirm an association of neuropathy with serum lipid levels, hypertension, or cigarette smoking. Hispanics were not at increased risk despite their greater risk of type 2 DM.[13] Likewise, ethnicity (white, black, Mexican-American) was not significantly associated with self-reported sensory neuropathy in the National Health Interview Survey.[19] In that study, the independent risk factors for sensory neuropathy among patients with type 2 DM were increasing duration of diabetes, hypertension, and high blood glucose; age, gender, insulin treatment, and height were not associated with diabetic neuropathy. Among type 2 diabetics in East Dorset, the independent predictors of neuropathy were age, alcohol consumption, height, HbA₁ levels, and retinopathy.[54] In rural Australia, the independent predictors of sensory neuropathy were duration of diabetes, age at diagnosis, plasma creatinine, insulin dose, and diastolic blood pressure (difference between erect and supine values).[23] In this study, a 5-year increase in the

TABLE 17.5 CHARACTERISTICS ASSOCIATED WITH DISTAL SYMMETRICAL POLYNEUROPATHY IN SUBJECTS 18 YEARS OR OLDER WITH TYPE 1 DIABETES MELLITUS

	Neuropathy		
	Present	*Absent*	*P*-value
Age (year, $\overline{X} \pm SD$)	34 ± 6	28 ± 6	<0.0001
Type 1 DM duration (year, $\overline{X} \pm SD$)	25 ± 6	18 ± 6	<0.0001
Sex (% men)	52	50	NS
Height (cm, $\overline{X} \pm SD$)	167 ± 9	167 ± 9	NS
HbA₁ (%, $\overline{X} \pm SD$)	10.5 ± 2.0	9.8 ± 2.0	<0.001
LDL cholesterol (mmol, $\overline{X} \pm SD$)	3.4 ± 1.0	2.9 ± 0.8	<0.001*
HDL cholesterol (mmol, $\overline{X} \pm SD$)	1.3 ± 0.3	1.4 ± 0.4	<0.01*
Triglycerides (mmol, $\overline{X} \pm SD$)	1.4 ± 1.0	1.1 ± 0.9	<0.01*
Fibrinogen (g/L, $\overline{X} \pm SD$)	3.1 ± 1.0	2.8 ± 0.9	<0.001
Alcohol use (%)	27	40	<0.05
Cigarette smoking (%)	60	35	<0.0001
Hypertension (%)	28	10	<0.0001
Macrovascular disease (%)	24	8	<0.0001
Proliferative retinopathy (%)	58	19	<0.0001
Overt nephropathy (%)	44	18	<0.0001

$\overline{X}$, sample mean; HbA₁, glycosylated hemoglobin; LDL, low-density lipoprotein; HDL, high-density lipoprotein; NS, not significant.
*Adjusted for age.
Modified from Maser RE, Steenkiste AR, Dorman JS, et al. Epidemiological correlates of diabetic neuropathy: Report from Pittsburgh Epidemiology of Diabetes Complications Study. Diabetes 1989; 38(11):1456.

TABLE 17.6 BASELINE CHARACTERISTICS IN PERSONS WITH TYPE 2 DIABETES BY NEUROPATHY STATUS, ALAMOSA AND CONEJOS COUNTIES, COLORADO, 1984–1986

	Neuropathy		
	Present	*Absent*	*P*-value
Age (years, $\overline{X}$)	61.7	58.6	0.026
Sex (% male)	49.4	41.0	0.21
Diabetes duration (years, $\overline{X}$)	13.4	8.3	<0.0001
Ethnicity (% Hispanic)	64.9	68.0	0.63
Systolic blood pressure (mm Hg, $\overline{X}$)	140.2	140.2	0.99
Height (cm, $\overline{X}$)	163.2	161.7	0.34
Glycohemoglobin (%, $\overline{X}$)	11.2	10.2	0.003
Insulin use (%)	73.0	42.4	<0.001
Peripheral vascular disease (%)	19.0	21.0	0.78
Retinopathy (% with preproliferative or proliferative)	36.0	13.0	<0.001
Nephropathy (% with microalbumin $\geq$ 200 μg/mL)	17.6	8.5	0.04
Cigarette use (%)			
Never	41.6	44.0	0.91
<20 pack-years	36.4	33.0	
$\geq$20 pack-years	22.1	23.0	
Prior alcohol use (%)			
Never	59.1	57.7	0.37
<20 g/wk	13.6	20.6	
>20 g/wk	27.3	21.7	
Cholesterol (mg/dL, $\overline{X}$)	222.1	225.5	0.60
Total HDL (mg/dL, $\overline{X}$)	43.4	44.2	0.67
Triglycerides (mg/dL, $\overline{X}$)	225.0	240.6	0.39
Fasting C-peptide (nmol/L, $\overline{X}$)	0.78	0.88	<0.03

$\overline{X}$, sample mean.
Modified from Franklin GM, Shetterly SM, Cohen JA, et al. Risk factors for distal symmetric neuropathy in NIDDM. The San Luis Valley Diabetes Study. Diabetes Care 1994; 17(10):1172.

duration of diabetes was about as potent a risk factor for neuropathy as a 10-year increase in age at diagnosis of diabetes. Duration of diabetes was also an important predictor of diabetic neuropathy in a Native American population.[44]

Many of these risk factors are correlated (e.g., hyperglycemia and insulin treatment or dosage), and it is not possible in observational studies to determine causality. However, definitive evidence that the association of hyperglycemia with neuropathy is a direct one is provided by data from the Diabetes Control and Complications Trial.[9] Among 1441 subjects with type 1 DM, intensive therapy (three or more daily insulin injections or continuous infusion guided by 4 or more daily glucose tests) compared with conventional therapy (one to two daily insulin injections) reduced the risk of any neuropathy by history or physical examination during 5 years of observation by 54% among 539 diabetic subjects in the primary prevention cohort (diabetes for 1 to 5 years and no retinopathy or microproteinuria) and by 61% among 622 subjects in the secondary prevention cohort (diabetes for 1 to 15 years, minimal to moderate proliferative retinopathy, and albuminuria less than 200 mg per 24 hours [0.0031 mmol/24 h]). There was an even more impressive 64% reduction in neuropathy confirmed by abnormal nerve conduction (abnormal conduction velocity, F-wave latency or amplitude in two or more of median, peroneal or sural nerves) or autonomic dysfunction (beat-to-beat heart rate variation during deep breathing or Valsalva or orthostatic hypotension), from 9.6 to 2.8% in the primary prevention cohort and from 16.9 to 6.7% in the secondary prevention cohort (Table 17.7). Nerve conduction velocities stabilized in the intensive treatment group but declined under conventional management, so the development of abnormal nerve conduction was reduced from 40.2 to 16.5% and from 52.4 to 32.7%, respectively, in the two patient strata. The analysis excluded 6% of the study cohort who had confirmed clinical neuropathy at baseline. Thus, there is strong evidence that some aspect of hyperglycemia can cause peripheral neuropathy: (1) intensive treatment was effective in lowering glucose levels over the 6.5-year average duration of study (mean HbA_{1c} levels 7.2 versus 9.1%); (2) neuropathy was reduced by intensive treatment, and this effect was similar across

TABLE 17.7 RISK FOR DEVELOPING DIABETIC NEUROPATHY AT 5 YEARS IN THE DIABETES CONTROL AND COMPLICATIONS TRIAL

Outcome	Primary Prevention Cohort (%)			Secondary Intervention Cohort (%)			Combined Cohorts (%)
	Conventional Therapy	*Intensive Therapy*	*Risk Reduction (95% CI)*	*Conventional Therapy*	*Intensive Therapy*	*Risk Reduction (95% CI)*	*Risk Reduction (95% CI)*
Confirmed clinical neuropathy*	9.6	2.8	71 (34–87)	16.9	6.7	61 (36–76)	64 (45–76)
Clinical neuropathy†	15.2	6.9	54 (22–73)	21.2	11.8	45 (20–62)	48 (29–62)
Abnormal nerve conduction	40.2	16.5	59 (44–70)	52.4	32.7	38 (25–48)	44 (34–53)
Abnormal autonomic function	5.5	2.4	56 (−11–83)	11.8	5.7	51 (16–72)	53 (24–70)

*Abnormal history, physical examination, or both, confirmed by unequivocally abnormal nerve conduction or autonomic nervous system function.
†Abnormal history, physical examination, or both.
Modified from The Diabetes Control and Complications Trial Research Group. Effect of intensive diabetes therapy on the development and progression of neuropathy. Ann Intern Med 1995; 122(8):561.

various subgroups of patients; and (3) the treatment was assigned randomly.

CONCLUSION

Despite the methodological problems enumerated in this chapter, which have been pervasive in diabetes research, there has been an improvement in the quality of data concerning the frequency of diabetic neuropathy and the etiologic factors that may be responsible. This has been brought about by use of standardized and validated tests in prospectively designed studies, use of control groups, better classification and staging of neuropathy, and a focus on population-based studies. Although there still is considerable variation in estimates of the prevalence, incidence, or morbidity in diabetic polyneuropathy from different studies, reasons for the discrepancies are becoming more evident. However, additional work is needed to better define specific varieties of diabetic neuropathy and to establish whether risk factors are the same for each one. Moreover, simple tallies of the different manifestations of diabetic neuropathy are no longer sufficient. Instead, it is necessary to quantify the severity of diabetic neuropathy and to assess its impact on patient function and quality of life. Reliable epidemiologic data about the subpopulation that is disabled by diabetic neuropathy would help focus pathophysiologic and therapeutic research where it could do the most good.

ACKNOWLEDGMENTS

The authors wish to thank Mrs. Mary Roberts for help in preparing the manuscript. Supported in part by research grants NS-14304 and AR-30582 from the National Institutes of Health, United States Public Health Service.

References

1. Bauer ML. Characteristics of persons with diabetes. Vital and Health Statistics: Characteristics of Persons with Diabetes, U.S. July 1964–June 1965. PHS No. 1000-Series 10, No. 40, p 1, 1967.
2. Bender AP, Sprafka JM, Jagger H, et al. Incidence, prevalence, mortality and population-based profile of diabetes mellitus in Wadena, Minnesota, 1981. Minn Med 1983; 66(4):251.
3. Bharucha NE, Bharucha AE, Bharucha EP. Prevalence of peripheral neuropathy in the Parsi community of Bombay. Neurology 1991; 41(8):1315.
4. Chronic symmetric symptomatic polyneuropathy in the elderly: A field screening investigation in two Italian regions. I: Prevalence and general characteristics of the sample. Italian General Practitioner Study Group (IGPSG). Neurology 1995; 45(10):1832.
5. Dahl-Jørgensen K, Brinchmann-Hansen O, Hanssen K, et al. Effect of near normoglycaemia for two years on progression of early diabetic retinopathy, nephropathy, and neuropathy: The Oslo study. BMJ 1986; 293(6556):1195.
6. U.S. Department of Health, Education, and Welfare. Diabetes Data. Compiled 1977. National Institutes of Health. DHEW Publication No. NIH 78-1468. Washington, DC, U.S. Government Printing Office, 1978.
7. Dyck PJ, Kratz KM, Karnes JL, et al. The prevalence by staged severity of various types of diabetic neuropathy, retinopathy, and nephropathy in a population-based

cohort: The Rochester Diabetic Neuropathy study. Neurology 1993; 43(4):817.

8. Dyck PJ, Davies JL, Litchy WJ, et al. Longitudinal assessment of diabetic polyneuropathy using a composite score in the Rochester Diabetic Neuropathy Study cohort. Neurology 1997; 49:229–239.

9. Effect of intensive diabetes therapy on the development and progression of neuropathy: The Diabetes Control and Complications Trial Research Group. Ann Intern Med 1995; 122(8):561.

10. Ellenberg M. The deep reflexes of old age. JAMA 1960; 174(5):468.

11. Factors in development of diabetic neuropathy: Baseline analysis of neuropathy in feasibility phase of diabetes control and complications trial (DCCT). The DCCT Research Group. Diabetes 1988; 37(4):476.

12. Franklin GM, Kahn LB, Baxter J, et al. Sensory neuropathy in non–insulin-dependent diabetes mellitus: The San Luis Valley Diabetes Study. Am J Epidemiol 1990; 131(4):633.

13. Franklin GM, Shetterly SM, Cohen JA, et al. Risk factors for distal symmetric neuropathy in NIDDM: The San Luis Valley Diabetes Study. Diabetes Care 1994; 17(10):1172.

14. Fraser DM, Campbell IW, Ewing DJ, et al. Peripheral and autonomic nerve function in newly diagnosed diabetes mellitus. Diabetes 1977; 26(6):546.

15. Fry IK, Hardwick C, Scott GW. Diabetic neuropathy: A survey and follow-up of 66 cases. Guy's Hospital Reports 1962; 111(1–4):113.

16. Geiss LS, Herman WH, Smith PJ. Morality in non-insulin-dependent diabetes. In Harris MI, Cowie CC, Stern MP, et al (eds): Diabetes in America, ed 2. Bethesda, MD, National Institutes of Health, NIH Publication No. 95-1468, 1995, p 233.

17. Graves EJ. Detailed diagnoses and procedures, National Hospital Discharge Survey, 1991. National Center for Health Statistics Hyattsville, MD, DHHS Publication No. PHS 94-1776, Vital Health Stat 13(115), 1994.

18. Harris MI. Epidemiology of diabetes mellitus among the elderly in the United States. Clin Geriatr Med 1990; 6(4):703.

19. Harris M, Eastman R, Cowie C. Symptoms of sensory neuropathy in adults with NIDDM in the U.S. population. Diabetes Care 1993; 16(11):1446.

20. Holman RR, Dorman TL, Mayon-White V, et al. Prevention of deterioration of renal and sensory-nerve function by more intensive management of insulin-dependent diabetic patients: A two year randomized prospective study. Lancet 1983; 1(8318):204.

21. Huse DM, Oster G, Killen AR, et al. The economic costs of non–insulin-dependent diabetes mellitus. JAMA 1989; 262(19):2708.

22. Kaplan MH, Feinstein AR. A critique of methods in reported studies of long-term vascular complications in patients with diabetes mellitus. Diabetes 1973; 22(3):160.

23. Knuiman MW, Welborn TA, McCann VJ, et al. Prevalence of diabetic complications in relation to risk factors. Diabetes 1986; 35(12):1332.

24. Kozak LJ, Moien M. Detailed diagnoses and surgical procedures for patients discharged from short-stay hospitals. United States, 1983. Vital and Health Statistics, Series 13, No. 82. Data from the National Health Survey, DHHS Publication No. PHS 85-1743. Washington, DC, U.S. Government Printing Office, March 1985.

25. Kriska AM, LaPorte RE, Patrick SL, et al. The association of physical activity and diabetic complications in individuals with insulin-dependent diabetes mellitus:

The epidemiology of diabetes complications study—VII. J Clin Epidemiol 1991; 44(11):1207.

26. Lauritzen T, Frost-Larsen K, Larsen H-W, et al. Two-year experience with continuous subcutaneous insulin infusion in relation to retinopathy and neuropathy. Diabetes 1985; 34(suppl 3):74.

27. Lloyd CE, Becker D, Ellis D, et al. Incidence of complications in insulin-dependent diabetes mellitus: A survival analysis. Am J Epidemiol 1996; 143(5):431.

28. Martin MM. Diabetic neuropathy: A clinical study of 150 cases. Brain 1953; 76(part 3):594.

29. Maser RE, Steenkiste AR, Dorman JS, et al. Epidemiological correlates of diabetic neuropathy: Report from Pittsburgh Epidemiology of Diabetes Complications Study. Diabetes 1989; 38(11):1456.

30. Maser RE, Laudadio C, DeCherney GS: The effects of age and diabetes mellitus on nerve function. J Am Geriatr Soc 1993; 41(11):1202.

31. Mayne N. Neuropathy in the diabetic and non-diabetic populations. Lancet 1965; 2(7426):1313.

32. Melton LJ III, Ochi JW, Palumbo PJ, et al. Sources of disparity in the spectrum of diabetes mellitus at incidence and prevalence. Diabetes Care 1983; 6(5):427.

33. Melton LJ III, Palumbo PJ, Dwyer MS, et al. Impact of recent changes in diagnostic criteria on the apparent natural history of diabetes mellitus. Am J Epidemiol 1983; 117(5):559.

34. Melton LJ III, Ochi JW, Palumbo PJ, et al. Referral bias in diabetes research. Diabetes Care 1984; 7(1):12.

35. Mincu I. Micro- and macroangiopathies and other chronic degenerative complications in newly detected diabetes mellitus. Rev Roum Med 1980; 18(2):155.

36. National Center for Health Statistics. Vital Statistics of the United States, 1991, vol II, Mortality, part A. Washington, DC, Public Health Service, DHHS Publication No. PHS 96-1101, 1996.

37. Neil HAW, Thompson AV, Thorogood M, et al. Diabetes in the elderly: The Oxford Community Diabetes Study. Diabetic Med 1989; 6(7):608.

38. Nilsson SE, Nilsson JE, Frostberg N, et al. The Kristianstad survey II. Acta Med Scand 1967; suppl 469:5.

39. O'Brien PC, Dyck PJ. Procedures for setting normal values. Neurology 1995; 45(1):17.

40. Palumbo PJ, Elveback LR, Whisnant JP. Neurologic complications of diabetes mellitus: Transient ischemic attack, stroke, and peripheral neuropathy. Adv Neurol 1978; 19:593.

41. Pecoraro RE, Reiber GE, Burgess EM. Pathways to diabetic limb amputation: Basis for prevention. Diabetes Care 1990; 13(5):513.

42. Pirart J. Diabetes mellitus and its degenerative complications: A prospective study of 4,400 patients observed between 1947 and 1973. Part 1. Diabetes Care 1978; 1(3):168.

43. Pirart J. Diabetes mellitus and its degenerative complications: A prospective study of 4,400 patients observed between 1947 and 1973. Part 2. Diabetes Care 1978; 1(4):252.

44. Rate RG, Knowler WC, Morse HG, et al. Diabetes mellitus in Hopi and Navajo Indians: Prevalence of microvascular complications. Diabetes 1983; 32(10):894.

45. Reiber GE, Boyko EJ, Smith DG. Lower extremity foot ulcers and amputations in diabetes. In Harris MI, Cowie CC, Stern MP, et al (eds): Diabetes in America, ed 2. Bethesda, MD, National Institutes of Health, NIH Publication No. 95-1468, 1995, p 409.

46. Reichard P, Nilsson B-Y, Rosenqvist U. The effect of long-term intensified insulin treatment on the development of microvascular complications of diabetes mellitus. N Engl J Med 1993; 329(5):304.

47. Rothenberg RB, Olsen CL, Schnure JJ, et al. The community ecology of diabetes patient classification and practice characteristics. Diabetes Care 1985; 8(suppl 1):87.

48. Savettieri G, Rocca WA, Salemi G, et al. Prevalence of diabetic neuropathy with somatic symptoms: A door-to-door survey in two Sicilian municipalities. Neurology 1993; 43(6):1115.

49. Sayetta RB, Murphy RS. Summary of current diabetes-related data from the National Center for Health Statistics. Diabetes Care 1979; 2(2):105.

50. Service FJ, Daube JR, O'Brien PC, et al. Effect of blood glucose control on peripheral nerve function in diabetic patients. Mayo Clin Proc 1983; 58(5):283.

51. Songer TJ. Disability in diabetes. *In* Harris MI, Cowie CC, Stern MP, et al (eds): Diabetes in America, ed 2. Bethesda, MD, National Institutes of Health, NIH Publication No. 95-1468, 1995, p 259.

52. Thomas PK, Tomlinson DR. Diabetic and hypoglycemic neuropathy. *In* Dyck PJ, Thomas PK, Griffin JW, et al (eds): Peripheral Neuropathy, ed 3. Philadelphia, WB Saunders Co, 1993, p 1219.

53. Veglio M, Sivieri R. Prevalence of neuropathy in IDDM patients in Piemonte, Italy. Diabetes Care 1993; 16(2):456.

54. Walters DP, Gatling W, Mullee MA, et al. The prevalence of diabetic distal sensory neuropathy in an English community. Diabetic Med 1992; 9(4):349.

55. West KM. Epidemiology of Diabetes and Its Vascular Lesions. New York, Elsevier North-Holland, 1978.

Chapter 18

Diabetic Polyneuropathy

James B. Dyck • Peter James Dyck

CHARACTERISTICS AND DIAGNOSIS IN BRIEF

Diabetic polyneuropathy (DPN) typically begins as a generalized asymptomatic dysfunction of peripheral nerve fibers. The most common early dysfunction is abnormality of nerve conduction (nerve conduction abnormality) or a reduction of the heartbeat response to deep breathing (heartbeat deep breathing abnormality) or to the Valsalva maneuver (heartbeat Valsalva abnormality). The first clinical signs that develop after or concurrently with the nerve conduction abnormality or heartbeat deep breathing abnormality are decrease or loss of ankle reflexes and decrease or loss of vibration sensation of the great toes. With more severe involvement, patients develop varying degrees and kinds of pan-modality sensory loss of the toes, feet, and distal legs; muscle stretch reflex abnormality; autonomic abnormalities; and weakness of small foot muscles and of ankle dorsiflexor muscles.

In a given patient, these abnormalities develop at different rates and degrees, depending on total hyperglycemic exposure and other applicable risk factors. In some patients, no abnormalities develop; in others, more severe abnormalities develop. Symptoms may occur with any degree of neuropathic impairment or may not occur at all. Generally, symptoms develop only after onset of the functional abnormalities and mild clinical impairments. Symptoms are of two kinds. Negative symptoms resulting from neural hypofunction include loss of tactile and other mechanoreceptor sensations, sensory ataxia, loss of thermal and pain sensations, autonomic impairments such as impotence in the male, gastroparesis, sudomotor loss, muscle weakness, and atrophy. Positive symptoms probably resulting from neural hyperfunction are prickling (pins and needles), a tightly wrapped feeling, retained sock or cotton wool feeling under toes or feet, or pain (lancinating, surges, burning, or deep ache). Tenderness to compression of calf muscles (pressure myalgia) was commonly reported by early investigators. Positive motor symptoms are cramps that typically occur in the calves. Generally, autonomic symptoms do not lend themselves to being classified as positive or negative because hyperactivity may in some cases be inhibiting of the action of the end organ, and some autonomic phenomena are caused by factors other than neural hyperactivity or hypoactivity.

The diagnosis of DPN can be made with some certainty when the following criteria have been met:

1. The patient has diabetes mellitus (DM) by National Diabetes Data Group criteria or other accepted criteria.
2. Diabetes mellitus has caused prolonged chronic hyperglycemia.
3. The patient has a predominantly distal symmetrical sensorimotor polyneuropathy of the lower limbs.
4. Other causes of neurologic disease and sensorimotor polyneuropathy and other varieties of diabetic neuropathy have been excluded, for example, diabetic lumbosacral radiculoplexus neuropathy (DLSRPN) (also called diabetic amyotrophy, proximal diabetic neuropathy, Bruns Garland syndrome, or femoral neuropathy), diabetic thoracolumbar radiculoneuropathy (DTLRN), diabetic autonomia, oculomotor neuropathy, and upper limb mononeuropathies (median neuropathy of the wrist [MNW] or ulnar neuropathy of the elbow [UNE]).
5. Diabetic retinopathy or nephropathy is approximately similar in severity to polyneuropathy.

Insistence on these five criteria will prevent spuriously diagnosing DPN when it is not present. Also, use of these criteria may avoid not recognizing another, perhaps treatable, neurologic disorder masquerading as DPN. It is not uncommon (approximately 5 to 10%) for the neurologic findings in a diabetic patient to be from another cause than DPN. Patients with DM may also have a combination of DPN and other varieties of diabetic neuropathy, or they may have DPN and other neurologic problems. Each of these different neurologic disorders may contribute to the neurologic symptoms and impairments of a given patient.

To illustrate, a patient may have an upper limb mononeuropathy (MNW, carpal tunnel syndrome, UNE, or other upper limb mononeuropathy), lower extremity symptoms from another cause such as DLSRPN, DTLRN, DPN, or lumbar radiculopathy from intervertebral disk disease. The physician must, therefore, learn to apportion which symptoms and signs come from which diabetic disease or other type of neuropathy or neurologic disease. The presence or absence and stage of diabetic retinopathy should be confirmed by an ophthalmologist.

Because DPN may be partially or wholly preventable by excellent glycemic control, the severity of DPN must be measured sensitively, accurately, and reproducibly. The assessment of DPN is too often perfunctory and unreliable. Footwear may not be removed during a neurologic examination, or, if the footwear is removed, the ensuing neurologic examination is not performed carefully and lacks accuracy. To address these problems, we developed a series of standard testing instruments to assess the symptoms and neuropathic impairments: the Neuropathy Impairment Score (NIS) and the NIS of Lower Limbs (LL).[36, 37, 45] We also developed uniform approaches and testing standards to assess for vibration detection threshold (VDT), cooling detection threshold (CDT),[41, 44, 46, 93] and heat-pain (HP) thresholds using computer systems. Quantitative autonomic testing is also available.[44, 84]

Two approaches are available to judge severity of DPN: a staging approach and composite score of impairment.[35, 37, 40, 42]

Staging of DPN may be performed with or without use of nerve conduction, quantitative sensory testing (QST), or heartbeat deep breathing. For detailed staging, as shown here, the tests referred to above are needed.

N0 = no polyneuropathy. Less than N1a.
N1a = asymptomatic polyneuropathy as recognized by nerve conduction abnormality (≥99th or ≤1st, whichever applies) in at least two nerves or heartbeat deep breathing abnormality (<1st), caused by DPN. If a percentile abnormality of a

composite score (for example, NIS[LL] + 7 tests) is used, it should be ≥97.5th.

N1b = N1a criteria plus neurologic examination abnormality, for example, NIS(LL) ≥2 points or abnormality (≥99th) on quantitative sensory testing of VDT, CDT, or HP:5 (an intermediate heat-pain response).

N2a = symptomatic mild DPN. Sensory, autonomic, or motor symptoms caused by DPN. Neuropathic impairment is the same or more than N1a. Patient has less than 50% weakness of ankle dorsiflexor muscles (able to walk on heels).

N2b = symptomatic severe DPN. Neuropathic impairment is the same or more than N1a. Patient has 50% or greater weakness of ankle dorsiflexor muscles (unable to walk on heels).

N3 = disabling DPN as defined in the section entitled Clinical Syndrome and Staging of Severity.

A *composite score* of the NIS(LL) plus a given number of test abnormalities may be used (for example, 4 to 9 tests) to score overall neurologic impairment.[37] Transformed point values are used for percentile abnormalities of tests: <95th = 0, ≥95th to 99th = 1, ≥99th to 99.9th = 2, and ≥99.9th = 3. In the NIS(LL) + 7 composite score, the transformed point values for VDT (percentile abnormality), obtained by computer-assisted sensory testing, is substituted for the clinical evaluation, and transformed point values from heartbeat deep breathing and five nerve conduction attributes are added to this score (Table 18.1). From a study of the Rochester Diabetic Neuropathy Study (RDNS) cohort, the 97.5th percentile value of NIS(LL) + 7 tests is approximately 4.5 points. This value, therefore, may be used as a minimum criteria for DPN.

HISTORY OF DESCRIPTIONS OF CLINICAL MANIFESTATIONS

Early Descriptions of Symptomatic Diabetic Neuropathy of All Types

Marchal de Calvi[31] and Rollo[108] are credited with early descriptions of diabetic neuritis. Marinian and Bouchard[87] and Buzzard[18] observed that knee reflexes were frequently decreased or absent in DM. Althaus[1] noted the similarity of some cases with DM to patients with tabes dorsalis—hence, the term *pseudotabes diabetica*. Leyden[81] reported three varieties of "neuritis": (1) hyperesthetic or neuralgic (painful), (2) paralytic (motor), and (3) ataxic. Pavy[98, 99] emphasized spontaneous pain in lower limbs, especially at night. Auche[5] and Pryce[104] reviewed previously reported cases. Auche reviewed 11 patients with symptomatic neuropathy. The individual case histories are presented in brief because they provide information about onset, course and outcome, symptoms, and individual variability that may be lost in summary statements. They also provide information on natural history before the availability of insulin. These early accounts include most of the varieties of diabetic neuropathy now recognized. Only symptomatic cases were included.

Cases 1 to 4 probably had DPN. *Case 1:* a 56-year-old man was in good health until 18

TABLE 18.1   FREQUENCY, SENSITIVITY, AND SPECIFICITY OF VARIOUS MINIMAL CRITERIA FOR DIABETIC POLYNEUROPATHY USING THE COMPOSITE SCORE (NIS(LL) + 7 TESTS) AS THE GOLD STANDARD

Criteria	Frequency of DPN (%)	Sensitivity (%)	Specificity (%)
1. NIS(LL) + 7 tests	58/195 = 29.7	58/58 = 100	137/137 = 100*
2. Abn ankle reflex	48/195 = 24.6	35/58 = 60.3	124/137 = 90.5
3. Abn vibration sensation (toe)	15/195 = 7.7	10/58 = 17.2	132/137 = 96.4
4. Point 2 + 3	53/195 = 27.2	36/58 = 62.1	120/137 = 87.6
5. Point 2 + VDT	74/195 = 37.9	48/58 = 82.8	111/137 = 81.0
6. NIS(LL)	58/195 = 29.7	40/58 = 69.0	119/137 = 86.9
7. ≥ 2 tests abn	73/195 = 37.4	51/58 = 87.9	115/137 = 83.9
8. ≥ 2 tests abn 1 NC or QAT	70/195 = 35.9	51/58 = 87.9	118/137 = 86.1
9. ≥ 1 nerve with NC abn	112/195 = 57.4	54/58 = 93.1	79/137 = 57.7
10. ≥ 2 nerves with NC abn	59/195 = 30.3	47/58 = 81.0	125/137 = 91.2
11. ≥ 3 nerves with NC abn	33/195 = 16.9	30/58 = 51.7	134/137 = 97.8

DP, diabetic polyneuropathy; NIS(LL), Neuropathy Impairment Score of Lower Limbs; Abn, abnormal; VDT, vibration detection threshold; NC, nerve conduction; QAT, quantitative autonomic testing.
*NIS(LL) + 7 tests is the gold standard.

months before his death when he developed excessive thirst; polyuria; deadness, numbness, and pains in his legs; abdominal pains; and vomiting. A corn of the sole of the foot developed into a plantar ulcer. He died in diabetic coma. At postmortem examination, peripheral nerve fiber degeneration was found. *Case 2:* a 74-year-old woman had experienced excessive thirst for 10 years—an indication of the duration of her DM. She had shooting pains in the foot and then an ulcer of the heel. She experienced painful muscle cramps, especially at night. She developed gangrene of the right third and fourth toes. *Case 3:* a 50-year-old woman with DM since age 44 developed excessive tiredness, weakness of legs, intense itching, and painful tingling of feet and hands 3 years before death. Teased nerve fibers obtained at postmortem examination were undergoing axonal degeneration. *Case 4:* a 19-year-old man who had experienced increased thirst, hunger, weight loss, and glycosuria for 3 months. He developed violent cramps of his calf muscles and diminished sensation.

Cases 5, 6, and 9 probably had DLSRPN. *Case 5:* a 55-year-old man (case of Leyden[81]) had DM and then intense pain in the lower limbs, which was associated with paralysis that later improved. *Case 6* (case of Leyden[81]): a patient who had mild DM and developed severe pain and paralysis of the lower limbs. Later, the pain and eventually the paralysis improved. *Case 9* (case of Auche[5]): a 47-year-old diabetic man suddenly developed intense pain in anterior thighs (L more than R) and pressure-induced muscle pain (pressure allodynia). The pain "became atrocious" and "intolerable at night." Because of thigh weakness, he could not walk up and down stairs. By 2 months, the pain had disappeared, but the paralysis and atrophy persisted for a long time.

Case 7 probably had two varieties of diabetic neurologic complications—DTLRN and DPN. *Case 7* (patient of Charcot[21]): a 35-year-old diabetic man, developed pain in the region of his kidneys that radiated around his body (DTLRN). He also developed excessive burning and weakness of dorsiflexion of his feet (R more than L). *Case 8* (Buzzard[18]): the patient had intense pains in thighs, legs, and feet, followed by "muscle paralysis" (probably DLSRPN and DPN) and weakness and atrophy of thenar and hypothenar muscles of his hands (either DPN or MNW and UNE). Cases 10 and 11 both probably had brachial plexus neuropathies. *Case 10* (Althaus[1]): a 48-year-old man, awakened one night with pain in his shoulder

that radiated to the elbow. The pain disappeared in 3 weeks, but weakness persisted for a long time. *Case 11* (Buzzard as cited by Auche[5]): the patient had left upper extremity pain and weakness.

Bruns[16] described four patients with "neuritic paralysis" affecting femoral muscles (similar to cases 5, 6, and 9). Diabetic lumbosacral radiculoplexus neuropathy is described in more detail in Chapter 35.

Kraus[75] classified diabetic neuropathies into polyneuritis or mononeuritis and motor, sensory, or cranial type.

Later Reports of Symptomatic Diabetic Neuropathy

In later reports, the emphasis generally was on review of series of hospital or clinic patients with symptomatic neuropathy. Because these were usually problem cases, it is difficult to know whether the neuropathy was related to DM. Generally, it was assumed that the variety of neuropathy was causally associated with DM.

Although different varieties of diabetic neuropathy were described in the late 19th century, they were not usually considered to be different disorders from DPN until recent times. Good early descriptions of DLSRPN were provided in Case 9 of Auche,[5] later cases by Bruns,[16] and much later cases of Garland.[55] Only with electrophysiologic[8, 19] and postmortem[106] or biopsy studies[7] was the patchy involvement caused by ischemia of the lumbosacral plexus and lower limb nerves and inflammatory vasculopathy identified.[46b, 112] Patients with DTLRN were described by Charcot[21] and later by others.[8] Even today, this condition has not been adequately studied.

An important early study of autonomic nerve abnormalities in DM is that of Rundles.[111] Many authors contributed to descriptions of the various autonomic manifestations in DM: diarrhea,[6] neurogenic bladder with retention,[56, 72] Argyll-Robertson pupils,[117] postural hypotension, nocturnal diarrhea, altered sweat distribution,[82] paroxysmal diarrhea, impotence, paralysis of bladder,[56, 73] anhidrosis,[66] vasomotor abnormality,[100] and various other autonomic abnormalities.[7, 10, 14, 15, 71, 74, 86, 88, 89, 111, 114, 134, 135] Although tachycardia had been observed by Eichhorst,[48] others described sensory loss and other complications: cardiac denervation (Wheeler and Watkins[130]), Charcot's joints (Boehm[11] and Jordan[71]), sensory symptoms without ataxia (Bosanquet and Henson[12]), and decreased vibratory threshold using quantitative sensory testing (Steiness[121]). Nerve conduction abnormalities were described by Downie and Newell,[32] Mulder and coworkers,[91] Skillman and associates,[116] Lawrence and Locke,[80] Gilliatt and Willison,[57] LaMontagne and Buchtal,[78] and Buchtal and Rosenfalck.[17]

Woltman and Wilder[135] attributed DPN to atherosclerosis and ischemia. They were impressed by the evident atherosclerosis and patchy loss of nerve fibers of lower limb nerves. Whereas some of the previous studies had emphasized that DPN usually followed diabetic neglect, these patients were often old and did not appear to have a severe metabolic disturbance. Woltman and Wilder's conclusion that diabetic peripheral neuropathy is caused by atherosclerosis no longer appears credible. The nerves studied were taken from amputated limbs removed because of peripheral vascular disease and ischemia; the regions called fiber loss in some cases were not areas of ischemic injury but were unrecognized Renaut's corpuscles (structures found in healthy nerve). In addition, DPN may occur in patients without evident peripheral vascular disease.

Jordan[71] reviewed 226 persons with diabetic neuropathy. He divided these patients into three groups. Group 1: 34 patients with neuritic symptoms (pain) but few neurologic signs. Group 2: 72 patients who had poor glycemic control and chronic neuropathy characterized by symptoms (pain; cramps; and paresthesia, especially at night) and "degenerative" neurologic signs (hyporeflexia; areflexia; muscle weakness, especially in legs; tenderness of nerves and muscles; sensory loss; and abnormal pupillary responses). Their neuropathy tended to progress. Group 3: 120 patients who had acute and severe symptoms and findings of "neuritis." This group tended to improve over weeks to months and may have included patients with DLSRPN. The recognition that positive neuropathic symptoms (prickling, lancinating pains, hyperesthesia, or hyperalgesia) may occur with few signs of neuropathy is an important observation.

At the University of Michigan, Rundles[111] reviewed 125 patients with symptomatic neuropathy. Symptoms of neuropathy usually did not develop for 5 years after the diagnosis of DM. Whereas earlier investigators observed that patients who developed neuropathy had typically lost weight and had poor glycemic control, many of Rundles' patients with neuropathy were well nourished and had glycosuria and acidosis infrequently. The view that

neuropathy could develop in patients with relatively mild metabolic derangement was shared by several other investigators (Woltman and Wilder,[135] Root and Rogers,[109] and Joslin and Root[73]). However, on closer inspection, 11 of Rundles' patients had previously had diabetic coma—perhaps an indication that metabolic control was hardly ideal in some of these patients. Rundles believed that decreased or absent muscle stretch reflexes were the most reliable sign of DPN. He attributed gastrointestinal dysfunction to metabolic derangement. Symptoms consisted of anorexia, nausea and vomiting, severe constipation, and chronic diarrhea (sometimes after meals and sometimes at night). About one fifth of the group had genitourinary disturbances—impotence in the male, urinary retention, and sphincter disturbances.

Rundles presented five patients in detail.

Case 1: a 49-year-old woman with symptoms of DM (fatigue, excessive thirst, and increased appetite) for 1 year. She had lost weight from 196 to 156 pounds in 4 years. Insulin treatment was refused and she lost another 20 pounds. She then developed aching and cramping of leg muscles. Sweating was decreased over her feet. Sharp shooting pains were reported in the legs. Her feet felt cold and numb; they tingled and were clumsy. For night pain in the feet, she used a hot pad. She became constipated. Her fingers became numb, tingled, and were clumsy. Knee and ankle reflexes were absent, and vibration and pinprick were diminished in the feet. A starch-iodine test revealed decreased sweating over the feet. With insulin treatment, symptoms were markedly improved, but the neuropathic findings remained unchanged.

Case 2: a 19-year-old man with DM was admitted to the hospital with symptoms of chronic fatigue, severe aching muscles, numbness and tingling of feet and legs, and severe shooting pains. He had ankle swelling. He was reported to be "a severely neglected diabetic patient." Thereafter, he developed constipation and urinary retention, with a flaccid, enlarged bladder with weak contraction. Muscle stretch reflexes were absent. With more rigorous insulin treatment, bladder function improved but neuropathic findings remained unchanged.

Case 3: a 14-year old boy who had DM for 5 years. His symptoms of neuropathy followed a period of weight loss and began with leg cramps, dribbling of urine, watery diarrhea, pain in the scrotum, and cutaneous hyperesthesia. He was discharged unimproved.

Case 4: a 43-year-old man with DM who had stopped using insulin for 6 to 8 months, during which time his weight decreased from 180 to 160 pounds. He then developed weak legs, numbness, tingling, and shooting pains. In addition, he developed diarrhea, urgency of urination, dizzy spells caused by postural hypotension, Argyll Robertson pupils, decreased tendon reflexes, muscle tenderness, skin hypersensitivity, and vibration loss. With insulin treatment, the neuropathic pain improved.

Case 5: a complicated case; the patient had neurosyphilis and DM.

Martin,[88] like Rundles,[111] presented a selected series of diabetic patients with symptoms and signs of diabetic neuropathy. He believed that diabetic neuropathy occurred most commonly in diabetic patients whose metabolic control had been neglected, especially in older people whose metabolic disorder had escaped recognition. Diabetic polyneuropathy usually developed after a prolonged period of chronic hyperglycemia. He attributed neuropathic foot lesions (plantar ulcers and Charcot's joints) to sensory neuropathy and not to atherosclerosis. Many of the patients who developed DPN had not attended diabetic clinics for years.

In a review of diabetic neuropathy, Garland[55] classified diabetic neuropathies into diabetic sensory neuropathy, diabetic amyotrophy, mixed sensory and motor syndromes, and diabetic autonomic syndromes.

Characteristic Patterns of Diabetic Polyneuropathy Manifestations From Epidemiologic Studies

Descriptions of series of patients with problems (the preceding sections) are of value in characterizing advanced cases of the disorder. They tend, however, to focus on worst cases and unusual manifestations. To get a better idea of what usually happens, it is necessary to consider what happens in representative prevalence cohorts. However, as Melton and Dyck discuss in Chapter 17, cross-sectional and longitudinal data on DPN are unsatisfactory in many respects and for a variety of reasons. In this section, we review some of the studies and attempt to provide a more representative view of the characteristic features of DPN based on epidemiologic studies.

Mulder and colleagues[91] evaluated 103 serially examined and consenting ambulatory diabetic patients who attended diabetic clinics at Mayo Clinic Rochester. "By chance" none of these patients "had peripheral neuropathy as a major complaint." They were independently evaluated for clinical evidence of DPN (examination of muscle stretch reflexes, sensation, and muscle weakness) and for nerve conduction abnormality. Patient ages ranged from 11 to 79 years, and duration of DM ranged from onset of DM to 37 years. Two major insights resulted from the study. (1) Associated neurologic diseases were not uncommon and were caused by multiple sclerosis, essential tremor, protruded intervertebral disk, hemiplegia from cerebral infarct, syphilis, myxedema, and hyperthyroidism. (2) Fifty-six of 103 (54%) patients had neuropathy of various kinds as determined by clinical or electromyographic criteria; 31 (30%) had diffuse polyneuropathy; 12 (12%) had mononeuropathy; and 4 (4%) had mononeuropathy and polyneuropathy. In the 16 persons with mononeuropathy, 29 nerves were affected—13 common peroneal nerves at the fibular head, 9 median nerves at the wrist (MNW), 5 ulnar nerves at the elbow (UNE), 1 femoral nerve, and 1 lateral femoral cutaneous nerve. As will be discussed subsequently, the frequency of associated neurologic disorders and the frequency distribution of types of neuropathy is not unlike what was found later by Palumbo and associates[96] and Dyck and colleagues.[42]

Fagerberg[51] examined more than 300 diabetic patients from three medical centers near Göteborg between the years 1952 and 1958. The criteria for diabetic neuropathy were (1) at least two neuropathic signs or (2) one neuropathic sign if it was pronounced or typical. Equivocal abnormalities were not to be included. Symptoms alone were not sufficient for the diagnosis of neuropathy. Sixty-three percent of patients were judged to have neuropathy. The authors found a statistically significant association among retinopathy, neuropathy, and nephropathy—confirmed by a later author.[42] The incidence of DPN increased with greater duration of DM.

Pirart[101, 102] reported on serial evaluation of 4400 patients with DM from Brussels Hospitals and Clinics between the years 1947 and 1973. Initially, neuropathy was judged based on decreased or absent ankle reflexes. Later, decreased vibration sensation of the foot was added. The severity of DPN was not judged. Varieties of diabetic neuropathy were not classified. The data show that the frequency of decreased ankle reflexes and decreased vibration sensation increased with duration of DM.

A study by Palumbo and associates[96] addressed the prevalence, incidence, and survival of patients with neurologic complications (transient ischemic attacks, stroke, and varieties of peripheral neuropathy) based on a retrospective review of the medical records of patients with DM (n = 1028) living in Rochester, MN. The study is noteworthy because it is population-based and because of the quality of the neurologic data. Nearly all inhabitants of the town were evaluated at Mayo Clinic, and information was compiled in one dossier-type medical record used by all health care providers in the region. Investigators classified all varieties of neuropathies encountered. The epidemiologic approaches used were good. Based on clinical diagnosis (presumably most symptomatic), 108 of 1028 (10.5%) had neuropathy; of these, 78 (72%) had distal polyneuropathy, 13 (12%) had carpal tunnel syndrome (MNW); 6 (6%) had another type of mononeuropathy, and 11 (10%) other neuropathies. Autonomic neuropathy was found in three patients with DPN. The frequency of neuropathy was increased in patients with poor diabetic control. They concluded that the most common type of neuropathy in DM is distal polyneuropathy and that frequency increased with duration of DM.

Of those patients with DM attending three Sheffield hospitals, the percentage with neuropathic symptoms (numbness, paresthesia, altered temperature sensation, weakness, or a history of painless foot ulceration) was similar to the experience in Rochester, approximately 10%.[92] For a 6-month period, all diabetic patients attending these three hospitals were asked about symptoms and foot ulcers that had been present for at least 6 weeks. Patients with foot ulcers had significantly decreased vibration and thermal sensation when compared with neuropathy patients without foot ulcers; autonomic function was not found to be different.

A study similar to that done in Sheffield was performed in Limerick. During a 1-year period, 800 patients with DM (336 type 1, 464 type 2)[94] were surveyed to identify the morbidity from the various forms of diabetic neuropathy. In 100 nondiabetic control subjects, 2% had loss of feeling and 7% had restless legs. In the diabetic patients, 13% had pain or paresthesia, 7% had loss of feeling, and 2% had neuropathic ulcers. In addition, 0.8% had DLSRPN; 0.1%, oculomotor palsy; 0.1%, peroneal nerve palsy; 20%, erectile impotence; and 1%, symptomatic postural hypotension. Overall, 22.9% of the population had symptoms of neuropathy—higher than in the Sheffield study and in the RDNS. Univariate analysis showed that neuropathy was associated with various factors, such as age and retinopathy in types 1 and 2 DM, and with duration of diabetes, proteinuria, hypertension, and ischemic heart disease in type 1 DM.

Harris and coworkers[69] used the 1989 U.S. National Health Interview Survey to identify 2829 persons with DM in a representative survey of 84,572 persons in the United States 18 years or older. The questionnaire was also given to a representative sample of 20,037 subjects without DM. Patients were asked whether they had, during the past 3 months, experienced numbness or loss of feeling in the hands or feet other than from hands or feet falling asleep; painful sensations or tingling in the hands or feet, not including normal foot aches from standing or walking for long periods; or decreased ability to feel hot or cold. If any of these questions were answered positively, the patient was considered to have symptoms of sensory neuropathy. Symptoms of sensory neuropathy occurred in 30.2% of patients with type 1 DM and in 36% of men and 39.8% of women with type 2 DM. In the control group, sensory symptoms occurred in 9.8% of men and 11.8% of women. These results would suggest that about 20% of diabetic patients have sensory symptoms suggestive of diabetic neuropathy or mononeuropathy. Prevalent symptoms were related to duration of DM, hypertension, and hyperglycemia. The study is notable for its size, its representation of the United States population, use of an adequate control population, and statistical treatment. There are some weaknesses: (1) it is unclear how sensitive and specific the test instrument was at identifying diabetic neuropathies; (2) the test instrument does not discriminate among varieties of neuropathy (symptoms in the hands probably result from MNW or UNE); and (3) the results appear to overestimate the frequency of symptomatic neuropathy when compared with results of studies cited previously and the RDNS (see subsequent section).

We assessed the prevalence and severity (by stages and by continuous measures of severity) of varieties of diabetic neuropathies in Rochester's diabetic population.[42, 43] Important features of this study (RDNS) are listed below.

1. The study had high ascertainment of DM because most inhabitants are medically evaluated at least every 2 to 3 years. Patients generally had fasting plasma glucose determinations performed at such examinations, and, as mentioned

previously, this medical information is recorded in a common medical record available for analysis.

2. The patients who agreed to participate in the RDNS were not significantly different in comorbidity from nonparticipants.

3. Diabetes mellitus was defined by National Diabetes Data Group criteria.

4. Minimal criteria and staged and continuous measures of severity were used to identify and quantitate major varieties of neuropathy.

5. End points of neuropathy were expressed as percentile values (specific for test, site, age, sex, and other applicable physical characteristics) based on study of a representative healthy subject cohort, drawn from the same community from which patients with neurologic diseases, neuropathy, and diseases known to predispose to neuropathy were excluded.

6. Neuropathies were prospectively and comprehensively evaluated and classified.

As shown in Figure 18.1, approximately half of the diabetic patients (47.6%) had DPN as defined by the criteria of at least two abnormalities (≥99th or ≤1st percentile, whichever applied) from the five evaluations (symptoms, impairments, nerve conduction abnormality, QST abnormality, and quantitative autonomic test [QAT] abnormality).[44, 93] Approximately 13% had symptoms, and an even smaller percentage had stage N2B (50% or greater weak-

ness of ankle dorsiflexor muscles [inability to walk on heels]). The frequency of DPN increased with duration of diabetes (Fig. 18.2). Using univariate analysis, many risk factors were found to be associated with severity of DPN. Using multivariate analysis, the main risk factors were identified as total hyperglycemia exposure, 24-hour proteinuria and type of DM (type 1).

Thomas and Tomlinson published a worthwhile review of diabetic neuropathy in 1993.[126]

SEPARATION FROM OTHER VARIETIES OF DIABETIC NEUROPATHIES

Diabetic neuropathy is heterogenous. Diabetic polyneuropathy is sufficiently distinctive from other varieties of diabetic neuropathy (DLSRPN,[5, 8, 10, 15, 16, 19, 20, 22–26, 34, 55, 61, 63, 67, 81, 83, 105–107, 115, 122, 124, 127, 134] DTLRN,[8, 13, 53, 68, 123] and oculomotor neuropathy [4, 33, 47, 60, 110, 139]) to be considered a different disorder. These disorders differ in their anatomicopathological distribution of involvement, course, association with variety of diabetes mellitus, risk factors, and outcome. All the other varieties of diabetic neuropathy, except for DPN, appear acutely or subacutely and tend to have a monophasic course. Generally, the other varieties appear to have only a weak association with total hyperglycemic exposure and may occur more frequently in type 2 DM than in type 1 DM. For some of these other varieties (such as DLSRPN), an inflammatory angiitis and ischemia appear to be involved.

Early accounts of DLSRPN were those of Leyden,[81] Auche,[5] Bruns,[16] and Garland.[55] More recent accounts were those of Calverley and Mulder,[19] Bastron and Thomas,[8] Raff and coworkers,[106] Chokroverty and colleagues,[25] Barohn and associates,[7] Said and colleagues,[112] and Dyck and colleagues.[46b] Several investigators emphasized DTLRN.[8, 53, 68, 123] Early accounts of oculomotor neuropathy were reported by various authors.[47, 60, 110, 139] The ischemic basis of oculomotor neuropathy was discussed by Dreyfus and colleagues[33] and Asbury and associates.[4]

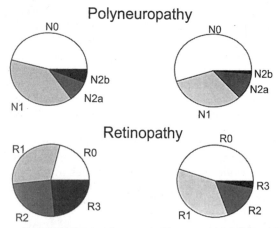

■ Figure 18.1 A diagrammatic representation of Rochester, Minn, diabetic patients with type 1 DM *(left)* and type 2 DM *(right)* who had different stages of severity of neuropathy *(top)* and retinopathy *(bottom)*. For both complications, there is a more severe distributon of stages of the complication in type 1 DM than in type 2 DM.

CLINICAL SYNDROME AND STAGING OF SEVERITY

We suggest that the diagnosis of DPN rests on five cardinal features.

1. Presence of DM.

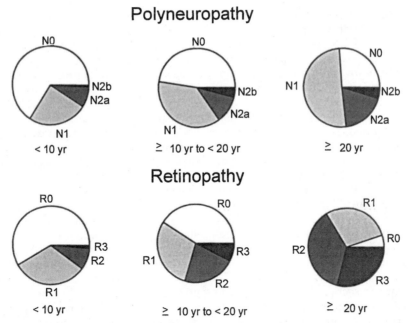

■ **Figure 18.2** The change in the stage distribution of neuropathy *(top)* and retinopathy *(bottom)* with increasing duration of diabetes mellitus.

2. Sufficient chronic hyperglycemia exposure.
3. A characteristic pattern of neuropathy consisting of a symmetrical distal lower limb sensorimotor polyneuropathy (DPN).
4. An association with diabetic retinopathy or nephropathy.
5. Exclusion of other neurologic diseases or neuropathies, and exclusion of other varieties of diabetic neuropathy, such as oculomotor neuropathy, DLSRPN, MNW, UNE, and DTLRN.

In type 1 DM, distal symmetrical sensorimotor polyneuropathy (DPN) usually develops only in patients who have had chronic and prolonged hyperglycemia for several years. Typically, in type 2 DM, DPN also develops only after years of poor glycemic control. However, occasionally in type 2 DM, DPN may already be present at the time of recognition of DM. It is assumed that chronic hyperglycemia was present, but unrecognized, for long periods of time in those patients with type 2 DM who already have DPN at the time of diagnosis of their DM. In type 2 DM, the true time of onset of DM is seldom precisely known, whereas in type 1 DM, it usually is known.

The fully expressed syndrome is a symmetrical distal lower limb sensorimotor polyneuropathy with a variable degree of autonomic involvement. Almost without exception, clinical involvement is restricted to the distal extremities of the lower limbs. By contrast, electrophysiologic abnormality affects nerves diffusely. The clinical sensorimotor syndrome is poorly distinguished from many other varieties of sensorimotor polyneuropathy, such as inherited, immune (Sjögren's syndrome), toxic (alcohol, medicinal), metabolic (uremia, hepatic, and others), and malnutrition. These causes of neuropathy must be excluded.

An important diagnostic point is that DPN is usually associated with some degree of diabetic retinopathy or nephropathy.[42, 51] There is a caveat. Retinopathy cannot be assumed to be absent unless it has been adequately searched for with the pupils dilated and by an ophthalmologist. Nephropathy cannot be assumed to be absent without evaluation of 24-hour urine protein (or microalbumin) or plasma creatinine. In the RDNS cohort of 380 community-based patients with DM, highly significant associations were found between patients with polyneuropathy and retinopathy ($P < 0.001$) and with nephropathy ($P = 0.003$). Other varieties of neuropathy other than DPN are not associated with diabetic retinopathy or nephropathy.[42] There may be patients with DPN who may not have diabetic retinopathy or nephropathy, but this is thought to be uncommon and other causes for th neuropathy should be sought. Conversely, a sensorimotor polyneuropathy in a diabetic patient may result from a cause other than DM, even when diabetic retinopathy or nephropathy is present.

The diagnosis of DPN (especially severe DPN) should not be assumed simply because of an association with prolonged hyperglycemia—other neurologic disorders and neuropathies must be excluded. Whisnant and Love[131] reported a case of spinal cord ependymoma that went unrecognized for a long period of time because the neurologic syndrome was assumed to be completely caused by DPN. In the RDNS, we incorrectly attributed a patient's neurologic manifestations to DPN when, in fact, they were caused by spinal stenosis. The clue was the severity of the sensorimotor involvement without eye or kidney complications. The variety of conditions that need to be considered and the approaches that need to be used are outlined in Chapter 31.

In the subsequent sections, we discuss the progression of DPN through various stages of severity. The criteria for different stages of severity came from cross-sectional and longitudinal studies of the RDNS cohort. The first approach to staging is to find accurate and reproducible minimal criteria for the diagnosis of DPN. It is self-evident that the frequency of abnormality depends on which test(s) are used, criteria for abnormality, and the criteria for DPN. Thus, the percentage of patients with DM and neuropathy will increase with using less stringent criteria for test abnormality—for example, from the $\geq$99th, to the $\geq$97.5th, and to the $\geq$95th percentile (or from the $\leq$1st, to the $\leq$2.5th, and to the $\leq$5th percentile, whichever applies). Likewise, the percentage of patients with abnormality increases if one decreases the number of tests or nerves that must be abnormal, that is, abnormality in three nerves, to two nerves, or to one nerve.

Because of the great variability in the sensitivity of tests, frequency of abnormality also depends on the test(s) chosen for the diagnosis of DPN. This variability among tests and among different criteria for the diagnosis of DPN was seen in studies of the RDNS cohort. There is a considerable difference in sensitivity among the following neuropathy tests: nerve conduction abnormality, heartbeat deep breathing abnormality or heartbeat Valsalva abnormality, QST abnormality, NIS, and Neuropathy Symptom Score (NSS).[37, 40] The frequency of test abnormalities was highest for nerve conduction and heartbeat deep breathing or heartbeat Valsalva, followed by abnormality of ankle reflexes and VDT abnormalities, and then toe extensor or ankle dorsiflexor muscle

weakness or cooling or heat-pain loss of the foot.[37, 40] These observations were exploited to set minimal criteria for the diagnosis of DPN (see Table 18.1) and for staging DPN severity.

Having set an appropriate minimal criteria for DPN, it was possible to logically subdivide asymptomatic DPN patients into those with abnormality of neuropathic tests only (nerve conduction abnormality, heartbeat deep breathing abnormality, or heartbeat Valsalva abnormality [stage N1a]) and those who additionally had neurologic signs, such as absent ankle reflex or muscle weakness (but less than stage N2b), or raised VDT (stage N1b). We reasoned that symptomatic (stage N2) was a more severe stage than asymptomatic (stage N1) DPN. Inability to walk on heels (or 50% or greater weakness of ankle dorsiflexor muscles bilaterally in obese or elderly people) was found to be a useful and reproducible criterion to divide stage N2 DPN into two categories of severity—stage N2a (able to walk on heels) and stage N2b (unable to walk on heels).[40] We developed a list of sensory, autonomic, and motor criteria to designate a category called disabling DPN (stage N3). The following discussion of the stages of DPN is slightly modified and improved based on new insights from the RDNS.[37]

Stage N0. No evidence for DPN. The minimal criteria for DPN (two or more abnormal [$\geq$99th or $\leq$1st, whichever applies] tests, one being nerve conduction or heartbeat deep breathing) or a percentile level ($\geq$97.5th) have not been met. The composite score NIS(LL)+7 tests is useful for this purpose, but NIS(LL)+3–9 tests would also serve well.

Stage N1a. Minimal criteria for DPN have been fulfilled (criteria 7, 8, 10, or 11 (Table 18.2) or NIS(LL)+3–9 tests $\geq$97.5th), but the patient does not have clinical abnormalities (decreased ankle reflexes or decreased vibration sensation). The patient may have an asymptomatic abnormality of nerve conduction, heartbeat deep breathing, or heartbeat Valsalva. With nerve conduction abnormality, conduction velocities or distal latencies are usually abnormal before compound muscle or sensory action potentials. Heartbeat deep breathing or Valsalva abnormalities are also very early functional abnormalities in DPN. Because these are sensitive markers of functional abnormality, conservative minimal criteria for abnormality of attributes of nerve conduction or heartbeat deep breathing or Valsalva should be used, that is,

TABLE 18.2 MINIMAL CRITERIA FOR DIABETIC POLYNEUROPATHY

Criteria	Definition
1	Symptomatic polyneuropathy not defined.[5]
2	$\geq$ 2 neuropathic signs or $\geq$ 1 neuropathic sign (if "pronounced or typical").[51]
3	Abnormality of nerve conduction.[32, 91, 116]
4	Abnormality of neurologic examination and NC abn.[91]
5	Abnormality of vibration detection threshold.[121]
6	Abnormality of ankle reflexes (and later of clinical vibration sensation).[101, 102]
7	$\geq$ 2 abnormalities from among (1) symptoms; (2) neuropathic impairment; (3) NC abn; (4) quantitative sensory test (QST abn); or (5) quantitative autonomic test (QAT abn) abnormality. Symptoms were to be evaluated by a physician using Neuropathy Symptom Score or Neuropathy Symptoms and Change. Impairment was to be judged by a performance of a standard neurologic examination and scoring weakness, reflexes, and sensation of great toe or index finger, e.g., the Neuropathy Impairment Score (NIS) or NIS of lower limbs (NIS[LL]). To be abnormal attributes of NC ($\geq$ 99th or $\leq$ 1st, whichever applies) should be found in $\geq$ 2 nerves and not be caused by another process, e.g., entrapment neuropathy. For QST abn, the abnormality ($\geq$ 99th) could be of vibration or cooling detection threshold or heat-pain (HP:0.5 or HP:5 response). For QAT abn, the abnormality could be of heartbeat with deep breathing or Valsalva ($\leq$ 1st).[40]
8	$\geq$ 2 abnormalities from among the five evaluations (listed in criterion 7 above), but 1 of the abnormalities must be NC abn or QAT abn.[40]
9	Morphometric and teased fiber abnormalities.[38]
10	An abnormality of NC (as defined above) or heartbeat with deep breathing or Valsalva.[37]
11	$\geq$ 97.5th percentile of NIS(LL) + 7 tests (see Table 18.1).[37]

NC abn, nerve conduction abnormality; QST, quantitative sensory test; QAT, quantitative autonomic test.

$\geq$99th or $\leq$1st percentile, whichever applies. To ensure that the abnormality is not from a mononeuropathy and caused by a polyneuropathy, nerve conduction abnormality should be observed in at least two nerves, and it should not be the same nerve on opposite sides (for example, bilateral median nerve conduction abnormality as in MNW).

Nerve conduction abnormality or heartbeat deep breathing or Valsalva abnormality are important minimal criteria for DPN because they are quantitative and objective (responses cannot be willed) measures. Standard approaches to evaluate them are available, and results can be compared with normal values for nerve, attribute, age, sex, height, weight, and body mass index.[44, 93] Generally, they are not thought to be as clinically meaningful as symptoms, neuropathic impairments, or quantitative sensory loss. We have proposed several minimal criteria for DPN using nerve conduction and heartbeat deep breathing or Valsalva (see Table 18.2). If the composite score NIS(LL)+7 tests is used for level of abnormality, we suggest it be $\geq$97.5th.

Stage N1b. The criteria for stage N1b proposed here are slightly changed from ones published earlier. The new criteria state that the patient should meet minimal criteria for DPN (criteria 7, 8, 10, or 11) (see Table 18.2), but in addition have neuropathic abnormality (for example, decreased or absent ankle reflexes [$\geq$99th] or NIS(LL)+3–9 tests $\geq$97.5th and/or abnormality of vibratory sensation of the great toes), but not have symptoms of DPN. To be accepted as abnormal, muscle stretch reflexes should be elicited with a sufficiently strong blow to elicit stretch of the gastrocnemius-soleus muscle using an appropriate reflex hammer (the Troemner hammer or the Queen Square hammer). For patients 50 to 69 years old, normal or reduced ankle reflexes are graded 0, and when absent are graded 1. For patients 70 years or older, normal, reduced, or absent ankle reflexes are graded 0 because 5% or greater of normal persons of this age have absent ankle reflexes. Vibration sensation is influenced by site, age, and weight. Therefore, it is not a simple matter for the examining physician to judge whether vibration sensation of the toe is normal, decreased, or absent. It is essential to begin by using an adequately designed tuning fork. We recommend the tuning fork made by Riverbank Laboratory (distributed by V. Mueller in Chicago; length 25 cm; made from ½ in. × 1¼ in. aluminum alloy standard stock; 156 Hz with counterweights). For a more reliable assessment of abnormality of vibration sensation, it is preferable to use a computerized system, such as CASE IV. Using such a system, it is possible to provide precisely shaped and quantified stimuli, given at defined magnitudes (steps) of intensity, using validated algorithms of testing and finding threshold. One can express results in μm of displacement, natural log (ln) of μm, normal deviates, percentiles specific for test, anatomical site, age, gender, and physical variables. With the general availability of personal computers, it is possible to express results as a percentile value specific for test, anatomical site, age, gender, and physical variables. In clinical practice, unequivocal decrease or absence of ankle reflexes (when reliably assessed) not explained by another neurologic disease or old age usually indicates stage 1b DPN (or a higher stage). Other neurologic signs unaccompanied by neuropathic symptoms may indicate stage 1b DPN as well.

How does one stage the patient who has unequivocally reduced ankle reflexes or raised vibration threshold of the toe, but who does not have abnormal nerve conduction abnormality or heartbeat deep breathing abnormality or heartbeat Valsalva abnormality criteria? We suggest that the patient be staged as normal (N0) for reasons of specificity. This should not occur frequently.

Stage N2 DPN. Four conditions must be met: (1) minimal criteria for DPN must be met, as given for stage N1a; (2) the pattern must be a lower limb symmetrical length-dependent sensorimotor polyneuropathy; (3) the patient must have positive or negative neuropathic symptoms caused by DPN; and (4) these symptoms must be attributable to DPN.

Symptoms of DPN are classified as negative (such as dead-type numbness or weakness) or positive (such as prickling or burning). Symptoms accompanying DPN vary according to anatomical location, kind, severity, constancy, change over time, associations, and response to treatment. Accurate information about these characteristics is useful for diagnosing, characterizing, and judging severity. As discussed in Chapter 8, the features of the symptoms have value in differential diagnosis. Thus, symptoms in the hands usually have different implications than those in the feet. We have found that symptoms of weakness and atrophy or prickling or loss of sensation in the hands in patients with DM are generally caused by carpal tunnel syndrome (MNW) or UNE or both, whereas altered reflexes and abnormal conduction velocity may be caused by a generalized neuropathic process.[46a] Also, the pain typical of DPN generally occurs in the toes and feet, but it may also occur in the legs. Pain in the thighs is more often caused by DLSRPN. The pain of

DPN is of several kinds: short-lived (lasting seconds or minutes) sticking or lancinating, burning, tightly wrapped (such as in the toes or feet), deep aching in calf, cold aching, boring, and restless leg discomfort. The severity is extremely variable, from mild discomfort lasting for only short intervals of time to severe and persistent discomfort. Any of the pains described above can occur in DPN. Typically, they are in the toes, feet, ankles, and distal legs. Some patients and physicians emphasize the night occurrence. Frequently, an "asleep" numbness (like "a hand gone asleep"), an excessive feeling of "coldness," "burning," and "asleep prickling" may accompany the pain. Excessive tenderness (such as excessive pain from walking on pebbles) may be evidence of hyperalgesic polyneuropathy. Generally, there is a poor association between severity of positive symptoms (such as pain) and neuropathic impairment. In many patients, the positive symptoms appear to be a transitory phase (for weeks, months, or years) followed by insensitivity. Other patients (perhaps as common or more common than the former) develop insensitivity without developing positive symptoms, but this observation needs further study. The idea that DPN is usually a painful condition is wrong—most patients with DPN do not have pain.

Negative sensory symptoms are perhaps more common than positive sensory symptoms. Thus, decreased tactile recognition of texture, size, or shape of objects with the feet is a common symptom. Another symptom is inability to recognize hot from cold with the feet. Still another is decreased ability to recognize cuts, bruises, and injuries as painful. On inquiry, the patient might recognize decreased autonomic function—decreased sweating, vasomotor changes in feet, impotence in the male (usually before loss of ability to ejaculate). Visceral autonomic neuropathy symptoms may be increased satiety, abdominal fullness, frank vomiting of retained gastric contents, diarrhea (typically unexplained after meals and at night), and sphincter alterations, such as urinary retention. Muscle weakness, if it occurs, is usually bilateral toe dorsiflexion weakness and then bilateral foot drop. It is an important marker of severity of DPN. As mentioned already, weakness of the thigh (collapse of the lower limb at the knee) usually is attributable to DLSRPN, and weakness of hands, to upper limb mononeuropathies (MNW and UNE). The degree of muscle weakness of ankle dorsiflexion appears to be a reproducible marker for dividing mild and severe DPN. In the RDNS, we found that DPN with 50% or more weakness of ankle dorsiflexion was often associated with neuropathic symptoms and with more severe neuropathic impairments.

Stage N2a. Symptomatic DPN with less than 50% weakness of ankle dorsiflexion.

Stage N2b. Symptomatic DPN with 50% or more weakness of ankle dorsiflexion.

Patients with stages N2b and N3 (disabling) DPN usually have definite or advanced diabetic retinopathy or nephropathy. Typically, these patients have advanced preproliferative or proliferative retinopathy. They usually have had preventative retinal laser treatment. Not uncommonly, they may have loss of vision caused by macular edema and advanced proliferative disease with vitreous hemorrhage or traction macular detachment or cataracts. Varying degrees of kidney function, up to frank uremia, may be encountered in this group. Also, at this stage it is not uncommon to have complications related to premature atherosclerosis—coronary, cerebrovascular, and peripheral vascular disease. Complications related, in part, to insensitivity—plantar ulcers, Charcot joints, and other mutilating acropathies—may also occur.

Stage N3. Disabling DPN. Occurrence of any of the following 10 motor, sensory, or autonomic conditions, judged to be the result of diabetic neuropathy, results in the diagnosis of the neuropathy as stage N3.

Motor
  Symptoms of muscle weakness, confirmed by examination, of sufficient severity that the patient is unable to walk independently.
Sensory
  Symptoms of sensory loss of sufficient severity, confirmed by examination, that the patient cannot walk independently because of sensory ataxia.
  Absence of feeling in hands so that the patient is disabled.
  Symptoms of pain, having the characteristics of neuropathic pain, that is disabling. The following criteria have to be fulfilled.
    A. The patient has previously attended physicians for pain relief.
    B. Work and recreational activities have been curtailed by at least 25% because of pain.

C. Medication for pain relief has been taken on a continuing ($\geq$50% of days) basis for at least 6 weeks.
Autonomic
  Gastric atony, as demonstrated by gastric retention tests and by exclusion of other gastric or psychiatric causes of emesis, causing emesis of retained ($\geq$ 18 hours) food at least once weekly for at least 6 weeks.
  Urinary retention as demonstrated by manometric evidence of detrusor hyperactivity, necessitating continuous use of a catheter for 6 weeks or longer and not caused by psychiatric disturbance or urinary bladder disease.
  Urinary incontinence caused by loss of sphincter function, necessitating continuous ($\geq$ 50% of time) use of diapers or leg urinal for at least 6 weeks and not caused by psychologic or bladder disease.
  Rectal incontinence caused by loss of anal sphincter function of at least 6 weeks' duration and not caused by psychiatric or rectal disease.
  Diarrhea to the degree that it causes weight loss ($\geq$ 5 kg) and steatorrhea (10 mg or more per 24 hours) not caused by psychiatric disturbance, laxative abuse, or other bowel disease.
  Symptomatic lightheadedness or fainting caused by orthostatic hypotension ($\geq$ 30 mm Hg systolic) with concomitant blood pressure drop, present continuously (lightheadedness or fainting weekly) for at least 6 weeks.

PAINFUL POLYNEUROPATHY WITH WEIGHT LOSS

Archer and coworkers[3] described an acute painful neuropathy with weight loss that they consider to be a clinical entity separate from DPN. They believe the syndrome to be similar to the cases of diabetic neuropathic cachexia described by Ellenberg.[49] Actually, some early workers[5, 71, 111] emphasized that weight loss might be a precursor of sensory polyneuropathy. In the first edition of this textbook, Thomas and Brown[125] describe the acute painful neuropathy as a separate neuropathy from DPN. In a personal communication to us, Watkins takes the position that acute painful diabetic neuropathies (DLSRPN, DTLRN, and painful small fiber neuropathy with weight loss) run an entirely separate course, distinct from that of DPN. He suggests that these painful neuropathies are distinctive because they are not associated with duration and severity of DM, tend to occur in men, are more common in NIDDM than in IDDM, and have a monophasic course usually over months. Severity of pain is not closely related to the severity of the neurologic impairment, and weight loss is a concomitant that is regained as the pain leaves.

We agree that DLSRPN and DTLRN (and we would add oculomotor neuropathy and diabetic autonomia) are disorders that should not be lumped in with DPN. We are less clear that acute painful small fiber polyneuropathy with weight loss is a separate disorder from DPN for the following reasons: weight loss and small-fiber symptoms are frequently a phase of DPN, and the clinical hallmarks appear to be overlapping with DPN. Further studies are needed.

TESTS USEFUL FOR THE DETECTION AND CHARACTERIZATION OF DIABETIC POLYNEUROPATHY

This is covered in Chapter 8.

MINIMAL CRITERIA FOR THE DIAGNOSIS OF DIABETIC POLYNEUROPATHY

This topic is discussed in the previous section entitled Clinical Syndrome and Staging of Severity.

Here we describe in more detail why individual tests are not adequate as minimal criteria and why a composite score or staging is better to express overall characteristics and severity. In a series of studies of the RDNS cohort, we have assessed which tests, combination of tests, clinical scores, or composite scores are most sensitive, specific, reproducible, and characterizing of overall impairment. We came to the following conclusions.

1. There is no one test (nerve conduction abnormality, heartbeat deep breathing abnormality, or heartbeat Valsalva abnormality) or clinical sign (decreased ankle reflexes or vibration sensation of the foot) that reliably serves as a minimal criteria for DPN.
2. To characterize the diverse neuropathic symptoms, impairments, and pathologic alteration of sensory, autonomic, and motor nerve fibers, it is necessary to quantitate these diverse items and express abnormality as a composite score.

3. A suitable composite score for neuropathic impairment is NIS(LL)+7 tests (see Tables 18.1 and 18.2); other composite scores that could be considered are NIS(LL)+3–9 tests.
4. A reasonable minimal criteria for abnormality is a defined percentile abnormality, for example, 97.5th percentile of NIS(LL)+3–9 tests, based on study of a suitable healthy subject cohort
5. The composite score (for example, NIS[LL]+7 tests) and the minimal criterion for abnormality (for example, 97.5th percentile) may be used in staging (to determine the severity of a patient's DPN).

What is an appropriate minimal criteria for DPN when NIS(LL)+7 tests or another composite score cannot be derived? Table 18.1 provides some alternative possibilities. Using NIS(LL)+7 tests as the gold standard, the order (sensitivity and specificity) of the criteria were (best to worst): criterion 8 ($\geq$ 2 test abnormal, 1 nerve conduction or QAT) (88% and 86%); criterion 7 ($\geq$ 2 test abnormal) (88% and 84%); criterion 10 ($\geq$ 2 nerves with nerve conduction abnormality) (81% and 91%); criterion 4 (abnormal ankle reflex and abnormal vibration sensation) (62% and 88%)]; and criterion 2 (abnormal ankle reflexes) (60% and 91%). The other criteria considered in Table 18.2 had lower sensitivities and specificities.

ASSESSING SEVERITY OF DIABETIC POLYNEUROPATHY

Severity is the sum of all the sensory, autonomic, and motor symptoms and impairments caused by DPN. As we discuss in our recent publication,[37] up to this time surveys of diabetic cohorts generally have identified the magnitude of DPN simply by frequency of occurrence, often using imprecise and variable minimal criteria for the diagnosis of DPN. A much better assessment of DPN demands not only that the disorder be reliably identified, but also that its overall severity be characterized and quantitated.

There are several approaches to scale severity of symptoms, impairment, both symptoms and impairments, and outcome. All four have value and are described in this section.

Symptoms need to be measured because they bother patients, but by themselves they are not a good measure of severity of DPN. Symptoms may be reported without neuropathy being present; they tend to come and go and do not correlate well with severity of impairment. Symptoms will frequently worsen without the neuropathy worsening.

Of the three quantitative approaches to assess severity of symptoms we have developed (Neuropathy Symptom Score [NSS],[45] Neuropathy Symptom Profile [NSP],[39] and Neuropathy Symptoms and Change [NSC],[37] NSC is the best measure of symptoms because (1) it tallies the number of symptoms; (2) it assesses severity—the tally of symptoms multiplied by severity (1 = slight, 2 = moderate, and 3 = severe); and (3) it assesses change (as compared with a defined previous time (same, better [1 = slight, 2 = moderate, and 3 = much], or worse [−1 = slight, −2 = moderate, and −3 = much]).

Severity of DPN is best assessed by overall neuropathic impairment or by a staged assessment of symptoms and impairments.[37] The NIS[45] or the NIS(LL) is a composite score of overall impairment. Although it is a standard test in the sense that a standard number of items of the neurologic examination are performed, the scaling approach is defined and is approximately linear. It has been tested and validated in healthy subjects and disease trials, but the judgments that physicians make may not be standardized. The results might be quite variable depending on physician training, experience, and care they take with the examination. To illustrate, physicians need to judge whether a muscle is weak (1 to 4) as compared with what is normal considering the muscle tested, age, sex, height, weight, and physical fitness. But how accurately and reproducibly can neurologists or general physicians make the necessary judgments? Using trained neurologists, reproducibility may be high.[43]

There are two approaches to quantitate overall severity—use of a composite score and staging. The NIS(LL) + 7 test (or NIS(LL) + 3–9 tests) uses the composite score approach. In the NIS(LL) + 7 tests, transformed points for percentile abnormality of VDT is substituted for the clinical vibratory examination. To this are added transformed points for percentile abnormality of heartbeat variation with deep breathing and attributes of nerve conduction. All the tests are expressed as NIS point transformations based on percentile abnormality considering age, sex, and various physical attributes. The abnormal limit (the 97.5th percentile value) for the NIS(LL) + 7 tests is approximately 4.5 points. This measure has been found to provide a good minimal criteria for diagnosis of DPN and is also a good continuous measure of severity of impairment. There is not an

overestimate of the frequency of DPN because of the error of multiple measurements when a composite score is used.[37, 93]

Staged severity of DPN provides a measure of severity combining symptoms and impairments. (See Introduction and Clinical Syndrome and Staging of Severity.)

COURSE OF DIABETIC POLYNEUROPATHY

There is some information on longitudinal change in the frequency of markers of diabetic polyneuropathy[27, 35, 42–44, 54, 62, 69, 77, 79, 94, 95, 97, 101, 102, 128] but little information on longitudinal change in overall severity of DPN using a composite score or staging and based on representative population-based cohorts. The change in frequency of markers of DPN was based on such dichotomous measures as normal or decreased vibratory perception at the lateral malleolus or toe, decreased ankle reflexes, or abnormal nerve conductions. Knowing the change in frequency of DPN, by one of the above listed markers, is of some value, but it provides only limited information because these markers are not reliable markers of DPN and provide little information about characteristics, severity, disease progression, and outcome. For these purposes, a composite score of impairment (for example, NIS(LL) + 7 tests) or staging is preferable.

Use of markers of DPN provided some information about the course of DPN. Pirart[101, 102] found that the frequency of polyneuropathy (as judged by decreased ankle reflexes and vibration sensation) among diabetic patients attending Brussels hospitals and diabetic clinics increased with duration of diabetes. He inferred that complications of nerve, kidney, and eye were related and caused by chronic hyperglycemia. In a study of 71 type 2 diabetic patients for 5 years, Hillson and colleagues[70] found a slight deterioration of vibratory sensation of the feet, measured by bioesthesiometry. Factors that related to this decrease were initial sensory threshold, age, gender, mean fasting plasma glucose, and failure to lose weight.

Another way in which the course of DPN can be assessed is following the neuropathic end points used in the placebo arm of the double-blind, controlled clinical drug trial. The results from such trials are disappointing because they are so inconsistent. Several reasons may explain this variability: (1) patients were usually highly selected for a given study, and different kinds of patients were selected for different studies; (2) clinical responses were biased toward improvement because of a patient's or a physician's expectation that the experimental drug would be efficacious (a placebo effect); or (3) lack of use of standard tests, adequate reference values, or composite scores. Florkowski and associates[52] randomly assigned 54 type 1 and 2 diabetic patients with symptoms of pain, numbness, or paresthesia into treatment with an aldose reductase inhibitor (ARI) or a placebo for a period of 24 weeks. In the placebo group, they found no statistically significant worsening of tibial nerve conduction velocity. In another ARI (tolrestat) study of symptomatic DPN,[85] investigators reported symptoms and motor nerve conduction velocities to have improved in the placebo-treated patients during a 6-month period, whereas vibration sensation at the wrist worsened. The improvement of pain and paresthesia by approximately 0.8 and 0.6 points, respectively, on a 4-point scale in the placebo group is hard to explain except perhaps as a placebo effect, whereas the improvement of all motor nerve conduction velocities in the tolrestat and placebo groups (by as much as 5.9 ± 1.6 percent [$P < 0.001$] for the placebo peroneal motor nerve conduction velocity) should not be subject to placebo effect; this is hard to explain and is unlikely to be correct. In the Sorbinil Retinopathy Trial Research Group study,[118] the frequency of clinically diagnosed polyneuropathy rose from 15% at 1 year to 30% at 4 years. Also difficult to understand is the nerve conduction worsening at 4 years, for example, by 2.3 m/sec for median motor nerve conduction velocity (MNCV) and by 0.3 m/sec for peroneal MNCV. Comparable values for compound muscle action potential decreased by 1.0 mV for the median and 1.1 mV for the peroneal nerves. In another ARI trial, investigators found small degrees of worsening for cardiovascular autonomic test results.[58, 59] Because the values in these latter studies were not corrected for age and physical variables, one should not assume that all of the worsening was caused by DM, but at least the direction of the change and its magnitude are similar to what we found.

Information about change in polyneuropathy over time also came from intervention trials of glycemic control. In a 1994 study from Oslo,[2] 45 patients with type 1 DM, 18 to 42 years old, were assigned into three treatment groups using insulin (infusion by pump, multiple injections, or twice daily injections [conventional treatment]). The trial was for 4 years,

and thereafter the patients could choose their treatment for the next 4 years. These investigators compared nerve conduction values after 8 years and found a striking difference in worsening of neuropathic end points for the twice daily injection (poor glycemic control) group. To illustrate, whereas the tibial MNCV had decreased by 3.9 m/sec in patients whose average hemoglobin A_{1C} (HbA_{1C}) had been controlled below 10%, it had decreased by 6.8 m/sec for the group whose HbA_{1C} had averaged 10% or greater. The effect appeared to be greater in lower than in upper limb nerves. Likewise, they found a significantly greater decrease of heartbeat deep breathing or heartbeat response to standing in patients whose average HbA_{1C} was 10% or greater. In the Diabetes Control and Complications Trial (DCCT),[27, 126] only patients with type 1 DM without or with mild background retinopathy were included for longitudinal study. The percentage of patients who developed "evident polyneuropathy" and abnormalities of nerve conduction were significantly lower in the near euglycemic group than in the conventionally treated-group. They did not estimate overall severity or stage of DPN.

We studied a representative cohort of approximately 200 community diabetic patients longitudinally for times of 2 to 10 years.[37] We comprehensively assessed for nerve, eye, and kidney complications; large vessel complications; and risk factors that might be implicated. Because we assumed that the frequency and severity of DPN increased with duration of DM, we tested the relative ability of the different evaluations, tests, or composite scores to reflect this worsening. We found that overall, diabetic patients worsened by 0.34 NIS(LL)+7 test points per year, whereas diabetic patients with neuropathy worsened by 0.85 NIS(LL)+7 test points per year. To provide an idea of the degree of magnitude that this represents, one should recall that 1 point change is equivalent to a 25% change in one muscle's strength, a 50% change in one reflex, or a 50% change of one modality of sensation at one site (of the muscles, reflexes, and modalities of sensation tested in the NIS). To this point change from the neurologic examination, we add selected test results of nerve conduction, QST, and QAT abnormalities. The transformations that are made, from percentile to point abnormality, are shown in Table 18.3.

Based on these data, we have been able to estimate power to perform a controlled clinical trial based on 2-year follow-up data of RDNS

TABLE 18.3 COMPARISON OF THE CHANGE PER YEAR (SLOPE) EXPRESSED AS A NORMAL DEVIATE OR POINTS AND MONOTONICITY OF WORSENING (MEAN R) FOR THE LONGITUDINAL RDNS COHORT NORMAL DEVIATE (FROM RDNS-HS COHORT)[37]

	Normal Deviate					
	Magnitude			*Monotonicity**		
Test	*Mean Slope*	P	*T Groups†*	*Mean R‡*	P	*T Groups*
U SNDL‡	0.239	0.0001	A	0.492	0.0001	A
VDT	0.203	0.0001	A,B	0.453	0.0001	A,B
T MNDL	0.167	0.0001	B,C,D	0.448	0.0001	A,B
P MNCV	0.164	0.0001	B,C,D	0.389	0.0001	A,B,C
U MNDL	0.142	0.0001	B,C,D,E	0.400	0.0001	A,B,C
P MNDL	0.140	0.0001	C,D,E,F	0.493	0.0001	A
U MNCV	0.105	0.0001	D,E,F,G	0.227	0.0001	D
HB DB	0.089	0.0001	E,F,G	0.271	0.0001	C,D
T MNCV	0.079	0.0001	F,G	0.230	0.0001	D
S SNAP	0.063	0.0001	G	0.303	0.0001	B,C,D
U F-wave	0.050	0.0001	G	0.195	0.0001	D
HB Valsalva	0.044	0.0069	G	0.236	0.0001	D
T F-wave	0.044	0.0012	G	0.192	0.0001	D
ΣSNAP§	0.043	0.0005	G	0.178	0.0001	D
NIS(LL)+7	0.188	0.0001	A,B,C	0.273	0.0001	C,D
	Points (Equivalent to NIS Points)					
U MNDL	0.068	0.0001	B	0.234	0.0001	A,B
U SNDL‡	0.067	0.0001	B	0.179	0.0001	B,C
P MNCV	0.055	0.0001	B	0.170	0.0001	B,C,D
U MNCV	0.054	0.0001	B	0.145	0.0001	B,C,D,E
HB Valsalva	0.046	0.0007	B	0.129	0.0001	C,D,E
VDT	0.045	0.0001	B	0.132	0.0001	B,C,D,E
ΣSNAP§	0.034	0.0007	B	0.100	0.0013	C,D,E
S SNAP	0.034	0.0001	B	0.141	0.0001	B,C,D,E
HB DB	0.034	0.0036	B	0.111	0.0002	C,D,E
	Points (Equivalent to NIS Points)					
T MNCV	0.028	0.0037	B	0.110	0.0012	C,D,E
T MNDL	0.025	0.0001	B	0.109	0.0001	C,D,E
U CMAP	0.017	0.0341	B	0.044	0.1227	E
P CMAP	0.016	0.0110	B	0.070	0.0079	D,E
ΣCMAP	0.015	0.0565	B	0.076	0.0159	D,E
U F-wave	0.015	0.0557	B	0.069	0.0217	D,E
P MNDL	0.013	0.0352	B	0.054	0.0039	E
T CMAP	0.011	0.1261	B	0.055	0.0414	E
NIS(LL)+7	0.339	0.0001	A	0.337	0.0001	A

U, ulnar; T, tibial; P, peroneal; S, sural; SNDL, sensory nerve distal latency; MNDL, motor nerve distal latency; MNCV, motor nerve conduction velocity; SNAP, sensory nerve action potential; CMAP, compound muscle action potential; VDT, vibration detection threshold; HB DB, heartbeat with deep breathing; HB Valsalva, heartbeat with Valsalva; ΣCMAP, summated compound muscle action potentials of ulnar, peroneal, and tibial nerves; ΣSNAP, summated sensory nerve action potentials of ulnar and sural nerves.
*Monotonicity, as evaluated by the Spearman correlation coefficient.
†Points, Neuropathy Impairment Score (NIS), or NIS lower limb (NIS[LL]) points or values equivalent to NIS points as described in ref. 37.
‡Left palmar.
§RDNS-HS data are based on a study of more than 300 healthy subjects from Rochester, Minn.[44]

diabetic patients 65 years or older with polyneuropathy (≤97.5th NIS[LL]+7). Using data on subjects with data at baseline and 4 years, the mean and SD of the changes in 29 subjects (no outliers) were 3.28 and 4.74, respectively. Based on these results, we estimate that a 4-year study would require 45 patients per arm to achieve power of .90 to detect a treatment effect that eliminates progression of disease; a clinically meaningful effect can be expected to be observed at approximately 2.4 years.

Based on the calculations provided above, we would conservatively project that a clinical trial involving these types of patients should extend for a period of at least 3 years and include approximately 70 to 100 patients per arm to have a high probability of demonstrating a clinically meaningful effect of a therapy.

Various attributes of nerve conduction; VDT as measured by CASE IV using the 4, 2, and 1 algorithm; and decrease in heartbeat with deep breathing provided the best measures of worsening having the greatest monotonicity and magnitude.

The outcome of diabetic patients varies considerably depending on duration of DM, degree of glycemic control, development of kidney dysfunction, and type of DM (see Chapter 17). At a given age or at death, patients with DM, therefore, may have no evidence of DPN or varying stages of it. From prevalence studies, the frequency of diabetic patients with symptoms is approximately 13%, and this is approximately the same in types 1 and 2 DM. In Figures 18.1 and 18.2, we show the frequency distribution of stages of DPN and retinopathy in the RDNS cohort.

ASSOCIATION OF DIABETIC RETINOPATHY, NEPHROPATHY, AND POLYNEUROPATHY

Fagerberg[51] found a statistically significant association between the occurrence of retinopathy, nephropathy, and polyneuropathy in a diabetic cohort. This question was restudied in the RDNS.[42] This cohort of 380 diabetic patients is thought to be representative of diabetic patients in the community, at least for patients younger than 70 years. In this cohort, we carefully classified diabetic neuropathies and excluded other varieties of neurologic disease and neuropathy. We found a highly significant statistical association for the three complications (retinopathy, nephropathy, and neuropathy).

There are now three lines of evidence that the three diabetic complications have a similar metabolic-microvessel-hypoxic genesis: (1) the complications are statistically associated; (2) there appears to be a striking similarity in the functional and structural alterations of microvessels; and (3) prospective studies of hyperglycemic control appear to have the same preventive effect on all three diabetic complications.

PATHOLOGY OF DIABETIC POLYNEUROPATHY

This is discussed by Giannini and Dyck in Chapter 19.

PATHOGENESIS OF DIABETIC POLYNEUROPATHY

As we discuss in our review of the pathology of diabetic neuropathy,[38] the marked heterogeneity of natural history, disease, association, pathologic alteration, and biochemical derangement in diabetic neuropathy makes it highly likely that it is made up of different disorders with different underlying mechanisms. There probably are at least four mechanisms implicated in the different diabetic neuropathies: metabolic-microvessel derangement (hyperglycemic), immune, compression, and hypoglycemia.

The metabolic-microvessel derangement (hyperglycemic) may be the responsible mechanism for DPN, retinopathy, and nephropathy. In diabetic patient cohorts, the complication of neuropathy, retinopathy, and nephropathy are closely associated. The microvessel alterations are similar in the three complications. In nerves, retina, and kidney of diabetic patients, altered permeability of microvessels appears to precede or accompany overt complications. The endoneurial microvessels changes typical of DPN include pericyte degeneration, basement membrane reduplication, and degeneration of endoneurial microvessels. The changes precede and are associated with severity of DPN. Whereas in retinopathy and nephropathy the proximate causes of retinal and kidney injury are known, it is not as evident in nerve. In retina, an early lesion is transudation of fluorescein followed by focal expansion of microvessels (berry aneurysm), edema, and ischemia, and neovascularization (possibly in response to hypoxia). These changes can be prevented and probably even reversed by prolonged periods of near-euglycemia. A somewhat similar sequence of events occurs in the diabetic kidney.

Intervention trials have shown that this deleterious sequence of events can be inhibited, perhaps prevented, and even improved by prolonged rigorous control of hyperglycemia.

The data, therefore, suggest that DPN could be prevented if euglycemia could be reliably maintained. It seems unlikely that present modes of treatment—continuous subcutaneous insulin infusion (by a preprogrammed pump) or multiple daily injections of insulin—will result in euglycemia without also developing hypoglycemic episodes. It is possible, however, that improved plasma glucose monitoring and insulin delivery approaches will be found that will prevent the development of DPN and avoid hypoglycemia. Pancreas or pancreas-renal transplantation are generally not available for the prevention of early diabetic complications because of lack of availability of tissue, high frequency and severity of complications from surgery, viral infections, toxicity of immunosuppressants, and high cost. The idea has grown that it might be possible to tolerate a higher degree of hyperglycemia if one or several crucial intermediate metabolic derangements could be prevented or rectified by an additional treatment in addition to rigorous glycemic control. Unfortunately, rigorous glycemic control is frequently associated with hypoglycemic episodes with the attendant risk of hypoglycemic injury to nerves.

It has not been settled how hyperglycemia causes nerve injury, but there is some information on the subject. The two general hypotheses that we have explored are:

hyperglycemia → metabolic derangement → microvessel dysfunction → nerve fiber alterations

or

hyperglycemia → metabolic derangement → injury of Schwann cells or nerve fibers

As discussed in Chapters 19 to 27, the postulated metabolic derangement is not agreed on either, but possibilities include derangements of the polyol pathway, glycosylation of proteins, abnormalities of phospholipids, oxygen free-radical stress, deficiency of growth factors, and others. There is still no compelling data that use of ARIs, prevention of glycosylation of proteins (such as with methylguanidine), addition of supplemental fatty acids (for example, an enriched source of linolenic acid, such as evening primrose oil), antioxidants (vitamin E or α-lipoic acid), or growth factors (such as nerve growth factor) can be used to offset the needs for rigorous glycemic control.

As we discuss elsewhere, the observation of lymphocyte infiltrates[76, 137] in some patients with DPN raises the question whether immune mechanisms may also be involved in pathogenesis. In considering the evidence for such involvement, we note that for cases with DPN, the degree of inflammation was often not severe and some of the studies were not adequately controlled. Younger and colleagues[137] showed increased vascular and perivascular inflammation in nerves of DPN and DLSRPN when compared with control nerves. An argu-

ment against immune factors being a primary cause of DPN is the epidemiologic evidence that total hyperglycemic exposure (for example, HbA_{1C} × duration of DM in type 1 DM is the major risk factor for DPN[41a]) and that near euglycemia appear to inhibit development of DPN.[2, 28, 29, 113]

We do not wish to discuss the pathogenesis of other varieties of diabetic neuropathies, but it is evident that DLSRPN is commonly associated with frank perivascular inflammation (sometimes unequivocal necrotizing vasculitis) and multifocal fiber loss. The disorder tends to improve with time. Said and colleagues,[112] who first described the inflammation in this condition, attributed it to ischemia and vasculitis in the severe forms and to metabolic derangement in the milder forms. We have recently reviewed the pathologic alterations of sural nerves in this condition and found evidence that microscopic vasculitis appears to underlie the condition.[46b] It may be that thoracolumbar radiculoneuropathy and some multiple mononeuropathies likewise have an immune genesis.

We have also found that symptomatic involvement of upper limb nerves are generally caused by compression injury at entrapment points, such as at the wrist (MNW) and elbow (UNE).[46a] Whether it is caused by nerve vulnerability or to a greater degree of compression or repeated injury from stiffer or increased collagen volume has not been shown.

SPECIAL EVALUATIONS AND TESTS

These are discussed in detail in Chapter 8.

RISK FACTORS FOR DIABETIC POLYNEUROPATHY

Previous epidemiologic studies have identified putative risk factors that might relate to the development of DPN, but with the exception of chronic hyperglycemia, these studies did not identify a consistent list of risk factors. The reasons for this inconsistency may be that (1) the cohort was not representative of community diabetic patients; (2) DPN was not adequately characterized at regular intervals and quantitated using a comprehensive composite score based on standard and appropriate reference values; and (3) risk factors were not prospectively studied using reliable test measurements at regular intervals of time and not associated with intercurrent disease.

In a cross-sectional study of 145 diabetic patients and 46 control patients, Gregersen[62] found that duration of DM and poor glycemic control were related to the occurrence of DPN determined from motor nerve conductions of ulnar and peroneal nerves. Pirart,[101, 102] in a cross-sectional and longitudinal study of more than 4000 diabetic patients attending Brussels hospitals and clinics, concluded that poor glycemic control related to the occurrence of decreased ankle reflexes and decreased vibration sensation of the foot. He noted that sex, family history of diabetes mellitus, age, or obesity were not risk factors for DPN. In untreated type 2 DM, Porte and colleagues[103] found that glycemic control as measured by fasting plasma glucose or HbA_{1C} correlated with degree of slowing of nerve conduction.

Studying 79 patients with type 1 DM and 20 controls aged 16 to 19 years, Young and associates[136] found that abnormality of nerve conduction and heartbeat variation with deep breathing were associated with poor chronic glycemic control as measured by HbA_{1C}. Hillson and coworkers,[70] studying vibratory perception threshold (VPT) in 71 type 2 diabetic patients, found that initial sensory threshold, age, gender, mean fasting plasma glucose, and failure to become thinner were associated with an abnormal VPT. Also studying VPT, Sosenko and associates[119, 120] found in patients with type 1 DM that this threshold was unrelated to HbA_{1C} in younger patients, but in older patients VPT was related to level of HbA_{1C} and to duration of DM. In a later study of VPT in 200 diabetic patients and 22 control subjects, the same authors found that VPT was related to height, duration of DM, and age. In 67 diabetic patients, Weinberg and Pfeifer[129] found that symptomatic neuropathy was associated with heart rate and with duration of DM. Using the judgment of "clinically detectable neuropathy," neurologists in the DCCT[28–30] found that the factors related to DPN were older age, longer duration of DM, and male gender. It is unclear what criteria neurologists actually used to make the judgment of who had DPN.

In a study from Children's Hospital in Pittsburgh of a cohort of patients with type 1 DM and clinically diagnosed DPN, Maser and associates[90] identified the following multivariate risk factors: duration of DM, HbA_{1C}, smoking, and low density lipoproteins. In a further study of 100 patients with type 1 DM and 51 healthy subjects and using staging of DPN, Ziegler and coworkers[138] found that abnormality of tibial nerve somatosensory evoked po-

tentials depended on stage of DPN more than on glycemic control or duration of DM. In the San Luis Valley Diabetic Study of 277 patients with type 2 DM given a "standard neurologic history and examination," Franklin and colleagues[54] found that increasing age, longer duration of diabetes, higher value of HbA_{1C}, and insulin use were the multivariate factors that related to DPN.

In the RDNS, Dyck and associates[41a] found that the risk factors for DPN are different for type 1 and type 2 DM. For the two groups combined, they are (in order of magnitude): ln (HbA_{1C} × duration of DM); HbA_{1C}; 24-hour protein and type of DM.

The role of total hyperglycemic exposure as a risk factor for DPN has now been established in controlled clinical trials. In a seminal early study of C peptide–deficient diabetic (type 1 DM) patients with abnormality of nerve conduction, patients were randomly assigned into two treatment groups.[113] One group continued on conventional treatment, and the other group was given insulin continuously. At entry, the patients were not different in level of hyperglycemia, neuropathic impairment, VDT using CASE IV, or nerve conduction abnormality. At 4 months, there was a striking difference in glycemic control between the rigorous and conventional treatment groups (fasting plasma glucose 5.3 versus 9.9 mmol/L and HbA_{1C} 8.5 versus 10.7%), and neuropathic end points were not significantly different between groups. By 8 months, however, attributes of nerve conduction ($P = 0.03$) and VDT ($P = 0.002$) were significantly better in the rigorous treatment group.

In a second intervention trial, Amthor and associates[2] randomly assigned 45 patients with type 1 DM to continuous infusion of insulin or multiple injections of insulin or conventional control for a period of 4 years. For the succeeding 4 years, patients could remain on the same schedule or cross over. At 8 years, patients were divided into two groups—those whose mean HbA_{1C} had averaged less than 10% and those whose mean HbA_{1C} had been 10% or more. Thirty-three patients had average HbA_{1C} of 9.0%, and 12 had an average of 10.9%. Peroneal motor nerve conduction velocity had worsened by an average of 2.2 ± 5.3 m/sec in the first group and by 4.8 ± 4.9 m/sec in the second group ($P < .01$). Comparable values for the posterior tibial nerve were 3.9 ± 5.1 m/sec and 6.8 ± 5.7 m/sec ($P < 0.05$).

In a third large study (DCCT),[28] insulin-taking diabetic patients were selected by the criteria of no or mild retinopathy and randomly assigned into continuation of conventional treatment or rigorous treatment using continuous insulin infusion or multiple daily subcutaneous injections of insulin. The end point for DPN was "clinically evident DPN" and change in nerve conduction. By the first criteria, rigorous control of glycemia reduced the development of clinically evident DPN. Nerve conductions were significantly better in the rigorous group as compared with the conventionally treated group.

These three studies, therefore, provide compelling evidence that rigorous control of glycemia inhibits the development of DPN.

TREATMENT

Because chronic hyperglycemia exposure appears to be the most important risk factor for DPN, the first approach to prevention or amelioration of DPN is to maintain plasma glucose in or as near as possible to euglycemia without inducing hypoglycemia. For strategy of how this should be done, see Chapter 2.

We believe that it is difficult, perhaps impossible, for some patients to achieve euglycemia. Therefore, it would be desirable to modulate the adverse metabolic consequences related to such chronic hyperglycemia. Conceptually, one would like to normalize the metabolic derangements consequent to chronic hyperglycemia and to test whether this would inhibit development of diabetic complications. Whether such normalization could favorably offset the deleterious effect of hyperglycemia is still unknown. Oral supplemental of *myo*-inositol in dosages of 1 g/day, 3 g/day, and 6 g/day did not appear to be efficacious.[64, 65] A series of ARIs have been tried; in experimental diabetes they appear to have a favorable effect on conduction velocity, but in human studies their effectiveness has not been proved. With the introduction of improved ARI, further trials are in progress (see Chapter 22). Agents to inhibit glycation of proteins have been considered, but evidence that they are effective in preventing or improving polyneuropathy is not available. Supplementation of the diet with an enriched source of the fatty acid linolenic acid (evening primrose oil) has been tried and appeared to show a beneficial effect. Antioxidants, such as vitamin E or α-lipoic acid, have been tried. In Germany, α-lipoic acid has been extensively prescribed as an intravenous solution for painful neuropathy with claimed efficacy.[85] In a double-blind trial, it affected symptoms favorably.

References

1. Althaus J. On sclerosis of the spinal cord, including locomotor ataxy, spastic spinal paralysis and other system diseases of the spinal cord: Their pathology, symptoms, diagnosis, and treatment, London, Green & Company, 1885.
2. Amthor K-F, Dahl-Jorgensen K, Berg TJ, et al. The effect of 8 years of strict glycaemic control on peripheral nerve function in IDDM patients: The Oslo Study. Diabetologia 1994; 37:579.
3. Archer AG, Watkins PJ, Thomas PK, et al. The natural history of acute painful neuropathy in diabetes mellitus. J Neurol Neurosurg Psychiatry 1983; 46:491.
4. Asbury AK, Aldredge H, Hershberg R, et al. Oculomotor palsy in diabetes mellitus: A clinico-pathological study. Brain 1970; 93:555.
5. Auche MB. Des alterations des nerfs périphériques. Arch Med Exp Anat Pathol 1890; 2:635.
6. Bargen JA, Bollman JL, Kepler EJ. The "diarrhea of diabetes" and steatorrhea of pancreatic insufficiency. Proc Staff Meet Mayo Clin 1936; 11:737.
7. Barohn RJ, Sahenk Z, Warmolts JR, et al. The Bruns-Garland syndrome (diabetic amyotrophy) revisited 100 years later. Arch Neurol 1991; 48:1130.
8. Bastron JA, Thomas JE. Diabetic polyradiculopathy: Clinical and electromyographic findings in 105 patients. Mayo Clin Proc 1981; 56:725.
9. Berner JH Jr. Orthostatic hypotension in diabetes mellitus. Acta Med Scand 1952; 143:336.
10. Bloodworth JMB, Epstein M. Diabetic amyotrophy: Light and electron microscopic investigation. Diabetes 1967; 16:181.
11. Boehm HJ Jr. Diabetic Charcot joint: Report of a case and review of the literature. N Engl J Med 1962; 267:185.
12. Bosanquet FD, Henson RA. Sensory neuropathy in diabetes mellitus. Folia Psychiatry Neurol 1957; 60:107.
13. Bouton AJ, Angus E, Ayyar DR, et al. Diabetic thoracic polyradiculopathy presenting as abdominal swelling. Br Med J 1984; 289:798.
14. Bowen BD, Aaron AH. Gastric secretion in diabetes mellitus. Arch Intern Med 1926; 37:674.
15. Bradley WG, Chad D, Verghese JP. Painful lumbosacral plexopathy with elevated erythrocyte sedimentation rate: A treatable inflammatory syndrome. Ann Neurol 1984; 15:457.
16. Bruns L. Uber neuritische Lahmungen beim Diabetes Mellitus. Berl Klin Wochenschr 1890; 27:509.
17. Buchtal F, Rosenfalck A. Sensory conduction from digit to palm and from palm to wrist in the carpal tunnel syndrome. J Neurol Neurosurg Psychiatry 1971; 34:243.
18. Buzzard F. Illustrations of some less known forms of peripheral neuritis, especially alcoholic monoplegia and diabetic neuritis. Br Med J 1890; 1:1419.
19. Calverley JR, Mulder DW. Femoral neuropathy. Neurology 1960; 10:963.
20. Casey EB, Harrison MJG. Diabetic amyotrophy: A follow-up study. Br Med J 1972; 1:656.
21. Charcot M. Sur un cas de paraplégie diabetique. Arch Neurol 1890; 19:318.
22. Chokroverty S. Proximal nerve dysfunction in diabetic proximal amyotrophy. Arch Neurol 1982; 39:403.

23. Chokroverty S. AAEE case report 13: Diabetic amyotrophy. Muscle Nerve 1987; 10:679.

24. Chokroverty S, Reyes MG, Rubino FA. Bruns-Garland syndrome of diabetic amyotrophy. Trans Am Neurol Assoc 1977; 102:1.

25. Chokroverty S, Reyes MG, Rubino FA, et al. The syndrome of diabetic amyotrophy. Ann Neurol 1977; 2:181.

26. Choudhury AKR, Mukerjee AB, Choudhury NKR. Diabetic amyotrophy. J Indian Med Assoc 1973; 61:37.

27. DCCT Research Group: The effect of intensive treatment of diabetes on the development and progression of long-term complications in insulin-dependent diabetes mellitus. N Engl J Med 1993; 329:977.

28. DCCT Research Group: The Diabetes Control and Complications Trial (DCCT): Design and methodologic considerations for the feasibility phase. Diabetes 1986; 35:530.

29. DCCT Research Group: The effect of intensive diabetes therapy on the development and progression of neuropathy. Ann Intern Med 1995; 122:561.

30. DCCT Research Group: Effect of intensive diabetes treatment on nerve conduction in the diabetes control and complications trial. Ann Neurol 1995; 38:869.

31. de Calvi M. Recherches sur les Accidents Diabétiques. Paris, 1864.

32. Downie AW, Newell DJ. Sensory nerve conduction in patients with diabetes mellitus and controls. Neurology 1961; 11:876.

33. Dreyfus RM, Hakim S, Adams RD. Diabetic ophthalmoplegia: Report of a case with postmortem study and comments on vascular supply of human oculomotor nerve. Arch Neurol Psychiatry 1957; 77:337.

34. Dyck PJ. Resolvable problems in diatetic neuropathy. J NIH Res 1990; 2:57–62.

35. Dyck PJ. Detection, characterization, and staging of polyneuropathy: Assessed in diabetics. Muscle Nerve 1988; 11:21.

36. Dyck PJ. Quantitating severity of neuropathy. In Dyck PJ, Thomas PK, Griffin JW, et al (eds): Peripheral Neuropathy. Philadelphia, WB Saunders, 1993, p 686.

37. Dyck PJ, Davies JL, Litchy WJ, et al. Longitudinal assessment of diabetic polyneuropathy using a composite score in the Rochester Diabetic Neuroapthy Study cohort. Neurology 1997; 49:229.

38. Dyck PJ, Giannini C. Pathologic alterations in the diabetic neuropathies of humans: A review. J Neuropathol Exp Neurol 1996; 55:1181.

39. Dyck PJ, Karnes J, O'Brien PC, et al. Neuropathy symptom profile in health, motor neuron disease, diabetic neuropathy, and amyloidosis. Neurology 1986; 36:1300.

40. Dyck PJ, Karnes JL, O'Brien PC, et al. The Rochester Diabetic Neuropathy Study: Reassessment of tests and criteria for diagnosis and staged severity. Neurology 1992; 42:1164.

41. Dyck PJ, Karnes JL, O'Brien PC, et al. Detection thresholds of cutaneous sensation in humans. In Dyck PJ, Thomas PK, Griffin J, et al (eds): Peripheral Neuropathy. Philadelphia, WB Saunders, 1993, p 706.

41a. Dyck PJ, Kratz KM, Davies JL, et al. Risk factors for severity of diabetic polyneuropathy: Prospective and intensive longitudinal assessment of a population-based cohort in Rochester, Minn. In preparation.

42. Dyck PJ, Kratz KM, Karnes JL, et al. The prevalence by staged severity of various types of diabetic neuropathy, retinopathy, and nephropathy in a population-based cohort: The Rochester Diabetic Neuropathy Study. Neurology 1993; 43:817.

43. Dyck PJ, Kratz KM, Lehman KA, et al. The Rochester Diabetic Neuropathy Study: Design, criteria for types of neuropathy, selection bias, and reproducibility of neuropathic tests. Neurology 1991; 41:799.

44. Dyck PJ, Litchy WJ, Lehman KA, et al. Variables Influencing Neuropathic Endpoints: The Rochester Diabetic Neuropathy Study of Healthy Subjects (RDNS-HS). Neurology 1995; 45:1115.

45. Dyck PJ, Sherman WR, Hallcher LM, et al. Human diabetic endoneurial sorbital, fructose, and myo-inositol related to sural nerve morphometry. Ann Neurol 1980; 8:590.

46. Dyck PJ, Zimmerman IR, O'Brien PC, et al. Introduction of automated systems to evaluate touch-pressure, vibration, and thermal cutaneous sensation in man. Ann Neurol 1978; 4:502.

46a. Dyck PJB, Harper CM, Dyck PJ. Paresthesia, pain, and weakness in hands of diabetic patients attributable to mononeuropathies or radiculopathy, not polyneuropathy: The Rochester (RDNS) and Pancreas and Renal Transplant (MC-PRI) studies. In preparation.

46b. Dyck PJB, Norell J, Dyck PJ. The role of ischemia and microvasculitis in diabetic lumbosacral radiculoplexus neuropathies. In preparation.

47. Eareckson VO, Miller JM. Third nerve palsy with sparing of the pupil in diabetes mellitus. Arch Ophthalmol 1952; 47:607.

48. Eichhorst H. Beitrage zur Pathologie der Nerven und Muskeln. 3. Neuritis diabetica und ihre Beziehungen zum fehlenden Patellarsehnenreflex. Virchows Arch Pathol Anat Physiol 1892; 127:1.

49. Ellenberg M. Diabetic neuropathic cachexia. Diabetes 1974; 23:418.

50. Ewing DJ, Burt AA, Campbell IW, et al. Vascular reflexes in diabetic autonomic neuropathy. Lancet 1973; December 15, p 1354.

51. Fagerberg S-E. Diabetic neuropathy: A clinical and histological study on the significance of vascular affections. Acta Med Scand 1959; 164(suppl 345):1.

52. Florkowski CM, Rowe BR, Nightingale S, et al. Clinical and neurophysiological studies of aldose reductase inhibitor ponalrestat in chronic symptomatic diabetic peripheral neuropathy. Diabetes 1991; 40:129.

53. Frank B, Klingelhofer J, Benecke R, et al. Die thorakoabdominelle Manifestation der diabetischen Neuropathie. Nervenarzt 1988; 59:393.

54. Franklin GM, Shetterly SM, Cohen JA, et al. Risk factors for distal symmetric neuropathy in NIDDM. The San Luis Valley Diabetes Study. Diabetes Care 1994; 17:1172.

55. Garland H. Neurological complications of diabetes mellitus: Clinical aspects. Proc R Soc Med 1960; 53:137.

56. Gill RD. The diabetic (cord) bladder. J Urol 1936; 36:730.

57. Gilliatt RW, Willison RG. Peripheral nerve conduction in diabetic neuroapthy. J Neurol Neurosurg Psychiatry 1962; 25:11.

58. Giugliano D, Acampora R, Marfella R, et al. Tolrestat in the primary prevention of diabetic neuropathy. Diabetes Care 1995: 18:536.

59. Giugliano D, Marfella R, Quatraro A, et al. Tolrestat for mild diabetic neuropathy: A 52-week, randomized, placebo-controlled trial. Ann Intern Med 1993; 118:7.

60. Goldstein JE, Cogan DG. Diabetic ophthalmoplegia with special reference to the pupil. Arch Ophthalmol 1960; 64:592.

61. Goodman JI. Femoral neuropathy in relation to diabetes mellitus: Report of 17 cases. Diabetes 1954; 3:266.

62. Gregersen G. Diabetic neuropathy: Influence of age, sex metabolic control, and duration of diabetes on motor conduction velocity. Neurology 1967; 17:972.

63. Gregersen G. Diabetic amyotrophy: A well-defined syndrome? Acta Med Scand 1969; 185:303.

64. Gregersen G, Bertelsen B, Harbo H, et al. Oral supplementation of myoinositol: Effects on peripheral nerve function in human diabetics and on the concentration in plasma, erythrocytes, urine and muscle tissue in human diabetics and normals. Acta Neurol Scand 1983; 67:164.

65. Gregersen G, Borsting H, Theil P, et al. Myoinositol and function of peripheral nerves in human diabetics: A controlled clinical trial. Acta Neurol Scand 1978; 58:241.

66. Guttmann L. Topographic studies of disturbance of sweat secretion after complete lesions of peripheral nerves. J Neurol Neurosurg Psychiatry 1940; 3:197.

67. Hamilton CR Jr, Dobson HL, Marshall J. Diabetic amyotrophy: Clinical and electronmicroscopic studies in 6 patients. Am J Med 1968; 256:81.

68. Harati Y, Niakan E. Diabetic thoracoabdominal neuropathy. Arch Intern Med 1986; 146:1493.

69. Harris M, Eastman R, Cowie C. Symptoms of sensory neuropathy in adults with NIDDM in the U.S. population. Diabetes Care 1993; 16:1446.

70. Hillson RM, Hockaday TDR, Newton DJ. Hyperglycaemia is one correlate of deterioration in vibration sense during the 5 years after diagnosis of Type 2 (non-insulin-dependent) diabetes. Diabetologia 1984; 26:122.

71. Jordan WR. Neuritis manifestations in diabetes mellitus. Arch Intern Med 1936; 57:307.

72. Jordan WR, Crabtree HH. Paralysis of the bladder in diabetic subjects. Arch Intern Med 1935; 55:17.

73. Joslin EP, Root HF. The protein of the cerebrospinal fluid in diabetic neuropathy. Tr A Am Physicians 1939; 54:251.

74. Joslin EP, Root HF, White P, et al. The Treatment of Diabetes Mellitus. London, Henry Kimpton, 1952.

75. Kraus WM. Involvement of the peripheral neurons in diabetes mellitus. Arch Neurol Psychiatry 1922; 7:202.

76. Krendel DA, Costigan DA, Hopkins LC. Successful treatment of neuropathies in patients with diabetes mellitus. Arch Neurol 1995; 52:1053.

77. Kumar S, Ashe HA, Parnell LN, et al. The prevalence of foot ulceration and its correlates in type 2 diabetic patients: A population-based study. Diabetic Med 1994; 11:480.

78. LaMontagne A, Buchthal F. Electrophysiological studies in diabetic neuropathy. J Neurol Neurosurg Psychiatry 1970; 33:442.

79. LaPorte RE, Tajima N, Dorman JS, et al. Differences between blacks and whites in the epidemiology of insulin-dependent diabetes mellitus in Allegheny County, Pennsylvania. Am J Epidemiol 1986; 123:592.

80. Lawrence DG, Locke S. Motor nerve conduction velocity in diabetes. Arch Neurol 1962; 7:365.

81. Leyden E. Die Entzundung der peripheren Nerven. Deut Militar Zeitsch 1887; 17:49.

82. List CF, Peet MM. Sweat secretion in man. II. Anatomic distribution of disturbances in sweating associated with lesions of the sympathetic nervous system. Arch Neurol Psychiatry 1938; 40:37.

83. Locke S, Lawrence DG, Legg MA. Diabetic amyotrophy. Am J Med 1963; 34:775.

84. Low PA. Clinical Autonomic Disorders: Evaluation and Management. Boston, Little, Brown, 1993.

85. Macleod AF, Boulton AJM, Owens DR, et al. A multi-centre trial of the aldose-reductase inhibitor tolrestat, in patients with symptomatic diabetic peripheral neuropathy. Diabete Metab 1992; 18:14.

86. Marble A, White P, Bogan IK, et al. Enlargement of the liver in diabetic children. Arch Intern Med 1938; 62:740.

87. Marinian: Contgribuzione-allo-studio clinico deiriflessi tendinei. Rivista Clinica di Bologna, 1884.

88. Martin MM. Diabetic neuropathy: A clinical study of 150 cases. Brain 1953; 76:594.

89. Martin MM. Involvement of autonomic nerve fibres in diabetic neuropathy. Lancet 1953; 1:560.

90. Maser RE, Steenkiste AR, Dorman JS, et al. Epidemiological correlates of diabetic neuropathy: Report from Pittsburgh epidemiology of diabetes complications study. Diabetes 1989; 38:1456.

91. Mulder DW, Lambert EH, Bastron JA, et al. The neuropathies associated with diabetes mellitus: A clinical and electromyographic study of 103 unselected diabetic patients. Neurology 1961; 11:275.

92. Newrick PG, Boulton AJM, Ward JD. The distribution of diabetic neuropathy in a British clinic population. Diabetes Res Clin Pract 1986; 2:263.

93. O'Brien PC, Dyck PJ. Procedures for setting normal values. Neurology 1995; 45:17.

94. O'Hare JA, Abuaisha F, Geoghegan M. Prevalence and forms of neuropathic morbidity in 800 diabetics. Ir Med J 1994; 163:132.

95. Orchard TJ, Dorman JS, Maser RE, et al. Factors associated with avoidance of severe complications after 25 years of IDDM: Pittsburgh Epidemiology of Diabetes Complications Study I. Diabetes Care 1990; 13:741.

96. Palumbo PJ, Elveback LR, Chu C-P, et al. Diabetes mellitus: Incidence, prevalence, survivorship, and causes of death in Rochester, Minnesota, 1945–1970. Diabetes 1976; 25:566.

97. Palumbo PJ, Elveback LR, Whisnant JP. Neurologic complications of diabetes mellitus: Transient ischemic attack, stroke, and peripheral neuropathy. Adv Neurol 1978; 19:593.

98. Pavy FW. Introductory address to the discussion of the clinical aspect of glycosuria. Lancet 1885; 2:1085.

99. Pavy FW. On diabetic neuritis. Lancet 1904; 2:17.

100. Pfeiffer M, Cook D, Brodsky J, et al. Quantitative evaluation of cardiac parasympathetic activity in normal and diabetic man. Diabetes 1982; 31:339.

101. Pirart J. Diabetes mellitus and its degenerative complications: A prospective study of 4,400 patients observed between 1947 and 1973. Diabetes Care 1978; 1:168.

102. Pirart J. Diabetes mellitus and its degenerative complications: A prospective study of 4,400 patients observed between 1947 and 1973. Part 2. Diabetes Care 1978; 1:252.

103. Porte D Jr, Graf RJ, Halter JB, et al. Diabetic neuropathy and plasma glucose control. Am J Med 1981; 70:195.

104. Pryce TD. On diabetic neuritis with a clinical and pathological description of three cases of diabetic psuedo-tabes. Brain 1893; 16:416.

105. Raff MC, Asbury AK. Ischemic mononeuropathy and mononeuropathy multiplex in diabetes mellitus. N Engl J Med 1968; 279:17.

106. Raff MC, Sangalang V, Asbury AK. Ischemic mononeuropathy multiplex associated with diabetes mellitus. Arch Neurol 1968; 18:487.

107. Redwood DR. Diabetic amyotrophy: Importance of good diabetic control. Br Med J 1962; 2:521.

108. Rollo J. Cases of Diabetes Mellitus. London, 1798.

109. Root HF, Rogers MH. Diabetic neuritis with paralysis. N Engl J Med 1930; 202:1049.
110. Rucker WC. Paralysis of the third, fourth, and sixth cranial nerves. Am J Ophthalmol 1958; 46:787.
111. Rundles RW. Diabetic neuropathy: General review with report of 125 cases. Medicine (Baltimore) 1945; 24:111.
112. Said G, Goulon-Goeau C, Lacroix C, et al. Nerve biopsy findings in different patterns of proximal diabetic neuropathy. Ann Neurol 1994; 35:559.
113. Service FJ, Rizza RA, Daube JR, et al. Near normoglycaemia improved nerve conduction and vibration sensation in diabetic neuropathy. Diabetologia 1985; 28:722.
114. Shumacker HB. Sympathetic denervation of the feet and legs occurring spontaneously or as a result of disease. Bull Johns Hopkins Hosp 1942; 71:1.
115. Skanse B, Gydell K. A rare type of femoral-sciatic neuropathy in diabetes mellitus. Acta Med Scand 1956; 155:463.
116. Skillman TG, Johnson EW, Hamwi GJ, et al. Motor nerve conduction velocity in diabetes mellitus. Diabetes 1961; 10:46.
117. Smith MD. Diabetic neuropathy with Argyll-Robertson pupils: Report on two cases. Glasgow Med J 1949; 30:181.
118. Sorbinil Retinopathy Trial Research Group: The Sorbinil Retinopathy Trial: Neuropathy results. Neurology 1993; 43:1141.
119. Sosenko JM, Boulton AJM, Kubrualy DB, et al. The vibratory perception threshold in young diabetic patients: Associations with glycemia and puberty. Diabetes Care 1985; 8:605.
120. Sosenko JM, Gadia MT, Fournier AM, et al. Body stature as a risk factor for diabetic sensory neuropathy. Am J Med 1986; 80:1031.
121. Steiness IB. Diabetic neuropathy. Acta Med Scand 1963; 394:15.
122. Subramony SH, Wilbourn AJ. Diabetic proximal neuropathy: Clinical and electromyographic studies. J Neurol Sci 1982; 53:293.
123. Suhler K, Parhofer K, Richter WO, et al. Diabetische Radikalopathie. Dtsch Med Wochenschr 1990; 115:1665.
124. Sullivan JF. The neuropathies of diabetes. Neurology 1958; 8:243.
125. Thomas PK, Brown MJ. Diabetic polyneuropathy. In Dyck PJ, Thomas PK, Asbury AK, et al (eds): Diabetic Neuropathy. Philadelphia, WB Saunders, 1987.
126. Thomas PK, Tomlinson DR. Diabetic and hypoglycemic neuropathy. In Dyck PJ, Thomas PK, Griffin JW, et al (eds): Peripheral Neuropathy. Philadelphia. WB Saunders, 1993, p 1219.
127. Tsairis P, Dyck PJ, Mulder DW. Natural history of brachial plexus neuropathy: Report on 99 patients. Arch Neurol 1972; 27:109.
128. Walters DP, Gatling W, Mullee MA, et al. The prevalence of diabetic distal sensory neuropathy in an English community. Diabetic Med 1992; 9:349.
129. Weinberg CR, Pfeifer MA. Development of a predictive model for symptomatic neuropathy in diabetes. Diabetes 1986; 35:873.
130. Wheeler T, Watkins PJ. Cardiac denervation in diabetes. Br Med J 1973; 4:584.
131. Whisnant JP, Love JG. Pitfall in diagnosis of diabetic "cord bladder." JAMA 1960; 174:147.
132. White P. Diabetes in youth. N Engl J Med 1941; 224:586.
133. Wilkins RW, Kolb LC. Vasomotor disturbances in peripheral neuritis. Am J Med Sci 1941; 202:216.
134. Williams IR, Mayer RF. Subacute proximal diabetic neuropathy. Neurology 1976; 26:108.
135. Woltman HW, Wilder RM. Diabetes mellitus: Pathological changes in the spinal cord and peripheral nerves. Arch Intern Med 1929; 44:576.
136. Young RJ, Ewing DJ, Clarke BF. Nerve function and metabolic control in teenage diabetics. Diabetes 1983; 32:142.
137. Younger DS, Rosoklija G, Hays AP, et al. Diabetic peripheral neuropathy: A clinicopathologic and immunohistochemical analysis of sural nerve biopsies. Muscle Nerve 1996; 19:722.
138. Ziegler D, Muhlen H, Dannehl K, et al. Tibial nerve somatosensory evoked potentials at various stages of peripheral neuropathy in insulin dependent diabetic patients. J Neurol Neurosurg Psychiatry 1993; 56:58.
139. Zorrilla E, Kozak GP. Ophthalmoplegia in diabetes mellitus. Ann Intern Med 1967; 67:968.

Chapter 19

Pathologic Alterations in Human Diabetic Polyneuropathy

Caterina Giannini • Peter James Dyck

INTRODUCTION

Of the varieties of neuropathy occurring in diabetes mellitus (DM), diabetic polyneuropathy (DPN) is the most common variety. This chapter focuses on the pathologic changes involving nerve fibers and interstitium in DPN and analyzes the relationship between pathologic and electrophysiologic and clinical findings. The pattern of fiber loss, the fiber class vulnerability, the evidence for or against axonal atrophy and degeneration, and primary or secondary myelin remodeling are discussed in detail. The striking pathologic alterations of microvessels found in DPN and their association with fiber abnormalities are described. Pathologic and epidemiologic findings point to microangiopathy and possibly ischemia as pathogenetic mechanisms.

Diabetic polyneuropathy, retinopathy, and nephropathy are common complications of DM. In the Rochester Diabetic Neuropathy Study (RDNS), a population-based cross-sectional and longitudinal epidemiologic study, DPN occurred in approximately 50% of diabetic patients and caused symptoms in approximately 13% of them.[25] Diabetic polyneuropathy is a chronic symmetrical sensorimotor and autonomic neuropathy occurring in patients with types 1 and 2 DM. It affects the lower limbs predominantly in a length-dependent distribution. It is the most common diabetic neuropathy disorder. Diabetic neuropathy includes a heterogeneous group of neuropathies with different natural histories, findings, and outcomes.[75] In addition to DPN, entities generally recognized include lumbosacral radiculoplexus neuropathy (LSRPN), thoracolumbar radiculoneuropathy (TLRN), diabetic autonomia (DA), median neuropathy at the wrist (MNW), ulnar neuropathy at the elbow (UNE), cranial III neuropathies (DCrIIIN), and hypoglycemic neuropathy. Underlying causes and mechanisms of these different disorders are probably different from DPN and will be discussed separately.

This chapter will focus on the pathologic changes involving nerve fibers and interstitium in DPN, analyze the associations between nerve fiber abnormalities and electrophysiologic and clinical findings, and suggest possible mechanisms of nerve fiber damage. There is evidence that chronic hyperglycemia and associated metabolic derangements are implicated in the pathogenesis of retinopathy, nephropathy, and neuropathy and that rigorous glycemic control can prevent or ameliorate DPN.[16, 17] Pathologic alterations of microvessels appear to be implicated in the cause of the diabetic retinopathy, nephropathy, and polyneuropathy.

DIABETIC POLYNEUROPATHY

Historical Aspects

Early reports of neurologic disorders in DM date to 1798, when John Rollo mentioned them in his book, *Cases of Diabetes Mellitus.*[6] The earliest description of peripheral nerve disorders in DM is credited to Marchal de Calvi who, in 1864, reported the occurrence of pain in the sciatic nerve distribution and the presence of peripheral areas of anesthesia in diabetic patients and hypothesized that these disturbances were the consequence of DM.[18] Reports of the diverse clinical manifestations of diabetic neuropathies followed: Bouchard (1884),[10] Althaus (1885),[3] Pavy (1887),[55] Pryce (1887 and 1893),[59, 60] and Leyden (1893).[47a] Leyden reported on the autopsy findings of cases of diabetic patients and associated the clinical abnormalities with the involvement of peripheral nerves. The first patient described by Pryce had perforating ulcers of feet and ataxia.[59] Leyden subdivided the clinical peripheral nerve involvement into three syndromes: hyperalgesic, motor or para-

lytic, and ataxic or pseudotabetic. Auche (1890)[5] and Buzzard (1890)[14] reported series of diabetic patients with neuropathy and postulated that nerve damage might relate to increased sugar concentration. Further reports and descriptions of clinical features of diabetic neuropathy followed the discovery and use of insulin.[41, 52, 64, 81] Rundles in his report of 125 cases of diabetic neuropathy (1945) writes: "It will be apparent from the discussion to follow that most diabetics who develop organic disease of peripheral nerves have had antecedent periods usually of months or years duration of grossly neglected or poorly managed treatment. There is strong evidence that the disordered metabolism of DM itself is the etiologic factor in this as well as other accompanying diabetic complications."[64] Among the early pathologic descriptions of peripheral nerve involvement an often quoted study is the one by Woltman and Wilder, who in 1929 published their findings in 10 cases of diabetic neuropathy, 4 studied post mortem and 6 from limbs amputated for ischemic gangrene.[81] The authors found prominent thickened sclerotic vessels close to and within nerve and attributed nerve fiber degeneration to the vascular pathology. Although the Marchi stain provided unequivocal evidence of nerve fiber degeneration, their finding of "isolated nerve bundles degeneration," often interpreted as infarcts, is questionable, because their illustration of focal sciatic nerve degeneration has the appearance of a Renaut's corpuscle.[16] It is difficult today to judge the validity of the pathologic changes reported by some earlier workers because histologic methods used were less advanced than they are today. To illustrate, Reske-Nielsen and Lundbaek reported a variety of findings in the spinal cord and peripheral nerves of 15 patients with juvenile diabetes who died after many years of diabetes (15 to 36 years).[62] They found neuronal degeneration at the spinal cord level involving anterior and posterior horns, varying degrees of loss and degeneration of myelin sheaths and axis cylinders at the root level (with posterior roots being more affected than ventral roots) and at the peripheral nerve level. They studied nerves from both upper and lower extremities. The pathologic changes were more severe in the peripheral nerves than in the spinal cord, appeared to be quite symmetrical, and were often more severe in the distal portion of the sciatic nerve and its branches. In spite of the extensive studies and nerve sampling it is difficult to fully rely on and to interpret some of the reported findings, for example, demyelination (simply decreased myelin staining on paraffin sections). These authors noted at all levels vascular changes in large and small vessels, with a characteristic homogenous periodic acid–Schiff (PAS) positive thickening of walls of small diameter vessels, as reported by Fagerberg.[31] They concluded that a metabolic disturbance of nervous tissue combined with a slowly developing angiopathy, rather than ischemia alone, may explain ganglion cell and nerve fiber changes. In a 1970 paper, Reske-Nielsen and colleagues reported marked degenerative changes and prominent regeneration of the neuromuscular endings in muscle biopsies from 8 patients with type 1 DM.[61]

Introduction of plastic sections with light and electron microscopic examination and use of quantitation radically changed the approaches and the understanding of nerve pathology in DPN. In the past 20 years, most pathologic studies have concentrated on sural nerve biopsies, permitting optimal and standardized fixation and light as well as ultrastructural studies. What follows is a review of the detailed studies performed assessing numbers and classes of fibers involved, the presence of demyelination and remyelination, degeneration and regeneration of fibers, axonal atrophy, nodal and paranodal abnormalities, and interstitial pathology.

Three-Dimensional Pattern of Nerve Fiber Alterations

Diabetic polyneuropathy is a chronic symmetrical sensorimotor polyneuropathy that usually begins after years of hyperglycemia. The changes of DPN are sufficiently stereotypic to be useful in staging. In a prevalence cohort (RDNS), no DPN (stage N0) was found in 46% of type 1 DM and 56% of type 2 DM patients. Characteristically, DPN begins without symptoms and with a slight reduction of nerve conduction, decreased heartbeat response to deep breathing, decreased vibration sensibility of the toes, and decreased ankle reflexes (39% and 32% in the RDNS cohort). The more severe symptomatic involvement occurs in fewer patients. In stage 2 neuropathy, patients experience loss of feeling, prickling or pain in the feet and legs, impotence, or other sensory and autonomic symptoms. Autonomic failure and mutilating acropathy may occur.[25] The clinical findings are usually restricted to legs and feet. Only in rare, severe cases are distal upper limb findings attributable to DPN. More often they

are caused by MNW or UNE. In the RDNS, 9% of type 1 DM patients had stage 2a neuropathy (<50% weakness of ankle dorsiflexion), and 6% had stage 2b (≥ 50% weakness). For type 2 DM patients, the figures were 12% and 1%.[23]

Although the clinical findings appear to predominate in the lower limbs, abnormalities of nerve conduction appear to be more generalized and affect both lower and upper limbs. Early postmortem studies confirmed the anatomical pattern of involvement of nerve fibers with the most severe fiber loss affecting distal sensory nerves of lower limbs.[19, 62] A gradual increase of changes from proximal to distal, more severe in the lower than in the upper limbs was reported. These studies were performed by using formalin-fixed, paraffin-embedded tissue with standard paraffin sections, a type of preparation that has a limited resolution and allows only a limited evaluation of nerve fiber pathology. In addition, although several peripheral nerves from upper and lower extremities were examined, no systematic study along the nerve length was performed and changes were not quantitated or controlled by use of reference values. These studies also did not allow a precise assessment of class of fiber involved and type of fiber pathology. Sugimura and Dyck were the first to find focal and multifocal fiber loss in the proximal sciatic nerve and more severe and diffuse loss distally in a patient with DPN, by studying sequential nerve blocks from proximal to distal.[72] In a subsequent study, Dyck and associates assessed morphometrically sections from defined proximal to distal levels of the lower limb nerves in 15 patients with DPN and compared them to 9 control patients who died of other diseases.[24] The objective of the study was to carefully determine number and size distribution of myelinated fibers (MFs) at defined proximal-to-distal levels and also to assess the spatial distribution of fiber density (Fig. 19.1; Table 19.1). They found that lumbar root density was either normal or slightly decreased. The decrease in density was slightly greater in segmental nerves, much greater in the sciatic nerve, and greatest in distal nerves (Fig. 19.2). Furthermore, to assess for focality and multifocality of MF loss, the index of dispersion among sampled frames, a measure of increased variability of fiber density among frames was determined (Tables 19.2 and 19.3).[24, 27] The presence of a higher index of dispersion starting in proximal nerves was interpreted as supportive of a focal or multifocal pattern of MF loss, similar to the one observed

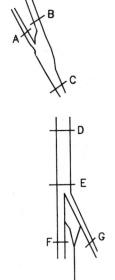

■ **Figure 19.1** The levels of the tissue collars of nerve tissue in a three-dimensional study of the spatial distribution of fiber degeneration and loss in diabetic neuropathy. The levels are: L5 ventral (A), dorsal (B), and segmental (C), proximal sciatic (D), distal sciatic (E), tibial (F), peroneal (G), and sural (H) nerves. Results of the number and spatial distribution of fibers are shown in Tables 19.1 to 19.3. (From Dyck, PJ, Karnes J, O'Brien P, et al. The spatial distribution of fiber loss in diabetic polyneuropathy suggests ischemia. Ann Neurol 1986; 19:440.)

TABLE 19.1 MEANS AND SIGNIFICANCE LEVELS OF NUMBER OF MYELINATED FIBERS/MM² IN DIABETICS WITH PERIPHERAL NEUROPATHY (% OF NORMAL)

	NID						Type 1 DM						Type 1 DM and NID					
	Without PVD		With PVD		All NID		Without PVD		With PVD		All Type 1		Without PVD		With PVD		All	
	Mean	P	Mean	P	Mean	P	Mean	P	Mean	P	Mean	P	Mean	P	Mean	P	Mean	P
							MF											
A	85	.171	78	.081	82	.066	113		99	.482	103	.402	91	.271	89	.167	90	.163
B	86	.071	78	.016	82	.014	128		96	.383	102	.422	93	.245	87	.103	89	.128
C	78	.063	80	.161	77	.032	68		68		68	.073	76	.034	76	.079	76	.011
D	99	.454	76	.015	89	.100	96	.420	85	.093	89	.177	98	.431	81	.016	89	.106
E	68	.003	52	.003	61	.000	78	.199	59	.040	65	.056	71	.022	56	.006	63	.005
F	68	.015	46	.001	58	.001	33		44	.012	42	.005	62	.008	45	.000	52	.001
G	61	.000	36	.000	50	.000	28		38	.002	36	.000	56	.000	37	.000	46	.000
H	39	.012	14	.008	29	.001	18		22	.004	21	.001	34	.002	15	.001	15	.000
							LMF											
A	84	.230	91	.314	87	.226	116		86	.248	92	.334	89	.297	89	.235	89	.237
B	49	.005	81	.089	64	.010	126		72	.084	83	.192	62	.034	77	.052	71	.128
C	85	.081	90	.243	87	.084	78		75		76	.038	84	.045	85	.114	84	.034
D	59	.002	38	.000	50	.000	42	.002	45	.000	44	.000	54	.000	42	.000	48	.000
E	40	.001	25	.000	33	.000	21	.004	29	.001	26	.000	34	.000	27	.000	30	.000
F	40	.005	24	.000	33	.000	30		15	.001	18	.000	39	.002	20	.000	28	.000
G	35	.000	19	.000	28	.000	21		16	.000	17	.000	32	.000	18	.000	25	.000
H	20	.002	5	.002	14	.000	9		8	.001	8	.000	16	.000	5	.000	11	.000

NID, non–insulin-dependent; DM, diabetes mellitus; PVD, peripheral vascular disease; MF, myelinated fiber;
LMF, large myelinated fiber.
Shaded areas are statistically different from controls ($P < .05$).

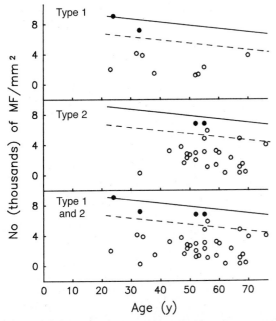

■ **Figure 19.2** The numbers of myelinated fibers (MF) per square millimeter of sural nerves of healthy subjects were regressed on age and lines fitted to the data. The 50th percentile is shown as a *solid line* and the 5th percentile line is shown as a *broken line*. The plotted values of the number of myelinated fibers per square millimeter against age in the sural nerves of patients with type 1, type 2, and combined diabetes mellitus have been overlaid. Diabetic patients without polyneuropathy are indicated by *solid symbols*. It is evident that values in most diabetics with neuropathy *(open symbols)* fall below the 5th percentile. (From Dyck PJ, Lais A, Karnes JL, et al. Fiber loss is primary and multifocal in sural nerves in diabetic polyneuropathy. Ann Neurol 1986; 19:425.)

in necrotizing vasculitis. Multifocality of nerve fiber loss in the lumbosacral trunk and the tibial nerve, but not in the sural nerve, was also observed by Johnson and colleagues in a postmortem study of 16 patients with DPN compared to a group of nondiabetic controls.[40] On the contrary, Llewelyn and coworkers,[49] studying sural nerves from diabetic patients, patients with inherited neuropathy (hereditary sensory and motor neuropathy, type 1 [HSMN 1]) and control nerves did not find the same degree of focal and multifocal MF loss found by Dyck and associates.[27] In addition, based on coefficient of variability and index of dispersion, the pattern of "nonuniform fiber loss" observed was identical in diabetic patients and patients with inherited neuropathy. They attributed the difference of their results mainly to the younger age of their patients as compared to the study by Dyck and associates.[27, 49] We note that the number of nerves these au-

thors studied in both disease and control groups was much smaller and that both coefficient of variability and index of dispersion were much smaller even in the control group. Because there was no difference in age of control subjects between the two studies, these results cannot be attributed to age. The results suggest that Llewelyn and coworkers must have used a larger frame area for studying coefficient of variability and index of dispersion, and this could make differences of fiber density among frames undetectable even if they were present. It is difficult for us to accept that the variability among frames is not different in DPN and inherited neuropathies because, in our experience, we have never encountered the striking degree of focal fiber loss seen in DPN in inherited neuropathy (Fig. 19.3).

Fiber Class Vulnerability

Loss of myelinated and unmyelinated fibers is readily apparent in transverse sections of patients with DPN.[7, 15, 24, 27, 40, 46, 49, 74, 79] Although based on symptoms and signs occurring in DPN, all classes of peripheral nerve fibers are usually functionally involved, and sometimes clinical involvement suggests the possibility of a selective involvement of large sensory, small sensory, or autonomic fibers.[75] These findings have led to the designation of such cases as different variants of DPN: for example, ataxic, hyperalgesic, autonomic, and large or small fiber DPN.

Pathologic studies do not support the idea of separate variants of DPN, but suggest that these so-called variants may be the extremes of a normal distribution of DPN. Dyck and associates, studying sural nerve biopsies, found that the ratio of small to large MFs, although more variable in DPN patients than in controls, did not show clustering of cases with large or small fiber loss.[27] Others have taken a different position. Said and colleagues, in a study of five cases of severe early-onset DPN in patients with type 1 DM, reported that the four patients with severe autonomic and sensory neuropathy showed a severe myelinated and unmyelinated fiber loss, no different from the fifth patient, who had muscle weakness and atrophy with sensory loss, but only little autonomic dysfunction.[65] Similar findings were previously reported by the same and other authors.[12, 48, 66] It should also be noted, as observed by Said and colleagues, that the predominance of involvement of subpopulations of fibers may not be easily assessed on

TABLE 19.2 MEANS AND SIGNIFICANCE LEVELS OF COEFFICIENT OF VARIATION (CV) OF DENSITIES AMONG FRAMES IN DIABETICS WITH PERIPHERAL NEUROPATHY (% OF NORMAL)

	NID						Type 1 DM						Type 1 DM and NID					
	Without PVD		With PVD		All NID		Without PVD		With PVD		All Type 1		Without PVD		With PVD		All	
	Mean	P	Mean	P	Mean	P	Mean	P	Mean	P	Mean	P	Mean	P	Mean	P	Mean	P
							MF											
A	155	.025	113	.398	137	.056	79		90	.365	88	.316	143	.060	102	.471	119	.177
B	119	.111	102	.446	111	.192	85		99	.458	96	.363	113	.183	100	.493	106	.308
C	120	.067	100	.490	113	.120	79		92		86	.038	112	.197	97	.302	106	.284
D	98	.413	101	.449	100	.480	79	.049	101	.473	93	.236	93	.188	101	.452	97	.353
E	105	.308	133	.027	177	.088	110	.316	123	.066	119	.117	106	.301	128	.025	118	.083
F	113	.183	126	.040	119	.070	126		196	.030	182	.038	116	.129	161	.050	141	.077
G	103	.391	115	.126	109	.219	130		138	.109	136	.087	108	.256	125	.114	117	.148
H	158	.007	274	.011	204	.020	190		231	.009	221	.005	162	.001	273	.002	212	.005
							LFM											
A	108	.361	108	.398	108	.348	92		94	.416	94	.399	105	.397	101	.481	103	.435
B	154	.033	122	.039	140	.035	102		132	.092	125	.115	145	.048	127	.056	135	.044
C	127	.035	113	.305	123	.066	129		165		147	.038	128	.019	130	.118	129	.028
D	163	.001	186	.002	173	.000	243	.000	226	.000	232	.000	186	.001	206	.003	197	.000
E	213	.007	286	.001	245	.001	290	.000	383	.008	352	.004	235	.001	334	.003	288	.002
F	248	.009	413	.052	321	.042	189		431	.005	383	.009	238	.008	422	.014	343	.018
G	228	.042	341	.006	278	.012	202		303	.018	278	.017	223	.033	325	.005	278	.008
H	264	.016	323	.001	288	.003	261		321	.000	306	.000	272	.002	325	.000	296	.000

NID, non–insulin-dependent; DM, diabetes mellitus; PVD, peripheral vascular disease; MF, myelinated fiber; LMF, large myelinated fiber.
Shaded areas are statistically different from controls (P < .05).

TABLE 19.3 MEANS AND SIGNIFICANCE LEVELS OF COEFFICIENT OF VARIATION (CV) OF DENSITIES AMONG FASCICLES IN DIABETICS WITH PERIPHERAL NEUROPATHY (% OF NORMAL)

	NID						Type 1 DM						Type 1 DM and NID					
	Without PVD		With PVD		All NID		Without PVD		With PVD		All Type 1		Without PVD		With PVD		All	
	Mean	P	Mean	P	Mean	P	Mean	P	Mean	P	Mean	P	Mean	P	Mean	P	Mean	P
							MF											
C	166	.068	122	.218	151	.082	147		144		146	.040	162	.055	129	.109	150	.055
D	93	.337	112	.252	101	.456	92	.361	113	.197	106	.315	93	.300	112	.153	103	.373
E	79	.108	125	.175	99	.481	174	.126	145	.116	158	.102	105	.436	137	.118	122	.240
F	67	.011	84	.163	74	.031	116		139	.147	134	.147	75	.052	112	.345	96	.431
G	104	.436	82	.212	94	.377	154		143	.120	146	.074	113	.299	108	.372	110	.314
H	101	.494	539	.075	276	.184	135		267	.014	234	.025	126	.267	422	.060	257	.134
							LMF											
C	163	.057	153	.049	160	.030	167		282		224	.017	164	.036	196	.024	176	.015
D	153	.067	233	.005	189	.012	205	.014	247	.011	233	.006	170	.019	240	.003	207	.005
E	177	.021	325	.006	243	.016	370	.002	345	.008	354	.002	232	.016	335	.003	345	.002
F	286	.016	385	.028	330	.016	249		588	.004	520	.007	280	.011	486	.006	398	.008
G	288	.025	329	.000	307	.003	247		429	.007	383	.008	281	.018	372	.001	330	.003
H	202	.110	559	.056	345	.097	148		524	.014	430	.031	210	.054	598	.017	383	.047

NID, non–insulin-dependent; DM, diabetes mellitus; PVD, peripheral vascular disease; MF, myelinated fiber; LMF, large myelinated fiber.
Shaded areas are statistically different from controls (P < .05).

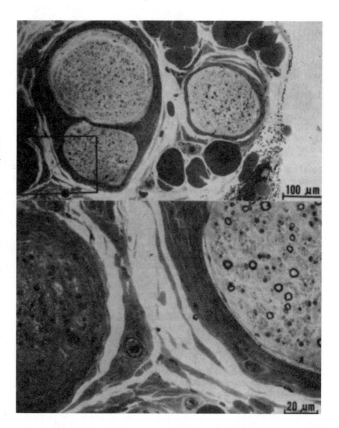

■ **Figure 19.3** A transverse section of the sural nerve of a patient with diffuse and focal loss of myelinated fibers. The rectangular *inset* is shown at a higher magnification below. Whereas the fascicle on the right shows a moderate number of myelinated fibers, the small fascicle on the left shows none. There is complete closure of an endoneurial vessel *(arrow)*. Such severe focal fiber loss without evident cause is itself presumptive evidence that ischemia may affect fiber loss of diabetic polyneuropathy. (From Dyck PJ, Lais A, Karnes JL, et al. Fiber loss is primary and multifocal in sural nerves in diabetic polyneuropathy. Ann Neurol 1986; 19:425.)

fiber histograms and a predominant involvement of small MFs may not be apparent on morphometric studies because of a large proportion of small regenerating fibers (Fig. 19.4). The function of these regenerating fibers cannot be determined from morphological studies.

Assessment of dysfunction (for example, clinical examination, quantitative sensory tests, and autonomic tests) may, therefore, provide a more accurate assessment of innervation and of selectivity of involvement by fiber size, but even here one must be careful to interpret re-

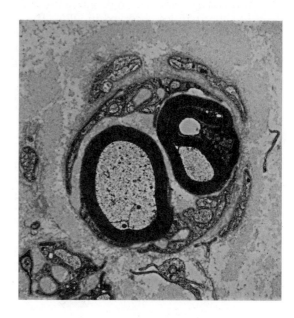

■ **Figure 19.4** Electron microscopic photograph illustrates a cluster composed of two regenerating myelinated fibers. Remnants of the original basement membrane are visible.

sults cautiously because innervation by class or size of fibers varies among tissues. For example, the finding of sensory loss of the toes and distal feet without muscle weakness cannot be interpreted as greater vulnerability of sensory than motor fibers because it could result from involvement of the distal part of the longest fibers and, therefore, sensory fibers innervating the skin of the toes would be more affected because motor fibers virtually end in muscles of the upper third of the leg. There is a second reason why it may be difficult to compare dysfunction of different classes of fibers. The sensitivity, specificity, and accuracy of tests to recognize dysfunction may be different for different fiber classes. Large-fiber dysfunction is perhaps more readily assessed by both physiologic and morphological tests than small-fiber dysfunction.

Axonal Degeneration Versus Segmental Demyelination

A variety of fiber abnormalities including axonal degeneration, regeneration, and segmental demyelination and remyelination have been reported in diabetic polyneuropathy. Early studies[4, 47, 72, 74] emphasized primary involvement of Schwann cells, resulting in demyelination and remyelination. These authors illustrated segmental demyelination and remyelination with onion bulb formation, and increased variability of internodal length. These findings were thought to be the consequence of repeated demyelination and a primary pathologic event in DPN. According to this view, myelin pathology was the primary explanation of the nerve conduction abnormalities observed in DPN. These observers also found axonal degeneration that was not quantitated. Vital and associates noted the coexistence of segmental demyelination and axonal degeneration in the same nerves.[79] In most cases, fiber loss of both myelinated and unmyelinated type were obvious. Regeneration was also noted. Behse and colleagues reported obvious loss of myelinated and unmyelinated fibers together with the phenomena of demyelination (rare) and remyelination (frequent) and concluded that loss of fibers, especially of large fibers was sufficient to explain the decreased conduction velocity.[7] In the study by Dyck and associates, the frequency of fiber pathologic abnormalities was assessed in sural nerve–teased fibers of a large group of diabetic patients with and without DPN and compared to control nerves (Fig. 19.5).[27]

The frequency of fibers undergoing axonal

degeneration and regeneration was more often abnormal in DPN patients as compared to controls than the frequency of segmental demyelination, demyelination and remyelination, and remyelination. The authors interpreted these findings together with the prominent multifocality of the pattern of fiber loss as evidence that axonal degeneration was primary in diabetes. Said and associates, in addition to finding decreased fiber density and axonal degeneration in the sural nerve of 5 patients with prominent small-fiber sensory loss, reported finding primary (random) and secondary (clustered to individual fibers) demyelination and remyelination.[66] These authors also reported the occurrence of fibers showing segmental demyelination proximally and axonal degenera-

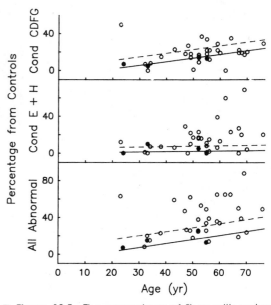

■ **Figure 19.5** The percentage of fibers with various pathologic abnormalities of sural nerves of controls were agressed on age and lines fitted to the data by the method of least squares. The 50th percentile is shown by the *solid line,* the 5th percentile by the *broken line.* Plotted values of diabetic nerves have been overlaid. Shown in the upper frame are percentages of teased fibers showing demyelination and remyelination; in the middle frame, those showing axonal degeneration and regeneration, and in the lower frame all teased fiber abnormalities (see text). The values shown as *solid symbols* are from diabetics without neuropathy; with one exception they are normal. Values in patients with neuropathy frequently fall within normal limits. Rates of de- and remyelination are not a good criterion by which to diagnose diabetic neuropathy. Teased fibers showing axonal degeneration and regeneration is better but not as good as numbers of myelinated fibers per square millimeter. (From Dyck PJ, Lais A, Karnes JL, et al. Fiber loss is primary and multifocal in sural nerves in diabetic polyneuropathy. Ann Neurol 1986; 19:425.)

tion distally and suggested that the two processes may be linked at least in some fibers.

Axonal Atrophy

There is evidence from human and experimental neuropathies that secondary demyelination and axonal degeneration may be linked through axonal atrophy, a process of progressive attenuation of axon caliber that manifests itself as a decreased axon/myelin ratio. In the permanent axotomy model, in which transected fibers are prevented from successful regeneration, proximal stump fibers undergo axonal atrophy and sequentially develop myelin wrinkling, paranodal demyelination, remyelination and axonal degeneration.[20] A similar sequence has been observed in uremic polyneuropathy, Friedreich's ataxia and other metabolic and inherited conditions.[22, 26] The hypothesis that axonal atrophy might also occur in DPN and precede demyelination and axonal degeneration appeared as an appealing explanation for the complex changes nerve fibers undergo in DPN. In addition, the findings of axons smaller than normal in experimental diabetes, although their origin was not entirely agreed upon (maldevelopment, axonal atrophy, or shrinkage), appeared to support the hypothesis.[39, 53, 73] Furthermore, the finding of reduced axonal flow associated with proximal enlargement and distal atrophy of axons in diabetic rats appeared to provide a possible link between metabolic abnormalities and structural changes.[53] Sugimura and Dyck first tested the hypothesis of axonal atrophy by using morphometric methods in human sural nerve biopsy specimens from diabetic patients with and without DPN and measuring myelin thickness (myelin spiral length) and axonal caliber.[71] The control nerves were from ambulatory healthy volunteers carefully evaluated to exclude patients with polyneuropathy or neurologic disease. They did not find evidence of axonal atrophy in large fibers. Other authors[67, 68] have repeatedly reported the occurrence of a decreased axon/myelin ratio of large MF in DPN. In all these studies, however, only a small group of control nerves was studied, and these were obtained either at autopsy or from organ donors and were therefore not adequate for the evaluation of fiber size and axon/myelin ratio. We have recently restudied the question of whether axonal atrophy occurs in DPN using more sural nerves from both healthy subjects and diabetic patients with and without DPN and using improved morphometric end points to assess fiber size.[29] Regression lines of the natural logarithm (ln) of axonal area on

number of myelin lamellae were assessed separately for subpopulations of fibers. Small (<80 myelin lamellae) and large (>80 myelin lamellae) MFs were separated to eliminate the influence of axonal regeneration and/or remyelination on regression lines covering the entire spectrum of fiber sizes. Inclusion of MF with thin myelin, relative to axonal caliber, could spuriously tilt a regression line so as to suggest atrophy of large fibers even when it was not present. In diabetic nerves, even for large MFs, the most reliable group on which to recognize atrophy, the common regression lines of ln axonal area on number of myelin lamellae were not significantly different from control nerves

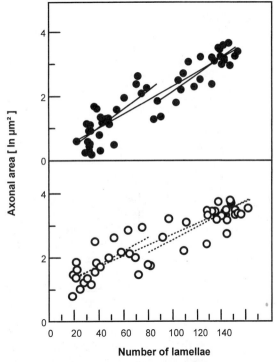

■ **Figure 19.6** Each point represents the plotted value of the natural log (ln) of axonal area on number of myelin lamellae of a transverse section of a myelinated fiber of a control (*top*) and diabetic (*bottom*) sural nerve. Regression lines were fitted to the data for small (<80 lamellae), large (≥80 lamellae), and all myelinated fibers. As described in the text, among the transformations of axonal area (mm²) on number of lamellae considered, ln axonal area provided the best fit. For each nerve evaluated in this study, similar regression lines were generated. Comparison of these regression lines among the three groups (healthy subjects, diabetic patients with polyneuropathy, and diabetic patients without polyneuropathy) formed the basis of the analysis to answer the question whether axonal atrophy occurs in diabetic polyneuropathy. Axonal atrophy was not found. (From Engelstad JK, Hokanson JL, Giannini C, et al. No evidence for axonal atrophy in human diabetic polyneuropathy. J Neuropathol Exp Neurol 56:255, 1997.)

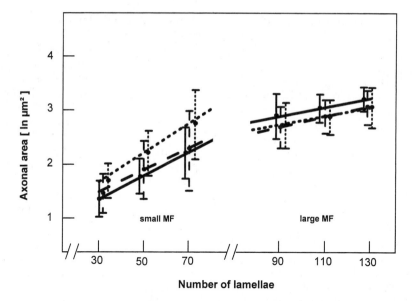

■ **Figure 19.7** Common regression lines of ln axonal area on number of myelin lamellae of myelinated fibers of sural nerves for the three groups (healthy subjects *(solid lines)*, diabetic patients with polyneuropathy *(dotted lines)*, and diabetic patients without polyneuropathy *(large dashed lines)*) and for small (<80 lamellae), and large (≥80 lamellae) myelinated fibers were estimated from the intercepts and slopes of individual nerves. These common regression lines and ISD are shown at various intercepts. The difference among groups for large fibers was not statistically significant. This provides no evidence for axonal atrophy in diabetic polyneuropathy. (From Engelstad JK, Hokanson JL, Giannini C, et al. No evidence for axonal atrophy in human diabetic polyneuropathy. J Neuropathol Exp Neurol 56:255, 1997.)

(Fig. 19.6 and 19.7). The common regression line of index of circularity on number of myelin lamellae, an index that is decreased in axonal atrophy, was not significantly different from control nerves. Last, the rate of adaxonal sequestration, which may be an indirect indicator of atrophy, was not increased in diabetic nerves. All these findings do not support the hypothesis that axonal atrophy occurs in human DPN. Axonal atrophy therefore cannot be advocated as the preceding event to myelin remodeling and axonal degeneration observed in DPN. Perhaps a more rapid mechanism may lead to fiber degeneration.

Onion Bulb Formation

Onion bulbs are the hallmark of hypertrophic neuropathy and are encountered in several varieties of inherited and acquired neuropathies[20] and also in DPN.[6] Onion bulbs are frequently encountered in nerves of diabetic patients. Their presence may be indicative of repeated episodes of demyelination and remyelination. Alternatively, one cannot exclude that they might result from combined events of axonal degeneration and regeneration.

Axoglial Dysjunction

Abnormalities of nerve conduction with decreased amplitude and conduction velocity (CV) and increased distal latency are an early feature of DPN affecting both motor and sensory fibers of upper and lower limbs. Functional and/or structural changes of nodes of Ranvier, specialized regions of the axolemma involved in saltatory nerve conduction, could contribute to decreased CV. Axoglial dysjunction was reported by Sima and coworkers as the typical and perhaps unique pathologic abnormality in experimental and human diabetic DPN linking the abnormalities of the polyol pathway and of *myo*-inositol metabolism to abnormalities of nodal cations and to decreased nerve conduction.[67, 68]

We recently critically reviewed the concept of axoglial dysjunction and found that there is ambiguity about its definition, the approaches used had not been validated, the change is not unique to DPN, and the link between metabolic events and structural changes remains uncertain.[34] Nodes of Ranvier are the points of abutment of two contiguous Schwann cells, each responsible for a paranode of adjacent internodes (Fig. 19.8). The terminal loops of the

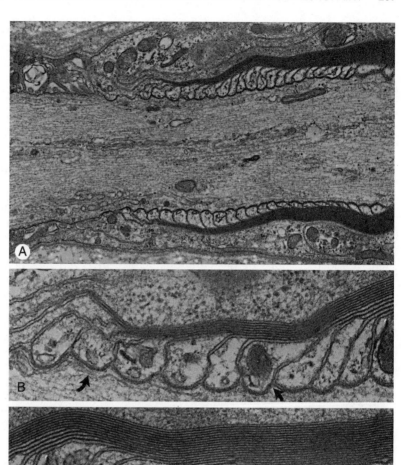

■ **Figure 19.8** *A*, The paranodal morphology of a node from a small-diameter fiber (23 lamellae of myelin). *B* and *C*, The upper heminode is shown at high magnification. Even in this optimal plane of section through the center of the node, only a small percentage of loops can be identified as showing transverse bands (9 of 23; loops with definite transverse bands as identified at this magnification ×60,000 and with the help of a magnifying lens, are indicated by *arrows*). In the other loops, minimal deviation from a perpendicular plane of section precludes their assessment. These electron micrographs demonstrate the importance of careful evaluation of serial sections and sufficiently high magnifications to address the question of axoglial dysjunction as presently defined. Original magnification: *A*, ×17,000; *B* and *C*, ×60,000. (From Giannini C, Dyck PJ. Axoglial dysjunction: A critical appraisal of definition, techniques, and previous results. Micros Res Tech 1996; 34:442.)

myelin lamellae end on both sides of the node, forming a specialized complex anchoring the edges of single myelin lamellae to the axolemma. Each terminal loop in contact with the axolemma acquires glial membrane specializations, morphologically described as transverse bands.[9, 45, 63] Transverse bands are considered to be ultrastructurally similar to gap junctions in other tissues. These structures, together with the desmosome-like junctions and tight junctions between adjacent Schwann cell loops form the axoglial junctional complex and separate nodal from internodal axolemma.[37] The sodium channels necessary for the generation of action potentials are segregated in the axolemma of the node of Ranvier. The paranodal complex is different for small (type I) and large (type II) fibers.[56]

The term *axoglial dysjunction* was first introduced by Sima and coworkers to indicate the loss of transverse bands between terminal loops of myelin and axolemma in the paranode of MFs in experimental and human DPN.[67, 68] The absence and/or loss of transverse bands had actually been described before by others during development and in pathologic conditions other than DPN.[1, 2, 8, 9, 38, 83] Sima and coworkers hypothesized that the lesion, characteristic in their opinion, of DPN might be the structural counterpart of various metabolic abnormalities (decrease in *myo*-inositol content and Na^+K^+-ATPase pump deficiency) leading to low CV. Quantitative morphometric assessment of axoglial dysjunction, as illustrated by these authors is, in our opinion, inadequate and not sufficiently rigorous to establish with certainty whether it occurs in DPN. An unequivocal definition of axoglial dysjunction is lacking. There is insufficient quantitative information on the structural variability of the para-nodes of large and small MFs, during development and aging, with axonal atrophy, with demyelination and remyelination, and in various disease conditions. Quantitative assessment of axoglial dysjunction appears to be a prohibitively time-consuming process requiring assessment of serial (or serial skip) ultra-structural sections at high magnification to evaluate if a myelin loop does or does not make contact with the axolemma at different levels of the node (Fig. 19.9). Certain technical problems would have to be overcome to quantitatively test the hypothesis: (1) sampling a representative number of small and large MFs and (2) for large fibers, how to sample a sufficient number of loops of the paranode. It is unlikely that axoglial dysjunction, assuming that it occurs in DPN, is specific for DPN. It may be a nonspecific reflection of demyelination and remyelination. Absence of transverse bands has been reported in different experimental and human pathologic conditions causing active demyelination and remyelination.[1, 2, 38, 83] In remyelination, the phenomenon seems to recapitulate the acquisition of junctions during development and primary myelination.[9] The mechanism underlying detachment of loops during demyelination, if by direct injury to the junctional components or by injury to the Schwann cell, remains unclear.

The hypothesis of Sima and coworkers that loss of transverse bands in the axoglial junctional complexes relate to paranodal swelling, as a result of *myo*-inositol and Na^+K^+-ATPase deficiency, cannot be accepted without more critical evidence.

Microangiopathy

The complications of diabetic retinopathy, nephropathy, and polyneuropathy are statistically associated in the same patients. Because microvascular alterations play a role in the retina and kidney complications, they may also be involved in DPN. Fagerberg first drew attention to the abnormalities of the microvascular wall with the deposition of strongly positive PAS material.[31] With the use of the electron microscope, a variety of structural abnormalities of endoneurial microvessels have been reported in diabetes and DPN, including endothelial cell hyperplasia,[76] capillary closure,[21] thrombosis,[77] thickening or reduplication of capillary wall basement membranes,[78] endothelial and pericyte degeneration,[80] and endothelial fenestration and dysjunction.[40, 58, 69, 80]

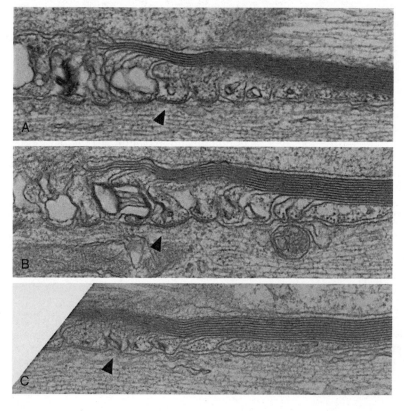

■ **Figure 19.9** These electron micrographs illustrate a paranode at three serial levels in a sural nerve biopsy from a diabetic 48-year-old patient. In *C*, part of the paranode is covered by a grid bar. Loss of transverse bands is apparent in many loops. As indicated by the *arrows*, one loop that shows transverse bands in *A* and *B* is lacking it in *C*. This illustrates that axoglial dysjunction might be judged as present in one plane of section and absent in another plane (focal discontinuity). Original magnification: *A* and *B*, ×49,500; *C*, ×38,500. (From Giannini C, Dyck PJ. Axoglial dysfunction: A critical appraisal of definition, techniques, and previous results. Micros Res Tech 1996; 34:436.)

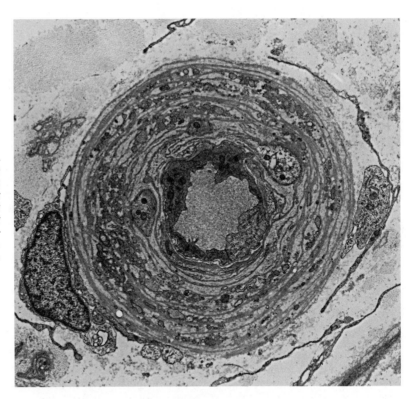

■ **Figure 19.10** This microvessel shows severe basement membrane reduplication and a very high number of cellular debris among the basement membrane leaflets. Basement membrane leaflets are often incomplete and fragmented. Original magnification, ×14,000.

Dyck and associates in 1985 and Yasuda and Dyck in 1987 first morphometrically assessed the ultrastructural abnormalities of transversely cut endoneurial microvessels (Fig. 19.10) and found that the basement membrane area and the endothelial cell area were significantly increased in DPN and that these changes were associated with the neuropathologic abnormalities of MF.[22, 82] The frequency of luminal occlusion also appeared to be associated with DPN, but the assessment was based only on study of semithin sections.[22] The observation of increased basement membrane reduplication in DPN has been confirmed by others.[11, 12, 50, 51, 69] In more recent studies, we have also confirmed that basement membrane reduplication is increased in DM and DPN and is accompanied by pericyte degeneration and decrease of periendothelial cell coverage, a finding typical of diabetic retinopathy (see Fig. 19.10).[32] The functional implications of pericyte degeneration remains unclear. It has been demonstrated that pericytes have contractile properties and may contribute to maintenance of vascular shape.[70] They also inhibit endothelial cell proliferation in vitro.[54] Loss of pericytes has been advocated as a possible factor in stimulating endothelial cell proliferation in the retina.[30] Last, pericyte degeneration may precede the degeneration of the entire microvessel with formation of ghost

capillaries, a finding that we observed with low frequency in DPN.[32]

From our studies, it appears that microvascular wall transformation rather than degeneration and regeneration of microvessels is the main pathologic process in DPN with marked degenerative processes taking place in the vascular wall (Fig. 19.11). These changes, including thickening of the vascular wall, loss of pericytes, and endothelial cell separation resulting in intercellular gaps, may also be in keeping with alterations of the blood-nerve barrier. An alteration of the blood-nerve barrier was demonstrated by Poduslo and colleagues, who showed an increased transfer of immunoglobulin (Ig) G and IgM across the blood-nerve barrier in diabetic patients as compared to controls.[57] Microvascular density was not altered, and we could not support the earlier observation of an increased frequency of luminal occlusion, resulting in increase of intercapillary distance (Fig. 19.12).

The severity of the microvascular changes has been associated with the severity of DPN,[50, 82] and the vascular changes appear to precede the development of DPN.[33]

Putative Mechanisms

There is strong evidence that prolonged hyperglycemia and the associated metabolic de-

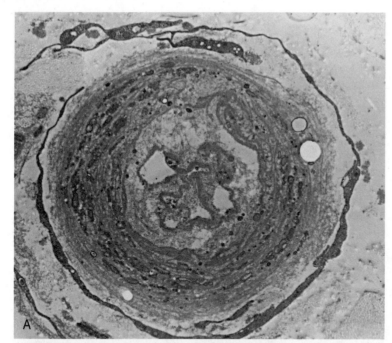

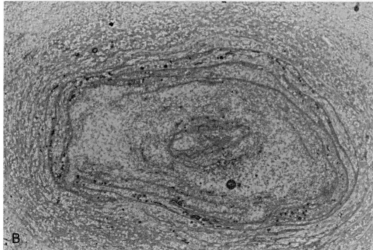

■ **Figure 19.11** *A* and *B,* Two microvessels undergoing complete degeneration (only 2 of 433 microvessels were observed in diabetic nerves, not observed in control nerves). Endothelial and periendothelial cell processes are not present. The lumen of the vessel has disappeared, substituted by a tortuous line of collapsed basement membranes. Multiple basement membrane layers and cellular debris remain in the outer part of the vessels. Similar microvessels have been described in diabetes in other tissues and called *acellular capillaries.* Original magnification: *A,* ×11,100; *B,* ×6100.

rangements can alter nerve function and induce DPN. It is now clear that euglycemia can in part or perhaps entirely prevent DPN,[17] whereas a return to normal after long-standing severe DPN is not possible even with long periods of euglycemia, for example, after pancreas transplantation.[43] As already discussed, there is evidence to support that nerve fiber loss is primary and generally severe in DPN. Incomplete regeneration following severe fiber loss may be caused by one or a combination of factors. Decreased regenerative activity, loss of Schwann cells, and breakdown of Schwann cell tubes as well as misdirection of regenerating fibers could all be responsible of defective re-generation. The frequently observed phenomena of demyelination and remyelination as well as onion bulb formation also point to the possibility that metabolism of Schwann cells may be deleteriously affected in a primary manner in DPN and result in damage to myelin and secondarily to axons. It is not settled if chronic hyperglycemia might lead directly to nerve fiber injury (axonal and/or neuronal and Schwann cells) or if it induces microvascular injury first and only secondarily nerve fiber injury.

Among the metabolic pathways altered in DM, the attention has been first directed to alterations of polyol pathways and more re-

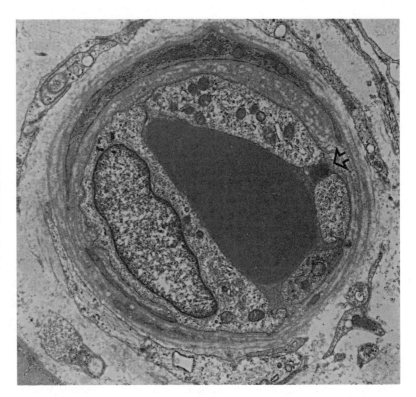

■ **Figure 19.12** This small endoneurial microvessel shows the presence of gap between two endothelial cell processes caused by loss of endothelial tight junctions. This finding was present in only a small number of microvessels (2 of 433 microvessels in diabetic nerves; not observed in control nerves). Original magnification, ×12,200.

cently of the phospholipids and fatty acid metabolism.[42, 67, 68] Alterations of the polyol pathways with accumulation of sorbitol and fructose as a result of inadequate utilization of glucose could be damaging to tissues. In experimental diabetes, accumulation of these sugars may explain the formation of diabetic cataract in which they represent the major component.[44] At present, however, the use of aldose reductase inhibitors, which could reverse this metabolic process, has not been shown to be effective in DPN. A decrease in tissue *myo*-inositol associated with a deficiency of the Na^+K^+-ATPase has been invoked to explain reduced nerve conduction velocity and axoglial dysjunction.[67, 68] However, a deficiency of endoneurial *myo*-inositol could not be demonstrated in sural nerves of insulin-treated patients with DPN.[28] Furthermore, a beneficial effect of oral *myo*-inositol supplementation in human diabetics was not found.[35, 36] More recently, attention has been directed to derangements of phospholipids and fatty acid metabolism. In a multicenter trial, a favorable effect on nerve conduction velocity was found by administration of large amounts of linolenic acid.[42] Chronic hyperglycemia also causes increase of glycosylation of protein and may result in tissue accumulation of highly insoluble

advanced glycation products causing metabolic derangements.[13]

Chronic hyperglycemia directly or through altered metabolic pathways may affect the integrity of nerve fibers (axons and/or Schwann cells). The fact that retinopathy and nephropathy, complications of DM in which microvascular disease is unequivocally involved, are strongly associated with DPN in studied cohorts of patients prompts consideration that microvascular disease may also be involved in causing DPN.[31] In the retina, the altered permeability of blood microvessels, the formation of microaneurysms, the presence of hemorrhage and of ischemic lesions all implicate vessel pathology in causing retinopathy. Similarly, in kidney, the glomerular alterations implicate microvessel pathology in diabetic renal failure. So, in peripheral diabetic nerves, the striking microvascular changes demonstrated, their association with neuropathic abnormalities of nerve fibers, and the evidence of frank focal nerve injury to both nerve fibers and perineurium point to microvascular pathology and possibly ischemia as pathogenetic mechanisms. Alteration of the blood-nerve barrier, resulting in alteration of the endoneurial microenvironment, may also ultimately contribute to nerve fiber damage.[57]

References

1. Allt G. Repair of segmental demyelination in peripheral nerve: An electron microscopic study. Brain 92:639, 1969.
2. Allt G. The node of Ranvier in experimental allergic neuritis: An electron microscope study. J Neurocytol 4:63, 1975.
3. Althaus J. On Sclerosis of the Spinal Cord, Including Locomotor Ataxy, Spastic Spinal Paralysis and Other System Diseases of the Spinal Cord: Their Pathology, Symptoms, Diagnosis, and Treatment. London, Green & Company, 1885.
4. Arne L. Neuropathie peripherique diabetique. Rev Neurol (Paris) 126:115, 1972.
5. Auche MB. Des alterations des nerfs peripheriques. Arch Med Exp Anat Pathol 2:635, 1890.
6. Ballin RHM, Thomas PK. Hypertrophic changes in diabetic neuropathy. Acta Neuropathol (Berl) 11:93, 1968.
7. Behse F, Buchthal F, Carlsen F. Nerve biopsy and conduction studies in diabetic neuropathy. J Neurol Neurosurg Psychiatry 40:1072, 1977.
8. Berthold CH, Skoglund S. Postnatal development of feline paranodal myelin-sheath segments. II. Electron microscopy. Acta Soc Med Ups 73:127, 1968.
9. Bertram M, Schroder JM. Developmental changes at the node and paranode in human sural nerves: Morphometric and fine-structural evaluation. Cell Tissue Res 273:499, 1993.
10. Bouchard M. Sur la perte des reflexes tendineux dans le diabete sucre. Progres Med 12:819, 1884.
11. Bradley J, Thomas PK, King RHM, et al. Morphometry of endoneurial capillaries in diabetic sensory and autonomic neuropathy. Diabetologia 33:611, 1990.
12. Britland ST, Young RJ, Sharma SK, et al. Relationship of endoneurial capillary abnormalities to type and severity of diabetic polyneuropathy. Diabetes 39:909, 1990.
13. Brownlee M, Cerami A, Vlassara H. Advanced glycosylation end products in tissue and the biochemical basis of diabetic complications. N Engl J Med 318:1315, 1988.
14. Buzzard F. Illustrations of some less known forms of peripheral neuritis, especially alcoholic monoplegia and diabetic neuritis. Br Med J 1:1419, 1890.
15. Chopra JS, Hurwitz LJ, Montgomery DAD. The pathogenesis of sural nerve changes in diabetes mellitus. Brain 92:391, 1969.
16. DCCT Research Group: The Diabetes Control and Complications Trial (DCCT): Design and methodologic considerations for the feasibility phase. Diabetes 35:530, 1986.
17. DCCT Research Group: The effect of intensive diabetes therapy on the development and progression of neuropathy. Ann Intern Med 122:561, 1995.
18. de Calvi, M. Recherches sur les Accidents Diabetiques. Paris, 1864.
19. Dolman CL. The pathology and pathogenesis of diabetic neuropathy. Bull NY Acad Med 43:773, 1967.
20. Dyck PJ, Giannini C, Lais A. Pathologic alterations of nerves. In Dyck PJ, Thomas PK, Low PA, et al (eds): Peripheral Neuropathy. Philadelphia, WB Saunders, 1993, p 514.
21. Dyck PJ, Hansen S, Karnes J, et al. Capillary number and percentage closed in human diabetic sural nerve. Proc Natl Acad Sci USA 82:2513, 1985.
22. Dyck PJ, Johnson WJ, Lambert EH, et al. Segmental demyelination secondary to axonal degeneration in uremic neuropathy. Mayo Clin Proc 46:400, 1971.
23. Dyck PJ, Karnes JL, O'Brien PC, et al. The Rochester Diabetic Neuropathy Study: Reassessment of tests and criteria for diagnosis and staged severity. Neurology 42:1164, 1992.
24. Dyck PJ, Karnes JL, O'Brien PC, et al. The spatial distribution of fiber loss in diabetic polyneuropathy suggests ischemia. Ann Neurol 19:440, 1986.
25. Dyck PJ, Kratz KM, Karnes JL, et al. The prevalence by staged severity of various types of diabetic neuropathy, retinopathy, and nephropathy in a population-based cohort: The Rochester Diabetic Neuropathy Study. Neurology 43:817, 1993.
26. Dyck PJ, Lais AC. Evidence for segmental demyelination secondary to degeneration in Friedreich's ataxia. In Kakulas BA (ed): Clinical Studies in Myology. Amsterdam, Excerpta Medica, 1973, p 253.
27. Dyck PJ, Lais A, Karnes JL, et al. Fiber loss is primary and multifocal in sural nerves in diabetic polyneuropathy. Ann Neurol 19:425, 1986.
28. Dyck PJ, Zimmerman BR, Vilen TH, et al. Nerve glucose, fructose, sorbitol, myo-inositol, and fiber degeneration and regeneration in diabetic neuropathy. N Engl J Med 319:542, 1988.
29. Engelstad JK, Hokanson JL, Giannini C, et al. No evidence for axonal atrophy in human diabetic polyneuropathy. J Neuropathol Exp Neurol 56:255, 1997.
30. Engerman RL. Pathogenesis of diabetic retinopathy. Diabetes 38:1203, 1989.
31. Fagerberg S-E. Diabetic neuropathy: A clinical and histological study on the significance of vascular affections. Acta Med Scand 164(suppl 345):1, 1959.
32. Giannini C, Dyck PJ. Ultrastructural morphometric features of human sural nerve endoneurial microvessels. J Neuropathol Exp Neurol 52:361, 1993.
33. Giannini C, Dyck PJ. Basement membrane reduplication and pericyte degeneration precede development of diabetic polyneuropathy and are associated with its severity. Ann Neurol 37:498, 1995.
34. Giannini C, Dyck PJ. Axoglial dysfunction: A critical appraisal of definition, techniques, and previous results. Micros Res Tech 34:436, 1996.
35. Gregersen G, Bertelsen B, Harbo H et al. Oral supplementation of myoinositol: Effects on peripheral nerve function in human diabetics and on the concentration in plasma, erythrocytes, urine and muscle tissue in human diabetics and normals. Acta Neurol Scand 67:164, 1983.
36. Gregersen G, Borsting H, Theil P, et al. Myoinositol and function of peripheral nerves in human diabetics: A controlled clinical trial. Acta Neurol Scand 58:241, 1978.
37. Harkin JC. A series of desmosomal attachments in the Schwann sheath of myelinated mammalian nerves. Z Zellforsch 64:189, 1964.
38. Hirano A, Cook SD, Whitaker JN, et al. Fine structural aspects of demyelination in vitro: The effects of Guillain-Barré syndrome. J Neuropathol Exp Neurol 30:249, 1971.
39. Jakobsen J. Axonal dwindling in early experimental diabetes. I. A study of cross sectioned nerves. Diabetologia 12:539, 1976.
40. Johnson PC, Doll SC, Cromey DW. Pathogenesis of diabetic neuropathy. Ann Neurol 19:450, 1986.
41. Jordan WR. Neuritis manifestations in diabetes mellitus. Arch Intern Med 57:307, 1936.
42. Keen H, Payan J, Allawi J, et al. Treatment of diabetic neuropathy with gamma-linolenic acid: The gamma-Linolenic Acid Multicenter Trial Group. Diabetes Care 16:8, 1993.

43. Kennedy WR, Navarro X, Goetz FC, et al. Effects of pancreatic transplantation on diabetic neuropathy. N Engl J Med 322:1031, 1990.
44. Kinoshita JH. Cataracts in galactosemia. Invest Ophthalmol 4:786, 1965.
45. Laatsch RH, Cowan WM. A structural specialization at nodes of Ranvier in the central nervous system. Nature 210:757, 1966.
46. Lambert EH, Dyck PJ. Compound action potentials of sural nerve in vitro in peripheral neuropathy. In Dyck PJ, Thomas PK, Griffin JW, et al (eds): Peripheral Neuropathy. Philadelphia, WB Saunders, 1993, p 672.
47. Lascelles RG, Thomas PK. Changes due to age in internodal length in the sural nerve in man. J Neurol Neurosurg Psychiatry 29:40, 1966.
47a. Leyden E: Beiträg zur Klinik des Diabetes Mellitus. Wien Med Wochenschr 43:926, 1893.
48. Llewelyn JG, Gilbey SG, Thomas PK, et al. Sural nerve morphometry in diabetic autonomic and painful sensory neuropathy: A clinicopathological study. Brain 114:867, 1991.
49. Llewelyn JG, Thomas PK, Gilbey SG, et al. Pattern of myelinated fibre loss in the sural nerve in neuropathy related to type 1 (insulin-dependent) diabetes. Diabetologia 31:162, 1988.
50. Malik RA, Newrick PG, Sharma AK, et al. Microangiopathy in human diabetic neuropathy: Relationship between capillary abnormalities and the severity of neuropathy. Diabetologia 32:92, 1989.
51. Malik RA, Veves A, Masson EA, et al. Endoneurial capillary abnormalities in mild human diabetic neuropathy. J Neurol Neurosurg Psychiatry 55(7):557, 1992.
52. Martin MM. Diabetic neuropathy: A clinical study of 150 cases. Brain 76:594, 1953.
53. Medori R, Autilio-Gambetti B, Monaco B, et al. Experimental diabetic neuropathy: Impairment of slow transport with changes in axon cross-sectional area. Proc Natl Acad Sci USA 82:7716, 1985.
54. Orlidge A, D'Amore PA. Inhibition of capillary endothelial cell growth by pericytes and smooth muscle cells. J Cell Biol 105:1455, 1987.
55. Pavy FW. Address on diabetes. Washington International Congress, 1887. Philadelphia, Medical News, p. 357, September 23, 1887.
56. Phillips DD, Hibbs RG, Ellison JP, et al. An electron microscopic study of central and peripheral nodes of Ranvier. J Anat 111:229, 1972.
57. Poduslo JF, Low PA, Windebank AJ, et al. Altered blood-nerve barrier in experimental lead neuropathy assessed by changes in endoneurial albumin concentration. J Neurosci 2:1507, 1982.
58. Powell HC, Rosoff J, Myers RR. Microangiopathy in human diabetic neuropathy. Acta Neuropathol (Berl) 68:295, 1985.
59. Pryce TD. Perforating ulcers of both feet associated with diabetes and ataxic symptoms. Lancet 2:11, 1887.
60. Pryce TD. On diabetic neuritis with a clinical and pathological description of three cases of diabetic psuedo-tabes. Brain 16:416, 1893.
61. Reske-Nielsen E, Gregersen G, Harmsen A, et al. Morphological abnormalities of the terminal neuromuscular apparatus in recent juvenile diabetes. Diabetologia 6:104, 1970.
62. Reske-Nielsen E, Lundbaek K. Pathological changes in the central and peripheral nervous system of young long-term diabetics. II. The spinal cord and peripheral nerves. Diabetologia 4:34, 1968.
63. Rosenbluth J. Glial membrane specializations in extraparanodal regions. J Neurocytol 7:709, 1978.
64. Rundles RW. Diabetic neuropathy: General review with report of 125 cases. Medicine (Baltimore) 24:111, 1945.
65. Said G. Goulon-Goeau C, Tchobroutsky G. Severe early-onset polyneuropathy in insulin dependent diabetes mellitus: A clinical and pathological study. N Engl J Med 326:1257, 1992.
66. Said G, Slama G, Salva J. Progressive centripetal degeneration of axons in small fibre diabetic polyneuropathy. Brain 106:791, 1983.
67. Sima AAF, Lattimer SA, Hagihashi S, et al. Axoglial dysjunction: A novel structural lesion that accounts for poorly-reversible nerve conduction slowing in the spontaneously-diabetic Bio-breeding rat. J Clin Invest 77:474, 1986.
68. Sima AAF, Nathaniel V, Bril V, et al. Histopathological heterogeneity of neuropathy in insulin-dependent and non-insulin-dependent diabetes, and demonstration of axoglial dysjunction in human diabetic neuropathy. J Clin Invest 81:349, 1988.
69. Sima AAF, Nathaniel V, Prashar A, et al. Endoneurial microvessels in human diabetic neuropathy: Endothelial cell dysjunction and lack of treatment effect by aldose reductase inhibitor. Diabetes 40:1090, 1991.
70. Sims DE. The pericyte: A review. Tissue Cell 18:153, 1986.
71. Sugimura K, Dyck PJ. Sural nerve myelin thickness and axis cylinder caliber in human diabetes. Neurology 31:1087, 1981.
72. Sugimura K, Dyck PJ. Multifocal fiber loss in proximal sciatic nerve in symmetric distal diabetic neuropathy. J Neurol Sci 53:501, 1982.
73. Thomas PK, Fraher JP, O'Leary D, et al. Relative growth and maturation of axon size and myelin thickness in the tibial nerve of the rat. 2. Effect of streptozotocin-induced diabetes. Acta Neuropathol (Berl) 79:375, 1990.
74. Thomas PK, Lascelles RG. The pathology of diabetic neuropathy. Q J Med 35:480, 1966.
75. Thomas PK, Tomlinson DR. Diabetic and hypoglycemic neuropathy. In Dyck PJ, Thomas PK, Griffin JW, et al (eds): Peripheral Neuropathy. Philadelphia, WB Saunders, 1993, p 1219.
76. Timperley WR, Boulton AJM, Davies-Jones GAB, et al. Small vessel disease in progressive diabetic neuropathy associated with good metabolic control. J Clin Pathol 38:1030, 1985.
77. Timperley WR, Ward JD, Preston FE, et al. Clinical and histological studies in diabetic neuropathy: A reassessment of vascular factors in relation to intravascular coagulation. Diabetologia 12:237, 1976.
78. Vital C, LeBlanc M, Vallat JM, et al. Ultrastructural study of peripheral nerve in 16 diabetics without neuropathy: Comparisons with 16 diabetic neuropathies and 16 non-diabetic neuropathies. Acta Neuropathol (Berl) 30:63, 1974.
79. Vital C, Vallat JM, LeBlanc M, et al. Peripheral neuropathies caused by diabetes mellitus: Ultrastructural study of 12 biopsied cases. J Neurol Sci 18:381, 1973.
80. Williams E, Timperly WR, Ward JD, et al. Electron microscopic studies of vessels in diabetic peripheral neuropathy. J Clin Pathol 33:462, 1980.
81. Woltman HW, Wilder RM. Diabetes mellitus: Pathological changes in the spinal cord and peripheral nerves. Arch Intern Med 44:576, 1929.
82. Yasuda H, Dyck PJ. Abnormalities of endoneurial microvessels and sural nerve pathology in diabetic neuropathy. Neurology 37:20, 1987.
83. Yu RCP, Bunge RP. Damage and repair of the peripheral myelin sheath and node of Ranvier after treatment with trypsin. J Cell Biol 64:1, 1975.

Chapter **20**

Glycemic Control

Douglas A. Greene • *Martin J. Stevens* • *Eva L. Feldman*

INTRODUCTION

Recent clinical, epidemiologic, and neurophysiologic studies in humans strongly favor the hypothesis that metabolic alterations stemming from insulin deficiency or hyperglycemia or both contribute to the pathogenesis of human diabetic neuropathy, although the responsible pathogenetic mechanism(s) remain unclear. The results of the Diabetes Control and Complications Trial (DCCT) clearly demonstrate the validity of this hypothesis for the pathogenesis of diabetic polyneuropathy in type 1 diabetes. Epidemiologic and clinical studies suggest that the relationship between metabolic control and the development of diabetic neuropathy is similar in type 2 diabetes, once the effects of age are removed. Thus, at present, the hallmark of treatment for diabetic neuropathy should be its prevention by improved metabolic control, using intensive therapy for type 1 diabetes and an expanding selection of drugs for type 2 diabetes. The precise role of intensive metabolic treatment in established diabetic neuropathy remains to be established, but the results of the DCCT suggest that intensive therapy in patients with early neuropathy does improve nerve function. Elucidation of the mechanisms linking hyperglycemia and other metabolic abnormalities associated with insulin deficiency to the development and progression of diabetic neuropathy should lead to new pharmacologic interventions in the future; at present, aldose reductase inhibitors are well tested, but their

297

clinical usefulness remains to be established[106] in definitive clinical trials.

HISTORICAL PERSPECTIVE

Whether improved glycemia control can prevent or ameliorate neuropathy is of importance to patients, neurologists, and diabetologists because neuropathy is common, may be associated with prolonged morbidity, may become more frequent as people live longer, and may be preventable or reversible with the improved modalities for the control of glycemia which are becoming available.

Committee on Health Care Issues, American Neurological Association. Does Improved Control of Glycemia Prevent or Ameliorate Diabetic Polyneuropathy? Ann Neurol 1986;19:288–290.

The results of the DCCT (Diabetes Control and Complications Trial) conclusively establish that intensive diabetes management in patients with insulin-dependent diabetes mellitus markedly reduces the risk for developing clinically overt, objectively confirmed diabetic polyneuropathy.

Diabetes Control and Complications Trial Research Group. The Effect of Intensive Diabetes Therapy on the Development and Progression of Neuropathy. Ann Intern Med 1995;122:661–568.

After Marchal de Calvi stated that diabetes caused rather than resulted from its neurologic concomitants,[98] the specific role of hyperglycemia in the cause and clinical course of diabetic neuropathy remained a hotly debated issue.[73] More than 100 years later, the results of the DCCT[17] unequivocally established the overriding importance of metabolic factors associated with insulin deficiency in the pathogenesis of clinically evident, objectively confirmed diabetic polyneuropathy in patients with type 1 diabetes mellitus (DM) (Fig. 20.1).

Before insulin became widely available about 75 years ago, few type 1 diabetic patients survived long enough to develop chronic complications; therefore, the various syndromes of diabetic neuropathy were noted infrequently.

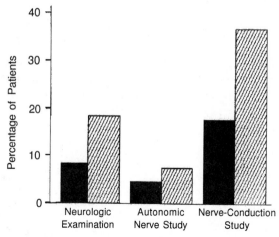

■ **Figure 20.1** The prevalence of abnormal clinical, autonomic, and nerve conduction examinations in patients in the Diabetes Control and Complications Trial (DCCT) with type 1 diabetes after 5 years of intensive (*solid bars*) or conventional (*hatched bars*) diabetes therapy. Only subjects with normal examinations at baseline were included in this analysis. Intensive diabetes therapy consisted of insulin administered either by multiple daily injections or chronic subcutaneous insulin infusion, adjusted on the basis of multiple daily self-measurement of blood glucose. (From DCCT Research Group. The effect of intensive treatment of diabetes on the development and progression of long-term complications in insulin-dependent diabetes mellitus. N Engl J Med 1993; 329:977.)

Neither the impetus nor the means for clinical exploration of the relationship between blood glucose and complications existed. In the subsequent 20 years, increasing numbers of insulin-treated patients developed nephropathy, neuropathy, and retinopathy. It became obvious that conventional insulin replacement therapy, which prolonged life and provided a sense of clinical well-being, provided little insurance against the development of chronic complications.[73] Accordingly, numerous studies were undertaken in the decades since World War II to explore the relationship between blood glucose control and the complications. Most of these efforts were thwarted by (1) the prolonged time course for the development of clinical complications, (2) inadequate methods for assessing diabetic control, (3) lack of effective treatment regimens to reduce blood glucose levels, and (4) poor understanding and primitive assessment of the complications themselves.[83] Within the past 20 years, new intervention strategies have evolved that can normalize or nearly normalize blood glucose fluctuations for prolonged periods in type 1 diabetic patients,[20, 52, 61, 88] and great strides have been made in our understanding and assessment of diabetic complications.[12, 62]

CONVENTIONAL AND "INTENSIVE" INSULIN TREATMENT FOR TYPE 1 DIABETES: THE DCCT EXPERIENCE

Shortly after the discovery of insulin and its dramatic lifesaving abilities by Banting and Best in 1922, it became obvious that chronic insulin treatment would be necessary to sustain health and well-being in type 1 diabetic patients. Rapid improvement in the purity of bovine and porcine insulin led to the final isolation of "soluble," or "regular," insulin in 1926, with its peak biologic action at 2 to 4 hours and its total duration of biologic action of 5 to 8 hours after subcutaneous injection. This insulin preparation required multiple daily injections, a characteristic considered to be an inconvenience at the time. Subsequent efforts were directed at prolonging or extending the action of injectable insulin, giving rise to the intermediate- and long-acting insulin preparations, which are now produced almost entirely in human rather than animal form by recombinant technology.

At the beginning of the DCCT, conventional therapy for type 1 diabetic patients in many countries used these insulin preparations singly or in combination in one or two daily injections to prevent ketoacidosis and the symptoms and caloric wastage of continuous glycosuria, while avoiding hypoglycemia. Although lifesaving, this therapy was not directed at the normalization of glucose and insulin kinetics. In contrast, "intensive" treatment, advocated by some but not all experts and practiced routinely in only a few countries in the pre-DCCT era, was designed to simulate the highly controlled negative feedback modulation of blood glucose provided by the normally functioning endocrine pancreas. This technique consists of a rigorous approach to insulin administration that combines multiple (three or more) daily insulin injections (MDI) or continuous subcutaneous insulin infusion (CSII or pump therapy); dosage adjustment is based on multiple daily blood glucose determinations performed by the patient.[20, 61, 80] Long-term achievement of near-normal blood glucose regulation is reliably documented by determination of glycosylated hemoglobin (HbA$_{1c}$), an integrated measurement of blood glucose fluctuations over time.[65] These techniques were used in the DCCT to produce statistically and physiologically significantly lower blood glucose fluctua-

tions that approached but did not attain levels maintained by nondiabetic individuals (Fig. 20.2).[20] The widespread application of these effective but labor-intensive techniques requires considerable skill on the part of the patient and a multidisciplinary specialized health care team,[20] which results in considerable cost to society[23] as well as significant inconvenience and risk (from hypoglycemia) for the patient.[22, 26, 96] Nevertheless, cognitive function does not appear to be adversely affected by intensive therapy despite the increased frequency of hypoglycemia.[27] Overall, reduction of glycemic exposure with intensive therapy[21] that substan-

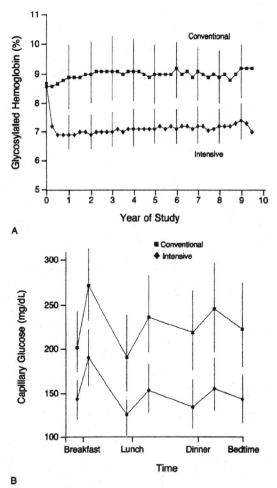

A

B

■ **Figure 20.2** Sequential measurement of glycosylated hemoglobin (HbA$_{1c}$) (*A*) and combined measurement of daily capillary blood glucose (*B*) in patients in the Diabetes Control and Complications Trial with type 1 diabetes receiving conventional or intensive therapy. (From DCCT Research Group. The effect of intensive treatment of diabetes on the development and progression of long-term complications in insulin-dependent diabetes mellitus. N Engl J Med. 1993; 329:977.)

tially reduces the risk of the development and progression of diabetic microvascular and neural complications of diabetes outweighs the risk of intensive therapy to an extent that should have lifelong benefit to patients with type 1 DM.[25] Current recommendations for treatment of type 1 diabetes specifies that the majority of patients should be treated with intensive therapy targeted at near-normal blood glucose and HbA_{1c} levels.[4, 5] Newer technologies under development may provide similar degrees of metabolic control at less risk of hypoglycemia in the future.[64]

RECENT ADVANCES IN THE METABOLIC TREATMENT OF TYPE 2 DIABETES

Until the final results of the United Kingdom Prospective Diabetes Study (UKPDS) are available,[103] the recommendations for glycemic targets in type 2 diabetes are derived essentially from the DCCT.[17] However, it is uncertain whether the DCCT results can or should be translated directly to type 2 diabetic subjects. In a Position Statement issued after the results of the DCCT were published, the American Diabetes Association stated that the benefits of good glycemic control in the prevention of microvascular diabetic complications should be equally applicable to type 2 diabetes because these complications are thought to arise by the same or similar mechanisms from underlying hyperglycemia or insulin deficiency.[3] However, the risks (principally in terms of macrovascular disease) of different modes of therapy in type 2 diabetes are uncertain. For example, high endogenous insulin levels have been cited as a risk factor for the development of macrovascular disease,[75] but large exogenous insulin doses have not been shown to have a deleterious effect on cardiovascular outcomes in subjects with type 2 diabetes thus far. One large multicenter study has attributed a significant reduction in mortality after myocardial infarction to aggressive treatment with insulin.[58]

Currently, the overall therapeutic strategy for type 2 diabetes is to achieve as near normal glycemic control as possible (preprandial plasma glucose, 80 to 120 mg/dL (4.4 to 6.7 mmol/L); bedtime plasma glucose, 100 to 140 mg/dL (5.6 to 7.8 mmol/L); HbA_{1c} less than 7%, with action suggested when the HbA_{1c} exceeds 8%),[3] while minimizing the risk of hypoglycemia. However, as discussed in the section on patients with type 1 DM, these goals must be individualized for each patient based on risk factors for hypoglycemia, comorbidities, and life expectancy. Appropriate strategies include diet, exercise and weight loss, oral hypoglycemic agents or insulin or both (with insulin doses increased as required [with no maximal ceiling]) to achieve glycemic control (see Fig. 20.2). The initial therapeutic approach usually comprises a 3-month trial of diet and exercise before the institution of pharmacological therapy, unless symptomatic hyperglycemia (e.g., polyuria or polydipsia) persists. Oral hypoglycemic agents should be considered if HbA_{1c} is not below 8%. Broadly speaking, *sulfonylureas* are the usual first-line therapy in lean patients, and a *biguanide* or α-*glucosidase inhibitor* should be considered as initial therapy in obese subjects. *Thiazolidinediones*, a new class of insulin-sensitizing agents, are currently approved in the United States only in conjunction with insulin therapy, although their indications may expand as new data emerge. They have been withdrawn in the United Kingdom because of the risk of hepatotoxicity. Any improvement in overall glycemic control, by whatever means, will decrease β-cell glucose toxicity, stimulate endogenous insulin production, and decrease peripheral insulin resistance; patients with type 2 diabetes whose metabolic control has improved may subsequently respond to therapies that were initially ineffective.

Sulfonylureas stimulate insulin secretion by sensitizing the beta cell to the prevailing blood glucose through their action on ATP-sensitive K^+ channels in the pancreatic beta cell. Some members of this class may also improve peripheral insulin sensitivity by unknown mechanisms. The fall in fasting glucose is usually approximately 60 mg/dL (3.3 mmol/L) (HbA_{1c} reduction of 1.5 to 2.0%).[48] Because the principal side effects are hypoglycemia and weight gain, they may not be the most suitable first-line therapy in obese patients with type 2 DM. Newer once-daily preparations of glipizide and glimepiride may be particularly efficacious in reducing fasting hyperglycemia and fasting hyperinsulinemia; glimepiride is approved for combination therapy with insulin and is purported to have greater insulin-sensitizing actions and a lower incidence of hypoglycemia.[7, 30, 102] Animal studies suggest that glimepiride may be more beta-cell–specific in its action on ATP-sensitive K^+ channels, with theoretically more insulin secretory action and less deleterious cardiovascular effects,[8] although this has yet to be established in long-term studies in humans. These newer long-acting sulfonyl-ureas with once-daily dosing may have a role in combination therapy with other oral antidiabetic agents such as metformin or acarbose.

Biguanides, such as metformin, lower blood glucose primarily by direct inhibition of hepatic glucose output[92] and so complement the action of sulfonylureas. Metformin does not stimulate insulin secretion, and accordingly, does not precipitate hypoglycemia when used alone. The fall in fasting and postprandial blood glucose on average is about 60 mg/dL (3.3 mmol/L) (HbA$_{1c}$ reduction of 1.5 to 2.0%).[38] Unlike insulin and sulfonylureas, metformin does not stimulate weight gain and so may be appropriate first-line therapy in the more obese patient. Because metformin is rapidly cleared through the kidneys (90% in 12 hours), it is contraindicated by renal impairment. A rare but serious side effect, lactic acidosis, occurs in 3:100,000 patient years, always in the setting of significant liver, cardiac, or renal failure. Tolerability is limited by gastrointestinal side effects, which are usually dose related and often temporary.

α-Glucosidase inhibitors, such as acarbose, are minimally absorbed but competitively inhibit pancreatic and mucosal glucosidase within the intestinal lumen, reducing the rate of carbohydrate digestion and absorption and, in so doing, decrease postprandial plasma glucose levels by about 50 mg/dL (2.8 mmol/L) and HbA$_{1c}$ by 0.8 to 1%.[49] Acarbose is useful as monotherapy, especially in obese patients, and in combination with sulfonylureas and, potentially, insulin.[29] Weight gain and hypoglycemia do not occur when acarbose is used alone. Tolerability is limited by flatulence, which appears to vary widely by region.

Thiazolidinediones are a new class of insulin-sensitizing agents whose mechanism of action appears distinct from all other drug classes. Their principal target appears to be the transcription factor peroxisome proliferator-activated receptor-γ (PPAR-γ), and their site of action may be skeletal muscle.[78, 109] Troglitazone is approved for use in combination with insulin therapy and decreases insulin resistance in the obese insulin-treated type 2 diabetic subject, thereby improving glycemic control (HbA$_{1c}$ reduction of 1.4%) and lowering exogenous insulin requirements (insulin dose reduction, 25 to 40%). As already stated, it has been withdrawn in the United Kingdom. No weight gain or hypoglycemia are observed with monotherapy.[78] A significant proportion of type 2 diabetic subjects who do not achieve adequate glycemic control on one oral agent alone may respond to combination oral therapy, although rigorous dose-response studies of combination therapy are lacking. Sulfonylurea plus metformin or acarbose in combination may result in a decrease of HbA$_{1c}$ from 1 to 1.7%. Although troglitazone is theoretically a useful agent in combination with a sulfonylurea or metformin, it is not yet approved for this use in the U.S.

Insulin therapy should be considered in any patient with type 2 diabetes who fails to achieve an HbA$_{1c}$ of less than 8% while receiving oral combination therapy. Insulin may be initiated as a single injection of intermediate-acting insulin at bedtime in combination with oral agents or as twice daily injection of intermediate-acting insulin alone or in combination with a rapid-acting insulin. Intensive insulin therapy, as practiced in the DCCT, is useful in selected patients with type 2 diabetes. Insulin therapy is generally required in type 2 diabetic patients in the setting of severe intercurrent infections, major surgery, pregnancy, hyperosmolar nonketotic states, and myocardial infarction.

EVIDENCE SUGGESTING A ROLE FOR HYPERGLYCEMIA IN THE PATHOGENESIS OF DIABETIC NEUROPATHY

The results of the DCCT implicate metabolic abnormalities present in moderately controlled type 1 diabetic patients that are correctable by intensive metabolic therapy in the pathogenesis of diabetic neuropathy.[17] Hyperglycemia itself, as measured by HbA$_{1c}$, is a reasonable candidate, given the curvilinear relationship between glycemic exposure and the development and progression of diabetic complications in the DCCT.[21] Insulin deficiency per se is not likely to explain the differential effects of intensive versus conventional therapy on the development of diabetic neuropathy, because the total insulin doses did not differ significantly between the two treatment groups.[20] Several old and new observations suggest a close relationship between hyperglycemia and the development and severity of diabetic neuropathy.

Retrospective Epidemiologic and Clinical Studies

Early epidemiologic studies of diabetic neuropathy were often flawed by inconsistencies in terminology, diagnostic criteria, and study populations (see Chapter 17).[110] For instance, isolated minor paresthesias in a diabetic patient were classified as diabetic neuropathy in some studies, whereas others used much more rigid criteria,[99] and surveys of practice-based clinic populations introduce substantial selection and referral biases. Pirart's unique 25-year prospective study of 4400 unselected patients in a diabetic clinic provides a classical and enduring clinical view of diabetic neuropathy.[71] Neuropathy, defined as loss of Achilles' or patellar reflexes or both combined with diminished vibratory sensation in the presence or absence of "more dramatic polyneuropathy or mono- or multineuropathy" was present in 12% of patients at the time diabetes was diagnosed, with prevalence increasing linearly with duration of diabetes to nearly 50% after 25 years.[71, 72] The prevalence and incidence of neuropathy, corrected for duration of diabetes, did not differ substantially as a function of age at diagnosis of diabetes in Pirart's patients, although he had few pediatric patients.[72] This suggests that neuropathy appears to occur with somewhat similar frequency in type 1 and type 2 diabetes despite fundamental differences in the pathogenesis of the underlying metabolic abnormality. In particular, despite substantial differences in circulating insulin levels between types 1 and 2 diabetes, the risk for neuropathy appears to be similar. This view has been confirmed by recent, population-based studies comparing the prevalence of neuropathy in types 1 and 2 diabetes (Table 20.1).[31, 37, 56, 59, 112] Given that diabetic neuropathy also occurs in secondary forms of diabetes (pancreatectomy, nonalcoholic pancreatitis, and hemochromatosis),[99] the risk of diabetic neuropathy appears to be independent of the underlying pathogenetic mechanisms responsible for diabetes and of the absolute degree of insulin deficiency; rather, it appears to be a function of the diabetic state itself. Hyperglycemia, present in all forms of diabetes, therefore emerges as an attractive candidate for a common essential component to the pathogenesis of diabetic neuropathy. Subtle distinctions in the histopathology of diabetic polyneuropathy in types 1 and 2 diabetes have been described,[10, 86] but their significance remains unclear at present (see Chapter 19).

Many studies have demonstrated that diabetic neuropathy appears to be related to the duration and degree of hyperglycemia. Clinically detectable diabetic neuropathy is rarely reported within the first 5 years of diabetes[33] except in type 2 patients, in whom preexisting asymptomatic hyperglycemia is difficult to exclude.[71, 72] The prevalence of diabetic neuropathy is therefore initially low but increases progressively with duration of diabetes.[11, 71, 72, 105] On the other hand, the clinical relationship between concurrent blood glucose control and the development of clinically overt diabetic neuropathy has been the subject of much controversy and misinterpretation. The notion that the onset of symptomatic neuropathy in diabetic patients uniformly follows a prolonged period of poor diabetic control is readily dismissed on the basis of clinical observation.[32] Conversely, the precipitation of acutely painful neuropathic symptoms (often unaccompanied by significant sensory deficits) after rapid improvement in metabolic control with insulin is a rare but well-described clinical event (*insulin neuritis*) that has been ascribed to acute vascular[95] or perhaps metabolic dysequilibrium.[11, 12] In the vast majority of cases, the development of clinically overt diabetic polyneuropathy represents a late stage in a chronic indolent progressive underlying degenerative process (*subclinical neuropathy*[2]). Therefore, temporal dissociation between the quality of glucose control and the appearance of neuropathic signs and symptoms is not unexpected and does not itself constitute an argument against the overall importance of hyperglycemia.

The frequency of clinical neuropathy in populations of diabetic patients is generally closely related to the duration and often the severity of hyperglycemia.[11, 12, 72, 105] Duration of diabetes and attained age consistently emerge as important risk factors for diabetic neuropathy,[31, 37, 56, 59, 112] whereas HbA$_{1c}$ emerges in some[37, 59]

TABLE 20.1 PREVALENCE OF DIABETIC NEUROPATHY IN POPULATION-BASED COHORTS OF TYPE 1 AND/OR TYPE 2 DIABETES AND CORRELATION WITH RISK FACTORS OF DIABETES DURATION AND HBA$_{1c}$

Reference	Prevalence of Neuropathy (%)			Risk Factors	
	All	Type 1	Type 2	Duration	HbA$_{1c}$
Dyck et al[31]*	61	66	59	Yes	—
Knuiman et al[56]†	25	25	25	Yes	No
Boulton et al[9]‡	29	23	32	Yes	—
Maser et al[59]	—	34	—	Yes	Yes
Franklin et al[37]	—	—	28	Yes	Yes

* Includes autonomic and focal neuropathies.
† Corrected for age (0 to 39 y at diagnosis) and diabetes duration (25 y).
‡ Not corrected for effect of age.

but not all[56] cross-sectional studies, perhaps because of fluctuation in this measure over time. Thus, neuropathy increases with duration and perhaps severity of hyperglycemia, but the onset of clinically overt diabetic neuropathy in an individual patient is unpredictable, neither necessarily reflecting concurrent metabolic control[110] nor following inexorably from even prolonged and severe hyperglycemia.[72] This somewhat loose individual association reflects to some extent the indolent and occult nature of the underlying nerve damage. It also suggests the presence of other independent pathogenetic variables, such as genetic, nutritional, toxic (for example, alcohol),[60] and mechanical (entrapment and compression)[11, 12] factors (see Chapter 36).

Short-Term Studies of Nerve Electrophysiology

As discussed in Chapter 16, nerve conduction slowing in diabetes is attributed to several types of abnormalities. Maximum motor and sensory nerve conduction velocity, primarily reflecting the integrity of the largest and most rapidly conducting nerve fibers, is only modestly decreased in human diabetes.[16] Type 1 diabetic patients with minimally detectable clinical diabetic neuropathy have only slightly more severe electrophysiologic abnormalities than slightly younger patients without clinical neuropathy.[16] (As discussed in Chapter 30, diffuse demyelination results in a marked decrease in maximal conduction velocity in a small subgroup of patients with diabetic neuropathy that may represent coexisting disorders.[39]) In acute animal diabetes, nerve conduc-

tion slowing without associated fiber loss, atrophy, or demyelination is attributed directly to biophysical alterations that are themselves indirect consequences of metabolic or vascular derangements in peripheral nerve (see Chapters 21 to 26), supporting but by no means establishing a role for metabolic alterations in the pathogenesis of human diabetic neuropathy.

Nerve conduction velocity is slightly reduced at the time of diagnosis of type 1 diabetes. This defect improves rapidly with institution of insulin therapy (Fig. 20.3A). However, the improvement declines rapidly with withdrawal of insulin therapy in a pattern consistent with an initial direct and reversible metabolic contribution to conduction slowing reminiscent of that purported to occur in diabetic animals (Fig. 20.3B).[47, 107] Initial improvement in conduction velocity is accompanied by decreased vibratory perception threshold, implying physiologic significance.[94] Nerve conduction velocity thereafter becomes progressively but modestly reduced in types 1 and 2 diabetes as a function of duration of disease.[34, 49] In patients with overt diabetic neuropathy, slowing of sensory conduction velocity correlates largely with loss of large myelinated fibers,[6] with only a small residual component attributable to other factors such as "metabolic" factors or demyelination. Hence, acute improvement of nerve conduction velocity after metabolic intervention in patients with neuropathy or established diabetes is necessarily limited to that component of conduction slowing not attributable to fiber loss. Nerve conduction velocity is inversely correlated with HbA_{1c}[40] and improves slightly but proportion-

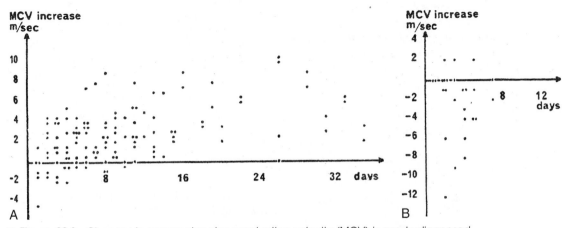

■ **Figure 20.3**   Changes in peroneal motor conduction velocity (MCV) in newly diagnosed type 1 diabetic patients after institution (*A*) and withdrawal (*B*) of insulin treatment.

ately with HbA_{1c} levels in response to conventional metabolic therapy in chronic stable type 2 diabetes.[41] Similarly, short-term intensive treatment significantly improves peripheral nerve conduction in type 1 diabetes.[41, 70, 82, 88]

Although these observations suggest a direct metabolic component to conduction slowing even in established diabetes, the time course of the response, extending over several weeks to months, does not exclude a significant contribution from structural repair. On the other hand, acute consistent effects of blood glucose normalization on nerve conduction would suggest direct metabolic contributions to nerve conduction slowing in human diabetes. Gallai and collaborators studied multiple motor and sensory nerve conduction velocities in 16 diabetic patients, 8 with and 8 without neuropathy, before and after 3 days of Biostator treatment.[38] Conduction velocity was improved in peroneal, tibial, and median sensory nerves in patients with (but not without) neuropathy after treatment. Service and associates studied 8 hyperglycemic type 1 diabetics before and after 72 hours of Biostator regulation and found improvement in ulnar sensory conduction velocity ($+3.2 \pm 1.4$ m/s) but no change in 24 other electrophysiologic parameters measured.[81] These inconsistent results could reflect either methodological limitations in the electrophysiologic techniques used or a marginal acute effect of blood glucose normalization on nerve conduction.

Troni and associates[101a] studied H-reflex conduction from the soleus muscle in 10 type 1 diabetic patients, aged 26.3 ± 9 (SD) years, with duration of diabetes more than 5 years (4 were described as "newly diagnosed") before and during 2 days of treatment with an external artificial pancreas (Biostator). The H-reflex conduction parameter was chosen by these authors on the basis of their previous demonstration that the day-to-day variation in this parameter was an order of magnitude less as compared with other conventional nerve conduction parameters. H-reflex conduction velocity (n-HCV) in m/s was taken as the mean of the difference of the H-reflex and M latencies bilaterally divided into twice the distance from the popliteal fossa to T11, corrected for rectal temperature. n-HCV was reduced in all 10 patients before Biostator regulation and was increased in all 10 from 1 to 3 m/s by 48 hours of Biostator treatment, with a mean increase of 1.66 m/s. However, normal n-HCV was achieved in only 1 patient. n-HCV also increased progressively during 6 months of in-

tensive insulin therapy in 12 other type 1 diabetic patients, with the greatest improvement occurring within the first week; the increase correlated closely with improvement in HbA_{1c}. These classical observations strongly suggested that a component of nerve conduction slowing in diabetic patients is rapidly reversible with metabolic therapy, probably reflecting a direct biochemical or biophysical contribution related to metabolic factors rather than structural abnormalities. Hence, nerve conduction impairment in diabetes appears to reflect a combination of processes in diabetic nerve—structural as well as functional—that cannot be easily resolved by standard electrophysiologic techniques.

One or more of these components appear to be related to metabolic alterations resulting from hyperglycemia or insulin deficiency or both. Conduction slowing is usually more pronounced in diabetic patients with clinically overt neuropathy, and the predictive value of conduction impairment for the subsequent development of diabetic neuropathy has been established in type 1 diabetes.[113] Nevertheless, none of these promising observations that metabolic intervention improves nerve conduction in diabetic patients establishes that such treatment will prevent or ameliorate diabetic neuropathy.

Uncontrolled Clinical Trials in Symptomatic Neuropathy

The isolated but unconfirmed reports of clinical improvements in diabetic neuropathy with intensive insulin therapy[9, 45, 100, 108] suggest a continuing role for the altered metabolism in established diabetic neuropathy. However, appropriately controlled studies of age- and sex-matched patients with similar type and duration of diabetic neuropathy are not available as of this writing.[73] These observations have led to the suggestion that a therapeutic trial of intensified insulin therapy may be indicated in cases of clinically overt diabetic neuropathy.[45] This enthusiasm must be tempered by recognition of the increased susceptibility to severe iatrogenic hypoglycemia that occurs in neuropathic diabetics as a result of autonomic impairment with its associated decreases in adrenergic counterregulatory mechanisms and delayed gastric emptying.[50, 79, 97]

Controlled Clinical Trials of Intensive Metabolic Therapy in Diabetic Neuropathy

Controlled randomized prospective clinical trials combining treatment strategies that consistently and predictably lower blood glucose with end points that reliably chart development and progression of clinically meaningful peripheral nerve disease such as the DCCT ultimately establish the efficacy of metabolic therapy in prevention and treatment of diabetic polyneuropathy. Several small studies for long-term randomized controlled prospective intervention trials using quantitative measures of nerve function (nerve conduction and quantitative sensory testing) heralded the DCCT results. Holman and associates[51] studied 74 type 1 diabetics randomly assigned to "usual" or intensified insulin and dietary therapy for 24 months. HbA$_{1c}$ was significantly lowered by intensive insulin therapy. Vibratory sensory threshold over both lateral malleoli and the medial border of the distal phalanx of both great toes was assessed at baseline and yearly thereafter with a biothesiometer. At the completion of the trial, mean vibratory threshold had increased in the conventionally treated group ($+2.0 \pm 5.7$ [SD] V) and *decreased* in the intensively treated group ($-0.9 + 4.5$ [SD] V; $2P = 0.026$). The authors concluded that intensive insulin therapy prevented deterioration of vibratory sensation that otherwise occurs in type 1 diabetic patients on conventional insulin therapy. Service and coworkers[82] studied type 1 diabetic patients randomly assigned either to conventional or CSII therapy. By 8 months, statistically significant differences in nerve conduction and vibratory threshold were found favoring the CSII-treated groups, supporting the observations of Holman and associates.[51] Similar results were reported by the Stockholm Diabetes Intervention Study, in which 5 years of intensive diabetes treatment preserved vibratory-perception threshold in type 1 diabetic patients.[76] If increasing vibratory-perception threshold or slowed nerve conduction or both are true harbingers of clinically overt neuropathy, then long-term intensive insulin therapy should delay or prevent the development of diabetic neuropathy.

Glucose Control and Autonomic Neuropathy

Cardiovascular diabetic autonomic neuropathy (DAN) has been implicated in the excess sudden cardiac death in diabetic patients.[35, 69, 74] Cardiovascular DAN, detectable at a subclinical stage in 40% of even newly diagnosed type 1 diabetics, confers a 5-year mortality of 16 to 53%,[35, 69, 74] with the highest mortality observed in advanced cases with symptomatic sympathetic denervation and orthostatic hypotension.[35] A clear beneficial effect of metabolic control on the development or progression of cardiac DAN would significantly improve overall prognosis for diabetes; however, such an effect has been difficult to demonstrate in a clinically meaningful way. Indeed, improved metabolic control has been reported to improve[53] or not to affect[87] DAN, leading to speculation that autonomic nerve function may be less responsive to improved glycemic control than somatic nerve function[114] (the effect of intensive metabolic therapy on the autonomic function in the DCCT is discussed in Chapter 17). Alternatively, autonomic function tests may be less sensitive and reliable than tests of somatic nerve function. The radiotracer C-11 hydroxyephedrine (HED) has recently been developed as a norepinephrine analogue for positron emission tomography (PET) to map sympathetic innervation.[1] The HED undergoes highly specific uptake and retention in the sympathetic nerve terminals,[1] which facilitates the quantitative regional characterization of sympathetic neuronal dysfunction and loss. In two young female subjects, HED PET was used to examine the effect of glycemic control on the progression of cardiac sympathetic DAN. The effect of intensive insulin therapy resulting in good glycemic control was assessed (average HbA$_{1c}$ approximately 7%) in a subject with extensive left ventricular sympathetic denervation. Abnormalities of HED retention originally affected 71% of the left ventricle in 1992, compared with 59% in 1995. In contrast, in the subject with poor glycemic control (average HbA$_{1c}$ approximately 10%) a small defect affecting only 11% of the left ventricle in 1991 progressed to involve 70% of the ventricle 4 years later. Thus good glycemic control is also important in the maintenance of cardiac sympathetic integrity, which may ultimately be of importance in the prevention of sudden cardiac death. Prospective studies with larger numbers of patients and correlation with cardiovascular outcomes will be required to validate these preliminary findings, which suggest that metabolic control may have dramatic effects on cardiac innervation in type 1 diabetes.

DIABETIC NEUROPATHY IN THE DCCT

The DCCT was designed to test whether intensive treatment in patients with type 1 diabetes would retard the development and progression of the chronic microvascular and neural complications of diabetes. Because the primary outcome was diabetic retinopathy, subjects were recruited, assigned, and randomized within 2 cohorts depending on baseline retinopathy status. All subjects had to be aged 13 to 39 years, with C-peptide deficient diabetes mellitus and an abnormal HbA_{1c}, and had to be free of renal impairment, hypertension, heavy alcohol consumption, or diabetic neuropathy that required pharmacologic treatment. Subjects had to prove themselves capable of undertaking a very demanding regimen of frequent blood glucose monitoring and complex insulin treatment regimens designed to attain near normoglycemia, but they had to be willing to accept randomization to conventional insulin treatment aimed merely at prevention of symptomatic hyperglycemia or hypoglycemia. Patients without photographic evidence of diabetic retinopathy, who were recruited into a primary prevention cohort, had to have a diabetes' duration of 5 years or less and a urinary albumin excretion rate less than 40 mg/24 h. Patients with photographic evidence of very mild to moderate nonproliferative diabetic retinopathy, who were recruited into a secondary intervention cohort, had to have a diabetes' duration of 15 years or less and a urinary albumin excretion rate less than 200 mg/24 h.[17] Subjects in the primary prevention and secondary intervention cohorts randomized to intensive therapy were initially hospitalized for institution of MDI or CSII therapy (between which they were able to switch during the course of the study) designed to maintain preprandial blood glucose below 120 mg/dL (6.7 mmol/L), postprandial blood glucose less than 180 mg/dL (10 mmol/L), weekly 3 a.m. blood glucose above 65 mg/dL (3.6 mmol/L), and HbA_{1c} less than 6.05%. All subjects received usual dietary and diabetes education. Their baseline characteristics are shown in Table 20.2.[17]

Neurologic assessment in the DCCT included a structured neurologic history and physical examination and nerve conduction studies (median and peroneal motor conduction velocity, amplitude and F-wave latency, and median and sural sensory conduction velocity and amplitude) performed by a neurologist at baseline, 5 years, and study end.[18] The examining neurologist was masked as to treatment group assignment. Cardiovascular autonomic nervous system (ANS) studies performed at baseline and every second year are described in Chapter 11. The primary neurologic end point was the development of clinical neuropathy confirmed by unequivocally abnormal nerve conduction or ANS testing (Table 20.3) in those subjects not exhibiting neuropathy at baseline.[18] A diagnosis of clinical neuropathy required the presence of at least two of the following: somatic or autonomic symptoms consistent with diabetic neuropathy, sensory deficits consistent with a distal symmetric polyneuropathy, or absent or decreased deep tendon reflexes consistent with a distal symmetric polyneuropathy (Table 20.3).[18]

Of the 1441 subjects randomized at 29 participating North American study centers, 99% completed the study, remaining on their assigned therapy 97% of the time for a mean follow-up period of 6.5 years until the study was terminated by an outside data monitoring committee.[17] HbA_{1c} values were comparable in the two treatment groups in the two cohorts at baseline and remained essentially unchanged in the conventional treatment groups (see Fig. 20.2A). HbA_{1c} fell by approximately 2% in the intensive treatment group within the first 6 months of the study and remained approximately 2% lower during the follow-up period (see Fig. 20.2A). This translated into a 33% reduction in mean blood glucose from approximately 230 mg/dL (12.8 mmol/L) in the conventional treatment groups to approximately 155 mg/dL (8.6 mmol/L) in the intensive treatment groups (see Fig. 20.2B).[17] A threefold increase in the incidence of severe hypoglycemia (defined by needing the assistance of another person) was associated with intensive therapy,[17] but was not associated with detectable deleterious effects on cognition[27] or quality of life.[26]

The presence and progression of diabetic retinopathy was assessed by biannual retinopathy staging by retinal fundus photographs and eye examination. Diabetic nephropathy was assessed by annual measures of urinary albumin excretion.[24] The primary retinal end point was a clinically significant "3-step" progression on retinal fundus photography sustained for at least 6 months, and secondary ocular end points included the development of macular edema, severe nonproliferative or proliferative retinopathy, and the need for laser photocoagulation. Renal end points included the development of microalbuminuria (>40 mg/24 h) or clinical-grade proteinuria (>300 mg/24 h). The relative risk reduction with intensive therapy for all end points except macular edema achieved statistical significance and ranged from 39 to 63% (Table 20.4).[17]

TABLE 20.2 BASELINE CHARACTERISTICS OF THE TWO DCCT STUDY COHORTS*

	Primary Prevention		Secondary Intervention	
Characteristic	Conventional Therapy (N = 378)	Intensive Therapy (N = 348)	Conventional Therapy (N = 352)	Intensive Therapy (N = 363)
Age (y)	26 ± 8	27 ± 7	27 ± 7	27 ± 7
Adolescents, 13–18 y (%)	19	16	9	10
Male sex (%)	54	49	54	53
White race (%)	96	96	97	97
Duration of IDDM (y)	2.6 ± 1.4	2.6 ± 1.4	8.6 ± 3.7	8.9 ± 3.8
Insulin dose (U/kg of body weight/day)	0.62 ± 0.26	0.62 ± 0.25	0.71 ± 0.24	0.72 ± 0.23
Glycosylated hemoglobin (%)†	8.8 ± 1.7	8.8 ± 1.6	8.9 ± 1.5	9.0 ± 1.5
Mean blood glucose (mg/dL)‡	229 ± 80	234 ± 86	232 ± 78	234 ± 81
Blood pressure (mm Hg)				
Systolic	114 ± 12	112 ± 11	116 ± 12	114 ± 12
Diastolic	72 ± 9	72 ± 9	73 ± 9	73 ± 9
Body weight (% of ideal)	103 ± 14	103 ± 13	105 ± 13	104 ± 12
Current smokers (%)	17	19	19	18
Serum cholesterol (mg/dL)	173 ± 35	176 ± 33	179 ± 32	178 ± 33
Serum triglycerides (mg/dL)	77 ± 57	75 ± 41	87 ± 44	87 ± 45
Serum HDL cholesterol (mg/dL)	51 ± 13	52 ± 13	49 ± 11	49 ± 12
Serum LDL cholesterol (mg/dL)	106 ± 30	109 ± 29	112 ± 28	112 ± 29
Absence of retinopathy (%)	100	100	0	0
Microaneurysms only (%)§	0	0	58	67
NPDR‖				
Mild	0	0	23	18
Moderate	0	0	19	15
Urinary albumin excretion (mg/24 h)	12 ± 8	12 ± 9	19 ± 24	21 ± 25
Creatinine clearance (mL/mm)	127 ± 28	128 ± 30	130 ± 30	128 ± 31
Clinical neuropathy (%)¶	2.1	4.9	9.4	9.4

* Plus-minus values are means ± SD. To convert values for glucose to millimoles per liter, multiply by 0.05551. To convert values for triglycerides to millimoles per liter, multiply by 0.05551. To convert values for cholesterol, low-density lipoprotein (LDL) cholesterol, and high-density lipoprotein (HDL) cholesterol to millimoles per liter, multiply by 0.02586.
† Mean value in nondiabetic persons, 5.05 ± 0.5%.
‡ Based on the mean value of seven determinations during a 24-hour period.
§ P = 0.01 by the Wilcoxon rank-sum test for the difference in the level of retinopathy at baseline between the treatment groups in the secondary-intervention cohort.
‖ NPDR, nonproliferative diabetic retinopathy. Mild NPDR was defined by the presence of microaneurysms plus mild-to-moderate retinal hemorrhages or hard exudates. Moderate NPDR was defined by the presence of microaneurysms plus any of the following: cotton-wool spots, mild intraretinal microvascular abnormalities or venous beading, or severe retinal hemorrhages.
¶ Defined as peripheral sensorimotor neuropathy on physical examination by the study neurologist plus either abnormal nerve conduction in two different peripheral nerves or unequivocally abnormal autonomic test results. P = 0.04 for the difference between groups in the primary-prevention cohort with respect to the baseline prevalence of clinical neuropathy.
From DCCT Research Group. The effect of intensive treatment of diabetes on the development and progression of long-term complications in insulin-dependent diabetes mellitus. N Engl J Med 1993; 329:977.

Prevention of Diabetic Neuropathy by Intensive Therapy in the DCCT

The beneficial effects of intensive therapy on the development of diabetic neuropathy was similar in magnitude to those on retinopathy and nephropathy. The risk of development of confirmed clinical neuropathy that was diagnosed by neurologic history and physical examination and confirmed by nerve conduction or autonomic function studies[18] at year 5 was reduced by 69% from 9.8 to 3.1% in the primary prevention cohort, and 57% from 16.1 to 7.0% in the secondary intervention cohort by intensive therapy, with an overall risk reduc-

tion of 60% (see Table 20.4).[17] Although patients with symptomatic neuropathy meriting treatment were excluded from the DCCT, confirmed clinical neuropathy was present in 92 of the 1441 subjects entering the DCCT. These comprised 2.1 and 4.9% of subjects randomized to conventional and intensive therapy, respectively, in the primary prevention cohort, and 9.4% of each randomization group in the secondary intervention cohort (Table 20.5).[18] Of the remaining 1349 randomized subjects without confirmed clinical neuropathy at baseline, 1161 completed the neurologic evaluation at year 5 (see Fig. 20.1 and Table 20.4). Intensive therapy reduced the risk of developing con-

TABLE 20.3 DCCT NEUROLOGIC END
POINT DEFINITIONS

Confirmed clinical neuropathy—a finding of definite
   clinical neuropathy by physical examination and
   history confirmed by unequivocal abnormality of nerve
   conduction or autonomic nervous system response as
   defined below
Clinical neuropathy—a definite diagnosis of peripheral
   diabetic neuropathy by clinical examination based on
   the presence of at least two of the following:
      Physical symptoms
      Abnormalities on sensory examination
      Absent or decreased tendon reflexes
Abnormal nerve conduction—at least one abnormal
   conduction attribute on each of at least two
   anatomically distinct peripheral nerves according to the
   following standards:
      Median nerve motor conduction
         Amplitude < 4.2 mV
         Conduction velocity < 49.0 m/s
         F-wave latency > 31.8 ms
      Median sensory nerve action potential
         Amplitude > 10.0 μV
         Conduction velocity < 48.0 m/s
      Peroneal nerve motor conduction
         Amplitude < 2.5 mV
         Conduction velocity < 40.0 m/s
         F-wave latency > 56.0 ms
      Sural nerve sensory action potential
         Amplitude < 5.0 μV
         Conduction velocity < 40.0 m/s
Abnormal autonomic response—any of the following
   indications of cardiac autonomic neuropathy:
      R-R variation (mean resultant) < 15.0
      R-R variation < 20.0 in combination with Valsalva
         ratio < 1.5
      Orthostatic hypotension caused by autonomic
         neuropathy as indicated by a decrease of at least
         10 mm Hg in diastolic blood pressure in postural
         studies confirmed by blunted norepinephrine
         response in plasma catecholamine specimens
Subclinical neuropathy—abnormal nerve conduction,
   autonomic nervous system response, or both without a
   definite diagnosis of peripheral neuropathy by clinical
   examination

From DCCT Research Group. The effect of intensive diabetes
therapy on the development and progression of neuropathy. Ann
Intern Med 1995; 122:561.

firmed clinical neuropathy, clinical neuropathy
(by history and physical examination), or subclinical neuropathy (as defined by abnormal
nerve conduction or ANS testing) in the primary prevention, secondary intervention, and
combined cohorts by 28 to 71% (Table 20.6).
The relative risk reduction with intensive therapy was similar in the two cohorts, despite the
longer duration of diabetes and the greater
retinal and renal disease burden of patients in
the secondary intervention cohort. (The development of abnormal autonomic nervous system [ANS] testing was a rare phenomenon in

the primary prevention cohort, and the effect
of intensive therapy did not achieve statistical
significance in this group [see Table 20.6].)
Thus, 5 years of improved metabolic control
with intensive diabetes therapy in patients
with type 1 diabetes with little or no evidence
of clinically significant secondary complications markedly reduced the risk of developing
clinically detectable diabetic neuropathy, abnormal nerve conduction, and abnormal autonomic nervous system tests. These results unequivocally implicate metabolic abnormalities
associated with insulin deficiency or hyperglycemia or both in the pathogenesis of diabetic
polyneuropathy in patients with type 1 diabetes mellitus.

Treatment of Diabetic Neuropathy by Intensive Therapy in the DCCT

The DCCT was not designed to test the efficacy
of intensive therapy in the treatment of diabetic
neuropathy. Because patients with clinically
troublesome diabetic neuropathy were excluded from enrollment in the DCCT, the efficacy of intensive therapy in the treatment of
symptomatic diabetic neuropathy could not be
evaluated. Indeed, the rarity at baseline of confirmed (only 92 subjects) or even unconfirmed
(134 subjects) clinical neuropathy precluded
meaningful evaluation of the effects of intensive therapy within these subgroups. A broader
subgroup consisting of 450 patients with at
least one abnormality on clinical examination
(among neuropathic symptoms, sensory deficits, and abnormal deep tendon reflexes) was
defined as having "possible or definite" clinical
neuropathy at baseline.[19] The frequency of abnormal nerve conduction was roughly twice
as great in patients with possible or definite
neuropathy compared with those without neuropathy.[19] The likelihood of having abnormal
nerve conduction was significantly reduced in
patients with possible or definite neuropathy
treated with intensive (37%) versus conventional (56%) therapy at 5 years ($P<0.001$), although this effect was more marked in the
primary prevention cohort (intensive, 24%;
conventional, 49%; $P<0.01$) versus the secondary intervention cohort (intensive, 48%; conventional, 63%; $P=$ NS). Nevertheless, statistically significant positive effects of intensive
versus conventional therapy on change in
nerve conduction measures over 5 years in patients with possible or definite neuropathy at
baseline were evident for median and peroneal
motor conduction velocities and F-wave laten-

TABLE 20.4 DEVELOPMENT AND PROGRESSION OF CHRONIC COMPLICATIONS OF DIABETES AND REDUCTION IN RISK WITH INTENSIVE THERAPY IN THE PRIMARY PREVENTION AND SECONDARY INTERVENTION COHORTS OF THE DCCT

Complications	Primary Prevention*			Secondary Intervention*			Both Cohorts†
	Conventional Therapy	Intensive Therapy	Risk Reduction	Conventional Therapy	Intensive Therapy	Risk Reduction	Risk Reduction
≥3-Step sustained retinopathy	4.7	1.2	76(62–85)‡	7.8	3.7	54(39–66)‡	63(52–71)‡
Macular edema§	—	—	—	3.0	2.0	23(−13–48)	26(−8–50)
Severe nonproliferative or proliferative retinopathy§	—	—	—	2.4	1.1	47(12–67)¶	47(15–67)¶
Laser treatment§‖	—	—	—	2.3	0.9	56(26–74)‡	51(21–70)¶
Urinary albumin excretion (mg/24 h)							
≥40	3.4	2.2	34(2–56)¶	5.7	3.6	43(21–58)‡	39(21–52)‡
≥300	0.3	0.2	44(−124–86)¶	1.4	0.6	56(18–76)¶	54(19–74)¶
Clinical neuropathy at 5 y**	9.8	3.1	69(24–87)¶	16.1	7.0	57(29–73)	60(38–74)‡

* Rates shown are absolute rates of the development and progression of complications per 100 patient-years. Risk reductions represent the comparison of intensive with conventional treatment, expressed as a percentage and calculated from the proportional-hazards model with adjustment for baseline values as noted, except in the case of neuropathy. Confidence interval is 95%.
† Stratified according to the primary-prevention and secondary-prevention cohorts.
‡ P ≤ 0.002 by the two-tailed rank-sum test.
§ Too few events occurred in the primary-prevention cohort to allow meaningful analysis of this variable.
¶ P < 0.04 by the two-tailed rank-sum test.
‖ Denotes the first episode of laser therapy for macular edema or proliferative retinopathy.
** Excludes patients with clinical neuropathy at baseline.
From DCCT Research Group. The effect of intensive treatment of diabetes on the development and progression of long-term complications in insulin-dependent diabetes mellitus. N Engl J Med 1993; 329:977.

TABLE 20.5   BASELINE NEUROLOGIC CHARACTERISTICS IN DCCT SUBJECTS

| | Primary Prevention Cohort | | Secondary Intervention Cohort | |
Variable	Conventional Therapy, n(%)	Intensive Therapy, n(%)	Conventional Therapy, n(%)	Intensive Therapy, n(%)
None	281(74.5)	264(76.3)	219(62.2)	216(59.5)
Decreased reflexes only	22(5.8)	18(5.2)	33(9.4)	38(10.5)
Symptoms only	14(3.7)	6(1.7)	7(2.0)	10(2.8)
Symptoms and reflexes	2(0.5)	0(0.0)	1(0.3)	2(0.6)
Sensory examination only	46(12.2)	35(10.1)	42(12.0)	43(11.8)
Sensory examination and reflexes	8(2.1)	17(4.9)	31(8.8)	37(10.2)
Sensory examination and symptoms	4(1.1)	3(0.9)	3(0.9)	5(1.4)
Sensory examination, reflexes, and symptoms	1(0.3)	3(0.9)	16(4.6)	12(3.3)
Definite clinical neuropathy*	17(4.5)	22(6.4)	46(13.1)	49(13.5)
Abnormal nerve conduction (in at least two distinct nerves)	82(21.8)	68(19.7)	168(47.7)	155(42.7)
Abnormal autonomic nervous system function	9(2.4)	9(2.6)	29(8.3)	19(5.3)
Confirmed clinical neuropathy†	8(2.1)	17(4.9)‡	33(9.4)	34(9.4)

* Defined by at least two of the following: symptoms consistent with peripheral neuropathy, abnormal sensory examination findings, or absent or decreased tendon reflexes.
† Defined as peripheral sensorimotor neuropathy on physical examination by a neurologist from the DCCT research group plus either abnormal nerve conduction in two different peripheral nerves or unequivocally abnormal autonomic nervous system test results.
‡ Difference between treatment groups in baseline prevalence in primary prevention cohort, P = 0.04.
From DCCT Research Group. The effect of intensive diabetes therapy on the development and progression of neuropathy. Ann Intern Med 1995; 122:561.

cies and for sural sensory amplitudes in the primary prevention and secondary intervention cohorts.[19] For peroneal motor conduction velocity, the magnitude of the positive treatment effect of intensive versus conventional therapy was 4.2 and 3.6 m/s in the primary prevention cohort without and with possible/ definite neuropathy and 2.3 and 3.0 m/s for the secondary intervention cohort without and with possible/definite neuropathy. An overall test of stochastic ordering of change in nerve conduction parameters was strongly positive for intensive versus conventional treatment in patients with and without possible/definite neuropathy at baseline,[19] Thus, although not designed to examine the question directly, the DCCT is consistent with the belief that intensive diabetes treatment may benefit patients with existing diabetic neuropathy, at least in its very earliest stage. This suggestion stands along with the unequivocal demonstration that intensive diabetes treatment designed to attain near normoglycemia in subjects with type 1 diabetes markedly reduces the risk of devel-

TABLE 20.6   RISK FOR DEVELOPING NEUROPATHY END POINTS AT YEAR 5 IN DCCT SUBJECTS IN THE PRIMARY, SECONDARY, OR COMBINED COHORTS AND RISK REDUCTION OF INTENSIVE VERSUS CONVENTIONAL THERAPY (NEAREST %)

| End Point | Primary Cohort (%) | | | Secondary Cohort (%) | | | Combined (%) |
	Conv	Inten	↓ Risk	Conv	Inten	↓ Risk	↓ Risk
Confirmed*	10	3	71†	17	7	61†	64†
Clinical	15	7	54†	21	12	45†	48†
Subclinical							
NC and ANS	1	0	—	4	2	48	—
NC or ANS	33	15	54†	40	29	28†	37†
NC only	40	17	59†	52	33	38†	44†
ANS only	6	2	56	12	6	51†	53†

* Confirmed clinical neuropathy, clinical neuropathy, abnormal nerve conduction (NC), and abnormal autonomic nervous system (ANS) testing are defined in Table 20.3.
† Conv, conventional; Inten, intensive. Confidence intervals do not overlap zero.
From DCCT Research Group. The effect of intensive diabetes therapy on the development and progression of neuropathy. Ann Intern Med 1995; 122:561.

oping clinically detectable, objectively confirmed diabetic polyneuropathy. As the secondary sequelae of diabetic polyneuropathy such as neuropathic foot ulceration, deformity, and amputation are ascribed to the neurologic impairment associated with the disease, the prevention of diabetic neuropathy in type 1 diabetic patients would be expected to prevent these disastrous clinical outcomes.[25]

The results of the DCCT clearly implicate hyperglycemia and related metabolic abnormalities as an overriding factor in the development of clinical neuropathy in type 1 diabetes. The similar temporal, anatomical, and clinical characteristics of polyneuropathy in types 1 and 2 diabetes would make extrapolation of this conclusion to type 2 diabetes not unreasonable. Ongoing large multicenter clinical trials in type 2 diabetes, such as the UKPDS,[103] will hopefully establish this directly in patients with type 2 diabetes. Extrapolation of these results to type 2 diabetes would greatly magnify the societal importance of intensive metabolic treatment designed to prevent diabetic neuropathy and its devastating clinical consequences. Successful prevention would remove or significantly diminish the clinical and economic impact of one of the most widespread and damaging neurologic disorders in developed nations.[25]

EFFECT OF REVERSAL OF THE DIABETIC STATE ON PERIPHERAL NEUROPATHY IN PATIENTS WITH ADVANCED DIABETIC COMPLICATIONS

Some perspective on the role of hyperglycemia and insulin deficiency in advanced diabetic neuropathy is provided by studies of peripheral nerve function in patients with type 1 diabetes undergoing successful pancreatic transplantation that results in near normoglycemia. Reestablishment of the euglycemic state in diabetic patients by pancreas transplantation has been practiced for more than 10 years.[55, 93, 104] Pancreas transplantation has been primarily reserved for patients with existing complications, including neuropathy. Early reports suggested that pancreas transplantation of neuropathic diabetic patients halted progression of neuropathy.[93, 104] This was confirmed by Kennedy and colleagues who carefully examined 61 patients before and at yearly intervals after transplantation.[55] Compared with a control group of type 1 insulin-dependent patients, patients who received pancreatic transplants had improve-

ment or stabilization of quantitative measurements of sensory, motor, and autonomic nervous system function.[55] In a separate study, detailed examinations of diabetic patients with autonomic neuropathy revealed that successful pancreas transplantation prevents progression of autonomic neuropathy[67, 68] and enhances long-term survival.[66, 67] Collectively, these reports suggest that reinstitution of the normoglycemic state by pancreas transplantation prevents progression of clinically advanced diabetic neuropathy, and may actually be associated with marginal improvement.[55, 67, 93] Thus, hyperglycemia or other metabolic consequences of insulin deficiency continue to contribute to the progression of diabetic peripheral neuropathy even at an advanced stages. However, complete restoration of normal glucose metabolism by pancreas transplantation is not associated with dramatic or complete reversal of advanced diabetic neuropathy, suggesting that a major component of advanced diabetic neuropathy is irreversible or poorly reversible despite complete euglycemia.

GLUCOSE AS A NEUROTOXIN

The mechanism(s) by which glucose, a vital metabolic fuel for the nervous system, at concentrations between 155 and 230 mg/dL (8.6 and 12.8 mmol/L) might confer a three-fold increase in the risk of developing peripheral neuropathy[17] continue to pose a perplexing challenge to medical biochemists.[63] Although abundant data from laboratory models suggest a wide range of glucose-associated biochemical, functional, and structural abnormalities in peripheral nerve and supporting tissue,[13, 14, 36, 90] evidence from diabetic patients is extremely limited, consisting primarily of clinical trials with aldose reductase inhibitors (see Chapter 22). These compounds inhibit the enzyme that in human and animal peripheral nerve converts glucose to sorbitol by an NADPH-linked reaction as a function of intracellular glucose content (with subsequent oxidation of sorbitol to fructose by sorbitol dehydrogenase).[101] Potent aldose reductase inhibitors that penetrate human sural nerve and block sorbitol formation have been shown to improve nerve conduction velocity in patients with diabetic neuropathy to an extent similar to that of intensive insulin therapy in the DCCT[42, 43] and, by standardized and validated morphometric techniques,[44] to reverse the progressive loss of myelinated nerve fibers in sural nerve biopsies[42] to an extent judged to be clinically meaningful

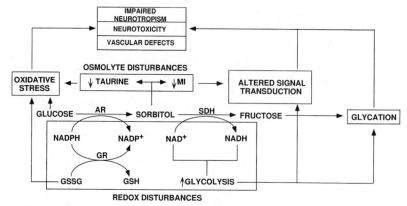

■ **Figure 20.4**   Hypothetical scheme by which glucose, by its metabolism through aldose reductase (AR) and sorbitol dehydrogenase (SDH), produces redox disturbances affecting glutathione reductase (GR) and glycolysis and osmolyte disturbances affecting taurine and *myo*-inositol (MI). The shift of glutathione from the reduced (GSH) to the oxidized (GSSG) form, combined with depletion of taurine (an endogenous antioxidant) and auto-oxidation of glucose, promotes oxidative stress. Depletion of *myo*-inositol and disturbed glycolysis impair signal transduction. Glycolytic disturbances and fructose accumulation promote nonenzymatic glycation. The combination of oxidative stress, impaired signal transduction, and nonenzymatic glycation produces secondary vascular defects, impairs neurotropism, and produces direct neurotoxicity in peripheral nerve.

and that parallels the clinical manifestations of diabetic polyneuropathy.[77] Studies in animals provide some suggestion that activation of the aldose reductase pathway may contribute to peripheral nerve damage by a cascade of pathways[14, 90] involving shifts in cytoplasmic and mitochondrial redox couples and osmolyte depletion (Fig. 20.4), leading to oxidative stress[91] (see Chapter 21) and signal transduction deficits involving nitric oxide,[85, 88] cyclic AMP[84] and prostanoids[111] (see Chapter 26), redistribution of nerve blood flow and ischemia,[14, 90] accelerated nonenzymatic glycation (via fructose)[57] (see Chapter 24), and impaired neurotrophism (see Chapter 27). The potential pathogenetic role of a parallel, interacting glucose-independent but insulin-sensitive metabolic abnormality involving defective fatty acid metabolism and deficiency of linolenic acid[14, 54] is reviewed in Chapter 25. These mechanisms thus provide a conceptual basis to explain chronic neurotoxic effects of insulin deficiency and hyperglycemia that may link metabolic control to the development and progression of diabetic neuropathy.

References

1. Allman KC, Stevens MJ, Wieland DM, et al. Noninvasive assessment of cardiac diabetic neuropathy by C-11 hydroxyephedrine and positron emission tomography. J Am Coll Cardiol 1993; 22:1425.

2. American Diabetes Association. Report and recommendations of the San Antonio conference on diabetic neuropathy: Consensus statement. Diabetes 1988; 37:1000.

3. American Diabetes Association. Implications of the Diabetes Control and Complications Trial. Diabetes Care 1993; 16:1517.

4. American Diabetes Association. Consensus statement: Diabetic neuropathy. Diabetes Care 1996; 19 (suppl 1):67.

5. American Diabetes Association. Consensus statement: Standardized measures in diabetic neuropathy. Diabetes Care 1996; 19(suppl 1):72.

6. Behse F, Buchthal F, Carlsen F. Nerve biopsy and conduction studies in diabetic neuropathy. J Neurol Neurosurg Psychiatry 1977; 40:1072.

7. Berelowitz M, Fischette C, Cefalu W, et al. Comparative efficacy of a once-daily controlled release formulation of glipizide and immediate-release glipizide in patients with NIDDM. Diabetes Care 1994; 17:1460.

8. Bijlstra PJ, Lutterman JA, Russel FGM, et al. Interaction of sulphonylurea derivatives with vascular ATP-sensitive potassium channels in humans. Diabetologia 1996; 39:1083.

9. Boulton AJ, Drury J, Clarke B, et al. Continuous subcutaneous insulin infusion in the management of painful diabetic neuropathy. Diabetes Care 1982; 5:386.

10. Bradley JL, Thomas PK, King RHM, et al. Myelinated nerve fiber regeneration in diabetic sensory polyneuropathy: Correlation with type of diabetes. Acta Neuropathologica 1995; 90:403.

11. Brown MJ, Asbury AK. Diabetic neuropathy. Ann Neurol 1984; 15:2.

12. Brown MJ, Greene DA. Diabetic neuropathy: Pathophysiology and management. *In* Asbury AK, Gilliatt RW (eds): Peripheral Nerve Disorders: A Practical Approach. London, Butterworth International Medical Reviews, 1984, pp 126–154.

13. Cameron NE, Cotter MA. Neurovascular dysfunction in diabetic rats: Potential contribution of autoxidation and free radicals examined using transition metal chelating agents. J Clin Invest 1995; 96:1159.
14. Cameron NE, Cotter MA, Hohman TC. Interactions between essential fatty acid, prostanoid, polyol pathway and nitric oxide metabolism in the neurovascular deficit of diabetic rats. Diabetologia 1996; 39:172.
15. DeFronzo RA, Goodman AM, the Multicenter Metformin Study Group. Efficacy of metformin in patients with non-insulin-dependent diabetes mellitus. N Engl J Med 1995; 333:541.
16. Diabetes Control and Complications Trial Research Group. Factors in development of diabetic neuropathy: Baseline analysis of neuropathy in feasibility phase of Diabetes Control and Complications Trial (DCCT). Diabetes 1988; 37:476.
17. Diabetes Control and Complications Trial Research Group. The effect of intensive treatment of diabetes on the development and progression of long-term complications in insulin-dependent diabetes mellitus. N Engl J Med 1993; 329:977.
18. Diabetes Control and Complications Trial Research Group. The effect of intensive diabetes therapy on the development and progression of neuropathy. Ann Intern Med 1995; 122:561.
19. Diabetes Control and Complications Trial Research Group. Effect of intensive diabetes treatment on nerve conduction in the Diabetes Control and Complications Trial. Ann Neurol 1995; 38:869.
20. Diabetes Control and Complications Trial Research Group. Implementation of conventional and intensive treatment in the Diabetes Control and Complications Trial. Diabetes Care 1995; 18:361.
21. Diabetes Control and Complications Trial Research Group. The relationship of glycemic exposure (HbA$_{1c}$) to the risk of development and progression of retinopathy in the Diabetes Control and Complications Trial. Diabetes 1995; 44:968.
22. Diabetes Control and Complications Trial Research Group. Adverse events and their association with treatment regimens in the Diabetes Control and Complications Trial. Diabetes Care 1995; 18:1415.
23. Diabetes Control and Complications Trial Research Group. Resource utilization and costs of care in the Diabetes Control and Complications Trial. Diabetes Care 1995; 18:1468.
24. Diabetes Control and Complications Trial Research Group. Effect of intensive therapy on the development of diabetic nephropathy in the Diabetes Control and Complications Trial. Kidney Int 1995; 47:1703.
25. Diabetes Control and Complications Trial Research Group. Lifetime benefits of intensive therapy as practiced in the Diabetes Control and Complications Trial. JAMA 1996; 276:1408.
26. Diabetes Control and Complications Trial Research Group. Influence of intensive diabetes therapy on quality of life outcomes in the DCCT. Diabetes Care 1996; 19:195.
27. Diabetes Control and Complications Trial Research Group. Effects of intensive diabetes therapy on neuropsychological function in adults in the Diabetes Control and Complications Trial. Ann Intern Med 1996; 124:379.
28. Diabetes Control and Complications Trial Research Group. Hypoglycemia in the DCCT. Diabetes 1997; 46:271.
29. Dimitriadis GD, Tessari P, Go VLW, et al. α-Glucosidase inhibition improves postprandial hyperglycemia and decreases insulin requirements in insulin-dependent diabetes mellitus. Metabolism 1985; 34:261.
30. Draeger E. Clinical profile of glimepiride. Diabetes Res Clin Pract 1995; 28(suppl):S139.
31. Dyck PJ, Kratz KM, Karnes JL, et al. The prevalence by staged severity of various types of diabetic neuropathy, retinopathy, and nephropathy in a population-based cohort: The Rochester Diabetic Neuropathy Study. Neurology 1993; 43:817.
32. Ellenberg M. Diabetic neuropathy: Clinical aspects. Metabolism 1976; 25:1627.
33. Eng GD, Hung W, August GP, et al. Nerve conduction velocity determinations in juvenile diabetes: Continuing study of 190 patients. Arch Phys Med Rehabil 1976; 57:1.
34. Eng GD, Nellington H, August GP. Nerve conduction velocity determination in juvenile diabetes. Mod Probl Paediatr 1975; 12:213.
35. Ewing DJ, Campbell IW, Clarke BF. The natural history of diabetic autonomic neuropathy. QJM 1980; 49:95.
36. Fernyhough P, Diemel LT, Brewster WJ, et al. Altered neurotrophin mRNA levels in peripheral nerve and skeletal muscle of experimentally diabetic rats. J Neurochem 1995; 64:1231.
37. Franklin GM, Shetterly SM, Cohen JA, et al. Risk factors for distal symmetric neuropathy in NIDDM: The San Luis Valley Diabetes Study. Diabetes Care 1994; 17:1172.
38. Gallai V, Agostini L, Rossi A, et al. Evaluation of the motor and sensory conduction velocity (MCV, SCV) in diabetic patients before and after a three-day treatment with the artificial beta cell (biostator). In Canal N, Pozza G (eds): Peripheral Neuropathies. New Amsterdam, Elsevier/North-Holland Biomedical Press, 1978, pp 287–289.
39. Gilliatt RW, Willison RG. Peripheral nerve conduction in diabetic neuropathy. J Neurol Neurosurg Psychiatry 1962; 25:11.
40. Graf RJ, Halter JB, Halar E, et al. Nerve conduction abnormalities in untreated maturity-onset diabetes: Relation to levels of fasting plasma glucose and glycosylated hemoglobin. Ann Intern Med 1979; 90:298.
41. Graf RJ, Halter JB, Pfeifer MA, et al. Glycemic control and nerve conduction abnormalities in non-insulin-dependent diabetic subjects. Ann Intern Med 1981;94:307.
42. Greene DA, Arezzo J, Brown M. Dose-related effects of the aldose reductase nerve conduction velocity and nerve fiber density in human diabetic neuropathy. Diabetes 1996; 45(suppl. 2):190A.
43. Greene DA, Arezzo JC, Klioze SS, et al. Results of a phase II multicenter study of zopolrestat in patients with peripheral diabetic polyneuropathy. Diabetologia 1996; 39(suppl 1):A35.
44. Greene DA, Brown MB. Validation of sural nerve fiber density and percent normal teased fibers as morphological endpoints in clinical trials of diabetic neuropathy. In Hotta N, Greene DA, Ward JD, et al (eds): Diabetic Neuropathy: New Concepts and Insights. Amsterdam, Excerpta Medica, 1995, pp 379–385.
45. Greene DA, Brown MJ, Braunstein SN, et al. Comparison of clinical course and sequential electrophysiological tests in diabetics with symptomatic polyneuropathy and its implications for clinical trials. Diabetes 1981; 30:139.
46. Gregersen G. Diabetic neuropathy: Influence of age, sex, metabolic control, and duration of diabetes on motor conduction velocity. Neurology 1967; 17:972.

47. Gregersen G. Variations in motor conduction velocity produced by acute changes of the metabolic state in diabetic patients. Diabetologia 1968; 4:273.
48. Groop LC. Sulfonylureas in NIDDM. Diabetes Care 1992; 15:737.
49. Hanefeld M, Fischer S, Schulze J, et al. Therapeutic potentials of acarbose as first-line drug in NIDDM insufficiently treated with diet alone. Diabetes Care 1991; 14:732.
50. Hoeldtke RD, Boden G, Shuman CR, et al. Reduced epinephrine secretion and hypoglycemia unawareness in diabetic autonomic neuropathy. Ann Intern Med 1982; 96:459.
51. Holman RR, Dornan TL, Mayon-White V, et al. Prevention of deterioration of renal and sensory-nerve function by more intensive management of insulin-dependent diabetic patients: A two-year randomised prospective study. Lancet 1983; 1:204.
52. Holman RR, Turner RC. The quest for normoglycaemia. Lancet 1976; 1:469.
53. Jakobsen J, Christiansen JS, Kristoffersen I, et al. Autonomic and somatosensory nerve function after 2 years of continuous subcutaneous insulin infusion in type 1 diabetes. Diabetes 1988; 37:452.
54. Keen H, Payan J, Allawi J, et al. Treatment of diabetic neuropathy with gamma-linolenic acid: The Gamma-Linolenic Acid Multicenter Trial Group. Diabetes Care 1993; 16:8.
55. Kennedy WR, Navarro X, Goetz FC, et al. Effects of pancreatic transplantation on diabetic neuropathy. N Engl J Med 1990; 322:1031.
56. Knuiman MW, Welborn TA, McCann VJ, et al. Prevalence of diabetic complications in relation to risk factors. Diabetes 1986; 35:1332.
57. Lal S, Szwergold BS, Taylor AH, et al. Metabolism of fructose-3-phosphate in the diabetic rat lens. Arch Biochem Biophys 1995; 318:191.
58. Malmberg K, Ryden L, Efendic S, et al. Randomized trial of insulin-glucose infusion followed by subcutaneous insulin treatment in diabetic patients with acute myocardial infarction (DIGAMI Study): Effects on mortality at one year. J Am Coll Cardiol 1995; 26:57.
59. Maser RE, Steenkiste AR, Dorman JS, et al. Epidemiological correlates of diabetic neuropathy: Report from Pittsburgh Epidemiology of Diabetes Complications Study. Diabetes 1989; 38:1456.
60. McCulloch DK, Campbell IW, Prescott RJ, et al. Effect of alcohol intake on symptomatic peripheral neuropathy in diabetic men. Diabetes Care 1980; 3:245.
61. Nathan DM. Management of insulin-dependent diabetes mellitus. Drugs 1992; 44:39.
62. Nathan DM. Detection and treatment of diabetic complications. In Raskin P (ed): Medical Management of Non-Insulin Dependent Diabetes, ed 3. Alexandria, VA, American Diabetes Association, 1994, pp 87–92.
63. Nathan DM. The pathophysiology of diabetic complications: How much does the glucose hypothesis explain? Ann Intern Med 1996; 124:86.
64. Nathan DM, Dunn FL, Bruch J, et al. Post-prandial insulin profiles with implantable pump therapy may explain decreased frequency of severe hypoglycemia, compared with subcutaneous intensive regimens in IDDM. Am J Med 1996; 100:412.
65. National Diabetes Data Group. Report of the expert committee on glycosylated hemoglobin. Diabetes Care 1984; 7:602.
66. Navarro X, Kennedy WR, Aeppli D, et al. Neuropathy and mortality in diabetes: Influence of pancreas transplantation. Muscle Nerve 1996; 19:1009.
67. Navarro X, Kennedy WR, Loewenson RB, et al. Influence of pancreas transplantation on cardiorespiratory reflexes, nerve conduction, and mortality in diabetes mellitus. Diabetes 1990; 39:802.
68. Navarro X, Kennedy WR, Sutherland DER. Autonomic neuropathy and survival in diabetes mellitus: Effects of pancreas transplantation. Diabetologia 1991; 34:S108.
69. O'Brien OA, McFadden JP, Corral RJM. The influence of autonomic neuropathy on mortality in insulin-dependent diabetes. QJM 1991; 290:295.
70. Pietri A, Ehle AL, Raskin P. Changes in nerve conduction velocity after six weeks of glucoregulation with portable insulin infusion pumps. Diabetes 1980; 29:668.
71. Pirart J. Diabetic neuropathy: A metabolic or a vascular disease? Diabetes 1965; 14:1.
72. Pirart J. Diabetes mellitus and its degenerative complications: A prospective study of 4,400 patients observed between 1947 and 1973. Diabetes Care 1978; 1:168.
73. Policy Statement of the Committee on Health Care Issues, American Neurological Association. Does improved control of glycemia prevent or ameliorate diabetic polyneuropathy? Ann Neurol 1986; 19:288.
74. Rathman W, Ziegler D, Jahnke M, et al. Mortality in diabetic patients with cardiovascular autonomic neuropathy. Diabetic Med 1993; 10:820.
75. Reaven GM, Laws A. Insulin resistance, compensatory hyperinsulinaemia and coronary heart disease. Diabetologia 1994; 37:948.
76. Reichard P, Nilsson B-Y, Rosenqvist U. The effect of long-term intensified insulin treatment on the development of microvascular complications of diabetes mellitus. N Engl J Med 1993; 329:304.
77. Russell JW, Karnes JL, Dyck PJ. Sural nerve myelinated fiber density differences associated with meaningful changes in clinical and electrophysiologic measurements. J Neurol Sci 1996; 135:114.
78. Saltiel AR, Olefsky JM. Thiazolidinediones in the treatment of insulin resistance and type 2 diabetes. Diabetes 1996; 45:1661.
79. Santiago JV, White NH, Skor DA, et al. Defective glucose counterregulation limits intensive therapy of diabetes mellitus. Am J Physiol 1984; 247:E215.
80. Schade DS, Santiago JV, Skyler JS, et al. Intensive Insulin Therapy. Princeton, NJ, Excerpta Medica, 1983.
81. Service FJ, Daube JR, O'Brien PC, et al. Effect of artificial pancreas treatment on peripheral nerve function in diabetes. Neurology 1981; 31:1375.
82. Service FJ, Rizza RA, Daube JR, et al. Near normoglycaemia improved nerve conduction and vibration sensation in diabetic neuropathy. Diabetologia 1985; 28:722.
83. Sherwin RS, Tamborlane WV. Metabolic control and diabetic complications. In Olessky JM, Sherwin RS (eds): Contemporary Issues in Endocrinology and Metabolism: Diabetes Mellitus, Management and Complications. New York, Churchill Livingstone, 1985, vol 1, pp 1–29.
84. Shindo H, Tawata M, Aida K, et al. The role of cyclic adenosine 3',5'-monophosphate and polyol metabolism in diabetic neuropathy. J Clin Endocrinol Metab 1992; 74:393.
85. Shindo H, Thomas TP, Larkin DD, et al. Modulation of basal nitric oxide-dependent cyclic-GMP production by ambient glucose, myo-inositol, and protein kinase C in SH-SY5Y human neuroblastoma cells. J Clin Invest 1996; 97:736.

86. Sima AA, Nathaniel V, Bril V, et al. Histopathological heterogeneity of neuropathy in insulin-dependent and non-insulin-dependent diabetes, and demonstration of axo-glial dysjunction in human diabetic neuropathy. J Clin Invest 1988; 81:349.

87. St Thomas' Diabetic Study Group. Failure of improved glycaemic control to reverse diabetic autonomic neuropathy. Diabet Med 1986; 3:330.

88. Steno Study Group. Effect of 6 months of strict metabolic control on eye and kidney function in insulin-dependent diabetics with background retinopathy. Lancet 1982; 1:121.

89. Stevens MJ, Dananberg J, Feldman EL, et al. The linked roles of nitric oxide, aldose reductase and, (Na+,K+)-ATPase in the slowing of nerve conduction in the streptozotocin diabetic rat. J Clin Invest 1994; 94:853.

90. Stevens MJ, Feldman EL, Greene DA. The aetiology of diabetic neuropathy: The combined roles of metabolic and vascular defects. Diabet Med 1995; 12:566.

91. Stevens MJ, Lattimer SA, Kamijo M, et al. Osmotically-induced nerve taurine depletion and the compatible osmolyte hypothesis in experimental diabetic neuropathy in the rat. Diabetologia 1993; 36:608.

92. Stumvoll M, Nurjhan N, Perrhello G, et al. Metabolic effects of metformin in non-insulin dependent diabetes mellitus. N Engl J Med 1995; 333:550.

93. Sutherland DER, Kendall DM, Moudry KC, et al. Pancreas transplantation in nonuremic, type 1 diabetic recipients. Surgery 1988; 104:453.

94. Terkildsen AB, Christensen NJ. Reversible nervous abnormalities in juvenile diabetics with recently diagnosed diabetes. Diabetologia 1971; 7:113.

95. Tesfaye S, Malik R, Harris N, et al. Arteriovenous shunting and proliferating new vessels in acute painful neuropathy of rapid glycaemic control (insulin neuritis). Diabetologia 1996; 39:329.

96. Teuscher A, Reinli K, Nathan DM, et al. Severe hypoglycaemia in the Diabetes Control and Complications Trial. Lancet 1994; 343:1098.

97. Teutsch SM, Herman WH, Dwyer DM, et al. Mortality among diabetic patients using continuous subcutaneous insulin-infusion pumps. N Engl J Med 1984; 310:361.

98. Thomas PK, Eliasson SG. Diabetic neuropathy. In Dyck PJ, Thomas PK, Lambert EH, et al (eds): Peripheral Neuropathy. Philadelphia, W.B. Saunders Company, 1984, pp 1773–1810.

99. Thomas PK, Ward JD, Watkins PJ. Diabetic neuropathy. In Keen H, Jarrett J (eds): Complications of Diabetes. London, Edward Arnold, 1982, pp 109–136.

100. Tolaymat A, Roque JL, Russo LS Jr. Improvement of diabetic peripheral neuropathy with the portable insulin infusion pump. South Med J 1982; 75:185.

101. Tomlinson DR, Willars GB, Carrington AL. Aldose reductase inhibitors and diabetic complications. Pharmacol Ther 1992; 54:151.

101a. Troni W, Carta Q, Cantello R, et al. Peripheral nerve function and metabolic control in diabetes mellitus. Ann Neurol 1984; 16:178.

102. Tsumura K. Clinical evaluation of glimepiride (HOE490) in NIDDM, including a double blind comparative study versus gliclazide. Diabetes Res Clin Pract 1995; 28 (suppl):S147.

103. Turner R, Cull C, Holman R, et al. A 9-year update of a randomized, controlled trial on the effect of improved metabolic control on complications in non-insulin-dependent diabetes mellitus. Ann Intern Med 1996; 124:136.

104. van der Vliet JA, Navarro X, Kennedy WR, et al. The effect of pancreas transplantation on diabetic polyneuropathy. Transplantation 1988; 45:368.

105. Ward JD. Abnormal processes in the nerve. In Brownless M (ed): Diabetes Mellitus. New York, Garland SPTPM Press, 1981, vol 4, pp 87–113.

106. Ward JD. Biochemical and vascular factors in the pathogenesis of diabetic neuropathy. Clin Invest Med 1995; 18:267.

107. Ward JD, Barnes CG, Fisher DJ, et al. Improvement in nerve conduction following treatment in newly diagnosed diabetics. Lancet 1971; 1:428.

108. White NH, Waltman SR, Krupin T, et al. Reversal of neuropathic and gastrointestinal complications related to diabetes mellitus in adolescents with improved metabolic control. J Pediatr 1981; 99:41.

109. Willson TM, Cobb JE, Cowan DJ, et al. The structure-activity relationship between peroxisome proliferator-activated receptor g agonism and the antihyperglycemic activity of thiazolidinediones. J Med Chem 1996; 39:665.

110. Winegrad AI, Morrison AD, Greene DA. Late complication of diabetes. In DeGroot LJ, et al (eds): Endocrinology. New York, Grune & Stratton, 1979, vol 2, pp 1041–1060.

111. Yasuda H, Sonobe M, Yamashita M, et al. Effect of prostaglandin E1 analogue TFC 612 on diabetic neuropathy in streptozocin-induced diabetic rats: Comparison with aldose reductase inhibitor ONO 2235. Diabetes 1989; 38:832.

112. Young MJ, Boulton AJM, Macleod AF, et al. A multicentre study of the prevalence of diabetic peripheral neuropathy in the United Kingdom hospital clinic populations. Diabetologia 1993; 36:150.

113. Young RJ, Macintyre CC, Martyn CN, et al. Progression of subclinical polyneuropathy in young patients with type 1 (insulin-dependent) diabetes: Associations with glycaemic control and microangiopathy (microvascular complications). Diabetologia 1986; 29:156.

114. Ziegler D, Dannehl K, Wiefels K, et al. Differential effects of near-normoglycaemia for 4 years on somatic nerve dysfunction and heart rate variation in type 1 diabetic patients. Diabetic Med 1992; 9:622.

Chapter 21

Role of Hypoxia, Oxidative Stress, and Excitatory Neurotoxins in Diabetic Neuropathy

Phillip A. Low • Kim K. Nickander • Luciano Scionti

INTRODUCTION

The pivotal role of hyperglycemia in the pathogenesis of diabetic neuropathy is well accepted. The roles of numerous other mechanisms are discussed in various chapters of this book. This chapter will focus on the interacting roles of ischemia and hypoxia, oxidative stress, and to a lesser extent, excitotoxic injury. We will discuss the roles of altered vasoregulation, resulting in a reduction in nerve blood flow (NBF), the generation of oxidative stress from ischemic and nonischemic mechanisms, and, briefly, the role of N-methyl-D-aspartate (NMDA) receptors in hyperalgesia. Finally, we will attempt to synthesize the information into a pathogenetic schema.

ISCHEMIA AND HYPOXIA

Diabetic neuropathy is a metabolic disorder with a significant effect on microvascular vasoreactivity. The endothelial cell is perceived as being a dynamic tissue manifesting perturbations in function of nitric oxide, endoneurial eicosanoids, advanced glycation end products, oxidative stress, growth factors, and neurotransmitters and neuromodulators. Endoneurial hypoxia is caused by a reduction in NBF and increased endoneurial vascular resistance,[15, 111] which begins by the first week of diabetes[15] and affects the cell body as well as the axon.[96] This reduction has been independently confirmed in a number of laboratories[14, 27, 105] using microelectrode H_2-polarography,[14, 59] laser Doppler flowmetry,[27, 105, 109] and iodoantipyrine.[96]

We first demonstrated a reduction in NBF in streptozotocin diabetic rats (duration of diabetes, 4 months) using microelectrode-hydrogen polarography.[111] The reduction in NBF was likely the result of microvascular changes or hemorheological changes because there was a marked increase in nerve vascular resistance to 170%.[66, 111] The reduced NBF could theoretically have been the result of reduced oxygen requirements caused by deranged metabolism of peripheral nerve[32] or the result of fiber loss. To resolve this issue, we measured endoneurial oxygen tensions using oxygen-sensitive microelectrodes. The ensuing oxygen histograms from sciatic nerve showed a significant shift into the hypoxic range in experimental diabetic neuropathy (EDN).[111] The critical oxygen tension in mammalian nerve is about 25 mm Hg,[61] so after 4 months of diabetes, the majority of nerve fibers were in a hypoxic state. Additional evidence was obtained from the demonstration that hypoxia per se will reproduce the lipid biosynthetic[122] and electrophysiologic abnormalities.[63] Subsequently, endoneurial oxygen tension was directly measured by oxygen microelectrode in human sural nerve of patients with diabetic neuropathy, and endoneurial hypoxia was found to be present.[80]

Peripheral nerve is susceptible to reduced oxygen tension, induced by increasing intercapillary distance, as in experimental nerve edema,[61, 89] or by reducing atmospheric oxygen tension.[63] In the former, edema has a particular topography, being maximal in the subperineurial area. Endoneurial oxygen tension and NBF reductions exactly paralleled the distribution of edema and of intercapillary distance, confirming that nerve was indeed susceptible to hypoxia.[61, 73] Reducing atmospheric oxygen (10%) will reproduce the conduction slowing, resistance to ischemic conduction failure,[63] and the pattern of impaired ^{14}C-acetate incorporation.[122]

Conversely, when diabetic rats were reared in an oxygen-enriched environment (40% oxygen), nerve conduction slowing and resistance to ischemic conduction failure were partly prevented. The levels of nerve free sugars (glucose, fructose, or sorbitol) were markedly increased in EDN. Oxygen supplementation resulted in no change in plasma glucose, but the endoneurial sugars returned toward normal (by 60, 30, and 34%, respectively). ^{14}C-acetate incorporation in EDN was 57% lower than controls. After oxygen supplementation, the changes were no longer significantly different from controls.[122] By combined high-performance thin-layer chromatography and fluorography, we found that proportionately less ^{14}C-acetate was incorporated into cholesterol and more into free fatty acids of diabetic nerves. Oxygen supplementation largely prevented these abnormalities.[122]

The increase in endoneurial oxygen with oxygen supplementation is too small to likely benefit established diabetic neuropathy. It is possible, however, to greatly enhance endoneurial oxygenation by hyperbaric oxygenation (HBO). We found that treatment with HBO (100% oxygen, 2.5 ata 2 h/d for 4 weeks) resulted in nerve hypermetabolism and will normalize the deficit in nerve action potential and resistance to ischemic conduction failure in well-established EDN.[62]

RHEOLOGICAL ALTERATIONS

In diabetes, the combination of increased whole blood or plasma viscosity, increased aggregability, and reduced red cell deformability results in a reduction of blood flow and stagnation hypoxia. Blood viscosity is increased in human and experimental diabetes,[37, 101] and there is reduced red cell deformability.[74] The increased aggregability[74] coupled with the reduced deformability leads to increased thixotropy of diabetic blood,[74] a phenomenon of increased resistance to acceleration of blood flow, resulting in increased shear stress to microvascular wall and leading to increased permeability and stimulation of synthesis of connective tissue.[74] Blood hematocrit is the major determinant of whole blood viscosity, but erythrocyte aggregability and deformability are also important contributors of blood viscosity.[25] Plasma or serum viscosity is increased in diabetics.[25, 37, 74] Plasma fibrinogen is increased[101] as is α_2-globulin, but albumin was reduced.[101]

VASOREGULATORY ALTERATIONS

Regional NBF is regulated by systemic blood pressure[65] and the balance between neural va-

TABLE 21.1 VASOREGULATION OF PERIPHERAL NERVE IN EXPERIMENTAL DIABETIC NEUROPATHY

	Site of Action	Sensitivity/Activity	Reference
Vasoconstrictors			
Norepinephrine	Epineurial α-adrenoreceptors	Increased	48, 126
Endothelin	Endothelial cell	Normal	13, 125
Vasopressin	Epineurial; ? endothelial	Normal	95
Vasodilators			
Calcitonin gene-related peptide	Endothelium	Normal or reduced	124
SP	Endothelium	Reduced	124
Nitric oxide	Endothelium	Reduced	12, 49
Prostaglandins	Endothelium	Reduced	50

SP, substance P.

soconstrictors and vasodilators (Table 21.1). Vasoconstriction is known to be mediated by epineurial α-adrenergic receptors[48, 126] and by endothelin receptors.[125] In a previous study, we reported a median effective concentration (EC_{50}) of $10^{-4.9}$ mol, based on a dose-response study of the epineurial application of norepinephrine (NE), a method that generates EC_{50} values about 2 orders of magnitude lower than intra-arterial methods.[48] The EC_{50} for endothelin, using identical methodology, was about 3 orders of magnitude lower, at 10^{-8} mol.[125] That these receptors are responsible for vasomotor tone is supported by the efficacy of specific antagonists in improving perfusion in EDN, including endothelin.[13] These potent vasoconstrictor actions are balanced by vasodilatation, mediated by calcitonin-gene related peptide,[124] substance P,[124] nitric oxide[10, 49] and the prostaglandins.[50]

The effects of vasopressin on NBF are interesting. It has a potency similar to endothelin, but it does not seem to be active in resting vasomotor tone nor is it responsible for the deficit in NBF in EDN. It could, however, presumably play a role in hypovolemic conditions or conditions of severe hypotension, when NBF is already reduced.

OXIDATIVE STRESS

There is considerable evidence of oxidative stress in EDN and human diabetic neuropathy. We will summarize the evidence in nonneural tissues in human diabetic neuropathy and EDN followed by data on neural tissue. Studies on nonneural tissues have been done on plasma, erythrocyte, and mainly heart, liver, kidney, and pancreas. These studies have focused on evidence of increased lipid peroxidation and alteration in the patterns of glutathione and of antioxidant enzymes.

Nonneural Tissue: Human Diabetes

Plasma levels of lipid peroxide are increased in human diabetes.[1, 41, 71, 97] The highest levels were found in patients with microvascular angiopathy and retinopathy or microalbuminuria, lowest in those diabetic patients without angiopathy,[17, 97] and normal in patients with well-controlled diabetes.[97] The relationship may relate to the observation that low-density lipoproteins of diabetic patients are significantly more oxidizable than controls, an abnormality that is correctable by 6 weeks of treatment with the antioxidant, probucol.[3] Presumably, diabetics with angiopathy, who have higher levels of low-density lipoproteins, will have the greatest lipid peroxidation.

Glutathione (GSH) is reduced in erythrocytes from patients with type 1 diabetes mellitus (DM), and oxidized glutathione (GSSG) is correspondingly increased.[76] In subsequent studies, reductions in the glutathione synthesizing enzyme, γ-glutamylcysteine synthetase, and the transport of thiol [S-(s,4-dintrophenyl)glutathione] in erythrocytes of patients with type 1 DM were demonstrated. These abnormalities were reversible with improved glycemic control. They also demonstrated that a high-glucose medium augments the toxicity of xenobiotics on K562 cells, associated with reduction in the enzyme and its mRNA.[123]

Erythrocyte cuprozinc superoxide dismutase is reduced in patients with type 2 DM.[71] This reduction is suggested to be mediated by the accumulation of intracellular H_2O_2.[56]

α-Tocopherol levels are reported to be reduced in the platelets[47, 56] and erythrocytes[29] but not plasma of patients with type 1 DM.

Wolff[117] has emphasized the role of decompartmentalized transitional metals in diabetic patients, in addition to the effects of hyperglycemia in producing auto-oxidative lipid peroxidation. Particular emphasis has been placed on copper and iron. Copper levels have been reported to be higher in diabetics than in normals and are highest in those with angiopathy.[70, 86]

Nonneural Tissue: Experimental Diabetes

Oxidative stress occurs in experimental diabetes induced by streptozotocin, alloxan, and diabetic BB Wistar rats. Lipid peroxidation in drug-induced diabetes appears to be the result of hyperglycemia, and not the agent, because the pattern of changes are not agent specific. Streptozotocin and alloxan cause similar changes, and additionally, the *spontaneously* diabetic BB Wistar rat shows virtually identical patterns of tissue antioxidant enzyme changes.[31] Furthermore, these alterations are preventable by insulin treatment.[7, 31, 115, 116] Therefore, the common mechanism of increased oxidative stress is diabetes and not its mode of induction.

Plasma and liver lipid peroxides are increased in streptozotocin- or alloxan-induced diabetes[71, 90] and improved by α-tocopherol supplementation.[90] Tissue levels of lipid peroxide, estimated by the thiobarbituric acid method, were increased in kidney and retina and accompanied by a reduction in fat-soluble antioxidants, as determined by the ferric chloride-bipyridyl reaction. These changes were eliminated by insulin treatment.[84]

Complex patterns of changes in antioxidant enzymes have been described in different tissues in streptozotocin diabetes.[115, 116] Liver and kidney have reduced catalase and superoxide dismutase. Glutathione peroxidase and GSH are reduced in liver; glutathione peroxidase is increased in kidney. Catalase and glutathione reductase are increased in heart and pancreas, and superoxide dismutase is also increased in pancreas.

One of the most common alterations is a reduction in cuprozinc superoxide dismutase. This reduction has been reported in numerous tissues, including erythrocyte,[22, 57, 71] liver,[57, 71] retina,[57] kidney, spleen, heart, testis, pancreas, and skeletal muscle in rats with streptozotocin or alloxan diabetes.[57, 71] The loss of superoxide dismutase appears to be a function of duration and severity of diabetes.[56]

α-Tocopherol is reported to be reduced in streptozotocin diabetes.[56] Our observations are that plasma α-tocopherol is variable and is greatly dependent on dietary intake; it can be increased in experimental diabetes because of polyphagia.[82]

Evidence of Oxidative Stress in Diabetic Peripheral Nerve and Free Radical Defenses of Peripheral Nerve

Peripheral nerve has a number of cytosolic and lipophilic antioxidant defenses whose actions are closely integrated (Table 21.2). These comprise a number of low molecular weight and enzymic antioxidant molecules. The key enzymatic scavengers are superoxide dismutase, catalase, glutathione peroxidase, and glutathione reductase. Glutathione is particularly important in that it is the main scavenger in the blocking of chain propagation.[83] The cytosolic and membrane antioxidants work in concert in a well-organized interacting chain. Ample activity of all components is needed to maintain these antioxidants in their reduced state. There is an enormous literature on free radical biology, but information on peripheral nerve, and in particular diabetic peripheral nerve, is quite limited.

Free radical defenses of peripheral nerve are reduced relative to brain and liver.[92, 93] Of great interest is the marked and selective reduction in antioxidant defenses in rodent sciatic nerve (Table 21.3). Reduced glutathione and GSH-containing enzymes scavengers (glutathione peroxidase and reductase) are only about 10% that of brain, whereas other enzymes such as superoxide dismutase are near normal.[92] Corresponding enzyme activities of these enzymes in brain are in turn about half that of liver.[93]

The diabetic state results in additional alterations in these defenses (Table 21.4). Cuprozinc superoxide dismutase is reduced in sciatic nerve of EDN, and this reduction is improved by insulin treatment.[60] Glutathione peroxidase is further reduced in EDN.[35] Hermenegildo et

TABLE 21.2 SOME FREE RADICAL DEFENSES OF PERIPHERAL NERVE

Cytosolic	
Ascorbate	Reduced glutathione
Urate	Glutathione peroxidase
Cysteine	Catalase
Glutathione	Superoxide dismutase
Transferrin	Glutathione reductase
Albumin	Membrane
β-Carotene	α-Tocopherol
Ceruloplasmin	

TABLE 21.3 ACTIVITIES OF ENZYMATIC FREE RADICAL SCAVENGERS IN PERIPHERAL NERVE RELATIVE TO BRAIN AND LIVER

Antioxidant	Nerve	% of Brain	Brain	Liver
GSH-GSSG	261.0 ± 24.0	10	2620.0 ± 124.0	
GSH-Px ($\to H_2O_2$)	6.4 ± 2.1	13	48.5 ± 5.5	74.9 ± 7.1
GSH-Px ($\to$ t-BOOH)	4.6 ± 1.4	9	50.3 ± 1.4	144.0 ± 16.9
GSSG reductase	2.7 ± 0.3	13	20.5 ± 0.6	56.3 ± 6.1
GST ($\to$ CDNB)	9.4 ± 2.4	4	232.5 ± 14.0	171.3 ± 55.4
GST ($\to$ 4-HNE)	5.4 ± 1.2	5	116.5 ± 10.4	345.2 ± 92.0
DT-diaphorase	9.9 ± 2.2			208.0 ± 49.9
SOD	93.8 ± 12.4			171.3 ± 55.4

GSH-GSSG, total glutathione; GSH-Px, glutathione peroxidase; t-BOOH, tert-butyl-hydroperoxide; GSSG reductase, glutathione disulfide reductase; GST, glutathione transferase; CDNB, 1-chloro-2,4-dinitrobenzene; 4-HNE, 4-hydroxy-2,3-trans-nonenol; SOD, superoxide dismutase. Results are expressed as nmol/min $\times$ mg protein, $\pm$ SEM.

Data from Romero FJ, Monsalve E, Hermenegildo C, et al. Oxygen toxicity in the nervous tissue: Comparison of the antioxidant defense of rat brain and sciatic nerve. Neurochem Res 1991; 16:157; Romero FJ, Segura-Aguilar J, Monsalve E, et al. Antioxidant and glutathione-related enzymatic activities in rat sciatic nerve. Neurotoxicol Teratol 1990; 12:603.

al[35] were able to regress glutathione peroxidase activity against blood glucose concentration, as shown in the equation

$$y = 69.3 - 0.9x$$

where y was enzyme activity as nmol/mg protein/minute and x was blood glucose in mmol (R=0.9). Plasma and leukocyte ascorbic acid are reduced, and oxidation of this antioxidant is increased.[40, 104] Reduced glutathione is reduced in diabetic nerves.[79, 82]

Free Radical Generation in Experimental Diabetic Neuropathy

There are a number of potential sources of increased free radical generation in diabetes:

1. Hyperglycemic auto-oxidative peroxidation
2. Ischemia
3. Increased mitochondrial leak
4. Catecholamine oxidation
5. Leukocytes

Hyperglycemia, by a process of auto-oxida-

TABLE 21.4 CHANGES IN ANTIOXIDANT DEFENSES IN EXPERIMENTAL DIABETIC NEUROPATHY

Antioxidant	Change	References
Superoxide dismutase (cuprozinc)	Reduced	60
Glutathione peroxidase	Reduced	35
Ascorbic acid content	Reduced	40, 104
Ascorbic oxidation	Increased	40, 104
Reduced glutathione	Reduced	79, 82

tion, in the presence of decompartmentalized trace transitional metals, can generate highly reactive oxidants and result in lipid peroxidation.[118] We have demonstrated, using an in vitro lipid peroxidation model (ascorbate-iron-EDTA preparation), that a high-glucose medium will result in lipid peroxidation in vitro vof brain and sciatic nerve. The addition of 20 mmol glucose to the incubation medium increased lipid peroxidation fourfold, confirming rapid and marked glucose-mediated auto-oxidative lipid peroxidation.[81] These studies confirm the observation in plasma of auto-oxidative glycation/oxidation.[4, 117] The relationship between oxidative glycation and free radical production has been explored.[36] Glucose auto-oxidation results in the production of protein reactive ketoaldehydes, hydrogen peroxide, and other highly reactive oxidants and in the fragmentation of proteins (indicative of free radical mechanisms). Glycation and oxidation are simultaneous and were considered to be inextricably linked.[36]

An NBF deficit of 50% in EDN[15, 79, 111] results in the generation of hypoxanthine, from adenosine triphosphate (ATP), and nicotinamide adenine dinucleotide phosphate (NADPH) (the cofactor) and conversion of the inactive enzyme to xanthine oxidase.[59, 72] The effects of oxidative stress depend on a balance among oxidative stress, pro-oxidant status, and free radical defenses.[33] Changes in all three areas occur in diabetic peripheral nerve. Diabetic pro-oxidant status is increased, because diabetic sciatic nerve has increased polyunsaturated fatty acids with excessive lipolysis.[122]

It has also been suggested that metals, especially copper, might be decompartmentalized or increased.[117] We have not been able to demonstrate this increase in diabetic nerves (P. A. Low et al., unpublished observations). We measured copper, iron, and manganese in EDN and found no significant difference. An increase in copper in human diabetic plasma has been found.[54]

The role of the leukocyte and of catecholamine oxidation is uncertain. Leukocytic infiltration is not a feature in most cases of diabetic neuropathy. In human diabetic neuropathy, there are some suggestions of an immune-mediated process, as suggested by the presence of iritis and inflammatory infiltrates in sympathetic ganglia.[26] Some forms of diabetic neuropathy, such as acute autonomic neuropathy and the subacute proximal neuropathies, might be associated with round cell infiltration.

Although there is good evidence that oxidative stress occurs in the diabetic state, the demonstration of lipid peroxidation alone is insufficient evidence for a free radical role in the etiopathogenesis of neuropathy. We propose that following four criteria should be satisfied before accepting that lipid peroxidation is mechanistically involved:

1. That an increase in lipid peroxidation in previously normal nerves results in neuropathy.
2. That an increase in lipid peroxidation in diabetic neuropathic nerves further worsens function.
3. That antioxidant improves or prevents neuropathy.
4. That this improvement or prevention is associated with an improvement in the indices of lipid peroxidation of peripheral nerve.

When weanling rats were fed an α-tocopherol deficient diet, plasma α-tocopherol became unmeasurable.[82] Endoneurial oxidative stress developed, as indicated by a reduction in GSH and increased lipid peroxidation (conjugated dienes, lipid hydroperoxides). These findings were associated with the development of a sensory neuropathy in previously normal nerves.[82] A second line of evidence derives from the worsening of neuropathy in EDN[82] associated with an increase in lipid peroxidation. The pro-oxidant primaquine caused conduction deficit in the hindlimb nerves of previously normal rats, a reduction in sciatic NBF, and endoneurial hypoxia; these deficits were prevented by treatment with the antioxidant probucol.[14]

Evidence of increased nerve lipid peroxidation is now available. Diabetic peripheral nerve has increased conjugated dienes,[60, 82] reduced GSH,[82] and reduced glutathione peroxidase.[92] Among the indices of increased oxidative stress in a chronic in vivo situation, malondialdehyde, conjugated dienes, and lipid hydroperoxides are increased in peripheral nerve of EDN,[60, 79, 82] and the increase is more consistent in lumbar dorsal root and superior cervical ganglia.[79, 82] The most reliable index of increased oxidative stress is reduction in GSH.[79, 82]

ANTIOXIDANTS

Several antioxidants have shown promise in the treatment of EDN (Table 21.5). Probucol, a powerful free radical scavenger,[42] normalizes NBF and electrophysiology.[14, 46] These workers also reported an improvement in nerve perfusion with 1% vitamin E diet.[46] α-Lipoic acid

TABLE 21.5 ANTIOXIDANTS AND EXPERIMENTAL DIABETIC NEUROPATHY

Antioxidant	Lipid Peroxidation	Nerve Blood Flow Deficit	NCS Deficit	Reference
Probucol	Not studied	Prevented	Prevented	14
α-Tocopherol	Not studied	Prevented	Prevented	14, 20, 46
α-Lipoic acid	Improved	Prevented	Prevented	79
Reduced glutathione	Not studied	Not studied	Partially prevented	8
Butylated hydroxytoluene	Not studied	Not studied	Prevented	16
Carvidilol	Not studied	Prevented	Prevented	19
Deferoximine	Not studied	Prevented	Prevented	18
Superoxide dismutase	Improved	Prevented	Partially prevented	With J. F. Poduslo, unpublished observations
β-Carotene	Not studied	Prevented	Prevented	20
Ascorbic acid	Not studied	Partially prevented	Partially prevented	20

■ **Figure 21.1** Nerve blood flow and nerve vascular resistance of control (Con), streptozotocin diabetic neuropathy (STZ), and animals supplemented with lipoic acid at doses of 20 mg/kg (STZ20), 50 mg/kg (Con50; STZ50), and 100 mg/kg (STZ100). Lipoic acid supplementation results in normal nerve blood flow and nerve vascular resistance. (From Nagamatsu M, Nicklander KK, Schmelzer JD, et al. Lipoic acid improves nerve blood flow, reduces oxidative stress, and improves distal nerve conduction in experimental diabetic neuropathy. Diabetes Care 1995; 18:1160–1167.)

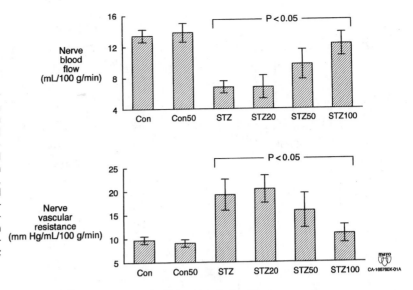

is a powerful lipophilic antioxidant.[9, 88] It also stimulates nerve growth factor[77] and promotes fiber regeneration in a culture system.[24] α-Lipoic acid will prevent the deficit in NBF (Fig. 21.1) and the distal electrophysiologic changes in EDN[79] (Fig. 21.2). These benefits are associated with improved indices of lipid peroxidation, the most sensitive of which is a prevention of the reduction in GSH (Fig. 21.3). Mild improvement in EDN has been reported after treatment with GSH.[8] One percent butylated hydroxytoluene for 2 months completely prevented the conduction deficit in EDN.[16] Carvedilol, an antioxidant and vasodilator, is reported to be efficacious in preventing the deficits in blood flow and conduction.[19] Cameron and Cotter[11] have reported improvement

in NBF and nerve conduction in EDN after treatment with the iron chelator deferoxamine. We have also found that modified SOD will prevent the deficit in NBF. However, a significant deficiency in most antioxidant studies in EDN is the lack of measurements of oxidative stress, so that it is not known if antioxidants, all of which have multiple mechanisms of action, improve neuropathy by their antioxidant or other properties.

N-METHYL-D-ASPARTATE RECEPTORS

There is no evidence of excitotoxic injury to peripheral nerve at the nerve trunk level. However, NMDA receptors at the nerve root entry zone (NREZ) may be vitally involved in the

■ **Figure 21.2** Digital nerve conduction velocity at 1 month *(top)* and 3 months *(bottom)* of supplementation with lipoic acid at 0 mg/kg (Con, STZ), 25 mg/kg (STZ25), 50 mg/kg (Con50; STZ50), and 100 mg/kg (STZ100). Lipoic acid supplementation improved conduction velocity (*, $P < 0.05$; **, $P < 0.01$; ***, $P < 0.001$). Con, control; STZ, streptozotocin diabetic neuropathy. (From Nagamatsu M, Nicklander KK, Schmelzer JD, et al. Lipoic acid improves nerve blood flow, reduces oxidative stress, and improves distal nerve conduction in experimental diabetic neuropathy. Diabetes Care 1995; 18:1160–1167.)

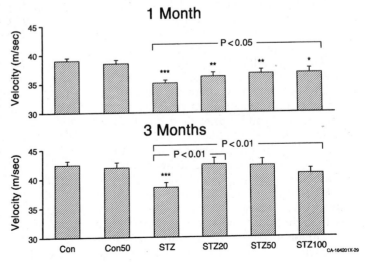

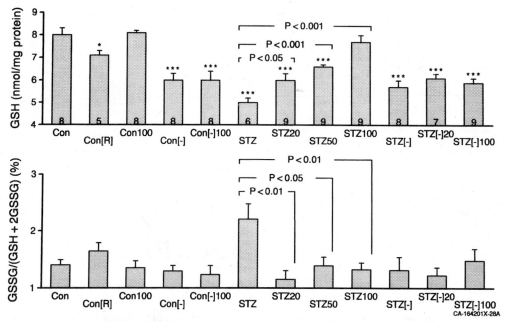

■ **Figure 21.3** Sciatic nerve reduced glutathione (GSH) concentrations, in controls (Con), on restricted caloric intake (Con(R)), streptozotocin diabetic (STZ), α-tocopherol depleted (−), and supplemented with lipoic acid at 20 mg/kg, 50 mg/kg, and 100 mg/kg. Lipoic acid supplementation resulted in a dose-dependent prevention of GSH. Significance of difference versus control, *$P < 0.05$; ***$P < 0.001$. (From Nagamatsu M, Nicklander KK, Schmelzer JD, et al. Lipoic acid improves nerve blood flow, reduces oxidative stress, and improves distal nerve conduction in experimental diabetic neuropathy. Diabetes Care 1995; 18:1160–1167.)

pathophysiology of painfulness.[23, 120] Three closely interlinked sites of sensitization (nerve axon/microenvironment, dorsal root ganglion [DRG], NREZ) may together be operative in producing hyperalgesia. The chronic constriction model results in increased norepinephrine, neuropeptide Y (NPY), and calcitonin gene-related peptide (CGRP) at the nerve lesion. Nerve blood flow is increased within the lesion but reduced at the lesion edge by more than 50%, a deficit that is sufficient to cause fiber degeneration.[51, 102] This increase in CGRP in the lesion is associated with reduced pain threshold.[5] Second, we found a large increase of NPY and CGRP by radioimmunoassay and immunocytochemistry in ipsilateral L5 dorsal root ganglion, but not in sympathetic ganglia. For instance, central sensitization requires peripheral inputs and can be prevented if peripheral input is blocked or absent.[23]

Rats with a chronic constriction injury to the sciatic nerve have been found to have small- to medium-sized, pyknotic, and hyperchromatic neurons (dark neurons) in spinal dorsal horn laminae I–III.[78] These hyperchromatic neurons were thought to be produced by an excitotoxic insult involving NMDA receptor activation subsequent to ectopic nociceptor discharge,

and that at least some dark neurons are inhibitory interneurons whose functional impairment or death contributes to a central state of hyperexcitability that underlies neuropathic hyperalgesia and allodynia. NMDA antagonists will prevent or reverse allodynia.[103, 110]

Pain models include the chronic constriction nerve trunk model of Bennett and Xie,[6] the root constriction model of Chung,[53] and the paw formalin injection model. A sustained afferent barrage from small nerve fibers is associated with spinal release of glutamate, prostaglandins, and aspartate[67] and results in a hyperalgesic state. There are close interactions among spinal NMDA, neurokinin 1 (NK1), and α-adrenoreceptors. There is also nitric oxide modulation and mediation by the spinal release of cyclo-oxygenase products.[121] The hyperalgesic state can be prevented by antinociceptive doses of cyclo-oxygenase inhibitors,[69] the α2-adrenoceptor agonist clonidine, or NMDA antagonists (such as MK-801). Intrathecal clonidine may act to diminish sympathetic outflow, whereas MK-801 blocks the NMDA receptor. The two separate mechanisms may account for the powerful synergy observed by Lee and Yaksh.[55] This hyperalgesic component appears initiated by the activation of a spinal NMDA receptor that, through the generation of nitric oxide, leads to the observed augmented processing of afferent input and the associated hyperalgesic component of the subsequent pain behavior.[68] Hyperalgesia is prevented by pretreatment with agents known to block afferent input (local anesthetics) or C-fiber transmitter release (opiates) or to act at one of several links to block a complex spinal cascade involving the NMDA receptor, nitric oxide synthase, and cyclo-oxygenase.[119]

Neuropathic animals that have thermal hyperalgesia had an ipsilateral decrease in substance P (SP) staining density without an accompanying change in CGRP staining density. MK-801-treated animals showed a dose-dependent attenuation of the thermal hyperalgesia, and the expected ipsilateral decrease in SP was prevented. MK-801 treatment in naive rats caused a global increase in SP and CGRP staining in the dorsal horn. The results suggest a functional interaction between excitatory amino acids and SP, with activation of NMDA receptors mediating depletion of SP in neuropathic animals. It is suggested that SP-containing interneurons are a target of the excitatory amino acids in the dorsal horn.[30]

Although nitric oxide–NMDA interactions can result in hyperalgesia, nitric oxide also produces a dose-dependent antinociceptive response in diabetic mice.[43] The antinociceptive effects were significantly antagonized by subcutaneous administration of naltrindole, a selective δ-opiate receptor antagonist, suggesting the involvement of activation of δ-opiate receptors. The hyperalgesic state in experimental diabetic rats is associated with increased spinal release,[45] reduced spinal levels of SP, and a significant increase in the number of binding sites for SP in dorsal spinal cord.[44] RP-67580, a specific tachykinin NK1 receptor antagonist, relieves chronic hyperalgesia in diabetic rats.[21]

PATHOGENESIS OF DIABETIC NEUROPATHY

The information in this chapter has been synthesized into a pathogenetic model of diabetic neuropathy[58, 59, 64] and is briefly summarized here (Fig. 21.4). Hyperglycemia results in a reduction in NBF, by altering vasoregulation of nerve microvessels, and increasing viscosity.[59] Microvascular vasoconstrictor tone is increased and vasodilator tone is reduced.[59, 64] Reduced vasodilator tone is caused by reduced endothelial activities of nitric oxide,[11, 49] CGRP, and SP.[28] Prostaglandin E_1 and prostacyclin generation

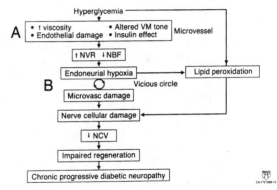

■ **Figure 21.4** Simplified pathogenetic model of diabetic neuropathy. *A* depicts changes in microvessel; *B* refers to vicious circle of changes. NVR, nerve vascular resistance; NBF, nerve blood flow; NCV, nerve conduction velocity; VM, vasomotor.

are also reduced.[100, 113] Increased vasoconstrictor tone is caused by increased α-adrenergic[2, 38, 75] and endothelin[14, 49, 107, 108] tone. The latter is possibly related to altered nitric oxide modulation. Insulin administration aggravates hypoxia by increasing arteriovenous shunt flow and reducing nutritive flow.[52] The ensuing endoneurial ischemia and increased nerve microvascular resistance result in endoneurial hypoxia. Hypoxia results in lipid peroxidation and a further reduction in vasomotor tone,[59] resulting in a vicious circle. Hyperglycemia per se causes lipid auto-oxidation/glycation.[117, 118] Nerve cellular damage and neuropathy results. Figure 21.5 expands on the mechanisms of dorsal root ganglion and radicular neuropathy. Lipid peroxidation is aggravated by a reduction in nerve growth factor.[34] Nerve growth

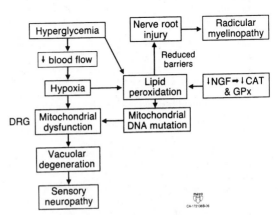

■ **Figure 21.5** Proposed mechanisms of changes in dorsal root ganglia and spinal roots in experimental diabetic neuropathy. DRG, dorsal root ganglion; NGF, nerve growth factor; CAT, catalase; GPx, glutathione peroxidase.

factor reduction will reduce, and its administration will restore, glutathione peroxidase and catalase.[85, 94] Lipid peroxidation effects are worsened in nerve root and dorsal root ganglion because the blood-nerve and perineurial barriers are lower at these sites,[39, 87] and a radicular myelinopathy ensues. We propose that the dorsal root ganglion pathology is caused by reduced oxygen species generated in mitochondria. The vacuoles observed in our study may be related to dysfunctional mitochondria.[106] Oxidative stress has been suggested to be a major pathogenetic mechanism in other states such as aging, and the mitochondrion is a selective focus of its action.[114] Mitochondrial DNA is unusually susceptible to oxidative damage[91] and leads to increased mutations; these dysfunctional mitochondria have increased reduced oxygen species leakage.[112] A vicious cycle of oxidative damage to inner membrane proteins (of mitochondria), leading to imbalances in the electron transport chain, resulting in increased superoxide and hydrogen peroxide production, which in turn further damages membrane proteins is suggested.[99] The physiologic alterations (reduced sensory threshold; spontaneous firing) in EDN could be the result of the sensory neuropathy and radiculopathy described above. A peripheral and distal involvement likely also exists, as suggested by denervation of skin and muscle[28] and gut.[98]

References

1. Ahlskog JE, Uitti RJ, Low PA, et al. No evidence for systemic oxidant stress in Parkinson's or Alzheimer's disease. Mov Disord 1995; 10:566.
2. Amenta D, Cavallot C, Collier WL, et al. Noradrenergic innervation of the superior mesenteric artery in streptozotocin-diabetic rats. Acta Histochem Cytochem 1987; 20:177.
3. Babiy AV, Gebicki JM, Sullivan DR, et al. Increased oxidizability of plasma lipoproteins in diabetic patients can be decreased by probucol therapy and is not due to glycation. Biochem Pharmacol 1992; 43:995.
4. Baynes JW. Role of oxidative stress in the development of complications in diabetes. Diabetes 1991; 40:405.
5. Bennett GJ. An animal model of neuropathic pain: A review. Muscle Nerve 1993; 16:1040.
6. Bennett GJ, Xie YK. A peripheral mononeuropathy in rat that produces disorders of pain sensation like those seen in man. Pain 1988; 33:87.
7. Bhimji S, Godin DV, McNeill JH. Insulin reversal of biochemical changes in hearts of diabetic rats. Am J Physiol 1986; 251:H670.
8. Bravenboer B, Kappelle AC, Hamers FPT, et al. Potential use of glutathione for the prevention and treatment of diabetic neuropathy in the streptozotocin-induced diabetic rat. Diabetologia 1992; 35:813.
9. Busse E, Zimmer G, Schopohl B, et al. Influence of α-lipoic acid on intracellular glutathione in vitro and in vivo. Arzneimittelforschung 1992; 42:829.
10. Cameron NE, Cotter MA. Effects of chronic treatment with a nitric oxide donor on nerve conduction abnormalities and endoneurial blood flow in streptozotocin-diabetic rats. Eur J Clin Invest 1995; 25:19.
11. Cameron NE, Cotter MA. Neurovascular dysfunction in diabetic rats: Potential contribution of autoxidation and free radicals examined using transition metal chelating agents. J Clin Invest 1995; 96:1159.
12. Cameron NE, Cotter MA. Rapid reversal by aminoguanidine of the neurovascular effects of diabetes in rats: Modulation by nitric oxide synthase inhibition. Metabolism 1996; 45:1147.
13. Cameron NE, Cotter MA. Effects of a nonpeptide endothelin-1 ETA antagonist on neurovascular function in diabetic rats: Interaction with the renin-angiotensin system. J Pharmacol Exp Ther 1996; 278:1262.
14. Cameron NE, Cotter MA, Archibald V, et al. Antioxidant and pro-oxidant effects on nerve conduction velocity, endoneurial blood flow and oxygen tension in non-diabetic and streptozotocin-diabetic rats. Diabetologia 1994; 37:449.
15. Cameron NE, Cotter MA, Low PA. Nerve blood flow in early experimental diabetes in rats: Relation to conduction deficits. Am J Physiol 1991; 261:E1.
16. Cameron NE, Cotter MA, Maxfield EK. Anti-oxidant treatment prevents the development of peripheral nerve dysfunction in streptozotocin-diabetic rats. Diabetologia 1993; 36:299.
17. Collier A, Rumley A, Rumley AG, et al. Free radical activity and hemostatic factors in NIDDM patients with and without microalbuminuria. Diabetes 1992; 41:909.
18. Cotter MA, Cameron NE. Correction of impaired sciatic nerve perfusion by desferrioxamine in diabetic rats (abstract). Diabetologia 1995; 38(suppl 1):898.
19. Cotter MA, Cameron NE. Neuroprotective effects of carvedilol in diabetic rats: Prevention of defective peripheral nerve perfusion and conduction velocity. Naunyn Schmiedebergs Arch Pharmacol 1995; 351:630.
20. Cotter MA, Love A, Watt MJ, et al. Effects of natural free radical scavengers on peripheral nerve and neurovascular function in diabetic rats. Diabetologia 1995; 38:1285.
21. Courteix C, Lavarenne J, Eschalier A. RP-67580, a specific tachykinin NK1 receptor antagonist, relieves chronic hyperalgesia in diabetic rats. Eur J Pharmacol 1993; 241:267.
22. Crouch R, Kimsey G, Priest DG, et al. Effect of streptozotocin on erythrocyte and retinal superoxide dismutase. Diabetologia 1978; 15:53.
23. Dickenson AH. NMDA receptor antagonists as analgesics. In Fields HL, Liebeskind JC (eds): Progress in Pain Research and Management. Seattle, IASP Press, 1994, vol 1, p 173.
24. Dimpfel W, Spuler M, Pierau F-K, et al. Thioctic acid induces dose-dependent sprouting of neurites in cultured rat neuroblastoma cells. Dev Pharmacol Ther 1990; 14:193.
25. Dintenfass L. Haemorheology of diabetes mellitus. J Pharmacol Exp Ther 1979; 278:1262.
26. Duchen LW, Anjorin A, Watkins PJ, et al. Pathology of autonomic neuropathy in diabetes mellitus. Ann Intern Med 1980; 92:301.
27. Emmons PR, Blume WT, DuShane JW. Cardiac monitoring and demand pacemaker in Guillain-Barre syndrome. Arch Neurol 1975; 32:59.

28. Fernyhough P, Diemel LT, Brewster WJ, et al. Deficits of nerve neuropeptide content coincide with a reduction in target tissue nerve growth factor messenger RNA in streptozotocin-diabetic rats: Effects of insulin treatment. Neuroscience 1994; 62:337.

29. Gandhi CR, Roychowdhury D. Effect of diabetes mellitus on activities of some glycolytic, hexose monophosphate and other enzymes of erythrocytes of different ages. Indian J Exp Biol 1982; 20:347.

30. Garrison CJ, Dougherty PM, Carlton SM. Quantitative analysis of substance P and calcitonin gene-related peptide immunohistochemical staining in the dorsal horn of neuropathic MK-801-treated rats. Brain Res 1993; 607:205.

31. Godin DV, Wohaieb SA, Garnett ME, et al. Antioxidant enzyme alterations in experimental and clinical diabetes. Mol Cell Biochem 1988; 84:223.

32. Greene DA, Lattimer SA. Impaired rat sciatic nerve sodium-potassium adenosine triphosphatase in acute streptozotocin diabetes and its correction by dietary myo-inositol supplementation. J Clin Invest 1983; 72:1058.

33. Halliwell B, Gutteridge JM. Free Radicals in Biology and Medicine. Oxford, Clarendon Press, 1985.

34. Hellweg R, Hartung HD. Endogenous levels of nerve growth factor (NGF) are altered in experimental diabetes mellitus: A possible role for NGF in the pathogenesis of diabetic neuropathy. J Neurosci Res 1990; 26:258.

35. Hermenegildo C, Raya A, Roma J, et al. Decreased glutathione peroxidase activity in sciatic nerve of alloxan-induced diabetic mice and its correlation with blood glucose levels. Neurochem Res 1993; 18:893.

36. Hunt JV, Wolff SP. Oxidative glycation and free radical production: A causal mechanism of diabetic complications. Free Radic Res 1991; 1:115.

37. Isogai Y, Iida A, Michizuki K, et al. Hemorheological studies on the pathogenesis of diabetic microangiopathy. Thromb Res 1976; 8:17.

38. Jackson CV, Carrier GO. Supersensitivity of isolated mesenteric arteries to noradrenaline in the long-term experimental diabetic rat. J Auton Pharmacol 1981; 1:399.

39. Jacobs JM, MacFarlane RM, Cavanagh JB. Vascular leakage in the dorsal root ganglia of the rat: Studies with horse-radish peroxidase. J Neurol Sci 1976; 29:95.

40. Jennings PE, Chirico S, Lunec J, et al. Vitamin C metabolites and microangiopathy in diabetes mellitus. Diabetes Res 1987; 6:151.

41. Kaji H, Kurasaki M, Ito K, et al. Increased lipoperoxide value and glutathione peroxidase activity in blood plasma of type 2 (non-insulin dependent) diabetic women. Klin Wochenschr 1985; 63:765.

42. Kalyanaraman B, Darley-Usmar VM, Wood J, et al. Synergistic interaction between the probucol phenoxyl radical and ascorbic acid in inhibiting the oxidation of low density lipoprotein. J Biol Chem 1992; 267:6789.

43. Kamei J, Iwamoto Y, Misawa M, et al. Antinociceptive effect of L-arginine in diabetic mice. Eur J Pharmacol 1994; 254:113.

44. Kamei J, Ogawa M, Kasuya Y. Development of supersensitivity to substance P in the spinal cord of the streptozotocin-induced diabetic rats. Pharmacol Biochem Behav 1990; 35:473.

45. Kamei J, Ogawa Y, Ohhashi Y, et al. Alterations in the potassium-evoked release of substance P from the spinal cord of streptozotocin-induced diabetic rats in vitro. Gen Pharmacol 1991; 22:1093.

46. Karasu C, Dewhurst M, Stevens EJ, et al. Effects of anti-oxidant treatment on sciatic nerve dysfunction in streptozotocin-diabetic rats: Comparison with essential fatty acids. Diabetologia 1995; 38:129.

47. Karpen CW, Cataland S, O'Dorisio TM, et al. Interrelation of platelet vitamin E and thromboxane synthesis in type I diabetes mellitus. Diabetes 1984; 33:239.

48. Kihara M, Low PA. Regulation of rat nerve blood flow: Role of epineurial alpha-receptors. J Physiol 1990; 422:145.

49. Kihara M, Low PA. Impaired vasoreactivity to nitric oxide in experimental diabetic neuropathy. Exp Neurol 1995; 132:180.

50. Kihara M, Low PA. Vasoreactivity to prostaglandins in rat peripheral nerve. J Physiol 1995; 484:463.

51. Kihara M, Zollman PJ, Schmelzer JD, et al. The influence of dose of microspheres on nerve blood flow, electrophysiology, and fiber degeneration of rat peripheral nerve. Muscle Nerve 1993; 16:1383.

52. Kihara M, Zollman PJ, Smithson IL, et al. Hypoxic effect of exogenous insulin on normal and diabetic peripheral nerve. Am J Physiol 1994; 266:E980.

53. Kim SH, Chung JM. An experimental model for peripheral neuropathy produced by segmental spinal nerve ligation in the rat. Pain 1992; 50:355.

54. Lacka B, Grzeszczak W, Strojek K, et al. Pro-oxidant–antioxidant imbalance in insulin-dependent diabetes mellitus (abstract). Diabetologia 1995; 38(suppl 1):A40.

55. Lee YW, Yaksh TL. Analysis of drug interaction between intrathecal clonidine and MK-801 in peripheral neuropathic pain rat model. Anesthesiology 1995; 82:741.

56. Loven DP, Oberley LW. Free radicals, insulin action and diabetes. In Oberley LW (ed): Superoxide Dismutase. Vol. III: Disease States. Boca Raton, CRC, 1985, p 151.

57. Loven DP, Schedl HP, Oberley LW, et al. Superoxide dismutase activity in the intestine of the streptozotocin-diabetic rat. Endocrinology 1982; 111:737.

58. Low PA. Recent advances in the pathogenesis of diabetic neuropathy. Muscle Nerve 1987; 10:121.

59. Low PA, Lagerlund TD, McManis PG. Nerve blood flow and oxygen delivery in normal, diabetic, and ischemic neuropathy. Int Rev Neurobiol 1989; 31:355.

60. Low PA, Nickander KK. Oxygen free radical effects in sciatic nerve in experimental diabetes. Diabetes 1991; 40:873.

61. Low PA, Nukada H, Schmelzer JD, et al. Endoneurial oxygen tension and radial topography in nerve edema. Brain Res 1985; 341:147.

62. Low PA, Schmelzer JD, Ward KK, et al. Effect of hyperbaric oxygenation on normal and chronic streptozotocin diabetic peripheral nerves. Exp Neurol 1988; 99:201.

63. Low PA, Schmelzer JD, Ward KK, et al. Experimental chronic hypoxic neuropathy: Relevance to diabetic neuropathy. Am J Physiol 1986; 250:E94.

64. Low PA, Suarez GA. Diabetic neuropathies (review). Baillieres Clin Neurol 1995; 4:401.

65. Low PA, Tuck RR. Effects of changes of blood pressure, respiratory acidosis and hypoxia on blood flow in the sciatic nerve of the rat. J Physiol 1984; 347:513.

66. Low PA, Tuck RR, Takeuchi M. Nerve microenvironment in diabetic neuropathy. In Dyck PJ, Thomas PK, Winegrad A, et al (eds): Diabetic Neuropathy. Philadelphia, WB Saunders, 1987, p 266.

67. Malmberg AB, Yaksh TL. Hyperalgesia mediated by spinal glutamate or substance P receptor blocked by spinal cyclooxygenase inhibition. Science 1992; 257:1276.

68. Malmberg AB, Yaksh TL. Spinal nitric oxide synthesis inhibition blocks NMDA-induced thermal hyperalgesia and produces antinociception in the formalin test in rats. Pain 1993; 54:291.

69. Malmberg AB, Yaksh TL. Cyclooxygenase inhibition and the spinal release of prostaglandin E2 and amino acids evoked by paw formalin injection: A microdialysis study in unanesthetized rats. J Neurosci 1995; 15:2768.

70. Mateo MCM, Bustamante JB, Cantalapiedra MAG. Serum zinc, copper and insulin in diabetes mellitus. Biomedicine 1978; 29:56.

71. Matkovics B, Varga SI, Szabo L, et al. The effect of diabetes on the activities of the peroxide metabolism enzymes. Horm Metab Res 1982; 14:77.

72. McCord JM. Oxygen-derived free radicals in postischemic tissue injury. N Engl J Med 1985; 312:159.

73. McManis PG, Low PA, Yao JK. Relationship between nerve blood flow and intercapillary distance in peripheral nerve edema. Am J Physiol 1986; 251:E92.

74. McMillan DE. The microcirculation in diabetes (review). Microcirc Endothelium Lymphatics 1984; 1:3.

75. Morff RJ. Microvascular reactivity to norepinephrine at different arteriolar levels and durations of streptozocin-induced diabetes. Diabetes 1990; 39:354.

76. Murakami K, Kondo T, Ohtsuka Y, et al. Impairment of glutathione metabolism in erythrocytes from patients with diabetes mellitus. Metabolism 1989; 38:753.

77. Murase K, Hattori A, Kohno M, et al. Stimulation of nerve growth factor synthesis/secretion in mouse astroglial cells by coenzymes. Biochem Mol Biol Int 1993; 30:615.

78. Nachemson AK, Bennett GJ. Does pain damage spinal cord neurons? Transsynaptic degeneration in rat following a surgical incision. Neurosci Lett 1993; 162:78.

79. Nagamatsu M, Nickander KK, Schmelzer JD, et al. Lipoic acid improves nerve blood flow, reduces oxidative stress, and improves distal nerve conduction in experimental diabetic neuropathy. Diabetes Care 1995; 18:1160.

80. Newrick PG, Wilson AJ, Jakubowski J, et al. Sural nerve oxygen tension in diabetes. BMJ 1986; 293:1053.

81. Nickander KK, McPhee BR, Low PA, et al. α-Lipoic acid: Antioxidant potency against lipid peroxidation of neural tissue in vitro and implications for diabetic neuropathy. Free Radic Biol Med 1996; 21:631.

82. Nickander KK, Schmelzer JD, Rohwer DA, et al. Effect of α-tocopherol deficiency on indices of oxidative stress in normal and diabetic peripheral nerve. J Neurol Sci 1994; 126:6.

83. Niki E. Antioxidants in relation to lipid peroxidation. Chem Phys Lipids 1987; 44:227.

84. Nishimura C, Kuriyama K. Alteration of lipid peroxide and endogenous antioxidant contents of retina of streptozotocin-induced diabetic rats: Effect of vitamin A administration. Jpn J Pharmacol 1985; 37:365.

85. Nistico G, Cirolo MR, Fiskin K, et al. NGF restores decrease in catalase activity and increases superoxide dismutase and glutathione peroxidase activity in the brain of aged rats. Free Radic Biol Med 1992; 12:177.

86. Noto R, Alicata R, Sfogliano LA. A study of cupremia in a group of elderly diabetics. Acta Diabetol 1983; 20:81.

87. Olsson Y. Topographical differences in the vascular permeability of the peripheral nervous system. Acta Neuropathol 1968; 10:26.

88. Packer L, Witt EH, Tritschler HJ. alpha-Lipoic acid as a biological antioxidant (review). Free Radic Biol Med 1995; 19:227.

89. Poduslo JF, Low PA, Nickander KK, et al. Mammalian endoneurial fluid: Collection and protein analysis from normal and crushed nerves. Brain Res 1985; 332:91.

90. Pritchard KA Jr, Patel ST, Karpen CW, et al. Triglyceride-lowering effect of dietary vitamin E in streptozocin-induced diabetic rats: Increased lipoprotein lipase activity in livers of diabetic rats fed high dietary vitamin E. Diabetes 1986; 35:278.

91. Richter C, Park JW, Ames BN. Normal oxidative damage to mitochondrial and nuclear DNA is extensive. Proc Natl Acad Sci USA 1988; 85:6465.

92. Romero FJ, Monsalve E, Hermenegildo C, et al. Oxygen toxicity in the nervous tissue: Comparison of the antioxidant defense of rat brain and sciatic nerve. Neurochem Res 1991; 16:157.

93. Romero FJ, Segura-Aguilar J, Monsalve E, et al. Antioxidant and glutathione-related enzymatic activities in rat sciatic nerve. Neurotoxicol Teratol 1990; 12:603.

94. Sampath D, Jackson GR, Werrbach-Perez K, et al. Effects of nerve growth factor on glutathione peroxidase and catalase in PC12 cells. J Neurochem 1994; 62:2476.

95. Sasaki H, Low PA. Extreme vasoreactivity of rat epineurial arterioles to vasopressin. Am J Physiol 1996; 271:H1307.

96. Sasaki H, Schmelzer JD, Zollman PJ, et al. Neuropathology and blood flow of nerve, spinal roots and dorsal root ganglia in longstanding diabetic rats. Acta Neuropathol 1997; 93:118.

97. Sato Y, Hotta N, Sakamoto N, et al. Lipid peroxide level in plasma of diabetic patients. Biochem J 1979; 21:104.

98. Schmidt RE, Plurad DA, Plurad SB, et al. Ultrastructural and immunohistochemical characterization of autonomic neuropathy in genetically diabetic Chinese hamsters. Lab Invest 1989; 61:77.

99. Shigenaga MK, Hagen TM, Ames BN. Oxidative damage and mitochondrial decay in aging. Proc Natl Acad Sci USA 1994; 91:10771.

100. Shindo H, Tawata M, Aida K, et al. Clinical efficacy of a stable prostacyclin analog, iloprost, in diabetic neuropathy. Prostaglandins 1991; 41:85.

101. Skovborg F, Nielsen AV, Schlichtkrull J, et al. Blood viscosity in diabetic patients. Lancet 1966; 1:129.

102. Sladky JT, Greenberg JH, Brown MJ. Regional perfusion in normal and ischemic rat sciatic nerves. Ann Neurol 1985; 17:191.

103. Smith GD, Wiseman J, Harrison SM, et al. Pre-treatment with MK-801, a non-competitive NMDA antagonist, prevents development of mechanical hyperalgesia in a rat model of chronic neuropathy, but not in a model of chronic inflammation. Neurosci Lett 1994; 165:79.

104. Som S, Basu S, Mukherjee D, et al. Ascorbic acid metabolism in diabetes mellitus. Metabolism 1981; 30:572.

105. Stevens EJ, Carrington AL, Tomlinson DR. Nerve ischaemia in diabetic rats: Time-course of development, effect of insulin treatment plus comparison of streptozotocin and BB models. Diabetologia 1994; 37:43.

106. Struys-Ponsar C, Florence A, Gauthier A, et al. Ultrastructural changes in brain parenchyma during normal aging and in animal models of aging. J Neural Transm Suppl 1994; 44:111.

107. Takahashi K, Ghatei MA, Lam HC, et al. Elevated plasma endothelin in patients with diabetes mellitus. Diabetologia 1990; 33:306.

108. Takeda Y, Miyamori I, Yoneda T, et al. Production of endothelin-1 from the mesenteric arteries of streptozotocin-induced diabetic rats. Life Sci 1991; 48:2553.

109. Takeuchi M, Low PA. Dynamic peripheral nerve metabolic and vascular responses to exsanguination. Am J Physiol 1987; 253:E349.

110. Tal M, Bennett GJ. Extra-territorial pain in rats with a peripheral mononeuropathy: Mechano-allodynia in the territory of an uninjured nerve. Pain 1994; 57:375.

111. Tuck RR, Schmelzer JD, Low PA. Endoneurial blood flow and oxygen tension in the sciatic nerves of rats with experimental diabetic neuropathy. Brain 1984; 107:935.

112. Turrens JF, Boveris A. Generation of superoxide anion by the NADH dehydrogenase of bovine heart mitochondria. Biochem J 1980; 191:421.

113. Ward KK, Low PA, Schmelzer JD, et al. Prostacyclin and noradrenaline in peripheral nerve of chronic experimental diabetes in rats. Brain 1989; 112:197.

114. Wilson PD, Franks LM. The effect of age on mitochondrial ultrastructure and enzymes. Adv Exp Med Biol 1975; 53:171.

115. Wohaieb SA, Godin DV. Alterations in free radical tissue-defence mechanisms in streptozotocin-induced diabetes in the rat. Diabetes 1987; 36:1014.

116. Wohaieb SA, Godin DV. Alterations in tissue antioxidant systems in the spontaneously diabetic (BB Wistar) rat. Can J Physiol Pharmacol 1987; 65:2191.

117. Wolff SP. Diabetes mellitus and free radicals. Br Med Bull 1993; 49:642.

118. Wolff SP, Jiang ZY, Hunt JV. Protein glycation and oxidative stress in diabetes mellitus and ageing. Free Radic Biol Med 1991; 10:339.

119. Yaksh TL. The spinal pharmacology of facilitation of afferent processing evoked by high-threshold afferent input of the postinjury pain state (review). Curr Opin Neurol Neurosurg 1993; 6:250.

120. Yaksh TL, Chaplan SR, Malmberg AB. Future directions in the pharmacological management of hyperalgesic and allodynic pain states: The NMDA receptor (review). NIDA Res Monogr 1995; 147:84.

121. Yaksh TL, Malmberg AB. Spinal actions of NSAIDS in blocking spinally mediated hyperalgesia: The role of cyclooxygenase products (review). Agents Actions Suppl 1993; 41:89.

122. Yao JK, Low PA. Improvement of endoneurial lipid abnormalities in experimental diabetic neuropathy by oxygen modification. Brain Res 1986; 362:362.

123. Yoshida K, Kirokawa J, Tagami S, et al. Weakened cellular scavenging activity against oxidative stress in diabetes mellitus: Regulation of glutathione synthesis and efflux. Diabetologia 1995; 38:201.

124. Zochodne DW, Ho LT. Influence of perivascular peptides on endoneurial blood flow and microvascular resistance in the sciatic nerve of the rat. J Physiol 1991; 444:615.

125. Zochodne DW, Ho LT, Gross PM. Acute endoneurial ischemia induced by epineurial endothelin in the rat sciatic nerve. Am J Physiol 1992; 263:H1806.

126. Zochodne DW, Low PA. Adrenergic control of nerve blood flow. Exp Neurol 1990; 109:300.

Chapter 22

Role of Aldose Reductase Inhibitors in the Treatment of Diabetic Polyneuropathy

David R. Tomlinson

INTRODUCTION

In 1959, Ruth van Heyningen published evidence that formation of sorbitol by aldose reductase contributed to the development of sugar cataracts in diabetes.[90] Seven years later the hypothesis linking sorbitol production to diabetes-induced damage was extended to peripheral nerve.[28] The first aldose reductase inhibitor was introduced to the scientific community in 1973.[16] So, why is it that, 25 years later, these drugs are not licensed for treatment or prevention of diabetes complications in Europe or North America? Read on and find out.

BIOCHEMISTRY OF ALDOSE REDUCTASE AND THE SORBITOL PATHWAY

Aldose reductase is the first enzyme of the sorbitol (or polyol) pathway (Fig. 22.1). It converts glucose to the sugar alcohol, sorbitol, using NADPH as a proton donor, and the sorbitol is then converted to fructose, using NAD^+ as a proton acceptor. Aldose reductase will also metabolize galactose (see Fig. 22.1).[51] Furthermore, the fact that the product of the action of aldose reductase on galactose—galactitol (dulcitol)—is not a substrate for sorbitol dehydro-

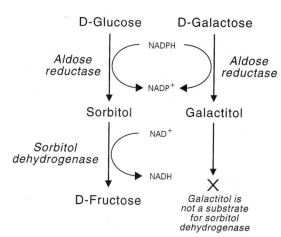

■ **Figure 22.1** The polyol (sorbitol) pathway, illustrating its physiologic mode, whereby glucose is converted to sorbitol and fructose, and an experimental alternative, in which orally administered galactose is converted to galactitol (dulcitol).

genase causes accumulation of the sugar alcohol at a faster rate and to a greater extent than occurs in diabetes. Activity can also be slaved to the dose of ingested galactose. For these reasons, galactose feeding has been used by several groups to study putative consequences of polyol pathway flux without other influences of diabetes mellitus.[16] However, the consequences of these two interventions may not always be similar.[95]

Under "physiologic" conditions, flux through this pathway is probably low in most tissues, though it has not been measured in vivo. Certainly, the measured level of sorbitol in most tissues is negligible,[44] and the affinity of aldose reductase for glucose is much lower than that of hexokinase. It is therefore likely that most intracellular glucose is phosphorylated and that the rate of sorbitol formation is low and matched by its clearance (Fig. 22.2). Neither sorbitol nor fructose crosses biologic membranes until significant concentration gradients are established and the affinities of sorbitol dehydrogenase and of fructokinase may also be relatively low. Thus, in hyperglycemia (or, strictly, cellular glucoplethora) steady-state flux through the entire pathway is associated with significant accumulations of the intermediates (see Fig. 22.2).

There are two situations that alter the dynamics of the pathway: an increase in the glucose concentration (as described in the previous paragraph and as occurs in some tissues in diabetes mellitus) or an increase in the amount of aldose reductase. Induction of the

enzyme occurs with osmotic stress, and this indicates its physiologic role.

PHYSIOLOGIC ROLE OF ALDOSE REDUCTASE

Renal tubular cells at the medullary extremity of the loop of Henle are bathed in hypertonic interstitial fluid. Compensation for this osmotic stress involves production of sorbitol from glucose by aldose reductase.[2] Exposure of kidney cells in culture to graded increments in tonicity of their culture medium provokes graded increases in the messenger RNA for aldose reductase, increases in enzyme protein, and increases in activity as revealed by increases in the rate of formation of sorbitol.[3] Sorbitol accumulates, providing the intracellular offsetting of the extracellular tonicity. Other osmolytes also contribute, in particular *myo*-inositol, betaine, and glycerophosphorylcholine; the amino acids taurine and aspartate may also be increased intracellularly after exposure to hypertonic extracellular fluid.[21, 53, 73] This phenomenon is not restricted to kidney cells; similar changes in vitro are seen in lens epithelium[6] and the retinal pigment epithelium.[53] It is therefore possible that the capacity to increase aldose reductase expression and produce graded amounts of sorbitol in response to hypertonicity is a highly conserved and fundamental property of all nucleated cells. The

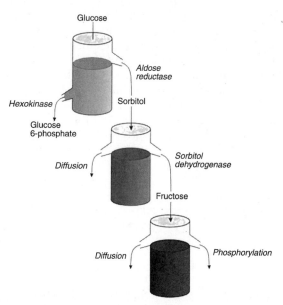

■ **Figure 22.2** The polyol pathway in diabetes, illustrating the factors determining steady-state flux (see text).

identity of the "osmosensor" that initiates this cellular reflex is a mystery.

The capacity to generate sorbitol also confers cryoprotection. There are examples of poikilotherms whose capacity to survive environments with seasonal subzero temperatures depends on generation of sorbitol via aldose reductase as an intracellular "antifreeze."[78] Interestingly, this property is being exploited for cryoprotection of erythrocytes[4] and, via transfection of the enzyme gene, for the freezing of plant tissues without distortion.[82] Thus, aldose reductase may be considered as an inducible enzyme whose physiologic role appears to be the production of electrically neutral solute with osmo- and cryo-protective properties in cells exposed to marked increases in the osmolality of their extracellular fluid or to ambient freezing conditions.

The importance of aldose reductase in diabetes mellitus stems from its potential as a pathogenetic mechanism. Thus, the related therapeutic strategy requires inhibition of the enzyme. The suggestions for a physiologic role indicate that the use of aldose reductase inhibitors as a therapeutic intervention in diabetes might constitute a potential compromise of cellular osmoregulation, particularly in the renal medulla. Interestingly, the treatment of osmotically stressed cells with aldose reductase inhibitors in the culture experiments described in the previous paragraphs produced surprising results. In cultured renal tubular cells, exposure to hypertonic medium in the presence of an aldose reductase inhibitor provoked an increase in the intracellular level of betaine and *myo*-inositol; the inhibitor precluded stimulation of sorbitol synthesis, but the increased intracellular milliosmoles constituted by the sum of betaine and *myo*-inositol compensated for the lack of sorbitol.[43] Thus, the capacity to recruit other osmolytes after inhibition of aldose reductase obviates compromise of cellular osmoprotection, when such drugs are used to inhibit aldose reductase in diabetes.

PATHOPHYSIOLOGIC CONSEQUENCES OF EXAGGERATED POLYOL PATHWAY FLUX

The concept that the polyol pathway might link hyperglycemia with dysfunction in diabetes energized some pharmaceutical companies to produce inhibitors of aldose reductase as drugs with the potential to combat diabetic complications. These provided the tools to enable the pragmatic demonstration of involvement of the pathway in diabetes-associated dysfunction. Perhaps because of this opportunity for research driven by pragmatism, it has taken much longer to forge links whereby increased flux through the polyol pathway predisposes tissues to biochemical defects that form the next stage in the pathway to the functional or structural defects that are the hallmarks of diabetic complications. Indeed, we still do not know which links are patent and important.

In the early years, studies concentrated on lenticular cataract formation and its association with sorbitol and fructose accumulation in diabetes,[16, 90] providing convincing evidence for an involvement of the pathway. Cataracts were also seen in galactose-fed rats,[16, 51] lending further support to this notion. It was generally assumed that the mechanism was simply osmotic attraction of water into the lens with consequent disaggregation of the lens fibers and formation of an opacity composed of disrupted fibers and water vacuoles.[50, 51] This simple concept of physical disruption as a result of inappropriate accumulation of intracellular osmolytes has not adapted to other tissues, except for the erythrocyte, in which water accumulation, driven by sorbitol and fructose, appears to increase turgor pressure, making the red cell less flexible and less compressible and probably contributing to impaired capillary flow in response to a normal perfusion pressure gradient.[10]

The next stage in the development of hypotheses appropriate to peripheral nerve came from a series of convergent observations. The oldest was the observation that exaggerated polyol pathway flux was associated temporally with depletion of *myo*-inositol in peripheral nerve.[74–77] The potential importance of this was emphasized by the finding that administration of large doses of *myo*-inositol to diabetic rats could prevent the development of slowed motor nerve conduction, linking biochemical and functional anomalies.[35] The availability of potent, selective aldose reductase inhibitors (ARIs) enabled the demonstration that these drugs could also prevent the development of the motor nerve conduction velocity (MNCV) deficit in diabetic[85] and galactosemic rats.[47] It was observed that ARIs prevented the development of depleted levels of *myo*-inositol in peripheral nerves concomitantly with their prevention of the MNCV deficit.[26, 31, 57] The known involvement of *myo*-inositol in the cycling of the second messenger system derived from membrane phosphoinositides provoked a hypothesis that attempted to explain these links in terms of regulation of Na^+/K^+-ATPase activity via phosphoinositide turnover. This mechanism proposed a translation of *myo*-inositol depletion to a reduced transmembrane Na^+ gradient at the node of Ranvier and a consequent slowing of passive Na^+ influx during saltatory conduction.[36, 37] Though this hypothesis has never been discredited, it has never been proved, and we await patch-clamping of nodal membrane for a proper resolution. Of course, the demonstration of effects of osmotic stress on cellular *myo*-inositol uptake (see previous section) now proves an adequate explanation for the link between polyol pathway flux and *myo*-inositol depletion in nerve. Thus, accumulation of sorbitol, driven by raised intracellular glucose in the absence of extracellular osmotic stress, as occurs in diabetes, would be expected to provoke a reciprocal attenuation of *myo*-inositol uptake to compensate for the osmotic effect of the sorbitol. This also explains the normalization of nerve *myo*-inositol levels on treatment of diabetic rats receiving an ARI.

It has been difficult to explain the increasingly complex and varied effects of ARIs in experimental diabetes either in terms of an osmotic hypothesis or in terms of interactions with *myo*-inositol. Indeed, there is accumulating evidence to suggest differential effects at different doses, which are associated with different degrees of inhibition of flux through the sorbitol pathway.[23] Most studies, including several by this author, have used a single dose of a given ARI and have monitored tissue levels of sorbitol and fructose as indicators of pharmacologic efficacy for the drug.[16, 48, 57, 66] Such an approach, with the end points of normalization of nerve sorbitol and near-normalization of fructose, will remove the cellular osmotic stress imposed by the pathway, as indicated by the fact that nerve *myo*-inositol levels are also normalized.[26, 57] Thus, any residual effects cannot be explained by either of the above hypotheses, and anomalies that resist ARI treatment, adjusted to meet the above-mentioned end points, have been judged to be unrelated to the polyol pathway.[87, 88] However, abolition of the accumulation of metabolites may not necessarily be equated with normalization of flux through the pathway; indeed, this represents a significant unknown feature of the polyol pathway, because it is so difficult to measure flux in a multicompartment system, as represented by peripheral nerve, in vivo. Figure 22.1 will remind the reader that the pathway con-

sumes both NADPH and NAD^+; these cofactors are used by other metabolic pathways, and it is entirely conceivable that their consumption by aldose reductase and sorbitol dehydrogenase might deprive some of these pathways to the detriment of nerve function. One example is the maintenance of adequate levels of reduced glutathione (GSH), as illustrated in Figure 22.3. Reduced glutathione is important in maintaining cellular redox potential in the reduced state, enabling cells to withstand oxi-

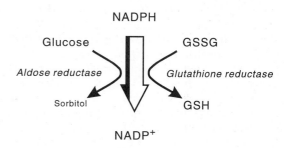

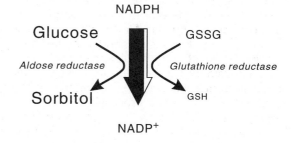

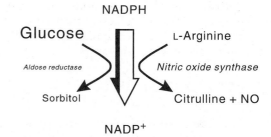

■ **Figure 22.3** Competition for NADPH between aldose reductase and glutathione reductase (*top*) and between aldose reductase and nitric oxide synthase (*bottom*).

dative stress. Obviously, there is cross-talk between GSH and other antioxidants, with clear evidence of mutual support between GSH and vitamin E in nerves of diabetic rats[61] and between GSH and α-lipoic acid.[65] Inhibition of aldose reductase clearly supports maintenance of GSH levels in diabetes, but this has only been clearly demonstrated in the lens.

The principle of piracy of protons from NADPH might also be expected to compromise nitric oxide production (see Fig. 22.3). The reduced sciatic nerve blood flow seen in diabetic rats is clearly derived for the most part from impaired endoneurial synthesis of nitric oxide, whereas the capacity of endoneurial vascular smooth muscle to respond to nitric oxide is not defective.[63] At the time of this writing, there is no clear demonstration that inhibition of aldose reductase normalizes endoneurial nitric oxide production. It is not possible to predict the clinical impact of disturbed endoneurial nitric oxide synthesis and reduced nerve blood flow. Recent examination of the potential involvement of reduced nerve blood flow in diabetic neuropathy has compiled evidence that is persuasive[83]; however, endoneurial ischemia is an unlikely candidate as a prime causative event. First, it is difficult to see how nerve trunk hypoxia could give the bias toward sensory defects in distal symmetrical diabetic neuropathy and even harder to explain many aspects of autonomic neuropathy on this basis. Second, the powerful arguments derived from rat experiments are frustrated by the observation that muscle wasting in nondiabetic rats also causes a profound reduction in sciatic nerve blood flow,[86] so the observation may offer a clear example of unrealistic animal modeling. It seems more likely that the clinical picture derives from primary insults unrelated to nerve blood flow and that the undoubted influence of axonal hypoxia is seen later in development of the condition. However, this subject is covered in Chapter 21. The point to be emphasized in relation to aldose reductase is that consumption of cofactors may have an important part to play in the disturbances derived from the polyol pathway.

SITES OF ALDOSE REDUCTASE ACTIVITY IN PERIPHERAL NERVE

Accumulation of sorbitol and fructose, indicating an active polyol pathway, occurs in peripheral nerve of diabetic rats,[28] nerve of diabetic individuals of other animal species,[9, 70] and in nerve samples from diabetic patients.[41, 59, 91] Although significant reductions in sorbitol[71] or sorbitol and fructose[20] have been reported in sural nerve biopsies after sorbinil treatment of diabetic patients, the location and extent of aldose reductase activity cannot be determined from such studies.

Aldose reductase activity in peripheral nerve is not subject to anterograde axonal transport,[13] implying that it is not expressed in the axon, at least under normal conditions. The Schwann cell location has now been confirmed by enzyme histochemistry[64] and immunohistochemistry.[54] At greater resolution, the enzyme is present in the paranodal cytoplasm of Schwann cells.[12] It is also demonstrable in pericytes and endothelial cells of endoneurial capillaries in peripheral nerve of BB rats.[12] More recently, intense immunostaining for aldose reductase has been found in the paranodal region and the Schmidt-Lanterman clefts as well as in the terminal expansions of paranodal myelin lamellae and nodal microvilli.[67]

FUNCTIONAL DEFICITS AND DIABETIC NEUROPATHY

It is important to distinguish between the very early manifestations of abnormal nerve function in diabetes and the chronic disorders that constitute diabetic neuropathy. The former may safely be referred to as subclinical neurologic dysfunction or even hyperglycemic neuropathy.[84] Thus, nerve conduction velocity is frequently abnormal in diabetic patients without neurologic symptoms or signs of neuropathy, and this conduction deficit may even be present at the time of diagnosis of diabetes itself.[38, 39] These subclinical abnormalities are valuable for the early correlation of disorders of biochemistry with those of function, but the critical questions are whether they are prognostic for the future development of neuropathic symptoms[25] and whether the latter may also be related to the early biochemical defects. Correlation of symptoms and nerve conduction anomalies with structural pathology in sural nerve biopsies revealed that abnormal vibration sense and conduction velocity showed predictive value for structural degeneration and for diagnosis of neuropathy.[19]

The slowing of peripheral nerve conduction velocity is of a clear metabolic origin[38, 39] and exhibits similar incidence and metabolic pathogenesis in patients and in diabetic models.[35] It is likely that a degree of conduction slowing persists but evolves, at least in some patients, from a reversible metabolic phenomenon into a structurally based dysfunction, which has not proved reversible with interventions currently available. We do not yet know whether these two superficially similar phenomena—acute and chronic slowing of conduction—are related.

EXPERIMENTAL STUDIES

Aldose reductase inhibition was first demonstrated to prevent the development of slowed nerve conduction in experimental diabetes in 1982 using the experimental inhibitor ICI 105552.[85, 100] Since that time, many studies have examined the effects of different inhibitors on conduction defects.[8, 11, 42, 48, 49, 60, 62, 68, 72, 98] These studies then gave rise to explorations of the relation between the conduction deficit and biochemical changes in the nerve as described earlier. Studies with aldose reductase inhibitors at longer durations of experimental diabetes demonstrate persistent but incomplete efficacy against decreased nerve conduction velocity,[17, 55, 80] indicating a partial involvement of the polyol pathway in the development of chronic neuronal dysfunction in diabetic animals. Chronic benefits from aldose reductase inhibitors may derive from beneficial actions against deficits in axonally transported proteins.[22, 58, 87, 93, 94, 96] It may be that the distal degenerative axonopathy of diabetic neuropathy develops as a consequence of progressive starvation of the neuronal extremities.

The most important structural studies have concentrated on effects of aldose reductase inhibition on ultrastructural abnormalities seen in long-term experimental diabetes. The reduced fiber occupancy, seen in sural nerves of untreated rats with long-term streptozotocin-induced diabetes, was prevented by 28 weeks of ponalrestat treatment.[97] Axon-fiber size ratio was also preserved in the ponalrestat-treated group. However, ponalrestat had no effect on unmyelinated nerve fiber structure revealed by morphometry. Beneficial effects on nerve ultrastructure have also been reported for up to 6 months of treatment with ponalrestat in the BB rat.[72] The treatment prevented structural abnormalities at the node of Ranvier but only partially preserved axonal integrity. The frequency of neuroaxonal dystrophy in the superior mesenteric sympathetic ganglia of rats with 8 months of streptozotocin diabetes has been found to be increased sevenfold compared with age-matched controls.[69] Sorbinil administration decreased but did not completely normalize this neuroaxonal dystrophy.

CLINICAL STUDIES

It is probably fair to suggest that Judzewitsch and colleagues[46] began the clinical saga of aldose reductase clinical trials in neuropathy with a randomized, double-blind crossover trial of sorbinil. The major finding was an increase in peroneal MNCV from 40.6 to 42.1 m/s in the treatment group ($P<0.05$ by comparison with placebo). Cessation of sorbinil treatment was associated with a decline in peroneal conduction velocity. A subcohort of the patients studied in the multicenter trial were examined to determine whether sorbinil treatment affected the pain sometimes associated with diabetic neuropathy,[45] and sorbinil relieved pain in 8 of 11 patients. Other trials have revealed modest benefits of sorbinil against pain, tendon reflex scores, diminished sural nerve action potential amplitude, and signs of autonomic dysfunction,[24, 40, 56, 79, 81, 99] whereas no effects of aldose reductase inhibition were seen in other studies.[14, 52]

These functional studies with sorbinil had used all available expertise in classical trial designs but had produced little to indicate real efficacy. It was clear in 1988—as it is today—that acceptable functional end points with proved prognostic value for neuropathy would change measurably only in very long trials. Another strategy to indicate efficacy and secure product registration was indicated with the morphometric approach of Sima and colleagues.[71] This came with a randomized, placebo-controlled, double-blind trial of sorbinil at 250 mg/d in diabetic patients, in which the major assessment was morphometric examination of sural nerve biopsies, taken at the start and after 1 year of the trial. Sorbinil-treated patients showed a 42% decrease in nerve sorbitol and a 3.8-fold increase in the percentage of regenerating myelinated nerve fibers, when compared with placebo-treated diabetics. Thus, it was suggested that sorbinil could improve the neuropathologic lesions of diabetic neuropathy.

Ponalrestat had been introduced through experimental studies as a potent inhibitor of aldose reductase,[89] and clinical trials began on the basis of satisfactory toxicity studies. In spite of this, trials published to date have indicated no significant efficacy against functional end points of neuropathy.[5, 27, 30]

Direct assessment of sural nerve sorbitol levels[34] showed that the aldose reductase inhibitor tolrestat was effective at clinical dosage against peripheral nerve aldose reductase. However, functional studies using classical trial design have produced no more clear indicators for tolrestat than they did for sorbinil. No direct demonstration of reduced sural nerve sorbitol levels has been published for ponalrestat treatment in humans.

A multicenter trial of tolrestat used patients with symptomatic diabetic neuropathy.[7] Of the four doses tested, only the highest dose (200 mg/d) showed any improvements over baseline and placebo. Improvement in paresthetic symptoms were seen at 1 year, but painful symptoms improved in placebo and active therapies. Tibial and peroneal MNCVs improved significantly with 1 year of treatment with this high dose of tolrestat. Long-term benefit (improvement at 24 weeks maintained until 52 weeks) was seen in 28% of treated patients compared with 5% on placebo. Tolrestat was well tolerated in this study, but 11% of patients taking 200 mg/d experienced dizziness. Another study[32] assessed the effects of 6 months of treatment with tolrestat on various abnormalities of autonomic nerve function. The results were more encouraging, with significant improvements in heart-rate responses to deep breathing, lying-to-standing, and in vibration-perception threshold.

The most encouraging evidence to date of any effect of an aldose reductase inhibitor on symptomatic peripheral neuropathy has come from a recent withdrawal study with tolrestat.[33] Patients who had been receiving tolrestat for 4 to 5 years were continued on tolrestat (200 or 400 mg/d) or placebo for 52 weeks. Pain was found to worsen significantly in placebo-treated patients compared with those taking tolrestat. Sensation in the finger and great toe were improved for patients remaining on tolrestat, and the effect reached significance for the great toe at 36 weeks of treatment. The MNCV, measured in the median and peroneal nerves, worsened in the placebo-treated group by 1 m/s but remained unchanged in the tolrestat-treated group. This ingenious functional trial design has been supported by another structural examination of efficacy for tolrestat by Sima and colleagues. As with the sorbinil study, tolrestat treatment was associated with a reduction in structural signs of axonal degeneration, reduced incidence of myelin abnormalities, and an increase in the structural evidence of regeneration in sural nerve biopsies.[34]

CONCLUSION

Studies on experimental diabetes give a reasonably clear picture. The value of this is compromised by questions of validity of the experimental models, with respect to complications in humans. We know that aldose reductase inhibitors attenuate or prevent slowed nerve conduction, reduced *myo*-inositol uptake, some deficits of axonal transport, and some aspects of distal degeneration in nerves of diabetic rats.

Early clinical trials were inconclusive, and the assessment of these drugs has been bedeviled by a perceived need to begin with symptomatic patients, whose deficits may prove to be irreversible even when agents of clearly demonstrable efficacy are available. More recently, efficacy of tolrestat against ultrastructural signs of degeneration in sural nerve biopsies with concomitant signs of stimulation of regeneration was demonstrated. There has also been an encouraging withdrawal study, in which replacement of tolrestat with a placebo after 4 to 5 years of treatment was associated with accelerated decline of function relative to the patients who remained on the drug. Thus, we have learned some lessons from clinical studies that should improve the evaluation of new compounds, and it is certainly clear that the pharmaceutical companies have recognized the need for trials of much longer duration than before. However, the identification of appropriate end points is back in the melting pot.[1] The validity and feasibility of some of those features of sural nerve biopsies that have been claimed to be sensitive to ARIs have recently been questioned,[18, 29] so that if the Food and Drug Administration continues to regard improvement of sural nerve structure as a significant end point, we will need a clear consensus as to what can and should be measured.

It still appears that these drugs may offer some benefit, but how extensive this will be remains to be determined. The notion that aldose reductase might participate in the pathogenesis of diabetic neuropathy was first raised in 1966.[28] Thus, the concept and some of the early inhibitors of the enzyme have long since passed through puberty with little consequence to show for growth and development. Two inhibitors have reached the market to date—epalrestat in Japan and tolrestat in some European and South American countries and Australia. Tolrestat was withdrawn from all markets in 1996 because of elevation of plasma levels of liver enzymes and possible hepatotoxicity. This latter property has precluded development of some other inhibitors, but it does not seem that hepatotoxicity is a *sine qua non* of aldose reductase inhibition because sorbinil—although it caused hypersensitivity reactions—was free from liver toxicity at doses that were clinically effective for aldose reductase inhibition. The other problem that has hampered the development of clinically useful ARIs is the requirement for suitable pharmacokinetics as well as effective inhibition. Indeed, discovery of an effective ARI, as judged by activity in vitro, poses few problems for modern medicinal chemists; the structural requirements for interaction with the enzyme are broad, and hundreds of active molecules have been synthesized and tested.[18] However, many of these active molecules do not readily permeate tissues and reach the site of the enzyme in vivo. Thus, it has become an important paradigm that in vivo efficacy be demonstrated in human tissue as a *prima facie* requirement for phase II clinical testing. Ponalrestat[92] was subject to extensive double-blind testing against functional variables and parameters, whereupon it was found to be largely ineffective in many trials. However, removal of sural nerve biopsies from a small cohort of patients demonstrated that the clinically used dose was ineffective in lowering nerve sorbitol and fructose levels (C Laudadio, personal communication). Elevation of the dose was presumably unacceptable because of other effects, so development was discontinued. The structural requirements for penetration into peripheral nerve have not been defined, so current development tactics require the identification of highly potent inhibitors, which are then tested for elevation of liver enzymes and in vivo tissue penetration and efficacy as soon as possible. There are still new inhibitors at all stages of development, with zopolrestat and zenarestsat in clinical trial at the time of writing, so we may yet see this concept evolve into therapeutic efficacy.

ACKNOWLEDGMENTS

I thank all those in the pharmaceutical industry who, by virtue of their efforts (intellectual and fiscal), have fostered research into this important topic. If aldose reductase inhibitors ultimately fail to achieve all that they once promised, it should be recorded that this concept has stimulated extensive high-quality research that will contribute eventually to the well-being of diabetic patients.

References

1. Albers JW, Andersen H, Arezzo JC, et al. Diabetic polyneuropathy in controlled clinical trials: Consensus report of the Peripheral Nerve Society. Ann Neurol 1995; 38:478.
2. Bagnasco SM, Balaban R, Fales HM, et al. Predominant osmotically active solutes in rat and rabbit renal medullas. J Biol Chem 1986; 261:5872.
3. Bagnasco SM, Murphy HR, Bedford JJ, et al. Osmoregulation by slow changes in aldose reductase and rapid changes in sorbitol flux. Am J Physiol 1988; 254:788.
4. Behr W, Doukas K, Lang H, et al. Is preservation of erythrocyte concentrates with added solutions an alternative to deep freezing in heart surgery autologous blood donation? Beitr Infusionsther 1990; 26:252.
5. Bertelsmann FW, Faes TJC, de Weerdt O, et al. Treatment of diabetic autonomic neuropathy with the aldose reductase inhibitor Statil. Diabetologia 1991; 34(suppl 2):A37.
6. Bondy CA, Lightman SL. Developmental and physiological pattern of aldose reductase mRNA expression in lens and retina. Mol Endocrinol 1989; 3:1417.
7. Boulton AJM, Levin SR, Comstock JP. A multicentre trial of the aldose-reductase inhibitor, tolrestat, in patients with symptomatic diabetic neuropathy. Diabetologia 1990; 33:431.
8. Calcutt NA, Tomlinson DR, Biswas S. Coexistence of nerve conduction deficit with increased Na(+)-K(+)-ATPase activity in galactose-fed mice: Implications for polyol pathway and diabetic neuropathy. Diabetes 1990; 39:663.
9. Calcutt NA, Willars GB, Tomlinson DR. Statil-sensitive polyol formation in nerve of galactose-fed mice. Metabolism 1988; 37:450.
10. Carandente O, Colombo R, Girardi AM, et al. Role of red cell sorbitol as determinant of reduced erythrocyte filtrability in insulin-dependent diabetics. Acta Diabetol 1982; 19:359.
11. Carrington AL, Ettlinger CB, Calcutt NA, et al. Aldose reductase inhibition with imirestat: Effects on impulse conduction and insulin-stimulation of Na^+/K^+-adenosine triphosphatase activity in sciatic nerves of streptozotocin-diabetic rats. Diabetologia 1991; 34:397.
12. Chakrabarti S, Sima AAF, Nakajima T, et al. Aldose reductase in the BB rat: Isolation, immunological identification and localization in the retina and peripheral nerve. Diabetologia 1987; 30:244.
13. Chandler CE, Miller LJ. Studies of aldose reductase using neuronal cell culture and ligated rat sciatic nerve. Metabolism 1986; 35:71.
14. Christensen JEJ, Varnek L, Gregersen G. The effect of an aldose reductase inhibitor (Sorbinil) on diabetic neuropathy and neural function of the retina: A double-blind study. Acta Neurol Scand 1985; 71:164.
15. Dvornik D. Aldose Reductase Inhibition. New York, Biomedical Information Corporation (McGraw-Hill), 1987.
16. Dvornik D, Simard-Duquesne N, Krami M, et al. Polyol accumulation in galactosemic and diabetic rats: Control by an aldose reductase inhibitor. Science 1973; 182:1146.
17. Dyck PJ. Hypoxic neuropathy: Does hypoxia play a role in diabetic neuropathy? N Engl J Med 1989; 320:57.
18. Dyck PJ, Giannini C. Pathologic alterations in the diabetic neuropathies of humans: A review. J Neuropathol Exp Neurol 1996; 55:1181.
19. Dyck PJ, Karnes JL, Daube J, et al. Clinical and neuropathological criteria for the diagnosis and staging of diabetic polyneuropathy. Brain 1985; 108:861.
20. Dyck PJ, Zimmerman BR, Vilen TH, et al. Nerve

glucose, fructose, sorbitol, myo-inositol, and fiber degeneration and regeneration in diabetic neuropathy. N Engl J Med 1988; 319:542.

21. Edmands S, Yancey PH. Effects on rat renal osmolytes of extended treatment with an aldose reductase inhibitor. Comp Biochem Physiol 1992; 103C:499.

22. Ekström PAR, Tomlinson DR. Impaired nerve regeneration in streptozotocin-diabetic rats: Effects of treatment with an aldose reductase inhibitor. J Neurol Sci 1989; 93:231.

23. Engerman RL, Kern TS. Aldose reductase inhibition fails to prevent retinopathy in diabetic and galactosemic dogs. Diabetes 1993; 42:820.

24. Fagius J, Brattberg A, Jameson S, et al. Limited benefit of treatment of diabetic polyneuropathy with an aldose reductase inhibitor: A 24-week controlled trial. Diabetologia 1985; 28:323.

25. Fedele D, Negrin P, Fardin P, Tiengo A. Motor conduction velocity (MCV) in insulin-dependent and non-insulin-dependent diabetics with and without clinical peripheral neuropathy. Diabet Metab 1980; 6:189.

26. Finegold D, Lattimer SA, Nolle S, et al. Polyol pathway activity and myo-inositol metabolism: A suggested relationship in the pathogenesis of diabetic neuropathy. Diabetes 1983; 32:988.

27. Florkowski CM, Rowe BR, Nightingale S, et al. Clinical and neurophysiological studies of aldose reductase inhibitor ponalrestat in chronic symptomatic diabetic peripheral neuropathy. Diabetes 1991; 40:129.

28. Gabbay KH, Merola LO, Field RA. Sorbitol pathway: Presence in nerve and cord with substrate accumulation in diabetes. Science 1966; 151:209.

29. Giannini C, Dyck PJ. Axoglial dysjunction: A critical appraisal of definition, techniques, and previous results. Microsc Res Tech 1996; 34:436.

30. Gill JS, Williams G, Ghatei MA, et al. Effect of the aldose reductase inhibitor, ponalrestat, on diabetic neuropathy. Diabet Metab 1990; 16:296.

31. Gillon KRW, Hawthorne JN, Tomlinson DR. Myo-inositol and sorbitol metabolism in relation to peripheral nerve function in experimental diabetes in the rat: The effect of aldose reductase inhibition. Diabetologia 1983; 25:365.

32. Giugliano D, Marfella R, Salvatore T, et al. A double-blind controlled study on the effect of tolrestat on diabetic autonomic neuropathy. Diabetologia 1991; 34(suppl 2):A152.

33. Gonen B, Bochenek WJ, Beg M, et al. The effect of withdrawal of tolrestat, an aldose reductase inhibitor, on signs, symptoms and nerve function in diabetic neuropathy. Diabetologia 1991; 34(suppl 2):A153.

34. Greene DA, Bochenek WJ, Harati Y, et al. Biochemical and morphometric response to tolrestat in human diabetic nerve. Diabetologia 1990; 33(suppl):A92.

35. Greene DA, De Jesus PVJ, Winegrad AI. Effects of insulin and dietary myoinositol on impaired peripheral motor nerve conduction velocity in acute streptozotocin diabetes. J Clin Invest 1975; 55:1326.

36. Greene DA, Lattimer SA. Action of sorbinil in diabetic peripheral nerve: Relationship of polyol (sorbitol) pathway inhibition to a myo-inositol-mediated defect in sodium-potassium ATPase activity. Diabetes 1984; 33:712.

37. Greene DA, Lattimer SA, Ulbrecht J, Carroll PB. Glucose-induced alterations in nerve metabolism: Current perspective on the pathogenesis of diabetic neuropathy and future directions for research and therapy. Diabetes Care 1985; 8:290.

38. Gregersen G. Diabetic neuropathy: Influence of age, sex, metabolic control and duration of diabetes on motor conduction velocity. Neurology 1967; 17:972.

39. Gregersen G. A study of the peripheral nerves in diabetic subjects during ischaemia. J Neurol Neurosurg Psychiatry 1968; 31:175.

40. Guy RJ, Gilbey SG, Sheehy M, et al. Diabetic neuropathy in the upper limb and the effect of twelve months sorbinil treatment. Diabetologia 1988; 31:214.

41. Hale PJ, Nattrass M, Silverman SH, et al. Peripheral nerve concentrations of glucose, fructose, sorbitol and myo-inositol in diabetic and non-diabetic patients. Diabetologia 1987; 30:464.

42. Hirata Y, Okada K. Relation of Na^+, K^+-ATPase to delayed motor nerve conduction velocity: Effect of aldose reductase inhibitor, ADN-138, on Na^+, K^+-ATPase activity. Metabolism 1990; 39:563.

43. Hohman TC, Kwon HM. Tolrestat blocks the glucose-induced down regulation of Na^+/myo-inositol co-transporter mRNA. Diabetologia 1992; 35(suppl 1):398.

44. Holcomb GN, Klemm LA, Dulin WE. The polyol pathway for glucose metabolism in tissues from normal, diabetic, and ketotic Chinese hamsters. Diabetologia 1974; 10:549.

45. Jaspan JB, Herold K, Maselli R, et al. Treatment of severely painful diabetic neuropathy with an aldose reductase inhibitor: Relief of pain and improved somatic and autonomic nerve function. Lancet 1983; 2:758.

46. Judzewitsch RG, Jaspan JB, Polonsky KS, et al. Aldose reductase inhibition improves nerve conduction velocity in diabetic patients. N Engl J Med 1983; 308:119.

47. Kamijo M, Basso M, Cherian PV, et al. Galactosemia produces ARI-preventable nodal changes similar to those of diabetic neuropathy. Diabetes Res Clin Pract 1994; 25:117.

48. Kikkawa R, Hatanaka I, Yasuda H, et al. Prevention of peripheral nerve dysfunction by an aldose reductase inhibitor in streptozotein-diabetic rats. Metabolism 1984; 33:212.

49. Kikkawa R, Hatanaka I, Yasuda H, et al. Effect of a new aldose reductase inhibitor, (E)-3-carboxymethyl-5-((2E)-methyl-3-phenylpropenylidene) rhodanine (ONO-2235), on peripheral nerve disorders in streptozotocin-diabetic rats. Diabetologia 1983; 24:290.

50. Kinoshita JH. Mechanisms initiating cataract formation. Invest Ophthalmol 1974; 13:713.

51. Kinoshita JH, Merola LO, Dikmak E. Osmotic changes in experimental galactose cataracts. Exp Eye Res 1962; 1:405.

52. Lewin IG, O'Brien IAD, Morgan MH, et al. Clinical and neurophysiological studies with the aldose reductase inhibitor, sorbinil, in symptomatic diabetic neuropathy. Diabetologia 1984; 26:445.

53. Lin L-R, Carper D, Yokoyama T, et al. The effect of hypertonicity on aldose reductase, alpha$_B$-crystallin, and organic osmolytes in the retinal pigment epithelium. Invest Ophthalmol Vis Sci 1993; 34:2352.

54. Ludvigson MA, Sorenson RL. Immunohistochemical localization of aldose reductase. I: Enzyme purification and antibody preparation—localization in peripheral nerve, artery and testis. Diabetes 1980; 29:438.

55. Malik RA, Masson EA, Sharma AK, et al. Hypoxic neuropathy: Relevance to human diabetic neuropathy. Diabetologia 1990; 33:311.

56. Martyn CN, Reid W, Young RJ, et al. Six-month treatment with sorbinil in asymptomatic diabetic neuropathy: Failure to improve abnormal nerve function. Diabetes 1987; 36:987.

57. Mayer JH, Tomlinson DR. Prevention of defects of axonal transport and nerve conduction velocity by oral administration of myo-inositol or an aldose reductase inhibitor in streptozotocin-diabetic rats. Diabetologia 1983; 25:433.

58. Mayer JH, Tomlinson DR, McLean WG. Slow orthograde axonal transport of radiolabelled protein in sciatic motoneurones of rats with short-term experimental diabetes: Effects of treatment with an aldose reductase inhibitor or myo-inositol. J Neurochem 1984; 43:1265.

59. Mayhew JA, Gillon KRW, Hawthorne JN. Free and lipid inositol, sorbitol and sugars in sciatic nerve obtained post-mortem from diabetic patients and control subjects. Diabetologia 1983; 24:13.

60. Miwa I, Kanbara M, Okuda J. Improvement of nerve conduction velocity in mutant diabetic mice by aldose reductase inhibitor without affecting nerve myo-inositol content. Chem Pharm Bull 1989; 37:1581.

61. Nickander KK, Schmelzer JD, Rohwer DA, et al. Effect of α-tocopherol deficiency on indices of oxidative stress in normal and diabetic peripheral nerve. J Neurol Sci 1994; 126:6.

62. Notvest RR, Inserra JJ. Tolrestat, an aldose reductase inhibitor, prevents nerve dysfunction in conscious diabetic rats. Diabetes 1987; 36:500.

63. Omawari N, Dewhurst M, Vo PA, et al. Deficient nitric oxide responsible for reduced nerve blood flow in diabetic rats: Effects of L-NAME, L-arginine, sodium nitroprusside and evening primrose oil. Br J Pharmacol 1996; 118:186.

64. Orosz SE, Townsend SF, Tornheim PA, et al. Localization of aldose reductase and sorbitol dehydrogenase in the nervous system of normal and diabetic rats. Acta Diabetol 1981; 18:373.

65. Packer L, Witt EH, Tritschler HJ. Alpha-lipoic acid as a biological antioxidant. Free Radic Biol Med 1995; 19:227.

66. Peterson MJ, Sarges R, Aldinger CE, et al. CP-45, 634: A novel aldose reductase inhibitor that inhibits polyol pathway activity in diabetic and galactosemic rats. Metabolism 1979; 28:456.

67. Powell HC, Garrett RS, Kador PF, et al. Fine-structural localization of aldose reductase and ouabain-sensitive, K(+)-dependent p-nitro-phenylphosphatase in rat peripheral nerve. Acta Neuropathol 1991; 81:529.

68. Price DE, Airey CM, Alani SM, et al. Effect of aldose reductase inhibition on nerve conduction velocity and resistance to ischemic conduction block in experimental diabetes. Diabetes 1988; 37:969.

69. Schmidt RE, Plurad SB, Sherman WR, et al. Effects of aldose reductase inhibitor sorbinil on neuroaxonal dystrophy and levels of myo-inositol and sorbitol in sympathetic autonomic ganglia of streptozotocin-induced diabetic rats. Diabetes 1989; 38:569.

70. Sekiguchi M, Watanabe K, Eto M, et al. Polyol pathway in tissues of spontaneously diabetic Chinese hamsters (Cricetulus griseus) and the effect of an aldose reductase inhibitor, ONO-2235. Comp Biochem Physiol 1991; 98:637.

71. Sima AAF, Bril V, Nathaniel V, et al. Regeneration and repair of myelinated fibers in sural-nerve biopsy specimens from patients with diabetic neuropathy treated with sorbinil. N Engl J Med 1988; 319:548.

72. Sima AAF, Prashar A, Zhang W-X, et al. Preventive effect of long-term aldose reductase inhibition (ponalrestat) on nerve conduction and sural nerve structure in the spontaneously diabetic Bio-Breeding rat. J Clin Invest 1990; 85:1410.

73. Stevens MJ, Lattimer SA, Kamijo M, et al. Osmotically-induced nerve taurine depletion and the compatible osmolyte hypothesis in experimental diabetic neuropathy in the rat. Diabetologia 1993; 36:608.

74. Stewart MA, Kurien MM, Sherman WR, et al. Inositol changes in nerve and lens of galatose fed rats. J Neurochem 1968; 15:941.

75. Stewart MA, Sherman WR, Anthony S. Free sugars in alloxan diabetic rat nerve. Biochem Biophys Res Commun 1966; 22:4.

76. Stewart MA, Sherman WR, Harris JT. Effects of galactose on levels of free myo-inositol in rat tissues. Ann NY Acad Sci 1969; 165:609.

77. Stewart MA, Sherman WR, Kurien MM, et al. Polyol accumulations in nervous tissue of rats with experimental diabetes and galactosaemia. J Neurochem 1967; 14:1057.

78. Storey KB, Miceli M, Butler KW, et al. 31P-NMR studies of the freeze-tolerant larvae of the gall fly, Eurosta solidaginis. Eur J Biochem 1984; 142:591.

79. Stornello M, Valvo EV, Scapellato L. Persistent albuminuria in normotensive non-insulin-dependent (type II) diabetic patients: Comparative effects of angiotensin-converting enzyme inhibitors and β-adrenoceptor blockers. Clin Sci 1992; 82:19.

80. Stribling D, Mirrlees DJ, Harrison HE, et al. Properties of ICI 128,436, a novel aldose reductase inhibitor, and its effects of diabetic complications in the rat. Metabolism 1985; 34:336.

81. Sundkvist G, Lilja B, Rosen I, et al. Autonomic and peripheral nerve function in early diabetic neuropathy: Possible influence of a novel aldose reductase inhibitor on autonomic function. Acta Med Scand 1987; 21:445.

82. Tao R, Uratsu SL, Dandekar AM. Sorbitol synthesis in transgenic tobacco with apple cDNA encoding NADP-dependent sorbitol-6-phosphate dehydrogenase. Plant Cell Physiol 1995; 36:525.

83. Tesfaye S, Malik R, Ward JD. Vascular factors in diabetic neuropathy. Diabetologia 1994; 37:847.

84. Thomas PK. Diabetic neuropathy: Models, mechanisms and mayhem. Can J Neurol Sci 1992; 19(1):1.

85. Tomlinson DR, Holmes PR, Mayer JH. Reversal by treatment with an aldose reductase inhibitor of impaired axonal transport and motor nerve conduction velocity in experimental diabetes mellitus. Neurosci Lett 1982; 31:189.

86. Tomlinson DR, Riaz S, Stevens EJ. Dependence of sciatic nerve blood flow on hind-limb muscle mass: An explanation for the deficits in nerve perfusion in experimental diabetes? Diabet Nutr Metab 1996; 9:258.

87. Tomlinson DR, Sidenius P, Larsen JR. Slow component-a of axonal transport, nerve myo-inositol, and aldose reductase inhibition in streptozocin-diabetic rats. Diabetes 1986; 35:398.

88. Tomlinson DR, Willars GB, Calthrop-Owen EF. Defects of axonal transport in experimental diabetes that are unrelated to the sorbitol pathway. Exp Neurol 1987; 96:194.

89. Tuffin DP, Dingle A, Sennitt CM, et al. Ponalrestat: A potent and selective inhibitor of bovine lens aldose reductase. Prog Lipid Res 1989; 290:221.

90. van Heyningen R. Formation of polyols by the lens of the rat with 'sugar' cataracts. Nature 1959; 184:194.

91. Ward JD, Baker RWR, Davis BH. Effect of blood sugar control on the accumulation of sorbitol and fructose in nervous tissues. Diabetes 1972; 21:1173.

92. Ward WH, Sennitt CM, Ross H, et al. Ponalrestat:

A potent and specific inhibitor of aldose reductase. Biochem Pharmacol 1990; 39:337.

93. Whiteley SJ, Townsend J, Tomlinson DR, et al. Fast anterograde axonal transport in wasted and non-wasted diabetic rats: Effects of aldose reductase inhibition. Diabetes Res Clin Pract 1986; 3:447.

94. Willars GB, Calcutt NA, Tomlinson DR. Reduced anterograde and retrograde accumulation of axonally transported phosphofructokinase in streptozotocin-diabetic rats: Effects of insulin and the aldose reductase inhibitor "Statil." Diabetologia 1987; 30:239.

95. Willars GB, Lambourne JE, Tomlinson DR. Does galactose feeding provide a valid model of the consequences of exaggerated polyol-pathway flux in peripheral nerve in experimental diabetes? Diabetes 1987; 36:1425.

96. Willars GB, Townsend J, Tomlinson DR, et al. Studies on peripheral nerve and lens in long-term experimental diabetes: Effects of the aldose reductase inhibitor statil. Metabolism 1988; 37:442.

97. Yagihashi S, Kamijo M, Ido Y, et al. Effects of long-term aldose reductase inhibition on development of experimental diabetic neuropathy: Ultrastructural and morphometric studies of sural nerve in streptozocin-induced diabetic rats. Diabetes 1990; 39:690.

98. Yasuda H, Sonobe M, Yamashita M, et al. Effect of prostaglandin E_1 analogue TFC 612 on diabetic neuropathy in streptozocin-induced diabetic rats: Comparison with aldose reductase inhibitor ONO 2235. Diabetes 1989; 38:832.

99. Young RJ, Ewing DJ, Clark BF. A controlled trial of sorbinil, an aldose reductase inhibitor, in chronic painful diabetic neuropathy. Diabetes 1983; 32:938.

100. Yue DK, Hanwell MA, Satchell PM, et al. The effect of aldose reductase inhibition on motor nerve conduction velocity in diabetic rats. Diabetes 1982; 31:789.

Chapter 23

Axonal Transport in Diabetic Neuropathy

S. Brimijoin

INTRODUCTION

This chapter deals with the possibility that diabetic neuropathy involves defects in intracellular motility that initiate or exacerbate a pathogenic chain of events. Cellular geometry makes neurons dependent on axonal transport of macromolecules, not only to sustain neurotransmission at distant synapses, but even to elaborate and maintain their peripheral processes. Anterograde axonal transport, from cell body toward the nerve terminals, is a ubiquitous, ATP-driven process with five or more phases, or *components*.[87, 88] A given component moves at a distinctive velocity, extending from about 1 mm/d (slow component-a) up to about 400 mm/d (fast transport). In addition, rapid retrograde transport delivers certain materials from the periphery to the cell body, at a unimodal rate of about 150 mm/d.

Different methods have contributed to our present understanding of axonal transport (Fig. 23.1). One method is based on stopping flow, either reversibly (local cooling) or irreversibly (nerve ligation). When this approach is coupled with specific neurochemical or immunochemical assays, one can measure the local accumulation of many individual substances. The accumulation is a direct index of the total flux of material along a nerve trunk and an indirect index of the actual velocity of trans-

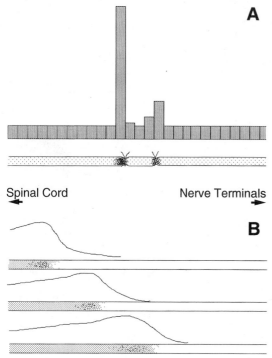

A

Spinal Cord ◄   Nerve Terminals ►

B

■ **Figure 23.1**   Methods for study of axonal transport. *A*, Nerve ligation. The qualitative pattern of accumulation of a typical rapidly transported protein in a doubly ligated nerve is illustrated. Accumulation above the proximal ligature indicates anterograde flux; accumulation below the distal ligature indicates retrograde flux; the interligature zone indicates mean resting concentration. The bar graph shows the relative amounts of material in successive nerve segments analyzed by quantitative assay for specific enzyme activity or protein immunoreactivity. *B*, Pulse radiolabeling. Profiles of radioactivity are illustrated at three successive times after injection of labeled precursor into spinal cord.

port. A second common method is based on pulse-labeling with radioactive protein or lipid precursors. Transport velocity is measured directly from the displacement of the wavefront of incorporated radioactivity as a function of time after introducing radiolabeling into spinal cord or ganglia. When the labeled samples are subjected to high-resolution separation by gel electrophoresis or other techniques, inferences about the nature of the transported material are also possible. A third method is based on optical techniques for direct visualization, typically with the aid of Nomarski video microscopy. This method has been used mainly in cell-free motility assays for studies of transport mechanism, but it can also be used with biopsied human peripheral nerve.

Application of such methods has yielded much information about the different compo-

nents involved in axonal transport. Each transport component or phase reflects the migration of a particular subset of axonal constituents. Examples are the slow-moving neurofilament proteins of slow component-a; the slightly faster moving glycolytic enzymes, actin, and soluble tubulin of slow component-b; and the rapidly transported proteins and lipids associated with synaptic vesicles.[30] The mechanism of the slower phases of transport remains obscure. Faster components of anterograde transport are propelled by microtubule-dependent kinesin ATPases.[9, 80] Several different classes of kinesin motors have been identified in the axons of brain and peripheral nerve, and each may play a specific role in anterograde transport.[11, 21, 56] An entirely separate ATPase motor protein, cytoplasmic dynein, appears to be responsible for rapid retrograde transport.[81, 83] Because of this biochemical diversity it is possible that a pathologic process such as diabetes might lead to selective impairment of one transport component. The result would be to deprive the neuronal extremities of a specific class of organelles and macromolecules or, perhaps equally significant, to cause local accumulations of these materials and thereby generate a characteristic structural abnormality. As yet, this possibility is more a hypothesis and goal for research than an explanation for the recognized features of diabetic neuropathy. Even so, it is worthwhile to consider what is known about the phases of transport and the different stages involved in delivery of proteins and lipids to the neuronal periphery.

The following stages of rapid axonal transport can be identified: (1) packaging of newly synthesized proteins into organelles and loading into the proximal axon; (2) distally directed, kinesin-driven motion (with occasional pauses and transient reversals); (3) arrival at the destination; (4) turnaround—a directional reversal possibly preceded by local incorporation (e.g., in axolemma) and retrieval; and (5) rapid dynein-driven retrograde transport. Not every protein follows the entire sequence, because metabolism or release may intervene. Nevertheless, there are multiple points at which the transport system could be attacked by toxicants or disease, with varying pathologic consequences.

Increased understanding of the physiologic role of axonal transport has aroused interest in the possibility that defects of motility underlie some types of peripheral neuropathy. Few would now argue that generalized failure of transport is a reasonable explanation for diabetic neuropathy, but there is evidence, reviewed in subsequent sections, suggesting that subtler transport disturbances *are* involved. Before turning to the specifics, it may be helpful to consider the general consequences of different transport defects.

ANTEROGRADE TRANSPORT DEFECTS

The most readily imagined type of transport malfunction is a reduction in speed. Some investigators seem to have been obsessed with demonstrating reduced transport rates in diseased nerve. As it happens, major slowing of rapid anterograde transport is rare, especially in the early stages of a disease process. Slow axonal transport appears more vulnerable to retardation, as will become apparent.

Normal axons have surplus capacity for rapidly transported materials and can compensate for reduced velocity by increasing the concentration of material in transit.[15, 17, 28] Hence, small changes in transport velocity are not by themselves physiologically relevant. The meaningful variable is the distal flux of material (amount moved per unit time). To reduce this flux may require extreme slowing or a simultaneous loss of carrying-capacity, for example, as a result of microtubular disorganization.

Delivery of materials to distant sites can also

be reduced, with minimal effects on average velocity, by lowering the probability of continued transport between one region and the next. Reasons could include partial disruption of microtubules, premature reversal of transport, or increased incorporation of transported material into fixed structures. Neurons are profoundly vulnerable to disturbances of this nature. Suppose that, in diabetes, the probability of continued transport over a 100 μm distance were reduced by as little as 0.03%. Cumulative probability of transport over a 1 meter distance (possible for long sensory nerves) would then drop to $(0.9997)^{10000} = 0.05$, a 95% reduction! That kind of transport defect would manifest itself as an altered profile of transported material, with normal displacement of the wavefront (Fig. 23.2). Such profiles have been noted with cytoskeletal proteins in the mutant diabetic mouse[84] and might also occur in human diabetes.

Any defect in anterograde transport that reduced the delivery of essential macromolecules would have important consequences. Depletion of synaptic vesicles and key synaptic proteins, for example, would cause long-term failure of transmission. On the other hand, failure to replenish modulatory neuropeptides, which also must be synthesized in the cell body, would alter the *character* of neurotransmission. That type of effect could be especially promi-

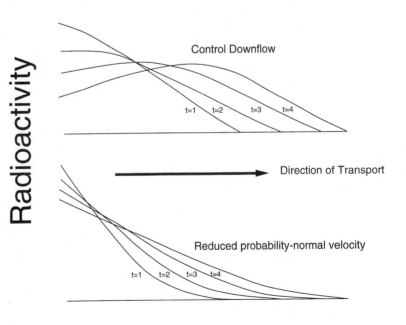

■ Figure 23.2 Effect of an axonal lesion that reduces "transport probability" without affecting maximal velocity. The *lower panel* illustrates an effect that has been observed with slow-transported proteins in streptozotocin-diabetic rats. t indicates time as a parameter.

nent at autonomic synapses, where peptides like neuropeptide Y (NPY), enkephalin, and vasoactive intestinal polypeptide (VIP) are released along with the classic transmitters, noradrenaline and acetylcholine. Neurotransmitter release would also be affected by loss of presynaptic receptors transported from the cell body, as claimed to occur in streptozotocin-diabetes.[44] Loss of transported membrane precursors and associated ion channels would compromise impulse conduction and the renewal of the axolemma. Reduced delivery of neurofilament proteins, which form skeletal elements that determine cross-sectional area,[34, 46] would produce axonal dwindling. Of course, deficits of neurotransmission, reduced impulse condition, and axonal dwindling are all features of the advanced stages of diabetic polyneuropathy.

TURNAROUND DEFECTS

Bray and associates[12] and Bisby[5, 6] first showed that of the protein rapidly transported to the periphery, half returns ultimately to nerve cell bodies by retrograde transport. This circulation involves directional reversal at the terminals or wherever fast transport is interrupted (there is apparently no turnaround of slow components). Impaired turnaround would generate local swellings packed with the membranous organelles that are normally removed by retrograde transport soon after their delivery by rapid anterograde transport (Fig. 22.3). Terminal and preterminal axons would be likely sites for such lesions. As will be discussed further, there is evidence that turnaround defects contribute to distal axonopathy in diabetes.

DEFECTS OF RETROGRADE AXONAL TRANSPORT

Rapid retrograde transport appears to reflect large particles, including multivesicular bodies and prelysosomal structures returning to the somata for disposal, and pinocytotic vesicles carrying trophic signals from the periphery. As mentioned previously, the mechanisms for rapid retrograde and anterograde transport are similar but not identical. Because different motors are involved, selective failure is possible. The result would probably resemble impaired turnaround, except that supply of extraneuronal trophic factors to nerve cell bodies would also be reduced. Moderate deficits of trophic factors would alter patterns of gene expression and protein synthesis, whereas severe deficits

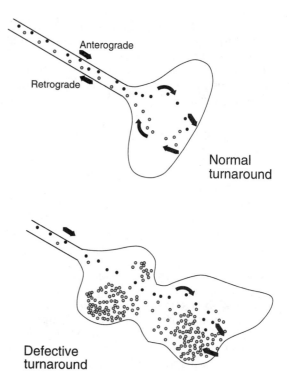

■ Figure 23.3 Turnaround defect. The *upper sketch* illustrates normal balance between delivery of fresh vesicular material (dark fill) by rapid anterograde transport of nerve endings, followed by turnaround and retrograde transport of ''used'' material (light fill). The *lower sketch* illustrates a failure of turnaround or retrograde transport, leading to local swellings filled with membranous structures. Turnaround defects are characteristic of some toxic neuropathies and, probably, diabetic neuropathy.

could cause atrophy and even cell death. There is some evidence for reduced retrograde transport of trophic factors in diabetes (see Axonal Transport in Diabetic Nerve).

POTENTIAL CAUSES OF TRANSPORT DEFECTS

Even a brief look of transport physiology suggests many ways in which diabetes could potentially impair axonal transport. Worth considering are local ischemia, inhibition of glycolysis or oxidative phosphorylation, disturbances in the amounts or organization of cytoskeletal proteins, interference with kinesin or dynein ATPases, and alterations of the ionic balance in axons.

Ischemia. Ischemia is a likely feature of diabetic neuropathy in view of the vascular disease that generally accompanies this disorder.[63] Local ischemia reduces the availability of oxygen and glucose together. Both are important in generating the ATP needed for rapid axonal transport.[60, 61, 66] Actually, transport is surprisingly resistant to moderate hypoxia,[57] although it is readily interrupted by local *anoxia.*[59] Nevertheless, ischemic impairment of transport has been demonstrated experimentally.[42] Furthermore, there are indications that diabetic nerve is particularly prone to the local ischemia associated with focal compression.[23] Therefore, this mechanism is a potential contributor to the peripheral neuropathy in advanced diabetes.

Impairment of Glycolysis or Oxidative Phosphorylation. Any deficiency of energy metabolism will tend to deplete cellular stores of ATP, which are critical for fast transport.[41, 60, 61] If ATP became limiting in the course of diabetes, even as a secondary phenomenon, fast transport would certainly be impaired, and probably other transport components as well. This pathogenic mechanism is worth considering in view of reports that the glycolytic enzymes, 6-phosphofructokinase and aldolase, accumulate at subnormal rates in ligated diabetic nerve.[89] As yet, there is no evidence that this phenomenon actually impairs glycolysis or oxidative phosphorylation in early diabetes, but secondary defects seem likely in later stages of neuropathy.

Cytoskeletal Disturbances. Antimitotic drugs, including colchicine and the vinca alkaloids vinblastine and vincristine, induce the disaggregation of microtubules and block axonal transport.[2, 3, 24, 26, 43] Such effects provided the initial evidence that microtubules are part of the machinery for transport, serving to direct the propulsive forces from extrinsic motors and to determine total transport capacity. Not surprisingly, peripheral neuropathy is the limiting side effect in the use of vinca alkaloids to treat leukemia,[85] probably because transport capacity is severely reduced by microtubular disaggregation.[8, 31] If diabetes did disturb the axonal cytoskeleton, a likely mechanism would be protein glycation. Studies in streptozotocin-treated rats have shown glycation of tubulin,[22] the basic subunit of microtubules, as well as actin,[62] another key cytoskeletal protein. As yet we do not know if these modifications lead to functional abnormalities.

Disturbances of Ionic Balance. Modern studies with permeabilized cells and reconstituted systems of kinesin, microtubules, and isolated organelles show that Mg^{2+}-ATP is suf-

ficient to support transport per se.[10, 81] However, fast transport depends at least indirectly on appropriate axonal cations. Ca^{2+} is important for the loading stage of fast transport and may also affect transport in a regulatory manner[14, 32, 52] Accordingly, long-term changes in levels of divalent cations might be pathologically significant, although the relevance to diabetes is uncertain.

EFFECTS ON TRANSPORT MOTORS

With cytoplasmic dynein and multiple kinesins as transport "motors" exhibiting different drug sensitivities,[82] the possibility of selective toxicity emerges. However, we know of no diseases in which selective attack on transport motors contributes to the pathogenesis of neuropathy, and there appear to have been no studies of kinesins in diabetes.

GENERAL EVIDENCE FOR TRANSPORT ABNORMALITIES IN HUMAN NERVE

If abnormalities of transport are likely causes of peripheral neuropathy in general, transport should be affected in actual diseases of human nerve, including diabetic neuropathy. Although protein radiolabeling is not appropriate in patients, axonal transport persists in vitro and has been studied in biopsied human nerves by enzyme redistribution and optical methods. The results of such experiments do provide a basis for supposing that transport abnormalities are associated with clinical neuropathies.

For enzyme redistribution experiments in human nerve, biopsy samples ligated at both ends are incubated in oxygenated physiologic salt solution; short pieces are later assayed for rapidly transported protein or neurotransmitter. So long as the total protein or transmitter is constant, the accumulation in the distal segment can be attributed to redistribution by anterograde axonal transport. The rate of accumulation reveals the transport flux, that is, the amount of material delivered per unit time. From the length of nerve that must contribute its content each hour to produce the accumulation, one calculates an overall average velocity of transport. Interpretation of this measure is limited by uncertainties about the size of the moving fraction.[16] In favorable cases one can estimate the moving fraction by observing the clearance of marker from the middle of the sample or by identifying a break in the course of accumulation. Even when this is not possible, the average velocity of transport is useful because it is independent of the number of axons in the sample. A reduced average velocity of transport implies an actual slowing or an increased proportion of stationary material. Either would point to an abnormality of transport as opposed to simple loss of fibers.

Several studies of enzyme redistribution in human sural nerve have used dopamine-β-hydroxylase (DBH) and acetylcholinesterase (AChE) as markers. These two enzymes respectively catalyze the biosynthesis of norepinephrine in adrenergic nerves and the hydrolysis of acetylcholine in cholinergic nerves. In biopsy samples from normal volunteers, both enzymes accumulate linearly for several hours.[18]

Some early work on hereditary peripheral neuropathies indicated that when the sensory system was involved, presumably together with sympathetic fibers, there were consistent reductions in DBH transport.[19, 20] More recently, Behrens and colleagues[4] reported complete failure of AChE accumulation in a case of myotonic dystrophy, even though enzyme content was more than 3 SD above the normal mean. In diabetic neuropathy, statistically significant reductions of enzyme content and of average transport velocity have been observed with DBH and with AChE. One recognizes that this information is insufficient to prove a primary pathogenic role for transport defects. Some of the findings, for example, might reflect end-stage axonal damage. However, the abnormalities of enzyme redistribution in neuropathic biopsies are consistent with fundamental disturbances of transport and they merit continued study.

Optical methods are well suited to analysis of transport kinetics in neuropathy. Nearly 20 years ago, differential interference contrast microscopy was applied to axonal transport in large myelinated sural nerve axons from cases of peroneal muscular atrophy, Friedreich's ataxia, and diabetic polyneuropathy.[40] Visible particles were transported in some axons of all samples studied and transport velocity varied considerably from case to case. Conclusions were limited because control biopsy specimens were not available. Another older optical study[58] examined motor nerves in intercostal muscles of patients with amyotrophic lateral sclerosis (ALS). Estimated transport velocity was 30% slower than in normal nerves from patients undergoing radical mastectomy. More recently, Breuer and coworkers used modern video-enhanced–contrast microscopy

and image processing to reexamine axonal transport in ALS.[13, 14] Retrograde and anterograde transport were evaluated statistically in the motor branch of the median nerve. Controls were mostly other somatic nerves from patients undergoing limb amputation for tumors, but the basic kinetics of transport appeared to be independent of nerve type. Interestingly, the only significant kinetic abnormality in ALS nerves was a 57% *increase* in speed of anterograde transport. On the other hand, analysis of traffic density showed a 70% decrease in the number of retrogradely moving organelles per second and per μm^2 of axoplasm. This result is especially interesting because anterograde traffic density was only slightly reduced. Therefore, total anterograde flux may have exceeded retrograde flux by a large margin. An imbalance between anterograde and retrograde traffic does not necessarily imply a defect in transport turnaround, but it may reflect an important biologic abnormality in ALS. To our knowledge, modern optical methods for analyzing intracellular motility have not yet been exploited for studies of diabetic neuropathy.

The data from enzyme and optical studies indicate that some human peripheral nerve diseases may well involve abnormalities of rapid axonal transport. To determine whether the functional abnormalities trigger the associated pathology or whether they merely reflect structural damage from other causes, animal models of neuropathy must be investigated. See Axonal Transport in Diabetic Nerve for current research in this area. Meanwhile, it is worth emphasizing that even a secondary failure of transport could determine the course of neuropathy by inducing axonal atrophy, deficits in axolemmal renewal, impaired nerve conduction, failure of synaptic transmission, degeneration of nerve terminals, loss of trophic interactions, and reactive changes in the perikaryon.

AXONAL TRANSPORT IN DIABETIC NERVE

Evidence for abnormalities of anterograde transport, transport turnaround, and retrograde transport are considered in this section.

Anterograde Transport

The literature shows disagreement about the status of rapid anterograde transport in experimental diabetes, but a few basic points can still be made: (1) it is unlikely that the diabetic state, in itself, leads quickly to a specific impairment of fast transport; (2) when fast transport is affected, the changes are modest, at least early in the course of diabetes; (3) there may be alterations in the total amount delivered per unit time for *some* substances in *some* nerves, perhaps because of changes in protein or peptide synthesis at the level of the cell body. Evidence for these statements is summarized in the following paragraphs.

Most studies based on pulse-radiolabeling techniques[1, 7, 64, 86] have demonstrated no changes in the velocity of fast transported protein, overall. Moderate slowing was observed in two studies, one in streptozotocin-diabetic rats[54] and one in spontaneously diabetic BB Wistar rats.[55] The effects were quantitatively minor, however.

Using the different method of nerve ligation to study specific, rapidly transported proteins in streptozotocin-diabetic rats, Schmidt and associates[71] originally reported slight reductions in flux of the enzyme, AChE. Another group made similar observations on alloxan-diabetic rats.[49] On the other hand, these findings were not confirmed in a third, rather comprehensive study. Thus, in rats examined at five different times, from 3 days to 4 months after induction of streptozotocin diabetes, Jakobsen and collaborators found normal anterograde and retrograde transport of AChE and DBH.[37] Later, Schmidt also reported normal fast anterograde transport of DBH in ileal mesenteric nerve of diabetic rats.[72] Therefore, the basic machinery for rapid axonal transport is able to deliver at least some proteins to the periphery at normal rates and in normal amounts.

Discrepancies have also arisen in studies of fast transported neuropeptides. For example, in ligated nerve of rats with 3 to 4 weeks of streptozotocin diabetes, substance P has been reported to accumulate at about half the normal rate.[65, 77] Apparently identical experiments by others, however, have shown no change in substance P transport at 3 days and significant *increases* at 1 and 3 months.[47] In any case, reduced transport was always accompanied by reduced peptide content in the unligated sciatic nerve and in the dorsal root ganglia. It is logical to infer that the true deficit was not in the transport system but in the production and export of peptide from sensory nerve cell bodies. Reduced synthesis and delivery could explain observations of a decreased substance P content in certain terminal fields, such as gut.[25, 29] Yet other end organs, such as cornea, show no change, and still others, such as iris,

show actual increases.[48] Evidently, more studies of peptide transport are needed to define the dynamics involved in diabetic nerve. By assessing production, delivery, and utilization together, we may hope to learn why peptide levels change in certain systems and what the functional implications are.

Studies of slow anterograde transport in experimental diabetes reveal changes that are more impressive and more consistent than those in rapid transport. The abnormalities are also more likely to stem from disturbances of the underlying transport machinery. Documented effects include a reduced accumulation of cytosolic enzymes such as choline acetyltransferase and phosphofructokinase, which move in slow component-b, and a retardation of the radiolabeled structural protein in slow component-a.[39, 45, 53, 71, 78, 84] Some of these defects are reversed or prevented by insulin, myoinositol, or aldose reductase inhibitors.[51, 76, 79] Such beneficial effects suggest that the transport abnormalities arise directly from defects in carbohydrate metabolism. On the other hand, aldose reductase inhibition seems not to improve slow axonal transport of all substances in diabetic nerve.[45, 78, 89] There is room for doubt, therefore, as to the precise pathogenic role of increased flux through the polyol pathway in diabetes, in terms of effects on this phase of axonal transport. The retardation and reduced flux of neurofilament protein are important nonetheless, and they probably explain the modest but definite axonal dwindling in experimental diabetes.[35, 36]

Mutant mice offer a genetic model of diabetes that avoids the issue of direct neurotoxicity. Transport of norepinephrine is reported to be markedly reduced in the adrenergic fibers of these animals.[27] The reduction is related to insulin deficiency rather than to hyperglycemia because it was corrected by insulin administration and was not seen in genetically related obese mice, which simultaneously displayed hyperglycemia and hyperinsulinemia.[27] Further work on this model has provided evidence for a defect in slow transport as well, with reduced average velocities of actin, tubulin and, especially, neurofilament subunits.[84]

Transport Turnaround and Retrograde Transport

Evidence is mounting to suggest that the characteristic abnormality of fast axonal transport, especially in toxicant-induced neuropathy, is impairment of transport reversal or retrograde transport. Transport turnaround also appears to be abnormal in experimental diabetes.

Abnormalities in the turnaround of rapidly transported proteins were demonstrated first in the experimental neuropathy induced by zinc pyridinethione (ZPT). Using the method of delayed nerve ligation after injecting radioactive amino acid into the spinal cord,[6] Sahenk and Mendell[69] showed a reduced return of labeled protein by retrograde transport in motor nerves of rats fed ZPT for 15 to 20 days. Further analysis indicated that ZPT caused a delay in onset of retrograde transport and a reduction in the amount of returning protein.[69] Parallel experiments failed to detect any consistent effect on fast anterograde transport; the occasional reductions of velocity did not correlate with the symptomatic severity of neuropathy. Sahenk and Mendell concluded that ZPT selectively impaired the turnaround of protein from anterograde to retrograde transport, thereby explaining the accumulation of branched tubular structures in distal axons.[68]

Axonal proteases have been implicated in transport turnaround, and there is evidence that ZPT interferes with this crucial mechanism. Thus, Schroer and associates[73] showed that protease treatment of synaptic vesicles from squid axoplasm converts their in vitro transport from anterograde to retrograde. Martz and coworkers[50] obtained evidence for proteolysis during turnaround in vivo, modifying the apparent mass of specific, vesicular proteins. Especially significant in the present context is the demonstration by Sahenk and Lasek[67] that protease inhibitors profoundly impair transport turnaround when applied directly to axonal tips and also induce organellar accumulations that closely resemble the lesions in ZPT neuropathy. Whether ZPT is itself a protease inhibitor has not yet been established.

Impaired turnaround also seems to be characteristic of experimental diabetes induced by streptozotocin. Jakobsen and Sidenius[38] found a significant reduction in the turnaround and retrograde transport of label associated with rapidly transported glycoconjugates in the sensory nerves of rats with streptozotocin diabetes. This reduction appeared within 1 day after onset of hyperglycemia[75] and persisted for at least 8 weeks.[38] Turnaround was restored when blood sugar was normalized by insulin treatment.[37] Hence, the defect was probably not a primary neurotoxic effect of streptozotocin, but a consequence of deranged carbohydrate metabolism. Interestingly, the turnaround of leucine-labeled material (encompassing essen-tially all transported protein) was much less affected than that of sugar-labeled glycoconjugates.[74] This discrepancy implies that a subset of proteins may be differentially affected in diabetes.

Observations on retrograde transport of ^{125}I-labeled nerve growth factor (^{125}I-NGF) argue in favor of a physiologically meaningful defect of retrograde transport in streptozotocin diabetes. Thus, after administration of ^{125}I-NGF in the hind paw, diabetic rats show a reduced accumulation of radiolabel in dorsal root ganglia and ligated sciatic nerve, as compared with control rats.[37] Schmidt and coworkers obtained similar results in comparable experiments on retrograde transport of exogenous ^{125}I-NGF in ligated ileal nerve.[70] They also showed that the effect persisted in normoglycemic media in vitro and was not reproduced when tissues from normal rats were incubated in hyperglycemic media. More recent experiments have demonstrated that the retrograde transport of *endogenous* NGF is also substantially reduced in a manner that correlates inversely with blood glucose levels.[33] Neural NGF receptors were also poorly saturated under these conditions (i.e., free of ligand). Therefore, one reason for reduced transport may be a deficit of NGF production in innervated tissues. Nevertheless, it appears likely that diabetes does impair turnaround or retrograde transport of at least some neuronal proteins. However, animals with chemically induced diabetes do not develop full-blown neuropathy, so it remains unclear whether defective turnaround plays an important role in the pathogenesis of human diabetic neuropathy.

CONCLUSION

One clear result of the past decade of studies is the increasing sophistication of our ideas about the relationship between axonal transport and diabetic nerve disease. Outright failure of transport would surely cause rapid degeneration and death of the nerve cell, but it is an unlikely cause of most forms of neuropathy. Often, the most important pathology of rapid transport appears to involve defects operating during transport reversal or at stages just before or after this event. In the case of slow transport, there is an emerging consensus that chemical modifications of neurofilament subunits contribute to the development of diabetic neuropathies. The challenge now is to develop fuller biochemical and molecular explanations of these phenomena.

References

1. Bajada S, Sharma AK, Thomas PK. Axoplasmic transport in vagal afferent fibers in normal and alloxan-diabetic rabbits. J Neurol Sci 1980; 47:365.

2. Banks P, Mayor D, Tomlinson D. Further evidence for the involvement of microtubules in the intra-axonal movement of noradrenaline storage vesicles. J Physiol (Lond) 1971; 219:755.

3. Banks P, Till R. A correlation between the effects of antimitotic drugs on microtubule assembly in vitro and the inhibition of axonal transport in noradrenergic neurons. J Physiol (Lond) 1975; 252:283.

4. Behrens MI, Torrealba G, Court J, et al. Axonal transport dysfunction in dystrophia myotonica. Acta Neuropathol (Berl) 1983; 62:157.

5. Bisby MA. Orthograde and retrograde axonal transport of labeled protein in motoneurons. Exp Neurol 1976; 50:628.

6. Bisby MA. Retrograde axonal transport of endogenous protein: Differences between motor and sensory axons. J Neurochem 1977; 28:249.

7. Bisby MA. Axonal transport of labelled protein and regeneration rate in nerves of streptozotocin-diabetic rats. Exp Neurol 1980; 69:74.

8. Bradley WG, Williams MH. Axoplasmic flow in axonal neuropathies. I: Axoplasmic flow in cats with toxic neuropathies. Brain 1973; 96:235.

9. Brady ST. A novel brain ATPase with properties expected for the fast axonal transport motor. Nature 1985; 317:73.

10. Brady ST, Lasek RJ, Allen RD. Video microscopy of fast axonal transport in extruded axoplasm: A new model for study of molecular mechanisms. Cell Motil 1985; 5:81.

11. Brady ST, Sperry AO. Biochemical and functional diversity of microtubule motors in the nervous system. Curr Opin Neurobiol 1995; 5:551.

12. Bray JJ, Kon EM, Breckenridge BM. Reversed polarity of rapid axonal transport in chicken motoneurons. Brain Res 1971; 33:560.

13. Breuer AC, Atkinson MB. Fast axonal transport alterations in amyotrophic lateral sclerosis (ALS) and in parathyroid hormone (PTH)-treated axons. Cell Motil Cytoskeleton 1988; 10:321.

14. Breuer AC, Lynn MB, Atkinson MS, et al. Fast axonal transport in amyotrophic lateral sclerosis: An intra-axonal organelle traffic analysis. Neurology 1987; 37:738.

15. Brimijoin S. On the kinetics and maximal capacity of the system for rapid axonal transport in mammalian neurones. J Physiol (Lond) 1979; 292:325.

16. Brimijoin S. Axonal transport in autonomic nerves: Views on its kinetics. In Kalsner S (ed): Trends in Autonomic Pharmacology. Baltimore, Urban and Schwarzenberg, 1982, p 17.

17. Brimijoin S. Microtubules and the capacity of the system for rapid axonal transport. Fed Proc 1982; 41:2312.

18. Brimijoin S, Capek P, Dyck PJ. Axonal transport of dopamine-beta-hydroxylase by human sural nerves in vitro. Science 1973; 180:1295.

19. Brimijoin S, Dyck PJ. Axonal transport of dopamine-beta-hydroxylase and acetylcholinesterase in human peripheral neuropathy. Exp Neurol 1979; 66:467.

20. Brimijoin S, Dyck PJ, Jakobsen J, et al. Axonal transport in human nerve disease and in the experimental neuropathy induced by p-bromophenylacetylurea. In Weiss DG, Gorio A (eds): Axoplasmic Transport in Physiology and Pathology. Berlin, Springer, 1982, p 124.

21. Coy DL, Howard J. Organelle transport and sorting in axons. Curr Opin Neurobiol 1994; 4:662.

22. Cullum NA, Mahon J, Stringer K, et al. Glycation of rat sciatic nerve tubulin in experimental diabetes mellitus. Diabetologia 1991; 34:387.

23. Dahlin LB, Meiri KF, McLean WG, et al. Effects of nerve compression on fast axonal transport in streptozotocin-induced diabetes mellitus: An experimental study in the sciatic nerve of rats. Diabetologia 1986; 29:181.

24. Dahlström A. Effect of colchicine on transport of amine storage granules in sympathetic nerves of the rat. Eur J Pharmacol 1968; 5:111.

25. Di Giulio AM, Tenconi B, La Croix R, et al. Denervation and hyperinnervation in the nervous system of diabetic animals. I: The autonomic neuronal dystrophy of the gut. J Neurosci Res 1989; 24:355.

26. Friede RL, Ho K-C. The relation of axonal transport of mitochondria with microtubules and other axoplasmic organelles. J Physiol (Lond) 1977; 265:507.

27. Giachetti A. Axoplasmic transport of noradrenaline in the sciatic nerves of spontaneously diabetic mice. Diabetologia 1979; 16:191.

28. Goldberg DJ, Schwartz JH, Sherbany AA. Kinetic properties of normal and perturbed axonal transport of serotonin in a single identified axon. J Physiol (Lond) 1978; 281:559.

29. Gorio A, Di Giulio AM, Tenconi B, et al. Peptide alterations in autonomic diabetic neuropathy prevented by acetyl-L-carnitine. Int J Clin Pharmacol Res 1992; 12:225.

30. Grafstein B, Forman D. Intracellular transport in neurons. Physiol Rev 1980; 60:1167.

31. Green LS, Donoso JA, Heller-Bettinge IE, et al. Axonal transport disturbances in vincristine-induced peripheral neuropathy. Ann Neurol 1977; 1:255.

32. Hammerschlag R. Is the intrasomal phase of fast axonal transport driven by oscillations of intracellular calcium? Neurochem Res 1994; 19:1431.

33. Hellweg R, Raivich G, Hartung HD, et al. Axonal transport of endogenous nerve growth factor (NGF) and NGF receptor in experimental diabetic neuropathy. Exp Neurol 1994; 130:24.

34. Hoffman PN, Lasek RJ. The slow component of axonal transport: Identification of major structural polypeptides of the axon and their generality among mammalian neurons. J Cell Biol 1975; 66:351.

35. Jakobsen J. Axonal dwindling in early experimental diabetes. I: A study of cross-sectioned nerves. Diabetologia 1976; 12:539.

36. Jakobsen J. Axonal dwindling in early experimental diabetes. II: A study of isolated nerve fibers. Diabetologia 1976; 12:547.

37. Jakobsen J, Brimijoin S, Skau K, et al. Retrograde axonal transport of transmitter enzymes, fucose-labeled proteins, and nerve growth factor in streptozotocin-diabetic rats. Diabetes 1981; 30:797.

38. Jakobsen J, Sidenius P. Decreased axonal flux of retrogradely transported glycoproteins in early experimental diabetes. J Neurochem 1979; 33:1055.

39. Jakobsen J, Sidenius P. Decreased axonal transport of structural proteins in streptozotocin diabetic rats. J Clin Invest 1980; 66:292.

40. Kirkpatrick JB, Stern LZ. Axoplasmic flow in human sural nerve. Arch Neurol 1973; 28:308.

41. Kirpekar SM, Prat JC, Wakade AR. Metabolic requirements for the intraaxonal transport of noradrenaline in the cat hypogastric nerve. J Physiol (Lond) 1973; 228:173.

42. Korthals JK, Korthals MA, Wisniewski HM. Peripheral nerve ischemia. Part 2: Accumulation of organelles. Ann Neurol 1978; 4:487.

43. Kreutzberg GW. Neuronal dynamics and axonal flow. IV: Blockade of intraaxonal enzyme transport by colchicine. Proc Natl Acad Sci USA 1969; 62:722.

44. Laduron PM, Janssen PF. Impaired axonal transport of opiate and muscarinic receptors in streptozocin-diabetic rats. Brain Res 1986; 380:359.

45. Larsen JR, Sidenius P. Slow axonal transport of structural polypeptides in rat, early changes in streptozocin diabetes, and effect of insulin treatment. J Neurochem 1989; 52:390.

46. Lasek RJ, Hoffman PN. The neuronal cytoskeleton, axonal transport and axonal growth. *In* Goldman R, Pollard T, Rosenbaum J (eds): Cell Motility. Cold Spring Harbor Press, Cold Spring Harbor Conferences on Cell Proliferation Series, 1976, vol 3, p 1021.

47. MacLean DB. Substance P and somatostatin content and transport in vagus and sciatic nerves of the streptozocin-induced diabetic rat. Diabetes 1987; 36:390.

48. Marfurt CF, Echtenkamp SF. The effect of diabetes on neuropeptide content in the rat cornea and iris. Invest Opthalmol Vis Sci 1995; 36:1100.

49. Marini P, Vitadello M, Bianchi R, et al. Impaired axonal transport of acetylcholinesterase in the sciatic nerve of alloxan-diabetic rats: Effect of ganglioside treatment. Diabetologia 1986; 29:254.

50. Martz D, Garner J, Lasek RJ. Protein changes during anterograde-to-retrograde conversion of axonally transported vesicles. Brain Res 1989; 476:199.

51. Mayer JH, Tomlinson DR. Prevention of defects of axonal transport and nerve conduction velocity by oral administration of myo-inositol or an aldose reductase inhibitor in streptozotocin-diabetic rats. Diabetologia 1983; 25:433.

52. McNiven MA, Ward JB. Calcium regulation of pigment transport in vitro. J Cell Biol 1988; 106:111.

53. Medori R, Autilio-Gambetti L, Monaco S, et al. Experimental diabetic neuropathy: Impairment of slow axonal transport with changes in cross-sectional area. Proc Natl Acad Sci USA 1985; 82:7716.

54. Meiri KF, McLean WG. Axonal transport of protein in motor fibres of experimentally diabetic rats: Fast anterograde transport. Brain Res 1982; 238:77.

55. Mendell JR, Sahenk Z, Warmolts JR, et al. The spontaneously diabetic BB Wistar rat: Morphologic and physiologic studies of peripheral nerve. J Neurol Sci 1981; 52:103.

56. Moore JD, Endow SA. Kinesin proteins: A phylum of motors for microtubule-based motility. Bioessays 1996; 18:207.

57. Nagata H, Brimijoin S, Low P, et al. Slow axonal transport in experimental hypoxia and in neuropathy induced by p-bromophenylacetylurea. Brain Res 1987; 422:319.

58. Norris FA Jr. Axon particle movement in motor neuron disease. Trans Am Neurol Assoc 1976; 101:1.

59. Ochs S. Local supply of energy to the fast axoplasmic transport mechanism. Proc Natl Acad Sci USA 1971; 68:1279.

60. Ochs S, Hollingsworth D. Dependence of fast axoplasmic transport in nerve on oxidative metabolism. J Neurochem 1971; 18:107.

61. Ochs S, Smith CB. Fast axoplasmic transport in mammalian nerve in vitro after block glycolysis with iodoacetic acid. J Neurochem 1971; 18:833.

62. Pekiner C, Cullum NA, Hughes JN, et al. Glycation of brain actin in experimental diabetes. J Neurochem 1993; 61:436.

63. Pirart J. Diabetic neuropathy: A metabolic or vascular disease? Diabetes 1965; 14:1.

64. Robinson JP, Tomlinson DR. Fast anterograde axonal transport of choline-containing lipids in rats with experimental diabetes. J Neurol Sci 1987; 81:93.

65. Robinson JP, Willars GB, Tomlinson DR, et al. Axonal transport and tissue contents of substance P in rats with long-term streptozotocin-diabetes. Effects of the aldose reductase inhibitor "statil." Brain Res 1987; 426:339.

66. Sabri MI, Ochs S. Relation of ATP and creatine phosphate to fast axoplasmic transport in mammalian nerve. J Neurochem 1972; 19:2821.

67. Sahenk Z, Lasek RJ. Inhibition of proteolysis blocks anterograde-to-retrograde conversion of axonally transported vesicles. Brain Res 1988; 460:199.

68. Sahenk Z, Mendell JR. Ultrastructural study of zinc pyridinethione-induced peripheral neuropathy. J Neuropathol Exp Neurol 1979; 38:532.

69. Sahenk Z, Mendell JR. Axoplasmic transport in zinc pyridinethione neuropathy: Evidence for an abnormality in distal turn-around. Brain Res 1980; 186:343.

70. Schmidt RE, Grabau GG, Yip HK. Retrograde axonal transport of [^{125}I] nerve growth factor in ileal mesenteric nerves in vitro: Effect of streptozotocin diabetes. Brain Res 1986; 378:325.

71. Schmidt RE, Matschinsky FM, Godfrey DA, et al. Fast and slow axoplasmic flow in sciatic nerve of diabetic rats. Diabetes 1975; 3:24.

72. Schmidt RE, Modert CW, Grabau GG. Orthograde and retrograde axonal transport of dopamine-b-hydroxylase in ileal mesenteric nerves of rats with chronic streptozotocin diabetes. Brain Res 1987; 410:142.

73. Schroer TA, Brady ST, Kelly RB. Fast axonal transport of foreign synaptic vesicles in squid axoplasm. J Cell Biol 1985; 101:568.

74. Sidenius P, Jakobsen J. Axonal transport in early experimental diabetes. Brain Res 1979; 173:315.

75. Sidenius P, Jakobsen J. Retrograde axonal transport: A possible role in the development of neuropathy. Diabetologia 1981; 20:110.

76. Tomlinson DR, Mayer JH. Reversal of deficits in axonal transport and nerve conduction velocity by treatment of streptozotocin-diabetic rats with myo-inositol. Exp Neurol 1985; 89:420.

77. Tomlinson DR, Robinson JP, Willars GB, et al. Deficient axonal transport of substance P in streptozocin-induced diabetic rats: Effects of sorbinil and insulin. Diabetes 1988; 37:488.

78. Tomlinson DR, Sidenius P, Larsen JR. Slow component-a of axonal transport, nerve myo-inositol, and aldose reductase inhibition in streptozocin-diabetic rats. Diabetes 1985; 35:398.

79. Tomlinson DR, Townsend J, Fretten P. Prevention of defective axonal transport in streptozocin-diabetic rats by treatment with "Statil" (ICI 128436), an aldose reductase inhibitor. Diabetes 1985; 34:970.

80. Vale RD, Reese TS, Sheetz MP. Identification of a novel force-generating protein, kinesin, involved in microtubule-based motility. Cell 1985; 42:39.

81. Vale RD, Schnapp BJ, Mitchison T, et al. Different axoplasmic proteins generate movement in opposite directions along microtubules in vitro. Cell 1985; 43:623.

82. Valee RB, Sheetz MP. Targeting of motor proteins. Science 1995; 271:1539.

83. Vallee RB, Shpetner HS, Paschal BM. The role of dynein in retrograde axonal transport. Trends Neurosci 1989; 12:66.

84. Vitadello M, Filliatreau G, Dupont JL, et al. Altered

axonal transport of cytoskeletal proteins in the mutant diabetic mouse. J Neurochem 1985; 45:860.

85. Weiss HD, Walker MD, Wiernik PH. Neurotoxicity of commonly used antineoplastic drugs. N Engl J Med 1974; 291:127.

86. Whitely SJ, Townsend J, Tomlinson DR, et al. Fast orthograde axonal transport in sciatic motoneurones and nerve temperature in streptozotocin-diabetic rats. Diabetologia 1985; 28:8471.

87. Willard M, Cowan WM, Vagelos PR. The polypeptide composition of intraaxonally transported proteins. Evidence for four transport velocities. Proc Natl Acad Sci USA 1974; 71:2183.

88. Willard M, Hulebak KL. The intraaxonal transport of polypeptide H: Evidence for a fifth (very slow) group of transported proteins in the retinal ganglion cells of the rabbit. Brain Res 1977; 136:289.

89. Willars GB, Calcutt NA, Tomlinson DR. Reduced anterograde and retrograde accumulation of axonally transported phosphofructokinase in streptozotocin-diabetic rats: Effects of insulin and the aldose reductase inhibitor "Statil." Diabetologia 1987; 30:239.

Chapter 24

Advanced Glycation End Products and Diabetic Peripheral Neuropathy

Michael Brownlee

INTRODUCTION

The Diabetes Control and Complications Trial (DCCT) established unequivocally that the effects of inadequate insulin action (as monitored by the level of hyperglycemia) are associated with the incidence of diabetic neuropathy. In this landmark study, the intensively treated groups had an overall incidence reduction of 64%.[17] The clinical manifestations of hyperglycemia-induced peripheral sensory neuropathy reflect the combined effects of microvascular and neuronal damage. Axonal degeneration occurs in a spatial distribution that suggests multifocal ischemia.[18, 58] Capillary closure is frequently observed in the vasa nervorum, and endoneurial blood flow and oxygen tension are reduced.[36] Thus, hyperglycemia-induced injury to peripheral nerve fibers in diabetes appears to be secondary to microvascular abnormalities. Once injury has occurred, axonal regrowth and myelination are markedly impaired,[41] and reduced gene expression or axonal transport is observed for neurotropins such as nerve growth factor (NGF) and neurotrophin-3 (NT-3).[60]

How does hyperglycemia induce these functional and morphologic changes? For the microvascular dysfunction that figures prominently in the initial damage of diabetic sensory nerve fibers, increasing evidence points to a major role for sugar-derived advanced glycation end products (AGEs), which form inside and outside cells as a function of glucose concentration. For the neuronal dysfunction that impairs nerve fiber regeneration, fewer mechanistic data exist, but there is suggestive evidence that excessive glycation may play an important role in this process as well.

ADVANCED GLYCATION END PRODUCTS FORM NONENZYMATICALLY FROM SUGAR-DERIVED INTERMEDIATES

Increases in AGE accumulation precede and are accompanied by histologic evidence of diabetic microvascular damage in retina and kidney.[3, 28, 42] In both animal and human diabetic peripheral nerve, levels of the AGE pentosidine are high, and there is increased cross-linking (see next section) of cytoskeletal protein fractions.[49, 50]

Advanced glycation end products may arise by several mechanisms. It has long been recognized that AGEs can be produced by autoxidation of the so-called Amadori product, a 1-amino-1-deoxyketose produced by the reaction of reducing sugars with protein amino groups.[17] This occurs via reactive dicarbonyl intermediates such as 3-deoxyglucosone. Recently, it has been shown that dicarbonyl AGE intermediates may also form from metal-catalyzed autoxidation of sugars, with glyoxal and arabinose as intermediates. Nonoxidative pathways also exist, the best studied of which involves generation of the reactive dicarbonyl methylglyoxal from triose phosphates formed during glycolysis.[1, 2, 5, 22, 25, 29, 32–34, 43, 44, 47, 66, 69] In vivo, the Amadori product appears to be the more significant precursor of AGEs,[67] whereas in vitro it appears that about 50% of the AGE carboxymethyllysine originates from Amadori product oxidation, and 50% by other pathways.[26] In cultured endothelial cells, however, increased methylglyoxal production accounts for all of the increase in AGE formation.[55] Glucose has the slowest rate of glycosylation product formation of any naturally occurring sugar. Thus, the rate of AGE formation by such intracellular sugars as fructose, glucose-6-phosphate, and glyceraldehyde-3-phosphate is considerably faster than the rate for glucose.[43] For this reason, the rate of intracellular AGE formation is much more rapid than the rate of AGE formation in the extracellular compartment.

The reactive dicarbonyl intermediates formed from Amadori products and from sugars react with protein amino groups to form a variety of AGEs. Increased levels of both 3-deoxyglucosone and methyglyoxal have been reported in diabetes.[1, 65, 70] A 2-oxoaldehyde reductase that has been isolated and cloned reduces 3-deoxyglucosone to 3-deoxyfructose. This enzyme appears to be identical to aldehyde reductase.[56] Glyoxalase I specifically converts methylglyoxal to D-lactate via the intermediate S-D-lactoylglutathione.[59] The nature and efficiency of such enzymes could be an important determinant of the amount of AGEs that form at any given level of blood glucose in both diabetic and nondiabetic patients. Inherited differences in the ability to enzymatically detoxify AGE-intermediates such as 3-deoxyglucosone and/or methylglyoxal may be one important genetic factor responsible for determining the impact of a given level of glycemia on diabetic complications.

There are three general mechanisms by which AGE formation may cause pathologic changes. First, extracellular AGEs alter matrix-matrix, matrix-cell, and cell-cell interactions. Second, AGE interactions with cellular receptors alter the level of gene expression for a variety of molecules involved in the genesis of vascular, and perhaps also neural pathology, by generation of reactive oxygen species and activation of the pleiotropic transcription factor NFκB. Third, rapid intracellular AGE formation by glucose, fructose, and more highly reactive metabolic pathway–derived intermediates can directly alter protein function in cells that do not require insulin for glucose transport, such as microvascular endothelial cells and neurons.

ADVANCED GLYCATION END PRODUCTS INTERFERE WITH NORMAL MATRIX-MATRIX, MATRIX-CELL, AND CELL-CELL INTERACTIONS

Formation of AGEs alters the functional properties of several important matrix molecules. Collagen was the first matrix protein used to demonstrate that glucose-derived AGEs form covalent, intermolecular bonds.[8, 35] On type I collagen, this cross-linking induces an expansion of the molecular packing.[57] Soluble plasma proteins such as low-density lipoprotein (LDL) and immunoglobulin (Ig) G are also covalently cross-linked by AGEs on collagen.[6, 7, 54] The luminal narrowing that characterizes diabetic vessels may arise, in part, from accumulation of subendothelial AGE-linked plasma proteins.

Formation of AGEs on type IV collagen from basement membrane inhibits lateral association of these molecules into a normal network-like structure by interfering with binding of the noncollagenous NC1 domain to the helix-rich domain.[61] In vitro AGE formation on intact glomerular basement membrane increases its permeability.[15]

Formation of AGEs on extracellular matrix not only interferes with matrix-matrix interactions, it interferes with matrix-cell interactions as well. Modification by AGEs of type IV collagen's cell-binding domains decreases endothelial cell adhesion, for example.[27] Modification by AGEs of either basement membrane components or whole retinal basement membrane causes reduced proliferation of retinal pericytes and increased proliferation of retinal endothelial cells; the same changes are observed in diabetic patients.[31] These AGE-induced abnormalities in extracellular matrix function alter the structure and function of intact vessels. The AGEs decrease elasticity in large vessels from diabetic rats, even after vascular tone is abolished, and increase fluid filtration across the carotid artery.[30] Defects in the vasodilatory response to nitric oxide correlate with the level of accumulated AGEs in diabetic animals because of dose-dependent quenching by AGEs. Formation of AGEs also appears to be responsible for the restricted hypotonic swelling of peripheral nerve myelin in diabetic animals, which reflects altered myelin membrane structure and interation.[37]

The decreased regenerative response of neurons to injury in diabetes may reflect, in part, AGE formation of laminin. Formation of AGE on laminin causes decreased polymer self-assembly, decreased binding to type IV collagen, and decreased binding of heparin sulfate proteoglycan.[14] Normally, interaction with a six–amino acid sequence in the A chain of the laminin molecule is necessary for nerve regeneration. When AGEs are present on the lysine residue of this sequence, neurite outgrowth is markedly reduced.[21]

ADVANCED GLYCATION END PRODUCT RECEPTORS MEDIATE PATHOLOGIC CHANGES IN GENE EXPRESSION

Specific receptors for AGEs were first identified on monocytes and macrophages. Protein binding of AGEs to this receptor stimulates macrophage production of interleukin-1, insulin-like growth factor I, tumor necrosis factor α, and granulocyte/macrophage colony-simulating

factor at levels that have been shown to increase glomerular synthesis of type IV collagen and to stimulate proliferation of both arterial smooth muscle cells and macrophages.[38, 62, 72]

Vascular endothelial cells also express AGE-specific receptors. A 35-kD and a 46-kD AGE-binding protein have been purified to homogeneity from endothelial cells.[46, 52, 53] The N-terminal sequence of the 35-kD protein was identical to lactoferrin, whereas the 46-kD protein was novel. A full-length 1.5-kb cDNA for the 46-kD protein was cloned and sequenced. This novel AGE-binding protein appears to be a member of the Ig superfamily, with 3 disulfide-bonded immunoglobulin homology units. In endothelial cells, AGE binding to its receptor induces changes in gene expression that include alterations in thrombomodulin, tissue factor, and vascular cell adhesion molecule 1.[20, 51, 63] These changes induce procoagulatory changes in the endothelial surface and increase the adhesion of inflammatory cells to the vessel wall. In addition, endothelial AGE-receptor binding appears to mediate in part the hyperpermeability induced by diabetes.[64]

The AGE-receptor appears to mediate signal transduction through the generation of oxygen free radicals. Reactive oxygen species are generated by AGE binding to endothelial cells. These reactive oxygen species activate the free radical–sensitive transcription factor NFκB, a pleiotropic regulator of many "response-to-injury" genes. This signal transduction cascade can be blocked by antibodies to either of the AGE-receptor components and by antibodies to AGEs themselves.[71] The antioxidant alpha lipoic acid blocks the AGE receptor–induced production of oxygen radicals and activation of NFκB in cultured endothelial cells,[4] which may explain its beneficial effect in the treatment of diabetic peripheral sensory neuropathy.[45, 73]

Intracellular AGE formation may also affect DNA function directly. The AGEs form on prokaryotic DNA in vitro and cause mutations and DNA transposition in bacteria and mammalian cells.[9–11, 39] Incubation of nucleotides with Amadori products or methylglyoxal yields N2-1-(1-carboxyethyl)guanine as a major AGE product.[48]

ADVANCED GLYCATION END PRODUCTS INCREASE MUCH MORE RAPIDLY INSIDE CELLS THAN OUTSIDE, ALTERING INTRACELLULAR PROTEIN FUNCTION

Advanced glycation end products have been thought to form only on long-lived extracellular macromolecules, since the rate of AGE formation from glucose is so slow that more rapidly turned over intracellular proteins would not exist long enough to accumulate them. Recently, however, it has been demonstrated that AGEs do, in fact, form on proteins in vivo. After only 1 week, AGE content increases 13.8-fold in endothelial cells cultured in high glucose–containing media.[23] This extremely rapid rate of AGE formation most likely reflects hyperglycemia-induced increases in intracellular glycolytic intermediates, which are much more reactive than glucose. Recently, we demonstrated[55] that hyperglycemia-induced increases in endothelial cell macromolecular endocytosis can be completely prevented by inhibition of methylglyoxal-derived intracellular AGEs. These data support the hypothesis that AGE modification of intracellular proteins can alter vascular cell function.

In diabetic rat brain, glycated tubulin exhibits less guanosine triphosphate (GTP)–induced polymerization than tubulin from nondiabetic controls.[68] In vitro, glycation profoundly inhibits GTP-dependent tubulin polymerization. These findings provide support for the notion that AGE-modification of cytoskeletal proteins interferes with axoplasmic transport of essential neurotrophic factors such as NGF in diabetes.[60]

PREVENTION OF NEUROPATHY BY AMINOGUANIDINE, AN INHIBITOR OF ADVANCED GLYCATION END PRODUCT FORMATION

Pharmacologic agents that specifically inhibit AGE formation have made it possible to investigate the role of AGEs in the development of diabetic complications in animal models. The hydrazine compound aminoguanidine was the first AGE inhibitor discovered,[8] and it has been by far the most extensively studied. Aminoguanidine reacts mainly with non–protein-bound dicarbonyl intermediates such as 3-deoxyglucosone[19] and methylglyoxal.[40] In addition to inhibiting AGE formation, aminoguanidine has been shown to inhibit the inducible form of nitric oxide synthase in vitro.[16] Aminoguanidine has been shown to prevent diabetes-induced changes in neuronal blood flow and concomitant electrophysiologic abnormalities (LOW 4). These effects of aminoguanidine appear to reflect an augmentation of nitric oxide, rather than an inhibition, perhaps by inhibiting nitric oxide–consuming free radicals generated by AGE formation.[12, 24]

In peripheral nerve of diabetic rats, both motor nerve and sensory nerve conduction velocity are decreased after 8 weeks of diabetes.[13] Nerve action–potential amplitude is decreased by 37%, and peripheral nerve blood flow is decreased by 57% after 24 weeks of diabetes.[36] Aminoguanidine treatment prevents each of these abnormalities of diabetic peripheral nerve function.[13, 36] Whether these effects reflect AGE inhibition or other pharmacologic properties of aminoguanidine remains to be determined. The place of aminoguanidine and other inhibitors of AGE formation in the treatment of diabetic peripheral sensory neuropathy must ultimately be defined by multicentered, randomized, double-blinded clinical studies. Positive effects of aminoguanidine treatment on diabetic microvascular disease in ongoing human trials would provide a strong rationale for undertaking such studies in the future.

References

1. Atkins TW, Thornally PH. Erythrocyte glyoxalase activity in genetically obese and streptozotocin diabetic mice. Diabetes Res 1989; 11:125–129.
2. Baynes JW, Thorpe SR, Murtiashaw MH. Nonenzymatic glycosylation of lysine residues in albumin. Methods Enzymol 1984; 106:88–98.
3. Beisswenger PJ, Makita Z, Curphey TJ, et al. Formation of immunochemical advanced glycosylation end products precedes and correlates with early manifestations of renal and retinal disease in diabetes. Diabetes 1995; 44:824–829.
4. Bierhaus A, Chevion S, Chevion M, et al. Advanced glycation end product-induced activation of NF-kappaB is suppressed by alpha-lipoic acid in cultured endothelial cells. Diabetes 1997; 46:1481–1490.
5. Brownlee M. Advanced products of non-enzymatic glycosylation and the pathogenesis of diabetic complications. In Rifkin H, Porte D Jr (eds): Diabetes Mellitus: Theory and Practice. New York, Elsevier, 1990, pp 279–292.
6. Brownlee M, Pongor S, Cerami A. Covalent attachment of soluble protein by nonenzymatically glycosylated collagen: Role in the in situ formation of immune complexes. J Exp Med 1983; 158:1739–1744.
7. Brownlee M, Vlassara H, Cerami A. Non-enzymatic glycosylation products on collagen covalently trap low-density lipoprotein. Diabetes 1985; 34:938–941.
8. Brownlee M, Vlassara H, Kooney T, et al. Aminoguanidine prevents diabetes-induced arterial wall protein cross-linking. Science 1986; 232:1629–1632.
9. Bucala R, Lee AT, Rourke L, et al. Transposition of an Alu-containing element induced by DNA-advanced glycosylation endproducts. Proc Natl Acad Sci USA 1993; 90:2666–2670.
10. Bucala R, Model P, Cerami A: Modification of DNA by reduced sugars: A possible mechanism for nucleic acid aging and age-related dysfunction in gene expression. Proc Natl Acad Sci USA 1984; 81:105–109.
11. Bucala R, Model R, Russl M, et al. Modification of DNA by glucose-6-phosphate induces DNA rearrangements in an E. coli plasmid. Proc Natl Acad Sci USA 1985; 82:8439–8442.

12. Cameron NE, Cotter MA. Rapid reversal by aminoguanidine of the neurovascular effects of diabetes in rats: Modulation by nitric oxide synthase inhibition. Metabolism 1996; 45:1147–1152.

13. Cameron NE, Cotter MA, Dines K, et al. Effects of aminoguanidine on peripheral nerve function and polyol pathway metabolites in streptozotocin-diabetic rats. Diabetologia 1992; 35:946–950.

14. Charonis AS, Reger LA, Dege JE, et al. Laminin alterations after in vitro nonenzymatic glycosylation. Diabetes 1988; 39:807–814.

15. Cochrane SM, Robinson GB. In vitro glycation of a glomerular basement membrane alters its permeability: A possible mechanism in diabetic complications. FEBS Letters 1995; 375:41–44.

16. Corbett JA, Tilton RG, Chang K, et al. Aminoguanidine, a novel inhibitor of nitric oxide formation, prevents diabetic vascular dysfunction. Diabetes 1992; 41:552–556.

17. Diabetes Control and Complications Trial Research Group. N Engl J Med 1993; 329:683–689.

18. Dyck PJ. Hypoxic neuropathy: Does hypoxia play a role in diabetic neuropathy? Neurology 1989; 39:111–118.

19. Edelstein D, Brownlee M. Mechanistic studies of advanced glycosylation end product inhibition by aminoguanidine. Diabetes 1992; 41:26–29.

20. Esposito C, Gerlach H, Brett J, et al. Endothelial receptor-mediated binding of glucose modified albumin is associated with increased monolayer permeability and modulation of cell surface coagulant properties. J Exp Med 1992; 170:1387–1407.

21. Federoff HJ, Lawrence D, Brownlee M. Non enzymatic glycosylation of laminin and the laminin peptide CIKVAVS inhibits neurite outgrowth. Diabetes 1993; 42:509–513.

22. Fu M-X, Wells-Knecht KJ, Blackledge JA, et al. Glycation, glycoxidation, and cross-linking of collagen by glucose: Kinetics, mechanisms and inhibition of late stages of the Maillard reaction. Diabetes 1994; 43:676–684.

23. Giardino I, Edelstein D, Brownlee M. Nonenzymatic glycosylation in vitro and in bovine endothelial cells alters basic fibroblast growth factor activity. J Clin Invest 1994; 94:110–117.

24. Giardino I, Fard AK, Hatchell DL, et al. Aminoguanidine inhibits ROS formation, lipid peroxidation, and oxidant-induced apoptosis. Diabetes 1998; 47:1114–1120.

25. Giardino I, Horiuchi S, Brownlee M. Accelerated formation of extracellular advanced glycation end products (AGE's) detected by a specific monoclonal antibody. Diabetes 1994; 43:320.

26. Glomb MA, Monnier VM. Mechanisms of protein modification by glyoxal and glycoaldehyde, reactive intermediates of the Maillard reaction. J Biol Chem 1995; 270:10017–10026.

27. Haitoglou CS, Tsilibary EC, Brownlee M, et al. Altered cellular interactions between endothelial cells and nonenzymatically glycosylated laminin/type IV collagen. J Biol Chem 1992; 267:12404–12407.

28. Hammes H-P, Martin S, Federlin K, et al. Aminoguanidine treatment inhibits the development of experimental diabetic retinopathy. Proc Natl Acad Sci USA 1991; 88:11555–11558.

29. Higgins PJ, Bunn HF. Kinetic analysis of the nonenzymatic glycosylation of hemoglobin. J Biol Chem 1981; 256:5204–5208.

30. Huijberts MSP, Wolffenbuttel BRH, Struijker Boudier HAJ, et al. Aminoguanidine treatment increases elasticity and decreases fluid filtration of large arteries from diabetic rats. J Clin Invest 1993; 92:1407–1411.

31. Kalfa TA, Gerritsen ME, Carlson EC, et al. Altered proliferation of retinal microvascular cells on glycated matrix. Invest Ophthalmol Vis Sci 1995; 36:2358–2367.

32. Kato H, Cho RK, Okitani A, et al. Responsibility of 3 deoxyglucosone for the glucose induced polymerization of proteins. Agric Biol Chem 1987; 51:683–687.

33. Kato H, Hayase F, Shin DB, et al. 3-Deoxyglucasone, an intermediate product of the Maillard reaction. In Baynes JW, Monnier VM (eds): The Maillard Reaction in Aging, Diabetes and Nutrition: An NIH Conference. New York, Alan R Liss, 1989, pp 69–84.

34. Kato H, Shin DB, Hayase F. 3,Deoxyglucasone cross links proteins under physiological conditions. Agric Biol Chem 1987; 51:2009–2013.

35. Kent MJC, Light ND, Bailey AJ. Evidence for glucose-mediated covalent cross-linking of collagen after glycosylation in vitro. Biochem J 1985; 225:745–752.

36. Kihara M, Schmelzer JD, Poduslo JF, et al. Aminoguanidine effects on nerve blood flow, vascular permeability, electrophysiology, and oxygen free radicals. Proc Natl Acad Sci USA 1991; 88(14):6107–6111.

37. Kirschner DA, Eichberg J. Restricted hypotonic swelling of peripheral nerve myelin in streptozotocin-induced diabetic rats. J Neurosci Res 1994; 38(2):142–148.

38. Kirstein M, Aston C, Hintz R, et al. Receptor-specific induction of insulin-like growth factor I in human monocytes by advanced glycosylation end product-modified proteins. J Clin Invest 1992; 90:439.

39. Lee AT, Cerami A. Elevated glucose 6-phosphate levels are associated with plasmid mutations in vivo. Proc Natl Acad Sci USA 1987; 84:8311–8314.

40. Lo TW, Selwood T, Thornalley PJ. The reaction of methylglyoxal with aminoguanidine under physiological conditions and prevention of methylglyoxal binding to plasma proteins. Biochem Pharmacol 1994; 48:1865–1870.

41. Longo FM, Powell HC, Lebeau J, et al. Delayed nerve regeneration in streptozotocin diabetic rats. Muscle Nerve 1986; 9:385–393.

42. Mitsuhashi T, Nakayama H, Itch S, et al. Immunochemical detection of advanced glycation end products in renal cortex from STZ induced diabetic rat. Diabetes 1993; 42:826–832.

43. Monnier V. Toward a Maillard reaction theory of aging. In Baynes JW, Monnier VM (eds): The Maillard Reaction in Aging, Diabetes and Nutrition: An NIH Conference. New York, Alan R Liss, 1989, pp 1–22.

44. Mortensen HB, Christophersen C. Glycosylation of human haemoglobin A in red blood cells studied in vitro: Kinetics of the formation and dissociation of haemoglobin A1c. Clin Chim Acta 1983; 134:317–326.

45. Nagamatsu M, Nickander KK, Schmelzer JD, et al. Lipoic acid improves nerve blood flow, reduces oxidative stress, and improves distal nerve conduction in experimental diabetic neuropathy. Diabetes Care 1995; 18:1160–1167.

46. Neeper M, Schmidt AM, Brett J, et al. Cloning and expression of RAGE: A cell surface receptor for advanced glycosylation end products of proteins. J Biol Chem 1992; 267:14998–15004.

47. Ohmori S, Mori M, Shiraha, K, et al. In Weiner H, Flynn TG (eds): Enzymology and Molecular Biology of Carbonyl Metabolism 2. New York, Alan R Liss, 1989, pp 397–412.

48. Papoulis A, al-Abed Y, Bucala R. Identification of N2-(1-carboxyethyl) guanine (CEG) as a guanine advanced glycosylation end product. Biochemistry 1995; 34:648–655.

49. Ryle C, Donaghy M. Non-enzymatic glycation of peripheral nerve proteins in human diabetics. J Neurol Sci 1995; 129(1):62–68.

50. Ryle C, Leow CK, Donaghy M. Nonenzymatic glycation of peripheral and central nervous system proteins in experimental diabetes mellitus. Muscle Nerve 1997; 20:577–584.

51. Schmidt AM, Hori O, Chen JX, et al. Advanced glycation endproducts interacting with their endothelial receptor induce expression of vascular cell adhesion molecule-1 (VCAM-1) in cultured human endothelial cells and in mice: A potential mechanism for the accelerated vasculopathy of diabetes. J Clin Invest 1995; 96:1395–1403.

52. Schmidt AM, Mora R, Cao K, et al. The endothelial cell binding site for advanced glycation endproducts consists of A complex: An integral membrane protein and a lactoferrin-like polypeptide. J Biol Chem 1994; 269:9882–9888.

53. Schmidt AM, Vianna M, Gerlach M, et al. Isolation and characterization of two binding proteins for advanced glycosylation end products from bovine lung which are present on the endothelial cell surface. J Biol Chem 1992; 267:14987–14997.

54. Sensi M, Tanzi P, Bruno RM, et al. Human glomerular basement membrane: Altered binding characteristics following in vitro non-enzymatic glycosylation. Ann NY Acad Sci 1986; 488:549–552.

55. Shinohara M, Thornalley PJ, Giardino I, et al. Overexpression of glyoxalase-I in bovine endothelial cells inhibits intracellular advanced glycation endproduct formation and prevents hyperglycemia-induced increases in macromolecular endocytosis. J Clin Invest; in press.

56. Takahashi M, Fujii J, Teshima T, et al. Identity of a major 3 deoxyglucosone reducing enzyme with aldehyde reductase in rat liver established by amino acid sequencing and cDNA expression. Gene 1993; 127:249–253.

57. Tanaka S, Avigad G, Brodsky B, et al. Glycation induces expansion of the molecular packing of collagen. J Mol Biol 1988; 203:495–505.

58. Tesfaye S, Malik R, Ward JD. Vascular factors in diabetic neuropathy. Diabetologia 1994; 37(9):847–854.

59. Thornalley PJ. The glyoxalase system: New developments towards functional characterization of a metabolic pathway fundamental to biological life. Biochem J 1990; 269:1–11.

60. Tomlinson DR, Fernyhough P, Diemel LT. Role of neurotrophins in diabetic neuropathy and treatment with nerve growth factors. Diabetes 1997; 46(suppl 2):S43–49.

61. Tsilbary EC, Charonis AS, Reger LA, et al. The effect of nonenzymatic glucosylation on the binding of the main noncollagenous NC1 domain to type IV collagen. J Biol Chem 1990; 263:4302–4308.

62. Vlassara H, Brownlee M, Monogue K, et al. Cachectin/TNF and IL-1 induced by glucose-modified proteins: Role in normal tissue remodeling. Science 1988; 240:1546–1548.

63. Vlassara H, Fuh H, Donnelly T, et al. Advanced glycation endproducts promote adhesion molecule (VCAM-1, ICAM-1) expression and atheroma formation in normal rabbits. Mol Med 1995; 1:447–456.

64. Wautier JL, Zoukourian C, Chappey O, et al. Receptor-mediated endothelial cell dysfunction in diabetic vasculopathy: Soluble receptor for advanced glycation endproducts blocks hyperpermeability in diabetic rats. J Clin Invest 1996; 97:238–243.

65. Wells-Knecht KJ, Lyons TJ, McCance DR, et al. 3-Deoxyfructose concentrations are increased in human plasma and urine in diabetes. Diabetes 1994; 43:1152–1156.

66. Wells-Knecht KJ, Zyzak DV, Litchfield JE, et al. Mechanism of autoxidative glycosylation: Identification of glyoxal and arabinose as intermediates in the autoxidative modification of proteins by glucose. Biochemistry 1995; 34:3702–3709.

67. Wells-Knecht MC, Thorpe SR, Baynes JW. Pathways of formation of glycoxidative products during glycation of collagen. Biochemistry 1995; 34:15134–15141.

68. Williams SK, Howarth NL, Devenny JJ, et al. Structural and functional consequences of increased tubulin glycosylation in diabetes mellitus. Proc Natl Acad Sci USA 1982; 79:6546–6550.

69. Wolff SP, Dean RT. Glucose autoxidation and protein modification: The potential role of autoxidative glycosylation in diabetes. Biochem J 1987; 245:243–252.

70. Yamada, H, Miyata S, Igaki N, et al. Increase in 3-deoxyglucosone levels in diabetic rat plasma: Specific in vivo determination of intermediate in advanced Maillard reaction. J Biol Chem 1994; 269:20275–20280.

71. Yan SD, Schmidt AM, Anderson GM, et al. Enhanced cellular oxidant stress by the interaction of advanced glycation end products with their receptors/binding proteins. J Biol Chem 1994; 269:9889–9897.

72. Yui S, Sasaki T, Araki N, et al. Induction of macrophage growth by advanced glycation end products of the Maillard reaction. J Immunol 1994; 152:1943–1949.

73. Ziegler D, Gries FA. Alpha-lipoic acid in the treatment of diabetic peripheral and cardiac autonomic neuropathy. Diabetes 1997; 46(suppl 2):S62–S66.

Chapter 25

Role of Linolenic Acid in Diabetic Polyneuropathy

Norman E. Cameron • Mary A. Cotter

INTRODUCTION

During the past 10 years, work on experimental models has established a role for altered ω-6 essential fatty acid metabolism in the etiology of nerve dysfunction in diabetes. The main effect relates to abnormal prostanoid synthesis, which contributes to impaired nerve perfusion. Basic findings have been extended to clinical trials of γ-linolenic acid (GLA)–containing oils, which showed improvements in nerve function and the absence of significant side effects. A rational framework exists to continue with this approach, using even more potent GLA-containing drugs, offering the possibility of greater therapeutic benefits.

ESSENTIAL FATTY ACIDS AND THEIR METABOLISM IN DIABETES

There are two types of essential fatty acids that, like vitamins, must be derived from the diet. The ω-6 fatty acid series begins with linoleic acid and the ω-3 series starts with α-linolenic acid. Essential fatty acids are necessary for normal membrane structure and fluidity, eicosanoid production, and the maintenance of the water permeability barrier of the skin. They are also important for cholesterol transport.[30]

The main pathways for linoleic acid and α-linolenic acid metabolism are outlined in Figure 25.1. Both fatty acids are processed by the same enzymes, which perform an alternating series of desaturation and elongation steps. The desaturation steps are relatively slow and therefore rate limiting. They are depressed under certain conditions, including aging, diabetes, excess alcohol consumption, liver disease, and in cancer cells. For diabetes, impairment of the delta-6 (δ-6) desaturation step is particularly important, the probable cause being a combination of effects from hyperglycemia, hypoinsulinemia, and oxidative stress, although the precise mechanism is not known in detail.[29] Lesser defects have also been described for δ-5 and δ-4 desaturase in diabetic rats.[50, 52] The ω-6 essential fatty acids appear to be physiologically more important than the ω-3 series, judging from the results of deprivation and dietary intervention studies in animals and humans.[30] In diabetic animals and human subjects, the δ-6 desaturation deficit typically results in elevated plasma and tissue levels of linoleic acid (the normal dietary source) coupled with a reduction in important ω-6 metabolites such as GLA, dihomo-GLA, and arachidonic acid (ARA).[27]

Most of the actions of essential fatty acids are mediated not by linoleic acid or α-linolenic acid, but by their metabolites. These are necessary for the normal structure and function of cell membranes and influence the microenvironment and activity of membrane-bound proteins such as receptors, ion channels, transporters, and ATPase pumps.

The essential fatty acids are precursors for eicosanoids: prostaglandins (PGs), thromboxanes (TXs), leukotrienes (LTs), and other oxygenated derivatives. Being an integral part of most species of diacylglycerol (DAG), essential fatty acids also participate in second messenger systems. Cyclo-oxygenase participates in the synthesis of prostanoids, the most physiologically important ones being derived from ARA; PGs D_2, E_2, $F_{2\alpha}$, I_2 (prostacyclin), and TXA_2. Dihomo-GLA is the source of series 1 prostanoids, of which PGE_1 may be important in diabetes, and series 3 prostanoids such as TXA_3 may be synthesized from eicosapentaenoic acid. Several of these prostanoids have vascular effects; PGs D_2, E_1, E_2, and I_2 cause vasodilation, and D_2, E_1, and I_2 inhibit platelet aggregation, whereas TXA_2 promotes platelet aggregation and vasoconstriction. Arachidonic acid can also be metabolized to epoxides via the cytochrome P-450 epoxygenase pathway. The 5,6-epoxide causes vasodilation and has been suggested to contribute to the regulation of vascular tone.[17]

The LTs, synthesized primarily from ARA via 5-lipoxygenase, participate in inflammatory responses. Leukotriene B_4, produced mainly by neutrophils, is a powerful chemotaxic agent for neutrophils and macrophages and causes upregulation of membrane adhesion molecules. The cysteinyl-LTs, C_4, D_4, E_4, and F_4, produce vasodilation in most vessels and increase vascular permeability. Other lipoxygenase derivatives may also be important in diabetic complications. The vascular complications in retina and kidney of diabetic rats have recently been linked to an increase in DAG stimulation of the β isoform of protein kinase (PK) C.[33] In skin, the ω-6 lipoxygenase derivative, 13-hydroxyoctadecadienoic acid, is incorporated into DAG to form an effective inhibitor of PKC-β, thus acting to regulate cell proliferation.[18] Arachidonic acid also has a second messenger function and can increase DAG kinase activity in neuronal membranes, thereby favoring DAG catabolism to reduce PKC stimulation.[53]

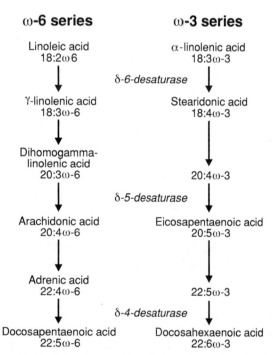

■ **Figure 25.1** An overview of the metabolism of ω-6 and ω-3 essential fatty acids. The nomenclature, for example, 18:2ω-6 for linoleic acid, refers to the number of carbon atoms in the molecule (18), the number of double bonds (2), and the series to which the molecule belongs (ω-6). The important enzymes for the desaturation stages are indicated in italics.

Thus, the δ-6 desaturation defect in diabetes limits the synthesis of vasoactive eicosanoids that could have significant consequences for nerve perfusion, and alters membrane properties and important second messenger systems that could deleteriously affect nerve function and its vascular supply. This is particularly unfortunate because the presence of double bonds makes unsaturated fatty acids a major target for damage by the elevated oxygen free radical activity in diabetes; thus, enhanced rather than reduced essential fatty acid availability is necessary. Two approaches have been taken to attempt to remedy the situation. One is to surmount the desaturation deficit by an increased linoleic acid intake. This has had some success in patients recently diagnosed with type 2 DM, in whom the development of retinopathy and coronary heart disease were reduced.[32] However, there is no information as to whether this approach could be successful in neuropathy. The second approach is to bypass the main δ-6 desaturase defect by dietary supplementation with a downstream metabolite, such as GLA. This has proved effective in both experimental models and clinical trials.

ESSENTIAL FATTY ACID EFFECTS ON NERVE FUNCTION AND PERFUSION IN EXPERIMENTAL DIABETES

Nerve Function

Julu[37] was the first to show that a daily dose of 1 mL/kg of evening primrose oil (EPO) largely prevented the development of sciatic motor and saphenous sensory conduction velocity deficits during a 5-week period in streptozotocin-induced diabetic rats. Evening primrose oil contains 70 to 75% linoleic acid and 8 to 10% GLA; therefore, treatment potentially combined both approaches outlined in the previous section. The effectiveness of EPO was confirmed in further studies by several groups.[11, 39, 58] Observations on nerve function were also extended to show that the development of elevated resistance to hypoxic conduction failure in diabetic rats was attenuated by EPO treatment,[11] but EPO did not alter the defective axonal transport of substance P–like immunoreactivity or the accumulation of polyol pathway metabolites in nerves.[58] In contrast, linoleic acid dietary supplementation had no effect on nerve function in diabetic rats,[11, 21, 22] suggesting that the GLA content was of primary importance for the mechanisms of EPO action. Further studies showed that EPO effects on

nerve function could be mimicked by an appropriate dose of pure GLA,[21] by the main GLA-containing triglyceride in EPO, di-linolein mono-GLA, and by the synthetic triglyceride, tri-GLA.[22] Thus, although the case for GLA being the active component of EPO can be strongly made in the context of nerve dysfunction in experimental diabetes, the choice of EPO for the early studies may have been somewhat fortuitous because the efficacy of natural oils does not closely correlate with their GLA content. Thus, a recent study on correction of motor and sensory nerve conduction velocity (NCV) in diabetic rats, ranked the effectiveness of EPO, fungal, borage, and black currant oils when equated for GLA.[24] The reason for this discrepancy is not fully understood; however, one confounding variable is that complex composition of these oils may cause interactions between different components. For example, black currant oil contains ω-3 components as well as GLA. In contrast to the ω-6 series, ω-3 essential fatty acids have only very modest effects on nerve conduction on their own and do not alter resistance to hypoxic conduction failure in diabetic rats. There is mutual competition between ω-6 and ω-3 series, with the ω-3 series exerting a larger inhibitory effect.[46] Cotreatment with fish oil (containing eicosapentaenoic acid) attenuates the beneficial actions of GLA on nerve function in experimental diabetes.[21]

Several hypotheses have been advanced to explain the effects of GLA and EPO in diabetic rats. These include neurochemical hypotheses based on second messenger or membrane actions of GLA metabolites[38, 58] and neurovascular hypotheses highlighting the effects of vasoactive prostanoids on nerve perfusion.[11]

Neurochemical Actions of Essential Fatty Acids

Neurochemical changes include altered sciatic nerve glycerophospholipid composition in diabetic rats, with a decline in arachidonyl-containing molecular species,[63] presumably as a consequence of the defective essential fatty acid desaturation. These species are normally a major source of DAG; such changes could therefore, also account for the reduced nerve content of this second messenger in diabetes.[62] The DAG activates PKC, as does the inositol triphosphate derived from phosphoinositide breakdown. In turn, PKC may phosphorylate a subunit of Na^+-K^+-ATPase to increase its activity. Depression of this putative mechanism in diabetes, exacerbated by a decreased nerve *myo*-inositol content, was postulated to reduce Na^+-K^+-ATPase activity that could cause conduction velocity deficits.[25] However, recent research has shown that the regulation of Na^+-K^+-ATPase activity by PKC is more complex. Although activation of PKC with phorbol esters corrects the decrease in Na^+-K^+-ATPase in cells exposed to high glucose, so does inhibition of PKC. It is possible that these apparently opposing PKC effects are mediated by different isoforms of the enzyme.[60] The nerve conduction deficits in diabetes have also been partially dissociated from Na^+-K^+-ATPase changes. Thus, conduction velocity may be reduced early in experimental diabetes, before any Na^+-K^+-ATPase alterations are apparent.[45] Treatment with vasodilators to increase nerve perfusion prevents the development of reduced conduction velocity but has no effect on the Na^+-K^+-ATPase deficit.[10] Treatment with EPO, although improving conduction velocity, did not increase Na^+-K^+-pump activity in nerves from diabetic rats. Rather, EPO caused a reduction,[47] perhaps reflecting a modulation of the PKC system or alterations in membrane fluidity. Thus, although ω-6 essential fatty acid treatment is likely to cause neurochemical effects in peripheral nerve, they probably do not explain the main actions of GLA and EPO against nerve dysfunction.

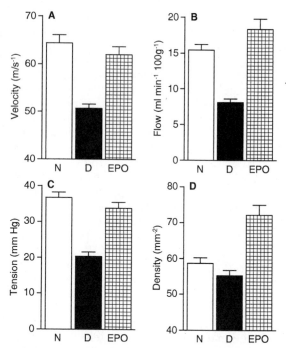

■ **Figure 25.2** Effects of streptozotocin-induced diabetes in rats and preventive evening primrose oil treatment on *A*, sciatic nerve motor conduction velocity, *B*, sciatic endoneurial blood flow, *C*, mean endoneurial oxygen tension, and *D*, endoneurial capillary density. N, nondiabetic group; D, 2-month diabetic group; EPO, 2-month diabetic group treated with evening primrose oil (1 g kg^{-1} d^{-1}). Data are mean + SEM.[6, 11, 12]

Vascular Actions of Essential Fatty Acids

Impaired nerve perfusion, leading to endoneurial hypoxia, occurs sufficiently early after the induction of diabetes to account for reduced nerve conduction velocity and the development of resistance to hypoxic conduction failure in rats.[5, 48] Similar neurovascular dysfunction is found in diabetic subjects with neuropathy.[57] In both cases, beneficial effects are found for treatment with peripheral vasodilators, for example, the angiotensin-converting enzyme inhibitor lisinopril.[5, 57] Because many of the prostanoid products of essential fatty acid metabolism have vasodilator or vasomodulator actions, they are potential candidates to explain EPO and GLA effects. Synthesis of prostacyclin by sciatic nerve epineurial and perineurial vessels is reduced by diabetes, mainly because of diminished ARA availability.[59] Chronic treatment of diabetic rats with EPO increases vasa nervorum prostacyclin production.[55] In addition to improving nerve function in diabetic rats (Fig. 25.2*A*), EPO corrects

impaired sciatic endoneurial blood flow (Fig. 25.2*B*), oxygen tension (Fig. 25.2*C*),[6, 16] and whole nerve red cell flux.[40, 56] Endoneurial blood flow deficits are also rapidly reversed (within 2 weeks) by treatment with pure GLA, dilinolein mono-GLA and tri-GLA.[7, 9, 22] In the longer term (1 to 2 months), the chronic elevation of perfusion caused by GLA and EPO treatment causes an increase in endoneurial capillary density (Fig. 25.2*D*).[11, 21] Although this effect is not necessary for the functional actions of GLA, it was also found for several other unrelated treatments that cause chronic vasodilation.[5] Interestingly, EPO also improves nerve function and capillary density in the galactosemic rat model of polyol pathway hyperactivity.[23]

The effects of EPO and GLA on nerve conduction velocity, resistance to hypoxic conduction failure, endoneurial blood flow, and capillary density in diabetic rats are completely blocked by cotreatment with a modest dose of a cyclo-oxygenase inhibitor.[12, 16, 22] This provides further support for the notion that the mediators are vasodilator prostanoids. The main candidate is prostacyclin because it is produced by vascular endothelium in much greater amounts than the other prostaglandins, although vasa nervorum is also sensitive to PGE_1 and $PGF_{2\alpha}$.[43] Prostaglandin E_1 has also been suggested to act directly on neuronal membranes to increase conduction velocity,[28] and pharmacologic doses of PGE_1 analogues improve nerve conduction velocity and Na^+-K^+-ATPase activity in diabetic rats.[54, 61] However, it is unlikely that PGE_1 is an important mediator of GLA effects in experimental diabetic neuropathy. Thus, treatment of diabetic rats with a mixture of fish oil and EPO or GLA had a detrimental effect on nerve function compared with EPO and GLA alone. The eicosapentaenoic acid in fish oil competes advantageously with ARA, the result being a buildup of dihomo-GLA. Dihomo-GLA is the precursor of PGE_1; fish oil admixture would therefore, be expected to improve GLA action if PGE_1 was important, contrary to the findings. The case for series 2 PGs is strengthened because EPO and GLA effects on nerve conduction velocity and blood flow in diabetic rats are mimicked by treatment with ARA-enriched oils.[19] Moreover, the ranking of the effects of complex natural GLA sources (EPO, fungal, borage, and black currant oils) on conduction velocity in diabetic rats agrees with that obtained for the ratio of 6-keto $PGF_{1\alpha}$/TXB_2 (the stable metabolites of prostacyclin and TXA_2, respectively) outflow from the mesenteric vascular bed in response to these oils.[36] Furthermore, prostacyclin analogues have similar effects to GLA on nerve conduction, resistance to hypoxic conduction failure, blood flow, and endoneurial capillary density in diabetic rats.[20, 31, 49]

Although much less effective than the ω-6 series, one of the potential vascular benefits of ω-3 essential fatty acids is that competitive interference with ARA metabolism results in preferential synthesis of TXA_3, which is much less potent for platelet aggregation and vasoconstriction than TXA_2.[46] However, at least in diabetic rats, increased platelet activation and TXA_2 synthesis do not appear to make a major contribution to nerve dysfunction; treatment with a TX receptor and synthase antagonist only marginally improved conduction velocity.[24] The potential advantages of ω-3 essential fatty acid treatment must be weighed against the disadvantages of inhibiting ω-6 metabolism. For example, in diabetic rats, prostacyclin analogues prevent the development of electroretinographic abnormalities,[31] but ω-3 essential

fatty acid treatment accelerates the progression of retinopathy.[26]

Thus, the data from experimental diabetes strongly support the view that ω-6 essential fatty acids are much more effective than ω-3 essential fatty acids and that the primary effect of ω-6 metabolites such as GLA is to compensate for reduced vasa nervorum prostacyclin synthesis, thereby improving nerve perfusion and the supply of oxygen to neurons and Schwann cells.

Interactions Between Prostanoid and Glucose-Induced Metabolic Defects

The neurovascular abnormalities in diabetes arise from a complex of changes in several systems. In addition to deficits in prostanoid synthesis, the endothelial nitric oxide (NO) system, which also causes vasodilation, is compromised by increased oxygen free radical production, the formation of advanced glycation end products, and polyol pathway activity.[1, 4, 41, 44] Appropriate treatments such as antioxidants, aminoguanidine, and aldose reductase inhibitors improve nerve perfusion and function in diabetic rats.[8, 14, 15] Free radical effects also promote endothelial vasoconstrictor synthesis, including endothelin-1 and angiotensin II.[5] Normally, these systems interact to provide an integrated local control of tissue perfusion. However, by disrupting several systems simultaneously, diabetes disengages this control and the balance is shifted toward vasa nervorum vasoconstriction. There are several examples of interactions between these systems. In nondiabetic rats, chronic treatment with moderate doses of cyclo-oxygenase or NO synthase inhibitors caused modest conduction velocity deficits. However, with joint treatment, there was a fivefold amplification of conduction effects compared with that expected for simple summation, suggesting that compensatory synergy between prostanoid and NO systems normally makes vasa nervorum relatively resistant to a single inhibitory action.[13] In diabetic rats, EPO treatment effects on nerve blood flow and conduction velocity involve an interaction with the NO system because they are attenuated by NO synthase inhibition.[16] This may be a result of the increase in blood flow promoted by GLA-stimulated prostanoid synthesis. Flow-induced shear stress enhances endothelial NO production,[51] causing further vasodilation to magnify the GLA effect. Consequently, blockade of NO synthesis reduces the total neurovascular action of GLA.

It may be possible to take advantage of these complex interactions to enhance the therapeutic effects of drug treatment by targeting more than one dysfunctional system. In diabetic rats treated with low doses of an aldose reductase inhibitor (to improve NO-mediated responses) and EPO (to stimulate prostanoid synthesis), the effects of individual treatments on conduction velocity and blood flow were very modest, but together there was about an eightfold increase in treatment efficacy.[16] Another example of such synergy was noted for joint treatment with a lipophilic antioxidant and GLA.[9] This approach led to the development of novel GLA-based compounds, such as ascorbyl-GLA, where the antioxidant, ascorbate, is attached to a GLA molecule.[7] Ascorbyl-GLA proved to have fourfold to fivefold greater effect than pure GLA on conduction velocity and blood flow in diabetic rats. Figure 25.3 shows the structure of ascorbyl-GLA and the synergistic interaction between both moieties for sciatic motor conduction velocity. Ascorbyl-GLA will soon be going into clinical trials for diabetic neuropathy.

CLINICAL TRIALS OF γ-LINOLENIC ACID

There have been three neuropathy trials using GLA in the form of EPO. The first was a pilot single-center randomized placebo-controlled study with 22 patients (about 50% had type 1 DM), 12 of whom received 360 mg of GLA daily for 6 months.[34, 35] This dose was sufficient to approximately halve the diabetic deficits in plasma GLA and arachidonic acid levels. During the 6-month period, there were significant improvements in symptoms, motor NCV and compound muscle action potential amplitude (median and peroneal nerves), sensory nerve action potential amplitude (median and sural nerves), and ankle thermal thresholds, against a background of modest deterioration in the placebo group. The second trial[42] was larger (111 patients, about 50% type 1 DM), multicenter, used a GLA dose of 480 mg/d and lasted for 12 months. Neurophysiologic tests revealed significant improvements in peroneal and median motor NCV of around 2 m/s compared with baseline in the treated group, whereas in the placebo group, there was deterioration of a similar magnitude. Compound muscle action potential and sensory nerve action potential amplitudes were significantly increased com-

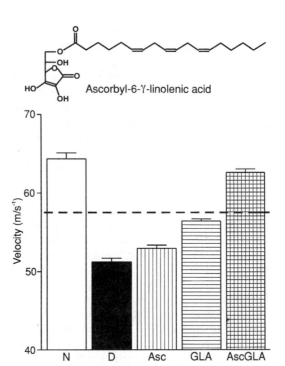

■ **Figure 25.3** Structure of ascorbyl-6-γ-linolenic acid and the effects of treatment on sciatic motor conduction velocity (histogram) in streptozotocin-induced diabetic rats. N, nondiabetic group; D, 8-week diabetic group; Asc, diabetic group treated with ascorbate (21 mg kg^{-1} d^{-1}) for 2 weeks after 6 weeks of untreated diabetes; GLA, diabetic group treated for 2 weeks with γ-linolenic acid (100 mg kg^{-1} d^{-1}) after 6 weeks of untreated diabetes; AscGLA, diabetic group treated with a matching dose of ascorbyl-6-γ-linolenic acid during the same period. The horizontal *dashed line* is the conduction velocity value predicted if the effects of ascorbate and γ-linolenic acid treatment were simply additive. This value was greatly exceeded in the AscGLA group, indicating a synergistic interaction between the two moieties of the drug. Data are mean + SEM.[7]

pared with baseline and placebo treatment and cold and hot thresholds were improved. Neurologic examination showed that muscle strength tended to increase compared with placebo. Tendon reflexes and sensation were improved compared with baseline and placebo in the leg and compared with placebo in the arm.

The third study,[2] which has recently been completed, had 291 patients and used a GLA dose of 480 mg/kg. It was placebo-controlled and double-blind for the first 12 months; then, in a subsequent 12-month period both active and placebo groups were treated with GLA. Results during the first 12 months were largely confirmatory of previous trials, for example, an approximate 1.3 m/s increase in motor NCV over baseline compared with an approximate

1.8 m/s deterioration with placebo. In the second year, there was further improvement in 8 of 28 variables for those patients treated with GLA during the first 12 months; for example, peroneal motor NCV increased by an additional 1.2 m/s. Those patients transferring from placebo to GLA showed a trend toward improvement for 18 of 28 variables. Thus, taken together, these trials demonstrate that GLA not only prevented the further progression of neuropathy during the treatment period but also caused a real improvement over baseline for a battery of tests. The trials showed that GLA was well tolerated, and no adverse events were attributed to treatment.

Species differences in essential fatty acid metabolism and the chronic nature of neuropathic changes in patients suggest that it may not be entirely appropriate to compare results from clinical trials with data from animal models. Nonetheless, the doses used in trials lie in the lowest quartile of the EPO and GLA NCV dose-response relationship for diabetic rats.[7, 22] An improvement of 0.5 to 2 m/s in NCV would be predicted from the rat data, which is comparable to the trial findings. This, coupled with the incomplete restoration of plasma GLA and metabolite levels in patients, suggests that a higher dose achieved using a more concentrated source of GLA or a compound such as ascorbyl GLA could potentially be more effective. However, the maximum extent of recovery that is possible from an existing clinical diabetic neuropathy remains unknown. None of the drug trials so far carried out (mainly using aldose reductase inhibitors (see Chapter 22) have used doses comparable to those found optimal in animal models.[3, 15] It is plausible that future trials of more potent and sophisticated GLA-containing preparations will answer key questions about the viability of treatment intervention versus preventive approaches to diabetic neuropathy.

References

1. Archibald V, Cotter MA, Keegan A, et al. Contraction and relaxation of aortas from diabetic rats: Effects of chronic anti-oxidant and aminoguanidine treatments. Naunyn Schmiedebergs Arch Pharmacol 1996; 353:584.
2. Boulton AJM, Ziegler D, Scarpello J, et al. A multicentre double-blind trial of gammalenic acid in diabetic peripheral sensorimotor neuropathy. Diabetologia 1997; 41(Suppl. 1):A32.
3. Cameron NE, Cotter MA. Dissociation between biochemical and functional effects of the aldose reductase inhibitor ponalrestat on peripheral nerve in diabetic rats. Br J Pharmacol 1992; 107:939.
4. Cameron NE, Cotter MA. Impaired contraction and relaxation in aorta from streptozotocin-diabetic rats: Role of polyol pathway activity. Diabetologia 1992; 35:1011.
5. Cameron NE, Cotter MA. The relationship of vascular changes to metabolic factors in diabetes mellitus and their role in the development of peripheral nerve complications. Diabetes Metab Rev 1994; 10:189.
6. Cameron NE, Cotter MA. Effects of evening primrose oil treatment on sciatic nerve blood flow and endoneurial oxygen tension in streptozotocin-diabetic rats. Acta Diabetol 1994; 31:220.
7. Cameron NE, Cotter MA. Comparison of the effects of ascorbyl γ-linolenic acid and γ-linolenic acid in the correction of neurovascular deficits in diabetic rats. Diabetologia 1996; 39:1047.
8. Cameron NE, Cotter MA. Rapid reversal by aminoguanidine of the neurovascular effects of diabetes in rats: Modulation by nitric oxide synthase inhibition. Metabolism 1996; 45:1147.
9. Cameron NE, Cotter MA. Interaction between oxidative stress and γ-linolenic acid in impaired neurovascular function of diabetic rats. Am J Physiol 1996; 271:E471.
10. Cameron NE, Cotter MA, Ferguson K, et al. Effects of chronic α-adrenergic receptor blockade on peripheral nerve conduction, hypoxic resistance, polyols, Na⁺-K⁺-ATPase activity, and vascular supply in STZ-D rats. Diabetes 1991; 40:1652.
11. Cameron NE, Cotter MA, Robertson S. Effects of essential fatty acid dietary supplementation on peripheral nerve and skeletal muscle function and capillarisation in streptozotocin-diabetic rats. Diabetes 1991; 40:532.
12. Cameron NE, Cotter MA, Dines KC, et al. The effects of evening primrose oil on peripheral nerve function and capillarization in streptozotocin-diabetic rats: Modulation by the cyclo-oxygenase inhibitor flurbiprofen. Br J Pharmacol 1993; 109:972.
13. Cameron NE, Cotter MA, Dines KC, et al. Pharmacological manipulation of vascular endothelium in non-diabetic and streptozotocin-diabetic rats: Effects on nerve conduction, hypoxic resistance and endoneurial capillarization. Diabetologia 1993; 36:516.
14. Cameron NE, Cotter MA, Archibald V, et al. Anti-oxidant and pro-oxidant effects on nerve conduction velocity, endoneurial blood flow and oxygen tension in non-diabetic and streptozotocin-diabetic rats. Diabetologia 1994; 37:449.
15. Cameron NE, Cotter MA, Dines KC, et al. Aldose reductase inhibition, nerve perfusion, oxygenation and function in streptozotocin-diabetic rats: Dose-response considerations and independence from a myo-inositol mechanism. Diabetologia 1994; 37:651.
16. Cameron NE, Cotter MA, Hohman TC. Interactions between essential fatty acid, prostanoid, polyol pathway and nitric oxide mechanisms in the neurovascular deficit of diabetic rats. Diabetologia 1996; 39:172.
17. Carroll MA, Schwartzman M, Capdevila J, et al. Vasoactivity of arachidonic acid epoxides. Eur J Pharmacol 1987; 138:281.
18. Cho Y, Ziboh VA. 13-Hydroxyoctadecadienoic acid reverses epidermal hyperproliferation via selective inhibition of protein kinase C-β activity. Biochem Biophys Res Commun 1994; 201:257.
19. Cotter MA, Cameron NE. Effects of dietary supplementation with arachidonic acid rich oils on nerve conduction and blood flow in streptozotocin-diabetic rats. Prostaglandins Leukot Essent Fatty Acids 1997; 56:337.
20. Cotter MA, Dines KC, Cameron NE. Prevention and

reversal of motor and sensory peripheral nerve conduction abnormalities in streptozotocin-diabetic rats by the prostacyclin analogue iloprost. Naunyn Schmiedebergs Arch Pharmacol 1993; 347:534.

21. Dines KC, Cotter MA, Cameron NE. Contrasting effects of treatment with ω-3 and ω-6 essential fatty acids on peripheral nerve function and capillarization in streptozotocin-diabetic rats. Diabetologia 1993; 36:1132.

22. Dines KC, Cotter MA, Cameron NE. Comparison of the effects of evening primrose oil and triglycerides containing γ-linolenic acid on nerve conduction and blood flow in diabetic rats. J Pharmacol Exp Ther 1995; 273:49.

23. Dines KC, Cotter MA, Cameron NE. Nerve function in galactosaemic rats: Effects of evening primrose oil and doxazosin. Eur J Pharmacol 1995; 281:303.

24. Dines KC, Cotter MA, Cameron NE. Effectiveness of natural oils as sources of γ-linolenic acid to correct peripheral nerve conduction velocity abnormalities in diabetic rats: Modulation by thromboxane A_2 inhibition. Prostaglandins Leukot Essent Fatty Acids 1996; 55:159.

25. Greene DA, Sima AAF, Stevens MJ, et al. Complications: Neuropathy, pathogenetic considerations. Diabetes Care 1992; 15:1902.

26. Hammes H-P, Weiss A, Führer D, et al. Acceleration of experimental diabetic retinopathy in the rat by omega-3 fatty acids. Diabetologia 1996; 39:251.

27. Holman RT, Johnson SB, Gerrard JM, et al. Arachidonic acid deficiency in streptozotocin-induced diabetes. Proc Natl Acad Sci USA 1983; 80:2375.

28. Horrobin DF, Durang LG, Manku MS. Prostaglandin E_1 modifies nerve conduction and interferes with local anaesthetic action. Prostaglandins 1977; 14:103.

29. Horrobin DF, Carmichael HA. Essential fatty acids in relation to diabetes. In Horrobin DF (ed): Treatment of Diabetic Neuropathy: A New Approach. Edinburgh, Churchill Livingstone, 1992, p 21.

30. Horrobin DF, Manku MS. Clinical biochemistry of essential fatty acids. In Horrobin DF (ed): Omega-6 Essential Fatty Acids: Pathophysiology and Roles in Clinical Medicine. New York, Wiley-Liss, 1990, p 21.

31. Hotta N, Koh N, Sakakibara F, et al. Effects of beraprost sodium and insulin on the electroretinogram, nerve conduction and nerve blood flow in rats with streptozotocin-induced diabetes. Diabetes 1996; 45:361.

32. Houtsmuller AJ, van Hal-Ferweda J, Zahn KJ, et al. Favourable influences of linoleic acid on the progression of micro- and macro-angiopathy in adult onset diabetes mellitus. Prog Lipid Res 1982; 20:377.

33. Ishii H, Jirousek MR, Koya D, et al. Amelioration of vascular dysfunctions in diabetic rats by an oral PKC β inhibitor. Science 1996; 272:728.

34. Jamal GA, Carmichael H, Weir AI. Gamma-linolenic acid in diabetic neuropathy. Lancet 1986; 1:1098.

35. Jamal GA, Carmichael H. The effects of gamma-linolenic acid on human diabetic peripheral neuropathy: A double-blind, placebo-controlled trial. Diabetic Med 1990; 7:319.

36. Jenkins DK, Mitchell JC, Manku MS, et al. Effects of different sources of gamma-linolenic acid on the formation of essential fatty acid and prostanoid metabolites. Med Sci Res 1988; 16:525.

37. Julu POO. Essential fatty acids prevent slowed nerve conduction velocity in streptozotocin diabetic rats. J Diabetes Complications 1988; 2:185.

38. Julu POO. Responses of peripheral nerve conduction velocities to treatment with essential fatty acids in diabetic rats: Possible mechanisms of action. In Horrobin DF (ed): Treatment of Diabetic Neuropathy: A New Approach. Edinburgh, Churchill Livingstone, 1992, p 41.

39. Julu POO, Mutamba A. Comparison of short-term effects of insulin and essential fatty acids on the slowed nerve conduction of streptozotocin diabetes in rats. J Neurol Sci 1991; 106:56.

40. Karasu C, Dewhurst M, Stevens EJ, et al. Effects of anti-oxidant treatment on sciatic nerve dysfunction in streptozotocin-diabetic rats: Comparison with essential fatty acids. Diabetologia 1995; 38:129.

41. Keegan A, Walbank H, Cotter MA, et al. Chronic vitamin E treatment prevents defective endothelium-dependent relaxation in diabetic rat aorta. Diabetologia 1995; 38:1475.

42. Keen H, Payan J, Allawi J, et al. Treatment of diabetic neuropathy with γ-linolenic acid. Diabetes Care 1993; 16:8.

43. Kihara M, Low PA. Vasoreactivity to prostaglandins of rat peripheral nerve. J Physiol 1995; 484:463.

44. Kihara M, Low PA. Impaired vasoreactivity to nitric oxide in experimental diabetic neuropathy. Exp Neurol 1995; 132:180.

45. Lambourne JE, Brown AM, Calcutt NA, et al. Adenosine triphosphatase in nerves and ganglia of rats with streptozotocin-induced diabetes or galactosaemia: Effects of aldose reductase inhibition. Diabetologia 1988; 31:379.

46. Lands WEM: Biochemistry and physiology of n-3 fatty acids. FASEB J 1992; 6:2530.

47. Lockett MJ, Tomlinson DR. The effects of dietary treatment with essential fatty acids on sciatic nerve conduction and activity of the Na^+/K^+ pump in streptozotocin-diabetic rats. Br J Pharmacol 1992; 105:355.

48. Low PA, Lagerlund TD, McManis PG. Nerve blood flow and oxygen delivery in normal, diabetic and ischemic neuropathy. Int Rev Neurobiol 1989; 31:355.

49. Ohno A, Kanazawa A, Tanaka A, et al. Effect of a prostaglandin I_2 derivative (Iloprost) on peripheral neuropathy of diabetic rats. Diabetes Res Clin Pract 1992; 18:123.

50. Peluffo RO, Ayala S, Brenner RR. Metabolism of fatty acids of the linoleic acid series in testicles of diabetic rats. Am J Physiol 1970; 218:669.

51. Pohl U, Herlan K, Huang A et al. EDRF-mediated shear-induced dilation opposes myogenic vasoconstriction in small rabbit arteries. Am J Physiol 1991; 261:H2016.

52. Poisson J-P. Comparative in vivo and in vitro study of the influence of experimental diabetes on rat liver linoleic acid 6- and 5-desaturation. Enzyme 1985; 34:1.

53. Rao KVR, Vaidyanathan VV, Sastry PS. Diacylglycerol kinase is stimulated by arachidonic acid in neural membranes. J Neurochem 1994; 63:1454.

54. Sonobe M, Yasuda H, Hisanaga T, et al. Amelioration of nerve Na^+-K^+-ATPase activity independently of *myo*-inositol level by PGE₁ analogue OP-1206•α-CD in streptozotocin-induced diabetic rats. Diabetes 1991; 40:726.

55. Stevens EJ, Carrington AL, Tomlinson DR. Prostacyclin release in experimental diabetes: Effects of evening primrose oil. Prostaglandins Leukot Essent Fatty Acids 1993; 49:699.

56. Stevens EJ, Lockett MJ, Carrington AL, et al. Essential fatty acid treatment prevents nerve ischaemia and associated conduction anomalies in rats with experimental diabetes mellitus. Diabetologia 1993; 36:111.

57. Tesfaye S, Malik R, Ward JD. Vascular factors in diabetic neuropathy. Diabetologia 1994; 37:847.

58. Tomlinson DR, Robinson JP, Compton AM. Essential

fatty acid treatment: Effects on nerve conduction, polyol pathway and axonal transport in streptozotocin diabetic rats. Diabetologia 1989; 32:655.

59. Ward KK, Low PA, Schmelzer JD, et al. Prostacyclin and noradrenaline in peripheral nerve of chronic experimental diabetes in rats. Brain 1989; 112:197.

60. Xia P, Kramer RM, King GL. Identification of the mechanism for the inhibition of Na^+, K^+-adenosine triphosphatase by hyperglycemia involving activation of protein kinase C and cytosolic phospholipase A_2. J Clin Invest 1995; 96:733.

61. Yasuda H, Sonobe M, Yamashita M, et al. Effect of prostaglandin E_1 analogue TFC 612 on diabetic neuropathy in streptozocin-induced diabetic rats: Comparison with aldose reductase inhibitor ONO 2235. Diabetes 1989; 38:832.

62. Zhu X, Eichberg J. 1,2-Diacylglycerol content and its arachidonyl-containing molecular species are reduced in sciatic nerve from streptozotocin-induced diabetic rats. J Neurochem 1990; 55:1087.

63. Zhu X, Eichberg J. Molecular species composition of glycerophospholipids in rat sciatic nerve and its alteration in streptozotocin-induced diabetes. Biochim Biophys Acta 1993; 1168:1.

Chapter **26**

Role of Antiprostaglandins in Diabetic Neuropathy

Hitoshi Yasuda • Ryuichi Kikkawa

INTRODUCTION

Prostaglandins (PGs) are physiologic substances that exert diverse and important pharmacologic and biologic actions,[5] including antiplatelet effects, vasodilator and membrane-fluidizing effects, and regulatory effects on tissue cyclic adenosine monophosphate (cAMP) levels and Na^+/K^+-ATPase activity. They act on many organs, including blood vessels and neurons, both of which are the most vulnerable target tissues in diabetic neuropathy. Functional and morphological abnormalities, which include decreased nerve blood flow (NBF),[41] leading to endoneurial hypoxia,[23] increased microvascular permeability (disrupted blood nerve barrier),[24, 30] thickening of microvascular walls including endothelial cells and their basement membrane,[44] and capillary closure,[9] have been reported in the endoneurial microvasculature of diabetic nerves. Vasotropic actions of PGs include vasodilation of arterioles, precapillary sphincters, and postcapillary venules; an antiplatelet action, and reduction in erythrocyte deformability. In addition, a direct effect of PGs on neurons and nerve fibers has also been noted in the central nervous system (CNS) and peripheral nervous system (PNS). The release of prostaglandin E_2 (PGE$_2$) in the hypothalamus has been proposed to explain the genesis of pyrogen-induced fever. Prostaglandin$_2$ is thought to be associated with the induction of sleep. Aside from these effects on the CNS, PGEs and prostacyclin (PGI$_2$) sensitize afferent nerve endings to chemical or mechanical stimuli by lowering the threshold of nociceptors or inhibiting the release of neurotransmitter from presynaptic nerve terminals. Thus, PGs have a crucial role in the regulation of vascular and neural function, and an antiprostaglandin effect is thought to be deleterious for PNS function.

PROSTAGLANDIN METABOLISM IN THE DIABETIC STATE

Synthesis of PG is known to be increased in renal glomeruli and the aorta of diabetic animals under high glucose concentrations in vitro. The increased glomerular filtration rate observed in experimental animals with a short duration of diabetes is partially caused by increased production of vasodilatory PGs. This increased PG synthesis has been attributed to a series of metabolic disruptions observed in the early stage of diabetes. Williamson proposed the concept *hyperglycemic pseudohypoxia*, in which the increased cytosolic ratio of free NADH/NAD$^+$ caused by hyperglycemia mimics the effects of true hypoxia on vascular and neural function; increased sorbitol pathway activity resulting from hyperglycemia results in an increase in the NADH/NAD$^+$ ratio, which increases de novo synthesis of diacylglycerol (DAG) and thereby protein kinase C (PKC) activity.[43] The increase in PKC activity and the subsequent increase in intracellular Ca^{2+} both enhance phospholipase A$_2$ activity, leading to mobilization of arachidonic acid from membrane phospholipid and a consequent increase in PG synthesis. Increased PGs and associated increases in superoxide and nitric oxide production all cause vasodilation and increased blood flow, leading to progressive vascular sclerosis through increased collagen synthesis, vascular scarring, decreased vascular compliance, etc. This scenario has been supported by a series of experiments on glomeruli from diabetic rats.

By contrast, decreased blood flow and glomerular filtration rate observed at more advanced stages of diabetes is attributed to a decreased ratio of vasodilator/vasoconstrictor PGs. Impaired contractile function of aortic rings from diabetic rabbits exposed to high glucose concentrations is associated with increased production of vasoconstrictor prostanoids. Thus, synthesized PGs vary with the severity and duration of hyperglycemia. Similarly, there is vigorous controversy about nerve DAG levels and PKC activity. Some investigators have reported that both are decreased.[19, 48] However, the observation that treatment with calphostin C, a PKC inhibitor, improves nerve Na$^+$/K$^+$-ATPase activity may suggest increased PKC activity in diabetic nerves.[11] Furthermore, the flux rather than the tissue level of DAG may be important. It remains uncertain whether these abnormalities of DAG levels and PKC activity depend on the duration and severity of diabetes.

On the other hand, PGE$_1$ synthetic systems have been known to be disrupted at several sites in the synthetic pathway in the diabetic state (Fig. 26.1). Prostaglandin E$_1$ is synthesized by ω-6 essential fatty acids such as linoleic acid and dihomo-γ-linolenic acid. At the first step in the metabolism of linoleic acid, its σ-6-desaturation to γ-linolenic acid is impaired.[13] For this reason, it has been proposed that γ-linolenic acid is likely to be beneficial in the management of complications of diabetes, including neuropathy.[18] This abnormality may well exist in diabetic nerve, leading to nerve dysfunction caused by decreased nerve blood flow and effects on myelin. Thus, the abnormality of ω-6 essential fatty acids metabolism might contribute to the pathogenesis of diabetic neuropathy.[15] In this sense, treatment with PGs, especially PGE$_1$, may well be warranted.

PROSTAGLANDINS AND PERIPHERAL NERVE

Prostaglandins exert significant effects on nerve fibers and vessels in the nervous system. Prostaglandin Es are released from sympathetically innervated tissues, and inhibition of local PG production is associated with an increase in the release of norepinephrine and subsequent effector responses induced by neural activity. Prostaglandins have also been reported to be involved in the propagation of action potentials. Blockade of PGE$_1$ synthesis in rats resulted in a reduction in nerve action potential amplitude that could be corrected by PGE$_1$.[12] Furthermore, PGEs and PGI$_2$ are known to lower nociceptor thresholds and to contribute to the generation of pain[5]; subdermal injections of PGE$_2$ in the rat foot lead to increases in the potentials evoked in sensory nerve branches by mechanical stimulation of the skin.[29]

The variability in the action of PGs partially appears to arise from the variety of mechanisms by which PGs exert their biologic effects;

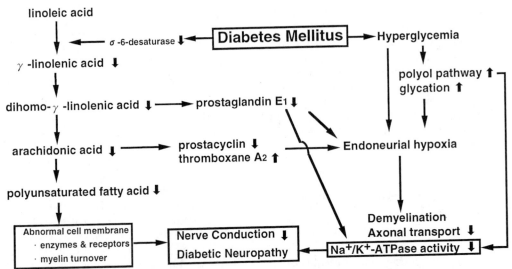

■ **Figure 26.1** The pathogenesis of diabetic neuropathy with special reference to the synthetic pathway of essential fatty acids to prostaglandins. (Data from Jamal GA. Pathogenesis of diabetic neuropathy: The role of the n = 6 essential fatty acids and their eicosanoid derivatives. Diabetic Med 1990; 7:574.)

a number of distinct receptors mediate their actions. The receptors have been named for the natural PG for which they have the greatest apparent affinity and have been divided into five main types, designated DP (PGD), FP (PGF), IP (PGI$_2$), TP (thromboxane, TXA$_2$) and EP (PGE). The PGE receptor has four subtypes, EP$_1$, EP$_2$, EP$_3$, and EP$_4$.[17] Each receptor has different second messenger systems and effects: EP$_1$ receptor activates calcium channels (smooth muscle contraction); IP, EP$_2$, and EP$_4$ receptors stimulate adenylate cyclase (smooth muscle relaxation); and the EP$_3$ receptor inhibits adenylate cyclase. Brain contains PGD$_2$ in high concentrations along with its receptors, especially EP$_3$ (EP$_1$ and EP$_4$) and DP. Dorsal root ganglion (DRG) neurons have been shown to have IP, EP$_1$, EP$_3$, and EP$_4$ receptors.[26] In the dorsal root and trigeminal ganglia of the mouse EP$_3$ receptor, messenger RNA has been demonstrated in about half of the neurons.[37] The hybridization signal for IP has also been reported to be expressed in about 40% of the neurons, in large and small neurons to the same degree, in mouse DRGs. The expression of IP receptor mRNA in small neurons may support the notion that PGI$_2$ causes hyperalgesia.[16] Approximately 70% γ-preprotachykinin (the substance P precursor) mRNA positive neurons have been reported to coexpress IP receptor mRNA. Therefore, IP receptor may have an important role in hyperalgesia in the substance P positive neurons. However, it is unknown whether the expression of each receptor might undergo any change in distribution or type frequency in diabetes.

Prostaglandins are known to exert a wide variety of actions to maintain local homeostasis in the body. They are released immediately after synthesis and act on the cell-surface receptors to elicit their actions. Thus, the source of PGs in the nervous tissue is thought to be the nerve tissue itself. Peripheral nerve has been known to use arachidonic acid for the formation of PGs.[10] Using [^{14}C]arachidonic acid, both desheathed rat nerve and homogenates have been shown to synthesize PGE$_2$, PGF$_{2\alpha}$, PGD$_2$, 6-ketoPGF$_{1\alpha}$, and TXB$_2$. Either the production of PGs or their effect on nerves might be changed in pathologic conditions, including diabetes. Although prostanoids are produced by every tissue in the body, Schwann cells may be one of the candidates in PNS. Schwann cells have been demonstrated to produce significant amounts of PGE$_2$ and TXA$_2$ in vitro.[7] Because the metabolism of Schwann cells is disrupted in diabetes, prostanoid synthesis might be disturbed in diabetes. However, it remains unsettled whether this leads to deleterious effects on nerve function. It has been postulated that decreased prostanoid synthesis could affect autoimmune inflammatory reactions in peripheral nerve diseases such as Guillain-Barré syndrome and chronic inflammatory demyelinating polyneuropathy.[7]

Vasoregulation in the PNS is thought to be

controlled by nitric oxide, prostanoids, angiotensin II, endothelin, etc.[3] Nitric oxide and prostanoids have a vasodilator effect, and angiotensin II and endothelin contribute to vasoconstriction. Cameron and coworkers reported that nondiabetic rats treated with the cyclooxygenase inhibitor flurbiprofen or the nitric oxide synthase inhibitor N-nitro-L-arginine (NOARG) at a low dose for 2 months caused very similar modest reductions in nerve conduction velocity (NCV).[2] By contrast, combination therapy with the two compounds produced a greater effect on NCV than predicted from a simple addition of their individual actions. Treatment with flurbiprofen and high-dose NOARG matched the NCV deficit found with untreated diabetes. Thus, vasodilator control may be regulated by mutually compensatory mechanisms and may provide a relative resistance to dysfunction of a single mechanism in normal nerves.

PROSTAGLANDINS AND DIABETIC NERVE

As described in the preceding section, it has been accepted that PG synthesis and metabolism are disturbed in several ways as a result of hyperglycemia and its associated metabolic defects. Prostaglandin metabolism in diabetic nerve is also subject to ischemic effects; diabetic nerves have been demonstrated to be ischemic and hypoxic as early as 1 week after the induction of diabetes.[20] Endoneurial ischemia-hypoxia results in the breakdown of ATP[1] to hypoxanthine and the generation of reducing equivalents, including NADPH. Intermittent ischemia, which is expected in diabetic nerves,[22] is deleterious because reperfusion after ischemia to the rat sciatic nerve was shown to result in reduced reflow and blood-nerve barrier impairment. Ischemia activates phospholipases, especially A_2, to break down membrane phospholipids and activate the arachidonic cascade and generate leukotrienes and PGs. This results in superoxide production by reduction of PGG_2 to PGH_2 by PG hydroperoxidase, producing superoxide via a side-chain reaction that uses NADH as a reducing cosubstrate. Although it has not been established that oxygen free radicals are increased in diabetic nerve, conjugated dienes, which are products of lipid peroxidation, were consistently increased in diabetic nerve,[21] consistent with increased oxygen free radical activity.

Because PGI_2 synthase is inactivated by superoxide but TX synthase is resistant to it, the PGI_2:TXA_2 ratio, which is considered important in the maintenance of vascular tone, is reduced in diabetes, favoring vasoconstriction and platelet aggregation in diabetes and further aggravating microvascular ischemia-hypoxia. The possibility that these events develop in diabetic nerve has been partially supported by Ward and coworkers, who demonstrated that 6-keto-$PGF_{1\alpha}$ ($6KPGF_{1\alpha}$), the stable metabolite of PGI_2, in the epineurium of rat sciatic nerve after 4 months of diabetes was reduced in the sciatic nerve.[42] Sciatic nerve sheath in vitro biosynthesis of $6KPGF_{1\alpha}$ was significantly reduced, but not in acute experimental diabetes. By contrast, nerves with reduced $6KPGF_{1\alpha}$ had an excessive response to arachidonic acid stimulation, suggesting that the reduced endogenous biosynthesis of PGI_2 is the result of reduced substrate availability, possibly because of the coexistent reduction in nerve norepinephrine content, because norepinephrine release results in the increased synthesis and release of PGI_2 metabolites by an α-receptor-mediated and calcium/calmodulin–dependent mechanism. It is unknown to what degree PGI_2 is important in regulating vasomotor control in diabetic nerve. However, the complete normalization of NCV and NBF in diabetic rats after administration of evening primrose oil (a γ-linolenic acid–rich natural source that converts to PGE_1) and the reduction of PGI_2 to untreated diabetic levels with the cyclo-oxygenase inhibitor flurbiprofen suggests that vasodilatory PGs play a significant role in maintaining nerve function in the diabetic state.[4]

EFFECTS AND MECHANISM OF ACTION OF PROSTAGLANDINS AND THEIR DERIVATIVES IN DIABETIC NEUROPATHY

In view of the vascular concept for the pathogenesis of diabetic neuropathy in which NBF is decreased and PG metabolism is disrupted, PGE_1 and PGI_2 and their derivatives are candidates for use as therapeutic agents in treating diabetic neuropathy. A number of experimental studies in animals have reported encouraging findings, whereas the results of human trials are somewhat less convincing (Table 26.1). Although essential fatty acids, which are partly converted to PGE_1 and PGI_2, have been reported to be effective for treating diabetic neuropathy in patients and experimental animals, this chapter does not deal with free fatty acids because their efficacy is considered in Chapter 25. It is not known whether PGE_1 or PGI_2 is

TABLE 26.1 EFFECTS OF PROSTAGLANDINS AND THEIR ANALOGUES ON CLINICAL AND EXPERIMENTAL DIABETIC NEUROPATHY

Compound	Clinical Improvement	Motor NCV	Sensory NCV	RHCF	NBF	Capillary Density	Morphometric Improvement	Na$^+$/K$^+$-ATPase Activity
Clinical Trial								
PGE$_1$	+	+	–					
PGI$_2$	(+)	(–)						
TXA$_2$ receptor/synthase inhibitor			(+)					
Experimental Study								
ω-6		+	+	+	+	+		
ω-3		Δ +	Δ +	–		–		
PGE$_1$ analogue		+	+	+	+		+	
PGI$_2$ analogue		+	+	+	+	+		+

Parentheses indicate that the clinical assessment is based on open trials. NCV, nerve conduction velocity; RHCF, resistance to hypoxic conduction failure; Δ +, improvement is significant but partial; NBF, nerve blood flow; PGE$_1$, prostaglandin E$_1$; PGI$_2$, prostacyclin; TXA$_2$, thromboxane A$_2$.
Data from Cameron NE, Cotter MA: The relationship of vascular changes to metabolic factors in diabetes mellitus and their role in the development of peripheral nerve complications. Diabetes Metab Rev 1994; 10:189.

more important for vasodilatory regulation of diabetic nerve and in terms of the treatment of diabetic neuropathy. The results of experimental studies using a combination of evening primrose oil and fish oil might provide some clues. Because the eicosapentanoic acid in fish oil inhibits the conversion of dihomo-GLA to arachidonic acid, the combination therapy enhances PGE_1 synthesis at the expense of PGI_2 production.[8] In this setting, the improvement in NCV produced by evening primrose oil was blunted with fish oil, suggesting that PGI_2 might be the primary mediator of their beneficial action.

Nevertheless, PGE_1 is the most frequently used agent among PGs for the treatment of diabetic complications, including diabetic neuropathy. Free PGE_1 (PGE_1 cyclodextrine [CD]) is the common form. However, this form of PGE_1 was thought to be completely metabolized in the lung in the first circulation. Although arterial infusion was initially used for the treatment with PGE_1, the intravenous route of administration has been widely used since its efficacy was recognized. Lipo-PGE_1, which is a drug preparation of PGE_1 incorporated into lipid microspheres similar in properties to liposomes, has been devised to explore more effective delivery systems. This form of PGE_1 is theoretically believed to collect on lesioned sites without being easily metabolized in the lung. In a randomized, single-blind, cross-over study comparing PGE_1-CD with lipo-PGE_1 in 20 patients with peripheral vascular diseases and diabetic neuropathy, Hoshi and colleagues found lipo-PGE_1 to be superior to PGE_1-CD in final global improvement and patient preference.[14]

Experimental Study

Analogues of PGE_1 (TFC-612 and OP 1206.αCD) and a PGI_2 analogue (iloprost) have been reported to prevent or to lessen decreases in motor nerve conduction velocity (MNCV), NBF, and myelinated nerve fiber diameter without affecting decreased body weight, hyperglycemia, abnormalities of sorbitol and *myo*-inositol metabolism in sciatic nerves of diabetic animals.[25, 33, 36, 38, 45] The improvement of the ischemic milieu in diabetic nerves was supported by a reduction in the lactate content of the endoneurium.[45] Analogues of PGE_1 were initially used to improve nerve function by means of restoring NBF in diabetic animals. Later, these compounds were found to restore decreased nerve Na^+/K^+-ATPase activity in-

dependent of NBF[47] and the *myo*-inositol content in isolated nerves from diabetic rats. The effect of PGE_1 and PGE_2 on cAMP content of normal peripheral nerve had already been reported by Kalix.[17] This improvement in enzyme activity parallels a recovery in cAMP, which is also decreased in diabetic nerves. Furthermore, both dibutyryl cAMP and aminophylline, which inhibits phosphodiesterase activity, and thereby increases cAMP content, can also improve nerve Na^+/K^+-ATPase activity. These observations suggest that the effect of PGE_1 analogues on Na^+/K^+-ATPase activity is mediated by cAMP (Fig. 26.2). Furthermore, the improvement of Na^+/K^+-ATPase activity in diabetic nerve with PGE_1 analogues can be blocked by pretreating isolated nerve preparations from diabetic animals with H8, a protein kinase A inhibitor, suggesting that protein kinase A mediates the effect. In addition to PGs and aminophylline, cilostazol, an antiplatelet drug, is known to increase NBF and also has the ability to inhibit phosphodiesterase activity, thereby increasing cAMP content.[40] Interestingly, aldose reductase inhibitors not only correct nerve sorbitol accumulation but also suppress nerve cAMP content.[32] This observation suggests that cAMP reduction and polyol metabolism in the sciatic nerve may be closely interrelated.

The significance of decreased cAMP content in the pathogenesis of diabetic neuropathy remains unclear, although increased nerve cAMP content corrects the decrease in nerve Na^+/K^+-ATPase activity that is thought to be essential for maintaining nerve function. The mecha-

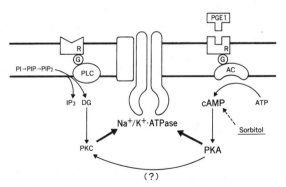

■ **Figure 26.2** Putative mechanisms by which nerve Na^+/K^+-ATPase activity is regulated in diabetic nerve. PGE_1, prostaglandin E_1; R, receptor; G, G protein; AC, adenylate cylase; PI, phosphatidylinositol; PIP, phosphatidylinositol 4-phosphate; PIP_2, phosphatidylinositol 4,5-biphosphate; IP_3, inositol triphosphate; PKC, protein kinase C; PKA, protein kinase A; cAMP, cyclic adenosine monophosphate.

nism by which cAMP content is decreased in diabetic nerves is controversial. Shindo and associates reported decreased adenylate cyclase activity in diabetic nerves,[34] whereas the authors failed to find any change in the activity of adenylate cyclase or phosphodiesterase, although a significantly lower response to isoproterenol was found in diabetic than in control nerves. The latter observation suggests that the transduction from receptor to adenylate cyclase, which regulates cAMP production, may be disturbed in diabetic nerve (personal unpublished data).

Although PGE_1 and its analogues exert a significant beneficial effect on nerve function, the effect is not complete. In view of the possible implication of multifactorial mechanisms, multiple-drug therapy with different mechanisms of action may have greater effects on diabetic neuropathy than single-drug therapy. Combination therapy with the aldose reductase inhibitor Statil and the PGE_1 analogue OP-1206.αCD for 2 months to streptozotocin-induced diabetic rats with 5 months' duration of diabetes improved abnormal nerve sorbitol and *myo*-inositol levels and normalized decreased MNCV and Na^+/K^+-ATPase activity.[46] In contrast, only incomplete improvement of MNCV and morphology of myelinated nerve fibers was obtained with OP-1206.αCD monotherapy.

Human Trials

Some PG trials have reported effective treatment of patients with diabetic neuropathy, although there are few positive double-blind trials. Toyota and associates reported the efficacy of lipo-PGE_1.[40] The effect of lipo-PGE_1 (10 μg/d) was compared with placebo and with a normal dose of a free PGE_1 preparation (PGE_1-CD, 40 μg/d) in well-controlled, double-blind studies that enrolled 364 diabetic patients with neuropathy and/or leg ulcers. The drugs were given intravenously for 4 weeks. Clinical improvement was noted in 62% of the lipo-PGE_1 group and 30% of the placebo group in Trial 1 (P <0.01). In Trial 2, 58% in the lipo-PGE_1 group and 37% in the PGE_1-CD group demonstrated clinical improvement (P <0.01). Motor nerve conduction velocity improved in the lipo-PGE_1 group in Trial 2 (P = 0.016). No serious adverse effects were noted in the patients receiving lipo-PGE_1 or placebo, whereas some patients developed local side effects in the PGE_1-CD group (P <0.01).

Many anecdotal reports have demonstrated an effect of PGE_1 and its derivatives on diabetic neuropathy. Diabetic patients with neuropathy who received PGE_1-CD intravenously for 4 weeks were reported to show a significant improvement in pain and hypesthesia and vibratory threshold both at the radial styloid process and the medial malleolus (n = 38).[35] Another study examined the effects of lipo-PGE_1 on subjective symptoms and hemodynamic effects in 20 patients with type 2 diabetic neuropathy.[27] Subjective symptoms were markedly improved. Furthermore, new real-time two-dimensional color Doppler echography showed that the cross-sectional area of the dorsalis pedis artery and the blood flow index increased significantly.

Lipo-PGE_1 was also reported to improve vibration threshold (6/14), which was measured by an SMV-5 vibrameter, and subjective symptoms (5/14) as early as 24 hours after a single drip infusion in some of 14 patients with type 2 DM and neuropathy, although NCV was not improved.[39]

An effect of iloprost, a stable PGI_2 analogue, on diabetic neuropathy has also been reported; an intravenous infusion of iloprost at a dose 10 μg twice daily relieved subjective symptoms but did not improve MNCV in an open nonrandomized trial.[31]

The thromboxane A_2 (TXA_2) dual blocker KDI-792 was reported to improve NCV and vibration threshold as well as deep skin temperature and skin blood flow in diabetics with neuropathy.[28] Simultaneously, urinary $6KPGF_{1α}$ increased significantly, suggesting that the compound increased PGI_2 production and thereby improved nerve function in patients with diabetic neuropathy.

References

1. Cameron NE, Cotter MA, Low PA. Nerve blood flow in early experimental diabetes in rats: Relation to conduction deficits. Am J Physiol 1991; 261:E1.
2. Cameron NE, Cotter MA, Dines KC, et al. Pharmacological manipulation of vascular endothelium in nondiabetic and streptozotocin-diabetic rats: Effects on nerve conduction, hypoxic resistance and endoneurial capillarization. Diabetologia 1993; 36:516.
3. Cameron NE, Cotter MA. The relationship of vascular changes to metabolic factors in diabetes mellitus and their role in the development of peripheral nerve complications. Diabetes Metab Rev 1994; 10:189.
4. Cameron NE, Cotter MA, Hohman TC. Interactions between essential fatty acid, prostanoid, polyol pathway and nitric oxide mechanisms in the neurovascular deficit of diabetic rats. Diabetologia 1996; 39:172.
5. Campbell WB. 24 Lipid-derived autacoids: Eicosanoids and platelet-activating factor. *In* Gilman AG, Rall TW, Nies A, et al (eds): The Pharmacological Basis of Therapeutics, ed 8. New York, Pergamon Press, 1990, p 600.

6. Coleman RA, Smith WL, Narumiya S. International union of pharmacology classification of prostanoid receptors: Properties, distribution, and structure of the receptors and their subtypes. Pharmacol Rev 1994; 46:205.

7. Constable AL, Armati PJ, Toyka KV, et al. Production of prostanoids by Lewis rat Schwann cells in vitro. Brain Res 1994; 635:75.

8. Dines KC, Cotter MA, Cameron NE. Contrasting effects of treatment with ω-3 and ω-6 essential fatty acids on peripheral nerve function and capillarization in streptozotocin-diabetic rats. Diabetologia 1993; 36:1132.

9. Dyck PJ, Hansen S, Karnes J, et al. Capillary number and percentage closed in human diabetic sural nerve. Proc Natl Acad Sci USA 1985; 82:2513.

10. Goswami SK, Gould RM. Prostanoid synthesis in peripheral nerve. Biochim Biophys Acta 1985; 834:263.

11. Hermenegildo C, Felipo V, Minana M-D, et al. Sustained recovery of Na^+-K^+-ATPase activity in sciatic nerve of diabetic mice by administration of H_7 or Calphostin C, inhibitors of PKC. Diabetes 1993; 42:257.

12. Horrobin DF, Durand LG, Manku MS. Prostaglandin E1 modifies nerve conduction and interferes with local anaesthetic action. Prostaglandins 1977; 14:103.

13. Horrobin DF. The roles of essential fatty acids in the development of diabetic neuropathy and other complications of diabetes mellitus. Prostaglandins Leukot Essent Fatty Acids 1988; 31:181.

14. Hoshi K, Mizushima Y, Kiyokawa-S, et al. Prostaglandin E_1 incorporated in lipid microspheres in the treatment of peripheral vascular diseases and diabetic neuropathy. Drugs Exp Clin Res 1986; 12:681.

15. Jamal GA. Pathogenesis of diabetic neuropathy: The role of the n-6 essential fatty acids and their eicosanoid derivatives. Diabetic Med 1990; 7:574.

16. Juan H: The pain enhancing effect of PGI_2. Agent Actions 1979; 9:204.

17. Kalix P. Prostaglandin E_1 raises the cAMP content of peripheral nerve tissue. Neurosci Lett 1979; 12:361.

18. Keen H, Payan J, Allawi J, et al. Treatment of diabetic neuropathy with γ-linolenic acid. Diabetes Care 1993; 16:8.

19. Kim J, Rushovich EH, Thomas TP, et al. Diminished specific activity of cystosolic protein kinase C in sciatic nerve of streptozocin-induced diabetic rats and its correction by dietary myo-inositol. Diabetes 1991; 40:1545.

20. Low PA, Ward K, Schmelzer JD, et al. Ischemic conduction failure and energy metabolism in experimental diabetic neuropathy. Am J Physiol 1985; 248:E457.

21. Low PA, Nickander KK. Oxygen free radical effects in sciatic nerve in experimental diabetes. Diabetes 1991; 40:873.

22. MacCord JM. Oxygen-derived free radicals in post ischemic tissue injury. N Engl J Med 1985; 312:159.

23. Newrick PG, Wilson AJ, Jakubowski J, et al. Sural nerve oxygen tension in diabetes. Br Med J 1986; 293:1053.

24. Ohi T, Poduslo JF, Dyck PJ. Increased endoneurial albumin in diabetic polyneuropathy. Neurology 1985; 35:1790.

25. Ohno A, Kanazawa A, Tanaka A, et al. Effect of a prostaglandin I_2 derivative (iloprost) on peripheral neuropathy of diabetic rats. Diabetes Res Clin Pract 1992; 18:123.

26. Oida H, Namba T, Sugimoto Y, et al. In situ hybridization studies of prostacyclin receptor mRNA expression in various mouse organs. Br J Pharmacol 1995; 116:2828.

27. Okuda Y, Mizutani M, Ogawa-M, et al. Hemodynamic effects of lipo-PGE1 on peripheral artery in patients with diabetic neuropathy: Evaluated by two-dimensional color Doppler echography. Diabetes Res 1993; 22:87.

28. Ono Y, Katoh M, Hirayama A, et al. Improvement in blood flow and diabetic neuropathy by thromboxane A_2 dual blocker KDI-792. Prostaglandins Leukot Essent Fatty Acids 1995; 53:139.

29. Pateromichelakis S, Rood JP. Prostaglandin E_2 increases mechanically evoked potentials in the peripheral nerve. Experientia 1981; 37:282.

30. Poduslo JF, Curran GL, Dyck PJ. Increase in albumin, IgG, and IgM blood-nerve barrier indices in human diabetic neuropathy. Proc Natl Acad Sci USA 1988; 85:4879.

31. Shindo H, Tawata M, Aida K, et al. Clinical efficacy of a stable prostacyclin analogue, iloprost, in diabetic neuropathy. Prostaglandins 1991; 41:85.

32. Shindo H, Tawata M, Aida K, et al. The role of cyclic adenosine 3',5'-monophosphate and polyol metabolism in diabetic neuropathy. J Clin Endocrinol Metab 1992; 74:393.

33. Shindo H, Tawata M, Onaya T. Cyclic adenosine 3',5'-monophosphate enhances sodium, potassium-adenosine triphosphatase activity in the sciatic nerve of streptozocin-induced diabetic rats. Endocrinology 1993; 132:510.

34. Shindo H, Tawata M, Onaya T. Reduction of cyclic AMP in the sciatic nerve of rats made diabetic with streptozotocin and the mechanism involved. J Endocrinol 1993; 136:431.

35. Shindo H, Tawata M, Inoue M, et al. The effect of prostaglandin E1.alpha CD on vibratory threshold determined with the SMV-5 vibrometer in patients with diabetic neuropathy. Diabetes Res Clin Pract 1994; 24:173.

36. Sonobe M, Yasuda H, Hisanaga T, et al. Amelioration of nerve Na^+-K^+-ATPase activity independently of myo-inositol level by PGE_1 analogue OP-1206.α-CD in streptozocin-induced diabetic rats. Diabetes 1991; 40:726.

37. Sugimoto Y, Shigemoto R, Namba T, et al. Distribution of the messenger RNA for the prostaglandin E receptor subtype EP3 in the mouse nervous system. Neuroscience 1994; 62:919.

38. Suzuki K, Saito N, Sakata Y, et al. A new prostaglandin E_1 analogue (TFC-612) improves the reduction in motor nerve conduction velocity in spontaneously diabetic GK (Goto-Kakizaki) rats. Prostaglandins 1990; 40:463.

39. Tawata M, Nitta K, Kurihara A, et al. Effects of a single drip infusion of lipo-prostaglandin E_1 on vibratory threshold in patients with diabetic neuropathy. Prostaglandins 1995; 49:27.

40. Toyota T, Hirata Y, Ikeda Y, et al. Lipo-PGE1, a new lipid-encapsulated preparation of prostaglandin E_1: Placebo- and prostaglandin E_1-controlled multicenter trials in patients with diabetic neuropathy and leg ulcers. Prostaglandins 1993; 46:453.

41. Tuck RR, Schmelzer JD, Low PA. Endoneurial blood flow and oxygen tension in the sciatic nerves of rats with experimental diabetic neuropathy. Brain 1984; 107:935.

42. Ward KK, Low PA, Schmelzer JD, et al. Prostacyclin and noradrenaline in peripheral nerve of chronic experimental diabetes in rats. Brain 1989; 112:197.

43. Williamson JR. Hyperglycemic pseudohypoxia and diabetic complications. Diabetes 1993; 42:801.

44. Yasuda H, Dyck PJ. Abnormalities of endoneurial mi-

crovessels and sural nerve pathology in diabetic neuropathy. Neurology 1987; 37:20.

45. Yasuda H, Sonobe M, Yamashita M, et al. Effect of prostaglandin E₁ analogue TFC 612 on diabetic neuropathy in streptozocin-induced diabetic rats: Comparison with aldose reductase inhibitor ONO 2235. Diabetes 1989; 38:832.

46. Yasuda H, Sonobe M, Hisanaga T, et al. A combination of the aldose reductase inhibitor, statil, and the prostaglandin E₁ analogue, OP1206.αCD, completely improves sciatic motor nerve conduction velocity in streptozocin-induced chronically diabetic rats. Metabolism 1992; 41:778.

47. Yasuda H, Maeda K, Sonobe M, et al. Metabolic effect of PGE1 analogue OP1206.αCD on nerve Na⁺-K⁺-ATPase activity of rats with streptozocin-induced diabetes is mediated via cAMP: Possible role of cAMP in diabetic neuropathy. Prostaglandins 1994; 47:367.

48. Zhu X, Eichberg J. 1,2-diacylglycerol content and its arachidonyl-containing molecular species are reduced in sciatic nerve from streptozocin-induced diabetic rats. J Neurochem 1990; 55:1087.

Chapter **27**

Growth Factors and Peripheral Neuropathy

Eva L. Feldman • Anthony J. Windebank

INTRODUCTION

Neuropathy is a common, frequently disabling complication of diabetes.[19] In a prospective study of more than 4400 diabetic patients, Pirart reported that approximately 10% of his patients had neuropathy at the time of diagnosis of their diabetes. After 25 years of diabetes, more than 50% of his diabetic patients were neuropathic.[87] In parallel, results from the Diabetes Control and Complications Trial (DCCT) clearly indicate that neuropathy correlates with the degree and duration of hyperglycemia.[23, 28, 29] In the Rochester diabetic study, 59% of patients with type 2 diabetes mellitus (DM) and 66% of patients with type 1 DM had a neuropathy.[31–33] Although the presence of neuropathy is ascribed to the diabetic state, the specific metabolic and vascular abnormalities that underlie the onset of neuropathy remain controversial and are the subject of active research.[43, 44] Potential etiologies include disruption of the polyol pathway, enhanced oxidative stress, vascular insufficiency, abnormal lipid or amino acid metabolism, advanced glycation products, or blunted growth factor action.[42, 44] It is unclear whether the primary effects of these metabolic or vascular abnormalities (or both) are on peripheral nervous system neurons or Schwann cells.[44] Importantly, secondary dysfunction of peripheral nervous system components, including the perineurium or extracellular matrix, may underlie the development of diabetic neuropathy.[44]

Although the pathogenesis of diabetic neuropathy is unknown, a growing body of research suggests that growth factors may be involved in the etiology of this common complication.[14, 56, 76, 82, 93, 107] Three main classes of growth factors are present in the peripheral nervous system and could play a role in the development of neuropathy: neurotrophins, insulin-like growth factors, and cytokine-like growth factors.[14, 56, 76, 82, 93, 107] In this chapter, we will review normal growth factor function, discuss the changes in growth factor function observed in the diabetic state, and summarize the therapeutic potential of growth factors in the treatment of diabetic neuropathy.

PERIPHERAL NERVOUS SYSTEM GROWTH FACTORS

Neurotrophins

Nerve growth factor (NGF) was described by Levi-Montalcini and Calissano.[70] Nerve growth factor is produced by target organs of sympathetic and neural-crest derived dorsal root ganglion sensory neurons, where levels of NGF messenger RNA parallel the density of innervation by NGF-sensitive neurons.[70, 106] During embryogenesis, 50% of dorsal root ganglion neurons are responsive to NGF. Most of these neurons represent nociceptive C fibers with small cell bodies and unmyelinated axons.[1] In the past 15 years, three additional growth factors with structural homology to NGF have been discovered[12, 74]: brain-derived neurotrophic factor (BDNF), neurotrophin-3 (NT-3), and neurotrophin-4/5 (NT-4/5). There is approximately 50% amino acid sequence homology among the family members, all of which have retained six critical cysteine residues.[74]

The neurotrophins bind to a family of tyrosine kinase receptors called Trk (tropomyosin-related kinase).[12, 53] Trk A is the high affinity NGF receptor, Trk B serves as the receptor for both BNDF and NT-4/5, and Trk C binds NT-3. In addition to the Trk receptors, a "low" affinity receptor for all the neurotrophins exists, termed p75. Trk B and C exist in truncated forms, devoid of the active kinase domain.[12]

Retrograde transport of neurotrophins from target organs to neuronal cell bodies is required for normal growth, maintenance, and regeneration of the peripheral nervous system.

In general, dorsal root ganglion neurons and primary sensory neurons derived from neural crest are responsive to NGF, BDNF, or NT-3, and cranial nerve sensory ganglia respond to BDNF or NT-3 but not NGF. During chick development, approximately 50% of the dorsal root ganglion neurons are NGF responsive, and 30 to 40% require BDNF.[74] Neurotrophin-3 appears to support primarily proprioceptive neurons and promotes the survival of muscle afferents.[17] Analyses of knockout mice have further confirmed the specific role of neurotrophins. Nerve growth factor–homozygous knockout mice have loss of all sympathetic neurons and small neural crest–derived sensory neurons (nociceptive C neurons).[24] Neurotrophin-3 knockout animals lack type Ia sensory afferents and muscle spindles, and BDNF and NT-4/5 null mutants lack all neural placode–derived sensory cranial ganglia.[20, 35, 100]

Insulin-like Growth Factors

A second family of growth factors, the insulin-like growth factors (IGF-I, IGF-II), are polypeptides with growth-promoting and insulin-like metabolic activities. The effects of IGFs on growth are mediated by the IGF-I receptor, a tyrosine kinase receptor.[27] Insulin-like growth factors and the IGF-I receptor are essential for normal growth.[25, 92] Insulin-like growth factors, which are abundant in the developing nervous system,[8, 66, 103] share many important neurotrophic properties with NGF. Insulin-like growth factors have neurotrophic actions in sensory,[57] sympathetic,[57, 121] and motor neurons[57] as well as in Schwann cells.[18] During neurite outgrowth, IGFs promote organization of the actin cytoskeleton,[67, 68] activation of focal adhesion proteins,[69] and expression of microtubular proteins and growth-associated proteins, such as GAP-43.[64] In parallel, IGFs also support Schwann cell mitogenesis[18] and promote nervous system myelination.[84]

Insulin-like growth factors are presently the only known neurotrophic factors, found in nerve and muscle, capable of supporting sensory and motor nerve regeneration in adult animals.[22, 40, 52, 54, 56, 72] In mice that have been genetically altered to overexpress IGF-I, brain mass is increased because of enhanced myelin production.[16] Disruption of IGF-I receptor expression in mice is lethal; autopsy reveals hypomyelination and small brains.[9] In both paradigms, no data are available on neuron counts or more detailed nervous system pathology.[9, 16]

Cytokine-like Growth Factors

Two cytokine-like growth factors, ciliary neurotrophic factor (CNTF)[95] and glial-derived neurotrophic factor (GDNF),[50, 101] have been localized within the peripheral nervous system. Ciliary neurotrophic factor is a member of the cytokine superfamily and is produced by Schwann cells.[79] Motor neurons serve as the major target for CNTF. Ciliary neurotrophic factor enhances avian motor neuron survival in vivo and in vitro and can rescue neonatal rat facial motor neurons from experimentally induced cell death.[86, 88, 96] Ciliary neurotrophic factor receptors have been localized throughout the nervous system during development and in adult tissues.[79, 102].

Glial-derived neurotrophic factor is a recently described neuronal growth factor in the transforming growth factor-β family. Glial-derived neurotrophic factor supports survival of motor neurons as well as subpopulations of sensory neurons in mouse, rat, and chick.[85] During development, GDNF is present in target tissue of motor neurons, and addition of GDNF during the period of neuronal apoptosis results in an increase in the number of surviving neurons.[85] After axotomy of the facial nerve, GDNF application promotes the survival of up to 92% of facial motor neurons and prevents normally occurring atrophy.[85, 119] Schwann cells are known to produce GDNF, and this locally available growth factor may aid in maintaining axon integrity.[114] The receptor for GDNF has only recently been described and is comprised of a glycosylphosphatidylinositol (GPI) linked α subunit (GDNFR-α) and the transmembrane protein Ret.[30, 61, 112, 113, 116] Expression of Ret is widespread during development and has been detected in the central and peripheral nervous systems[112, 115] as well as in the developing kidney.[30, 115, 116]

GROWTH FACTORS AND DIABETIC NEUROPATHY

Mounting evidence suggests that the roles of growth factors change during development; growth factors are required for survival of embryonic neurons, whereas their role in the adult is one of defining the neuronal and glial phenotype and promoting local regeneration.[74] For example, neurotrophins regulate the expression of phenotypic neuropeptides such as substance P and calcitonin gene-related peptide (CGRP) in adult dorsal root ganglion neurons[109] and, after nerve injury in the adult,

promote local neurite sprouting and regeneration.[26] The concept has emerged that potential blunting of these normal growth factor responses may play a role in the pathogenesis of nervous system diseases.[75] This may be especially true of diabetic neuropathy, where persistent hyperglycemia may decrease *growth factor synthesis* by target organs or supporting cells, disrupt *axonal transport* of growth factors to the neuronal cell body, alter *growth factor signaling* at the level of growth factor receptors or at more downstream signaling cascades, or promote *neuroglial cell death*.[14, 118] There are data that support each of these possibilities, and, in each case, NGF is the best studied of the growth factors.

Growth Factor Synthesis

Neurons that require NGF are commonly affected in diabetes. Injury of these neurons produces autonomic and sensory neuropathy. Evidence suggests that altered NGF production may play a role in the pathophysiology of these neuropathies. Endogenous NGF levels are reduced in sympathetically innervated target organs of streptozotocin-treated rats.[48] In streptozotocin-treated rats as well as genetically diabetic mice (C57BL/KsJ db/db), there is a decrease in NGF production[37, 63] that corresponds to a decrease in neuropeptide levels.[37] Patients with diabetic neuropathy have significantly lower levels of serum NGF than non-diabetic controls,[36] and it has been speculated that autoantibodies to NGF may play a role in autonomic neuropathy.[122] Decreased skin axon reflexes, mediated by small sensory fibers, correlate with loss of NGF expression in keratinocytes in patients with early diabetic neuropathy.[2, 3]

In adult rat sciatic nerve, NGF expression is regulated by axonal contact.[11, 62] After nerve injury in normal rodents, Schwann cells distal to the injury dramatically increase their production of NGF[51] and NGF receptors,[104, 105] reaching a maximum at 5 to 7 days. Interestingly, there is no change in p75 NGF receptor expression in sural nerve biopsy specimens from patients with diabetic neuropathy,[13] implying that Schwann cells from diabetics have lost normal neurotrophic responses to injury.

Less is known about the expression of the other neurotrophin family members in the diabetic state. One recent report found between 30 and 50% decrease in NT-3 and NT-4/5 gene expression in nerves from rodents with experimental diabetes, whereas BDNF was undetectable.[89] Leg muscles from diabetic rats are deficient in NT-3, and administration of NT-3 increases conduction velocity of sensory nerves.[109] Collectively, these data suggest that neurotrophin production, particularly NGF, is altered in diabetes, and such a disruption of normal neurotrophic factor production may contribute to the development of diabetic neuropathy.

There are multiple examples where the diabetic state in rodents and humans has led to altered IGF expression or action. Schwann cells from genetically diabetic rodents express lowered amounts of IGF-I and the IGF-I receptor.[120] In streptozotocin-treated rats, there is a decrease in serum IGF-I levels[34, 41, 120] and a reduction in IGF-I mRNA in sciatic nerve, liver, kidney, lung, and heart.[10, 58, 78, 117, 120] In humans, IGF-I and IGF-I receptor levels are decreased in diabetic patients with neuropathy, compared with those diabetics without neuropathy.[83] Although research is ongoing, there are few data yet on CNTF and GDNF production in diabetes.

Axonal Transport

The axonal transport of neurotrophins, especially NGF, has been well described. Nerve growth factor binds selectively to the terminal portions of sympathetic and neural crest–derived sensory neurons, and, after internalization, is transported by retrograde axonal flow to the cell bodies. Retrograde axonal transport of NGF is altered in streptozotocin-diabetic rats. Mesenteric nerves, which supply the alimentary tract, can develop a distal diabetic axonopathy. During experimentally induced diabetes, retrograde axonal transport of NGF along the mesenteric nerves to the superior mesenteric ganglion is reduced by approximately half.[77, 110] Similarly, NGF transport is decreased in diabetic somatic sensory neurons.[49, 60] These alterations in NGF transport form a subset of more widespread transport dysfunction in diabetes. Decreased axonal transport during experimentally induced diabetes has been reported for proteins, glycoproteins, and neurotransmitters.[110] These results suggest that impairment of axonal transport, especially the retrograde flow of neurotrophins, may play a role in the pathogenesis of diabetic neuropathy.

Signal Transduction of Growth Factors in Diabetes

Activation of phosphatidylinositol 4,5-biphosphate-specific phospholipase C produces inositol 1,4,5-trisphosphate (IP_3) and 1,2-diacylglycerol (DAG). Inositol 1,4,5-trisphosphate mediates intracellular calcium mobilization, and DAG increases the affinity of protein kinase C for calcium, resulting in kinase activation. In neural tissues, activation of muscarinic, cholinergic, adrenergic, histaminergic, or serotonergic receptors results in stimulation of phosphoinositide (PI) turnover.[38] Nerve growth factor has been shown to stimulate PI turnover in rat superior cervical ganglia[65] and PC12 cells,[111] and IGF-II stimulates IP_3 and DAG production in canine kidney.[90]

Alterations in PI metabolism are well documented in diabetes[44, 108] and are thought by many investigators to form the cornerstone of diabetic complications.[44] In contrast, much less is known about the potential role growth factors may play in these alterations. In human liver, acute exposure to insulin, IGF-I, and IGF-II has no effect on PI turnover, yet diabetic liver has increased PI turnover. Definitive experiments, examining growth factor–coupled PI turnover in multiple diabetic tissues, have not yet been done.

Deficient expression of neurotrophin-responsive genes also occurs in diabetic animals. Nerve growth factor regulates the expression of two neuropeptides: substance P and CGRP.[14] In diabetic rats, substance P and CGRP gene and protein levels are decreased in dorsal root ganglia and sciatic nerves[37, 94] but restored to normal levels with NGF, but not BDNF, administration.[37, 91] Although the exact mechanism(s) underlying altered neuropeptide levels remains unknown, the two most likely etiologies are either deficient NGF production or altered NGF signaling, caused by a change in receptor number or a change in downstream signaling. Additional studies are needed to address these important possibilities as well as the effects of the diabetic milieu on downstream signaling by all classes of growth factors.

Neuroglial Cell Death

One novel theory that may link growth factors with diabetic neuropathy suggests that chronic hyperglycemia induces apoptosis of Schwann cells as well as sensory and motor neurons. Glycemic-mediated death results in myelin loss, axon loss and the signs and symptoms of diabetic neuropathy. In vivo, short-term exposure to high glucose induces apoptosis of dorsal root ganglia neurons and Schwann cells in rats (Fig. 27.1). In vitro, chronic hyperglycemia and hyperosmotic exposure results in ap-

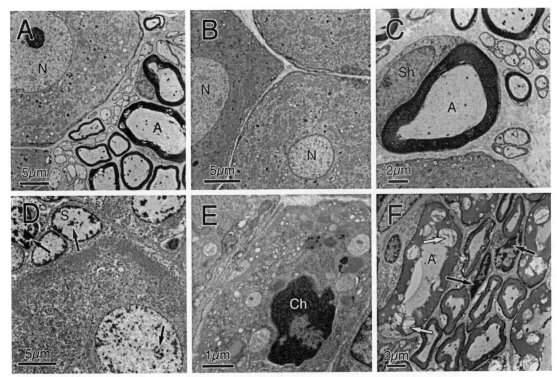

■ **Figure 27.1** Hyperglycemia in vivo induces apoptosis in dorsal root ganglion (DRG) neurons, satellite cells, and Schwann cells. Adult rats were infused with 100% dextrose or vehicle without dextrose. After 6 to 10 hours, they were fixation perfused and DRG removed as described in the methods section. *A–C*, Control animals. *D–F*, Glucose-infused animals. *A*, DRG neuron with normal nucleus (N) and distinct nucleolus. The myelinated axons (A) show normal axoplasmic volume, and myelin lamellae. *B*, Normal DRG neurons showing chromatin dispersed regularly throughout the nucleus (N). *C*, Normal myelinated axon (A) and adjacent Schwann cell (Sh) surrounded by normal unmyelinated axons. *D*, Initial chromatin condensation *(black arrows)* in a large DRG neuron and smaller satellite cells (S) consistent with early apoptotic changes (compare with control *A* and *B*). *E*, Advanced chromatin compaction (Ch), nuclear and cytoplasmic shrinkage with vacuolation in a DRG neuron, consistent with apoptosis. *F*, Myelinated axons (A) show shrinkage and disruption of the axoplasm with prominent vesiculation of the myelin lamellae *(white arrows)*. Schwann cells show distinct nuclear condensation *(black arrows)* and cytoplasmic shrinkage with preservation of the cell membrane, consistent with apoptotic cell death.

optosis of rat dorsal root ganglion neurons and well-differentiated human neuroblastoma cells.[80, 81, 98, 99] Interestingly, IGF-I can rescue rat and human neurons from hyperglycemic-coupled apoptosis,[80, 81, 98, 99] but NGF is ineffective.

GROWTH FACTOR TREATMENT OF DIABETIC NEUROPATHY

We have presented evidence that suggests that growth factor defects are present in diabetes and their collective interaction within the diabetic milieu may contribute to the development and progression of diabetic neuropathy. These findings have formed the basis of growth factor treatment trials in diabetic neuropathy. Currently, these treatments are initially testable on the diabetic rodent, an animal model of human diabetes.[97] A wide range of treatments in the diabetic rodent are linked to improved nerve conduction velocities or evoked amplitudes, improved nerve blood flow, or restoration of normal rates of axonal transport.[97]

Initial trials in rodents suggest NGF and IGF-I protect against the development of diabetic neuropathy and restore normal nerve function.[14, 55, 56, 59] Administration of IGF-I blocks the development of sensory neuropathy in diabetic rats and reverses impaired nerve regeneration.[123] In the streptozocin rat, NGF administration improves tail-flick thresholds[5] and ameliorates diabetes-induced decreases in neuropeptide levels in vivo[5, 37, 94] and in vitro.[91]

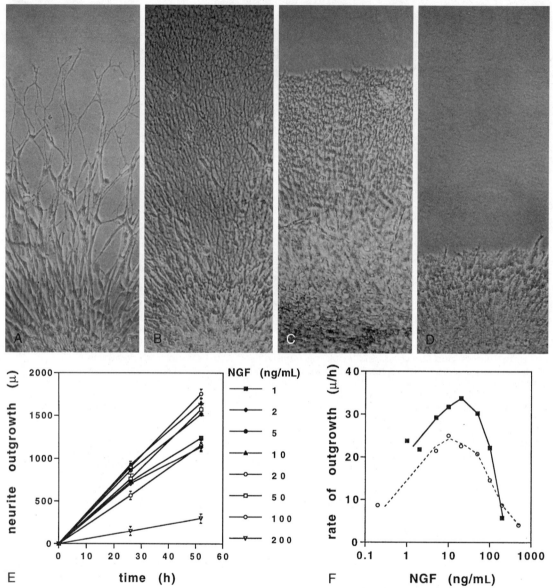

■ **Figure 27.2** Induction of neurite outgrowth from dorsal root ganglion (DRG) neurons. Dorsal root ganglions were removed from E15 rats and explanted onto a collagen surface. *A–D,* Neurite outgrowth in the presence of 1, 10, 50, and 200 ng/mL nerve growth factor (NGF), respectively. Images acquired by phase contrast microscopy were measured by a blinded observer. For each concentration, 9 to 12 separate explants were measured. Mean neurite outgrowth was measured for each concentration *(E)* and rate of growth calculated by linear regression using the method of least squares. This demonstrated a window of 2.5S mouse NGF-responsive neurite outgrowth *(F, closed squares).* At 24 hours, the inhibition by 100 ng/mL was significant ($P < .01$) and by 200 ng/mL was highly significant ($P < .001$). At 48 hours, 50, 100, and 200 ng/mL all produced highly significant ($P < .001$) inhibition. Significance was calculated by analysis of variance. The whole series was repeated on at least three occasions for each concentration, with similar results. *Open circles* and *dotted lines* represent identical experiments using rat DRG and rhNGF *(F).* (From Conti AM, Fischer SJ, Windebank AJ: Inhibition of axonal growth from sensory neurons by excess nerve growth factor. Ann Neurol 42:838–846, 1997.)

Diabetic rodents treated with NGF retain the ability to respond to noxious thermal stimuli and express normal neuropeptide levels.[5] Treatment with 4-methylcatechol, which stimulates endogenous NGF synthesis, also ameliorates the signs of neuropathy in streptozocin-treated rodents.[45] A preliminary clinical trial in humans suggests NGF may be effective in the treatment of diabetic neuropathy,[4] although its use may be limited by side effects.[1] Recent reports suggest that excess NGF may actually inhibit neurite outgrowth (Fig. 27.2), emphasizing that caution is needed in human clinical trials using growth factor therapy.[21]

Growth factors have also been widely used in animal models of neuropathies of nondiabetic origin. Administration of NT-3 prevents the behavioral, electrophysiologic, and morphological sequelae of pyridoxine- and cisplatin-mediated neuropathy,[39, 47] whereas IGF-I and NGF rescue rodents from cisplatin- and taxol-induced neuropathy.[6, 94] In humans, IGF-I is currently being administered in clinical trials to lung cancer patients treated with cisplatin in hopes of preventing the development of neuropathy. A phase 3 clinical trial has also shown that IGF-I is effective in the treatment of amyotrophic lateral sclerosis. Unfortunately, neither BDNF nor CNTF were effective in phase 3 clinical trials in the same patient population.[71] To date, there are no human clinical trials of NT-3, IGF-I, CNTF, or BNDF in diabetic neuropathy.

SUMMARY AND FUTURE DIRECTIONS

As we increase our understanding of the role of growth factors in the adult nervous system, we can better define their importance in the pathogenesis and treatment of diabetic neuropathy. Data suggest that aberrant expression and function of growth factors and growth factor receptors occurs in diabetes. In the past, most investigators directed their scientific efforts toward understanding the actions of NGF. However, with the discovery of NT-3 and BDNF as well as the recent promise of IGF-I and the cytokine-like growth factors, it is clear that several growth factors may be therapeutically important in diabetic neuropathy.[7, 14, 15, 46, 56, 73, 82] IGF-I, with its insulin-like metabolic activity as well as its growth-promoting properties, is an excellent candidate for the treatment of diabetic neuropathy.[55, 56, 123] The cytokine-like growth factors, especially GDNF, also hold special promise because of their unique distribu-

tion and function in the peripheral nervous system. As interest in growth factor therapies continues to escalate, it is likely that clinical trials with not only NGF but also other growth factors (BDNF, NT-3, IGF-I, GDNF) will become an important component of our efforts toward effectively treating diabetic neuropathy.

ACKNOWLEDGMENTS

The authors thank Judy Boldt for expert secretarial assistance and Jim Beals for photographic preparation.

Sources of Support: This work was supported by NIH NS32843 (E.L.F.), grants from the Juvenile Diabetes Foundation (E.L.F.) and the American Diabetes Association (E.L.F.), and NIH NS14304 (A.J.W).

References

1. Anand P. Nerve growth factor regulates nociception in human health and disease. Br J Anaesth 1995; 75:201.
2. Anand P. Neurotrophins and peripheral neuropathy. Philos Trans R Soc Lond B Biol Sci 1996; 351:449.
3. Anand P, Terenghi G, Warner G, et al. The role of endogenous nerve growth factor in human diabetic neuropathy. Nature Med 1996; 2:703.
4. Apfel SC, Adornato BT, Dyck PJ, et al. Results of a double-blind, placebo-controlled trial of recombinant human nerve growth factor in diabetic polyneuropathy (abstract). Ann Neurol 1996; 40:540.
5. Apfel SC, Arezzo JC, Brownlee M, et al. Nerve growth factor administration protects against experimental diabetic sensory neuropathy. Brain Res 1994; 634:7.
6. Apfel SC, Arezzo JC, Lipson L, et al. Nerve growth factor prevents experimental cisplatin neuropathy. Ann Neurol 1992; 31:76.
7. Apfel SC, Kessler JA. Neurotrophic factors in the therapy of peripheral neuropathy. Baillieres Clin Neurol 1995; 4:593.
8. Beck F, Samani NJ, Byrne S, et al. Histochemical localization of IGF-I and IGF-II mRNA in the rat between birth and adulthood. Development 1988; 104:29.
9. Beck KD, Powell-Braxton L, Widmer H-R, et al. *Igf1* gene disruption results in reduced brain size, CNS hypomyelination, and loss of hippocampal granule and striatal parvalbumin-containing neurons. Neuron 1995; 14:717.
10. Bornfeldt KE, Arnqvist HJ, Enberg B, et al. Regulation of insulin-like growth factor-I and growth hormone receptor gene expression by diabetes and nutritional state in rat tissues. J Endocrinol 1989; 122:651.
11. Bosch EP, Zhong W, Lim R. Axonal signals regulate expression of glia maturation factor-β in Schwann cells: An immunohistochemical study of injured sciatic nerves and cultured Schwann cells. J Neurosci 1989; 9:3690.
12. Bothwell M. Functional interactions of neurotrophins and neurotrophin receptors. Annu Rev Neurosci 1995; 18:223.
13. Bradley JL, Thomas PK, King RHM, et al. Myelinated nerve fibre regeneration in diabetic sensory polyneu-

ropathy: Correlation with type of diabetes. Acta Neuropathologica 1995; 90:403.

14. Brewster WJ, Fernyhough P, Diemel LT, et al. Diabetic neuropathy, nerve growth factor and other neurotrophic factors. Trends Neurosci 1994; 17:321.

15. Cameron NE, Cotter MA. Potential therapeutic approaches to the treatment or prevention of diabetic neuropathy: Evidence from experimental studies. Diabet Med 1993; 10:593.

16. Carson MJ, Behringer RR, Brinster RL, et al. Insulin-like growth factor I increases brain growth and central nervous system myelination in transgenic mice. Neuron 1993; 10:729.

17. Chalazonitis A. Neurotrophin-3 as an essential signal for the developing nervous system. Mol Neurobiol 1996; 12:39.

18. Cheng H-L, Randolph A, Yee D, et al. Characterization of insulin-like growth factor-I (IGF-I), IGF-I receptor and binding proteins in transected nerves and cultured schwann cells. J Neurochem 1996; 66:525.

19. Committee on Health Care Issues American Neurological Association. Does improved control of glycemia prevent or ameliorate diabetic neuropathy? Ann Neurol 1986; 19:288.

20. Conover JC, Erickson JT, Katz DM, et al. Neuronal deficits, not involving motor neurons, in mice lacking BDNF and/or NT4. Nature (Lond) 1995; 375:235.

21. Conti AM, Fischer SJ, Windebank AJ. Inhibition of axonal growth from sensory neurons by excess nerve growth factor. Ann Neurol 1997; 42:838–846.

22. Contreras PC, Steffler C, Yu EY, et al. Systemic administration of rhIGF-I enhanced regeneration after sciatic nerve crush in mice. J Pharmacol Exp Ther 1995; 274:1443.

23. Crofford OB. Diabetes control and complications. Annu Rev Med 1995; 46:267.

24. Crowley C, Spencer SD, Nushimura MC, et al. Mice lacking nerve growth factor display perinatal loss of sensory and sympathetic neurons yet develop basal forebrain cholinergic neurons. Cell 1994; 76:1001.

25. Daughaday WH, Rotwein P. Insulin-like growth factor I and II. Peptide, messenger ribonucleic acid and gene structures, serum, and tissue concentrations. Endocr Rev 1989; 10:(1) 68.

26. Davies AM. The neurotrophic hypothesis: Where does it stand? Philos Trans R Soc Lond B Biol Sci 1996; 351:389.

27. De Meyts P, Wallach B, Christoffersen CT, et al. The insulin-like growth factor-I receptor: Structure, ligand-binding mechanism and signal transduction. Horm Res 1994; 42:152.

28. Diabetes Control and Complications Trial Research Group. The effect of intensive treatment of diabetes on the development and progression of long-term complications in insulin-dependent diabetes mellitus. N Engl J Med 1993; 329:977.

29. Diabetes Control and Complications Trial Research Group. The effect of intensive diabetes therapy on the development and progression of neuropathy. Ann Intern Med 1995; 122:561.

30. Durbec P, Marcos-Gutierrez CV, Kilkenny C, et al. GDNF signalling through the Ret receptor tyrosine kinase. Nature 1996; 381:789.

31. Dyck PJ, Karnes JL, O'Brien PC. The Rochester Diabetic Neuropathy Study: Reassessment of tests and criteria for diagnosis and staged severity. Neurology 1992; 42:1164.

32. Dyck PJ, Kratz KM, Lehman KA. The Rochester Diabetic Neuropathy Study: Design, criteria for types

33. Dyck PJ, Litchy WJ, Lehman KA, et al. Variables influencing neuropathic endpoints: The Rochester Diabetic Neuropathy Study of Healthy Subjects. Neurology 1995; 45:1115.

34. Ekstrom AR, Kanje M, Skottner A. Nerve regeneration and serum levels of insulin-like growth factor-I in rats with streptozotocin-induced insulin deficiency. Brain Res 1989; 496:141.

35. Ernfors P, Lee K-F, Jaenisch R. Mice lacking brain-derived neurotrophic factor develop with sensory deficits. Nature (Lond) 1994; 368:147.

36. Faradji V, Sotelo J. Low serum levels of nerve growth factor in diabetic neuropathy. Acta Neurol Scand 1990; 81:402.

37. Fernyhough P, Diemel LT, Hardy J, et al. Human recombinant nerve growth factor replaces deficient neurotrophic support in the diabetic rat. Eur J Neurosci 1995; 7:1107.

38. Fisher SK, Heacock AM, Agranoff BW. Inositol lipids and signal transduction in the nervous system: An update. J Neurochem 1992; 58:(1)18.

39. Gao W-Q, Dybdal N, Shinsky N, et al. Neurotrophin-3 reverses experimental cisplatin-induced peripheral sensory neuropathy. Ann Neurol 1995; 38:30.

40. Glazner GW, Lupien S, Miller JA, et al. Insulin-like growth factor II increases the rate of sciatic nerve regeneration in rats. Neuroscience 1993; 54:791.

41. Graubert MD, Goldstein S, Phillips LS. Nutrition and somatomedin: XXVII. Total and free IGF-I and IGF binding proteins in rats with streptozocin-induced diabetes. Diabetes 1991; 40:959.

42. Greene DA, Lattimer SA, Sima AAF. Pathogenesis and prevention of diabetic neuropathy. Diabetes Metab Rev 1988; 4:201.

43. Greene DA, Sima A, Pfeifer MA, et al. Diabetic neuropathy. Annu Rev Med 1990; 41:303.

44. Greene DA, Sima AAF, Stevens MJ, et al. Complications: Neuropathy, pathogenetic considerations. Diabetes Care 1992; 15:1902.

45. Hanaoka Y, Ohi T, Furukawa S, et al. The therapeutic effects of 4-methylcatechol, a stimulator of endogenous nerve growth factor synthesis, on experimental diabetic neuropathy in rats. J Neurol Sci 1994; 122:28.

46. Hefti F. Neurotrophic factor therapy for nervous system degenerative diseases. J Neurobiol 1994; 25:1418.

47. Helgren ME, Cliffer KD, Torrento K, et al. Neurotrophin-3 administration attenuates deficits of pyridoxine-induced large-fiber sensory neuropathy. J Neurosci 1997; 17:372.

48. Hellweg R, Hartung H-D. Endogenous levels of nerve growth factor (NGF) are altered in experimental diabetes mellitus: A possible role for NGF in the pathogenesis of diabetic neuropathy. J Neurosci Res 1990; 26:258.

49. Hellweg R, Raivich G, Hartung H-D, et al. Axonal transport of endogenous nerve growth factor (NGF) and NGF receptor in experimental diabetic neuropathy. Exp Neurol 1994; 130:24.

50. Henderson CE, Phillips HS, Pollock RA, et al. GDNF: A potent survival factor for motoneurons present in peripheral nerve and muscle. Science 1994; 266:1062.

51. Heumann R, Korsching S, Bandtlow C, et al. Changes of nerve growth factor synthesis in nonneuronal cells in response to sciatic nerve transection. J Cell Biol 1987; 104:1623.

52. Houenou LJ, Li L, Lo AC, et al. Naturally occurring and axotomy-induced motoneuron death and its pre-

vention by neurotrophic agents: A comparison between chick and mouse. *In* van Pelt J, Corner MA, Uylings HBM, et al (eds): Progress in Brain Research. New York, Elsevier Science BV, 1994, pp 217–226.

53. Ip NY, Yancopoulos GD. Neurotrophic factors and their receptors. Ann Neurol 1994; 35(suppl):S13.

54. Ishii D, Marsh D. On the therapeutic potential for insulin-like growth factor use in motor neuron disease. Neurol 1993; 124:96.

55. Ishii DN. Insulin and related neurotrophic factors in diabetic neuropathy. Diabet Med 1993; 10(suppl)2:14S.

56. Ishii DN. Implication of insulin-like growth factors in the pathogenesis of diabetic neuropathy. Brain Res Rev 1995; 20:47.

57. Ishii DN, Glazner GW, Pu S-F. Role of insulin-like growth factors in peripheral nerve regeneration. Pharmacol Ther 1994; 62:125.

58. Ishii DN, Guertin DM, Whalen LR. Reduced insulin-like growth factor-I mRNA content in liver, adrenal glands and spinal cord of diabetic rats. Diabetologia 1994; 37:1073.

59. Ishii DN, Lupien SB. Insulin-like growth factors protect against diabetic neuropathy: Effects on sensory nerve regeneration in rats. J Neurosci Res 1995; 40:138.

60. Jakobsen J, Brimijoin S, Skau K, et al. Retrograde axonal transport of transmitter enzymes, fucose-labeled protein, and nerve growth factor in streptozotocin-diabetic rats. Diabetes 1981; 30:797.

61. Jing S, Wen D, Yu Y, et al. GDNF-Induced activation of the ret protein tyrosine kinase is mediated by GDNFRα, a novel receptor for GDNF. Cell 1996; 85:1113.

62. Johnson EM, Taniuchi M, DiStefano PA. Expression and possible function of nerve growth factor receptors on Schwann Cells. Trends Neurosci 1988; 111:299.

63. Kasayama S, Oka T. Impaired production of nerve growth factor in the submandibular gland of diabetic mice. Am J Physiol 1989; 257:E400.

64. Kim B, Leventhal PS, Saltiel AR, et al. Insulin-like growth factor-I-mediated neurite outgrowth in vitro requires mitogen-activated protein kinase activation. J Biol Chem 1997; 272:21268–21273.

65. Lakshmanan J. Post-synaptic PI-effect of nerve growth factor in rat superior cervical ganglia. J Neurochem 1979; 32:1599.

66. Lee JE, Pintar J, Efstratiadis A. Pattern of the insulin-like growth factor II gene expression during early mouse embryogenesis. Development 1990; 110:151.

67. Leventhal PS, Feldman EL. The tyrosine kinase inhibitor methyl 2,5-dihydroxycinnimate disrupts changes in the actin cytoskeleton required for neurite formation. Mol Brain Res 1996; 43:338.

68. Leventhal PS, Feldman EL. Insulin-like growth factors as regulators of cell motility: Signaling mechanisms. Trends Endocrinol Metab 1997; 8:1.

69. Leventhal PS, Shelden EA, Kim B, et al. Tyrosine phosphorylation of paxillin and focal adhesion kinase during insulin-like growth factor-I-stimulated lamellipodial advance. J Biol Chem 1997; 272:5214.

70. Levi-Montalcini R, Calissano P. Nerve growth factor as a paradigm for other polypeptide growth factors. Trends Neurosci 1986; 9:473.

71. Levine R, Stambler N, Charatan M, et al. A double-blind placebo-controlled clinical trial of subcutaneous recombinant human ciliary neurotrophic factor (rHCNTF) in amyotrophic lateral sclerosis. Neurol 1996; 46:1244.

72. Lewis ME, Vaught JL, Neff NT, et al. The potential of insulin-like growth factor-I as a therapeutic for the treatment of neuromuscular disorders. Ann NY Acad Sci 1993; 692:201.

73. Lindsay RM. Neurotrophic growth factors and neurodegenerative diseases: Therapeutic potential of the neurotrophins and ciliary neurotrophic factor. Neurobiol Aging 1994; 15:249.

74. Lindsay RM. Role of neurotrophins and trk receptors in the development and maintenance of sensory neurons: An overview. Philos Trans R Soc Lond B Biol Sci 1996; 351:365.

75. Lindsay RM, Wiegand J, Altar CA, et al. Neurotrophic factors: From molecule to man. Trends Neurosci 1994; 17:182.

76. Llewelyn JG. Diabetic neuropathy. Curr Opin Neurol 1995; 8:364.

77. Low PA, Tuck RR, Takeuchi M: Diabetic Neuropathy. Philadelphia, WB Saunders, 1987, p 276.

78. Luo J, Murphy LJ. Differential expression of insulin-like growth factor-I and insulin-like growth factor binding protein-1 in the diabetic rat. Mol Cell Biochem 1991; 103:41.

79. MacLennan AJ, Vinson EN, Marks L, et al. Immunohistochemical localization of ciliary neurotrophic factor receptor α expression in the rat nervous system. J Neurosci 1996; 16:621.

80. Matthews CC, Odeh HM, Feldman EL. Insulin-like growth factor-I is an osmoprotectant in human neuroblastoma cells. Neuroscience 1997; 79:525–534.

81. Matthews CC, Feldman EL. Insulin-like growth factor I rescues SH-SY5Y human neuroblastoma cells from hyperosmotic induced programmed cell death. J Cell Physiol 1996; 166:323.

82. McMahon SB, Priestley JV. Peripheral neuropathies and neurotrophic factors: Animal models and clinical perspectives. Curr Opin Neurobiol 1995; 5:616.

83. Migdalis IN, Kalogeropoulou K, Kalantzis L, et al. Insulin-like growth factor-I and IGF-I receptors in diabetic patients with neuropathy. Diabet Med 1995; 12:823.

84. Mozell RL, McMorris FA. Insulin-like growth factor I stimulates oligodendrocyte development and myelination in rat brain aggregate cultures. J Neurosci Res 1991; 30:382.

85. Oppenheim RW, Houenou LJ, Johnson JE, et al. Developing motor neurons rescued from programmed and axotomy-induced cell death by GDNF. Nature 1995; 373:344.

86. Oppenheim RW, Prevette D, Qin-Wei Y, et al. Control by embryonic motoneuron survival in vivo by ciliary neurotrophic factor. Science 1991; 252:1616.

87. Pirart J. Diabetes mellitus and its degenerative complications: A prospective study of 4,400 patients observed between 1947 and 1973. Diabetes Care 1978; 1:168.

88. Rabinovsky ED, Smith GM, Browder DP, et al. Peripheral nerve injury down-regulates CNTF expression in adult rat sciatic nerves. J Neurosci Res 1992; 31:188.

89. Rodriguez-Pena A, Botana M, Gonzalez M, et al. Expression of neurotrophins and their receptors in sciatic nerve of experimentally diabetic rats. Neurosci Lett 1995; 200:37.

90. Rogers SA, Hammerman MR. Insulin-like growth factor II stimulates production of inositol triphosphate in proximal tubular basolateral membranes from canine kidney. Proc Natl Acad Sci USA 1988; 85:4037.

91. Sango K, Verdes JM, Hikawa N, et al. Nerve growth factor (NGF) restores depletions of calcitonin gene-related peptide and substance P in sensory neurons from diabetic mice in vitro. J Neurol Sci 1994; 126:1.

92. Sara VR, Hall K. Insulin-like growth factors and their binding proteins. Physiol Rev 1990; 70:591.
93. Schmidt RE. The role of nerve growth factor in the pathogenesis and therapy of diabetic neuropathy. Diabet Med 1993; 10(suppl 2):10S.
94. Schmidt Y, Unger JW, Bartke I, et al. Effect of nerve growth factor on peptide neurons in dorsal root ganglia after taxol or cisplatin treatment and in diabetic (db/db) mice. Exp Neurol 1995; 132:16.
95. Sendtner M, Carroll P, Holtmann B, et al. Ciliary neurotrophic factor. J Neurobiol 1994; 25:1436.
96. Sendtner M, Kreutzberg GW, Thoenen H. Cilliary neurotrophic factor prevents the degeneration of motor neurons after axotomy. Nature 1990; 345:440.
97. Sima AAF, Stevens MJ, Feldman EL, et al. Animal models as tools for the testing of preventive and therapeutic measures in diabetic neuropathy. In Shafrir E (ed): Lessons From Animal Diabetes IV. Great Britain, Smith-Gordon, 1993, pp 177–191.
98. Singleton JR, Dixit VM, Feldman EL. Type I insulin-like growth factor receptor activation regulates apoptotic proteins. J Biol Chem 1996; 271:31791.
99. Singleton JR, Randolph AE, Feldman EL. Insulin-like growth factor I receptor prevents apoptosis and enhances neuroblastoma tumorigenesis. Cancer Res 1996; 56:4522.
100. Snider WD. Functions of the neurotrophins during nervous system development: What the knockouts are teaching us. Cell 1994; 77:627.
101. Springer JE, Mu X, Bergmann LW, et al. Expression of GDNF mRNA in rat and human nervous tissue. Exp Neurol 1994; 127:167.
102. Stahl N, Yancopoulos GD. The tripartite CNTF receptor complex: Activation and signaling involves components shared with other cytokines. J Neurobiol 1994; 25:1454.
103. Stylianopoulou F, Herbert J, Soares MB, et al. Expression of the insulin-like growth factor II gene in the choroid plexus and the leptomeninges of the adult rat central nervous system. Proc Natl Acad Sci USA 1988; 85:141.
104. Taniuchi M, Clark HB, Johnson EM. Induction of nerve growth factor receptor in Schwann cells after axotomy. Proc Natl Acad Sci 1986; 83:4094.
105. Taniuchi M, Clark HB, Schweitzer JB, et al. Expression of nerve growth factor receptors by Schwann cells of axotomized peripheral nerves: Utrastructural location, suppression by axonal contact, and binding properties. J Neurosci 1988; 8:664.
106. Thoenen H, Bandtlow C, Heumann R. The physiological function of nerve growth factor in the central nervous system: Comparison with the periphery. Rev Physiol Biochem Pharmacol 1987; 109:146.
107. Thomas PK. Growth factors and diabetic neuropathy. Diabet Med 1994; 11:732.
108. Thomas TP, Feldman EL, Nakamura J, et al. Ambient glucose and aldose reductase-induced *myo*-inositol depletion modulate basal and carbachol-stimulated inositol phospholipid metabolism and diacylglycerol accumulation in human retinal pigment epithelial cells in culture. Proc Natl Acad Sci USA 1993; 90:9712.
109. Tomlinson DR, Fernyhough P, Diemel LT. Neurotrophins and peripheral neuropathy. Philos Trans R Soc Lond B Biol Sci 1996; 351:455.
110. Tomlinson DR, Mayer JH. Defects of axonal transport in diabetes mellitus: A possible contribution to the aetiology of diabetic neuropathy. J Auton Pharmacol 1984; 4:59.
111. Traynor AE, Schubert D, Allen WR. Alterations of lipid metabolism in response to nerve growth factor. J Neurochem 1982; 39:1677.
112. Treanor JJS, Goodman L, de Sauvage F, et al. Characterization of a multicomponent receptor for GDNF. Nature 1996; 382:80.
113. Trupp M, Arenas E, Fainzilber M, et al. Functional receptor for GDNF encoded by the c-*ret* proto-oncogene. Nature 1996; 381:785.
114. Trupp M, Ryden M, Jornvall H, et al. Peripheral expression and biological activities of GDNF, a new neurotrophic factor for avian and mammalian peripheral neurons. J Cell Biol 1995; 130:137.
115. Tsuzuki T, Takahashi M, Asai N, et al. Spatial and temporal expression of the ret proto-oncogene product in embryonic, infant, and adult rat tissues. Oncogene 1995; 10:191.
116. Vega QC, Worby CA, Lechner MS, et al. Glial cell line-derived neurotrophic factor activates the receptor tyrosine kinase RET and promotes kidney morphogenesis. Proc Natl Acad Sci USA 1996; 93:10657.
117. Wuarin L, Guertin DM, Ishii DN. Early reduction in insulin-like growth factor gene expression in diabetic nerve. Exp Neurol 1994; 130:106.
118. Yagihashi S. Pathology and pathogenetic mechanisms of diabetic neuropathy. Diabetes Metab Rev 1995; 11:193.
119. Yan Q, Matheson C, Lopez OT. *In vivo* neurotrophic effects of GDNF on neonatal and adult facial motor neurons. Nature 1995; 373:341.
120. Yang H, Scheff AJ, Schalch DS. Effects of streptozotocin-induced diabetes mellitus on growth and hepatic insulin-like growth factor I gene expression in the rat. Metabolism 1990; 39(3):295.
121. Zackenfels K, Oppenheim RW, Rohrer H. Evidence for an important role of IGF-I and IGF-II for the early development of chick sympathetic neurons. Neuron 1995; 14:731.
122. Zanone MM, Banga JP, Peakman M, et al. An investigation of antibodies to nerve growth factor in diabetic autonomic neuropathy. Diabet Med 1994; 11:378.
123. Zhuang HX, Synder CK, Pu SF, et al. Insulin-like growth factors reverse or arrest diabetic neuropathy: Effects on hyperalgesia and impaired nerve regeneration in rats. Exp Neurol 1996; 140:198.

Mechanisms and Treatment of Pain

P. K. Thomas

INTRODUCTION

A variety of different pain syndromes may develop in patients with diabetic neuropathy, indicating that the underlying mechanisms are likely to be correspondingly diverse. Pain may be encountered as a symptom in relation to focal nerve lesions and to generalized polyneuropathies. In polyneuropathy, it may occur as an acute severe self-limiting disorder or as a persistent but fortunately less troublesome complaint. This chapter will review the various pain syndromes related to diabetic neuropathy, the possible underlying mechanisms for the pain, and the current approaches to treatment.

PAIN SYNDROMES IN DIABETIC NEUROPATHY

Focal and Multifocal Neuropathies

Pain is common in focal and multifocal diabetic peripheral nerve lesions. In isolated lesions of the third cranial nerve (see Chapter 33), it is experienced in approximately half of the cases.[112] It may precede the onset of paralysis by several days and is usually felt in a retro-ocular location or supraorbitally. Diabetic truncal or thoracoabdominal radiculoneuropathy (see Chapter 34) is often associated with pain in a dermatomal distribution around the lower trunk or abdomen, unilaterally or bilaterally.[53] Several contiguous dermatomes may be affected simultaneously.[90] Diabetic amyotrophy (proximal lower limb motor neuropathy; see Chapter 35) is often accompanied by pain felt in the thighs, unilaterally or bilaterally, lumbar region, and perineum. It is aching in character and is characteristically worse at night. Focal limb nerve lesions may be painful, particularly if acute in onset. Entrapment neuropathies are more common in patients with diabetes and may be responsible for pain, as in the painful nocturnal acroparesthesias of the carpal tunnel syndrome, burning pain over the anterolateral aspect of the thigh in meralgia paresthetica, or on the sole of the foot in the tarsal tunnel syndrome.

Polyneuropathies

Acute Painful Diabetic Neuropathy. Acute painful diabetic neuropathy[3] is a distinctive but uncommon syndrome. The pain is felt predominantly in the lower limbs but can be experienced widely, sometimes also affecting the upper limbs and trunk. It is burning or aching in quality with superimposed lancinating stabs and is often accompanied by widespread contact hyperesthesia of the skin. Accompanying sensory loss is often slight. The syndrome may be associated with profound weight loss[3, 20, 67] and has been described in diabetic girls with anorexia nervosa.[89] The syndrome is probably equivalent to "diabetic neuropathic cachexia," described by Ellenberg.[35] Acute painful diabetic neuropathy usually occurs in patients with type 1 diabetes mellitus (DM).[3, 20] It may follow the initiation of strict glycemic control.[50, 94] Abnormalities of nerve conduction are often remarkably slight. Loss of sural sensory nerve action potentials may be found.[3] In other patients, they may be preserved, as in the case described by Shimamura and associates[79] in whom spinal somatosensory evoked potentials were absent and cortical potentials were delayed, suggesting a disturbance of the centrally directed axons of the primary sensory neurons in the posterior columns.

Diabetic Sensory Neuropathy. This is the commonest form of diabetic neuropathy (see Chapters 17 and 30). It is usually of insidious onset. The precise frequency of pain in this syndrome is not established. Pain distally in the legs can be a presenting feature in cases of type 2 DM, or it may develop in established cases of diabetic sensory polyneuropathy, some of which show a small fiber or pseudosyringo-

myelic neuropathy with predominant pain and temperature sensory loss.[14, 81] The pain is felt predominantly distally in the lower limbs and is often most troublesome at night. It is usually aching or burning in quality with superimposed stabs. It can be persistent or intermittent, occurring over periods or weeks or months with intervening periods or freedom.

MECHANISMS OF PAIN IN DIABETIC NEUROPATHY

In general terms, pain can be separated into three broad categories. *Nociceptive* pain is the result of activation of pain receptors that normally signal tissue injury. *Neuropathic*, or dysesthetic, pain[6] arises from damage to the nervous system, leading to the generation of pain by abnormal physiologic mechanisms. *Psychogenic* pain results from affective or other psychiatric disorders. In neuropathies, the occurrence of pain can be nociceptive from activation of pain fibers in the nervi nervorum innervating the connective tissues of the nerves,[97] referred to as nerve trunk pain,[6] or represent dysesthetic pain caused by nerve fiber damage. Hyperesthesia may arise from selective large fiber damage,[17] but neuropathic pain appears to be the result of damage to small myelinated and unmyelinated axons[96] or sensitization of nociceptors.[23]

Possible mechanisms for pain in diabetic neuropathy are listed in Table 28.1.

Nerve Trunk Pain

It is highly likely that local pain may develop as a result of nerve ischemia in conditions such

TABLE 28.1   POSSIBLE MECHANISMS FOR PAIN IN DIABETIC NEUROPATHY

Nerve trunk pain
Dysesthetic pain
  Sensitization of nociceptor endings
  Active axonal degeneration
  Damage to A delta and C fibers
  Ectopic impulse generation by regenerating axons
  Ephaptic transmission
  Axonal atrophy
  Alterations in peripheral blood flow
  Glycemic control
  Abnormalities in dorsal root ganglia
  Changes in central nervous system caused by
    peripheral nerve damage
    Surround inhibition
    Presynaptic inhibition
    Postsynaptic inhibition
    Dorsal horn deafferentation

as polyarteritis nodosa. This has been proposed as the mechanism for pain occurring in some focal neuropathies in diabetes, in particular those of the third cranial nerve.[5] This explanation was partly based on the assumption that this nerve did not contain somatosensory afferent fibers. An alternative hypothesis has been advanced by Bertolomi and colleagues[9] that the pain arises from damage to trigeminal sensory fibers now shown to travel in the oculomotor nerve of humans and other mammals.[7, 8, 56] In sheep, it was established that these fibers innervate the cornea and upper eyelid and the extraocular muscles.[7, 8, 56] Despite this, it is usually not possible to demonstrate any sensory loss in patients with diabetic third nerve palsies. A diabetic patient observed personally who developed an acute spontaneous radial nerve lesion experienced pain in the upper arm and not in the sensory distribution of the nerve.[97] Local tenderness of a nerve trunk, for example, of the ulnar nerve in the cubital tunnel syndrome, reflects activation of local pain afferents.

Dysesthetic Pain

Sensitization of Nociceptor Endings. Lowering of the threshold for pain in response to normal stimuli has been demonstrated after physical and chemical injury to cutaneous nociceptors in humans.[101] This is probably the explanation for chronic hyperalgesia in some focal neuropathies[23] and in the ABC (angry backfiring nociceptor) syndrome described by Ochoa.[63] It is uncertain whether this mechanism is implicated in the production of pain in diabetic neuropathy.

Active Axonal Degeneration. Dyck and coworkers[32] examined the correlation between the occurrence of "painfulness" and the types of pathologic change observed in sural nerve biopsies from a series of 72 patients with peripheral neuropathy that only included 1 patient with diabetic neuropathy. Painfulness was found to be correlated more frequently with active nerve fiber degeneration than with other types of pathologic change. Active fiber breakdown was also present in biopsies from the patients with acute painful diabetic neuropathy reported by Archer and colleagues[3] and Castellanos and associates.[20] However, it is unlikely that pain is specifically related to acute axonal breakdown. Llewelyn and colleagues[51] and Britland and associates[13] failed to detect a correlation between the occurrence of pain and

active fiber breakdown in nerve biopsies from patients with diabetic sensory polyneuropathy. The series reported by Dyck and coworkers[32] included a high proportion of patients with vasculitic neuropathy that could have accounted for the correlation between pain and active fiber breakdown that was found.

Damage to A Delta and C Fibers. Thomas[96] analyzed the morphometric findings in nerve biopsies from a wide range of neuropathies. It was found that the occurrence of spontaneous pain was related to selective loss of small myelinated A delta fibers and unmyelinated C fibers or to loss of fibers of all diameters. Spontaneous pain was not a feature of neuropathies with selective large fiber sensory loss. The occurrence of pain was thus related to pathology affecting small fibers, although the nature of the mechanisms involved could not be specified.

Hyperalgesia in response to nonnoxious cutaneous stimulation may be painful (allodynia) and can be signaled by large fibers after nerve injury[17] or by sensitized C nociceptors.[23] Amplification of the severity of pain would be predicted as a result of abnormal multiplication of primary afferent impulses in nociceptor channels. This has been demonstrated for single C nociceptors in painful diabetic neuropathy.[64]

Ectopic Impulse Generation by Regenerating Axon Sprouts. The finding of evidence of regenerative sprouting in nerve biopsies from patients with painful small fiber diabetic neuropathy led Brown and colleagues[14] and Asbury and Fields[6] to suggest that ectopic generation of impulses by these sprouts might be responsible for the pain. Some support for this view had been provided by Wall and Gutnick,[105] who demonstrated ectopic impulse generation in sprouts from sensory axons in neuromas produced by sciatic nerve transection in rats. It was later shown that this phenomenon occurs in a high proportion of myelinated sensory fibers and also in unmyelinated axons.[31, 76] Llewelyn and colleagues[50] reported the nerve biopsy findings from a patient with acute painful diabetic neuropathy precipitated by the institution of strict glycemic control. The presence of profuse regenerative activity was taken to support an association between the occurrence of pain and axonal regeneration. Nevertheless, subsequent studies by Britland and associates[12] and Llewelyn and colleagues[51] failed to confirm a correlation between the number of regenerative clusters derived from myelinated fibers and the occurrence of pain in diabetic sensory neuropathy. In addition, Llewelyn and colleagues[51] found no correlation between pain and the diameter of unmyelinated axons. If pain were correlated with the regeneration of unmyelinated axons, a reduction in caliber would have been expected. Currently, therefore, there is little support for the concept that pain arises by the generation of ectopic impulses in regenerating axon sprouts. This conclusion is in accordance with the fact that nerve regeneration in humans is usually a painless process.

Ephaptic Transmission. This can be demonstrated between motor and sensory nerve fibers after acute peripheral nerve injury.[41] This is a short-lived phenomenon with a time course of minutes. At longer intervals after injury, ephapses are only demonstrable between a few fibers.[78] The development of ephapses between afferent sympathetic fibers and sensory afferents was advanced as an explanation for sympathetically mediated causalgia[31] and considered to provide a possible basis for its relief by sympathectomy. This hypothesis was subsequently adopted somewhat overenthusiastically. Nevertheless, there is good electrophysiologic evidence for ephaptic interaction between motor fibers in humans,[62, 73] and it is feasible that this might also occur in sensory fibers. So far there is no indication that ephapses are involved in the generation of pain in diabetic neuropathy.

Axonal Atrophy. Thomas and Scadding[99] raised the theoretical possibility that fiber shrinkage could be implicated in the generation of pain in diabetic neuropathy. After axotomy, axons undergo atrophy central to the site of transection.[2, 33] After reconnection with appropriate peripheral structures, fiber diameter is restored.[28] Larger myelinated nerve fibers regain their conduction velocity more rapidly than A delta fibers.[28] This would give rise to an altered temporal patterning of impulses that conceivably could have an effect on sensation. Although Britland and associates[12] reported a correlation between the occurrence of pain in diabetic neuropathy and axonal atrophy, other studies have failed to confirm that axonal atrophy is a feature of this neuropathy.[51, 92]

Peripheral Blood Flow. This may be increased in diabetic polyneuropathy as a consequence of autonomic involvement. Archer and associates[4] assessed peripheral blood flow in patients with acute painful diabetic neuropathy in comparison with severe nonpainful neuropathy. Blood flow was found to be elevated in both groups, but it was observed that it could only be reduced by sympathetic stimulation in those with painful neuropathy when it was accompanied by a reduction in the severity of the pain. The explanation for the reduction in pain was uncertain, but it was considered that either reduced temperature or reduced arteriovenous shunting[94] could be involved.

Glycemic Control. Morley and colleagues[61] investigated the acute relationship between pain thresholds and tolerance and blood glucose levels. Diabetic subjects showed lower stimulus thresholds and a lower tolerance for pain than nondiabetic subjects. They also found that glucose infusion in nondiabetic subjects reduced their pain thresholds and tolerance levels. In streptozotocin diabetic rats, Simon and Dewey[81] observed that hyperglycemia diminishes the antinociceptive effect of morphine, suggesting a possible influence of glucose on opiate receptors.

The peripheral nerves in streptozotocin diabetic rats are known to be hypoxic.[102] From in vitro studies in nondiabetic rat nerve, Schneider and colleagues[77] found that hyperglycemic but not normoglycemic hypoxia induced alterations in fast K^+ conductance and after potential, and this was related to axoplasmic acidification. It is possible that this mechanism could contribute to the occurrence of positive symptoms, including pain, in poorly controlled diabetic patients with hyperglycemic neuropathy.[99]

Abnormalities in Dorsal Root Ganglia. Dorsal root ganglia are normally highly sensitive to mechanical stimulation.[44] If the peripheral axons of dorsal root ganglion cells are transected, even if the axotomy is far distally, the cells generate impulses spontaneously.[106] This behavior is exhibited by large and small ganglion cells. Diabetic sensory polyneuropathy involves a distal axonal degeneration of dying-back type.[72] The possibility therefore arises that this could lead to the generation of ectopic impulses from dorsal root ganglion cells after interruption of axons signaling pain. Against this is the indication that diabetic sensory polyneuropathy may consist of a central-peripheral distal axonopathy,[107] so that the centrally directed axons of the dorsal root ganglion cells would be disconnected from the central nervous system (CNS). This consideration also applies to the possibility of pain arising from ectopic impulses in regenerating axon sprouts that was discussed earlier.

Changes in the Central Nervous System Caused by Peripheral Nerve Damage. A variety of changes in the CNS that follow peripheral nerve injury have been identified from experimental studies in animals. They have been used to provide possible interpretations for painful phenomena that follow peripheral nerve injury in humans. Such extrapolations have not been without criticism.[64] The main changes identified have been surround inhibition, presynaptic inhibition, postsynaptic inhibition, and dorsal horn deafferentation.

Surround Inhibition. The activity of many dorsal horn cells is influenced not only by the excitatory action of peripheral afferents but also by other afferents that have an inhibitory surround effect on the excitatory receptive field.[43] A reduction in afferent input from a neuropathy could thus lead to a reduction in surround inhibition and lead to hyperesthesia and hyperpathia that are a conspicuous feature of acute painful diabetic neuropathy.[3]

Presynaptic Inhibition. Afferent volleys of impulses to the dorsal horn give rise by presynaptic inhibition to prolonged depolarization of the terminals of the fibers that have transmitted the afferent volleys.[104] This is the mechanism of the dorsal horn potential. Such presynaptic inhibition gradually ceases after nerve section. A failure of this inhibition hypothetically might contribute to the development of pain in neuropathies.

Postsynaptic Inhibition. In the gate-control theory of pain promulgated by Melzack and Wall,[60] impulses traveling in large-caliber dorsal root afferents exert a facilitatory effect on neurons in the substantia gelatinosa of the dorsal horn. In turn, this exerts presynaptic inhibition on neurons that give rise to a centrally conducting transmission pathway signaling pain. Impulses traveling in small-caliber dorsal root nociceptive afferents have an inhibitory effect on the substantia gelatinosa neurons and a facilitatory effect on the transmission neurons. It was thus believed that the larger fiber input had the capability of closing the dorsal horn gating mechanism and inhibiting pain. Conversely, loss of these fibers would be pre-

dicted to lead to pain. However, observations on the pattern of nerve fiber loss in neuropathies does not support this proposed gating mechanism, which is probably an oversimplified view. Selective large fiber neuropathies, as already stated, are not painful.[96]

Dorsal Horn Deafferentation. Loss of afferent input to dorsal horn neurons is known to lead to an increase in their spontaneous activity. Some show high-frequency bursting discharges.[52] The upper limb pain that frequently follows brachial plexus avulsion injury has been attributed to dorsal horn deafferentation, and theoretically this could apply to pain from diabetic neuropathy, particularly if it involves a central-peripheral distal axonopathy.[107] Loss of dorsal root ganglion cells is not conspicuous.[30, 107]

TREATMENT OF PAINFUL DIABETIC NEUROPATHY

The control of pain in patients with diabetic neuropathy often constitutes a substantial management problem. As an initial requirement, it is essential to establish the nature of the neuropathy to be able to predict the anticipated natural history. Thus, pain from an acute third cranial nerve palsy or truncal radiculoneuropathy will be self-limiting, although cutaneous hyperesthesia in the latter can be persistent. Pain from the rare acute painful diabetic neuropathy, although highly distressing, can be expected to subside within about 6 months. Reassurance that it will ultimately remit is likely to make it easier for the patient to tolerate the pain. Recurrent or persistent pain in established sensory polyneuropathy is frequently difficult to control and is often complicated by secondary depression. Simple analgesics are usually ineffectual; the same also probably is true for more potent opioid analgesics.

Possible treatment options for pain in diabetic neuropathy are listed in Table 28.2.

Glycemic Control

The Diabetes Control and Complications Trial[29] firmly established that close glycemic control with multiple daily insulin injections or continuous insulin infusion will significantly reduce the risk of developing neuropathy in patients with type 1 DM and can also lead to improvement, although at the cost of a threefold increase in the occurrence of hypoglycemic at-

TABLE 28.2 TREATMENT OPTIONS FOR PAINFUL DIABETIC NEUROPATHY

Glycemic control
Tricyclic antidepressant drugs
    Amitriptyline, imipramine, clomipramine, desipramine
Selective serotonin reuptake inhibitors
    Paroxetine, citalopram, fluoxetine
Anticonvulsant and antiarrhythmic drugs
    Phenytoin, carbamazepine, gabapentin, lamotrigine,
      mexiletine, lidocaine
    Aldose reductase inhibitors
    Topical capsaicin
    Vasoactive substances
    Transdermal clonidine, prostacyclin analogues
Physical measures
    Transcutaneous electrical nerve stimulation, Opsite
      film, electrical spinal cord stimulation

---

tacks. For patients with chronic painful diabetic neuropathy, it is therefore important to ensure that glycemic control is optimized. This also applies to cases of acute painful diabetic neuropathy. Even in those in whom the syndrome is precipitated by the initiation or tightening of glycemic control,[50] this is not an indication to relax treatment. In those patients in whom the painful neuropathy is related to severe weight loss, control of glycemia is accompanied by weight gain and resolution of the painful neuropathy.[3, 20] Boulton and colleagues[11] found that continuous subcutaneous insulin infusion was beneficial in patients with severe painful neuropathy.

Tricyclic Antidepressant Drugs

The frequent association of depression with chronic painful diabetic neuropathy led to the use of tricyclic antidepressant drugs, either on their own or in combination with a phenothiazine.[26, 39] In early studies, Turkington[103] and Kvinesdal and colleagues[49] reported benefit using imipramine or amitriptyline, whereas other studies at this stage[69, 109] obtained less satisfactory responses. Subsequently, carefully controlled trials established that tricyclic antidepressant drugs are effective in alleviating painful neuropathy.[59] They are beneficial in patients with normal and depressed mood,[57] although the response is greater in those with associated depression.[59] A reduction in severity rather than abolition of the pain is usually achieved. The precise level of the neuraxis at which they exert their effect is uncertain, although it is probably by inhibiting norepinephrine uptake at synapses in central descending pain control systems.[10]

Beta-endorphin is an important modulator in central pain pathways. To assess whether endogenous opioid peptides are implicated in the action of imipramine (and paroxetine) in painful diabetic neuropathy, Sindrup and associates[86] measured the plasma concentration of β-endorphin in patients during a randomized placebo-controlled trial of these drugs. Despite a significant reduction in symptoms, both during imipramine and paroxetine treatment, β-endorphin levels remained unaltered. It was concluded that there was no evidence that endogenous opioid peptides are involved in the relief of pain produced by these drugs. In another study, Byas-Smith and coworkers[15] found that β-endorphin concentrations in cerebrospinal fluid appear to be reduced in patients with diabetic polyneuropathy but that this was not correlated with the presence of pain. It was suggested that this could be equated with the observation that opioid analgesics are of little, if any, help in alleviating diabetic neuropathic pain.

Chan and colleagues[22] attempted to measure the levels of methionine and leucine enkephalins in the cerebrospinal fluid of patients with painful and painless diabetic neuropathy. The results were highly variable and difficult to interpret and provided no useful information on the function of enkephalinergic pathways.

Both steady burning pain and lancinating pains are relieved by tricyclic drugs, and the response appears to be dose related. In the series reported by Max and associates[59] the patients who were able to tolerate larger doses (up to 150 mg at night) reported greater benefit. Sindrup and associates[83] assessed the blood levels of imipramine necessary to relieve neuropathic pain and found substantial individual variation. In patients who responded, considerable relief was obtained with blood levels below 100 nmol/L, but concentrations of 400 to 500 nmol/L were required to produce maximal benefit in all patients.

Desipramine produces fewer anticholinergic side effects than amitriptyline and is less sedative. It is effective in relieving pain in diabetic neuropathy[58] with a potency similar to that of amitriptyline,[59] but in a study by Sindrup and associates[84] it was somewhat less effective than clomipramine. A controlled trial of the tetracyclic antidepressant mianserin by Sindrup and associates[87] in painful diabetic neuropathy detected no benefit. It may be relevant that mianserin has no or only a slight inhibitory action on norepinephrine uptake.

It is advisable to commence treatment with

tricyclic drugs at a low dosage and to increase them gradually depending on the symptomatic response. Orthostatic hypotension and tachycardia may sometimes pose a problem, particularly in elderly patients. There is no current indication that phenothiazine drugs given in conjunction with a tricyclic antidepressant produce any additional benefit, and they carry the risk of inducing tardive dyskinesia. Reviews concerning the use of tricyclic antidepressant drugs in the treatment of neuropathic pain have been provided by Bryson and Wilde[16] and Low and Nelson.[54]

Selective Serotonin Reuptake Inhibitors

A further category of drug used in the treatment of depression is the selective serotonin reuptake inhibitors. Sindrup and associates, using paroxetine[82, 85] and citalopram,[88] reported alleviation of sensory symptoms in diabetic neuropathy. Max and coworkers,[59] however, found that fluoxetine only relieved pain if there was accompanying depression. Galer[38] suggested the use of nefazodone, a serotonin reuptake inhibitor, or venlafaxine, a serotonin/norepinephrine reuptake inhibitor, because they are better tolerated than tricyclic antidepressants. No controlled trials are available.

Anticonvulsant and Antiarrhythmic Drugs

The success of phenytoin and, more dramatically, carbamazepine, in relieving trigeminal neuralgia led to their more widespread application in the treatment of neuropathic pain, including diabetic neuropathy.[34] An early study by Chadda and Mathur[21] reported a favorable response with phenytoin, although this was not the experience of Saudek and associates.[75] Both were controlled studies. Somewhat better results were documented for carbamazepine,[71, 109] but the benefit was not spectacular. These anticonvulsant agents probably act by stabilizing neuronal membranes through an effect on sodium conductance, as is also likely for the class I antiarrhythmic drugs used in the treatment of cardiac arrhythmias. The newer anticonvulsant drugs gabapentin and lamotrigine have also been recommended[38] but controlled trials have not been reported.

Kastrup and coworkers[46, 47] treated painful diabetic neuropathy by the intravenous infusion of lidocaine with benefit. Iontophoretically administered lidocaine was found to be effective in the treatment of painful diabetic truncal neuropathy in a single case report.[65] Dejgård and associates[27] proposed the use of oral mexiletine in painful diabetic polyneuropathy. This drug was assessed in a double-blind trial by Stracke and associates.[91] A global assessment of pain demonstrated no significant benefit but, from a subgroup analysis, those patients experiencing stabbing or burning pain, heat sensations, or formication showed definite alleviation. A medium-dose level of 450 mg/d appeared to be appropriate; increases into the antiarrhythmic range did not result in a proportionate benefit. Side effects were insignificant, and no cardiovascular effects were noted. Individual cases of severely painful diabetic neuropathy, one with chronic distal painful neuropathy[1] and the other with diabetic truncal neuropathy,[48] have been stated to have been improved by mexiletine in anecdotal reports. In the former case, mexiletine treatment was preceded by intravenous lidocaine.

Aldose Reductase Inhibitors

The basis for the use of this class of drugs in the treatment of diabetic neuropathy is discussed in Chapter 22. They were introduced to prevent the accumulation of sorbitol in nerve, but most also have other effects. Jaspan and coworkers,[45] in an early open study on patients with severe painful diabetic neuropathy, reported benefit with the aldose reductase inhibitor sorbinil, which was later withdrawn because of side effects. Young and associates,[110] in a short-term double-blind placebo-controlled study, again using sorbinil, obtained a significant reduction in pain scores. Using another aldose reductase inhibitor, tolrestat, now also withdrawn because of side effects, Santiago and colleagues[74] found a significant improvement in pain scores in favor of the drug in a withdrawal study. However, with the same drug, Macleod and coworkers[55] found an equally marked improvement in pain scores in the treatment and placebo groups in a 6-month double-blind placebo-controlled study. A beneficial effect from aldose reductase inhibitors on pain in diabetic neuropathy still requires convincing demonstration.

Topical Capsaicin

The alkaloid capsaicin is the active agent that imparts the heat to chili peppers. It is believed to stimulate the neurons of unmyelinated C fibers selectively, causing the release of substance P and possibly other neurotransmitters from their endings. Subsequent depletion of stores of substance P is then considered to impair the transmission of impulses signaling pain to central pathways. This provides the rationale for its use in the treatment of painful states.[68] It has been advocated for the treatment of postherpetic neuralgia and painful diabetic neuropathy as a topical cutaneous application. Several studies that compared capsaicin cream with vehicle reported a significant benefit in favor of capsaicin.[18, 19, 93] Its use in painful truncal neuropathy has also been documented.[65]

Topical capsaicin gives rise to local stinging and burning discomfort, which some patients are unable to tolerate. This is most evident in the first week of application and then tends to subside. There are no serious systemic side effects. The beneficial results obtained have to be qualified by the fact that it is impossible to arrange a patient-blinded study because of the burning sensation that capsaicin cream produces. Watson[108] commented that the high placebo response rate in painful states may account for some of the salutory effects that have been obtained.

Vasoactive Substances

How far direct metabolic effects and indirect vascular changes are implicated in the causation of the diabetic neuropathies is still unresolved. Moreover, it is certainly possible that symptoms related to ischemia could be superimposed on an underlying metabolic neuropathy. Tesfaye and colleagues[94] have observed appearances that they interpreted as epineurial neovascularization in patients with painful diabetic neuropathy and findings suggesting the opening of epineurial arteriovenous shunts, possibly secondary to autonomic neuropathy. It was suggested that this could lead to a "steal" effect, rendering the endoneurium ischemic and leading to the occurrence of neuropathic pain.

On the assumption that vascular changes are important, the use of pentoxifylline was investigated by Cohen and Mathews[25] in a double-blind placebo-controlled study on painful diabetic distal sensory neuropathy. Pentoxifylline has been shown to improve the circulation through partially occluded vessels. No benefit was detected. The same was true for clonidine. Ziegler and associates,[111] on the other hand, reported encouraging preliminary results for transdermal clonidine. A subsequent two-stage study with an "enriched enrollment" design

was undertaken by Byas-Smith and associates.[15] This was a randomized double-blind cross-over study with transdermal clonidine. Apparent responders in the first stage were transferred to the second double-blind placebo-controlled "enriched enrollment" phase. This confirmed a response to clonidine. Administration of the α-adrenergic blocker phentolamine had no effect on the pain, suggesting that the relief produced by clonidine was not mediated by a reduction in sympathetic outflow. Analysis of the symptoms indicated that patients who described their pain as "sharp" and "shooting" had a greater chance of responding to clonidine.

Cyclandelate can improve the rheological properties of blood. Heimans and associates[42] assessed the effect of this preparation on patients with diabetic neuropathy, including the evaluation of pain scores, but detected no beneficial effects. Shindo and colleagues[80] conducted an open nonrandomized trial of the prostaglandin analogue iloprost given intravenously during a 2-month period, obtaining subjective relief of symptoms that included pain. A larger double-blind study was recommended.

Physical Measures

Transcutaneous electrical nerve stimulation was recommended by Thorsteinsson[100] and Ruiz and coworkers,[70] but it was not found to be helpful in the treatment of acute painful diabetic neuropathy by Archer and associates.[3] The use of Opsite film was explored by Foster and colleagues.[37] It was found to alleviate the pain associated with chronic painful neuropathy. Tesfaye and associates[95] recently assessed the use of electrical stimulation of the spinal cord and obtained benefit in 8 of 10 cases. It was recommended that this form of treatment should be considered in patients with painful neuropathy that has failed to respond to conventional measures.

Acupuncture has been recommended, but in personal cases who have chosen to have this form of treatment, no conspicuous benefit has been obtained. Care must be taken in the use of alternative therapies in patients with painful diabetic neuropathy with anesthetic feet. Ewins and associates[36] reported two patients with previously undiagnosed type 2 DM complaining of painful cold feet who were treated by the traditional Chinese therapy of moxibustion; they both developed painless ulceration at the sites of treatment on the feet and legs.

Combination Therapy

As pointed out by Ruiz and coworkers,[70] the difficulty in managing patients with painful diabetic neuropathy often leads to pluritherapy. Pfeifer and colleagues[66] advocate a treatment algorithm that depends on establishing the source of the pain. Thus, superficial pain is treated by capsaicin, deep pain with imipramine without or without mexiletine, and muscle pain by stretching exercises in combination with a nonsteroidal anti-inflammatory drug. This three-pronged approach, which depends on the ability of the clinician to identify the site of origin of the pain, was found to be highly successful.

References

1. Ackerman WE III, Colclough GW, Juneja MM, et al. The management of oral mexilitine and intravenous lidocaine to treat chronic painful symmetrical distal diabetic neuropathy. J Ky Med Assoc 1989; 89:500.
2. Aitken JT, Thomas PK. Retrograde changes in fibre size following nerve section. J Anat 1962; 96:121.
3. Archer AG, Watkins PJ, Thomas PK, et al. The natural history of acute painful diabetic neuropathy. J Neurol Neurosurg Psychiatry 1983; 46:491.
4. Archer AG, Roberts VC, Watkins PJ. Blood flow patterns in painful diabetic neuropathy. Diabetologia 1984; 27:563.
5. Asbury AK, Aldredge H, Hershberg R, et al. Oculomotor palsy in diabetes mellitus: A clinico-pathological study. Brain 1970; 93:555.
6. Asbury AK, Fields HL. Pain due to peripheral nerve damage: An hypothesis. Neurology 1984; 34:1587.
7. Bertolomi R, Veggetti A, Callegari E, et al. Afferent fibers and sensory ganglion cells within the oculomotor nerve in some mammals and man. 1: Anatomical investigations. Arch Ital Biol 1977; 115:355.
8. Bertolomi R, Calzà L, Lucchi ML. Peripheral territory and neuropeptides of the trigeminal ganglion neurons centrally projecting through the oculomotor nerve demonstrated by fluorescent retrograde double-labeling compared with immunocytochemistry. Brain Res 1991; 547:82.
9. Bertolomi R, D'Alessandro R, Manni E. The origin of pain in "ischemic-diabetic" third-nerve palsy. Arch Neurol 1993; 50:795.
10. Botney M, Fields HL. Amitriptyline potentiates morphine analgesia by a direct action on the central nervous system. Ann Neurol 1983; 13:160.
11. Boulton AJM, Drury J, Clarke B, et al. Continuous subcutaneous insulin infusion in the management of painful diabetic neuropathy. Diabetes Care 1982; 5:386.
12. Britland ST, Young RJ, Sharma AK, et al. Association of painful and painless diabetic polyneuropathy with different patterns of nerve fiber degeneration and regeneration. Diabetes 1990; 39:898.
13. Britland ST, Young RJ, Sharma AK, et al. Acute and remitting painful diabetic polyneuropathy: A comparison of peripheral nerve fibre pathology. Pain 1992; 48:361.
14. Brown MJ, Martin JR, Asbury AK. Painful diabetic

15. neuropathy: A morphometric study. Arch Neurol 1976; 33:164.
15. Byas-Smith MG, Max MB, Muir J, et al. Transdermal clonidine compared to placebo in painful diabetic neuropathy using a two-stage "enriched enrollment" design. Pain 1995; 60:267.
16. Bryson HM, Wilde MI. Amitriptyline: A review of its pharmacological properties and therapeutic use in chronic pain states. Drugs Aging 1996; 8:459.
17. Campbell JN, Raja SN, Meyer RA, et al. Myelinated afferents signal the hyperalgesia associated with nerve injury. Pain 1988; 32:89.
18. Capsaicin Study Group: Treatment of painful diabetic neuropathy with topical capsaicin: A multicentre, double-blind, vehicle-controlled study. Arch Intern Med 1991; 151:2225.
19. Capsaicin Study Group: Effect of treatment with capsaicin on daily activities of patients with diabetic neuropathy. Diabetes Care 1992; 15:159.
20. Castellanos F, Mascías J, Zabala JA, et al. Acute painful diabetic neuropathy following severe weight loss. Muscle Nerve 1996; 19:463.
21. Chadda VS, Mathur MS. Double blind study on the effects of diphenylhydantoin sodium on diabetic neuropathy. J Assoc Physicians India 1978; 26:403.
22. Chan AW, MacFarlane IA, Masson EA, et al. CSF enkephalins in diabetic neuropathy. Neuropeptides 1992; 22:125.
23. Cline MA, Ochoa J, Torebjörk HE. Chronic hyperalgesia and skin warming caused by sensitized C nociceptors. Brain 1989; 122:621.
24. Cohen KL, Lucibello FE, Chomiak M. Lack of effect of clonidine and pentoxifylline in short-term therapy of diabetic peripheral neuropathy. Diabetes Care 1990; 13:1074.
25. Cohen SM, Matthews T. Pentoxifylline in the treatment of distal diabetic neuropathy. Angiology 1991; 42:741.
26. Davis JL, Lewis SB, Gerich JE, et al. Peripheral diabetic neuropathy treated with amitriptyline and fluphenazine. JAMA 1977; 238:2291.
27. Dejgård A, Petersen P, Kastrup J. Mexiletine for treatment of chronic painful diabetic neuropathy. Lancet 1988; 1:9–11.
28. Devor M, Govrin-Lippmann R. Maturation of axonal sprouts after nerve crush. Exp Neurol 1979; 64:260.
29. Diabetes Control and Complications Trial Research Group. The effect of intensive treatment of diabetes on the development and progression of long-term complications in insulin-dependent diabetes mellitus. N Engl J Med 1993; 329:304.
30. Dolman CL. The morbid anatomy of diabetic neuropathy. Neurology 1963; 13:135.
31. Doupe J, Cullen CH, Chance GQ. Post-traumatic pain and the causalgic syndrome. J Neurol Neurosurg Psychiatry 1944; 7:33.
32. Dyck PJ, Lambert EH, O'Brien PC. Pain in peripheral neuropathy related to rate and kind of fiber degeneration. Neurology 1976; 26:466.
33. Dyck PJ, Lais AC, Karnes JL, et al. Permanent axotomy, a model of axonal atrophy and secondary demyelination and remyelination. Ann Neurol 1981; 9:575.
34. Ellenberg M. Treatment of diabetic neuropathy with diphenylhydantoin. NY State J Med 1968; 68:2653.
35. Ellenberg M. Diabetic neuropathic cachexia. Diabetes 1974; 23:418.
36. Ewins DL, Bakker K, Young MJ, et al. Alternative medicine: Potential dangers for the diabetic foot. Diabetic Med 1993; 10:980.

37. Foster AV, Eaton C, McConville DO, et al. Application of Opsite film: A new and effective treatment of painful diabetic neuropathy. Diabetic Med 1994; 11:768.

38. Galer BS. Neuropathic pain of peripheral origin: Advances in pharmacologic treatment. Neurology 1996; 45(suppl 9):S17.

39. Gomez-Perez FJ, Rull JA, Dies H, et al. Nortriptyline and fluphenazine in the symptomatic treatment of diabetic neuropathy: A double-blind cross-over study. Pain 1985; 23:395.

40. Govrin-Lippmann R, Devor M. Ongoing activity in severed nerves: Source and variation with time. Brain Res 1978; 159:406.

41. Granit R, Leksell L, Skoglund CR. Fibre interaction in injured or compressed region of nerve. Brain 1944; 67:125.

42. Heimans JJ, Drukarch B, Matthaei I, et al. Cyclandelate in diabetic neuropathy: A double-blind placebo-controlled, randomized, cross-over study. Acta Neurol Scand 1991; 84:483.

43. Hillmann P, Wall PD. Inhibitory and excitatory factors controlling lamina 5 cells. Exp Brain Res 1969; 9:284.

44. Howe F, Loeser JD, Calvin WH. Mechanosensitivity of dorsal root ganglia and chronically injured axons: A physiological basis for the radicular pain of nerve root compression. Pain 1977; 3:25.

45. Jaspan J, Maselli R, Herdd K, et al. Treatment of severely painful diabetic neuropathy with an aldose reductase inhibitor: Relief of pain and improved somatic and autonomic nerve function. Lancet 1983; 2:758.

46. Kastrup J, Angelo HR, Peterson P, et al. Treatment of chronic painful diabetic neuropathy with intravenous lidocaine infusion. BMJ 1986; 292:173.

47. Kastrup J, Bach FW, Peterson P, et al. Lidocaine treatment of painful diabetic neuropathy and endogenous opioid peptides in plasma. Clin J Pain 1989; 5:239.

48. Kubota K, Joshita Y, Tamura J, et al. Relief of severe diabetic truncal pain with mexilitine. J Med Clin Exp Theoret 1991; 22:307.

49. Kvinesdal B, Molin J, Frøland A, et al. Imipramine treatment of painful diabetic neuropathy. JAMA 1984; 251:1727.

50. Llewelyn JG, Thomas PK, Fonseca V, et al. Acute painful diabetic neuropathy precipitated by strict glycaemic control. Acta Neuropathol 1986; 72:157.

51. Llewelyn JG, Gilbey SG, Thomas PK, et al. Sural nerve morphometry in diabetic autonomic and painful sensory neuropathy. Brain 1991; 114:867.

52. Loeser JD, Ward AA. Some effects of deafferentation on neurons of the cat spinal cord. Arch Neurol 1967; 17:629.

53. Longstreth GF, Newcomer AD. Abdominal pain caused by diabetic radiculopathy. Ann Intern Med 1977; 86:166.

54. Low DR, Nelson JP. A review of antidepressants for the treatment of painful diabetic neuropathy. Pract Diabet Internat 1996; 13:15.

55. Macleod AF, Boulton AF, Owens DR, et al. A multicenter trial of the aldose-reductase inhibitor tolrestat in patients with symptomatic diabetic peripheral neuropathy. Diabet Metab 1992; 18:14.

56. Manni E, Bertolomi R, Petorossi VE, et al. Trigeminal afferent fibers in the trunk of the oculomotor nerve in lambs. Exp Neurol 1976; 50:465.

57. Max MB, Culnane M, Schafer SC, et al. Amitriptyline relieves diabetic neuropathy pain in patients with normal or depressed mood. Neurology 1987; 37:589.

58. Max MB, Kishore-Kumar R, Schafer SC, et al. Efficacy of desipramine in painful diabetic neuropathy: A placebo-controlled trial. Pain 1991; 45:3.

59. Max MB, Lynch SA, Muir J, et al. Effects of desipramine, amitriptyline, and fluoxetine on pain in diabetic neuropathy. N Engl J Med 1992; 326:1250.

60. Melzack R, Wall PD. Pain mechanisms: A new theory. Science 1965; 150:971.

61. Morley GK, Mooradian AD, Levine AL, et al. Mechanisms of pain in diabetic peripheral neuropathy: Effect of glucose on pain perception in humans. Am J Med 1984; 77:79.

62. Nielsen VK. Pathophysiology of hemifacial spasm. I: Ephaptic transmission and ectopic excitation. Neurology 1984; 34:418.

63. Ochoa JL. The newly recognized painful ABC syndrome: Thermographic aspects. Thermology 1986; 2:65.

64. Ochoa JL. Positive sensory symptoms in neuropathy: Mechanisms and aspects of treatment. In Asbury AK, Thomas PK (eds): Peripheral Nerve Disorders 2. Oxford, Butterworth Heinemann, 1995, pp 44–58.

65. Ogata K, Masaki T, Takoa F, et al. Therapeutic trials with topical capsaicin cream and iontophoretically applied lidocaine for diabetic painful truncal neuropathy. Clin Neurol 1996; 36:30.

66. Pfeifer MA, Ross DR, Schrager JP, et al. A highly successful and novel model for treatment of chronic painful diabetic peripheral neuropathy. Diabetes Care 1993; 16:1103.

67. Plewe G, Weimann A, Linnemann B, et al. Diabetic neuropathic cachexia. Diabet Stoffwech 1996; 5:143.

68. Rains C, Bryson HM. Topical capsaicin: A review of its pharmacological properties and therapeutic potential in post-herpetic neuralgia, diabetic neuropathy and osteoarthritis. Drugs Aging 1995; 7:17.

69. Romain LF. Treatment of peripheral diabetic neuropathy. JAMA 1978; 239:1037.

70. Ruiz V, Ybarra J, Desnueles J, et al. Pain challenge: Diabetic neuropathy. Med Hyg 1996; 54:820.

71. Rull JA, Quibrera R, Gonzalez-Millan H, et al. Symptomatic treatment of peripheral diabetic neuropathy with carbamazepine: Double-blind cross-over study. Diabetologia 1969; 5:215.

72. Said G, Slama G, Selva J. Progressive centripetal degeneration of axons in small fibre diabetic neuropathy. Brain 1983; 106:791.

73. Sanders DB. Ephaptic transmission in hemifacial spasm: A single-fiber EMG study. Muscle Nerve 1989; 12:690.

74. Santiago JV, Sönksen PH, Boulton AJ, et al. Withdrawal of the aldose reductase inhibitor tolrestat in patients with diabetic neuropathy: Effect on nerve function. J Diabetes Complications 1993; 7:170.

75. Saudek CD, Werns S, Reidenberg MM. Phenytoin in the treatment of diabetic symmetrical polyneuropathy. Clin Pharmacol Ther 1977; 22:196.

76. Scadding JW. Development of ongoing activity, mechanosensitivity and adrenaline sensitivity in severed peripheral nerve axons. Exp Neurol 1981; 73:345.

77. Schneider U, Quastoff S, Mitrović N, et al. Hyperglycaemic hypoxia alters after-potential and fast K^+ conductance of rat axons by cytoplasmic acidification. J Physiol 1993; 465:697.

78. Seltzer Z, Devor M. Ephaptic transmission in chronically damaged peripheral nerves. Neurology 1979; 29:1061.

79. Shimamura H, Baba M, Ozaki I, et al. Delayed somatosensory conduction in acute painful neuropathy of diabetes. Eur J Neurol 1996; 3:264.

80. Shindo H, Tawata M, Aida K, et al. Clinical efficacy of a stable prostacyclin analog, iloprost, in diabetic neuropathy. Prostaglandins 1991; 41:85.

81. Simon GS, Dewey WL. Narcotics and diabetes. I: The effect of streptozotocin-induced diabetes on the antinociceptive potency of morphine. J Pharmacol Exp Ther 1981; 218:318.

82. Sindrup SH, Gram LF, Brosen K, et al. The selective serotonin reuptake inhibitor paroxetine is effective in the treatment of diabetic neuropathy symptoms. Pain 1990; 42:135.

83. Sindrup SH, Gram LF, Sjøld T, et al. Concentration response relationship in imipramine treatment of diabetic neuropathy symptoms. Clin Pharmacol Ther 1990; 47:509.

84. Sindrup SH, Gram LF, Skjøld T, et al. Clomipramine vs desipramine vs placebo in the treatment of diabetic neuropathy symptoms. Br J Clin Pharmacol 1990; 30:683.

85. Sindrup SH, Grodum E, Gram LF, et al. Concentration response relationship in paroxetine treatment of diabetic neuropathy symptoms: A patient-blinded dose-escalation study. Ther Drug Monit 1991; 13:408.

86. Sindrup SH, Bach FW, Gram LF. Plasma beta-endorphin is not affected by treatment with imipramine or paroxetine in patients with diabetic sensory neuropathy syndromes. Clin J Pain 1992; 8:145.

87. Sindrup SH, Tixen C, Gram LF, et al. Lack of effect of mianserin on the symptoms of diabetic neuropathy. Eur J Pharmacol 1992; 43:251.

88. Sindrup SH, Bjerre U, Dejgaard A, et al. The selective serotonin reuptake inhibitor citalopram relieves the symptoms of diabetic neuropathy. Clin Pharmacol Ther 1992; 52:547.

89. Steele JM, Young RJ, Lloyd GG, et al. Clinically apparent eating disorders in young diabetic women: Associations with painful neuropathy and other complications. BMJ 1987; 294:859.

90. Stewart JD. Diabetic truncal neuropathy: Topography of the sensory defect. Ann Neurol 1989; 25:233.

91. Stracke H, Mayer UE, Schumacher HE, et al. Mexiletine in the treatment of diabetic neuropathy. Diabetes Care 1992; 15:1550.

92. Sugimura K, Dyck PJ. Sural nerve myelin thickness and axon cylinder caliber in human diabetes. Neurology 1981; 31:1087.

93. Tandan R, Lewis GA, Krusinski PB, et al. Topical capsaicin in painful diabetic neuropathy: Controlled study with long-term follow-up. Diabetes Care 1992; 15:8.

94. Tesfaye S, Malik R, Harris N, et al. Arteriovenous shunting and proliferating new vessels in acute painful neuropathy of rapid glycaemic control. Diabetologia 1996; 39:329.

95. Tesfaye S, Watt J, Benbow S, et al. Electrical spinal cord stimulation for painful diabetic peripheral neuropathy. Lancet 1996; 348:1669.

96. Thomas PK. The anatomical substratum of pain. Can J Neurol Sci 1974; 1:92.

97. Thomas PK. Painful neuropathies. In Bonica JJ, Liebeskind JC, Albe-Fessard DG (eds): Advances in Pain Research and Therapy. New York, Raven Press, 1979, pp 103–110.

98. Thomas PK, Tomlinson DR. Diabetic and hypoglycemic neuropathy. In Dyck PJ, Thomas PK, Griffin JW, et al (eds): Peripheral Neuropathy, ed 3. Philadelphia, WB Saunders, 1993, pp 1219–1250.

99. Thomas PK, Scadding JG. Treatment of pain in diabetic neuropathy. In Dyck PJ, Thomas PK, Asbury AK, et al (eds): Diabetic Neuropathy. Philadelphia, WB Saunders, 1987, pp 216–222.

100. Thorsteinsson G. Management of painful diabetic neuropathy. JAMA 1997; 238:2695.

101. Torebjörk HE, La Motte RH, Robinson CJ. Peripheral nerve correlates of magnitude of cutaneous pain and hyperalgesia: Simultaneous recordings of human sensory judgements of pain and evoked responses of nociceptor C fibers. J Neurophysiol 1984; 51:325.

102. Tuck RR, Schmelzer JD, Low PA. Endoneurial blood flow and oxygen tension in the sciatic nerve of rats with experimental diabetic neuropathy. Brain 1984; 107:935.

103. Turkington RW. Depression masquerading as diabetic neuropathy. JAMA 1980; 243:1147.

104. Wall PD. Excitability changes in afferent fibre terminations and their relation to slow potentials. J Physiol 1958; 142:1.

105. Wall PD, Gutnick M. Ongoing activity in peripheral nerves: The physiology and pharmacology of impulses originating in a neuroma. Exp Neurol 1974; 43:580.

106. Wall PD, Devor M. Sensory afferent impulses originate from dorsal root ganglia as well as from the periphery in normal and injured rat nerves. Pain 1983; 17:321.

107. Watkins PJ, Gayle C, Alsanjari N, et al. Severe sensory-autonomic neuropathy and endocrinopathy in insulin-dependent diabetes. Q J Med 1995; 88:795.

108. Watson CP. Topical capsaicin as an adjuvant analgesic. J Pain Symptom Manage 1994; 9:425.

109. Weddington WW Jr. Treatment of peripheral diabetic neuropathy. JAMA 1978; 239:1037.

110. Young RJ, Ewing DJ, Clarke BF. A controlled trial of sorbinil, an aldose reductase inhibitor, in chronic painful diabetic neuropathy. Diabetes 1983; 32:938.

111. Ziegler D, Lynch SA, Muir J, et al. Transdermal clonidine versus placebo in painful diabetic neuropathy. Pain 1992; 43:403.

112. Zorilla E, Kozak GP. Ophthalmoplegia in diabetes mellitus. Ann Intern Med 1967; 67:968.

Chapter 29

Plantar Neuropathic Ulcer and Charcot Joints: Risk Factors, Presentation, and Management

M. E. Edmonds • P. J. Watkins

INTRODUCTION

Foot problems in diabetes cause substantial misery, hospital bed occupancy, and time off from work. They account for 45% of all major amputations and absorb huge financial resources.[30] The prevalence of foot ulceration in a diabetic population in the United Kingdom is approximately 5%,[28] with an estimated incidence of new lesions of about 10% each year.[44] The risk of foot ulceration probably exists in the majority of patients with type 2 diabetes mellitus (DM) and long-standing type 1 DM patients because neuropathy develops insidiously and without symptoms in a high proportion, causing a range of sensory, autonomic, and vascular changes.

Foot ulceration with the dangerous intrusion by infection only occurs after some form of trauma, most commonly from normal walking, causing callus and excessively high pressures under the foot, but many other common or bizarre circumstances and practices can cause problems. Prevention of foot ulceration and reduction of amputation are eminently feasible and cost effective and should form an important aspect of diabetes care.

Charcot joints are much less common but not as rare as previously thought. They are now known to affect almost 10% of patients with neuropathy and more than 16% of those with a history of neuropathic ulceration.[6] A more specific small-fiber neuropathy may underlie their development by causing major vascular and bony changes, described subsequently.

This chapter will describe the risk factors, presentation, and management of the neuropathic ulcer and the Charcot joint. It will conclude with a brief description of the organization of diabetic foot care necessary to prevent and treat these problems and to reduce the risk of amputation.

NEUROPATHIC ULCERATION
Risk Factors
NEUROPATHY

The neuropathies associated with diabetes form a diverse group of conditions, some of which put the foot at risk. The reversible mononeuropathies and painful syndromes described elsewhere generally recover and do not lead to foot problems. The major risks come from the conventional distal symmetrical sensory neuropathies combined with autonomic failure, which result in diminished sensation and gross circulatory changes in the feet.

The sensory loss develops in a stocking distribution, progressing proximally. Most patients with neuropathy are without symptoms and thus unaware of the risk of trauma and ulceration. Those experiencing paresthesias are aware of neuropathy, although the symptom is in itself harmless, but only a minority complain of numb feet, and then the neuropathy is usually very severe. In cases of exceptional severity, motor neuropathy can cause an irreversible foot drop, leading to further risks.

Nerve fiber loss in neuropathy is not uniform and usually begins with damage to small myelinated and unmyelinated nerve fibers, resulting in diminished thermal and pain sensation together with autonomic decline and its effect in the vasculature. There are no symptoms at this stage, and in some cases this small-fiber neuropathy progresses as an independent entity, leading to almost complete loss of these sensory modalities, symptomatic autonomic neuropathy, and often Charcot joints as well. Furthermore, sympathetic failure causes a loss of sweating, which leads to dry, cracking skin that serves as a portal of entry for infection.

The circulatory changes are also considerable and play a role in foot pathology, as described in the next section.

Progression of neuropathy in most patients leads to decline of large-fiber function as well as small-fiber deficits, so that diminished light touch and vibration sensation is easily detected. Loss of joint position sense and motor deficits are rare indeed.

Having diagnosed neuropathy, it is important to ascertain whether the patient has lost protective pain sensation that could lead to susceptibility to foot ulceration. Two clinical investigations are useful, vibrometry and nylon monofilaments.

Vibration threshold can be measured using a hand-held biothesiometer (Biomedical Instrument Company, 15764 Munn Road, Newbury, Ohio 44065, USA). The risk of foot ulceration is increased threefold to fourfold when vibration exceeds 25 V, rising to 23-fold when it exceeds 42 V. Recently, a prospective study confirmed the importance of vibration threshold in the prediction of neuropathic foot ulceration.[44]

Nylon monofilaments test the threshold to pressure sensation. The filament is applied to the foot until it buckles, and the patient is asked if he or she can detect its presence. There are various diameters, but the crucial filament is a nylon probe calibrated to a thickness such that buckling occurs at 10 g linear pressure, which is the limit used to detect protective pain sensation.[6] If the patient does not detect the filament, then protective pain sensation is lost and the patient is at risk of developing foot ulcers.[7] Thus, the filaments seem to be a reliable, simple, easy-to-use, and inexpensive screening device for identifying diabetic patients at risk of foot ulceration.[24]

CIRCULATORY CHANGES IN NEUROPATHY

Sympathetic denervation of the peripheral arteries may occur quite early in the evolution of neuropathy and may have major effects on blood flow and vascular responses and cause structural changes in the arterial wall. Postural hypotension develops in the most advanced cases of autonomic neuropathy.

Sympathetic denervation causes loss of vasoconstrictor tone and peripheral vasodilatation, associated with opening of arteriovenous shunts.[16, 22, 42] Skin blood flow increases substantially (on average, to above five times normal), and this can occur in the absence of other clinical evidence of neuropathy.[1] These blood flow changes explain some of the clinical features of the neuropathic foot, notably the excessively warm skin, bounding pulses, and marked venous distension. Venous partial pressure of oxygen (PO_2) in the feet is increased because of arteriovenous shunting.[5] Capillary pressure is increased and may contribute to neuropathic edema, which can occasionally be severe and sometimes is reversed by administration of ephedrine.[18] However, nutritive capillary flow is not compromised by shunting and has been shown directly by television microscopy to be normal or even increased.[22] Bone blood flow is also elevated in these patients,[19] and this is thought to contribute to the osteopenia that predisposes to the development of Charcot ostoarthropathy.

Blood flow responses to various stimuli are also abnormal. Sympathetic stimulation (for example, by coughing or standing) normally induces peripheral vasoconstriction. Neuropathic patients show blunting of these responses, although to a variable degree. Most strikingly, heating the skin of the neuropathic foot can induce paradoxical vasoconstriction (in contrast to the normal vasodilation), probably because neuropathy has interrupted the local axon reflex that governs this response.[36] Maximal vasodilation is also reduced in these patients; this defect is partly attributable to the effects of hyperglycemia per se on the microvasculature, although failure of nitric oxide–dependent smooth muscle vasodilatation in neuropathy has been described.[29] Interestingly, increased blood flow in the neuropathic foot may sometimes by related to pain, and a reduction in blood flow can be associated with diminution of pain in these cases.[1]

Vascular sympathetic denervation can lead to degeneration of the smooth muscle of arteries, leading to medial calcification (Mönckeberg's arteriosclerosis) and stiffening of the arteries.[17] This calcification may assume the histologic characteristics of bone[21] and has a striking radiographic appearance. Vascular calcification does not usually cause major pathologic effects in the feet. However, long-term progression of calcification in conjunction with atherosclerosis of the distal vessels has been associated with gangrene of the toes.

PRESSURE

The presence of excessive pressure is a prerequisite for the development of a neuropathic ulcer. Cross-sectional studies have shown that foot pressures in neuropathic diabetic subjects are higher compared with nonneuropathic sub-

jects, and foot ulcers develop predominantly in areas of high pressure at sites where plantar callus has formed.[38] A prospective study demonstrated that high foot pressures are predictive of subsequent foot ulceration.[41] Plantar pressure can be measured with a number of commercially available systems. However, progress has not yet been reached to the point of positive identification of a threshold pressure at which ulceration would be likely to occur in an individual with loss of protective sensation. Furthermore, different systems for measuring pressure distribution yield different results in the same patient.[10] The presence of neuropathy, even in its very earliest form with relatively mild sensory defects, may itself predispose to elevated foot pressures, although elevated foot pressures are more likely to be present when the foot is deformed. Patients with foot ulcers tend to be heavier than those without ulcers, although weight does not itself necessarily cause high foot pressure. Although vertical forces are obviously important, horizontal or shear forces must also be instrumental in damaging the neuropathic foot, and the sites of healed ulcers have been shown to correspond to the sites of maximal shear forces.

Using pressure sensitive mats, measurement of vertical foot pressures has the potential to identify those patients at risk of foot ulceration. It can also measure appropriate reduction of pressure after callus removal, which can be as much as 30%, and monitor the efficacy of footwear needed to prevent further ulceration.

FOOT DEFORMITIES

Deformities result in bony prominences that lead to areas of high localized pressure. The response to such pressure is different in the neuropathic foot compared with the neuroischemic foot. In the neuropathic foot, the response to pressure is hyperkeratosis and callus formation with eventual ulceration. In the ischemic foot, pressure leads to direct tissue damage and ulceration.

Charcot Deformity. Bony changes in the metatarsal-tarsal region lead to two classical deformities: the rocker bottom deformity, in which there is displacement and subluxation of the tarsus downward, and the medial convexity, which results from displacement of the talonavicular joint or from tarsometatarsal dislocation. If these deformities are not accommodated in properly fitting footwear, ulceration at vulnerable pressure points often develops.

Hammer Toes. A hammer toe is a flexion deformity of the proximal interphalangeal joint. It often leads to ulcer formation on the dorsal surface of the toe.

Claw Toes. Claw toes are characterized by hyperextension of the metatarsophalangeal joints. They are often associated with pes cavus, and callosities often develop over the dorsal surface of the toes and on the plantar surface of the metatarsal heads or the tips of the toes.

Although claw toes may be related to small-muscle weakness caused by neuropathy, they are often unrelated, especially when the clawing is unilateral and associated with trauma or surgery of the forefoot.

Pes Cavus. Normally, the dorsum of the foot is domed because of the medial longitudinal arch that extends between the first metatarsal head and the calcaneus. When it is abnormally high, the deformity is called pes cavus, and the abnormal distribution of weight leads to excessive callus formation under the metatarsal heads.

Hallux Rigidus. Hallux rigidus leads to stiffness of the first metatarsophalangeal joint, with loss of dorsiflexion, and results in excessive forces on the plantar surface, causing callus formation.

Nail Deformities. Gross thickening or deformity of the nail is often seen in the neuropathic foot, and in severe cases of neuropathy, atrophy of the nail develops. Ingrowing toenails arise when the nail plate develops a convex deformity, putting pressure on the tissues at the nail edge. Callus builds up at the nail edge in response to the pressure and inflammation. As a result of ulceration and infection, usually after an episode of trauma, the nail penetrates into the flesh at the nail edge.

Deformities Related to Previous Trauma and Surgery. Deformities of the hip and fractures of the tibia or fibula lead to shortening of the leg and hence abnormal gait, which predisposes to foot ulceration.

Ray amputations are normally performed for digital sepsis in the neuropathic foot. They are usually very successful, but obviously disturb the biomechanics of the foot, leading to high pressure under the metatarsal heads of the adjacent rays.

Deformities Related to Limited Joint Mobility. Limitation of joint motion caused by glycation of connective tissue can lead to deformity and high plantar pressures. The normal foot has been described as a mobile adaptor, and when mobility is impaired, elevated plantar pressure during walking results. Limitation at the ankle joint produces a fixed plantar flexion deformity (equinus), which leads to high mechanical loads under the forefoot.[43]

CALLUS

Callus formation on the sole of the foot can lead to the development of exceptionally high pressures. Liquefaction of tissues deep to the callus leads in due course to ulceration. It is not known whether neuropathy itself accelerates callus development, but the deformed foot with its high pressure points certainly predisposes to callus formation, further accelerating the buildup of high pressure. In a study of 17 patients, peak plantar pressures were reduced after sharp débridement of callus by an average of 26%.[43] In addition, gait pattern is disturbed in patients with diabetic neuropathy, and this may alter the foot pressure distribution, making the foot more prone to the effects of high pressures, again leading to callus formation.[11]

A key aspect of prevention and treatment of neuropathic ulcers is podiatric attention to regular removal of callus and establishing measures to prevent its formation, as described in the management section.

EDEMA

Edema is a major factor predisposing to ulceration, both in the neuropathic and ischemic foot, often exacerbating a tight fit inside poorly fitting shoes, which should also be examined.

The presence of foot edema may not only underlie the development of foot ulcers when the shoes become too tight, but also could impede healing of established ulcers. Edema is common in elderly patients, but in diabetic patients there are additional reasons for its occurrence, either from neuropathy or less commonly from fluid retention or the nephrotic syndrome in patients with diabetic nephropathy.

Edema is a complication of severe diabetic neuropathy. It has long been recognized and was observed in 35 of 125 patients with neuropathy described by Martin.[25] It is not a rare phenomenon, although severe intractable edema resulting from neuropathy is exceptional. This form of edema probably results from the major hemodynamic abnormalities associated with neuropathy. Thus, the high blood flow, vasodilatation, and arteriovenous shunting resulting from sympathetic denervation lead to abnormal venous pooling. Recently, high venous pressures have been demonstrated in the neuropathic foot. Edema probably develops because of loss of the venivasomotor reflex, which normally occurs on standing and results in an increase in precapillary resistance: the inability of the foot to compensate for the rise in venous pressure would thus predispose to edema formation. Relief of edema by administration of the sympathomimetic agent ephedrine[18] lends further strength to the argument that sympathetic failure is the cause of edema.

Presentation

The most frequent complication of the neuropathic foot is the neuropathic ulcer. Its classic position is under the metatarsal heads, but it is more frequently found on the tips of the toes and occasionally on the dorsum of the toe, between the toes and on the heel. The neuropathic ulcer is usually surrounded by callus and is generally painless. The ulcers on the plantar surface of the feet are usually circular, with a punched out appearance, often penetrating to involve deep tissues including bone.

Neuropathic ulcers result from mechanical, thermal, or chemical injuries that are unperceived by the patient because of loss of pain sensation.

Direct mechanical injuries may result from treading on nails and other sharp objects, but the most frequent cause of ulceration from mechanical factors is the neglected callosity. This results from excess friction at the tips of the toes and from high vertical and shear forces under the plantar surface of the metatarsal heads on walking. The repetitive mechanical forces of gait eventually result in callosity formation, inflammatory autolysis, and subkeratotic hematomas. The callosities are painless and are often neglected by the patient. The presence of hemorrhage into a callus is a sign of early ulcer formation, with a 50% chance of finding an ulcer when it is removed.[31] Tissue necrosis occurs below the plaque of callus, resulting in a small cavity filled with serous fluid

that eventually breaks through to the surface with ulcer formation.

At this stage, infection usually supervenes, caused by organisms from the surrounding skin, usually *Staphylococcus aureus* or streptococci. If drainage is inadequate, cellulitis develops, with spread of sepsis to infect underlying tendons and bones and joints. Occasionally, staphylococci and streptococci are present together and can combine to produce a rampant cellulitis that extends rapidly through the foot, producing marked necrosis within only a few hours. Streptococci secrete hyaluronidase, which facilitates widespread distribution of necrotizing toxins from staphylococci. Enzymes from these bacteria are also angiotoxic and cause in situ thrombosis of vessels. If both vessels are thrombosed in the toe, then it becomes necrotic and gangrenous, which is probably the basis of "diabetic" gangrene, in which tissue necrosis is seen only a few centimeters away from a bounding dorsalis pedis pulse. In deep-seated infections, aerobic gram-negative organisms and anaerobic organisms flourish. Both aerobic and anaerobic organisms can rapidly infect the bloodstream and occasionally result in life-threatening bacteremia.

Severe sepsis in the diabetic foot is often associated with gas in the soft tissues. Subcutaneous gas may be detected by direct palpation of the foot, and the diagnosis is confirmed by the appearance of gas in the soft tissues on the radiograph. Although clostridial organisms have previously been held responsible for this presentation, nonclostridial organisms are more frequently the offending pathogens. These include *Bacteroides*, *Escherichia*, and anaerobic streptococci.

Fungal infections also occur but usually do not cause systemic upset. However, infections of toenails (tinea unguium) and interdigital spaces (tinea pedis) by such fungi as *Trichophyton* and *Candida albicans* can serve as portals of entry for bacteria.

In addition to mechanical injury, ulceration can also result from thermal or chemical injury. Thermal injuries cause direct trauma and damage to the skin epithelium. This often results from bathing feet in excessively hot water, the injudicious use of hot water bottles, resting the feet too close to a fire or radiator, or walking barefoot on hot sand. Chemical trauma can result from the use of keratolytic agents such as corn plasters. They often contain salicylic acid, which causes ulceration in the diabetic foot.

Management

The management of ulceration in the purely neuropathic foot falls into three parts: (1) removal of callus and local treatment; (2) eradication of infection; and (3) reduction of weight-bearing forces.

Removal of Callus. The callus that surrounds the ulcer must be removed by expert podiatry. Excess keratin should be pared away with a scalpel blade to expose the floor of the ulcer and allow efficient drainage of the lesion and re-epithelialization from the edges of the ulcer. A simple nonadhesive dressing should be applied, after cleaning the ulcer and surrounding tissue with saline. Use of wound healing growth factors is being explored, including platelet-derived growth factor, and recent studies have shown that it may speed healing in the neuropathic foot.[23]

Eradication of Infection. A bacterial swab should be taken from the floor of the ulcer after the callus has been removed. A superficial ulcer may be treated on an outpatient basis and oral antibiotics prescribed, according to the organism isolated, until the ulcer has healed. The patient should be instructed to carry out daily dressings of the ulcer.

If cellulitis or skin discoloration is present, the limb is threatened, and urgent hospital admission should be arranged. The limb should be rested, and the ulcer irrigated with 2% sodium hypochlorite solution. After blood cultures have been taken, intravenous antibiotics are administered to treat possible staphylococci, streptococci, gram-negative bacteria, and anaerobes (flucloxacillin, 500 mg every 6 hours, amoxicillin, 500 mg every 8 hours, ceftazidime, 1 g every 8 hours, and metronidazole, 500 mg every 8 hours). This antibiotic regimen may need revision after the results of bacterial cultures are available. Blood glucose may need to be controlled with an intravenous insulin pump.

In the neuropathic foot, it is important that all necrotic tissue be removed and abscess cavities drained surgically. If gangrene has developed in a digit, a ray amputation to remove that toe and part of its associated metatarsal bone is necessary and is usually very successful in the neuropathic foot.[20]

Reduction of Weight-Bearing Forces. Bedrest in the acute stages of ulceration is ideal and will obviously remove the weight-bearing forces to promote healing. Proper care should be taken of the heels, and foam wedges should be used to protect them from pressure in bed. However, bedrest is not always possible. In the short term, a total contact plaster cast (with minimum of padding) can be applied to "unload" the ulcer and reduce shear forces.[27] Other forms of cast have become popular, especially removable casts, such as the Scotch cast.[9] Padded hosiery may also help to relieve pressure. With regular rotation, these padded socks have been shown to reduce plantar pressures for at least 6 months.[40] In the long term, redistribution of weight-bearing forces can be achieved by special footwear fashioned from casts of the patient's foot. Insoles made of closed-cell polyethylene foams such as Plastazote have energy-absorbing properties. These can be heated and molded to the shape of the foot to cushion the plantar surface of the foot and to spread the forces of weight-bearing evenly. When subjected to wear and tear, Plastazote insoles can "bottom out," and it is now possible to use more durable materials such as Poron. Indeed, composite insoles are often made with an upper layer of polyethylene foam for total contact and a lower layer of microcell rubber for resilience.[12] When there has been previous ulceration, a rigid weight-distributing cradle is required, as well as cushioning, to relieve weight from high pressure areas and to transfer it to other less vulnerable areas. Traditionally, cork cradles have been used, but recently Plastazote cradles have been manufactured, often with "windows" cut out (and filled in with cushioning material such as Neoprene) for weight relief at these sites.

Molded insoles must be accommodated in extra-depth shoes. When the foot is not deformed, shoes fashioned from commercial lasts and available "off the shelf" can be used. If the patient has a foot deformity with healed neuropathic ulcers, it is necessary to make individual lasts from casts of the patient's foot. In either case, the heels must be low, and slipping is prevented by using lace ties. The forefoot should be broad and square, and the uppers should be of high-quality leather that will adapt to toe pressure.[37] When pressure points are not adequately relieved by cushioned insoles, it is necessary to modify the soles of the shoe. When the ulcer is under the plantar surface of the first toe, a rigid rocker sole allows the shoe to rock like a seesaw on a pivot under the center of the shoe, minimizing contact between the forefoot and floor during gait. If the ulcer is under the metatarsal heads, a metatarsal bar placed just proximal to the heads can reapportion weight-bearing forces along the shafts.

CHARCOT FOOT

Risk Factors

NEUROPATHY

The development of Charcot osteoarthropathy depends on peripheral autonomic and somatic defects. Recent studies have indicated a specific deficit of small-fiber function that progresses.[35] Indeed, this specific pattern of fiber loss is often present at the onset of Charcot joints, leading to the speculation that associated changes are responsible for this rare syndrome.

BLOOD FLOW

An adequate blood supply is necessary for the development of the Charcot joint. Indeed, the Charcot foot has been reported after successful arterial bypass surgery in the lower limb.[15] Sympathetic denervation of arterioles causes an increase of blood flow, which in turn causes rarefaction of bone, making it prone to damage even after minor trauma. Bone formation and structure are closely linked with vascular changes. Large venules containing rapid linear velocities of blood flow cause resorption of bone spicules.[26] In animals, the site of maximum bone calcium loss after paraplegia corresponds to areas of maximum blood flow, which may lead to increased resorption of bone.[39] Histologic studies of Charcot joints have shown marked increase in vascularity, with vessel dilatation and trabecula resorption by large numbers of osteoclasts.[8] Thus, increased bony blood flow can lead to bony resorption and susceptibility to fracture.

OSTEOPENIA

Bony resorption leads to osteopenia, with bone structure compromized by hyperemia caused by autonomic dysfunction.[45]

TRAUMA

Loss of sensation from somatic neuropathy permits abnormal mechanical stresses to occur, normally prevented by pain. Relatively minor trauma can then cause major destructive changes in susceptible bone.

RENAL TRANSPLANTATION

Isolated reports have shown an association between renal transplantation with long-term corticosteroid or other immunosuppressive treatment and the subsequent development of the Charcot foot.[13] After renal transplantation, diabetics have a much higher incidence of neurotrophic joint disease than the nontransplanted diabetic population. Of 18 patients with type 1 DM and severe neuropathic arthropathy of the ankle and tarsus, 14 had received a renal transplant before the Charcot foot was diagnosed, and none had a history of major trauma.

It remains unclear whether corticosteroid-induced osteoporosis or some other metabolic abnormality, which tends to weaken bone, was the underlying factor responsible for the development of bone and joint destruction in these patients.

Presentation

The most frequent location of the neuropathic joint is the tarsal-metatarsal region, followed by the metatarsophalangeal joints and then the ankle and subtalar joints.[32] The initial presentation is often a hot, swollen foot, which can be uncomfortable in up to one third of cases and is often misdiagnosed as cellulitis or gout. The precipitating event is usually a minor traumatic episode such as tripping. If the patient is seen within a few days, radiographs are often normal, although isotope bone scans may be grossly abnormal, with localized areas of high uptake representing excessive osteoblastic activity and heralding eventual radiologic abnormalities. A common early radiologic abnormality is fracture, which is followed by osteolysis, bony fragmentation, and finally joint subluxation and disorganization. In addition to fracture, erosions, periosteal new bone formation, and sclerosis are also prominent bony findings in the development of the Charcot joint. Sclerosis is usually associated with lucency in the heads of the metatarsals, the final appearance being similar to the Freiberg's infarction lesion associated with osteonecrosis of the epiphysis of the metatarsal head. These initial bony abnormalities eventually lead to secondary joint destruction, with subluxation of the metatarsophalangeal joints; dislocation of the tarsal, subtalar, and ankle joints, and fragmentation of bone and soft tissue calcification.[34]

The process of destruction takes place over a few months only and leads to two classic

deformities: the rocker bottom deformity, in which there is displacement and subluxation of the tarsus downward, and the medial convexity, which results from displacement of the talonavicular joint or from tarsometatarsal dislocation. If these deformities are not accommodated in properly fitting footwear, ulceration at vulnerable pressure points often develops.

Management

It is essential to make the diagnosis early, before extreme joint destruction has taken place. The initial presentation of unilateral warmth and swelling in a neuropathic foot after an episode of minor trauma is suggestive of a developing Charcot joint.

There is no definite treatment that halts the progression of the disease, but immobilization may help. Treatment consists of rest (ideally bedrest) or the avoidance of weight bearing by the use of crutches until the edema and local warmth have resolved. Alternatively, the foot can be put in a well-molded nonwalking plaster cast. Immobilization is continued until bony repair is complete, usually a period of 2 to 3 months. Recently, bisphosphonates have been used to inhibit osteoclastic activity, leading to a reduction in foot temperature and resolution of symptoms.[33]

CONCLUSION
Organization of Diabetic Foot Care: The Diabetic Foot Clinic

It is vital that there is close liaison between podiatrist, shoe fitter, physician, and surgeon in the care of the diabetic foot. Since 1981, diabetic foot problems have been treated within a special Diabetic Foot Clinic at King's College Hospital. It has provided intensive podiatry, close surveillance, prompt treatment of foot infection, and a footwear service by the attending shoe fitter. A 50% reduction in major amputations[20] has been achieved by adhering to four main strategies: (1) accurate diagnosis of the neuropathic syndromes of the diabetic foot; (2) rapid and appropriate treatment of foot lesions, including sepsis; (3) intensive follow-up of patients; and (4) prevention of foot lesions.

The ultimate aim is, of course, prevention, and this therapeutic goal must be reached through education of the patient in foot care and regular examination of the feet. Patients who develop foot lesions have significantly less knowledge of diabetes, including foot care.[14] Moreover, education reduces the number of major amputations in a diabetic clinic population.[2] Routine examination of the feet in diabetic patients is an important part of management to identify those at risk of ulceration and to prevent its occurrence. However, it is a commonly underutilized preventive measure.[3] The feet of diabetic patients must be carefully examined for the presence of deformities, callus formation, and neuropathy to institute effective measures. Optimum care of the diabetic foot is provided in a diabetic foot clinic where the skills of podiatrists, shoe fitters, and nurses receive full support from physicians and surgeons. Many lesions of the diabetic foot are avoidable, making patient education immensely important.

References

1. Archer AG, Watkins PJ, Roverts VC. Blood flow patterns in painful diabetic neuropathy. Diabetologia 1984; 27:563.
2. Assal J-P, Gfeller R, Ekoe J-M. Patient education in diabetes. *In* Bostrum H, Ljungstedt N (eds): Recent Trends in Diabetes Research. Stockholm, Almqvust & Wiksell, 1981, pp 276–290.
3. Bailey TS, Yu HM, Rayfield EJ. Patterns of foot examination in a diabetes clinic. Am J Med 1985; 78:371.
4. Birke JA, Sims DS. Plantar sensory threshold in the ulcerative foot. Lepr Rev 1986; S7:261.
5. Boulton AJM, Scarpello JHB, Ward JD. Venous oxygenation in the diabetic neuropathic foot: Evidence of arteriovenous shunting? Diabetologia 1982; 22:6.
6. Boulton AJM, Kubrusly DB, Bowker JH, et al. TI: Impaired vibratory perception and diabetic foot ulceration. Diabet Med 1986; 3:335.
7. Boulton AJM, Mueller MJ. Identifying patients with diabetes mellitus who are at risk for lower extremity complications: Use of Siemmens-Weinstein monofilaments. Phys Ther 1996; 76:68.
8. Brewer AC, Allman RM. Pathogenesis of the neurotrophic joint: Neurotraumatic vs neurovascular. Radiology 1981; 139:349.
9. Burden AC, Jones GR, Jones R, et al. Use of the "Scotchcast boot" in treating diabetic foot ulcers. BMJ 1983; 286:1555.
10. Cavanagh PR, Ulbrecht JS. Plantar pressure in the diabetic foot. *In* Sammarco GJ (ed): The Foot in Diabetes. Philadelphia, Lea & Febiger, 1991, pp 54–70.
11. Cavanagh PR, Derr JA, Ulbrecht JS, et al. Problems with gait and posture in neuropathic patients with insulin dependent diabetes mellitus. Diabet Med 1992; 9:469.
12. Chantelau E, Leisch A. Footwear, uses and abuses. *In* Boulton AJM, Connor H, Cavanagh PR (eds): The Foot in Diabetes. Chichester, John Wiley & Sons, 1994, pp 99–108.
13. Clohisy DR, Thompson RC. Fractures associated with neuropathic arthropathy in adults who have juvenile onset diabetes. J Bone Joint Surg [Am] 1988; 70:1192.
14. Delbridge L, Appleberg M, Reeve TS. Factors associated with the development of foot lesions in the diabetic. Surgery 1983; 93:78.

15. Edelman SV, Kosofsky EM, Paul RA, et al. Neuro-osteoarthropathy (Charcot's Joint) in diabetes mellitus following revascularisation surgery: Three case reports and a review of the literature. Arch Intern Med 1987; 147:1504.
16. Edmonds ME, Roberts VC, Watkins PJ. Blood flow in the diabetic neuropathic foot. Diabetologia 1982; 22:9.
17. Edmonds ME, Morrison N, Laws JW, et al. Medial arterial calcification and diabetic neuropathy. BMJ 1982; 284:928.
18. Edmonds ME, Archer AG, Watkins PJ. Ephedrine: A new treatment for diabetic neuropathic oedema. Lancet 1983; 1:548.
19. Edmonds ME, Clarke MB, Newton S, et al. Increased uptake of bone radiopharmaceutical in diabetic neuropathy. Q J Med 1985; 57:8433.
20. Edmonds ME, Blundell MP, Morris HE, et al. The diabetic foot: Impact of a foot clinic. Q J Med 1986; 232:763.
21. Edmonds ME, Zachary I, Foster A, et al. Diabetic tibial arteries show increased calcification associated with increased gene expression of matrix Gla protein. Diabet Med 1995; 12(suppl 2):515.
22. Flynn MD, Edmonds ME, Tooke JE, et al. Direct measurement of capillary blood flow in the diabetic neuropathic foot. Diabetologia 1988; 31:652.
23. Krupski WC, Reilly LM, Perez S, et al. A prospective randomized trial of autologous platelet derived wound healing factors for the treatment of chronic non healing wounds: A preliminary report. J Vasc Surg 1991; 14:526.
24. Kumar S, Fernando DJ, Veves A, et al. Semmes-Weinstein monofilaments: A simple, effective and inexpensive screening device for identifying diabetic patients at risk of foot ulceration. Diabetes Res Clin Pract 1991; 13:63.
25. Martin MM. Diabetic neuropathy. Brain 1953; 76:594.
26. McClugage SG, McCuskey RS. Relationship of the microvascular system to bone resorption and growth in situ. Microvasc Res 1973; 6:132.
27. Mueller MJ, Diamond JE, Sinacore DR, et al. Total contact casting in treatment of diabetic plantar ulcers. Diabetes Care 1989; 12:384.
28. Neil HAW, Thompson AV, Thorogood M, et al. Diabetes in the elderly: The Oxford community diabetes study. Diabet Med 1989; 6:608.
29. Pitei DL, Watkins PJ, Edmonds ME. NO-dependent smooth muscle vasodilatation is reduced in NIDDM patients with peripheral sensory neuropathy. Diabet Med 1997; 14:284.
30. Reiber GE. Diabetes foot care: Financial implications and practical guidelines. Diabetes Care 1992; 15(suppl 1):29.
31. Rosen RC, Davids MS, Bohanske LM. Haemorrhage into plantar callus and diabetes mellitus. Cutis 1985; 35:339.
32. Sanders LJ, Frykberg RG. Diabetic neuropathic osteoarthropathy: The Charcot foot. *In* Frykberg RG (ed): The High Risk Foot in Diabetes. New York, Churchill Livingstone, 1991, pp 227–238.
33. Selby PL, Young MJ, Boulton AJM. Pamidronate: A definitive treatment for diabetic Charcot neuroarthropathy? Diabet Med 1992; 9(suppl 2):A27.
34. Sinha S, Munichoodappa CS, Kozak GP. Neuroarthropathy (Charcot joints) in diabetes mellitus. Medicine (Baltimore), 1972; 51:191.
35. Stevens MJ, Edmonds ME, Foster AVM, et al. Selective neuropathy and preserved vascular responses in the diabetic Charcot foot. Diabetologia 1992; 35:148.
36. Stevens MJ, Edmonds ME, Foster AVM, et al. Paradoxical skin blood flow responses in the neuropathic foot: An assessment of the contribution of neuropathy and microangiopathy. Diabet Med 1992; 9:49.
37. Tovey FI. Establishing a diabetic shoe service. Pract Diabetes 1985; 2:5.
38. Ulbrecht JS, Norkitis A, Cavanagh PR. Plantar pressure and plantar ulceration in the diabetic neuropathic foot. *In* Kominsky SJ (ed): Medical and Surgical Management of the Diabetic Foot. St Louis, Mosby–Year Book, 1994, pp 29–45.
39. Verhas M, Martinello Y, Mone M, et al. Demineralisation and pathological physiology of the skeleton in paraplegic rats. Calcif Tissue Int 1980; 30:83.
40. Veves A, Masson EA, Fernando DJS, et al. Studies of experimental hosiery in diabetic neuropathic patients with high foot pressures. Diabet Med 1990; 7:324.
41. Veves A, Murray HJ, Young MJ, et al. The risk of foot ulceration in diabetic patients with high foot pressure: A prospective study. Diabetologia 1992; 35:660.
42. Watkins PJ, Edmonds ME. Sympathetic nerve failure in diabetes. Diabetologia 1988; 25:73.
43. Young MJ, Cavanagh PR, Thomas G, et al. The effect of callus removal on dynamic plantar foot pressures in diabetic patients. Diabet Med 1992; 9:55.
44. Young MJ, Bready JL, Veves A, et al. The prediction of diabetic neuropathic foot ulceration using vibration perception thresholds: A prospective study. Diabetes Care 1994; 17:557.
45. Young MJ, Marshall A, Adams JE, et al. Osteopenias, neurological dysfunction and the development of Charcot neuroarthropathy. Diabetes Care 1995; 18:34.

Section **IV**

Differential Diagnosis of Diabetic Neuropathies

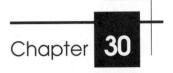

Chapter **30**

Classification of the Diabetic Neuropathies

Bruce V. Taylor • Peter James Dyck

INTRODUCTION

Almost from the time of the first descriptions of peripheral nerve involvement in diabetes mellitus (DM), it was obvious that different varieties of neuropathy occurred more frequently in diabetic patients than in the general population. This observation suggests (1) that DM is implicated in the pathogenesis of these neuropathies and (2) that different mechanisms probably account for different varieties of neuropathy. Table 30.1 provides a list of the varieties of neuropathy encountered in diabetic cohorts. Dyck and Giannini in 1996[10] concluded that there were nine principal clinical subtypes of neuropathy (Table 30.2). Many of the other described neuropathies are probably variants of these nine varieties.

Based on present information, these diabetic neuropathies perhaps fall into five mechanistic categories:

1. Metabolic-microvessel-hypoxic (for example, diabetic polyneuropathy [DPN])
2. Immune-vasculitic (for example, diabetic lumbosacral radiculoplexus neuropathy [DLSRPN])
3. Compression and repetitive injury (median neuropathy of the wrist [MNW] and ulnar neuropathy at the elbow [UNE])

TABLE 30.1 TYPES OF DIABETIC NEUROPATHY

Symmetrical Length-Dependent Neuropathy
Diabetic polyneuropathy (DPN)*—a symmetrical length-dependent sensorimotor polyneuropathy especially of the lower limbs, including some autonomic findings
Small-fiber diabetic polyneuropathy with weight loss†
Diabetic pandysautonomia‡
Hypoglycemic polyneuropathy‡
Asymmetrical Non–Length-Dependent Neuropathy
Diabetic lumbosacral radiculoplexus neuropathy (DLSRPN)—also called motor neuropathy, proximal diabetic neuropathy, diabetic amyotrophy, Bruns Garland syndrome, and femoral neuropathy*
Diabetic thoracolumbar radiculoneuropathy (DTLRN)—also called truncal radiculopathy*
Median neuropathy of the wrist (MNW)—also called carpal tunnel syndrome*
Ulnar neuropathy at the elbow (UNE)—also incorrectly called cubital tunnel syndrome*
Brachial plexus neuropathy‡
Oculomotor neuropathy*
Ischemic mononeuropathies of lower limbs

---

*Probably more frequent in patients with diabetes mellitus than in the general population.
†The variety described by Archer and Thomas.[1]
‡Insufficiently studied to know whether it is more frequent in patients with diabetes mellitus than in the general population.

4. Repeated hypoglycemia (insulin neuropathy)
5. Ischemia (for example, mononeuropathy of leg caused by peripheral vascular disease)

HISTORY

In the 19th century, it was realized that DM could be the cause of peripheral neuropathy and that this complication might result in serious symptoms and impairments but usually not death. Many of the now-recognized varie-

TABLE 30.2 CLINICAL SUBTYPES OF DIABETIC NEUROPATHY

Diabetic polyneuropathy (DPN)
Proximal diabetic neuropathy (PDN)
Truncal radiculopathy
Diabetic autonomia
Upper limb mononeuropathies: median neuropathy at the wrist (MNW) and ulnar neuropathy at the elbow (UNE)
Cranial nerve III neuropathy
Hypoglycemic polyneuropathy
Neuropathy caused by peripheral vascular disease

Data from Dyck PS, Giannini C. Pathologic alterations in the diabetic neuropathies of humans: A review. J Neuropathol Exp Neurol 1996; 55:1181.

ties of diabetic neuropathy were first described in the 19th century, including the first mention of pseudotabetic diabetic neuropathy in 1855 by Leval-Picquechef[21] and the lumbosacral plexus neuropathy varieties by Bruns[4] and Buzzard[6] in 1890. The awareness that diabetes could affect the peripheral nervous system in several distinct ways prompted the first attempts to classify diabetic neuropathy. The earliest classification, which appeared in the German literature in 1893 by Leyden,[22] divided diabetic neuropathies into hyperalgesia (painful), paralytic (motor), and ataxic forms. In 1893, Pryce[27] subdivided diabetic neuropathies into a predominantly sensory and a patchy motor form. Kraus in 1922[19] attempted the first pathologic classification from literature review and personal experience. However, many of the reviewed cases had concomitant tuberculosis or syphilis, making classification of the neuropathy of such cases problematic. He concluded that "extramedullary" involvement of the peripheral neurons (peripheral neuritis) had not been obtained from the review of the clinic and pathologic reports, in the literature or from his experience.

Jordon and Crabtree in 1935[18] suggested a classification based on the assumed mechanism of the development of symptoms. They separated neuralgic and myalgic varieties of neuropathy that responded to correction of hyperglycemia from other forms (including forms with pain, paresthesia, and paresis) that did not and therefore were caused by circulatory disturbances. They inferred that patients in the latter group were suffering from ischemic lesions of peripheral nerve, whereas the more distal sensory neuropathies were caused by metabolic disturbance. Sullivan in 1958[30] believed that there were really two major types of diabetic neuropathy: a distal symmetrical sensory neuropathy and a proximal motor neuropathy. The proximal motor variety was later shown usually to also have a prominent distal sensory component with much pain.[3] Because of the awareness of focal neuropathies occurring in diabetes, Fry and colleagues in 1962[15] suggested that a third category of isolated peripheral nerve lesions be included, and Gilliatt in 1965[16] added a fourth category of purely autonomic neuropathy.

Bruyn and Garland in 1970[5] proposed a more comprehensive classification that essentially revolved around the same question of symmetrical predominantly sensory and distal polyneuropathy and asymmetrical predominantly motor and other proximal neuropathies.

TABLE 30.3 CLASSIFICATION OF DIABETIC NEUROPATHY

Symmetrical Distal Polyneuropathies
Sensory or sensorimotor polyneuropathy
Autonomic neuropathy
Symmetrical proximal lower limb motor
  neuropathy
Asymmetrical Neuropathies
Cranial neuropathy
Trunk radiculopathy or mononeuropathy
Limb—plexus or mononeuropathy
Multiple mononeuropathies
Entrapment neuropathies
Ischemic nerve injury
Asymmetrical neuropathy and distal symmetrical
  polyneuropathy
Mixed forms

Data from Dyck PJ, Karnes J, O'Brien PC: Diagnosis, staging, and classification of diabetic neuropathy and associations with other classifications. *In* Dyck PJ, Thomas PK, Asbury A, et al (eds): Diabetic Neuropathy. Philadelphia, WB Saunders, 1987, p 36.

Dyck and associates in 1987[11] subdivided diabetic neuropathies into symmetrical and asymmetrical and listed varieties under each of these headings (Table 30.3). Based on studies of a prevalence cohort (Rochester Diabetic Neuropathy Study [RDNS]), diabetic patients who have received combined pancreas-renal transplantation, and patients referred to us, we now think that an improved classification is possible (see Table 30.1).

The classification by Thomas and Tomlinson in 1993[32] divided diabetic neuropathies into symmetrical, asymmetrical, and mixed forms (Table 30.4). The first group consisted of distal symmetrical polyneuropathies, and the second, focal and multifocal neuropathies. The first group included all the distal symmetrical sensory and autonomic varieties of diabetic neuropathy. The second group included diabetic proximal neuropathy (diabetic amyotrophy),

TABLE 30.4 CLASSIFICATION OF DIABETIC NEUROPATHY

Symmetrical Polyneuropathies
Sensory or sensorimotor polyneuropathy
Autonomic neuropathy
Symmetrical proximal lower limb motor
  neuropathy
Focal and Mutifocal Neuropathies
Cranial neuropathy
Trunk and limb mononeuropathies
Asymmetrical lower limb motor neuropathy
Mixed forms

Data from Thomas PK, Tomlinson DR. Diabetic and hypoglycemic neuropathy. *In* Dyck PJ, Thomas PK, Griffin JW, et al (eds): Peripheral Neuropathy, ed 3. Philadelphia, WB. Saunders, 1993.

isolated cranial nerve palsies, thoracolumbar radiculopathies, brachial plexopathies, and entrapment neuropathies. The justification for including autonomic neuropathy with the distal symmetrical sensory polyneuropathies is because results of thermoregulatory sweat testing in most patients with autonomic neuropathy demonstrate a length-dependent loss of sweating. Watkins and Thomas think (personal communication, 1997) that there may be an additional subtype, a symmetrical, painful small-fiber polyneuropathy usually preceded or accompanied by weight loss. We think an improved classification based on natural history, epidemiologic studies, and putative mechanisms is now possible (see Table 30.1).

Dyck and Giannini in 1996[10] suggested that there may be five fundamentally different mechanisms implicated in varieties of diabetic neuropathy. Chronic hyperglycemia and associated metabolic derangement is perhaps common to most varieties of diabetic neuropathy, but the association is strongest for DPN. These might be identified as:

1. Metabolic derangement, altered microvessel function and structure, and hypoxia (as found in DPN, retinopathy, and nephropathy)
2. Immune derangement and necrotizing vasculitis (as occurs in DLSRPN, diabetic thoracolumbar radiculoneuropathy [DTLRN], and diabetic brachial plexus radioculoneuropathy [DBPRN])
3. Compression and repetitive nerve injury (MNW, UNE)
4. Hypoglycemia (insulin neuropathy)
5. Peripheral vascular disease and ischemia (ischemic nerve injury)

This classification does not include the subacute painful sensorimotor neuropathy with weight loss described by Archer and associates in 1983.[1]

BASIS OF CLASSIFICATION

There is increasing evidence that diabetic neuropathy is heterogeneous. Historically, some authors have not agreed with this point of view. Pirart[26] stated in 1965 that no classification beyond the broad rubric of diabetic neuropathy was possible. Ellenberg in 1964[13] came to similar conclusions when he likened diabetes to syphilis and noted that with the wane of the great imitator, diabetes would take its mantle.

A stumbling block to a useful classification

of diabetic neuropathy is the presence of mixed pictures, in particular the presence of distal sensory neuropathy in a patient who subsequently develops a second focal neuropathy. This was noted in 85 of 105 patients with proximal diabetic neuropathy reported by Bastron and Thomas in 1981.[3]

We suggest that classification should be based on (1) natural history (onset, course, clinical features, and outcome), (2) anatomico-pathological characteristics, (3) underlying mechanism, (4) risk factors, and (5) response to treatment. If one can recognize different syndromes by these criteria, then classification is necessary and useful.

Based on review of the medical literature, our experience with several hundred diabetic patients followed for more than a decade, a longitudinal study of approximately 100 diabetic patients with end-stage complications undergoing pancreas and renal transplants, and many problematic diabetic patients referred to us, we are convinced that diabetic neuropathy is heterogeneous and made up of definable discrete syndromes.

Many neurologic disorders and neuropathies occurring in patients with DM are simply associated by chance, because DM and neurologic disease are both common. Many (perhaps up to 8%) of neuropathies and neurologic disorders occurring in diabetic patients probably are not causally related to DM—they simply occur by chance in patients with DM.[12] In this situation, the two disorders are not therefore mechanistically linked. It should be appreciated that none of the neuropathic patterns of neuropathy, thought to be mechanistically associated with DM, are completely unique. Symmetrical length-dependent sensorimotor polyneuropathy, asymmetrical lumbosacral plexus neuropathy, carpal tunnel syndrome, and UNE occur unassociated with DM. The arguments that DM is involved in pathogenesis of these varieties is based on the knowledge that they occur more frequently in DM than in the population at large and that they can be linked to a postulated mechanism of diabetic neuropathy—the latter still not proved. It should be appreciated that the association with DM has convincingly been made only for DPN and perhaps for lumbosacral plexus neuropathies and CTS, but not for most of the other varieties of neuropathy. This is not to say that such associations do not exist; they have not been adequately proved.

A troublesome situation arises when there is an admixture of diabetic neuropathies, neurologic disease of other cause, and atherosclerotic complications in the same patient—a not uncommon situation. A long-standing diabetic patient may have a distal DPN, develop a superimposed lumbosacral plexus neuropathy and carpal tunnel syndrome, and also have peripheral vascular disease. We think it inappropriate to force these different syndromes into one, even though overlap of impairment may not be discriminated.

CLASSIFICATION

It is perhaps useful to classify diabetic neuropathies by whether they are causally associated with DM, by the putative underlying mechanism, and by clinical syndromes. As discussed previously and in Chapter 8, it is always necessary to ask whether the neuropathic symptoms and findings in a diabetic patient, even though typical of diabetic neuropathy, are in fact caused by DM. Whisnant and Love report a patient whose neuropathic symptoms and findings were caused not by DPN but by a spinal cord ependymoma.[33] In the RDNS, we had a patient whose severe neuropathy was caused by spinal stenosis. The clinical manifestation of patients with inherited neuropathy is commonly attributed to DPN.

In a previous section, we listed five putative mechanisms that are probably implicated in diabetic neuropathies. Because in no instance are these mechanisms understood well, and because prevention or treatment is only incompletely known by mechanism, this is not a very useful classification.

The classification we prefer is given in Table 30.1. In the following paragraphs, we provide characterizing information to distinguish varieties. For additional information, see Chapters 8, 17, and 32 to 38.

Diabetic Polyneuropathy. This is a symmetrical length-dependent sensorimotor polyneuropathy that typically begins with an abnormality of nerve conduction or an abnormality of reduced response of the heartbeat to deep breathing. Usually, at a somewhat later time, loss of ankle reflexes and decrease of vibration perception in the toes develop. This is followed by greater sensory loss, and autonomic involvement develops in the feet and legs. In more severe cases, weakness of toe extension, ankle dorsiflexion, and toe flexion develop. Visceral autonomic symptoms of impotence in the male, gastroparesis, diarrhea, or sphincter dysfunction may occur at any stage of severity, but they tend to be more typical of severe impairment. The process develops and progresses insidiously, with many patients having some degree of dysfunction or impairment and only a minority developing symptoms of muscle weakness or visceral autonomic involvement. Symptoms may occur at any point of the worsening impairment but seldom occur during early stages of functional impairment. Sensory symptoms tend to be those related to hypofunction and hyperfunction. Autonomic symptoms generally are associated with the more severe stage of involvement (see Chapters 38, 39, and 40).

Should pseudotabetic diabetica (large fiber) and hyperalgesic (small fiber) polyneuropathies be distinguished as separate entities? As discussed in Chapter 17, we do not think so. In our experience, examples of polar involvement (large or small fiber) are encountered, but after careful clinical and electrophysiological assessment, there is typically involvement of both large and small fibers.

Should painful polyneuropathy associated with weight loss and cachexia be considered a separate neuropathic disorder?[1] Even from early times (see historical section of Chapter 17), weight loss was a frequent precursor or concomitant of DPN (including painful neuropathy). It may be that evidence will be found for a mechanism underlying weight loss independent of poor metabolic control, which would lead one to label this disorder unique.

Should visceral autonomic neuropathy be considered a separate entity? We have taken the position that it should be included with DPN if it appears to be a progression of severe distal symmetrical polyneuropathy. An acute or subacute visceral dysautonomia without or with minimal sensorimotor polyneuropathy and with a self-limited course probably should not be included with diabetic sensorimotor polyneuropathy.

Diabetic-Uremic Polyneuropathy. When diabetic patients develop uremia, DPN—which is usually already present in mild or moderate severity—tends to become more severe. It is not possible in this case to reliably separate the component causing DPN from that causing uremic polyneuropathy.

Diabetic-Hypoglycemic Polyneuropathy. It is likely, and perhaps probable, that repeated severe hypoglycemia leads to nerve injury indistinguishable from DPN. In patients with islet cell tumors, a sensorimotor polyneuropathy may develop that is indistinguishable from DPN (see section on Hypoglycemic Neuropathy in Chapter 32).

Diabetic Lumbosacral Radiculoplexus Neuropathy. Also called proximal diabetic neuropathy, diabetic amyotrophy, and femoral neuropathy (see Chapter 17), DLSRPN appears to be a distinct disorder, separate from DPN, by reason of disease association (more prevalent in type 2 DM), total hyperglycemia exposure (less related), course (it tends to be monophasic), and pathologic reaction (associated with an inflammatory angiopathy). It tends to be unilateral or asymmetrical. Not infrequently, it is associated with DTLRN. Although insufficiently studied, it appears to be more common in diabetic patients than in the general population.

Diabetic Thoracolumbar Radiculoneuropathy. The disorder occurs in the general population. Although not studied critically, it appears to be more common in diabetic cohorts. In single cases, we have encountered mononuclear cell infiltrates on biopsy of spinal ganglia.

Median Neuropathy of the Wrist. There appears to be reasonably strong evidence that MNW (carpal tunnel syndrome) occurs more frequently in diabetic cohorts than in the general population. As discussed elsewhere, we assume that diabetic nerves are more vulnerable to compression, stretch, or repeated trivial injury or that diabetic nerve is injured more because of thickened or stiffer surrounding structures—assuming that the injury rate of diabetics is not greater than in other patients.

Ulnar Neuropathy at the Elbow. There is as yet no rigorous information that compression (or repeat injury) of the ulnar nerve at the elbow is more frequent in diabetic patients than in the population at large, but from our preliminary analysis, it is likely to be.

Peripheral Vascular Ischemic Injury. Lower limb ischemic gangrene is known to be associated with nerve (and other tissue) injury. Peripheral vascular diseases occur earlier and more severely in patients with DM.

UNUSUAL VARIETIES OF DIABETIC NEUROPATHY

One of the problems of classification of diabetic neuropathy is what to do about unusual neuropathies associated with DM. These include diabetic cachexia, symmetrical distal and proximal demyelinating motor neuropathy, chronic inflammatory demyelinating polyradiculoneuropathy, acute and subacute visceral neuropathies, treatment-related neuropathies such as hypoglycemic neuropathy (insulin neuritis), brachial plexus neuropathy, and acute polyneuritis following diabetic ketoacidosis. These diffuse neuropathic disorders are uncommon and may represent chance associations with the far more prevalent condition of diabetes, or they may represent unusual variants of better documented diabetic neuropathies. They may occur as a result of the treatment of diabetes.

Diabetic Cachexia and Polyneuropathy

Cachexia and weight loss may be associated with symptomatic neuropathy.[2, 23, 28] Generally, the weight loss and polyneuropathy were attributed to poor glycemic control. This constellation of findings was reemphasized by Ellenberg in 1974[14] (also see Auche[2]). Subsequently, nine cases were described by Archer in 1983,[1] all of whom had severe painful diabetic neuropathy of acute onset associated with precipitous weight loss. All the patients were male and lost an average of 12.6 kg or 16.5% of body weight. The pain was of continuous burning quality and experienced principally in the legs. Sensory loss was noted, but it was generally mild, was not always present, and did not correlate well with the area of pain. Loss of reflexes was not always present. The severe manifestations subsided in all cases within 10 months and in most cases by 6 months. The course and findings in these patients were not unlike what was described by early workers. Sural nerve biopsies revealed active degeneration of myelinated nerve fibers with no clear inflammation. These cases may well represent one end of the spectrum of a length-dependent sensory predominant neuropathy with principal involvement of pain fibers, the same mechanism that causes DPN. Alternatively, it may be that weight loss and polyneuropathy are extreme manifestations of DLSRPN (from involvement of L5 and S roots, plexuses, and nerves); we think this is the most likely explanation.

Distal and Proximal Symmetrical Motor Neuropathy

Case reports have appeared in the literature describing the subacute onset of progressive distal motor neuropathy with albumino-cytologic disassociation within the cerebrospinal fluid. These symptoms are similar, in all or some respects, to those in acute inflammatory demyelinating polyradiculoneuropathy or chronic inflammatory demyelinating polyradiculoneuropathy (CIDP).[8] Some of these cases appear to have responded to treatment with either plasma exchange or intravenous immunoglobulin. Six cases were reported by Krendel and colleagues in 1995,[20] all of whom responded to immune-modulating therapy. Some of these cases may well represent chance occurrence of acute or chronic inflammatory demyelinating neuropathies in the diabetic population. Some of the patients may have had bilateral DLSRPN and, therefore, were identified as having CIDP. Whether there is an increased tendency for the occurrence of acute inflammatory demyelinating polyneuropathies or CIDP in diabetic patients is unclear. However, patients with these types of neuropathy appear to run the same clinical course as those without diabetes and therefore should be treated in a similar manner.[20]

Hypoglycemic Neuropathy

The development of a length-dependent symmetrical sensorimotor neuropathy predominantly affecting the lower limbs on repeated hypoglycemia was reported by Danta in 1969.[9] Rat models have shown that it takes severe degrees of hypoglycemia to induce axonal degeneration.[29, 34] Hypoglycemic neuropathy may be seen in patients with insulin-secreting islet cell tumors as well as in insulin-treated diabetics and insulin-abusing patients. Reports of muscle wasting and weakness after prolonged hypoglycemia are recorded.[9, 17, 24, 31]

Treatment-Related Neuropathies (Insulin Neuritis)

The development of an acute painful sensory neuropathy after beginning insulin therapy was initially noted by Caravati in 1933.[7] This may reflect a chance occurrence of neuropathy or the unmasking of a preexisting neuropathy. The slow amelioration of symptoms with continuing therapy may suggest that insulin neuritis is a distinct entity.[31]

Polyneuritis After Acute Diabetic Ketoacidosis

Ozrer and associates in 1959[25] reported two patients who developed a primarily motor polyneuropathy with facial diplegia after acute diabetic ketoacidosis. Both patients had elevated cerebrospinal fluid protein levels that returned toward normal after resolution of the neuropathy, which occurred in 2 to 3 weeks.

Acute and Subacute Visceral Neuropathy

Diabetes can affect the autonomic nervous system in many ways. With autonomic involvement in a length-dependent manner, neuropathy is detectable in many patients without symptoms, using sensitive measures of autonomic function such as the thermoregulatory sweat test.[32]

Transient acute-onset visceral autonomic neuropathies have been reported and are often referred to as diabetic autonomia.[10, 32] In addition a constellation of visceral autonomic symptoms, including gastroparesis, diarrhea, postural hypotension, Argyll Robertson pupils, impotence, and bladder atony, may occur with the development of proximal diabetic neuropathy and or worsening of the length-dependent distal sensory and autonomic neuropathies.[32]

Although some features of autonomic dysfunction are transient, most are permanent. The transient symptoms may well represent a monophasic non–length-dependent neuropathy, as in DLSRPN, and the development of subacute progressive visceral neuropathies may well represent the progression of a length-dependent autonomic neuropathy in association with DPN.

CONCLUSION

Using the classification and nomenclature of diabetic neuropathy from Table 30.1, it is possible to subdivide the heterogeneous grouping of diabetic neuropathies into subgroups that are potentially clinically relevant, allowing clinically and mechanistically distinct entities to be separated. It is important to be aware that the various diabetic neuropathies can occur in isolation or together. Whether to add or subtract other neuropathies associated with diabetes should be decided on the basis of a clear mechanistic link to DM. After this link is demonstrated or disproved, it should be determined that the neuropathies do not represent a subtype or variant of a recognized subtype.

References

1. Archer AG, Watkins PJ, Thomas PK, et al. The natural history of acute painful neuropathy in diabetes mellitus. J Neurol Neurosurg Psychiatry 1983; 46:491.
2. Auche MB. Des alterations des nerfs peripheriques. Arch Med Exp Anat Pathol 1890; 2:625.
3. Bastron JA, Thomas JE. Diabetic polyradiculopathy: Clinical and electromyographic findings in 105 patients. Mayo Clin Proc 1981; 56:725.
4. Bruns L. Über neuritische Lähmungen beim Diatebetes Mellitus. 1890; 27:509.
5. Bruyn GW, Garland H. Neuropathies of endocrine origin. In Vinken PJ, Bruyn GW (eds): Handbook of Clinical Neurology. Amsterdam, North Holland Publishing Company, 1970, p 29.
6. Buzzard F. Illustrations of some less known forms of peripheral neuritis, especially alcoholic monoplegia and diabetic neuritis. BMJ 1890; 1:1419.
7. Caravati CM. Insulin neuritis: A case report. Va Med 1933; 59:745.
8. Cornblath DR, McArthur JC, Kennedy PG, et al. Inflammatory demyelinating peripheral neuropathies associated with human T-cell lymphotropic virus type III infection. Ann Neurol 1987; 21:32.
9. Danta G. Hypoglycemic peripheral neuropathy. Arch Neurol 1969; 21:121.
10. Dyck PJ, Giannini C. Pathologic alterations in the diabetic neuropathies of humans: A review. J Neuropathol Exp Neurol 1996; 55:1181.
11. Dyck PJ, Karnes J, O'Brien PC. Diagnosis, staging, and classification of diabetic neuropathy and associations with other classifications. In Dyck PJ, Thomas PK, Asbury A, et al (eds): Diabetic Neuropathy. Philadelphia, WB Saunders, 1987, p 36.
12. Dyck PJ, Kratz KM, Karnes JL, et al. The prevalence by stages severity of various types of diabetic neuropathy, retinopathy, and nephropathy in a population-based cohort: The Rochester Diabetic Neuropathy Study. Neurology 1993; 43:817.
13. Ellenberg M. Diabetic neuropathy, with special reference to visceral neuropathy. Adv Intern Med 1964; 12:11.
14. Ellenberg M. Diabetic neuropathic cachexia. Diabetes 1974; 23:418.
15. Fry IK, Hardwick C, Scott GW. Diabetic neuropathy: A survey and follow-up of 66 cases. Guy's Hosp Rep 1962; 111:113.
16. Gilliatt RW. Clinical aspects of diabetic neuropathy. In Cumings JN, Kremer M (eds): Biochemical Aspects of Neurological Disorders. Oxford, Blackwell, 1965, p 117.
17. Harrison KJG. Muscle wasting after prolonged hypoglycaemic coma: Case report with electrophysiological data. J Neurol Neurosurg Psychiatry 1976; 39:465.
18. Jordon WR, Crabtree HH. Paralysis of bladder in diabetic subjects. Arch Intern Med 1935; 55:17.
19. Kraus WM. Involvement of the peripheral neurons in diabetes mellitus. Arch Neurol Psychiatry 1922; 7:202.
20. Krendel DA, Costigan DA, Hopkins LC. Successful treatment of neuropathies in patients with diabetes mellitus. Arch Neurol 1995; 52:1053.
21. Leval-Picquechef L. Des Pseudo-tabes. Lille, Imprinterie Desclee, de brouver et Cie, 1855.
22. Leyden E. Beitrag sur Klinik des diabetes mellitus. Wien Med Wochenschr 1893; 43:926.
23. Martin MM. Diabetic neuropathy: A clinical study of 150 cases. Brain 1953; 76:594.
24. Mulder DW, Bastron JW, Lambert EH. Hyperinsulin neuropathy. Neurology 1956; 6:627.
25. Ozrer RR, Richard NG, Schumaker OP. Acute polyneuritis following diabetic acidosis. Ohio State Med J 1959; 55: 1521.
26. Pirart J. Diabetic neuropathy: A metabolic or a vascular disease. Diabetes 1965; 14:1.
27. Pryce TD. On diabetic neuritis with a clinical and

pathological description of three cases of diabetic pseudo-tabes. Brain 1893; 16:416.

28. Rundles RW. Diabetic neuropathy: General review with report of 125 cases. Medicine (Baltimore) 1945; 24:111.

29. Sidenius P, Jakobsen J. Peripheral neuropathy in rats induced by insulin treatment. Diabetes 1983; 32:383.

30. Sullivan JF. The neuropathies of diabetes. Neurology 1958; 8:243.

31. Thomas PK. Metabolic neuropathy. J R Coll Physicians Lond 1973; 7:154.

32. Thomas PK, Tomlinson DR. Diabetic and hypoglycemic neuropathy. *In* Dyck PJ, Thomas PK, Griffin JW, et al (eds): Peripheral Neuropathy, ed 3. Philadelphia, WB Saunders, 1993, p 1219.

33. Whisnant JP, Love JG. Pitfall in diagnosis of diabetic "cord bladder." JAMA 1960; 174:47.

34. Yasaki S, Dyck PJ. Spatial distribution of fiber degeneration in acute hypoglycemic neuropathy in rat. J Neuropathol Exp Neurol 1991; 50:681.

Chapter 31

Differential Diagnosis of Diabetic Neuropathies

Ian A. Grant • Peter James Dyck

INTRODUCTION

No variety of diabetic neuropathy is unique in its clinical features, electrophysiologic manifestations, or pathologic findings. Diabetic individuals are subject to the same diverse group of conditions capable of producing neuropathy as are those without diabetes. This point is illustrated by the findings of the Rochester Diabetic Neuropathy Study, in which 10% of diabetic patients had neuropathy (or a polyradiculopathy causing a neuropathic pattern of deficits) of nondiabetic etiology.[89] Thus, neurologic symptoms and impairments must be shown to be caused by diabetes mellitus (DM) and not to another disease.

We have outlined a sequential approach to differential diagnosis, in which consideration is given to symptoms, deficits, clinical course, laboratory abnormalities, and evidence of associated disease. The importance of the initial step—careful classification of neuropathic pattern—cannot be overstated, because this immediately focuses the differential diagnosis and the subsequent investigations necessary to establish the cause. At each step, one is encouraged to consider whether the features are characteristic of a form of diabetic neuropathy or if an alternative diagnosis must be entertained. Such an algorithm is likely to be useful in minimizing the chance of a previously unrecognized disorder being overlooked and in

415

achieving an acceptable level of time- and cost-effectiveness.

Although peripheral neuropathy is recognized as a common complication of DM by most physicians, diagnosis is not always straightforward. Many factors contribute to misdiagnosis. First, most patients are cared for by primary care practitioners who may have limited experience with neurologic disorders. Second, symptoms of neuropathy may be mild or nonspecific and attributed to nonneurologic causes; this is particularly true of the focal and multifocal neuropathies (discussed later), which may go unrecognized even by experienced neurologists. Finally, the most common form of neuropathy in diabetic patients—a distal, predominantly sensory polyneuropathy—has no unique features, producing a clinical picture whose possible causes are many and varied. Nonetheless, a careful consideration of each patient's history, physical findings, laboratory abnormalities, and associated diseases will almost always allow a correct diagnosis of diabetic neuropathy or of those other disorders that mimic it.

Various approaches can be taken in the evaluation of peripheral neuropathy of unknown cause. The best specific approach varies according to a number of factors, including the experience of the physician and resources of the facility performing the assessment. In general, we advocate a sequential algorithm that has been described.[82, 83] The advantage of this approach, which emphasizes the history and physical examination, is its methodical progression from a large, undifferentiated list of possibilities, through a progressively shorter list, to the correct underlying disorder(s). In doing so, resources are used efficiently and the chance of the correct diagnosis being overlooked is minimized. This approach, which provides the basis for the following sections, can be applied to the evaluation of any case of peripheral nerve disease but is adapted here for the specific assessment of neuropathy in the diabetic patient.

The initial part of this chapter outlines a general approach for the assessment and classification of peripheral neuropathies, with emphasis on evaluation of the diabetic patient. Subsequent sections address the major diagnostic possibilities that must be considered before diagnosing specific varieties of diabetic neuropathy, that is, diabetic polyneuropathy (DPN) and specific focal and multifocal neuropathies; diabetic lumbosacral plexus neuropathy (DLSPN), diabetic truncal radiculopathy (DTR), and diabetic oculomotor neuropathy (DON).

GENERAL PRINCIPLES OF DIFFERENTIAL DIAGNOSIS
Anatomical Pattern of Neuropathy

The specific anatomical pattern of peripheral nerve involvement should be the initial consideration in differential diagnosis. Accurate characterization of pattern allows an often unmanageably large list of diagnostic possibilities to be quickly narrowed to a more focused set. However, it should be recognized that more than one pattern of neuropathy (i.e., polyneuropathy and superimposed mononeuropathy such as carpal tunnel syndrome) may coexist in a given diabetic patient.

The most common pattern of neuropathy in diabetes is a distal symmetric *polyneuropathy*[206] in which sensory symptoms and deficits predominate and are initially confined to distal lower limb sites, with gradual spread to more proximal sites and to the distal upper limbs as the process advances. Weakness is minimal or absent until much later and, like sensory loss, affects the distal lower limbs initially. Tendon areflexia is common at the ankles, less common at the knees, and uncommon in the upper limbs except in severe cases. In general, this pattern implies the simultaneous involvement of many nerves, with the longest fibers preferentially affected. This may result from (1) the length-dependent degeneration of the most distal portions of axons, (2) the summation of numerous multifocal axonal lesions, or (3) segmental demyelination. Although the recognition of a polyneuropathy pattern is important, the number of potential causes is extensive (Table 31.1) and includes a large number of inherited and acquired diseases. Further diagnostic steps are almost always necessary to establish a cause and are discussed in subsequent sections.

Mononeuropathy refers to a disorder confined to a single peripheral nerve. Mononeuropathies are frequently seen in the setting of diabetes. Focal neuropathies may coexist with polyneuropathy and should always be considered when symptoms are asymmetrical or intermittent or involve the upper limbs.

The most common form is median neuropathy at the wrist (carpal tunnel syndrome [CTS]). Although disagreement exists, CTS probably occurs more often in the diabetic population than in the general population.[64, 206] Apart from diabetes, CTS frequently occurs in

TABLE 31.1 DIABETIC POLYNEUROPATHY: DIFFERENTIAL DIAGNOSIS

Inherited
Hereditary motor and sensory neuropathies
Hereditary sensory and autonomic neuropathies
Spinocerebellar degeneration
Familial amyloid polyneuropathy
Fabry's disease
Tangier disease

Acquired
Inflammatory
  Sensory polyganglionopathy
    Paraneoplastic
    Associated with connective tissue disease
      Sjögren syndrome
      Sicca complex
      Idiopathic
Vasculitis
  Nonsystemic
  Systemic
Chronic inflammatory demyelinating
  polyradiculoneuropathy
Monoclonal gammopathy
  Monoclonal gammopathies of unknown significance
  Multiple myeloma
  Amyloidosis (primary)
Infectious
  Tabes dorsalis
  Lyme
  Leprosy
  Human immunodeficiency virus
Metabolic
  Uremia
  Hypothyroidism
Nutritional
  Vitamin B deficiency
  Alcohol
Toxic
  Drugs
  Heavy metals
  Industrial agents

individuals who perform repetitive hand movements, often in an occupational setting.[25] Other risk factors include pregnancy; arthritis (rheumatoid and osteoarthritis); uremia; endocrine conditions, such as hypothyroidism and acromegaly; amyloidosis; and inherited tendency to pressure palsy.

Ulnar neuropathy at the elbow may also be more common in diabetic patients than in controls.[111] In patients with ulnar neuropathy, tardy ulnar palsy[208] (a sequel of remote arm fracture), entrapment in the cubital tunnel,[106] and chronic compression at the elbow or, rarely, the wrist should be considered. True mononeuropathies in the lower limbs, such as peroneal neuropathy at the fibular head, can occur in diabetic patients, but there is no convincing evidence that their incidence is higher than in nondiabetics.

With involvement of these or other nerves, an inherited tendency to pressure palsies is possible.[17] This disorder, inherited as an autosomal dominant trait,[54] should be suspected when the neuropathy follows trivial trauma, although often no such history can be obtained. Other suggestive points are a history of recurrent focal neuropathy, clinical or electrodiagnostic signs of a mild polyneuropathy, foot deformities such as pes cavus, and a positive family history. Slowly progressive motor deficit over months to years suggests nerve sheath tumor (schwannoma, neurofibroma) or focal hypertrophic neuropathy (perineuroma).[142]

The term *multiple mononeuropathies* (mononeuritis multiplex) refers to the simultaneous or stepwise involvement of two or more discrete peripheral nerves. This pattern is widely regarded as common in diabetic patients, an assumption that is only partly correct. The term multiple mononeuropathy could be applied to several distinctive syndromes common in (but not restricted to) diabetic patients, such as lumbosacral polyradiculoplexopathy or truncal radiculopathy, which are discussed separately. However, apart from these specific examples, multiple mononeuropathy is not a common pattern; Fraser and colleagues found clinical and electromyographic (EMG) evidence of such in only 5 of 51 diabetic patients with symptomatic mononeuropathies.[111]

Necrotizing vasculitis should be considered in all cases. Vasculitic neuropathy may accompany a systemic disorder, such as polyarteritis nodosa,[60] Churg-Strauss syndrome,[57] Wegener's granulomatosis,[76] or cryoglobulinemia,[157] or may be confined to peripheral nerve (nonsystemic vasculitic neuropathy).[80] Other causes of multiple mononeuropathies include infections such as leprosy, human immunodeficiency virus (HIV)[69] (itself often vasculitic in nature[112]), and Lyme disease[221]; sarcoidosis; multifocal motor neuropathy with conduction block; and inherited tendency to pressure palsy. Diagnosis frequently rests on clinical and laboratory evidence of associated systemic disease and by nerve biopsy.

Polyradiculoneuropathy is used to describe a more or less symmetrical pattern in which proximal and distal nerve segments are involved simultaneously, that is, root, plexus, and peripheral nerve are affected by a process that to some degree involves the entire length of nerve. Often, motor deficits predominate and may involve proximal muscles in addition to distal ones. Diagnosis is supported by electrophysiologic studies showing neurogenic changes or denervation in paraspinal and limb girdle muscles. Nerve conduction studies may indicate that a demyelinating process is involved. The most important causes are the inflammatory demyelinating neuropathies—Guillain-Barré syndrome and chronic inflammatory demyelinating polyradiculoneuropathy. Polyradiculoneuropathy may also occur in association with monoclonal gammopathy,[68] chronic hepatitis, HIV infection,[61] amyloidosis, and acute intermittent porphyria.

True polyradiculoneuropathy is seldom, if ever, caused by diabetes alone. A patient with DM may develop acute or chronic inflammatory demyelinating polyradiculoneuropathy or the diseases referred to above, but it is not clear that they occur more frequently in diabetic patients than in the general population. However, the term is sometimes loosely used in reference to proximal asymmetric diabetic neuropathy (see Chapter 35). In our opinion, the term is also used incorrectly by some clinicians when needle electromyography reveals fibrillation potentials in the paraspinal muscles of a diabetic patient whose clinical and electrophysiologic picture is otherwise that of a distal polyneuropathy. Although paraspinal fibrillation potentials have been reported in 10 to 13% of patients with DPN,[16, 250] they are usually mild in severity and limited in distribution. These changes could reflect root damage caused by diabetes, but they could also be caused by other factors such as spondylosis or muscle trauma. Therefore, use of the term polyradiculoneuropathy in such cases is of questionable value.

Proximal symmetrical neuropathy has been used by some authors to describe patients in whom motor or sensory involvement is confined to the proximal limbs or trunk. This pattern may occur in inflammatory demyelinating neuropathies, Tangier disease, and in most forms of infantile and childhood-onset spinal muscular atrophy.

Population of Neurons or Fibers Affected

Consideration of the population of neurons or fibers affected can further narrow the list of diagnostic possibilities. Population refers to the relative involvement of motor, sensory, and autonomic neurons or their axons. With sensory involvement, a further distinction can be made between the degree of large and small fiber involvement. Large fiber loss can be inferred from impairment of vibration and joint-posi-

tion sense, sensory ataxia, and (in severe cases) pseudoathetosis as well as electrophysiologic evidence of loss of large myelinated fibers (decreased or absent sensory nerve action potentials or mild slowing of conduction velocity in sensory nerves). Small fiber loss is suggested by impairment of pain and temperature sensation and preserved sensory nerve action potentials unless simultaneous large fiber loss is present. Autonomic fibers are commonly affected together with small somatic fibers, but may be affected in isolation. Autonomic involvement is suggested by clinical or laboratory evidence of sweating abnormalities (anhidrosis, hypohidrosis, or hyperhidrosis), cardiovascular phenomena (orthostatic hypotension, heart rate abnormalities), impotence, gastrointestinal dysmotility (gastric stasis, constipation, or diarrhea), or pupillary abnormalities such as a tonic pupil.

Early diabetic polyneuropathy usually involves sensory fibers predominantly or exclusively; the relative degree of large versus small fiber dysfunction is quite variable and both typically occur to some degree. Infrequently, patients may present with burning pain and selective impairment of small fiber function (the "pseudosyringomyelic" pattern)[232] or selective large fiber loss ("pseudotabetic" form).

Purely or predominantly sensory neuropathy with mainly large fiber involvement should raise the possibility of immunoglobulin M (IgM) monoclonal gammopathy,[121] a subset of malignant and nonmalignant inflammatory sensory polyganglionopathies, certain toxins (e.g., cisplatin,[224] pyridoxine,[235] and methyl mercury), uremia, vitamin B_{12} deficiency, and the spinocerebellar ataxias. Selective small fiber sensory involvement is typical of hereditary sensory and autonomic neuropathy (HSAN) type 1, Fabry disease,[204] and amyloidosis. Mixed large and small fiber deficits are consistent with a large number of disorders, including inflammatory sensory polyganglionopathies, many toxins, hypothyroidism, and leprosy. Pure motor neuropathies are rare and suggest the spinal muscular atrophies, multifocal motor neuropathy with conduction block, acute motor axonal neuropathy, and, very rarely, lead toxicity.

Clinical motor deficits occur late in DPN, although subclinical abnormalities of motor nerve conduction may occur at an early stage. A predominance of motor involvement is common in DLSPN, but has only rarely been reported in symmetrical polyneuropathy; Timperley and associates[263] described severe distal motor deficits and denervation in the majority of 10 diabetic patients, in whom sensory loss was minimal. The presence of asymmetry and proximal involvement in most, and vascular pathology in sural nerve in all, are reminiscent of DLSPN and raise the possibility that polyradiculoplexopathy (affecting sacral plexus more than the more typical lumbar plexus pattern) was present rather than a true length-dependent polyneuropathy.

Autonomic dysfunction is variable; although consistently present in late neuropathy, it may be the sole initial manifestation in a minority of patients.

Clinical Course

The tempo of onset of neuropathy and its subsequent clinical course are often helpful in determining cause. Diabetic polyneuropathy is usually gradual in onset; patients may have difficulty in pinpointing the exact beginning of symptoms. The subsequent course is typically very slowly progressive; deficits worsen over time, but commonly remain mild 10 years or more after onset. Symptoms, in contrast, tend to fluctuate over time with little overall worsening.

An acute or subacute onset occurs in an uncommon small-fiber painful diabetic polyneuropathy with weight loss.[7, 99] This is characterized by initial abrupt weight loss, followed by burning pain in the feet. These symptoms are accompanied by few objective neurologic deficits or abnormalities of nerve conduction. Depression and impotence are often associated. Typically, symptoms resolve over months with rigorous glycemic control. An acute onset has also been described after initiation of insulin treatment.[46] Acuteness of onset and rapid progression of distal sensory symptoms, with or without relapse and remission, is seen in some cases of Guillain-Barré syndrome,[71] many toxic neuropathies (most notably those caused by arsenic and thallium, in which limb pain may be severe), and a subset of inflammatory sensory polyganglionopathies. An acute, symmetrical, painful neuropathy may also result from necrotizing vasculitis, although weakness and some degree of asymmetry are usually present. A relapsing and remitting course can occur in chronic inflammatory demyelinating polyradiculoneuropathy and other inflammatory demyelinating neuropathies, porphyria, Tangier disease,[102] and lumbosacral spondylosis (neurogenic claudication).

In contrast, a subacute onset and monophasic course is typical of the focal and multifocal neuropathies of diabetes and in many of the disorders that mimic them; these are discussed separately.

Family History

Careful consideration should be given to the possibility of an unrecognized inherited neuropathy. The most important reason for failure to diagnose inherited neuropathy is simply the clinician's failure to consider the possibility. Once considered, certain historical points support the diagnosis; these are discussed in the section on inherited neuropathy. By far, the most important step is a thorough family history. Careful questioning of the index patient, including information regarding consanguinity, may provide sufficiently detailed and specific information to allow a presumptive diagnosis. The presence of neuropathy in relatives is often unsuspected, with neuropathic symptoms attributed to arthritis or old age. Questioning of family members should be performed if possible, but need not always be done face to face; a simple telephone interview with relatives may provide useful information. Examination, electrodiagnostic studies, and occasionally genetic testing of relatives are necessary, however, for definitive documentation. Construction of a pedigree can clarify the inheritance pattern, particularly in large kindreds in whom the condition is incompletely expressed.

Features of Underlying Diabetes

DURATION OF DIABETES

It is useful to consider the known duration of diabetes when a patient has symptoms compatible with DPN. The prevalence of DPN increases with increasing duration of diabetes. Pirart[210] followed more than 4000 patients for up to 25 years, including 2795 from the time of diagnosis of diabetes. The prevalence of peripheral neuropathy, as judged by decreased ankle reflexes and later by decreased vibration sensation, increased from 7.5% at the time of diagnosis to 45% at 20 to 25 years. Incidence was also found to increase over time, from 3 cases per 100 per year to 19 cases per 100 per year after 25 years. Prevalence at the time of diagnosis of diabetes was much lower in patients younger than 40 years than in older patients, but this was interpreted as resulting from a longer period of unrecognized diabetes in the older group. Palumbo and associates[207] identified all 995 cases of maturity-onset diabetes free of neuropathy in Rochester, Minnesota, between 1945 and 1969; these patients were followed for approximately 20 years. The actuarially estimated cumulative incidence of polyneuropathy was 4% by 5 years, rising to 15% at 20 years. The median time between diagnosis of diabetes and diagnosis of polyneuropathy and mononeuropathy was 9 years. These studies indicate that neuropathy is more likely to be attributable to diabetes the longer diabetes has been present.

However, this relationship is not absolute. A major confounding factor is the long period of unrecognized disease that may precede diagnosis, especially common in type 2 diabetes mellitus. The interval between onset and diagnosis can be several decades. This is illustrated by the study of Mincu,[187] who found that the prevalence of neuropathy varied according to the duration of symptoms of underlying diabetes; a prevalence of 4% was found in patients diagnosed after diabetic symptoms of 5 months or less versus 19% in those with symptoms with a duration longer than 15 months. Prevalence also varied according to diabetic type— 1.4% in juvenile-onset diabetic patients versus 14.1% in maturity-onset cases. These two observations are probably related to a longer duration of unrecognized diabetes in the maturity-onset group.

Taken together, these studies suggest that one should consider duration of diabetes in judging the likelihood of neuropathy being diabetic in cause and that care should be taken not to underestimate duration in newly diagnosed diabetic patients, particularly those with type 2 disease.

RELATIONSHIP TO MICROVASCULAR COMPLICATIONS

Three major forms of end-organ damage complicate diabetes: neuropathy, retinopathy, and nephropathy. These complications share certain histologic characteristics that are reviewed elsewhere in this book. Determination of the presence or absence of retinal and renal disease is useful in judging the likelihood of neuropathy being diabetic in origin.

These three complications are statistically co-associated.[103] Pirart[210] found that all three complications occurred together more frequently than expected by chance, with a high degree of significance. Neuropathy was found to be especially likely in patients with nephropathy;

in his series, 89 cases of neuropathy occurred per 100 cases with nephropathy. Co-association was also found by Fagerberg.[103] Additional evidence comes from the Rochester Diabetic Neuropathy Study, a cross-sectional, longitudinal, population-based study following 380 diabetic patients.[89] Polyneuropathy was found to be highly associated with retinopathy and nephropathy (retinopathy and nephropathy were also associated with each other, an observation that has prompted all three complications to be collectively referred to as "triopathy"). However, other forms of neuropathy (mononeuropathies, proximal asymmetrical neuropathy) were not associated with microvascular complications.

In our practice, we apply this information by screening for renal and retinal disease in all diabetic patients with peripheral neuropathy (specific tests are discussed in the section on laboratory investigations). Although demonstrating retinopathy or nephropathy does not prove that neuropathy is diabetic in cause, it does provide a measure of increased statistical likelihood of such. Conversely, the absence of other microvascular complications should prompt the clinician to at least consider the possibility of another underlying disorder.

RELATIONSHIP TO GLYCEMIC CONTROL

There is evidence that polyneuropathy occurs more often in the setting of chronic, severe hyperglycemia. Pirart grouped his patients into those with good, fair, and poor glycemic control based on postprandial and fasting blood sugars, degree of glycosuria, and occurrence of ketoacidosis. It was found that incidence and prevalence of neuropathy was highest in the group with poor control. However, this and other older studies suffer from limitations in the accurate day-to-day monitoring of blood glucose levels, making interpretation difficult.

More recent studies have largely overcome these limitations. The Diabetes Control and Complications Trial[73] prospectively followed 1400 patients for a mean of 6.5 years, comparing conventional insulin treatment (one or two injections daily) and intensive treatment (three or more injections or continuous subcutaneous infusion). All patients had type 1 diabetes. Neuropathy was diagnosed based on clinical, electrophysiologic, and objective autonomic parameters. Among patients free of neuropathy at outset, the prevalence of neuropathy at 5 years was 9.6% in the conventionally treated group versus 2.8% with intensive treatment, a

71% reduction in risk. The most likely explanation for this finding is that the improved glycemic control resulting from intensive treatment limited the subsequent development of neuropathy. However, it is possible that other unrecognized factors in the intensive treatment group besides blood glucose levels accounted for this difference.

Associated Disease

A careful history with review of systems and a general physical examination may provide evidence that a disorder other than diabetes is causing the neuropathy in a patient with DM. Diabetic patients are susceptible to the same diseases (such as cancer or inherited disorders) that may cause neuropathy in anyone, with an increased risk of specific disorders (e.g., uremia and hypothyroidism[105, 127]) with neuropathic complications. Because other neurologic disease or neuropathies may occur in perhaps 5 to 8% of patients in diabetic cohorts,[89] it is necessary to actively exclude other neurologic disease or neuropathy in a patient with DM.

Constitutional symptoms such as severe weight loss or fatigue can occur secondary to diabetes, but they also raise the possibility of underlying malignancy, amyloidosis, thyroid disease, and chronic infection. Recent flulike symptoms or gastrointestinal symptoms such as diarrhea occur in antecedent viral or bacterial infections with acute or chronic inflammatory demyelinating neuropathies. Gastrointestinal symptoms, especially abdominal pain, are also important clues to chronic heavy metal toxicity (arsenic, lead, and thallium, mainly in acute cases) and in exacerbations of acute intermittent porphyria. It should be noted that such symptoms can also occur secondary to diabetes-related autonomic neuropathy. A history of exposure to neurotoxic substances should be sought. In particular, a medication history should be taken, with emphasis on antineoplastic, antiretroviral, and antibiotic agents.

On physical examination, lymphadenopathy may point to unsuspected carcinoma, lymphoma, or sarcoidosis that might be the putative cause of neuropathy. Inspection of the skin may provide clues to a large number of disorders: palpable purpura or ulcerations in vasculitis; Raynaud's phenomenon in vasculitis or connective tissue disease; hyperpigmentation in POEMS (*p*olyneuropathy, *o*rganomegaly, *e*ndocrinopathy, *M* protein, and *s*kin abnormalities) syndrome; hyperkeratosis, exfoliation or erythema of the palms and soles in arsenic

poisoning; nail changes (Mees lines) in arsenic or thallium poisoning; and angiokeratomata of the buttocks, groin, or scrotum in Fabry's disease. Hair loss is characteristic of thallium toxicity. Inspection of the mouth and pharynx may reveal orange discoloration of the tonsils in Tangier disease or macroglossia in primary amyloidosis. A careful funduscopic examination, preferably performed by an eye-care physician after pupillary dilatation, is important for several reasons; the finding of diabetic retinopathy increases the probability of associated complications including neuropathy, and pigmentary retinopathy suggests Refsum's disease, abetalipoproteinemia, and certain forms of inherited spinocerebellar ataxia. On abdominal examination, organomegaly may support chronic liver disease, amyloidosis, POEMS syndrome, or metastatic cancer. Musculoskeletal deformities of the feet are typical of chronic neuropathies beginning early in life, usually because of an inherited disorder. On neurologic examination, signs of neurologic involvement beyond pure neuropathy may suggest a diagnosis: spasticity in multiple system atrophy, deficiencies of vitamin B_{12} or E, and adrenomyeloneuropathy; parkinsonism or other extrapyramidal signs in multiple system atrophy; cerebellar signs in multiple system atrophy, abetalipoproteinemia and Refsum's disease; myopathic muscle weakness (not always easily distinguished clinically from neurogenic weakness) in hypothyroidism and with colchicine use[163] and delayed relaxation of tendon reflexes in hypothyroidism.

Laboratory Investigations

Laboratory tests are useful in confirming clinical suspicions regarding many causes of neuropathy, and they may sometimes point to a clinically unsuspected process by serendipity or a "shotgun" approach to testing.

Tests of diabetic control and complications are often useful. A marked elevation of glycosylated hemoglobin (HbA_{1C}) implies chronically poor glycemic control and provides some degree of support for a diabetic etiology. However, symptomatic polyneuropathy may occur despite adequate control. Similarly, proteinuria implying nephropathy also supports a diabetic basis for neuropathy provided other causes of proteinuria are excluded.

The extent of hematologic testing can range from a few limited, focused tests to an extensive evaluation. Even if diabetes is documented, it is reasonable to perform at least the following in addition to routine tests such as complete blood count and serum chemistries:

- Serum and urine protein electrophoresis, with immunoelectrophoresis if a monoclonal protein is found.
- Thyroid function tests.
- Liver function tests.
- Limited serologic testing for rheumatic disease. It should be noted that in the absence of clinical evidence of connective tissue disease, the low yield of antinuclear antibody, rheumatoid factor, SS-A, and similar tests limit their usefulness. The significant rate of antinuclear antibody false-positivity, especially in older patients, should limit its use where no clinical manifestations of connective tissue disease are present.
- Vitamin B_{12} level.

The following tests are often useful but are not performed in every patient:

- Serology for infectious agents (syphilis, Lyme, HIV, hepatitis viruses)
- Serum lipid profile (Tangier disease and abetalipoproteinemia)
- Chest radiograph (obtained in most patients)
- Metastatic bone survey (osteosclerotic myeloma, multiple myeloma, or metastatic disease)
- Urine heavy metal screen

Where the history and clinical findings suggest a specific diagnosis, consider:

- Abdominal fat aspirate or biopsy of other tissues for amyloid
- Lumbosacral spine imaging (magnetic resonance imaging [MRI] or computed tomography [CT]–myelography) to rule out spondylosis, disk herniation, or malignancy
- Biochemical/enzymatic testing for specific inherited disorders
- Molecular genetic testing (hereditary motor and sensory neuropathy [HMSN] type 1 and 3, hereditary tendency to pressure palsy, spinocerebellar ataxia (SCA) 1 and 3)

Nerve biopsy is a useful technique for the diagnosis of many causes of neuropathy. However, biopsy is seldom if ever necessary merely to establish the presence of neuropathy (regardless of cause), because this determination can usually be made on clinical, electrophysiologic, and other grounds. When the history, neuropathic pattern based on clinical findings, electrophysiology, and laboratory tests all strongly support diabetes and show evidence of no other underlying disease, nerve biopsy is generally unnecessary. Biopsy is best reserved for those patients in whom (1) there is clinical or paraclinical evidence for a disorder other than diabetes, (2) the disorder(s) being considered is capable of causing diagnostically relevant histologic changes in nerve, and (3) identification of the disorder is likely to influence subsequent investigations or treatment. In certain cases, biopsy is performed despite a secure diagnosis of diabetic neuropathy, for the purpose of grading severity of fiber loss or other changes, usually for research purposes. With few exceptions, the sural nerve is chosen because of its distal site and tendency for early involvement, ease of electrodiagnostic study, relative ease to obtain, and trivial sensory deficit caused by its removal.

Removal, preparation, and interpretation of nerve tissue is best performed at a center experienced in these techniques. In general, adequate information can be obtained using a limited number of histologic methods. Paraffin sections allow the detection of a variety of interstitial changes (inflammation, infection, vascular changes, amyloid) and provide a rough estimate of myelinated fiber numbers if myelin stains such as Luxol fast blue are used. Antibodies are available for the immunohistochemical study of various leukocyte and interstitial markers in paraffin-embedded tissue. Epoxy-embedded semithin sections of osmicated tissue offer a much higher resolution image of myelinated fibers, allowing an accurate determination of number and size of fibers, regenerating clusters, and fiber degeneration. Although requiring a degree of skill and experience to prepare, teased fibers provide excellent visualization of fiber degeneration and myelin changes (demyelination and remyelination, reduplication), which are readily quantified. Although not routinely necessary, electron microscopy is used to examine unmyelinated fibers and to detect abnormal storage material.

In the sural nerve, common findings in distal symmetric diabetic polyneuropathy include alterations of myelinated and unmyelinated fibers and interstitium. Fiber changes include decreased fiber density,[90, 262] alterations in size distribution, axonal degeneration, and a mild increase in segmental demyelination and remyelination.[19] Interstitial changes typical of diabetes include pericyte degeneration and endoneurial perivascular basement membrane reduplication.[114]

The major role of nerve biopsy is in ruling

out other causes of neuropathy. Those disorders most likely to be diagnosed on the basis of histopathologic changes in nerve are those reflected by distinctive interstitial pathology, including:

- Necrotizing vasculitis: vessel wall destruction and inflammation, vascular fibrinoid necrosis, hemorrhage
- Amyloidosis: amorphous acellular material with apple-green birefringence under polarized light
- Leprosy: acid-fast mycobacteria, granulomatous inflammation
- Sarcoidosis: noncaseating granulomata, perineuritis

Nerve biopsy is also useful in distinguishing diabetic neuropathy from:

- Inflammatory demyelinating neuropathies
- Other inflammatory neuropathies
- Many inherited disorders, especially
  - Those with characteristic fiber changes—HMSN I, III (hypertrophic changes), inherited tendency to pressure palsy (myelin reduplication), HMSN IIb (axonal spheroids)
  - Those with abnormal inclusion material—metachromatic leukodystrophy (stored sulfatide)

Changes in myelinated fibers are seldom diagnostic of themselves but often suggest or support a specific diagnosis. Focal or multifocal fiber loss can occur in diabetes,[90, 175] but marked focality is suggestive of ischemia, as in necrotizing vasculitis,[86] and can be seen in inflammatory sensory polyganglionopathies and inflammatory demyelinating neuropathies. Axonal degeneration in DPN is usually low grade and chronic. Active, early axonal degeneration suggests a more acute or subacute process and is more typical of DLSPN, vasculitis, acute polyganglionopathies, recent toxic exposure, and cases of inflammatory demyelinating neuropathies with secondary axon loss. Similarly, segmental demyelination is usually mild in diabetes[19, 97]; more prominent demyelination should raise a question of inflammatory demyelinating neuropathies, monoclonal gammopathies of unknown significance, osteosclerotic myeloma, and HMSN type I.

A reasonable indication for nerve biopsy is the suspicion of vasculitis or another disorder characterized by inflammation in nerve. The latter group is large and includes connective tissue diseases such as systemic lupus erythematosus, Sjögren's syndrome, and rheumatoid arthritis; monoclonal gammopathy; and eosinophilia-myalgia syndrome. It is critical to realize that small epineurial and endoneurial perivascular mononuclear cell collections are a common, nonspecific finding that may occur as a result of fiber degeneration, rather than as a primary pathologic event. Slight inflammation is not uncommon in DPN and should therefore be interpreted with caution. The severity of the inflammation (particularly relative to the degree of axonal degeneration or segmental demyelination) must be considered in judging its significance.

Examination of spinal fluid may provide important information, but must be interpreted with caution in diabetic patients. Ives[141a] noted elevated protein in 68% of diabetic patients with symptoms or signs of neuropathy; protein may be elevated even in patients without neuropathy. In addition, the degree of protein elevation is not well correlated with neuropathic severity. In most cases, however, the elevation is modest and a marked (>2 g/L) increase should prompt a search for another cause. The protein concentration is almost always raised in proximal asymmetrical diabetic neuropathy[42] and is usually raised in inflammatory demyelinating neuropathies, infection (syphilis, HIV, Lyme), granulomatous disease (sarcoid), and meningeal carcinomatosis.

Age

Studies of diabetic neuropathy vary widely in their criteria for the diagnosis of neuropathy. Many studies include patients on the basis of minimal criteria, such as symptoms alone, a single clinical abnormality such as the absence of ankle jerks, or abnormalities of nerve conduction alone.[87] In day-to-day practice, criteria used for diagnosis may be similarly nonspecific. For this reason, it is important to be aware of the degree to which normal aging is associated with clinical and electrodiagnostic changes that, taken in isolation, could lead to a questionable diagnosis of neuropathy.

The effect of age on nerve conduction parameters is well established.[43, 95, 155, 222, 247, 253] This has been found for most nerves studied in the upper and lower limbs. With increasing age, after maturity, one sees a decrease in sensory nerve and compound muscle action potential amplitudes, decreased conduction velocities, and increased distal latencies. Sensory nerve responses may be most subject to change with age. Stetson and colleagues found a 5 mV decrease in median sensory antidromic amplitude per decade,[247] and a sural response is often unobtainable in patients older than 60 years. Some studies suggest that conduction velocity may be more age dependent than other variables[94, 222] in most nerves, although for the sural nerve, amplitude is probably the most age sensitive.

Similarly, cutaneous sensory thresholds increase with advancing age. This has relevance for the bedside examination and for the clinical use of quantitative sensory tests. Using the latter approach, the Rochester Diabetic Neuropathy Study assessed vibration and cooling thresholds at multiple sites in about 400 healthy subjects between the ages of 18 and 74 years.[94] Both thresholds were positively correlated with age to a high degree. The inability to detect vibration on the toe cannot, therefore, be confidently attributed to disease in elderly individuals without corroborating evidence. The use of loss of ankle reflexes as a marker of neuropathy is also untrustworthy in the elderly; in the same study, hyporeflexia or areflexia at the ankle was present in more than 5% of healthy individuals older than 50 years, rising to almost 30% after age 70 years. In persons in whom maximal stimulation (to elicit a reflex or vibratory sensation) cannot be used to detect abnormality, one may need to test a more proximal site (knee reflex or lateral leg).

DIFFERENTIAL DIAGNOSIS OF DIABETIC POLYNEUROPATHY

This section discusses the differential diagnosis of distal symmetric polyneuropathy so often encountered in diabetic patients. It is not intended as a comprehensive review of polyneuropathy. Rather, it is an attempt to cover those disorders that are of greatest relevance, because of their common occurrence, clinical similarity to diabetic polyneuropathy, or both.

Uremia

This cause of neuropathy is particularly important because of the high prevalence of chronic renal failure in diabetic patients. Uremic neuropathy can occur at any age and is more common in females.[9] Incidence estimates vary widely, from 10 to 83%[33]; 60% of dialysis patients have evidence of neuropathy, although this is subclinical in the majority.[30, 214]

Uremic neuropathy shares many features with DPN. It is usually a distal symmetric polyneuropathy involving the lower extremities before the upper extremities. Sensory features predominate, usually beginning with pain, paresthesias, or dysesthesias in the feet.[10, 198] Although pain, particularly burning feet, was emphasized in the older literature as a classic complaint,[267] this is probably not the case[198]; Asbury and associates have stated that pain is less prominent in uremic than diabetic neuropathy.[10] Sensory deficits may be absent despite severe symptoms, generally occurring only with advanced uremia (creatinine clearance <5 mL/min).[147] Large-fiber deficits predominate, with loss of ankle jerks and vibration sense in the feet.[195] Small-fiber deficits are less common, with clinical loss of pain and temperature sensation in only 0 to 2.1% in Thomas's series.[260] Other common symptoms include cramps[194] and restless legs.[198, 260]

As with diabetes, predominantly motor neuropathy can rarely occur. McGonigle and colleagues described four young male patients with renal failure who developed a rapidly progressive, motor, greater than sensory, polyneuropathy or polyradiculoneuropathy after initiation of dialysis.[184] Hypertension or sepsis was also present. Electrophysiologic studies showed absent responses or slowed conduction velocities, with denervation in distal more than proximal muscles. Two patients improved markedly after renal transplantation, and a third after charcoal hemoperfusion. The authors suggested that nerve ischemia, triggered by hypertension or sepsis, might underlie the neuropathy; certain features are also shared with the syndrome of critical illness polyneuropathy described by Bolton and coworkers.[32]

Autonomic neuropathy may also occur, usually in patients with somatic neuropathy.[156, 243] This appears to be asymptomatic in most cases,[33] and even subclinical dysautonomia has been questioned.[183] Autonomic neuropathy may be responsible for some cases of dialysis-related hypotension.[156] A series comparing diabetic and nondiabetic uremic patients found that dysautonomia was more frequent and more severe in the former group.[136] Therefore, the presence of symptomatic autonomic neuropathy in a patient with diabetes and renal failure is more likely caused by diabetes.

Electrophysiologic abnormalities are a sensitive indicator of nerve involvement and precede clinical neuropathy.[72, 196, 197] Sensory and motor conduction are affected, with reduced amplitude responses, prolonged distal latencies, and reduced conduction velocities; the latter change is proportionate to the serum creatinine level.[146] Dispersion of motor responses is sometimes present, and F-wave latencies are usually prolonged.[30] Needle examination is normal in mild cases, with evidence of denervation found in distal muscles in advanced neuropathy.[31]

Pathologic features on sural nerve biopsy are nonspecific. These include demyelination (paranodal and segmental), internodal remyelination, axonal degeneration, and a reduction in number of myelinated and unmyelinated fibers. These changes are most severe distally,[10, 85, 262] where axonal atrophy leads to secondary myelin changes and subsequent axonal degeneration. The latter process does not appear to occur in diabetes, but its demonstration requires detailed morphologic studies that are not feasible in the routine assessment of nerve biopsies; it is therefore not of practical use in distinguishing uremic neuropathy from that caused by diabetes.

Uremic neuropathy tends to progress slowly over months without treatment. With institution of dialysis, most patients stabilize or improve slowly,[29, 146, 197] and improvement is the rule after renal transplantation.[31] Response to treatment is therefore the most reliable indicator of the etiology of the neuropathy.

In unpublished studies from the RDNS cohort, we have found that renal failure is a risk factor for DPN. This result implies that it may not be possible to distinguish the impairment, or some of the impairment, of DM from uremia.

Hypothyroidism

Focal neuropathy, typically carpal tunnel syndrome,[215] and diffuse polyneuropathy[92, 193] occur in the setting of hypothyroidism. Thyroid disease is important to consider in diabetic patients, given the probable association between these two diseases; the prevalence of hypothyroidism among diabetic patients is up to 4%.[105, 127] Although uncommon today because of early treatment, hypothyroid polyneuropathy is occasionally seen. The major symptoms are tingling paresthesias and lancinating pain with little demonstrable sensory deficit.[62] Subjective weakness is common, but objective weakness unusual; when present, care should be taken to exclude a myopathy. Delayed relaxation of deep tendon reflexes is characteristic. Nerve conduction abnormalities involve mainly sensory fibers, with either unobtainable sensory nerve action potentials or reduced sensory amplitudes and conduction velocities.[108, 212] Needle EMG may reveal mild denervation in distal muscles. Pathologic changes in

sural nerve include loss of large myelinated fibers, demyelination and remyelination on teased fiber preparations, and accumulations of glycogen granules within Schwann cells and axons.[91, 185, 212]

Diagnosis is suggested by other clinical features of hypothyroidism and by the distinctive reflex changes and is confirmed by the response to thyroid replacement, which results in marked improvement in symptoms and electrophysiologic abnormalities.[92, 185]

Immunologically Mediated Disorders

NECROTIZING VASCULITIS

Vasculitic neuropathy typically presents as single or multiple mononeuropathies, which may progress in a stepwise fashion. With confluence of multifocal lesions, a more diffuse neuropathy often occurs, and a symmetric polyneuropathy is the presenting pattern in approximately 20% of cases.[80, 231] Motor and sensory symptoms and deficits generally result, and pain, which may be burning in character, is common.[162]

In the majority of cases, the neuropathy is but one component of a systemic disorder. A complete classification of the vasculitides has been proposed by the American College of Rheumatology.[140] Neuropathy most frequently occurs in the setting of (1) the polyarteritis nodosa (PAN) group of disorders, including Churg-Strauss syndrome (allergic angiitis and granulomatosis) and (2) the vasculitides occurring secondary to collagen vascular diseases, such as rheumatoid arthritis, Sjögren's syndrome, and systemic lupus erythematosus (SLE). The neuropathy may be the initial manifestation of the disease or may occur in a patient in whom a systemic disorder is already recognized.

Diagnostic clues include nonspecific constitutional complaints such as fatigue, malaise, fever, and weight loss. Other clinical manifestations depend on the specific underlying disease. Polyarteritis nodosa can affect almost any organ, most often the kidney, muscles, gastrointestinal tract, and skin.[65] Churg-Strauss syndrome produces similar features, but has a higher frequency of lung involvement with asthma and peripheral eosinophilia. In Wegener's granulomatosis, vasculitis of the upper and lower respiratory tract produces symptoms such as nasal discharge and pain, cough, and hemoptysis, and glomerulonephritis may result in renal failure. A specific collagen vascular disease may be inferred from features such as arthritis, sicca complex, or serositis. Central nervous system manifestations such as encephalopathy, focal deficits, and seizures are common in SLE and PAN, and blindness and stroke are the usual neurologic complications of temporal (giant cell) arteritis in which neuropathy is unusual.[47]

Laboratory abnormalities may aid in diagnosis. Nonspecific hematologic abnormalities such as leukocytosis, anemia, thrombocytosis, elevated erythrocyte sedimentation rate, and hypergammaglobulinemia are common in most of these disorders, whereas eosinophilia is suggestive of Churg-Strauss syndrome. Individual serologic tests are not specific for any disease, but the profile of serologic abnormalities may support a particular disorder. Examples include rheumatoid factor, anti-nuclear antibody (positive in more than 95% of patients with SLE), and antibodies to extractible nuclear antigens SS-A and SS-B (positive in 40 to 75% of primary SS patients).[188] Hepatitis B surface antigenemia is frequently present in PAN. Antineutrophil cytoplasmic antibodies are sensitive and specific for Wegener's granulomatosis when present in a cytoplasmic staining pattern (c-ANCA) using indirect immunofluorescence.[244] Definitive diagnosis requires demonstration of vasculitis on biopsy of nerve. A presumptive diagnosis can be made based on biopsy of other tissues, which may provide greater sensitivity than nerve biopsy; in a series of patients with vasculitis neuropathy, Said and associates found diagnostic changes in 80% of muscle biopsies versus 53% of superficial peroneal nerve biopsies.[231]

In a subset of patients, necrotizing vasculitis involves nerve exclusively, without demonstrable involvement of other tissues over extended periods of follow-up. This condition, termed *nonsystemic vasculitic neuropathy* by Dyck and colleagues,[80] does not differ in its neurologic features from other causes of vasculitic neuropathy except that its severity is milder, its course more indolent, and its outlook much better.

MONOCLONAL GAMMOPATHY

The presence of a monoclonal protein (M protein) in serum is relatively common in older patients and exhibits an age-related prevalence. An M protein may result from an underlying lymphoproliferative disorder such as multiple myeloma, Waldenstrom's macroglobulinemia, amyloidosis, or lymphoma. If these disorders can be excluded, the patient is considered to have a monoclonal gammopathy of unknown significance. This diagnosis requires that several conditions be met: a serum M protein concentration less than 3 g/dL that remains stable over time; less than 5% plasma cells in the bone marrow; minimal or no M protein in the urine; and absence of lytic bone lesions, hypercalcemia, and uremia. Monoclonal gammopathy of unknown significance is present in 3% of patients older than 70 years.[12, 165]

Neuropathy associated with monoclonal gammopathy of unknown significance is a chronic, symmetrical, sensorimotor polyneuropathy or polyradiculoneuropathy that usually begins in the fifth decade or later and progresses slowly.[121] Males are more commonly affected. Positive sensory symptoms and sensory ataxia are frequent. The M protein is of the IgM class more often than IgG or IgA; when IgM is present, sensory ataxia and severe nerve conduction abnormalities are more common than when the M protein is of another class.

Nerve conduction studies usually reveal motor and sensory abnormalities indicative of a combination of axon loss and demyelination. Dispersion of compound muscle action potentials with proximal stimulation and F-wave prolongation are sometimes present. Evidence of denervation on needle examination is common in distal muscles. Examination of spinal fluid shows an increased protein concentration in 85% of patients. The finding of a serum M protein necessitates other investigations to exclude hematologic malignancy; these include serum chemistry including calcium, urine protein electrophoresis, and skeletal survey.

A therapeutic trial may be helpful in establishing the cause of neuropathy. In anecdotal reports, patients with neuropathy associated with monoclonal gammopathy of unknown significance may respond to a variety of immunomodulatory treatments, including prednisone, azathioprine, and alkylating agents.[152] In addition, a prospective, double-blind study comparing plasma exchange to sham exchange in 40 patients demonstrated clinical and electrophysiologic improvement with plasma exchange. The improvement was largely confined to patients with IgG and IgA gammopathy.

Multiple myeloma is more likely if there is bone pain, anemia, hypercalcemia, renal insufficiency, hyperuricemia, or lytic bone lesions. The most common neurologic complications are radiculopathy or cauda equina compression caused by an epidural mass, but sensorimotor polyneuropathy occurs in up to 13% of patients.[273] Polyneuropathy is much more common in patients with osteosclerotic myeloma. An M protein, usually IgG or IgA, is present in three fourths of patients.[152] These patients are young (mean age, 47 years[273]) and may have POEMS syndrome. This includes hepatomegaly, hypogonadism, diabetes mellitus, skin hyperpigmentation, hypertrichosis, and peripheral edema. The frequent occurrence of glucose intolerance (in 25 to 50% of cases[249]) should be borne in mind in assessing neuropathy in diabetic patients. One or more osteosclerotic bone lesions representing plasmacytomas occur in vertebrae, ribs, pelvis, and long bones. Electrophysiologic findings usually suggest a demyelinating neuropathy (or polyradiculoneuropathy), with or without a component of axonal degeneration.

INFLAMMATORY SENSORY POLYGANGLIONOPATHY

Purely or predominantly sensory neuropathy can result from a variety of disease processes that damage sensory ganglia, alone or in conjunction with involvement of other areas of the nervous system and nonneural tissues. Symptoms result from dysfunction or loss of primary sensory neurons whose cell bodies are located in dorsal root and trigeminal ganglia. Causes include inherited disorders, such as the spinocerebellar ataxias, and acquired disorders, including infections (e.g., tabes dorsalis), infiltration by malignancy, and toxic exposure. Inflammatory injury of sensory and autonomic ganglia can occur in the absence of such conditions, either as an isolated process or as a remote effect of a systemic disease. These can be conveniently subdivided into malignant (paraneoplastic) and nonmalignant forms.

The clinical features are similar in both forms. Symptoms and signs may reflect predominantly large-fiber dysfunction with paresthesias and sensory ataxia, small-fiber dysfunction with pain, dysesthesias and analgesia, or a combination of the two[241]; a mixed picture is most common. Autonomic symptoms, especially those of gastrointestinal dysmotility such as cramps and nausea, may be prominent. Sensory deficits reflect the fiber population affected, and loss of tendon reflexes is common. Weakness is absent or trivial. The neuropathic pattern is variable; patchy involvement of ganglia results in an asymmetrical distribution of deficits, often involving the trunk or upper limbs, or, with trigeminal involvement, the face. However, a distal symmetrical pattern confined to the lower limbs can also occur, making distinction from DPN difficult.

The clinical course varies from an abrupt onset and rapid progression to severe impairment within days, to a slowly progressive or static course over 10 years or more. A more aggressive course may be slightly more common in the malignant form.

Patients with associated cancer usually have small cell lung carcinoma.[63, 139, 160] Other histologic types of lung cancer and Hodgkin's disease are less commonly associated.[139] Among nonmalignant disease associations, the most important are Sjögren's syndrome[109, 129] and paraproteinemia.[67]

Polyganglionopathy should be considered in cases of sensory neuropathy, particularly when there is asymmetry, early proximal limb, upper limb, truncal, or facial involvement or a rapid course. Associated systemic symptoms, such as fatigue and weight loss, or respiratory symptoms may provide a clue regarding an occult malignancy. Sicca complex (dryness of the eyes and mouth) occurs in Sjögren's syndrome, in which it is typically symptomatic and associated with other clinical and serologic markers of rheumatic disease. However, asymptomatic sicca is an underrecognized occurrence in many cases of sensory neuropathy that, if objectively documented, provides useful evidence of an inflammatory disorder.[124] Confirmation of ocular sicca requires demonstration of decreased tear production via the Schirmer test and corneal or conjunctival dryness revealed by rose bengal staining. Salivary involvement is established by demonstration of lymphocytic infiltration of minor salivary glands. Serologic testing for antineuronal nuclear antibodies (ANNA-1, anti-Hu) is useful in detecting small cell lung carcinoma,[126, 171] whereas antibodies to extractible nuclear antigens are consistent with Sjögren's syndrome. Electrophysiologic studies typically show absent or low-amplitude sensory nerve action potentials despite normal or minimally abnormal motor studies and needle examination.[129] Sural nerve biopsy often reveals loss of myelinated fibers that may be profound.[84, 279]

Amyloidosis

Deposition of insoluble amyloid fibrils causes organ dysfunction involving nerve, skeletal muscle, heart, kidney, and other tissues to a varying degree. Neuropathy occurs in two major types of amyloidosis: primary and familial.

Primary amyloidosis is caused by the synthesis of monoclonal immunoglobulin light chains by an autonomous clone of plasma cells. In its usual isolated form, men older than 65 years are most often affected.[166] A similar disorder occurs in the setting of multiple myeloma or lymphoma. Neuropathic involvement is of three types. The most common pattern is a symmetrical polyneuropathy in which distal lower limb sensory symptoms including pain are the major initial complaints.[154] Symptoms of autonomic dysfunction such as orthostatic hypotension and impotence are common in advanced disease and may be the presenting problem. Distal muscle weakness and wasting occur late. The course is usually relentlessly progressive, culminating in death from renal or cardiac failure. Carpal tunnel syndrome is a second, less common form of neuropathy and may be an isolated finding; in the majority of cases in which amyloid is found histologically in tenosynovium after carpal tunnel release, systemic disease is absent.[164] Infrequently, a predominantly motor polyradiculoneuropathy with electrophysiologic features of axonal degeneration occurs.

Familial amyloid polyneuropathy (FAP) is a heterogeneous group of inherited disorders in which a mutant form of a normal nonimmunoglobulin-related protein is produced, principally by the liver. Three such proteins have been described. Transthyretin (TTR) is involved in most cases, with more than 40 described mutations in the gene located on chromosome 18. Age at onset of symptoms varies according to the specific mutation, usually occurring in the third or fourth decade in the most common form (TTR met 30). Patients develop a predominantly sensory polyneuropathy as in primary amyloidosis, but dysautonomia and loss of pain and temperature sensation may be particularly severe, and other features including vitreous opacities, cerebellar ataxia, and pyramidal tract dysfunction may occur.[5] Two other proteins have been described in families with FAP. Apolipoprotein A-I mutations are associated with early renal failure in addition to polyneuropathy similar to that already described. Mutations in the gelsolin gene result in a distinctive syndrome of corneal lattice dystrophy and cranial neuropathies unlike any syndrome associated with diabetes.[186]

Diagnostic clues include early prominent dysautonomia and constitution symptoms such as weight loss and fatigue, particularly in the primary form. Suggestive clinical findings include macroglossia, purpura, and hepatomegaly in primary amyloidosis and acral skin ulcers or signs of eye or cranial nerve involvement (see above) in FAP. The family history may be informative. Laboratory testing should include serum and urine protein electrophoresis or, preferably, immunoelectrophoresis; the latter reveals a monoclonal protein in either blood or urine in two thirds of cases. Echocardiography is useful in identifying cardiac involvement, and proteinuria, found in 80% of patients with amyloidosis, provides evidence of renal disease. Definitive diagnosis depends on the demonstration of amyloid protein in nerve or other tissue such as abdominal fat or rectal mucosa. The simplest technique involves staining the tissue with Congo red, which imparts a green birefringence under polarized light. Immunohistochemical approaches can also be used in identifying the type of amyloid fibril, such as TTR or light chain (kappa or lambda).

Toxic Exposure

Toxins are an uncommon cause of neuropathy, but recognition of these disorders is crucial because removal of the offending substance is usually followed by clinical improvement.

Drugs are the most frequent cause of toxic neuropathy seen by internists and neurologists. A large number of agents in current use have neuropathic toxicity; these are listed in Table 31.2. The most common pattern is a distal, symmetrical, predominantly sensory polyneuropathy that may be difficult to distinguish from DPN on purely clinical grounds. A careful medication history is therefore necessary, focusing on antineoplastic, anti-infective and anti-inflammatory agents, which are frequent offenders.

Heavy metal toxicity is less common than drug-induced neuropathy. Arsenic exposure is most often related to attempted homicide or suicide, but it can also occur in workers involved in copper or lead smelting, with consumption of contaminated well water, or in cocaine abusers who may be exposed to arsenic in the drug's diluent.[176] Diagnosis is most straightforward with acute, large exposures, which cause prominent gastrointestinal symptoms such as abdominal cramps, nausea, and vomiting. Neuropathy begins within a few days to 3 weeks later with distal sensory complaints such as tingling paresthesias, numbness, and burning pain,[169] followed by weak-

TABLE 31.2 IMPORTANT DRUGS THAT CAUSE
PERIPHERAL NEUROPATHY

*Predominantly sensory**
Predominantly large fiber
   Cisplatin[70]
   Pyridoxine[235]
Mixed or variable
   Isoniazid[203]
   Metronidazole[35]
   Nucleoside analogues (ddI, ddC)[23, 158]
   Phenytoin[180] (rarely symptomatic)
   Taxol[174]

Predominantly motor
Dapsone[132]
Sensorimotor
Amiodarone[110]
Gold[150]
Nitrofurantoin[178, 205]
Suramin[167]
Vinca alkaloids[48] (motor features often predominate)

*May include minor clinical or electrophysiologic motor
abnormalities.

ness soon after. Chronic exposure produces a less dramatic illness, but similar features are present. Clues to the diagnosis include the gastrointestinal symptoms, skin and nail changes, and the finding of pancytopenia on hematologic testing. Nerve conduction studies may transiently suggest a demyelinating neuropathy, but evolve to a picture of axonal loss.[75] Confirmation requires the demonstration of toxic levels of arsenic in urine, hair, or nails.

Thallium toxicity is rare and occurs mainly with exposure to older insecticides and rodenticides.[13] As with arsenic, acute exposure produces gastrointestinal symptoms and a painful distal neuropathy; tendon reflexes are usually preserved and weakness is rarely prominent. Autonomic involvement is common; tachycardia, hypertension, and anhidrosis may occur.[50] Diagnostic clues include the presence of alopecia beginning 2 to 4 weeks after exposure, cutaneous lesions similar to those seen in arsenic poisoning, and signs of central nervous system dysfunction such as a confusional state, seizures, ataxia, and choreoathetosis. Diagnosis rests on demonstration of thallium in urine.

Alcohol and Nutritional Factors

Chronic alcohol abuse is associated with the development of a peripheral neuropathy from incompletely understood mechanisms that may include a direct toxic effect, dietary B vitamin deficiencies, or both.[18, 107, 272] Symptoms are symmetrical and generally begin in the feet,

often with burning or lancinating pain; dysesthesias and paresthesias also occur. Allodynia to superficial touch and, in some cases, deep palpation is characteristic.[271] Sensory loss involves all modalities. Gait ataxia sometimes occurs and is caused by proprioceptive impairment or cerebellar atrophy. Weakness and muscle atrophy, present in more advanced cases, begin in the distal lower extremities and occasionally spread to the thighs and hands.

Diagnosis requires documentation of the patient's alcohol consumption and nutritional status. Neuropathy is more likely to develop in individuals who obtain most of their calories from carbohydrates in the alcoholic beverage, resulting in vitamin deficiency.[271] There may be physical signs of chronic liver disease such as hepatomegaly or a hard, shrunken liver; spider angiomas; palmar erythema; gynecomastia, and Dupuytren's contractures of the palmar fascia. Neurologic assessment may reveal evidence of central nervous system injury in the form of withdrawal symptoms, midline cerebellar ataxia or, in patients with Korsakoff's syndrome, amnesia. Laboratory studies such as serum transaminase and γ-glutamyltransferase are useful in identifying hepatic dysfunction. There are no distinctive features on electrophysiologic or pathologic testing; both show abnormalities in keeping with a length-dependant axonal neuropathy affecting sensory fibers predominantly.[18, 49, 274]

Deficiencies of specific vitamins also cause peripheral neuropathy, although most are mainly of historical interest in Western countries. Thiamine deficiency produces a polyneuropathy (dry beriberi) whose features are indistinguishable from those of alcoholic neuropathy. Accompanying features may include those of Wernicke's encephalopathy (delirium, ophthalmoplegia, and gait ataxia), Korsakoff's syndrome, or cardiac failure (wet beriberi). Measurement of erythrocyte transketolase activity is useful in diagnosing thiamine deficiency if blood is obtained before replacement therapy is begun.[275]

Other deficiency states are rarely encountered. Niacin deficiency causes pellagra, in which neuropathy may accompany gastrointestinal symptoms, a hyperkeratotic rash, and neuropsychiatric changes; the neuropathy, which does not respond to niacin replacement, may actually be caused by deficiencies of other vitamins.[245] Pyridoxine (vitamin B$_6$) deficiency is seen almost exclusively in patients taking the antituberculous agent isoniazid.[24] Vitamin B$_{12}$ deficiency occurs because of malabsorption in patients with pernicious anemia, gastrectomy, or disease of the terminal ileum. Neuropathy is typically overshadowed in these patients by other features of a multiple system degeneration, particularly myelopathy (subacute combined degeneration of the spinal cord); extensor plantar responses and Lhermitte's sign are common.[225] Optic neuropathy and mental changes including depression and delirium may also occur. Vitamin E deficiency, caused by intestinal disease or inherited disorders of vitamin absorption or transport, causes a spinocerebellar syndrome.[134, 190]

Inherited Neuropathy

Inherited disorders form a large and heterogeneous group of causes of peripheral neuropathy. Many are associated with known metabolic defects that may be identified by appropriate laboratory testing. A larger group, and one that contains entities more likely to cause confusion with DPN, is not associated with a metabolic marker, although the genetic bases of these diseases are increasingly well understood. These have been classified by Dyck as HMSN and HSAN according to their clinical and electrophysiologic features and patterns of inheritance.[78]

Certain generalizations can be made about the clinical features of inherited neuropathies that aid in differential diagnosis. Most inherited neuropathies are insidious in onset, beginning in childhood or early adulthood, with slow progression over years and decades; the indolent nature of the disorder is often such that the patient may be unable to accurately pinpoint the onset of symptoms and may underappreciate the degree of impairment. Symptoms may lead to neurologic referral only in late adulthood, with a long-standing process suspected only when specific questioning uncovers a history of clumsiness, abnormal gait, or inability to perform at the level of one's peers as a child. The nature of sensory symptoms is also helpful; prickling paresthesias occur less often in inherited disorders than in acquired ones.[96] On examination, foot deformities such as pes cavus and hammer toes are common in HMSN, and acral ulcerations, whitlows, and destructive arthropathy occur in severe cases of HSAN.[137, 269]

The HMSN have been divided into numerous subtypes that have been reviewed in detail.[81] The two most common forms, designated HMSN I and II, are most relevant in the differential diagnosis of DPN. Expression is highly variable; within affected families, many individuals never seek medical attention. Reasons for doing so are often nonspecific and include gait disturbance, leg weakness, muscle wasting, or foot deformity.

The distinctive clinical picture of fully expressed disease is one of the peroneal muscular atrophy phenotype. The principle features are distal muscle weakness and wasting, initially in toe extensors and foot dorsiflexors, with more diffuse weakness extending to the thighs and hands as the disease progresses. Distal leg atrophy may produce an "inverted champagne bottle" appearance, and foot deformities such as pes cavus and hammer toes are a hallmark feature; these may be the only manifestation of the condition, may be the reason the patient seeks medical attention, or may suggest the diagnosis to the alert clinician evaluating an unrelated complaint. Sensory symptoms are seldom volunteered, and positive symptoms such as "pins-and-needles" paresthesias should prompt consideration of an acquired disorder.[82] Sensory loss may be mild or undetectable despite pronounced weakness; when present, all modalities are usually involved in a distal pattern. Soft tissue complications such as skin ulceration are uncommon. Enlarged, and especially increased firmness, of nerves is found in HMSN I; this is best appreciated in the greater auricular nerve, the median and ulnar nerves in the arm, and the peroneal nerve at the fibular head. Symptomatic dysautonomia rarely occurs, although laboratory testing may reveal evidence of sudomotor,[145] cardiovascular,[39] or pupillary dysfunction.[26]

Electrophysiologic abnormalities form the basis for the division of HMSN into its major subtypes. HMSN I (the hypertrophic form) is characterized by marked slowing of motor and sensory conduction velocities, typically less than 30 ms, and prolonged distal latencies.[93] Dispersion of the evoked response is not a feature; its presence suggests an acquired demyelinating disorder. Nerve conduction tests are useful for screening family members, particularly children, in whom unequivocal slowing precedes clinical signs.[91] HMSN II (the axonal or neuronal form) is characterized by reduced amplitude motor and sensory responses, with normal or mildly reduced conduction velocities in keeping with the degree of axonal loss. In either type, no responses may be obtained, particularly on testing lower limb nerves.

Pathologic findings in sural nerve in HMSN I are distinctive. Fascicular area is increased.

The number of myelinated fibers is decreased, and their size distribution is abnormal with a decrease in large fibers.[79] The fiber is surrounded by concentric layers of Schwann cell processes, a structure referred to as an onion-bulb formation.[77] Teased fiber studies reveal both demyelination and remyelination. Sural nerve biopsy in HMSN II also reveals a decreased number of myelinated fibers and an abnormal size distribution, but hypertrophic changes are rare or absent, and teased fiber studies show an increased number of fibers undergoing axonal degeneration in the distal portion of the nerve.

Inheritance of HMSN I and II is heterogeneous; autosomal dominant inheritance is most common, but recessive and X-linked patterns have been documented. Recent molecular genetic advances have led to further subclassification of these disorders based on the identity of the mutant gene. HMSN Ia is associated with a large duplication, or, less often, a point mutation in the gene for peripheral myelin protein-22 (PMP-22) on chromosome 17p11.2.[181, 223] Testing for the duplication is commercially available. HMSN Ib is associated with point mutations in the gene for a second myelin protein, P0, located on chromosome 1q22-23.[135] The genetic basis of HMSN I in yet other families, collectively HMSN Ic, is undetermined. Linkage studies have established chromosomal localization for certain forms of HMSN II.[21]

The HSAN types I to V are heterogeneous with respect to age of onset, type and severity of symptoms, degree of somatic versus autonomic involvement, and mode of inheritance. For practical purposes, only HSAN I is likely to be confused with DPN. It is characterized by autosomal dominant inheritance,[88, 137] with onset in the second to fourth decade and subsequent slow progression. Symptoms and signs are mainly sensory, symmetrical, and distal, beginning in the lower extremities. Pain, most often burning or aching in quality, is common and may be the only manifestation of disease.[95] Lancinating pain is less common. Examination reveals distal hypalgesia for pain and temperature, with other modalities affected in some individuals.[256] Tendon reflexes are decreased or absent, most consistently the ankle jerks. Autonomic dysfunction is variable and often inconspicuous. Muscle weakness occasionally occurs in distal leg muscles, but is never prominent. Foot deformities such as pes cavus and hammer toes, so characteristic of the hereditary motor and sensory neuropathies, may be present. Soft tissue complications, although not invariable, are a classic feature; these range from plantar ulcers (over pressure points, typically the metatarsal heads or the interphalangeal joints) to neurogenic arthropathy, osteomyelitis and bone resorption. The site of ulcerations is not helpful in differential diagnosis; ulcers occur at the same sites in DPN.[98] Uncommon variants of HSAN present with associated neurologic abnormalities such as deafness, amyotrophy, spastic paraparesis, or restless legs.

Inherited Disorders With Known Metabolic Defects

Fabry's disease results from a deficiency of the lysosomal enzyme ceramide trihexosidase (α-galactosidase).[36] The resultant defect in sphingolipid breakdown leads to accumulation of ceramide trihexoside in nerve, blood vessel, kidney, skin, and other tissues. The disease is inherited as an X-linked recessive trait, and most patients are males, presenting by the third decade of life. A sensory neuropathy manifests as burning pain and allodynia in the feet and hands; distal anhidrosis is also present. Objective sensory deficits are mild or absent. Other features include ischemic stroke, myocardial infarction, renal failure, hypertension, and corneal clouding. A particularly important diagnostic clue is the presence of angiokeratoma corporis diffusum, appearing as a red maculopapular rash on the scrotum, abdomen, or buttocks; angiokeratomata should be looked for in any male patient with painful peripheral neuropathy. However, Fabry's disease may rarely cause neuropathic symptoms in female carriers.[37] Nerve conduction studies are either normal or show mild slowing of conduction velocities and prolonged distal latencies.[238] Sural nerve biopsy may reveal loss of small myelinated and unmyelinated fibers, and storage material can be demonstrated by electron microscopy.[204] Diagnosis rests on demonstration of reduced enzyme activity in leukocytes or cultured skin fibroblasts.

Tangier disease is a rare disorder of plasma lipid transport caused by a deficiency of α-lipoproteins. Plasma cholesterol and high-density lipoprotein concentrations are very low, but triglyceride levels are normal.[11] Symptomatic neuropathy occurs in one third of patients and is quite variable in its features. Weakness is common and often asymmetrical and may fluctuate in severity; prominent distal upper limb weakness and sensory loss may mimic syringomyelia.[115] A chronic, distal sensory polyneuropathy has also been described. Cranial neuropathy, typically presenting as diplopia, sometimes develops. Orange or yellow discoloration of the tonsils is a distinctive sign of this disorder in children. Nerve biopsy reveals lipid deposits in Schwann cell cytoplasm, but diagnosis is usually made based on plasma lipoprotein analysis.

DIFFERENTIAL DIAGNOSIS OF DIABETIC LUMBOSACRAL PLEXUS NEUROPATHY

Having established that the neuropathic pattern is one of a proximal asymmetrical neuropathy, that is, polyradiculopathy or polyradiculoplexopathy involving the lower limbs, and having confirmed this pattern by electrophysiologic tests as described, the differential diagnosis is narrowed considerably. It is often necessary to exclude disorders affecting primarily the nerve roots, the lumbosacral plexus, and occasionally the femoral nerve.

Disorders of the Lumbosacral Plexus

MALIGNANCY

Malignancy may involve the lumbosacral plexus in one of two ways. Extension of tumor arising from a pelvic organ may cause direct compression of the plexus; this most often results from cervical or colorectal carcinoma. Alternatively and less commonly, a distant tumor may metastasize to retroperitoneal lymph nodes. The initial symptom is usually pain in the low back, hip, or pelvis, radiating to leg.[144, 251, 257] In contrast with DLSPN, the pain is usually insidious in onset and may or may not radiate into the thigh. Generally, pain is followed by weakness and sensory loss over weeks to months.[143] Bowel and bladder involvement is common as the tumor grows. There is a tendency to involve the sacral plexus more often than the lumbar plexus, a point that contrasts with DLSPN, although selective upper plexus involvement can also occur.[143] In one third of patients, pain precedes other neurologic symptoms by at least 3 months; the course is therefore more prolonged than usually seen in DLSPN. On physical examination, leg edema may occur because of compression of the inferior vena cava or iliac veins, lymphatics, or both. Rectal examination may reveal a palpable mass. Retroperitoneal lymphoma may cause a LSPN in a patient with DM.

Confirmation is by imaging of the pelvis.

Computed tomography reveals a tumor mass in up to 96% of patients[144] and may also reveal bony involvement or lymphadenopathy. The relative usefulness of MRI has not been addressed.

RADIATION

Patients treated with radiotherapy to the lumbosacral plexus may have a proximal neuropathy similar to DLSPN. This complication is relatively rare. The diagnosis should be considered in any patient with cancer who has received radiotherapy and subsequently develops new neurologic symptoms in the lower limbs, bearing in mind that recurrent tumor is more likely. Symptoms develop after a delay of 1 month to 31 years, with a median of 5 years.[257] In contrast to DLSPN, the initial symptom is usually painless weakness; pain develops later, if at all, and is seldom severe. Other characteristic features are a tendency to have bilateral involvement, initial involvement of distal muscles, and a very slow course, with some patients exhibiting only mild weakness 5 years after the onset of symptoms.

As with pelvic tumor, electrophysiologic studies indicate an axonal process. The presence of myokymia favors radiation-induced plexopathy; in one series, myokymia was seen in 12 of 20 patients with radiation-induced plexopathy versus none of 30 patients with tumor.[257] Computed tomography or MRI is useful to rule out the current tumor, although radiation-induced soft tissue changes may be difficult to distinguish from the tumor. Both (radiation scarring and recurrent tumor) may also occur together.

RETROPERITONEAL HEMORRHAGE

Retroperitoneal hemorrhage usually occurs in the setting of anticoagulant treatment,[101] hemophilia,[1] thrombocytopenia, disseminated intravascular coagulation, and ruptured abdominal aortic aneurysm. In anticoagulated patients, it occurs more often with heparin use than with warfarin.[55, 182] Bleeding into the psoas muscle may involve only the lumbar plexus, and the patient may have acute pain in the groin, radiating to the leg and thigh. The pain is increased with movement. Typically, there is weakness of the quadriceps and iliopsoas, loss of the ipsilateral knee jerk, and sensory loss in the distribution of the femoral, obturator, and lateral femoral cutaneous nerves. The acuteness of the motor deficit helps distinguish this disorder from DLSPN, with maximal deficit typically within 24 hours. Occasionally, bleeding is confined to the iliacus compartment, resulting in femoral neuropathy.[280]

Most experience with diagnosis is by CT.[230] Rapid diagnosis may be important because anecdotal reports suggest that outcome may be improved by emergency surgical decompression.[38, 280]

RETROPERITONEAL ABSCESS

Pyogenic abscess may arise from a vertebra, perinephric tissues, or gastrointestinal tract.[133] Occasionally, hematogenous spread from a distant site occurs. Clinical clues include nonspecific symptoms of bacterial infection such as fever and chills and a demonstrated primary site of infection. The neurologic presentation is similar to but less acute than that described for retroperitoneal hemorrhage.

DRUG ABUSE

Lumbosacral plexopathy is well described in heroin addicts. Although incompletely understood, the mechanism probably involves rhabdomyolysis and infarction in pelvic and lower limb muscles, leading to elevated pressure within fascial compartments. These patients mainly have pelvic or proximal lower limb pain, with mild to moderate weakness and sensory loss and occasionally impairment of bowel and bladder function. Presentation is more acute than in DLSPN, but the usual monophasic course with gradual recovery over weeks to months may cause confusion with the latter. Laboratory abnormalities include elevated muscle enzymes. Magnetic resonance imaging of the pelvis has revealed enlarged, swollen muscles in some cases. Biopsy of affected muscle reveals nonspecific necrosis.

ANEURYSM

An acute ischemic or compressive plexopathy has been described in the setting of abdominal aortic aneurysm. Plexopathy may occur in the postoperative period after attempted repair[66] or after spontaneous aneurysmal rupture.[34, 220] Less often, a plexopathy develops without actual rupture.[277] The key clinical clue is the presence of signs of unilateral or bilateral limb ischemia, present in most cases. An aneurysm of the common or internal iliac artery may also cause plexopathy that, in contrast to the above, may develop subacutely or chronically. Pain is the major symptom and is felt in the buttock, hip, or leg, and it is sometimes accompanied by swelling of the ipsilateral buttock when the aneurysm extends through the sciatic notch.[112]

OTHER CAUSES

Plexopathy has been described after intramuscular injection into the buttock. The mechanism is probably accidental injection into a gluteal artery, triggering retrograde thrombosis to the iliac artery and resulting in ischemia of the plexus. Pain develops within minutes to hours after injection, and the buttock is generally bruised and edematous.

Segmental zoster paresis occurs in 5% of patients with zoster.[258] Older patients (mean age, 62 years) are affected in most cases. Paresis is always followed by cutaneous zoster, after an interval of 1 day to 5 weeks. In Thomas and Howard's series, a lower extremity was affected in 16 of 61 patients.[258] Diagnosis is based primarily on the recognition of the characteristic dermatomal eruption, which is often inconspicuous.

Disorders of the Cauda Equina

The major disorders of spinal nerve roots or cauda equina that may mimic DLSPN are presented in Table 31.3.

TABLE 31.3 PROXIMAL ASYMMETRICAL DIABETIC NEUROPATHY: DIFFERENTIAL DIAGNOSIS

Plexopathies
Pelvic tumor
Radiation
Retroperitoneal hemorrhage
Retroperitoneal abscess
Aneurysm
Drug abuse
Idiopathic lumbosacral plexus neuropathy

Radiculopathies
Disk herniation
Lumbar stenosis
Tumor
   Epidural (usually metastatic)
   Intradural
      Primary
      Meningeal carcinomatosis
Infection
   Lyme
   Cytomegalovirus
   Segmental zoster paresis

Local pathology
Osteoarthritis of the hip
Trochanteric bursitis

SPONDYLOSIS

The most important group consists of spondylosis and degenerative disk disease of the lumbar spine. Spondylosis refers to a series of interrelated structural changes of the spine, including dehydration and bulging of intervertebral disks with loss of disk height, vertebral osteophyte formation, and facet joint hypertrophy, resulting in stenosis of the spinal canal and intervertebral foramina. Spondylosis preferentially affects the L-5 and S-1 levels, but it is typically a multilevel process that may also be severe in the upper lumbar spine. Neurologic symptoms result from compression of nerve roots in the cauda equina or intervertebral foramina. The course is usually chronic,[266] continuing for many years. Low back pain, probably of mechanical origin[151] is the most common symptom; lower extremity pain without clear radicular features is also common. The most characteristic syndrome resulting from spondylosis is that of neurogenic claudication[151] in which lower extremity pain and weakness with or without sensory symptoms is reliably provoked by walking and relieved by sitting and other activities involving flexion of the lumbar spine. This syndrome is unlikely to be confused with DLSPN, but difficulty may arise in less typical cases in which back or limb pain develops subacutely, accompanied by quadriceps weakness.[122]

Factors favoring the presence of lumbosacral spondylosis include age older than 60 years,[173] male sex (in some but not all series),[211, 270] prominence of back pain, long-standing symptoms unaccompanied by significant objective deficits, and an indolent rather than monophasic course. Examination typically reveals limited lumbar range of movement. There may be signs of one or more lumbosacral radiculopathies, but commonly the neurologic examination is normal.[58]

Imaging studies are basic to diagnosis. Computed tomography with myelography is the traditional standard modality. Myelographic findings vary from indentation or amputation of one or more nerve roots or an hour-glass configuration of the thecal sac to complete obstruction of the subarachnoid space.[268] Computed tomography is useful for revealing canal dimensions, soft tissues including disk material, and compression fractures.[28, 239] However, most authorities now consider MRI the modality of choice because of its ability to image the entire spine in multiple planes, its superiority in delineating soft tissues including neural structures,[235] its noninvasive nature, and the avoidance of ionizing radiation. Where bony changes must be defined clearly, however, CT remains the modality of choice.

DISK DISEASE

Herniation of a lumbar intervertebral disk is a well-recognized cause of acute focal neurologic symptoms. In contrast to spondylosis, acute disk herniation is mainly a disease of patients under age 40 years. The majority occur at the L4–5 or the L5–S1 levels.[233]

In its classic form, the clinical picture is distinctive and unlikely to cause confusion with DLSPN. Patients complain of a combination of acute or subacute low-back pain and radicular pain (sciatica). The latter most typically involves the posterior thigh and usually extends below the knee,[20] although thigh pain may be prominent with upper lumbar disk herniations. Onset is typically acute, particularly in relation to activity. Weakness and sensory symptoms such as tingling paresthesias may occur, their location determined by the nerve root involved. Characteristically, pain is exacerbated by maneuvers that increase lumbar flexion, such as sitting or bending forward and by increases in intra-abdominal pressure, such as coughing, sneezing, or bowel movements. Physical examination often reveals local back tenderness or muscle spasm, scoliosis, and loss of lumbar lordosis. Neurologic deficits are variable and relate to the severity and a level of nerve root compression, when present. The straight leg raising test places the L5 and S1 roots under stretch and may be useful in confirming compression of either of these roots.

Confusion with DLSPN is more likely in cases of upper lumbar disk herniation. Albert and associates[3] described 141 patients with disk herniations between the L1–2 and L3–4 levels. Most occurred at the L3–4 level. In contrast to patients with the more common lower lumbar syndromes, these individuals were older (mean age, 52 years) and were predominantly male. Thigh pain was a common symptom, although specific patterns of pain and neurologic deficits were variable, particularly sensory deficits. These patients were also somewhat unusual by virtue of their chronic course; one quarter had pain for more than 6 months at the time of diagnosis. Further difficulty was caused by the high false-negative rate of imaging studies, especially myelography. Other authors have noted similar features with respect to age[4] and variability of symptoms.[179]

Imaging studies are required to confirm disk herniation. Myelography, the traditional gold standard, has largely been replaced by CT and MRI.[281] Magnetic resonance imaging is preferred, given the soft tissue nature of the protruding disk material and for the other reasons outlined previously. The diagnostic accuracy of MRI has been shown to be equal to CT and equal or superior to myelography.[189] Computed tomography (with or without myelography) remains useful in patients in whom MR is equivocal, in older patients with significant bony pathology, and in patients in whom MR is contraindicated or cannot be tolerated. It should be noted, however, that with the high sensitivity and increasing availability of MR scanning, a high prevalence of asymptomatic disk protrusions and other degenerative changes has been recognized.[27] One must therefore take care to not attribute symptoms of DLSPN to unrelated imaging findings.

PRIMARY TUMORS

The most common primary spinal tumors are ependymomas and neurofibromas. Less common types include meningiomas, lipomas, schwannomas, dermoids, hemangioblastomas, and paragangliomas. Patients with these tumors usually present with a combination of low-back pain and sciatica. Although a chronic course is usual, an acute presentation occasionally occurs. Patients typically complain of constant pain that worsens with recumbency and at night. Magnetic resonance imaging of the spine is diagnostic in most cases.

SECONDARY TUMORS

Metastatic disease occurs in either the epidural or intradural compartment. Most epidural tumors are metastatic and extend from a vertebral body or epidural soft tissue. Those within a vertebra most often originate from breast, prostate, or lung, whereas those arising within epidural soft tissues spread from lung, kidney, lymphoma, or multiple myeloma. A history of cancer is obviously important, but only half of all patients carry this diagnosis at the time of presentation.[246] Regarding symptoms, back pain is almost universal and is the presenting symptom in up to 96% of patients.[116] Pain may be local, radicular, or referred to nearby regions such as the hip and is often worse with recumbency. The course is highly variable; neurologic

symptoms develop from a few days to 3 years after back pain.[14] The course seems to be more protracted with breast and prostate cancer and shortest with renal cell tumors. Motor and sensory deficits are caused by compression of individual roots, cauda equina, or spinal cord. Once present, weakness usually progresses rapidly to paraplegia without intervention.[125]

The majority (70%) involve the thoracic spine (see section on diabetic truncal radiculopathy). However, the lumbar spine may also be involved, manifesting as upper lumbar radiculopathy and quadriceps weakness.

As with other types of lesions in this region, MRI has largely replaced CT-myelography as the diagnostic modality of choice. The ability of MR to identify noncontiguous disease is particularly important.

Intradural metastases may take the form of a single solid tumor, but meningeal carcinomatosis is more common, occurring in 5 to 8% of all solid tumors[119, 209] and in 5 to 29% of non-Hodgkin's lymphoma. A previous history of cancer is more common than with epidural disease, present in 85% of patients.[51] The causative tumor is most often adenocarcinoma from breast,[255, 276] lung, melanoma, or non-Hodgkin's lymphoma. The mode of presentation is highly variable. Back or limb pain may be the presenting feature as in DLSPN, but patients may also initially complain of limb weakness, sensory disturbances, or a combination of the above.[255, 276] Intracranial disease is often present concurrently, producing changes in mental status or cranial neuropathies.

Spinal fluid analysis is the most important diagnostic test and is abnormal in 97% of patients.[276] Nonspecific changes include increased opening pressure, increased protein concentration, decreased glucose concentration, and pleocytosis. Cytology is positive in 50% of first examinations, rising to 85% if three samples are obtained.[130] In certain cases, tumor markers such as carcinoembryonic antigen are useful. The imaging study of choice is MRI with gadolinium contrast; this often identifies meningeal enhancement.[52, 56] Coexisting epidural and intramedullary disease may also be identified.

Disorders of the Femoral Nerve

Femoral neuropathy must be differentiated from more proximal lesions of the lumbar plexus or L2–4 nerve roots. This distinction is often difficult to make. In true femoral neuropathy, findings are confined to femoral-innervated muscles (the quadriceps, iliacus, sartorius, and pectineus) and to cutaneous areas supplied by the anterior and medial cutaneous nerves of the thigh and the saphenous nerve (the anterior and inferomedial thigh, medial leg, and medial foot). Adductor weakness must be excluded because its presence indicates either a plexus lesion or simultaneous involvement of the obturator nerve. The quadriceps reflex is decreased or absent. Back pain is rarely a feature and suggests a root lesion.

Diabetes is the most common associated disease in most series.[45, 120] Other causes include trauma such as penetrating wounds, surgery (most often abdominal hysterectomy or renal transplantation), and femoral artery puncture. Nerve compression adjacent to the iliacus muscle has been described secondary to hematoma,[280] abscess,[2] and acute infarction in intravenous drug abusers.[149] Radiotherapy has been implicated,[168] but more often produces plexopathy. In a minority of cases, no cause can be found.

Electrophysiologic studies are invaluable in localization. Femoral motor and saphenous sensory nerve conduction studies may be useful but are sometimes technically problematic. Needle examination is most helpful in confirmation of involvement of femoral-innervated muscles and exclusion of plexus and root involvement. Both MRI and CT of the lumbar spine and pelvis can be performed to exclude a structural lesion.

Local Musculoskeletal Pathology

Local nonneurologic disorders may occasionally present in a fashion that mimics DLSPN. Disease of the hip is most likely to do so. Osteoarthritis usually presents as slowly progressive, partly exertional pain. Confusion with DLSPN is most likely when osteoarthritis presents acutely[237] and when the location of pain is referred to the thigh, knee, buttock, or groin.[278] On examination, a Trendelenburg sign may be present. Gait is typically antalgic and stiff with excessive hip rotation. Range of movement is decreased; internal rotation and abduction are lost early,[278] and flexion contracture is common. Palpation may reveal local tenderness or crepitus. The straight leg raising test may be falsely positive.

Radiologic confirmation is by plain x-ray studies. Findings include bony sclerosis, joint space narrowing, osteophytosis, or cyst formation. It should be recognized that such changes are also common in asymptomatic patients,[148] increasing in frequency with increasing age.

Radiologic changes should therefore be interpreted in light of the clinical syndrome.

Other diseases of the hip may present in a similar manner. These include septic arthritis, rheumatoid arthritis, calcium pyrophosphate disease (pseudogout), aseptic necrosis of the femoral head, and hip fracture.

DIFFERENTIAL DIAGNOSIS OF DIABETIC TRUNCAL RADICULOPATHY

Diabetic truncal radiculopathy is a distinctive but often misdiagnosed syndrome. A common reason for misdiagnosis is the failure to consider the diagnosis. Kikta and associates[159] reviewed 30 patients with thoracic radiculopathy of any cause; diabetes was the only identifiable disorder in 21. Such patients are usually middle aged and have type 2 diabetes, although a requirement for insulin is common.[99, 159, 248] An association with retinopathy and nephropathy has generally not been found.[99, 159] Diagnosis is made difficult by the lack of a clear radicular pattern in most patients; multiple contiguous levels are often involved, and bilateral symptoms are not uncommon.[159, 248, 252] Other clues to a diabetic cause include the frequent finding of a more diffuse polyneuropathy, either clinically or by nerve conduction studies, and the occasional finding of other focal neuropathies. Accompanying weight loss is common.[177] Examination may reveal hyperalgesia, hypesthesia, or a combination of the two in affected areas. Abdominal weakness is often present and may occasionally extend to adjacent proximal limb muscles. A monophasic course is typical; in Ellenberg's series, symptoms usually resolved within 3 months.

The EMG finding of neurogenic abnormalities in paraspinal muscles[159] confirms nerve root involvement. Thermoregulatory sweat testing often reveals segmental anhidrosis that may be more widespread than suggested by symptoms and may also reveal symmetrical distal anhidrosis of the lower limbs caused by coexistent polyneuropathy.[104]

In patients with subacute onset of unilateral truncal pain, the first priority is to rule out visceral pathology, including myocardial infarction, cholecystitis, and biliary colic. A history of trauma or vigorous exertion may suggest rib fracture or chest wall muscle strain.

When visceral disease has been excluded, thoracic disk herniation should be considered. Herniation at this level is uncommon, comprising fewer than 1% of symptomatic disk herniations.[8, 22] Patients usually are seen in the fourth to sixth decades.[6, 228] There is a male predominance in some series.[6] Most patients complain of back pain; radiation of pain around the torso is less common, occurring in 9 to 65%.[6, 74] Symptoms are often present for months or even years,[8] possibly because of underdiagnosis. Disk herniation should be suspected when there is accompanying gait difficulty or lower limb spasticity, weakness, or sensory disturbance, signs of a simultaneous compressive myelopathy.[240] Other clues include a history of trauma, particularly a fall onto extended legs of buttocks.[205] The imaging modality of choice is MRI.[40, 53]

Zoster should also be considered, especially in the elderly[218] and in patients with impaired cell-mediated immunity, including those taking immunosuppressive drugs, organ transplant recipients, and patients with solid tumors,[229] lymphoid malignancies, and HIV infection.[117, 138] The eruption consists of erythematous macules or papules that progress to vesicles, with crusting and eventual clearing over 2 to 3 weeks. A thoracic dermatome is involved in 60%, usually confined to a single dermatome. Chest or abdominal wall weakness occurs less often than with DLSPN, in 0.5 to 31% of patients.[131, 258] Objective sensory loss is usual in painful areas.[200, 201]

Series and case reports have suggested that diabetes may be a predisposing factor for zoster.[41, 44, 192] However, the only large population-based study to address this question found that diabetes was no more common in patients with zoster than in the general population and that these patients did not have an increased risk of developing diabetes over a prolonged period of follow-up. Also, zoster was not found to differ in severity in patients with diabetes and in controls. It was concluded that diabetes is not a risk factor for zoster.[217]

DIFFERENTIAL DIAGNOSIS OF DIABETIC OCULOMOTOR NEUROPATHY

Cranial mononeuropathies involving any of the three ocular motor nerves (oculomotor, abducens, and trochlear) can occur in diabetic individuals. Of these three, the oculomotor nerve (third cranial nerve) is most commonly affected. The clinical features of this disorder and pathologic evidence for a vascular (ischemic) etiology are reviewed in detail in Chapter 33.

Certain key clinical features will be empha-

sized here for the purpose of differential diagnosis. Diabetic oculomotor palsy generally affects persons older than age 50 years with type 2 DM; it may be the presenting manifestation of the diabetes. Pain is present in the majority of cases, but may be absent. Unilateral oculomotor palsy may be partial or complete. Sparing of pupillary function is widely accepted as a hallmark feature, but is not invariable, occurring in approximately 70 to 85% of lesions of ischemic cause.[128, 226] Bilateral simultaneous involvement or involvement of multiple nerves on the same side is unusual and should prompt a search for another cause. Diabetic oculomotor palsy is self-limited in most cases, improving over weeks and usually resolving within 3 months; a prolonged or progressive course justifies investigation.

An identical clinical syndrome occurs in nondiabetic individuals with hypertension or atherosclerosis, both of which may result in small vessel disease and nerve ischemia.[215, 226] Cases reported in the setting of temporal arteritis presumably reflect a similar mechanism.[123]

The differential diagnosis of acquired oculomotor palsy is extensive. Lesions may damage the oculomotor nucleus (located in the midbrain tegmentum anterior to the periaquaductal gray matter), or the fascicles of the nerve as they pass through the midbrain, the subarachnoid space, the cavernous sinus, or the orbit.

Nuclear lesions are rare. Responsible lesions are usually infarcts, tumors, or demyelinating plaques. This site of involvement is suggested by the finding—not invariably present—of ptosis and weakness of elevation of the contralateral eye, related to the origin of lid elevator fibers from a single midline nucleus, and to the unique innervation of the superior rectus by crossed fibers.

Damage to intra-axial fascicles within the midbrain is caused by a similar group of disorders. Diagnosis is guided by the presence of other neurologic signs of brain stem dysfunction. Weber's syndrome consists of oculomotor palsy and contralateral hemiplegia, caused by a lesion of the cerebral peduncle. In Benedikt's syndrome there is contralateral tremor or choreoathetosis, related to damage to the red nucleus. Depending on the precise extent of injury, other findings, including contralateral ataxia and hemisensory loss, may also be present with midbrain lesions.

The most important consideration in differential diagnosis is nerve compression in the subarachnoid space by aneurysm. Typically, the aneurysm arises from the posterior communicating artery at its junction with the internal carotid artery. When nerve compression occurs after aneurysmal rupture and subarachnoid hemorrhage, diagnosis is rarely difficult. Pain is prominent and headache is often sudden and excruciating. Focal neurologic deficits, decreased level of consciousness, or both may be present. In this situation, the oculomotor palsy is usually complete and the pupil is dilated and unreactive. Unfortunately, pupil sparing has been described in up to 5% of cases[161, 191, 202]; in such cases, ophthalmoplegia is typically incomplete. Partial third-nerve palsy also occurs with compression from an unruptured aneurysm.[15] In the opinion of most clinicians, any case of oculomotor palsy with pupillary involvement should be investigated promptly with angiography or another high-resolution imaging study; complete external oculomotor palsy with pupil sparing in a patient older than age 50 years may be followed closely for signs of progression.[118]

A cavernous sinus lesion should be excluded when oculomotor palsy is accompanied by signs of involvement of other ipsilateral ocular nerves or the ophthalmic division of the trigeminal nerve, the latter resulting in pain or numbness of the face. Third-nerve involvement is commonly incomplete. A coexistent Horner's syndrome may result in apparent pupil sparing. Causes include carotid aneurysm; metastases from lung, breast, prostate, or lymphoma[213, 259]; extension of extracavernous tumors such as meningiomas and pituitary adenomas; and sphenoid sinus mucoceles.[199] The Tolosa-Hunt syndrome is characterized pathologically by granulomatous inflammation of the sinus,[141, 264] with a tendency to spontaneous remissions; steroid responsiveness has been demonstrated.[141, 242] In diabetic patients, mucormycosis infection should be borne in mind; signs include facial pain, proptosis, and bloody rhinorrhea.[219] Diagnosis of cavernous sinus lesions requires CT or MRI, with angiographic confirmation if aneurysm is suspected.

Occasional cases are caused by intra-orbital lesions such as tumor, pseudotumor, and trauma. As with cavernous sinus lesions, oculomotor dysfunction is often incomplete, the abducens and trochlear nerves are usually involved, and proptosis is common. Orbital ultrasound and CT or MRI are the imaging modalities of choice.

Myasthenia gravis must also be considered in any patient with painless diplopia. Ptosis is particularly common, but weakness in other extraocular muscles is not necessarily limited to those innervated by the oculomotor nerve. Pupillary responses are normal. Weakness may begin in one eye but eventually becomes bilateral. Variability of deficits over the course of a day and day-to-day is characteristic,[59] and fatigue with sustained use may be seen. Examination may reveal weakness in other cranial muscles, such as orbicularis oculi, or in proximal limb muscles. Reversal of ptosis with the intravenous injection of Tensilon (edrophonium hydrochloride) provides evidence of abnormal neuromuscular transmission, but interpretation is sometimes difficult and false negatives are not uncommon. Single-fiber electromyography is useful in equivocal cases. Serum antibodies to acetylcholine receptor are present in 50 to 71% of individuals with purely ocular myasthenia.[170, 172, 234]

References

1. Aggeler PM, Lucia SP. The neurologic complications of hemophilia. J Nerv Ment Dis 1944; 99:475.
2. Aichroth P, Rowe-Jones DC. Iliacus compartment compression syndrome. Br J Surg 1971; 58:833.
3. Albert TJ, Balderston RA, Heller JG, et al. Upper lumbar disc herniations. J Spine Dis 1993; 6:351.
4. An HS, Vaccaro A, Simeone FA, et al. Herniated lumbar disc in patients over the age of fifty. J Spine Dis 1990; 3:143.
5. Andrade C. A peculiar form of peripheral neuropathy. Brain 1952; 75:408.
6. Arce CA, Dohrmann GJ. Thoracic disc herniation: Improved diagnosis with computed tomographic scanning and a review of the literature. Surg Neurol 1985; 23:356.
7. Archer AG, Watkins PJ, Thomas PK, et al. The natural history of acute painful neuropathy in diabetes mellitus. J Neurol Neurosurg Psychiatry 1983; 46:491.
8. Arseni C, Nash F. Protrusion of thoracic intervertebral discs. Acta Neurochir 1963; 11:3.
9. Asbury AK. Uremic neuropathy. In Dyck PJ, Thomas PK, Lambert EH (eds): Peripheral Neuropathy. Philadelphia, WB Saunders, 1975, p 982.
10. Asbury AK, Victor M, Adams RD. Uremic polyneuropathy. Arch Neurol 1963; 8:413.
11. Assmann G, Smootz E, Adler K, et al. The lipoprotein abnormality in Tangier disease: Quantitation of A apoproteins. J Clin Invest 1977; 59:565.
12. Axelsson U, Bachmann R, Hallen J. Frequency of pathological proteins (M-components) on 6,995 sera from an adult population. Acta Med Scand 1966; 179:235.
13. Bank WJ. Thallim. In Spencer PS, Schaumberg HH (eds): Experimental and Clinical Neurotoxicology. Baltimore, Williams & Wilkins, 1980, p 570.
14. Barron KD, Hirano A, Araki S. Experiences with metastatic neoplasms involving the spinal cord. Neurology 1959; 9:91.
15. Bartleson JD, Trautmann JC, Sundt TM Jr. Minimal oculomotor nerve paresis secondary to unruptured intracranial aneurysm. Arch Neurol 1986; 43:1015.
16. Bastron JA, Thomas JE. Diabetic polyradiculopathy: Clinical and electromyographic findings in 105 patients. Mayo Clin Proc 1981; 56:725.

17. Behse F. Hereditary neuropathy with liability to pressure palsies: Electrophysiological and histopathological aspects. Brain 1972; 95:777.
18. Behse F, Buchthal F. Alcoholic neuropathy: Clinical electrophysiological and biopsy findings. Ann Neurol 1977; 2:95.
19. Behse F, Buchthal F, Carlsen F. Nerve biopsy and conduction studies in diabetic neuropathy. J Neurol Neurosurg Psychiatry 1977; 40:1072.
20. Bell GR. Diagnosis of lumbar disc disease. Semin Spine Surg 1989; 1:8.
21. Ben Othmane K, Middleton LT, Loprest LJ, et al. Localization of a gene (CMT2A) for autosomal dominant Charcot-Marie-Tooth disease type 2 to chromosome 1p and evidence of genetic heterogeneity. Genomics 1993; 17:370.
22. Benson MK, Byrnes DP. The clinical syndromes and surgical treatment of thoracic intervertebral disc prolapse. J Bone Joint Surg 1975; 57:471.
23. Berger AR, Arezzo JC, Schaumburg HH, et al. 2',3'-dideoxycytidine (ddC) toxic neuropathy: A study of 52 patients. Neurology 1993; 43:358.
24. Biehl JP, Vilter RW. Effects of isoniazid on pyridoxine metabolism. JAMA 1954; 156:1549.
25. Birbeck MQ, Beer TC. Occupation in relation to the carpal tunnel syndrome. Rheumatol Rehabil 1975; 14:218.
26. Bird TD, Reenan AM, Pfeifer M. Autonomic nervous system function in genetic neuromuscular disorders: Hereditary motor-sensory neuropathy and myotonic dystrophy. Arch Neurol 1984; 41:43.
27. Boden SD, David DO, Dina TS, et al. Abnormal magnetic resonance scans of the lumbar spine in asymptomatic subjects: A prospective investigation. J Bone Joint Surg 1990; 72:403.
28. Bolender NF, Schonstrom NS, Spengler DM. Role of computed tomography and myelography in the diagnosis of central spinal stenosis. J Bone Joint Surg 1985; 67:240.
29. Bolton CF. Electrophysiologic changes in uremic neuropathy after successful renal transplantation. Neurology 1976; 26:152.
30. Bolton CF. Peripheral neuropathies associated with chronic renal failure (review). Can J Neurol Sci 1980; 7:89.
31. Bolton CF, Baltzan MA, Baltzan RB. Effects of renal transplantation on uremic neuropathy. N Engl J Med 1971; 284:1170.
32. Bolton CF, Gilbert JJ, Hahn AF, et al. Polyneuropathy in critically ill patients. J Neurol Neurosurg Psychiatry 1984; 47:1223.
33. Bolton CF, Young GB. Neurological Complications of Renal Disease. Boston, Butterworths, 1990, p 77.
34. Bolton PM, Blumgart LH. Neurological complications of ruptured abdominal aortic aneurysm. Br J Surg 1972; 59:707.
35. Bradley WG, Karlsson IJ, Rassol CG. Metronidazole neuropathy. Br Med J 1977; 2:610.
36. Brady RO. Enzymatic defect in Fabry's disease. N Engl J Med 1967; 276:1163.
37. Brady RO. Fabry disease. In Dyck PJ, Thomas PK, Griffin JW, et al (eds): Peripheral Neuropathy. Philadelphia, WB Saunders, 1993, p 1169.
38. Brantigan JW, Owens ML, Moody FG. Femoral neuropathy complicating anticoagulant therapy. Am J Surg Pathol 1976; 132:108.
39. Brooks AP. Abnormal vascular reflexes in Charcot-Marie-Tooth disease. J Neurol Neurosurg Psychiatry 1980; 43:348.
40. Brown CW, Deffer PA Jr, Akmakjian J, et al. The natural history of thoracic disc herniation. Spine 1992; 17:S97.
41. Brown GR. Herpes zoster: Correlation of age, sex, distribution, neuralgia, and associated disorders. South Med J 1976; 69:576.
42. Bruyn GW, Garland H. Neuropathies of endocrine origin. In Vinken PJ, Bruyn GW (eds): Handbook of Clinical Neurology. Amsterdam, North Holland Publishing Company, 1970, p 29.
43. Buchthal F, Rosenfalck A, Trojaborg W. Electrophysiological findings in entrapment of the median nerve at wrist and elbow. J Neurol Neurosurg Psychiatry 1974; 37:340.
44. Calandra P, Lisi P. Skin and diabetes. II: Incidence of diabetes in a group of patients with herpes zoster. Ital Gen Rev Dermatol 1974; 11:207.
45. Calverley JR, Mulder DW. Femoral neuropathy. Neurology 1960; 10:963.
46. Caravati CM. Insulin neuritis: A case report. Va Med 1933; 59:745.
47. Caselli RJ, Daube JR, Hunder GG, et al. Peripheral neuropathic syndromes in giant cell (temporal) arteritis. Neurology 1988; 38:685.
48. Casey EB, Jellife AM, LeQuesne PM, et al. Vincristine neuropathy: Clinical and electrophysiological observations. Brain 1973; 96:69.
49. Casey EB, LeQuesne PM. Electrophysiological evidence for a distal lesion in alcoholic neuropathy. J Neurol Neurosurg Psychiatry 1972; 35:624.
50. Cavanagh JB, Fuller NH, Johnson HR, et al. The effects of thallium salts, with particular reference to the nervous system changes: A report of three cases. Q J Med 1974; 43:293.
51. Chamberlain MC. Current concepts in leptomeningeal metastasis. Curr Opin Oncol 1992; 4:533.
52. Chamberlain MC, Sandy AD, Press GA. Leptomeningeal metastasis: A comparison of gadolinium-enhanced MR and contrast-enhanced CT of the brain. Neurology 1990; 40:435.
53. Chambers AA. Thoracic disk herniation. Semin Roentgenol 1988; 23:111.
54. Chance PF, Alderson MK, Leppig KA, et al. DNA deletion associated with hereditary neuropathy with liability to pressure palsies. Cell 1993; 72:143.
55. Chiu WS. The syndrome of retroperitoneal hemorrhage and lumbar plexus neuropathy during anticoagulant therapy. South Med J 1976; 69:595.
56. Chua SL, Goh PS, Tan LK. Magnetic resonance imaging of leptomeningeal metastases to the spine. Singapore Med J 1993; 34:253.
57. Chumbley LC, Harrison EG Jr, DeRemee RA. Allergic granulomatosis and angiitis (Churg-Strauss syndrome): Report and analysis of 30 cases. Mayo Clin Proc 1977; 52:477.
58. Ciricillo SF, Weinstein PR. Lumbar spinal stenosis. West J Med 1993; 158:171.
59. Cogan DG. Myasthenia gravis: A review of the disease and a description of lid twitch as a characteristic sign. Arch Ophthalmol 1965; 74:217.
60. Cohen RD, Conn DL, Ilstrup DM. Clinical features, prognosis, and response to treatment in polyarteritis. Mayo Clin Proc 1980; 55:146.
61. Cornblath DR, McArthur JC, Kennedy PG, et al. Inflammatory demyelinating peripheral neuropathies associated with human T-cell lymphotropic virus type III infection. Ann Neurol 1987; 21:32.
62. Crevasse LE, Logue RB. Peripheral neuropathy in myxedema. Ann Intern Med 1959; 50:1433.

63. Croft PB, Henson RA, Urich H, et al. Sensory neuropathy with bronchial carcinoma: A study of four cases showing serological abnormalities. Brain 1965; 88:501.
64. Cseuz KA, Thomas JE, Lambert EH, et al. Long-term results of operation for carpal tunnel syndrome. Mayo Clin Proc 1966; 41:232.
65. Cupps TR, Fauci AS. The Vasculitides. Philadelphia, WB Saunders, 1981, p 29.
66. D'Amour ML, Lebrun LH, Rabbat A, et al. Peripheral neurological complications of aortoiliac vascular disease. Can J Neurol Sci 1987; 14:127.
67. Dalakas MC. Chronic idiopathic ataxic neuropathy. Ann Neurol 1986; 19:545.
68. Dalakas MC, Engel WK. Polyneuropathy with monoclonal gammopathy: Studies of 11 patients. Ann Neurol 1981; 10:45.
69. Dalakas MC, Pezeshkpour GH. Neuromuscular diseases associated with human immunodeficiency virus infection. Ann Neurol 1988; 23(suppl):S38.
70. Daugaard GK, Petrera J, Trojaborg W. Electrophysiological study of the peripheral and central neurotoxic effect of cis-platin. Acta Neurol Scand 1987; 76:86.
71. Dawson DM, Samuels MA, Morris J. Sensory form of acute polyneuritis. Neurology 1988; 38:1728.
72. Del Campo M, Bolton CF, Lindsay RM. The value of electrophysiologic studies in assessing peripheral nerve function during optimal hemodialysis (abstract). Muscle Nerve 1983; 6:533.
73. Diabetes Control and Complications Trial Research Group. The effect of intensive diabetes therapy on the development and progression of neuropathy. Ann Intern Med 1995; 122:561.
74. Dietze DD Jr, Fessler RG. Thoracic disc herniations. Neurosurg Clin North Am 1993; 4:75.
75. Donofrio PD, Wilbourn AJ, Albers JW, et al. Acute arsenic intoxication presenting as Guillain-Barre-like syndrome. Muscle Nerve 1987; 114:120.
76. Drachman DA. Neurological complications of Wegener's granulomatosis. Arch Neurol 1963; 8:145.
77. Dyck PJ. Histologic measurements and fine structure of biopsied sural nerve: Normal, and in peroneal muscular atrophy, hypertrophic neuropathy, and congenital sensory neuropathy. Mayo Clin Proc 1966; 41:742.
78. Dyck PJ. Inherited neuronal degeneration and atrophy affecting peripheral motor, sensory, and autonomic neurons. In Dyck PJ, Thomas PK, Lambert EH (eds): Peripheral Neuropathy. Philadelphia, WB Saunders, 1975, p 825.
79. Dyck PJ, Beahrs OH, Miller RH. Peripheral nerves in hereditary neural atrophies: number and diameters of myelinated fibers. Presented at the Sixth International Congress of Electroencephalography and Clinical Neurophysiology. Vienna, Sept 5, 1965.
80. Dyck PJ, Benstead TJ, Conn DL, et al. Nonsystemic vasculitic neuropathy. Brain 1987; 110:843.
81. Dyck PJ, Chance P, Lebo R, et al. Hereditary motor and sensory neuropathies. In Dyck PJ, Thomas PK, Griffin JW, et al (eds): Peripheral Neuropathy. Philadelphia, WB Saunders, 1993, p 1094.
82. Dyck PJ, Dyck PJB, Chalk CH. The 10 P's: A mnemonic helpful in characterization and differential diagnosis of peripheral neuropathy. Neurology 1992; 42:14.
83. Dyck PJ, Dyck PJB, Grant IA, et al. Ten steps in characterizing and diagnosing patients with peripheral neuropathy. Neurology 1996; 47:10.
84. Dyck PJ, Gutrecht JA, Bastron JA, et al. Histologic and teased fiber measurements of sural nerve in disorders of lower motor and primary sensory neurons. Mayo Clin Proc 1968; 43:81.
85. Dyck PJ, Johnson WJ, Lambert EH, et al. Segmental demyelination secondary to axonal degeneration in uremic neuropathy. Mayo Clin Proc 1971; 46:400.
86. Dyck PJ, Karnes J, O'Brien P, et al. Spatial pattern of nerve fiber abnormality indicative of pathologic mechanisms. Am J Pathol 1984; 117:225.
87. Dyck PJ, Karnes JL, O'Brien PC, et al. The Rochester Diabetic Neuropathy Study: Reassessment of tests and criteria for diagnosis and staged severity. Neurology 1992; 42:1164.
88. Dyck PJ, Kennel AJ, Magal IV, et al. A Virginia kinship with hereditary sensory neuropathy: Peroneal muscular atrophy and pes cavus. Mayo Clin Proc 1965; 40:685.
89. Dyck PJ, Kratz KM, Karnes JL, et al. The prevalence by staged severity of various types of diabetic neuropathy, retinopathy, and nephropathy in a population-based cohort: The Rochester Diabetic Neuropathy Study. Neurology 1993; 43:817.
90. Dyck PJ, Lais A, Karnes JL, et al. Fiber loss is primary and multifocal in sural nerves in diabetic polyneuropathy. Ann Neurol 1986; 19:425.
91. Dyck PJ, Lambert EH. Lower motor and primary sensory neuron diseases with peroneal muscular atrophy. I: Neurologic, genetic, and electrophysiologic findings in hereditary polyneuropathies. Arch Neurol 1968; 18:603.
92. Dyck PJ, Lambert EH. Polyneuropathy associated with hypothyroidism. J Neuropathol Exp Neurol 1970; 29:631.
93. Dyck PJ, Lambert EH, Mulder DW. Charcot-Marie-Tooth disease: Nerve conduction and clinical studies of a large kinship. Neurology 1963; 13:1.
94. Dyck PJ, Litchy WJ, Lehman KA, et al. Variables influencing neuropathic endpoints: The Rochester Diabetic Neuropathy Study of Healthy Subjects (RDNS-HS). Neurology 1995; 45:1115.
95. Dyck PJ, Low PA, Stevens JC. "Burning feet" as the only manifestation of dominantly inherited sensory neuropathy. Mayo Clin Proc 1983; 58:426.
96. Dyck PJ, Oviatt KF, Lambert EH. Intensive evaluation of unclassified neuropathies yields improved diagnosis. Ann Neurol 1981; 10:222.
97. Dyck PJ, Sherman WR, Hallcher LM, et al. Human diabetic endoneurial sorbital, fructose, and myo-inositol related to sural nerve morphometry. Ann Neurol 1980; 8:590.
98. Edmunds ME, Watkins PJ. Management of the diabetic foot. In Dyck PJ, Thomas PK, Asbury AK, et al (eds): Diabetic Neuropathy. Philadelphia, WB Saunders, 1987, p 208.
99. Ellenberg M. Diabetic neuropathic cachexia. Diabetes 1974; 23:418.
100. Ellenberg M. Diabetic truncal mononeuropathy: A new clinical syndrome. Diabetes Care 1978; 1:10.
101. Emery S, Ochoa J. Lumbar plexus neuropathy resulting from retroperitoneal hemorrhage. Muscle Nerve 1978; 1:330.
102. Engel WK, Dorman JD, Levy RI, et al. Neuropathy in Tangier disease. Arch Neurol 1967; 17:1.
103. Fagerberg S-E. Diabetic neuropathy: A clinical and histological study on the significance of vascular affections. Acta Med Scand 1959; 164(suppl 345):1.
104. Fealey RD. The thermoregulatory sweat test. In Low PA (ed): Clinical Autonomic Disorders. Boston, Little, Brown and Co, 1993, p 225.
105. Feely J, Isles TE. Screening for thyroid dysfunction in diabetics. Br Med J 1979; 1:1678.

106. Feindel W, Stratford J. The role of the cubital tunnel in tardy ulnar palsy. Can J Surg 1958; 1:287.
107. Fennelly J. Peripheral neuropathy of the alcoholic. I: Aetiological role of aneurin and other B-complex vitamins. Br Med J 1964; 5420:1290.
108. Fincham RW, Cape CA. Neuropathy in myxedema: A study of sensory nerve conduction in the upper extremities. Arch Neurol 1968; 19:464.
109. Font J, Valls J, Cervera R, et al. Pure sensory neuropathy in patients with primary Sjögren's syndrome: Clinical, immunological, and electromyographic findings. Ann Rheum Dis 1990; 49:775.
110. Fraser AG, McQueen IN, Watt AH, et al. Peripheral neuropathy during long-term high-dose amiodarone therapy. J Neurol Neurosurg Psychiatry 1985; 48:576.
111. Fraser DM, Campbell IW, Ewing DJ, et al. Mononeuropathy in diabetes mellitus. Diabetes 1979; 28:96.
112. Geelen JA, deGraaff R, Biemans RG, et al. Sciatic nerve compression by an aneurysm of the internal iliac artery. Clin Neurol Neurosurg 1985; 87:219.
113. Gherardi R, Lebargy F, Gaulard P, et al. Necrotizing vasculitis and HIV replication in peripheral nerves. N Engl J Med 1989; 321:685.
114. Giannini C, Dyck PJ. Ultrastructural morphometric abnormalities of sural nerve endoneurial microvessels in diabetes mellitus. Ann Neurol 1994; 36:408.
115. Gibbels E, Schaefer HE, Runne U, et al. Severe polyneuropathy in Tangier disease mimicking syringomyelia or leprosy: Clinical, biochemical, electrophysiological, and morphological evaluation, including electron microscopy of nerve, muscle, and skin biopsies. J Neurol 1985; 232:283.
116. Gilbert RW, Kim JH, Posner JB. Epidural spinal cord compression from metastatic tumor: Diagnosis and treatment. Ann Neurol 1978; 3:40.
117. Gilden DH, Dueland AN, Cohrs R, et al. Preherpetic neuralgia. Neurology 1991; 41:1215.
118. Gittenger JW Jr. Non-myasthenic ophthalmoplegias. *In* Lessell S, van Dalen JTW (eds): Neuro-ophthalmology. Amsterdam, Elsevier Science Publishers, 1984, p 262.
119. Gonzalez-Vitale JC, Garcia-Bunuel R. Meningeal carcinomatosis. Cancer 1976; 37:2906.
120. Goodman JI. Femoral neuropathy in relation to diabetes mellitus: Report of 17 cases. Diabetes 1954; 3:266.
121. Gosselin S, Kyle RA, Dyck PJ. Neuropathy associated with monoclonal gammopathies of undetermined significance. Ann Neurol 1991; 30:54.
122. Grabias S. Current concepts review: The treatment of spinal stenosis. J Bone Joint Surg 1980; 62:308.
123. Graham E, Holland A, Avery A, et al. Prognosis in giant-cell arteritis. BMJ 1981; 282:269.
124. Grant IA, Hunder GG, Homburger HA, et al. Peripheral neuropathy associated with sicca complex. Neurology 1997; 48:855.
125. Grant R, Papadopoulos SM, Greenberg HS. Metastatic epidural spinal cord compression. Neurol Clin 1991; 9:825.
126. Graus F, Elkon KB, Cordon-Cardo C, et al. Sensory neuronopathy and small cell lung cancer: Antineuronal antibody that also reacts with the tumor. Am J Med 1986; 80:45.
127. Gray RS, Clarke BF. Primary autoimmune diabetes mellitus (letter). BMJ 1978; 2:1715.
128. Green WR, Hackett ER, Schlezinger NS. Neuro-ophthalmologic evaluation of oculomotor nerve paralysis. Arch Ophthalmol 1964; 72:154.
129. Griffin JW, Cornblath DR, Alexander E, et al. Ataxic sensory neuropathy and dorsal root ganglionitis associated with Sjögren's syndrome. Ann Neurol 1990; 27:304.
130. Grossman SA, Moynihan TJ. Neoplastic meningitis. Neurol Clin 1991; 9:843.
131. Gupta SK, Helal BH, Kiely P. The prognosis in zoster paralysis. J Bone Joint Surg 1969; 51:593.
132. Gutmann L, et al. Dapsone motor neuropathy: An axonal disease. Neurology 1976; 26:514.
133. Hardcastle JD. Acute non-tuberculous psoas abscess: Report of 10 cases and review of the literature. Br J Surg 1970; 57:103.
134. Harding AE, Muller DP, Thomas PK, et al. Spinocerebellar degeneration secondary to chronic intestinal malabsorption: A vitamin E deficiency syndrome. Ann Neurol 1982; 12:419.
135. Hayasaka K, Himoro M, Sato W, et al. Charcot-Marie-Tooth neuropathy type 1B is associated with mutations of the myelin P0 gene. Nat Genet 1993; 5:31.
136. Heidbreder E, Schafferhans K, Heidland A. Autonomic neuropathy in chronic renal insufficiency: Comparative analysis of diabetic and nondiabetic patients. Nephron 1985; 41:50.
137. Hicks EP. Hereditary perforating ulcer of the foot. Lancet 1922; 1:319.
138. Hirschmann JV. Herpes zoster. Semin Neurol 1992; 12:322.
139. Horwich MS, Cho L, Porro RS, et al. Subacute sensory neuropathy: A remote effect of carcinoma. Ann Neurol 1977; 2:7.
140. Hunder GG, Arend WP, Bloch DA, et al. The American College of Rheumatology 1990 criteria for the classification of vasculitis: Introduction. Arthritis Rheum 1990; 33:1065.
141. Hunt WE, Meagher JN, LeFever HE. Painful ophthalmoplegia: Its relation to indolent inflammation of the cavernous sinus. Neurology 1961; 11:56.
141a. Ives ER. Protein content in the cerebrospinal fluid of diabetic patients. Bull Los Angeles Neurol Soc 1957; 22:95–111.
142. Iyer VG, Garretson HD, Byrd RP, et al. Localized hypertrophic involving the tibial nerve. Neurosurgery 1988; 23:218.
143. Jaeckle KA. Nerve plexus metastases. Neurol Clin 1991; 9:857.
144. Jaeckle KA, Young DF, Foley KM. The natural history of lumbosacral plexopathy in cancer. Neurology 1985; 35:8.
145. Jammes JL. The autonomic nervous system in peroneal muscular atrophy. Arch Neurol 1972; 27:213.
146. Jebsen RH, Tenckhoff H, Honet JC. Natural history of uremic polyneuropathy and effects of dialysis. N Engl J Med 1967; 277:327.
147. Jennekens FG, Mees EJ, van der Most van Spijk D. Clinical aspects of uremic polyneuropathy. Nephron 1971; 8:414.
148. Jorring K. Osteoarthritis of the hip: Epidemiology and clinical role. Acta Orthop Scand 1980; 51:523.
149. Kaku DA, So YT. Acute femoral neuropathy and iliopsoas infarction in intravenous drug abusers. Neurology 1990; 40:1317.
150. Katrak SM, Pollock M, O'Brien CP, et al. Clinical and morphological features of gold neuropathy. Brain 1980; 103:671.
151. Katz JN, Dalgas M, Stucki G, et al. Diagnosis of lumbar spinal stenosis. Rheum Dis Clin North Am 1994; 20:471.
152. Kelly JJ, Adelman LS, Berkman E, et al. Polyneuropathies associated with IgM monoclonal gammopathies. Arch Neurol 1988; 45:1355.

153. Kelly JJ Jr, Kyle RA, Miles JM, et al. Osteosclerotic myeloma and peripheral neuropathy. Neurology 1983; 33:202.

154. Kelly JJ Jr, Kyle RA, O'Brien PC, et al. The natural history of peripheral neuropathy in primary systemic amyloidosis. Ann Neurol 1979; 6:1.

155. Kemble F. Conduction in the normal adult median nerve: The different effect of aging in men and women. Electromyogr Clin Neurophysiol 1967; 7:275.

156. Kersh ES, Kronfield SJ, Unger A, et al. Autonomic insufficiency in uremia as a cause of hemodialysis-induced hypotension. N Engl J Med 1974; 290:650.

157. Khella SL, Frost S, Hermann GA, et al. Hepatitis C infection, cryoglobulinemia, and vasculitis neuropathy: Treatment with interferon alfa: Case report and literature review. Neurology 1995; 45:407.

158. Kieburtz KD, Seidlin M, Lambert JS, et al. Extended follow-up of peripheral neuropathy in patients with AIDS and AIDS-related complex treated with dideoxyinosine. J Acquir Immune Defic Syndr 1992; 5:60.

159. Kikta DG, Breuer AC, Wilbourn AJ. Thoracic root pain in diabetes: The spectrum of clinical and electromyographic findings. Ann Neurol 1982; 11:80.

160. Kimmel DW, O'Neill BP, Lennon VA. Subacute sensory neuronopathy associated with small cell lung carcinoma: Diagnosis aided by autoimmune serology. Mayo Clin Proc 1988; 63:29.

161. Kissel JT, Burde RM, Klingele TG, et al. Pupil-sparing oculomotor palsies with internal carotid-posterior communicating artery aneurysms. Ann Neurol 1983; 13:149.

162. Kissel JT, Slivka AP, Warmolts JR, et al. The clinical spectrum of necrotizing angiopathy of the peripheral nervous system. Ann Neurol 1985; 18:251.

163. Kuncl RW, Duncan G, Watson D, et al. Colchicine myopathy and neuropathy. N Engl J Med 1987; 316:1562.

164. Kyle RA, Eilers SG, Linscheid RL, et al. Amyloid localized to tenosynovium at carpal tunnel release: Natural history of 124 cases (Review). Am J Clin Pathol 1989; 91:393.

165. Kyle RA, Finkelstein S, Elveback LR, et al. Incidence of monoclonal proteins in a Minnesota community with a cluster of multiple myeloma. Blood 1972; 40:719.

166. Kyle RA, Greipp PR. Amyloidosis: Clinical and laboratory features in 229 cases. Mayo Clin Proc 1983; 58:665.

167. La Rocca RV, Meer J, Gilliatt RW, et al. Suramin-induced polyneuropathy. Neurology 1990; 40:954.

168. Laurent LE. Femoral nerve compression syndrome with paresis of the quadriceps muscle caused by radiotherapy of malignant tumors: A report of four cases. Acta Orthop Scand 1975; 46:804.

169. LeQuesne PM, McLeod JG. Peripheral neuropathy following a single exposure to arsenic: Clinical course in four patients with electrophysiological and histological studies. J Neurol Sci 1977; 32:437.

170. Lefvert AK, Bergstrom K, Matell G, et al. Determination of acetylcholine receptor antibody in myasthenia gravis: Clinical usefulness and pathogenetic implications. J Neurol Neurosurg Psychiatry 1978; 41:394.

171. Lennon VA. Paraneoplastic autoantibodies: The case for a descriptive generic nomenclature (Review). Neurology 1994; 44:2236.

172. Lennon VA, Howard FM. Serologic diagnosis of myasthenia gravis. In Nakamura R (ed): Clinical Laboratory Molecular Analysis. Orlando, Grune & Stratton, 1985, p 29.

173. Lipson SJ. Clinical diagnosis. Semin Spine Surg 1989; 1:143.

174. Lipton RB, Apfel SC, Dutcher JP, et al. Taxol produces a predominantly sensory neuropathy. Neurology 1989; 39:368.

175. Llewelyn JG, Thomas PK, Gilbey SG, et al. Pattern of myelinated fibre loss in the sural nerve in neuropathy related to type 1 (insulin-dependent) diabetes. Diabetologia 1988; 31:162.

176. Lombard J, Levin IH, Weiner WJ. Arsenic intoxication in cocaine abuse (letter). N Engl J Med 1989; 320:869.

177. Longstreth GF, Newcomer AD. Abdominal pain caused by diabetic radiculopathy. Ann Intern Med 1977; 86:166.

178. Loughridge LW. Peripheral neuropathy due to nitrofurantoin. Lancet 1962; 1:1133.

179. Love JG, Walsh MN. Protruded intervertebral disks. JAMA 1938; 111:396.

180. Lovelace RE, Horwitz SJ. Peripheral neuropathy in long-term diphenylhydantoin therapy. Arch Neurol 1968; 18:69.

181. Lupski JR, de Oca-Luna RM, Slaugenhaupt S, et al. DNA duplication associated with Charcot-Marie-Tooth disease type 1A. Cell 1991; 66:219.

182. Mant MJ, O'Brien BD, Thong KL, et al. Hemorrhagic complications of heparin therapy. Lancet 1977; 1:1133.

183. Mathias CJ, Naik RB, Warren DJ, et al. Autonomic neuropathy (letter). Arch Intern Med 1983; 143:1635.

184. McGonigle RJ, Bewick M, Weston MJ, et al. Progressive, predominantly motor, uremic neuropathy. Acta Neurol Scand 1985; 71:379.

185. Meier C, Bischoff A. Polyneuropathy in hypothyroidism: Clinical and nerve biopsy study of 4 cases. J Neurol 1977; 215:103.

186. Meretoja J. Familial systemic paramyloidosis with lattice dystrophy of the cornea, progressive cranial neuropathy, skin changes, and various internal symptoms: A previously unrecognized heritable syndrome. Ann Clin Res 1969; 1:314.

187. Mincu I. Micro- and macroangiopathies and other chronic degenerative complications in newly detected diabetes mellitus. Medecine Interne 1980; 18:155.

188. Moder KG. Use and interpretation of rhematologic tests: A guide for clinicians. Mayo Clin Proc 1996; 71:391.

189. Modic MT, Masaryk T, Boumphrey F, et al. Lumbar herniated disk disease and canal stenosis: Prospective evaluation by surface coil MR, CT, and myelography. AJR 1986; 147:757.

190. Muller DP, Lloyd JK, Wolff OH. Vitamin E and neurological function. Lancet 1983; 1:225.

191. Nadeau SE, Trobe JD. Pupil sparing in oculomotor palsy: A brief review. Ann Neurol 1983; 13:143.

192. Neu I, Rodiek S. Significance of diabetes mellitus in the activation of the varicella zoster virus. MMWR 1977; 119:543.

193. Nickel SN, Frame B. Neurologic manifestations of myxedema. Neurology 1958; 8:511.

194. Nielsen VK. The peripheral nerve function in chronic renal failure. I: Clinical symptoms and signs. Acta Med Scand 1971; 190:105.

195. Nielsen VK. The peripheral nerve function in chronic renal failure. Acta Med Scand 1972; 191:287.

196. Nielsen VK. The peripheral nerve function in chronic renal failure. VI: The relationship between sensory and motor nerve conduction and kidney function, azotemia, age, sex, and clinical neuropathy. Acta Med Scand 1973; 194:455.

197. Nielsen VK. The peripheral nerve function in chronic

renal failure. VII: Longitudinal course during terminal renal failure and regular hemodialysis. Acta Med Scand 1974; 195:155.

198. Nielsen VK, Winkel P. The peripheral nerve function in chronic renal failure. 3: A multivariate statistical analysis of factors presumed to affect the development of clinical neuropathy. Acta Med Scand 1971; 190:119.

199. Nugent GR, Sprinkle P, Bloor BM. Sphenoid sinus mucoceles. J Neurosurg 1970; 32:443.

200. Nurmikko T. Clinical features and pathophysiologic mechanisms of postherpetic neuralgia. Neurology 1995; 45:S54.

201. Nurmikko T, Bowsher D. Somatosensory findings in postherpetic neuralgia. J Neurol Neurosurg Psychiatry 1990; 53:135.

202. O'Connor PS, Tredici TJ, Green RP. Pupil-sparing third nerve palsies caused by aneurysm (letter). Am J Ophthalmol 1983; 95:395.

203. Ochoa J. Isoniazid neuropathy in man: Quantitative electron microscope study. Brain 1970; 93:831.

204. Ohnishi A, Dyck PJ. Loss of small peripheral sensory neurons in Fabry disease: Histologic and morphometric evaluation of cutaneous nerves, spinal ganglia, and posterior columns. Arch Neurol 1974; 31:120.

205. Otani K, Yoshida M, Fujii E, et al. Thoracic disc herniation: Surgical treatment in 23 patients. Spine 1988; 13:1262.

206. Palumbo PJ, Elveback LR, Whisnant JP. Neurologic complications of diabetes mellitus: Transient ischemic attack, stroke, and peripheral neuropathy. Adv Neurol 1978; 19:593.

207. Palumbo PJ, Elveback LR, Whisnant JP. Neurologic complications of diabetes mellitus: Transient ischemic attack, stroke, and peripheral neuropathy. In Schoenberg BS (ed): Advances in Neurology. Neuroepidemiology: A Tribute to Bruce Schoenberg. New York, Raven Press, 1978, vol 19, p 593.

208. Panas P. Sur une cause peu connue de paralysie du nerf cubital. Arch Gen de Med 1878; 2:5.

209. Patchell RA, Posner JB. Neurologic complications of systemic cancer. Neurol Clin 1985; 3:729.

210. Pirart J. Diabetes mellitus and its degenerative complications: A prospective study of 4,400 patients observed between 1947 and 1973. Diabetes Care 1978; 1:168.

211. Pleatman CW, Lukin RR. Lumbar spinal stenosis. Semin Roentgenol 1988; 23:106.

212. Pollard JD, McLeod JG, Honnibal TG, et al. Hypothyroid polyneuropathy: Clinical, electrophysiological and nerve biopsy findings in two cases. J Neurol Sci 1982; 53:461.

213. Post MJ, Mendez DR, Kline LB, et al. Metastatic disease to the cavernous sinus: Clinical syndrome and CT diagnosis. J Comput Assist Tomogr 1985; 9:115.

214. Preswick G, Jeremy D. Subclinical polyneuropathy in renal insufficiency. Lancet 1964; 2:731.

215. Purnell DC. Carpal-tunnel syndrome associated with myxedema. Arch Intern Med 1961; 108:151.

216. Raff MC, Asbury AK. Ischemic mononeuropathy and mononeuropathy multiplex in diabetes mellitus. N Engl J Med 1968; 279:17.

217. Ragozinno MW, Melton LJ, Kurland LT. Herpes zoster and diabetes mellitus: An epidemiological investigation. J Chronic Dis 1983; 36:501.

218. Ragozzino MW, Melton LJ III, Kurland LT, et al. Population-based study of herpes zoster and its sequelae. Medicine (Baltimore) 1982; 61:310.

219. Rangel-Guerra R, Martinez HR, Saenz C. Mucormycosis: Report of 11 cases. Arch Neurol 1985; 42:578.

220. Razzuk MA, Linton RR, Darling RC. Femoral neuropathy secondary to ruptured abdominal aortic aneurysms with false aneurysms. JAMA 1967; 201:817.

221. Reik L. Borrelia burgdorferi infection: A neurologist's perspective. Ann NY Acad Sci 1988; 539:1.

222. Rivner MH, Swift TR, Crout BO, et al. Toward more rational nerve conduction interpretations: The effect of height. Muscle Nerve 1990; 13(3):232.

223. Roa BB, Garcia CA, Suter U, et al. Charcot-Marie-Tooth disease type 1A: Association with a spontaneous point mutation in the PMP22 gene. N Engl J Med 1993; 329:96.

224. Roelofs RI, Hrushesky W, Rogin J, et al. Peripheral sensory neuropathy and cisplatin chemotherapy. Neurology 1984; 34:934.

225. Roos D. Neurological complications in patients with impaired vitamin B12 absorption following partial gastrectomy. Acta Neurol Scand 1978; 69:1.

226. Rucker CW. The causes of paralysis of the third, fourth, and sixth cranial nerves. Am J Ophthalmol 1966; 61:1293.

227. Rush JA, Younge BR. Paralysis of cranial nerves III, IV and VI: Cause and prognosis in 1,000 cases. Arch Ophthalmol 1981; 99:76.

228. Russell T. Thoracic intervertebral disc protrusion: Experience of 67 cases and review of the literature. Br J Neurosurg 1989; 3:153.

229. Rusthoven JJ, Ahlgren P, Elhakim T, et al. Varicella-zoster infection in adult cancer patients: A population study. Arch Intern Med 1988; 148:1561.

230. Sagel SS, Siegel MJ, Stanley RJ, et al. Detection of retroperitoneal hemorrhage by computed tomography. AJR 1977; 129:403.

231. Said G, Lacroix-Ciaudo C, Fugimura H, et al. The peripheral neuropathy of necrotizing arteritis: A clinico-pathological study. Ann Neurol 1988; 23:461.

232. Said G, Slama G, Salva J. Progressive centripetal degeneration of axons in small fibre diabetic polyneuropathy. Brain 1983; 106:791.

233. Salter RB. Textbook of Disorders and Injuries of the Musculoskeletal System. Baltimore, Williams & Wilkins, 1983, p 228.

234. Sanders DB, Howard JF, Massey JM. Seronegative myasthenia gravis (abstract). Ann Neurol 1987; 22:126.

235. Schaumburg H, Kaplan J, Windebank A, et al. Sensory neuropathy from pyridoxine abuse: A new megavitamin syndrome. N Engl J Med 1983; 309:445.

236. Schnebel B, Kingston S, Watkins R, et al. Comparison of MRI to contrast CT in the diagnosis of spinal stenosis. Spine 1989; 14:332.

237. Schon L, Zuckerman JD. Hip pain in the elderly: Evaluation and diagnosis. Geriatrics 1988; 43:48.

238. Sheth KJ, Swick HM. Peripheral nerve conduction in Fabry disease. Ann Neurol 1980; 7:319.

239. Simeone FA, Rothman RH. Clinical usefulness of CT scanning in the diagnosis and treatment of lumbar spine disease. Radiol Clin North Am 1983; 21:197.

240. Singounas EG, Kypriades EM, Kellerman AJ, et al. Thoracic disc herniation: Analysis of 14 cases and review of the literature. Acta Neurochir 1992; 116:49.

241. Smith BE. Inflammatory sensory polyganglionopathies (Review). Neurol Clin 1992; 10:735.

242. Smith JL, Taxdal DS. Painful ophthalmoplegia: The Tolosa-Hunt syndrome. Am J Ophthalmol 1961; 61:1466.

243. Solders G, Persson A, Gutierrez A. Autonomic dysfunction in non-diabetic terminal uremia. Acta Neurol Scand 1985; 71:321.

244. Specks U, Wheatley CL, McDonald TJ, et al. Anticytoplasmic autoantibodies in the diagnosis and follow-up of Wegener's granulomatosis. Mayo Clin Proc 1989; 64:28.

245. Spies TD, Vilter RW, Ashe WF. Pellagra, beriberi and riboflavin deficiency in human beings. JAMA 1939; 113:931.

246. Stark RJ, Henson RA, Evans SJ. Spinal metastases: A retrospective survey from a general hospital. Brain 1982; 105:189.

247. Stetson DS, Albers JW, Silverstein BA, et al. Effects of age, sex, and anthropometric factors on nerve conduction measures. Muscle Nerve 1992; 15(10):1095.

248. Stewart JD. Diabetic truncal neuropathy: Topography of the sensory deficit. Ann Neurol 1989; 25:233.

249. Stewart PM, McIntyre MA, Edwards CR. The endocrinopathy of POEMS syndrome. Scott Med J 1989; 34:520.

250. Streib EW, Sun SF, Paustian FF, et al. Diabetic thoracic radiculopathy: Electrodiagnostic study. Muscle Nerve 1986; 9:548.

251. Stubgen JP. Neuromuscular disorders in systemic malignancy and its treatment. Muscle Nerve 1995; 18:636.

252. Sun SF, Streib EW. Diabetic thoracoabdominal neuropathy: Clinical and electrodiagnostic features. Ann Neurol 1981; 9:75.

253. Tackmann W, Kaeser HE, Magun HG. Comparison of orthodromic and antidromic sensory nerve conduction velocity measurements in the carpal tunnel syndrome. J Neurol 1981; 224:257.

254. Takatsuki K, Sanada I. Plasma cell dyscrasia with polyneuropathy and endocrine disorder: Clinical and laboratory features of 109 reported cases. Jpn J Clin Oncol 1983; 13:543.

255. Theodore WH, Gendelman S. Meningeal carcinomatosis. Arch Neurol 1981; 38:696.

256. Thevenard A. L'acropathie ulcero-mutilante familiale. Acta Neurol Belg 1953; 53:1.

257. Thomas JE, Cascino TL, Earle JD. Differential diagnosis between radiation and tumor plexopathy of the pelvis. Neurology 1985; 35:1.

258. Thomas JE, Howard FM Jr. Segmental zoster paresis: A disease profile. Neurology 1972; 22:459.

259. Thomas JE, Yoss RE. The paresellar syndrome: Problems in determining etiology. Mayo Clin Proc 1970; 45:617.

260. Thomas PK. Screening for peripheral neuropathy in patients treated by chronic hemodialysis. Muscle Nerve 1978; 196:396.

261. Thomas PK, Hollinrake K, Lascelles RG, et al. The polyneuropathy of chronic renal failure. Brain 1971; 94:761.

262. Thomas PK, Lascelles RG. The pathology of diabetic neuropathy. Q J Med 1966; 35:480.

263. Timperley WR, Boulton AJM, Davies-Jones GAB, et al. Small vessel disease in progressive diabetic neuropathy associated with good metabolic control. J Clin Pathol 1985; 38:1030.

264. Tolosa EJ. Periarteritic lesions of the carotid siphon with the clinical features of a carotid infraclinoid aneurysm. J Neurol Neurosurg Psychiatry 1961; 11:56.

265. Toole JF, Parrish ML. Nitrofurantoin polyneuropathy. Neurology 1973; 23:554.

266. Turner JA, Ersek M, Herron L, et al. Surgery for lumbar spinal stenosis: Attempted meta-analysis of the literature. Spine 1992; 17:1.

267. Tyler HR. Neurologic disorders in renal failure (Review). Am J Med 1968; 44:734.

268. Uden A, Johnsson KE, Jonsson K, et al. Myelography in the elderly and the diagnosis of spinal stenosis. Spine 1985; 10:171.

269. Van Epps C, Kerr HD. Familial lumbosacral syringomyelia. Radiology 1940; 160:173.

270. Verbiest H. Pathomorphologic aspects of developmental lumbar stenosis. Orthop Clin North Am 1975; 6:177.

271. Victor M. Polyneuropathy due to nutritional deficiency and alcoholism. *In* Dyck PJ, Thomas PK, Lambert EH, et al (eds): Peripheral Neuropathy. Philadelphia, WB Saunders, 1984, p 1899.

272. Victor M, Adams RD. On the etiology of the alcoholic neurologic diseases with special reference to the role of nutrition. Am J Clin Nutr 1961; 9:379.

273. Walsh JC. The neuropathy of multiple myeloma: An electrophysiological and histochemical study. Arch Neurol 1971; 25:404.

274. Walsh JC, McLeod JG. Alcoholic neuropathy: An electrophysiological and histological study. J Neurol Sci 1970; 10:457.

275. Warnock LG. Transketolase activity of blood hemolysate, a useful index for diagnosing thiamine deficiency. Clin Chem 1975; 21:432.

276. Wasserstrom WR, Glass JP, Posner JB. Diagnosis and treatment of leptomeningeal metastases from solid tumors: Experience with 90 patients. Cancer 1982; 49:759.

277. Wilberger JE Jr. Lumbosacral radiculopathy secondary to abdominal aortic aneurysms: Report of three cases. J Neurosurg 1983; 58:965.

278. Wilson MG, Poss R. Osteoarthritis of the hip. *In* Moskowitz RW, Howell DS, Goldberg VM, et al (eds): Osteoarthritis: Diagnosis and Medical/Surgical Management. Philadelphia, WB Saunders, 1992, p 621.

279. Windebank AJ, Blexrud MD, Dyck PJ, et al. The syndrome of acute sensory neuropathy: Clinical features and electrophysiologic and pathologic changes. Neurology 1990; 40:584.

280. Young MR, Norris JW. Femoral neuropathy during anticoagulant therapy. Neurology 1976; 26:1173.

281. Yussen PS, Swartz JD. The acute lumbar disc herniation: Imaging diagnosis. Semin Ultrasound CT MR 1993; 14:389.

Section V
Hypoglycemic Polyneuropathy

Chapter **32**

Hypoglycemic Polyneuropathy

Shunji Yasaki • *Johannes Jakobsen* • *Peter James Dyck*

INTRODUCTION

Distal symmetrical polyneuropathy of the extremities may develop in patients with insulinoma. This has been attributed to hypoglycemia because the neuropathy improves after tumor removal. Sensorimotor symptoms in the distal extremities also occurs with insulin shock therapy, and the putative mechanism is hypoglycemia. Further support for the idea that hypoglycemia can induce neuropathy comes from the experimental observation that multiple injections of exogenous insulin result in peripheral nerve injury. The suggestion has been made that strict glycemic control in humans, to the degree that it causes hypoglycemic episodes, may relate to the development of painful diabetic neuropathy. This explanation gains support from the observation that insulin-treated diabetic animals had higher frequencies of fiber degeneration than did untreated diabetic animals and controls. Because hypoglycemia occurs commonly among diabetics, especially in patients treated with insulin or with oral hypoglycemic agents, and because hypoglycemic unawareness develops in some diabetic patients,[10] hypoglycemia may be a risk factor for diabetic neuropathy. Severe hypoglycemia may also impair central nervous system function and structure.

In animal experiments, insulin-induced hypoglycemia may cause axonal nerve fiber degeneration, but to do so it must be severe (1.5 mmol/L) and of long duration (12 hours).[55] Axonal degeneration is the characteristic fiber alteration, and it predominates in central fascicular regions of peripheral nerves. Prolonged intermittent severe hypoglycemia may cause cell body changes of anterior horns of spinal cord and dorsal root ganglia as well as damage of nerve fibers. Decreased fast anterograde axonal transport, reduced nerve blood flow, and generalized deficiency of energy substrate in nerves may contribute to produce the neuropathy.

HISTORY

Prolonged severe hypoglycemia causes brain damage and rarely also causes damage of the peripheral nervous system in humans.[25] The pathogenesis of hypoglycemic neuropathy needs further clarification. When it was discovered in 1921 that insulin therapy could rescue patients from diabetic coma, it became clear that excessive insulin could produce severe cerebral dysfunction.[3, 12] Enthusiasm for the benefits of insulin had to be balanced against the central nervous system injury caused by insulin-induced hypoglycemia.[53]

During the following years, it was observed that paresthesias in fingers and toes, which might be symptoms of a peripheral neuropathy, could also follow and were perhaps attributable to onset of insulin therapy or insulin coma.[8, 53, 56] These reports were anecdotal without clarification of underlying mechanisms.

When the first large studies of peripheral neuropathy in diabetes mellitus (DM) appeared in the middle decades of the 20th century, a new and vaguely defined category of diabetic neuropathy was introduced, a so-called insulin neuritis. Neuropathic symptoms developed soon after institution of insulin therapy in 8 of 98 of Jordan's,[27] 20 of 125 of Rundles',[43] and 8 of 150 of Martin's[32] patients with DM. In addition to the effect of hypoglycemia, a toxic effect of insulin had to be considered. Rundles' writing about the treatment of insulin neuritis states that "persistence in the use of insulin will lead to a good clinical result, if good diabetic regulation is thereby obtained."

Thus, the term *insulin neuritis* gained some popularity and even appeared in textbooks. Recently, the existence of this entity was reemphasized; nerve fiber degeneration apparently unrelated to hypoglycemia was observed in diabetic rats treated with insulin for a few weeks.[44] However, we have not found credible scientific evidence that insulin itself induces peripheral polyneuropathy apart from its effect on hypoglycemia in conventionally treated diabetic patients. It is conceivable, however, that repeated bouts of hypoglycemia could induce or worsen diabetic polyneuropathy.

In 1946, Silfveskiöild described two patients with insulinoma who developed paresis of the hands and feet, atrophy of the hand muscles, and absence of ankle reflexes after hypoglycemic attacks.[47] He called this neuropathy *polyneuritis hypoglycemia*. In 1956, Mulder and colleagues used the term *hyperinsulin neuropathy* for the syndrome of distal muscular atrophy and paresthesias associated with hypoglycemia in patients with pancreatic adenoma.[35] Danta called the condition *hypoglycemic peripheral neuropathy*, and reported two patients with benign islet cell adenoma of the pancreas who developed tingling and numbness in hands and forearms and around the mouth and tongue, weakness and wasting of hands and legs (small muscles), and absent tendon reflexes.[11]

It has been shown experimentally that severe hypoglycemia can induce a peripheral neuropathy in nondiabetic rats.[45, 55]

CLINICAL FEATURES

Neuromuscular Symptoms Associated With Pancreatic Islet Cell Tumors

Most of our knowledge of neuromuscular syndromes associated with hypoglycemia is from study of patients with pancreatic islet adenomas or adenocarcinomas. These syndromes appear to be associated with recurrent or severe hypoglycemic episodes.

Since 1928, among the thousands of patients treated for insulinoma, only 32 cases with peripheral neuropathy have been reported. Danta reviewed 22 reported cases (2 of his own cases) of peripheral neurologic symptoms in association with spontaneous hypoglycemia.[11] A 1982 literature review included 29 cases.[25] Since then, 4 additional cases have been described.[9, 10, 26, 50] A symmetrical predominantly motor polyneuropathy was associated with hypoglycemia in a young woman with type I multiple endocrine neoplasia syndrome with multiple insulinomas and parathyroid adenomas.[9] After surgical removal of the insulinomas, the clinical condition improved.[9]

A characteristic and easily recognizable clinical sign of hypoglycemic neuropathy is atrophy of the small muscles of the hand. In photographs of hands, thenar, hypothenar, and interosseous atrophy of the hands was illustrated in several reports.[10, 11, 20]

The prominence of hand atrophy has led some to think that hypoglycemic neuropathy is predominantly motor.[22] On the other hand, initial manifestations are usually sensory.[6, 35] Early complaints are burning and tingling sensations in hands and feet.[35] Later, these painful paresthesias are accompanied by distal and symmetric weakness and wasting of the distal muscles of the upper and lower extremities.[35] The frequency of symptoms and clinical signs of neuropathy are given in Table 32.1.[24] The lower frequency of sensory rather than of motor symptoms might be ascribed to the severity of cerebral involvement, which could lead to underreporting of sensory disturbances.[35]

After removal of the insulinoma, neuromuscular symptoms and signs usually improve, but muscular atrophy or paresthesias may persist.[9, 50]

Electrophysiologic and Pathologic Findings in Patients With Insulinomas

Electromyographic studies were performed in 12 of the reported 32 cases, and denervation was found in all.[9, 25, 50] Nerve conduction velocities were within normal limits in three patients,[9, 11, 29] slightly abnormal in two,[20, 50] and moderately abnormal in three.[11, 25, 26] The muscle action potential amplitudes of motor nerves were reduced. Sensory nerve action potentials were absent.[50] F wave latencies of upper and lower limb muscles were either normal or slightly prolonged.[9, 25, 50] The electrophysiologic features were interpreted as indicating axonal sensorimotor neuropathy. The process was thought to be an axonopathy or a neuronopathy.

TABLE 32.1   INCIDENCE OF SYMPTOMS AND SIGNS OF A NEUROMUSCULAR DISORDER ASSOCIATED WITH INSULINOMA*

Symptom or Sign	No. of Patients Affected (%)
Early complaints of paresthesias	19 (59.4)
Muscular weakness and atrophy	29 (90.6)
"Glove and stocking" loss of sensation	7 (21.9)
Sensory impairment	9 (28.1)
Absent or diminished tendon reflexes	16 (50)

*In 32 cases in the literature.[9, 25, 26, 50]

After removal of the insulinoma, some degree of recovery occurred. This improvement was interpreted as favoring a peripheral nerve locus by one group[20] and an anterior horn cell locus by another group.[29] The finding of only minor alterations of conduction velocity and large-amplitude motor unit potentials with recovery is in keeping with a proximal lesion, for example, anterior horn cells.[20]

There are only two reports of histologic findings in the spinal cords of patients with insulinomas.[34, 51] In the first case, loss of anterior horn cells was observed, but dorsal root ganglia and peripheral nerves appeared normal.[34] In the second case, in which muscular atrophy of hands and legs had been observed in a patient with a pancreatic tumor, hypoglycemia was never demonstrated, but anterior horn cells were decreased and the ulnar nerve was partially demyelinated (loss of myelinated fibers).[51]

In recent reports, sural nerve biopsies were studied in patients with a typical insulinoma syndrome.[25, 50] Axonal degeneration was recognized in all cases. Myelinated nerve fiber loss exceeded 30%, no signs of segmental demyelination or remyelination were recognized in the first biopsied patient, and it was concluded that the condition was a peripheral neuropathy caused by axonal injury.[25]

The histologic studies in the muscles showed fiber atrophy indicative of denervation.[9, 23, 35]

The pathologic alterations in hypoglycemic neuropathy have been similar to that in diabetic polyneuropathy, but the microvasculopathy was not found in the former.

Neuromuscular Symptoms After Insulin Shock Therapy

Because insulin shock therapy was introduced for treatment of psychiatric conditions in 1933, some degree of brain damage has been reported.

Despite the extensive use of insulin coma therapy in psychiatric patients, only a few reports of neuromuscular complications have been reported. Transient painful paresthesias in hands and feet as well as sensory impairment in the fingers were observed after a series of shocks in two patients.[7] In a consecutive series of 103 patients, 10 complained of numbness and tingling in hands and feet, with objective loss of sensation in only one case.[49] In a prospective study of 24 young schizophrenic patients before and after an average of 40 treatments, 13 patients experienced paresthesias in fingers and toes, 7 showed unsteady gait, 2 had a stocking-type superficial hypalgesia, and 2 demonstrated decreased strength during a dynamometer performance.[58] The patients were specifically asked about abnormal cutaneous sensations and blurring of vision, which may have led patients to report more or less severe symptoms than actually occurred. Among the patients with paresthesias, four felt peculiar sensations over the chest and upper part of the back and experienced paresthesias in the region of the face, particularly of the nose. This distribution of neurologic symptoms is typical of a peripheral neuropathy.

All in all, studies in humans of hypoglycemia induced by insulinomas or insulin shocks have not convincingly demonstrated the occurrence of peripheral neuropathy. The symptomatology of these patients, however, suggests it.

ANIMAL EXPERIMENTS
Nondiabetic Animals

The physiologic, histopathologic, and biochemical alterations in insulin-induced hypoglycemic neuropathy have been studied in nondiabetic animals. Recent studies focused on the change of axonal transport, spatiotemporal distribution of fiber degeneration in the peripheral nerve and spinal cord, deranged nerve energy metabolism, and change of nerve blood flow in acute hypoglycemia.

AXONAL TRANSPORT IN ACUTE HYPOGLYCEMIC NEUROPATHY

Sidenius and Jakobsen found that the amount of material transported in the nerve was decreased as compared with the amount in the sensory ganglion after a few hours of insulin-induced acute hypoglycemia in rats.[46] When the rats were exposed to sustained hypoglycemia for 3 days before the transport experiment, no changes in axonal transport occurred. From these results, they considered that the metabolism of peripheral nerve, similar to the brain during starvation studies, can adapt to glucose deprivation. This study also showed that hypoglycemia rather than hyperinsulinism was responsible for the fast anterograde axonal transport abnormality.[46]

DURATION AND SEVERITY OF HYPOGLYCEMIA NEEDED TO INDUCE NEUROPATHY

The least degree and duration of hypoglycemia needed to induce nerve fiber degeneration in experimental animals given repeated and excessive amounts of insulin over time has been difficult to determine. Furthermore, it is uncertain whether nerve damage is caused by mechanisms other than hypoglycemia. Sidenius and Jakobsen[45] demonstrated sciatic nerve fiber degeneration in male Wistar rats in which hypoglycemia (blood glucose, 2.5 mmol/L) was induced by giving multiple subcutaneous injections of insulin for a period of 72 hours. Other investigators reported that a period of 4 weeks of hypoglycemia (blood glucose, 2.0 mmol/L) was needed to induce tibial nerve fiber degeneration in male Sprague-Dawley rats.[41] Because multiple injections of insulin over the course of several days were used, it was not possible to have close surveillance of the glycemic level, behavior, partial pressure of oxygen, partial pressure of carbon dioxide, temperature, and metabolic status to judge the duration and severity of hypoglycemia needed to produce neuropathy and to ensure that it was not caused by another mechanism, such as hypoxia. Whether anemia, hypoxia,[5] hypothermia,[28, 52] or altered rheological abnormalities[14, 21] induced by hypoglycemia might be sufficiently severe to induce nerve damage was at least a theoretical possibility.

In an experimental model of hypoglycemic neuropathy, Yasaki and Dyck achieved reproducible levels of hypoglycemia within a single period sufficient to induce various severities of neuropathy without inducing seizures or death.[55] In 23 rats subjected to severe and sustained hypoglycemic (1.4 ± 0.2 mmol/L, mean SEM) for various times up to 11 hours, the frequency of axonal degeneration of teased myelinated fibers (0 to 1%) was not different from that of controls.[55] In nine young rats made severely hypoglycemic (1.4 ± 0.2 mmol/L) for various times for 12 or more hours, the frequency of fiber degeneration was significantly higher than in controls ($P<0.01$) and increased to as high as 26% (Figs. 32.1 and 32.2).[55] By contrast, in five older rats made hypoglycemic (1.5 ± 0.1 mmol/L) for various times for 12 or more hours, the frequency of fiber degeneration was not different from that of controls.[55] Age of rats (young) and duration and severity of hypoglycemia were risk factors for fiber degeneration. General anesthesia, mechanical ventilation, and maintenance of normal partial pressure of oxygen, partial pressure of carbon dioxide, temperature, and fluid balance were needed to perform this study and to isolate the factor of hypoglycemia.[55]

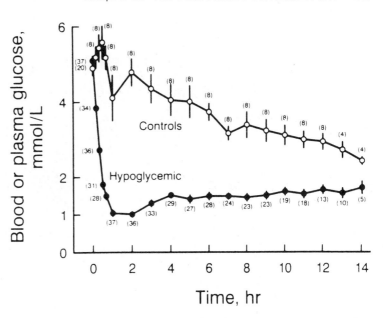

■ **Figure 32.1** The average plasma glucose values of rats that survived in the hypoglycemic group *(closed circles)* and ventilated control group *(open circles)*. The vertical lines extending upward and downward from the symbol each represent 1 SEM. The numbers within parentheses represent the number of rats. The number of rats decreased from left to right because of different durations of hypoglycemia. (From Yasaki S, Dyck PJ. Duration and severity of hypoglycemia needed to induce neuropathy. Brain Res 1990; 531:8. With permission of Elsevier Science–NL, Amsterdam, The Netherlands.)

FUNCTIONAL CLASS AND SPATIAL DISTRIBUTION OF FIBER DEGENERATION IN ACUTE HYPOGLYCEMIC NEUROPATHY

Some investigators have suggested preferential injury of motor neuron somas[20, 51] and others of peripheral nerves[13, 29, 42] in hypoglycemic neuropathy. The questions have not been finally settled.[13] Yasaki and Dyck assessed neuron class vulnerability and the spatial distribution of fiber degeneration in proximal-to-distal levels of peripheral nerves, different levels of fasciculus gracilis, neuron somas of lumbar motor neuron columns, and spinal ganglia.[56] In nine rats with sustained severe hypoglycemia (1.4 ± 0.2 mmol/L) for various times from 12 to 18 hours, axonal degeneration, dark axons, and attenuated axons were encountered in sciatic, common peroneal, and tibial nerves (Fig. 32.3).[56] In rats showing the highest frequencies of fiber degeneration, degenerating fibers were encountered in central fascicular regions of the proximal tibial nerves in two of three rats, of the distal sciatic nerves in three rats, and of proximal common peroneal nerves in two of three rats (Fig. 32.4).[56] This fiber degeneration was in central fascicular regions of the mid-thigh level of distal sciatic, proximal tibial, and proximal common peroneal nerves, which are watershed zones of poorest perfusion.[37] These results raise the question of ischemic damage, but the results were mild, making interpretation uncertain. In the rat hypoglycemic for 18 hours, neuron somas of motor columns and spinal ganglia occasionally demonstrated peripheral Nissl substance and eccentric nuclei, suggesting central chromatolysis (Fig. 32.5).[56]

Somal degeneration was not observed. No other pathologic changes were observed in the spinal cord. Perhaps these observations suggest that the major and primary abnormality is

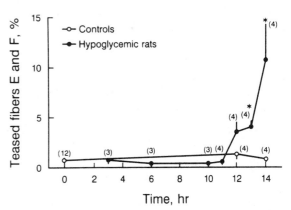

■ **Figure 32.2** The mean ± SEM of the percent of teased fibers of peroneal nerve undergoing axonal degeneration (condition E) and remyelination (condition F) in hypoglycemic rats *(solid circles)* and ventilated control group *(open circles)*. The numbers of rats for each duration of hypoglycemia or mechanical ventilation in the case of controls are given in parentheses. There is a striking increase in the mean percentage of fibers showing abnormality after 11 hours of hypoglycemia. Significance of differences between unventilated controls and hypoglycemic groups was assessed using Student's two sample *t* test (*P <0.002). In rats hypoglycemic for 12 or more hours, a statistically significant positive association was found between duration of hypoglycemia and frequency of fiber abnormality (r = 0.595; P <0.002). (From Yasaki S, Dyck PJ. Duration and severity of hypoglycemia needed to induce neuropathy. Brain Res 1990; 531:8. With permission of Elsevier Science–NL, Amsterdam, The Netherlands.)

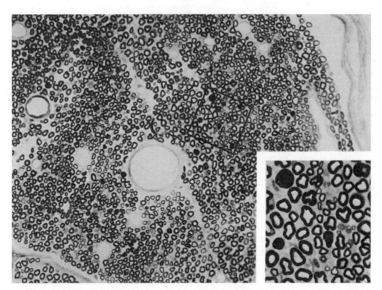

■ **Figure 32.3** Transverse semithin epoxy section stained with methylene blue of proximal tibial nerve of rats 7 days after 18 hours of hypoglycemia to show fiber degeneration. Throughout sections are abnormal degenerating myelinated fiber profiles. The *insert* (shown as square on low-power section) shows axonal atrophy, infolded myelin loop, and obvious axonal degeneration. Bar = 20 m. (From Yasaki S, Dyck PJ. Spatial distribution of fiber degeneration in hypoglycemic neuropathy in rat. J Neuropathol Exp Neurol 1991; 50(6):681. Reproduced with permission from the Journal of Neuropathology and Experimental Neurology.)

Nerve	Control rat	12-hour hypoglycemic rat	13-hour hypoglycemic rat	18-hour hypoglycemic rat
Proximal sciatic				
Distal sciatic				
Proximal common peroneal				
Proximal tibial				
Distal tibial				

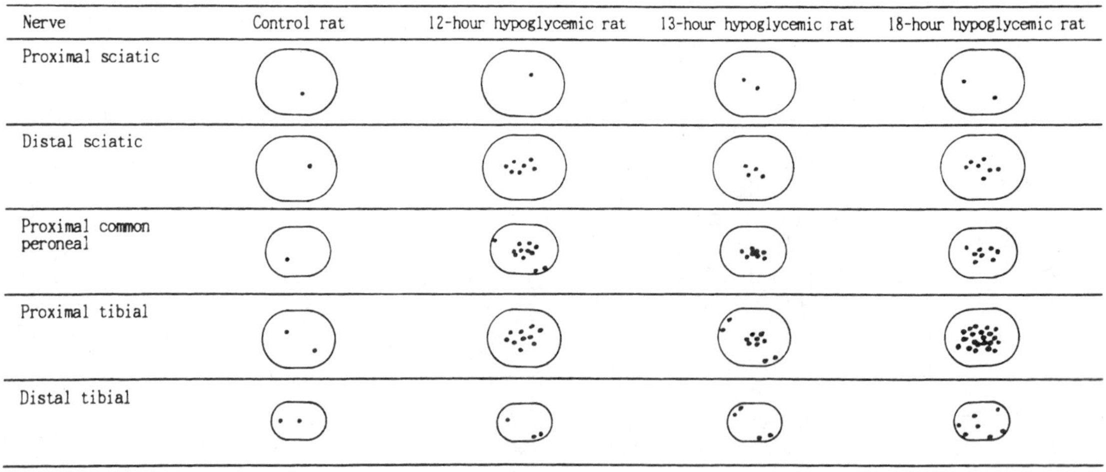

■ **Figure 32.4** Drawings of transverse semithin epoxy sections of proximal and distal sciatic, proximal common peroneal, proximal and distal nerves of a mechanically ventilated control rat for 14 hours and rats hypoglycemic for 12, 13, and 18 hours 7 days after experiments. Degenerating fibers and ''attenuated axon'' are indicated by dots. Note central fascicular fiber degeneration in most nerves at mid-thigh level. The proximal sciatic nerves of hypoglycemic rats did not show abnormal frequencies of fiber degeneration beyond what was seen in a control rat. (From Yasaki S, Dyck PJ: Spatial distribution of fiber degeneration in hypoglycemic neuropathy in rat. J Neuropathol Exp Neurol 1991; 50(6):681. Reproduced with permission from the Journal of Neuropathology and Experimental Neurology.)

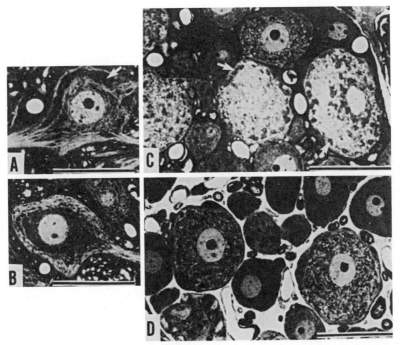

■ **Figure 32.5** Semithin epoxy sections stained with methylene blue of right fifth lumbar enlargements and lumbar dorsal root ganglia of rats 7 days after 18 hours of hypoglycemia and a control rat that was mechanically ventilated for 14 hours. *A,* Lower motor neurons of anterior horn of right fifth lumbar enlargements from a rat hypoglycemic for 18 hours. Peripheral Nissl substance is seen *(arrow)* in a rat hypoglycemic for 18 hours. *B,* A rat that was mechanically ventilated for 14 hours. *C,* Neuron cell bodies of right fifth lumbar dorsal root ganglia from a rat hypoglycemic for 18 hours. Peripheral Nissl substance is seen *(arrows)*, but neuronal cell death is not demonstrated in the rat hypoglycemic for 18 hours. *D,* A control rat that was mechanically ventilated for 14 hours. Bars = 50 m. (From Yasaki S, Dyck PJ. Spatial distribution of fiber degeneration in hypoglycemic neuropathy in rat. J Neuropathol Exp Neurol 1991; 50(6):681. Reproduced with permission from the Journal of Neuropathology and Experimental Neurology.)

in the axon, not in motor neuron columns of the anterior horn of spinal cord or spinal ganglia in hypoglycemic nerve injury. These observations also suggest two hypotheses: (1) the fiber degeneration in hypoglycemia might be caused by an energy substrate insufficiency or (2) the energy substrate might be lowest with or without a local hypoxia, especially in mid-thigh level of nerves.[56]

EFFECT OF ACUTE HYPOGLYCEMIA ON NERVE ENERGY METABOLISM

Because the peripheral nerve, unlike brain, does not autoregulate nerve blood flow,[16] the level of nerve glucose may be regulated by decreasing consumption. Insulin has no effect on glucose metabolism.[17] The brain depends on glucose for almost all of its energy source. The neural elements of peripheral nerve are also probably dependent on glucose for their major substrates for energy production.[18] Because adenosine triphosphate (ATP) and phosphocreatine (P-creatine), major sources of high-energy phosphate in tissue, are usually produced from glucose by aerobic glycolysis, finding comparable levels of endoneurial ATP and P-creatine and endoneurial glucose in hypoglycemic rats is not unexpected. Energy substrate for function of nerve fiber, especially anterograde fast axonal transport, may be locally supplied in the peripheral nerve.[39] In acute insulin-induced hypoglycemic rats, endoneurial nerve glucose and ATP were significantly decreased from those of controls in the sciatic, tibial, and peroneal nerves, especially in the distal sciatic, proximal tibial, and proximal peroneal nerves after 12 hours of hypoglycemia.[57] At these mid-thigh level of nerves, endoneurial lactate decreased initially for several hours and then increased up to at most 124.4% of that of controls 12 hours after onset of hypoglycemia.[57]

The first decrease of lactate is reasonable because ketone bodies, lactate, or other substances are used for maintaining the homeostasis of glucose metabolism when severe hypoglycemia occurs. The increase of nerve lactate after 12 hours of severe hypoglycemia suggests that local severe depletion of energy substrates and ischemia may occur especially at the watershed zones of poorest perfusion of nerves after long duration of severe hypoglycemia. These conditions of decrease in energy metabolites and ischemia may contribute to nerve fiber degeneration.

EFFECT OF ACUTE HYPOGLYCEMIA ON NERVE BLOOD FLOW

The peripheral nerve is vascularized segmentally by epineurial blood vessels and each fascicle by perineurial and endoneurial microvessels.[30] Blood flow in the proximal sciatic nerve is supplied by gluteal arteries, and distal nerves are supplied by branches of the femoral artery.[33, 36, 48] Experimental studies severely decreasing nerve blood flow and nerve oxygen tension (for example, by embolization or ligation of the arteries) in rats induces central fascicular injury of the distal sciatic nerves.[33, 37, 38] Recent studies on experimental insulin-induced acute hypoglycemic neuropathy in rats showed that axonal degeneration may also occur in central fascicular distributions at the mid-thigh level of nerves, suggesting that this metabolic neuropathy is similar to ischemic neuropathy and that nerve blood flow of this level of nerves may be reduced during hypoglycemia.[56] In fact, nerve blood flow in the sciatic nerves was significantly reduced to approximately 32 to 42% of controls at 120 minutes of acute insulin-induced hypoglycemic rats using the hydrogen clearance[1] or laser Doppler technique (Fig. 32.6).[19] It is known that acute hypoglycemia evokes glucose counter-regulation and that increased activity of adrenaline causes peripheral vasoconstriction, presumably mediated via adrenergic receptors.[59] Because the peripheral nervous system does not autoregulate nerve blood flow, an increased sympathetic nerve function or other vasoconstrictive factors may play a role in vasoconstriction of the peripheral nerves in acute hypoglycemic rats. It is hypothesized that ischemic or hypoxic mechanisms are one of the major reasons underlying hypoglycemic neuropathy. Recently, increase of nitric oxide or prostacyclin production has been reported in insulin-induced hypoglycemic rats[19] and in humans infused with insulin experimentally.[40] These findings raise the possibility that the increase of these vasodilators might be an antagonistic reaction against the decreased peripheral blood flow induced by activated adrenergic function in acute hypoglycemia for maintaining the endoneurial microcirculation in severe hypoglycemic condition.

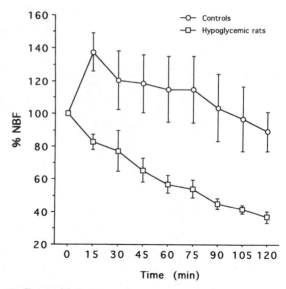

■ **Figure 32.6** The average percent of sciatic nerve blood flow (NBF) in the normoglycemic control rats and in insulin-induced hypoglycemic (blood glucose: 2.02–2.08 mmol/L in average) rats for 120 minutes (n = 5 for each). Nerve blood flow was measured by laser Doppler. In hypoglycemic rats, NBF significantly reduced to 36.8% of that in controls at 120 minutes ($P<0.003$) by Bonferroni/Dunn's multiple comparison test. (From Hata A. Effect of nitric oxide on sciatic nerve blood flow in acute hypoglycemic rats. St Marianna Med J 1996; 24(4):370.)

Diabetic Animals

Because hypoglycemia may occur frequently and to severe degrees, especially in humans with brittle diabetes mellitus, it may be that such repeated hypoglycemia is a risk factor for diabetic polyneuropathy.[2, 15]

The effect of insulin treatment on peripheral nerve morphology has been examined in four animal studies. An early study showed that axonal dwindling could be prevented by strict insulin treatment for a few weeks.[19] In the three other studies this effect was not obtained, but a slight and significant increase in number of isolated fibers with histologic signs of axonal degeneration was found.[31, 44, 54] Similar structural alterations are not present in untreated streptozocin diabetes.[23] Various explanations

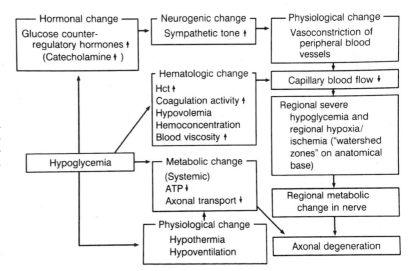

■ **Figure 32.7** Suggested pathogenesis of acute hypoglycemic neuropathy in nondiabetic animals. Hct, hematocrit.

for the occurrence of axonal degeneration in the insulin-treated rats are suggested in the reports, but no answers were provided. In none of the reports is it mentioned whether regression analysis of the relation between degree of axonal damage and glycemia or dose of insulin was performed. In one study, data are provided that allow such an analysis.[31] If hyperglycemia is expressed as a lower limit of the blood glucose values provided, the result is that the degree of axonal degeneration correlates inversely with the glucose levels ($r = -0.64$; $P<0.001$; n = 24). This observation points to an association between axonal degeneration and episodes of hypoglycemia.

In a study on fast anterograde axonal transport during hypoglycemia in streptozocin-diabetic rats, a decrease of the amount transported was observed, similar to nondiabetic rats.[46] This reduction in transport of axon membrane material and axolemmal complexes might be closely related to structural breakdown of the axon during hypoglycemia.

MECHANISM OF HYPOGLYCEMIC NEUROPATHY

The mechanism of hypoglycemic neuropathy is still unclear. It seems likely that decreased energy metabolism and reduction of axonal transport may be implicated. Other physiologic changes, such as hypothermia and hypoventilation, and rheological changes, such as hemoconcentration and hyperviscosity, may contribute to the mechanism. Whether the nerve ischemia or hypoxia play a role in the chronic or intermittent hypoglycemia in patients with

insulinoma is not yet known. The effect of excitatory amino acids, which are postulated to induce damage of the central nervous system in severe hypoglycemic condition, on the peripheral nerve seems unlikely so far because these excitatory neurotoxins are thought to preferentially affect dendrites and somas but not axon trunks of nerve.[4, 16] The suggested pathogenesis of acute hypoglycemic neuropathy in nondiabetic animals is shown in Figure 32.7.

The mechanism of this neuropathy in patients with pancreas islet cell tumors is still not clarified because of its rare incidence in humans. But considering the mechanisms of acute insulin-induced hypoglycemic neuropathy in nondiabetic animals, it is suggested that prolonged or intermittent severe hypoglycemic attacks may produce (1) disruption of nerve energy metabolism and axonal transport or (2) alternation of microvascular ischemia and reperfusion in peripheral nerves.

The role of other reactive factors, such as cytokines activated from the insult of severe hypoglycemia, in this neuropathy are not known so far.

References

1. Akanuma T. Effect of acute hypoglycemia on peripheral nerve blood flow in rats. St Marianna Med 1993; 21(4):623.
2. Arias P, Kerener W, Zier H, et al. Incidence of hypoglycemia episodes in diabetic patients under continuous subcutaneous insulin infusion and intensified conventional insulin treatment: Assessment by means of semiambulatory 24-hour continuous blood glucose monitoring. Diabetes Care 1985; 8(1):134.

3. Baker AB. Cerebral damage in hypoglycemia: A review. Am J Psychiatry 1939; 96(7):109.

4. Bird SJ. Specificity of neurotoxins. In Coyle JT, Bird SJ, Evans RH, et al (eds): Excitatory amino acid neurotoxins: Selectivity, specificity, and mechanisms of action. Neurosci Res Program Bull 1981; 19(1):381.

5. Borgstrom L, Norberg K, Siesjö BK. Glucose consumption in rat cerebral cortex in normoxia, hypoxia, and hypercapnia. Acta Physiol Scand 1976; 96(4):569.

6. Bruyn GW, Garland H. Neuropathies of endocrine origin. In Vinken PJ, Bruyn GW (eds): Handbook of Clinical Neurology. Amsterdam, North Holland Publishing Co, 1970, vol 8, p 52.

7. Buckmann I. Beriberisymptome bei der hypoglykamietherapie der schizophrenie. Nervenarzt 1937; 10(8):412.

8. Caravati CM. Insulin neuritis: A case report. Va Med Monthly 1933; 59(10):745.

9. Conri C, Ducloux G, Lagueny A, et al. Polyneuropathie au cours d'un syndrome polyendocrinien de type I. Presse Med 1990; 19(6):247.

10. Daggett P, Nabarro J. Neurological aspects of insulinomas neuritis. Postgrad Med J 1984; 60(9):577.

11. Danta G. Hypoglycemic peripheral neuropathy. Arch Neurol 1969; 21(8):121.

12. De Morsier G, Bersot H. Cerebral disorders in provoked hyperinsulinemia. Am J Psychiatry Suppl 1938; 94(1):143.

13. Dyer KR, Messing A. Peripheral neuropathy associated with functional islet cell adenoma in SV40 transgenic mice. J Neuropathol Exp Neurol 1989; 48(4):399.

14. Frier B M, Corrall RJM, Davidson N, et al. Peripheral blood cell changes in response to acute hypoglycemia in man. Eur J Clin Invest 1983; 13(1):33.

15. Gale E. Causes of hypoglycaemia. Br J Hosp Med 1985; 35(3):159.

16. Greenamyre JT. The role of glutamate in neurotransmission and in neurologic disease. Arch Neurol 1986; 43(10):1058.

17. Greene DA, Winegrad AI, Carpentier J-L, et al. Rabbit sciatic nerve fascicle and "endoneurial" preparations for in vitro studies of peripheral nerve glucose metabolism. J Neurochem 1979; 33(11):1007.

18. Greene DA, Winegrad AI. In vitro studies of the substrates for energy production and the effects of insulin on glucose utilization in the neural components of peripheral nerve. Diabetes 1979; 28(10):878.

19. Hata A. Effect of nitric oxide on sciatic nerve blood flow in acute hypoglycemic rats. St Marianna Med 1996; 24(4):370.

20. Harrison MJG. Muscle wasting after prolonged hypoglycemic coma. Case report with electrophysiological data. J Neurol Neurosurg Psychiatry 1976; 39(5). 465.

21. Hilsted J, Bone-Petersen F, Norgaard M-B, et al. Haemodynamic changes in insulin-induced hypoglycaemia in normal man. Diabetologia 1984; 26(5):328.

22. Hypoglycemic peripheral neuropathy (editorial). Lancet 1982; 2(6):1447.

23. Jakobsen J. Early and preventable changes of peripheral nerve structure and function in insulin-deficient diabetic rats. J Neurol Neurosurg Psychiatry 1979; 42(6):509.

24. Jakobsen J, Sidenius P. Hypoglycemic neuropathy. In Dyck PJ, Thomas PK, Asbury AK, et al (eds): Diabetic Neuropathy. Philadelphia, WB Saunders, 1987, p 94.

25. Jaspan JB, Wollman RL, Bernstein L, et al. Hypoglycemia peripheral neuropathy in association with insulinoma: Implication of glucopenia rather than hyperinsulinism. Medicine 1982; 61(1):33.

26. Jayasinghe KSA, Nimalasuriya A, Dharmadasa K. A case of insulinoma with peripheral neuropathy. Postgrad Med J 1983; 59(3):189.

27. Jordan WR. Neuritic manifestations in diabetes mellitus. Arch Intern Med 1936; 57(5):307.

28. Kedes LH, Field JB. Hypothermia: A clue to hypoglycemia. N Engl J Med 1964; 271(10):785.

29. Lambert EH, Mulder DW, Bastron JW. Regeneration of peripheral nerves with hyperinsulin neuropathy. Neurology 1960; 10(9):851.

30. Lundborg G. The intrinsic vascularization of human peripheral nerves: structural and functional aspects. J Hand Surg 1979; 4(1):34.

31. Mandelbaum JA, Felten DL, Westfall SG, et al. Neuropathic changes associated with insulin treatment of diabetic rats: electron microscopic and morphometric analysis. Brain Res Bull 1983; 10(4):377.

32. Martin MM. Diabetic neuropathy: A clinical study of 150 cases. Brain 1953; 76(6):594.

33. McManis PG, Low PA: Factors affecting the relative viability of centrifascicular and subperineurial axons in acute peripheral nerve ischemia. Exp Neurol 1988; 99(1):84.

34. Moersch FP, Kernohan JW. Hypoglycemia: Neurologic and neuropathologic studies. Arch Neurol Psychiatry 1938; 39(2):242.

35. Mulder DW, Bastron JW, Lambert EH. Hyperinsulin neuropathy. Neurology 1956; 6(9):627.

36. Nobel W. Observations on the microcirculation of peripheral nerves. Bibl Anat 1968; 10(10):316.

37. Nukada H, Dyck PJ. Microsphere embolization of nerve capillaries and fiber degeneration. Am J Pathol 1984; 115(5):275.

38. Nukada H, Dyck PJ, Karnes JL. Spatial distribution of capillaries in rat nerves: correlation to ischemic damage. Exp Neurol 1985; 87(2):369.

39. Ochs S. Energy metabolism and supply of P to the fast axoplasmic transport mechanism in nerve. Federation Proc 1974; 33(1):1049.

40. Polderman KH, Stehouwer CDA, van Kamp GJ, et al. Effects of insulin infusion on endothelium-derived vasoactive substances. Diabetologia 1996; 39(11):1284.

41. Potter CG, Sharma AK, Britland ST, et al. Hypoglycemia neuropathy in experimental diabetes (abstract). Peripheral Neuropathy Association of America 1988:57.

42. Rosner L, Elstad R. The neuropathy of hypoglycemia. Neurology 1964; 14(1):1.

43. Rundles RW. Diabetic neuropathy. General review with reports of 125 cases. Medicine 1945; 24(1):111.

44. Sharma AK, Duguid IGM, Blanchard DS, et al. The effect of insulin treatment on myelinated nerve fiber maturation and integrity and on body growth in streptozotocin-diabetic rats. J Neurol Sci 1985; 67(4):285.

45. Sidenius P, Jakobsen J. Peripheral neuropathy in rats induced by insulin treatment. Diabetes 1983; 32(4):383.

46. Sidenius P, Jakobsen J. Anterograde fast component of axonal transport during insulin-induced hypoglycemia in nondiabetic and diabetic rats. Diabetes 1987; 36(7):853.

47. Silfveskiöild BP. "Polyneuritis hypoglycemia": Late peripheral paresis after hypoglycemic attacks in two insulinoma patients. Acta Med Scand 1946; 125(12):502.

48. Sladky JT, Greenberg JH, Brown MJ. Regional perfusion in normal and ischemic rat sciatic nerves. Ann Neurol 1985; 17(2):191.

49. Stern K, Dancey TE, McNaughton FL. Sensory disturbances following insulin treatment of psychoses. J Nerv Ment Dis 1942; 95(2):183.

50. Tintore M, Montalban J, Cervera C, et al. Peripheral neuropathy in association with insulinoma: Clinical

features and neuropathology of a new case. J Neurol Neurosurg Psychiatry 1994; 57(8):1009.

51. Tom MI, Richardson JC. Hypoglycemia from islet cell tumor of pancreas with amyotrophy and cerebrospinal nerve cell changes: A case report. J Neuropathol Exp Neurol 1951; 10(1):57.

52. Tomlinson DR, James PJ. Impaired orthograde axonal transport in acute hypoglycemia, an effect mediated via hypothermia. Med Biol 1984; 62(1):34.

53. Wauchope GM. Critical review: Hypoglycemia. Q J Med 1933; 2(1):117.

54. Westfall SG, Felten DL, Mandelbaum JA, et al. Degenerative neuropathy in insulin-treated diabetic rats. J Neurol Sci 1983; 61(1):93.

55. Yasaki S, Dyck PJ. Duration and severity of hypoglycemia needed to induce neuropathy: Brain Res 1990; 531(1):8.

56. Yasaki S, Dyck PJ. Spatial distribution of fiber degeneration in hypoglycemic neuropathy in rat. J Neuropathol Exp Neurol 1991; 50(6):681.

57. Yasaki S, Dyck PJ. Effect of acute hypoglycemia on energy metabolism in rat peripheral nerve (abstract). Neurology 1991; 41(suppl 1)(3):206.

58. Ziegler DK. Minor neurologic signs and symptoms following insulin coma therapy. J Nerv Ment Dis 1954; 120(7–8):75.

59. Zochodne DW, Low PA. Adrenergic control of nerve blood flow. Exp Neurol 1990; 109(9):300.

Chapter **33**

Cranial Neuropathy in Diabetes Mellitus

Benn E. Smith

INTRODUCTION

Isolated cranial neuropathy is a recognized peripheral nerve complication of diabetes mellitus. Although cranial neuropathies are not unique to patients with this disease, they often occur in older individuals with long-standing diabetes. As a result, cranial mononeuropathy frequently coexists with other diabetes complications, including polyneuropathy. The most common clinical syndrome is acute to subacute onset of painful ocular mononeuropathy (cranial nerve [CN] III, IV, or VI), followed by complete or partial recovery over weeks to a few months. Other established syndromes include facial neuropathy and, less commonly, single or multiple cranial neuropathies often associated with serious infection.

OCULAR NEUROPATHIES

Clinical Features

The features of diabetic ocular palsies have been reviewed in many case series. Building on the previous series of Rucker[53] and Rush and Younge,[54] Richards and colleagues[50] reported 4278 cases of acquired oculomotor, abducens, and trochlear neuropathies from the Mayo Clinic, of which 103 were ascribed to diabetes. Goldstein and Cogan compiled 22 cases of diabetic ophthalmoplegia in 20 patients, focusing on pupillary involvement.[29] Zorilla and Kozak contributed an additional 27 episodes of diabetic ophthalmoplegia in 24 patients.[77] Teuscher and Meienberg described 19 patients with diabetes or impaired glucose tolerance with oculomotor palsy.[67] Watanabe and colleagues reported 11 palsies affecting the third or sixth cranial nerves among a population of 1961 diabetics patients.[71]

Epidemiology. To date, no rigorous population-based incidence studies have been reported that estimate the frequency of diabetic ocular mononeuropathy. In the series of Rucker, Rush, and Richards, abducens neuropathy was the most common mononeuropathy, followed by oculomotor and then trochlear neuropathy, although it is likely that the incidence of trochlear neuropathy is underestimated given the subtleties of the clinical findings.[50, 53, 54] Diabetes has been linked to oculomotor palsy in 3 to 36% of cases,[29, 50, 67] and 2 to 3% of fourth and sixth cranial nerve palsies were found in diabetic patients by Richards and colleagues.[50] Diabetic ocular mononeuropathy is a syndrome primarily affecting older diabetics with preexisting polyneuropathy, although cases of diabetes presenting with this syndrome have been documented.[21, 60] In the pediatric series of Kodsi and Younge, 160 ocular palsies were reported in 160 individuals between the ages of 0 and 17 years, none of whom were found to have diabetes mellitus or impaired glucose tolerance.[39] The sex ratio for all causes of acquired ocular motor palsy group in the Mayo Clinic series was 1:2 (M:F), although the gender ratio was not reported specifically for the diabetic subgroup. Among the patients reported by Goldstein and Cogan[29] and those by Teuscher and Meienberg,[67] the M:F ratio fell in the 1:0 to 1:1 range; Watanabe and colleagues described seven men and three women.[71]

Symptoms/Signs/Presentations. The typical presentation of diabetic oculomotor palsy is acute onset, usually over hours, of ipsilateral headache, often refractory to analgesics, and diplopia with ptosis, sparing the pupil. The headache may be periorbital, retro-orbital, frontal, temporal, or involve the entire side of the head. Although pupillary dysfunction is unusual in diabetic oculomotor neuropathy, occurring in 14 to 18% of cases,[29, 53] and complete iridoplegia even rarer, mydriasis can be seen in this disorder, mimicking structural ophthalmoplegia from aneurysm, tumor, or other mass

lesion. Recovery is complete or near complete, often occurring over a period of a few days to a few months. Aberrant regeneration is quite uncommon. Recurrence is infrequent. Nuchal rigidity and impairment of consciousness are absent.

Laboratory Findings. The presence of impaired glucose tolerance may be the only abnormality found on testing of a patient with acute ocular palsy. In those with long-standing diabetes, the fasting blood sugar and glycosylated hemoglobin are likely to be abnormal. Indicators of nephropathy, such as microalbuminuria, or of retinopathy, including the characteristic lesions on optic funduscopy, may be absent. Computed tomography (CT) and magnetic resonance imaging (MRI) studies are often unremarkable, being used primarily to exclude the presence of blood in the subarachnoid space or space-occupying lesions resulting in compression of posterior fossa or basal structures. Hopf and Gutmann reported 11 consecutive cases of diabetic oculomotor palsy, 10 of whom had abnormal masseter reflexes and 3 of whom showed small regions of increased T2 signal by MRI scanning in the mesencephalon, leading to the idea that in some cases this neuropathy might be related to small vessel ischemic infarction in the brainstem.[34] Cerebrospinal fluid studies and conventional as well as MR angiography are normal.

Anatomy/Pathophysiology

The oculomotor nerve conveys approximately 23,000 myelinated fibers (in a bimodal diameter frequency distribution with peaks at 5.1 and 11.1 μm) from the midbrain to the orbit[57] (Fig. 33.1). Sunderland and Hughes and later Kerr and Hollowell described the distribution of autonomic fibers in the third cranial nerve, noting that the pupillomotor fibers course near the surface of the nerve in a dorsomedial position.[37, 64] Although branches from the cervical sympathetic trunk are described as communicating with the ophthalmic nerve in the cavernous sinus, to my knowledge no such arrangement has been documented for the oculomotor nerve. A number of workers described sensory ganglion cells or afferent fibers in the oculomotor nerve,[30, 66] and morphological studies have shown bundles of small diameter myelinated fibers traveling in the epineurium of the third nerve in the cavernous sinus that appear to be absent in the subarachnoid course of the nerve[57] (Fig. 33.2). If these are of trigeminal

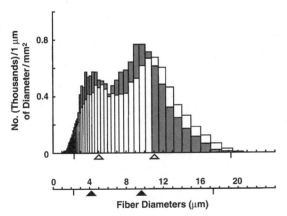

■ **Figure 33.1** Summated histograms of myelinated fiber diameter of oculomotor nerves from control subjects *(open bars)* and diabetic subjects *(gray bars)* show that the peaks in nerves of diabetic patients are at smaller diameters than those of control nerves. *Open arrows* indicate the positions of control diameter peaks, and *closed arrows* indicate the diabetic diameter peaks. (From Smith BE, Dyck PJ. Subclinical histopathological changes in the oculomotor nerve in diabetes mellitus. Ann Neurol 1992; 32:376.)

origin, the pain associated with diabetic ocular palsy would be more readily explained.

Four cases of diabetic oculomotor palsy have been studied histopathologically.[6, 20, 70, 73] These workers undertook painstaking serial sections of the oculomotor nerves to shed light on the underlying pathophysiology in this disorder. The first three used paraffin sections alone; Usui and associates used plastic-embedded semithin sections.[70] As a result of these investigations, a mechanism of focal ischemia resulting in segmental demyelination followed by remyelination has been the accepted pathophysiologic model in diabetic oculomotor palsy for more than 25 years. Parkinson described the vascular anatomy of the oculomotor nerve, noting the proximal third is supplied by branches from the posterior circle of Willis, the middle third by twigs from the meningohypophyseal trunk, and the distal third by recurrent branches of the ophthalmic artery.[47] The pathologic study of Asbury and coworkers showed a region of centrifascicular myelin stain pallor in the region between the posterior and middle vascular territories of the third nerve, leading these investigators to postulate that an ischemic event in that region leading to segmental demyelination could account for many of the clinical and pathologic features of diabetic ophthalmoplegia[6] (Fig. 33.3). Smith and Dyck undertook a postmortem histopathologic study of the oculomotor nerves in eight

diabetic subjects who did not have a history of ocular palsy, comparing these with 15 nondiabetic control third cranial nerves.[57] The main finding was microfasciculation of edge fibers in parts of the fascicles of half the diabetics but in none of the control nerves, perhaps representing subclinical injury of unknown cause, possibly from ischemia (Fig. 33.4). The idea that vascular injury is responsible for proximal asymmetrical lower limb diabetic neuropathy is supported by the work of Raff and coworkers[49] and Asbury.[7]

Differential Diagnosis

According to Richards and previous workers in Rochester, Minnesota, the causes of 1918 cases of abducens palsy were undetermined (26.2%), neoplasm (21.5%), head trauma (15.0%), vascular (12.5%, divided between 3.3% diabetes, 1.6% hypertension, 0.8% atherosclerosis, and 6.8% other), aneurysm (3.0%), and other (21.7%). For 1225 cases of oculomotor palsy, the causes were undetermined (23.9%), vascular (19.9%, divided between 3.3% diabetes, 1.3% hypertension, 0.4% atherosclerosis, and 14.9% other), aneurysm (15.8%), head trauma

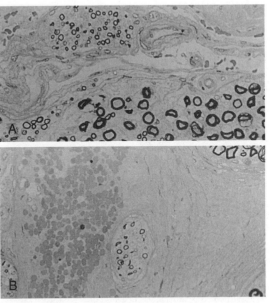

■ **Figure 33.2** Transverse sections of oculomotor nerves from *(A)* control and *(B)* diabetic subjects illustrate isolated fascicles of small myelinated fibers. (Paraphenylenediamine-stained semithin (0.75 μm) transverse epoxy sections of aldehyde-fixed and osmium tetroxide–fixed nerve, ×440.) (From Smith BE, Dyck PJ. Subclinical histopathological changes in the oculomotor nerve in diabetes mellitus. Ann Neurol 1992; 32:376.)

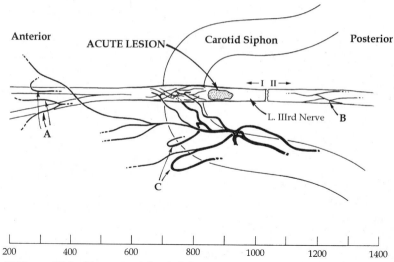

■ **Figure 33.3** Diagram of the left third nerve and its vascular supply. The three arterial branches supplying the nerve consist of recurrent vessels from the ophthalmic artery (A), branches from the posterior circle of Willis (B), and the meningohypophyseal trunk (C). The acute lesion occurs in the midcavernous portion of the nerve and may lie in a watershed zone between the meningohypophyseal trunk territory and the region supplied by branches from the posterior circle of Willis. (From Asbury AK, et al. Oculomotor palsy in diabetes mellitus: A clinicopathological study. Brain 1970; 93:555.)

(14.7%), neoplasm (12.5%), and other (13.2%). In the trochlear palsy group of 578 cases, the causes were undetermined (32.2%), head trauma (29.2%), vascular (17.8%, divided between 2.1% diabetes, 2.1% hypertension, 1.7% atherosclerosis, and 11.9% other), neoplasm (4.8%), aneurysm (0.9%), and other (15.1%).

The category of "other" included congenital, neurosurgical, multiple sclerosis, stroke, meningoencephalitis, caroticocavernous fistula, myasthenia gravis, migraine, hydrocephalus, nonaneurysmal subarachnoid hemorrhage, and other conditions.[50, 53, 54] A history of preceding ocular palsy or Bell's palsy makes diabetes

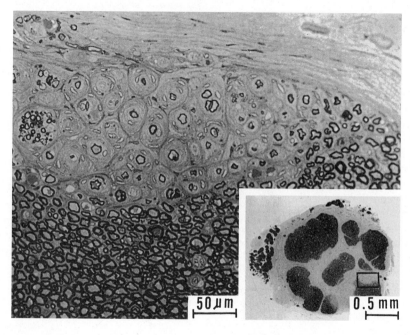

■ **Figure 33.4** Transverse section of oculomotor nerve from a diabetic subject showing microfasciculation of edge fibers in the intracavernous course of the nerve. (Paraphenylenediamine-stained semithin (0.75 μm) transverse epoxy sections of aldehyde-fixed and osmium tetroxide–fixed nerve, ×440, inset ×20.)

more likely. The differential diagnosis of monocular mydriasis includes aneurysm of the posterior circle of Willis, uncal herniation, orbital trauma or closed head injury, migraine, benign tonic pupil (Adie pupil), chemical mydriasis (pharmacologic or environmental), and early syphilis.[35] The causes of unilateral ptosis include levator dehiscence, congenital or hereditary ptosis, aneurysmal oculomotor palsy, diabetic oculomotor palsy, myasthenia gravis, myotonic dystrophy, trauma, Horner syndrome, and, less commonly, ophthalmoplegic migraine, giant cell arteritis, multiple sclerosis, sarcoidosis, varicella zoster infection, and syphilis.[35] Zorilla and Kozak made the observation that nondiabetic causes of oculomotor palsy may sometimes occur in diabetics, reporting 18 such subjects, including 6 patients with myasthenia gravis, 2 each with Graves' ophthalmopathy, ophthalmic zoster, and central demyelinating disease, and 1 patient each with various neoplasms, brain stem infarcts, and other conditions.[77]

Treatment

The principal aim of treatment in patients with diabetic cranial neuropathy, as in diabetic patients in general, is consistent regulation of the fasting blood glucose levels in the 100 to 150 mg/dL (5 to 8 mmol/L) range, with control of additional cardiovascular risk factors, including tobacco use, dyslipidemia, excessive body weight, hypertension, and lack of exercise. In the absence of complete ptosis, semitransparent adhesive tape can be applied to the eyeglass lens on the side of the ocular neuropathy, an economical strategy for suppressing diplopia during the recovery phase of the illness.

Prognosis

The outlook for diabetic ocular palsy is favorable. In the Mayo Clinic series, data on time to recovery for ocular palsies for all causes (diabetic and nondiabetic) were available on 248 patients. In the vascular subset, 71.7% recovered completely or partially by 4 to 6 weeks; the recovery rate in the group with aneurysms was 47.4%; and in those with neoplasms, 28.5%.[50] Goldstein and Cogan described a mean time to recovery of 2^1/$_2$ months in diabetic oculomotor palsy, with 5 of 20 cases having a recurrent ophthalmoplegia.[29]

FACIAL NEUROPATHY

Idiopathic facial neuropathy, often designated Bell's palsy after the 19th century British physician who described the anatomy of the seventh cranial nerve,[10] has been associated with diabetes mellitus by many workers,[2, 4, 40, 48] although the status of diabetes as a prognostic factor for recovery from facial neuropathy remains controversial.

Clinical Features

Epidemiology. Korczyn first studied the relationship between diabetes mellitus and facial neuropathy in a series of 130 patients reporting impaired glucose intolerance in 66%.[40] Aminoff and Miller found a frequency of 6% in 70 Bell's palsy patients referred to a tertiary center in London during a 20 month period.[5] Among 395 Bell's palsy patients from northern California, Adour and coworkers reported overt diabetes mellitus or impaired glucose tolerance in 10.7%, noting that 45% of nondiabetic and 76% of diabetic subject showed clinically complete paralysis.[4] Pecket and Schattner found diabetes mellitus in 39% of cases.[48] Abraham-Inpijn and colleagues studied 147 patients with Bell's palsy, reporting 48.8% with diabetes mellitus or impaired glucose tolerance,[2] and 5 years later performed regression analysis of prognostic factors associated with recovery in 200 Bell's palsy patients, reporting that severity of paralysis at onset and elevated mean arterial pressure (but not diabetes mellitus) were predictive of poorer recovery at 1 year.[3]

Symptoms/Signs/Presentations. The most common presentation of Bell's palsy is acute onset of unilateral weakness of the upper and lower muscles of facial expression, often with pain and less often sensory symptoms in the ear, and variably, taste disturbance or hyperacusis. Physical findings include variable degrees of unilateral facial weakness. This is accompanied by preservation of strength of muscles of mastication, normal sensation, abnormal corneal reflex on the affected side, and ipsilateral widening of the palpebral fissure, sometimes with corneal irritation caused by incomplete lid closure. The clinical findings are similar whether or not the palsy is associated with diabetes mellitus, although Pecket and Schattner reported a much lower frequency of taste disturbance in diabetic individuals—14% (7 of 49 patients)—versus Bell's palsy patients with normal glucose tolerance—83% (64 of 77 patients).[48] This may reflect a more distal site of disease in diabetic facial mononeuropathy beyond the chorda tympani branch.

Laboratory Findings. Facial compound muscle action potential (CMAP) amplitude values recording over the nasalis muscle are reduced to absent in facial neuropathy.[62] Trigeminal "blink reflex" studies may show prolongation of the ipsilateral R1 and R2 latencies or absence of one or more of these waveforms.[38] Magnetic resonance imaging of the posterior fossa performed with gadolinium may show enhancement of the affected seventh nerve.[45, 69] Apart from elevated blood glucose determinations, serologic tests including Lyme disease, human immunodeficiency virus (HIV) infection, and sarcoidosis are negative or normal.

Anatomy/Pathophysiology

The facial nerve enters the internal auditory canal and traverses the temporal bone, giving off the chorda tympani branch distal to the geniculate ganglion before exit through the stylomastoid foramen. The seventh nerve then gains the stylomastoid foramen after passing through the fallopian canal, branching after exit to supply ipsilateral facial muscles. In Bell's palsy, the site of disease is thought to be in the intratemporal course of the nerve where edema leads to compression and further damage to fibers in the vicinity. Pathologic studies in Bell's palsy unassociated with diabetes mellitus have found evidence of disease throughout the intratemporal course of the nerve, but the clinical observation of sparing of taste function in diabetics with this cranial mononeuropathy suggests a local process distal to the chorda tympani branch. Sunderland and Cossar observed that there are three arteries supplying the facial nerve before exit from the stylomastoid foramen.[65] A loop of the anterior inferior cerebellar artery, which usually gives off the labyrinthine artery, supplies the proximal portion of the nerve with fine branches as far distal as the geniculate ganglion. One or more petrosal branches of the middle meningeal artery enter the facial canal near the geniculate ganglion, branching to feed the nerve proximally and as distal as the stylomastoid foramen. The stylomastoid branch of the posterior auricular artery enters the stylomastoid foramen and travels a short distance before bifurcating into an ascending branch, which extends to the geniculate ganglion, and a descending branch, which exits from the stylomastoid foramen and accompanies the posterior auricular nerve. They noted that at least two vessels supply each segment of the facial nerve in its intratemporal bone course.[65] It

seems unlikely that there is a region of vascular vulnerability between these overlapping territories within the temporal bone. It remains to be seen whether such a region of tenuous vascular supply exists distal to the chorda tympani branch of the facial nerve, similar to the arterial border zone in the oculomotor nerve between the posterior circle of Willis and the meningohypophyseal artery.

Differential Diagnosis

The differential diagnosis of Bell's palsy associated with diabetes mellitus (DM) includes idiopathic facial neuropathy, trauma (skull fracture, neurosurgery), varicella zoster infection, chronic otitis media, neoplasm, Lyme disease, human immunodeficiency virus infection, and sarcoidosis.

Treatment

The focus of therapy in any neuropathy associated with DM is careful regulation of the fasting blood glucose to a range between 100 and 150 mg/dL (5 and 8 mmol/L). Whether the Bell's palsy is associated with DM or not, many clinicians treat Bell's palsy of less than 1 week of duration with a short course of prednisone, typically for 10 to 14 days, with appropriate monitoring for significant exacerbations of blood glucose levels. Careful examination for exposure keratopathy is mandatory so that appropriate lubrication and nocturnal lid taping may be instituted, and, in severe cases where the eye is sore or irritated, ophthalmologic evaluation may be needed for consideration of temporary marginal tarsorrhapy to protect the cornea from ulceration.

Prognosis

There is consensus that the severity of Bell's palsy at the time of maximal deficit is an adverse prognostic factor.[26, 58] Electrophysiologic testing more than 4 to 6 days after onset by assessment of the facial CMAP amplitude recording over the nasalis muscle is predictive of the likelihood of return of function.[13, 68] If the CMAP amplitude is greater than 30% of the lower limit of normal, the prognosis is excellent. With CMAP value between 30 and 10% of the lower limit of normal, the outlook is guarded. With a CMAP amplitude less than 10% of the lower limit of normal, there is little chance of meaningful return of function.[13, 68] Little agreement exists on other prognostic factors in Bell's palsy. Some workers report that diabetes mellitus is a poor prognostic factor,[4] whereas others find no such association.[3] An additional adverse prognostic factor is elevated arterial blood pressure.[2, 3]

CRANIAL NEUROPATHIES ASSOCIATED WITH LIFE-THREATENING INFECTION

Although rare, two serious infective syndromes are closely associated with diabetes mellitus and often affect single or multiple cranial nerves. Rhinocerebral mucormycosis (RM) and malignant external otitis (MEO) carried high mortality rates in the past, a situation that has been improved somewhat when these treatable syndromes are recognized earlier in the course of disease. Recent reviews of RM[22, 43, 59] and MEO[15, 28, 36, 51, 59] provide more detailed accounts of these syndromes.

Rhinocerebral Mucormycosis

CLINICAL FEATURES

Epidemiology. Rhinocerebral mucormycosis is a distinctive disorder with the overwhelming majority of reported cases occurring in individuals with DM, often poorly controlled, and frequently with concurrent diabetic ketoacidosis (DKA). Diabetics with RM without ketosis typically have markedly elevated serum glucose levels and significant dehydration.[59]

Symptoms/Signs/Presentations. The most common presentation of RM is abrupt onset of fever, headache, and malaise, accompanied soon after by periorbital pain, swelling, and induration. Necrosis of nasal or nasopharyngeal mucosa follows, giving rise to the characteristic black turbinate, often with a bloody nasal discharge.[59] With invasion of the orbit and vascular compromise of the optic nerve, a high proportion of patients experience visual loss. With cavernous sinus involvement, CN III, IV, VI, and V_1 may be affected, resulting in total ophthalmoplegia, upper hemifacial sensory loss, and chemosis and proptosis of the affected eye with engorgement of retinal veins. As the disease progresses, acute contralateral hemiparesis signals thrombosis and eventual occlusion of the internal carotid artery, which may be followed rapidly by meningeal extension, obtundation, and death.

Laboratory Findings. In addition to marked elevation of serum glucose levels and arterial

blood gas findings of metabolic acidosis, sinus radiographs and CT scans demonstrate nodular thickening of the nasal mucosa, sometimes with air-fluid levels. Magnetic resonance imaging may be the most sensitive modality for detecting early meningeal extension and cerebral involvement, and MR angiography may provide evidence for compromise of vascular channels such as the internal carotid artery or venous sinuses without resorting to the invasive technique of conventional angiography. Histologic confirmation is the diagnostic method of choice in RM. Biopsy of a necrotic blackened mucosal lesion with demonstration of nonseptate branching hyphae on hematoxylin-eosin or by periodic acid–Schiff or methenamine silver techniques is diagnostic. Unfortunately, routine cultures of the affected mucosa or blood are seldom helpful.[59] Even in the face of clinical and imaging evidence of meningeal disease, cerebrospinal fluid studies may be normal or fail to document more than nonspecific protein elevation and mild pleocytosis.

ANATOMY/PATHOPHYSIOLOGY

The organisms responsible for RM are common fungi of the class Zygomycetes and order Mucorales from four genera: *Mucor*, *Rhizopus*, *Rhizomucor*, and *Absidia*. Although these organisms frequently are found in bread and fruit molds, they appear to cause disease in man when airborne spores from the environment colonize the upper respiratory mucosa of susceptible individuals, most often those with hyperglycemia and DKA.[59] As the infection takes hold, the filamentous form of the fungus gives rise to the formation of hyphae, that exhibit a particular tropism for vascular structures. When vessel walls are invaded, thrombosis, ischemia, and hemorrhage ensue, with infarction and necrosis of the surrounding tissues, including adjacent cranial nerves.

TREATMENT/PROGNOSIS

The key to survival of the patient with RM is prompt recognition. Correction of hyperglycemia and ketoacidosis should be undertaken as in any individual with DKA. The treatment is then surgical and medical, with extensive débridement of affected tissues and intravenous amphotericin B therapy. Surgical excision of affected tissues is critical, even to the point of orbital exenteration (Fig. 33.5). Amphotericin B is given in high doses (1.0 to 1.5 mg/kg/day) to a total dose of 2 to 4 g.[59] Without

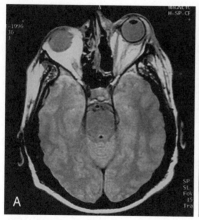
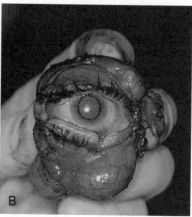

■ **Figure 33.5** *A*, Transverse T1-weighted magnetic resonance image of a 57-year-old diabetic man with biopsy proved left periorbital mucormycosis, showing proptosis and stranding of the intraconal retro-orbital fat consistent with cellulitis. *B*, Surgical pathology specimen after left orbital exenteration in the same patient. (Courtesy of Stephen F. Bansberg, M.D., Department of Otorhinolaryngology, Mayo Clinic Scottsdale.)

treatment, patients with RM invariably deteriorate and die within days. Blitzer and Lawson reported that of 170 cases of RM, untreated diabetics suffered a mortality rate of 63%, but only 17% died when treated with timely aggressive débridement and parenteral amphotericin administration.[12] Despite early recognition and aggressive therapeutic interventions, the mortality of RM remains close to 50%. Survivors of this devastating illness often require extensive reconstructive plastic surgery because of the disfigurement resulting from extensive tissue necrosis.[59]

Malignant External Otitis

CLINICAL FEATURES

Epidemiology. Malignant external otitis occurs almost exclusively in diabetes mellitus. Of 291 reported MEO cases in the last three decades, 85% have been diabetic, the mean age is 68 years (range, 11 to 92 years), and the sex ratio (M:F) is 2:1.[8, 15, 17–19, 31, 36, 41, 44, 52, 57, 75, 76] The rarity of this condition has doubtless contributed to the lack of population-based epidemiologic studies, such as rigorous analysis of prognostic covariates. Nonetheless, in addition to diabetes and advanced age, alleged adverse risk factors raised in the literature include hearing aids, swimming, aqueous irrigation of the external auditory canal, and perhaps empirical use of antibiotics ineffective against *Pseudomonas aeruginosa*.[52]

Symptoms/Signs/Presentations. The most frequent presenting symptom of MEO is ear pain, reported in 208/227 cases (92%).[8, 15, 17–19, 31, 36, 41, 44, 52, 57, 75, 76] Other findings include otorrhea, local swelling and tenderness of periauricular tissues, headache, and cranial nerve palsies. Initial neurologic manifestations occur 1 to 3 months after onset and may consist of facial palsy, most commonly, or other cranial neuropathies such as the tenth, eleventh, or other nerves. Disease of CN III, V, VI, VII, VIII, X, XI, and XII, sometimes with bilateral involvement, has been reported. Otoscopy typically shows a lobulated mass of erythematous granulation tissue, in an edematous inflamed external canal, without involvement of the tympanic membrane. Neurologically, isolated facial neuropathy is the most common finding, with other cranial nerves being involved less frequently. General examination can be surprisingly benign, often without signs of systemic infection such as fever or nuchal rigidity; laboratory studies usually fail to show leukocytosis or ketoacidosis.

Laboratory Findings. *Pseudomonas aeruginosa* is isolated in the vast majority of cultures from external ear exudates or biopsy material in MEO. Fewer than 1% of nonimmunocompromised adult patients are found to have other causative organisms.[52] Electrophysiologic investigation, including facial nerve conduction studies, trigeminal "blink" reflex testing, and masseter reflex studies may provide evidence of involvement of CN V or VII.[62] Imaging studies that may be useful in MEO include plain films, CT, and MRI. Skull films are usually normal early in the course of disease, with bony changes of osteomyelitis becoming evident at more advanced stages. Contrast CT scans are more sensitive in detecting subtle evidence of bone destruction, and MRI with gadolinium enhancement is the modality of choice for demonstrating meningeal or neural tissue involvement.[27]

ANATOMY/PATHOPHYSIOLOGY

Untreated, and frequently despite aggressive therapy, the infection of MEO can spread from the external auditory canal, leading to mastoiditis, osteomyelitis of the skull base, multiple cranial neuropathies, sinus thrombosis, and fatal meningitis. *Pseudomonas aeruginosa* is an aggressive gram-negative bacillus, thought to cause necrosis of infected tissues by suppression of polymorphonuclear leukocytes and inhibition of fibroblast growth factors to which diabetics appear to be more susceptible.[9, 24, 59]

TREATMENT/PROGNOSIS

The mainstay of treatment for MEO is inpatient intravenous antibiotic therapy in tandem with débridement of necrotic tissues in the affected external ear region. Empirical treatment with an aminoglycoside (such as tobramycin) and a third generation beta-lactam (such as ticarcillin) is instituted until the results from microbiologic studies on the patient's isolate(s) are available. In the past, aggressive surgical débridement was sometimes performed, although there is no convincing evidence that this approach is more effective than more conservative local débridement. The primary adverse prognostic factors in MEO are delay in diagnosis, inadequate antibiotic or surgical treatment (more often the former), and extension of disease outside of the external ear, as evidenced by involvement of the meninges or multiple lower cranial nerves. The mean mortality rate before 1980 was 30%,[15, 18, 75] whereas the mean mortality rate since 1980 is 10%.[2, 8, 17, 19, 31, 36, 41, 44, 52, 55, 76] Earlier recognition and more rapid institution of therapy are thought to explain the improvement in survival. Onset of ear or preauricular pain and headache with an abnormally elevated erythrocyte sedimentation rate in the 3 to 12 months after discontinuation of antibiotics for MEO may herald recrudescent disease, which is thought to erupt from inaccessible foci of osteomyelitis.[51] Relapse rates of up to one fourth of patients have been reported.

GUSTATORY FACIAL SWEATING

Gustatory sweating[1, 14, 63, 72] consists of profuse symmetrical sweating over the face, scalp, and neck that develops within minutes of eating food, especially strong tasting, spicy, or acid food that provokes salivation. Its causation is uncertain, but aberrant reinnervation in the territory of supply of the superior cervical ganglion has been suggested.[72] It is rarely a distressing symptom, and patients may respond by avoiding foods that provoke this phenomenon. If treatment is required, benefit may be obtained by taking an antimuscarinic drug such as propantheline hydrochloride or poldine methylsulfate before meals or on occasions when the sweating could be socially embarrassing.

OTHER CRANIAL NERVE SYNDROMES

Individual case reports of other cranial neuropathies appear from time to time in the diabetes literature, but these are unusual. Olfactory dysfunction has been reported in diabetic patients, although localization of the responsible lesion(s) has not been elucidated.[74] Of considerably greater clinical significance is the increased incidence of optic neuropathy in the diabetic population, which is beyond the scope of this discussion.[46] Trigeminal sensory neuropathy does not appear to related. It remains to be established whether diabetes is associated with an increased susceptibility to trigeminal neuralgia, and case reports linking the two are rare.[16, 23] Hearing loss in diabetics has been attributed to peripheral involvement of the eighth cranial nerve.[25, 42] The vagus nerve is commonly affected as part of diffuse diabetic autonomic neuropathy[33] and rarely in isolation.[32] Unusual cases of vocal cord paralysis caused by mononeuropathy of the recurrent laryngeal branch have also been described.[11, 56, 61] Multiple cranial nerves can be affected by local processes in the diabetic, including ischemia or infection in the cavernous sinus (CN II, III, IV, V, or VI) or by inflammatory disease of the skull base (CN VIII, IX, X, XI, or XII).

CONCLUSION

A number of characteristic cranial nerve syndromes have been described in association with diabetes mellitus, the most frequent being extraocular palsy thought to be on the basis of segmental ischemia resulting in focal demyelination, although some cases have been attributed to small central nervous system lesions affecting the general somatic efferent cell column and its connections in the brainstem. There appears to be an increased rate of facial neuropathy in diabetes mellitus, which clinically is nearly indistinguishable from Bell's palsy in nondiabetic individuals, including similar prognosis for recovery. Less common, although much more serious, are two diabetic syndromes associated with multiple cranial neuropathies, RM and MEO, conditions with mortality rates of 10 to 50%. For these life-threatening infections, rectifying hyperglycemia, instituting aggressive early parenteral antibiotic administration, and débriding necrotic tissues remain the first-line treatment strategies.

References

1. Aagenaes O. Neurovascular examinations on the lower extremities in young diabetics, with special reference to autonomic neuropathy. Copenhagen, C Hamburgers Bogtrykkeri, 1962.
2. Abraham-Inpijn L, Devriese PP, Hart AA. Predisposing factors in Bell's palsy: A clinical study with reference to diabetes mellitus, hypertension, clotting mechanism and lipid disturbance. Clin Otolaryngol 1982; 7:99.
3. Abraham-Inpijn L, Oosting J, Hart AA. Bell's palsy: Factors affecting prognosis in 200 patients with reference to hypertension and diabetes mellitus. Clin Otolaryngol 1987; 12:349.
4. Adour K, Bell DN, Wingerd J. Bell palsy. Arch Otolaryngol 1974; 99:114.
5. Aminoff MJ, Miller AL. The prevalence of diabetes mellitus in patients with Bell's palsy. Acta Neurol Scand 1972; 48:381.
6. Asbury AK, Aldredge H, Hershberg R, et al. Oculomotor palsy in diabetes mellitus: A clinicopathological study. Brain 1970; 93:555.
7. Asbury AK. Proximal diabetic neuropathy. Ann Neurol 1977; 2:179.
8. Babiatzki A, Sadé J. Malignant external otitis. J Laryngol Otol 1987; 101:205.
9. Bagdade JD, Root RK, Bulger RJ. Impaired leukocyte function in patients with poorly controlled diabetes. Diabetes 1974; 23:9.
10. Bell C. On the nerves: Giving an account of some experiments on their structure and function which lead to a new arrangement of the system. Phil Trans R Soc Lond 1821; 111:398.
11. Berry H, Blair RL. Isolated vagus nerve palsy and vagal mononeuritis. Arch Otolaryngol 1980; 106:333.
12. Blitzer A, Lawson W. Patient survival factors in paranasal sinus mucormycosis. Laryngoscope 1980; 90:635.
13. Boongird E, Vejjajiva A. Electrophysiologic findings and prognosis in Bell's palsy. Muscle Nerve 1978; 1:461.
14. Bronshrag MM. Spectrum of gustatory sweating with especial reference to its presence in diabetics with autonomic neuropathy. Am J Clin Nutr 1978; 31:307.
15. Chandler JR. Malignant external otitis. Laryngoscope 1968; 78:1257.
16. Collis JS, Wallace TW. Tic douloureux and diabetes mellitus. Cleve Clin Q 1968; 35:155.
17. Corey JP, Levandowski RA, Panwalker AP. Prognostic implications for therapy for necrotizing external otitis. Am J Otol 1985; 6:353.
18. Dinapoli RP, Thomas JE. Neurologic aspects of malignant external otitis: Report of three cases. Mayo Clin Proc 1971; 46:339.
19. Doroghazi RM, Nadol JB, Hyslop NE, et al. Invasive external otitis: Report of 21 cases and review of the literature. Am J Med 1981; 71:603.
20. Dreyfus PM, Hakim S, Adams RD. Diabetic ophthalmoplegia. Arch Neurol Psychiatry 1957; 77:337.
21. Ellenberg M. Diabetic neuropathy presenting as the initial clinical manifestation of diabetes. Ann Intern Med 1958; 49:620.
22. Ferguson BJ, Mitchell TG, Moon R, et al. Adjunctive hyperbaric oxygen for treatment of rhinocerebral mucormycosis. Rev Infect Dis 1988; 10:551.
23. Finestone AJ, Choudhry M, Shenkin HA. Trigeminal neuralgia and diabetes mellitus. J Med Soc New Jersey 1970; 67:269.
24. Fontan PA, Amura CR, Buzzola FR, et al. Modulation of human polymorphonuclear leukocyte chemotaxis and superoxide anion production by Pseudomonas aeruginosa exoproducts, IL-1 beta, and piroxicam. FEMS Immunol Med Microbiol 1995; 10:139.
25. Friedman SA, Schulman RH, Weiss S. Hearing and diabetic neuropathy. Arch Intern Med 1975; 135:573.
26. Gavilan C, Gavilan J, Rashad M, et al. Discriminant analysis in predicting prognosis of Bell's palsy. Acta Otolaryngol (Stockh) 1988; 106:276.
27. Gherini SG, Brackman DE, Bradley WG. Magnetic resonance imaging and computerized tomography in malignant external otitis. Laryngoscope 1986; 96:542.
28. Giamarellou H. Malignant otitis externa: The therapeutic evolution of a lethal infection. J Antimicrob Chemother 1992; 30:745.
29. Goldstein JE, Cogan DG. Diabetic ophthalmoplegia with special reference to the pupil. Arch Ophthalmol 1960; 64:592.
30. Gray H. Anatomy of the human body. Clemente CD (ed). Philadelphia, Lea & Febiger, 1985, p 1156.
31. Grobman LR, Ganz W, Casiano R, et al. Atypical osteomyelitis of the skull base. Laryngoscope 1989; 99:671.
32. Guy RJC, Dawson JL, Garrett JR, et al. Diabetic gastroparesis from autonomic neuropathy: Surgical considerations and changes in vagus nerve morphology. J Neurol Neurosurg Psychiatry 1984; 47:686.
33. Hilsted J, Low PA. Diabetic autonomic neuropathy. In Low PA (ed): Clinical Autonomic Disorders. Boston, Little, Brown, 1993, pp 423–443.
34. Hopf HC, Gutmann L. Diabetic 3rd nerve palsy: Evidence for a mesencephalic lesion. Neurology 1990; 40:1041.
35. Joffe WS. Cranial nerve disease: Int Ophthalmol Clin 1967; 7:823.
36. Johnson MP, Ramphal R. Malignant external otitis: Report on therapy with ceftazidime and review of therapy and prognosis. Rev Infect Dis 1990; 12:173.
37. Kerr F, Hollowell OW. Location of pupillomotor and accommodation fibers in the oculomotor nerve: Experimental studies on paralytic mydriasis. J Neurol Neurosurg Psychiatry 1964; 27:473.
38. Kimura J, Giron LT Jr, Young SM. Electrophysiological study of Bell palsy: Electrically elicited blink reflex in assessment of prognosis. Arch Otolaryngol 1976; 102:140.
39. Kodsi SR, Younge BR. Acquired oculomotor, trochlear, and abducent cranial nerve palsies in pediatric patients. Am J Ophthalmol 1992; 14:568.
40. Korczyn AD. Bell's palsy and diabetes mellitus. Lancet 1971; 1:108.
41. Lang R, Goshen S, Kitzes-Cohen R, et al. Successful treatment of malignant external otitis with oral ciprofloxacin: Report of experience with 23 patients. J Infect Dis 1990; 161:537.
42. Makishima K, Tanaka K. Pathological changes of the inner ear and central auditory pathways in diabetics. Ann Otol Rhinol Laryngol 1971; 80:218.

43. McNulty JS. Rhinocerebral mucormycosis: Predisposing factors. Laryngoscope 1982; 92:1140.
44. Meyers BR, Mendelson MH, Parisier SC, et al. Malignant external otitis: Comparison of monotherapy vs. combination therapy. Arch Otolaryngol Head Neck Surg 1987; 113:974.
45. Millen SJ, Daniels D, Meyer G. Gadolinium-enhanced magnetic resonance imaging in facial nerve lesions. Otolaryngol Head Neck Surg 1990; 102:26.
46. Moro F, Doro D. Diabetic optic neuropathies: Clinical features. Metab Pediatr System Ophthalmol 1986; 9:71.
47. Parkinson D. A surgical approach to the cavernous portion of the carotid artery: Anatomical studies and case report. J Neurosurg 1965; 23:474.
48. Pecket P, Schattner A. Concurrent Bell's palsy and diabetes mellitus: A diabetic mononeuropathy? J Neurol Neurosurg Psychiatry 1982; 45:652.
49. Raff MC, Sangalang V, Asbury AK. Ischemic mononeuropathy multiplex associated with diabetes mellitus. Arch Neurol 1968; 18:487.
50. Richards BW, Jones FR, Younge BR. Causes and prognosis in 4,278 cases of paralysis of the oculomotor, trochlear, and abducens cranial nerves. Am J Ophthalmol 1992; 113:489.
51. Rubin J, Yu VL. Malignant external otitis: Insights into pathogenesis, clinical manifestations, diagnosis, and therapy. Am J Med 1988; 85:391.
52. Rubin J, Yu VL, Kamerer DB, et al. Aural irrigation with water: A potential pathogenic mechanism for inducing malignant external otitis. Ann Otol Rhinol Laryngol 1990; 99:117.
53. Rucker CW. The causes of paralysis of the third, fourth, and sixth cranial nerves. Am J Ophthalmol 1966; 61:293.
54. Rush JA, Younge BR. Paralysis of cranial nerves III, IV, and VI: Cause and prognosis in 1000 cases. Arch Ophthalmol 1981; 99:76.
55. Salit IE, McNeely DJ, Chait G. Invasive external otitis: Review of 12 cases. Can Med Assoc J 1985; 132:381.
56. Schecter GL, Kostianovsky M. Vocal cord paralysis in diabetes mellitus. Trans Am Acad Ophthalmol Otolaryngol 1972; 76:729.
57. Smith BE, Dyck PJ. Subclinical histopathological changes in the oculomotor nerve in diabetes mellitus. Ann Neurol 1992; 32:376.
58. Smith IM, Heath JP, Murray JA, et al. Idiopathic facial (Bell's) palsy: A clinical survey of prognostic factors. Clin Otolaryngol 1988; 13:17.
59. Smitherman KO, Peakock JE. Infectious emergencies in patients with diabetes mellitus. Med Clin N Am 1995; 79:53.
60. Snydacker D. Diabetic neuropathy as a cause of extraocular muscle palsy. Trans Am Acad Ophthalmol 1958; 62:704.
61. Sommer DD, Freeman JL. Bilateral vocal cord paralysis associated with diabetes mellitus: Case reports. J Otol 1994; 23:169.
62. Stevens JC, Smith BE. Cranial reflexes. In Daube JR (ed): Clinical Neurophysiology. Philadelphia, FA Davis, 1996, pp 321–335.
63. Stuart DD. Diabetic gustatory sweating. Ann Intern Med 1978; 89:223.
64. Sunderland S, Hughes ESR. Pupilloconstriction pathway and the nerves to the ocular muscles in man. Brain 1946; 69:301.
65. Sunderland S, Cossar DF. The structure of the facial nerve. Anat Rec 1953; 116:147.
66. Taren JA. An anatomic demonstration of afferent fibers in the IV, V, and VI cranial nerves of the Macaca mulatta. Am J Ophthalmol 1964; 58:408.
67. Teuscher AU, Meienberg O. Ischaemic oculomotor nerve palsy. J Neurol 1985; 232:144.
68. Thomander L, Stålberg E. Electroneurography in the prognostication of Bell's palsy. Acta Laryngol (Stockh) 1981; 92:221.
69. Tien R, Dillon WP, Jackler RK. Contrast-enhanced MR imaging of the facial nerve in 11 patients with Bell's palsy. AJNR 1990; 11:735.
70. Usui Y, Mukoyama M, Hashizume M, et al. Diabetic ophthalmoplegia: A clinicopathologic study of the first case in Japan. Clin Neurol 1989; 29:442.
71. Watanabe K, Hagura R, Akanuma Y, et al. Characteristics of cranial nerve palsies in diabetic patients. Diabetes Res Clin Pract 1990; 10:19.
72. Watkins PJ. Facial sweating after food: A new sign of autonomic neuropathy. BMJ 1973; 1:583.
73. Weber RB, Daroff RB, Mackey EA. Pathology of oculomotor palsy in diabetes. Neurology 1970; 20:835.
74. Weinstock RS, Wright HN, Smith DU. Olfactory discrimination in diabetes mellitus. Physiol Behav 1993; 53:17.
75. Wilson DF, Pulec JL, Linthicum FH. Malignant external otitis. Arch Otolaryngol 1971; 93:419.
76. Yu VL, Stoehr G, Rubin J, et al. Efficacy of oral ciprofloxacin plus rifampin for therapy of malignant otitis externa (abstract 188). In Proceedings of the 27th Interscience Conference on Antimicrobial Agents and Chemotherapy. New York, American Society of Microbiology, 1987.
77. Zorilla E, Kozak G. Ophthalmoplegia in diabetes mellitus. Ann Intern Med 1967; 67:968.

Chapter **34**

Diabetic Truncal Radiculoneuropathy

P. J. Watkins • *P. K. Thomas*

INTRODUCTION

Diabetes causes distinctive neuropathies that either progress or remit.[18, 19] The commonest neuropathy is a diffuse, symmetrical sensory and autonomic neuropathy that is a classical diabetic complication, slowly progressing with duration of diabetes and associated with other diabetic complications. In striking contrast, radiculoneuropathies, often associated with severe pain, have a relatively acute onset, run a clearly defined course, and remit, usually completely, within 6 to 18 months, generally without recurring at a later time. These radiculoneuropathies are commoner in older diabetic men and occur in patients with type 1 and type 2 diabetes mellitus (DM). They are unrelated to the duration of diabetes or to other diabetic complications and may be the presenting feature of diabetes itself. Painful radiculopathy as a presenting feature of diabetes is uncommon but well recognized. Diabetic radiculoneuropathies affecting thoracic nerve roots occur infrequently and may give rise to localized abdominal pain, leading to extensive investigation to rule out intra-abdominal pathologies. Thoracic radiculoneuropathy with abdominal muscle bulging is rare and to our knowledge has been described in only four reports.

The designation *truncal neuropathy* has been used in more than one sense. These different usages need to be clearly distinguished. As with other distal length-related neuropathies, in more severe examples of diabetic sensory polyneuropathy, sensory loss develops over the midline of the lower anterior trunk and, with advance of the neuropathy, gradually spreads laterally around the abdominal wall in a symmetrical manner.[20] This has to be distinguished from focal truncal thoracoabdominal neuropathy, which is the subject of this chapter. Although it has been referred to as truncal radiculopathy, the precise localization of the pathologic changes is still uncertain. In view of this, the condition is referred to here as *diabetic radiculoneuropathy*.

Diabetic truncal radiculoneuropathy is not rare: Asbury[1] pointed out that between 1977 and 1987, more than 150 cases had been reported in the North American literature alone. He concluded that the more frequent documentation in recent years probably reflects increased recognition rather than a greater incidence of this syndrome. Early reports of focal diabetic truncal radiculoneuropathy were made by Schulz,[14, 15] Wessely and Schnaberth,[21] Ellenberg,[6] and Sun and Streib.[17] Similar cases were included in the series of patients with proximal lower limb motor neuropathy collected by Bastron and Thomas.[2] Schulz[15] and Longstreth and Newcomer[9] drew attention to the presentation of these cases with abdominal pain, and Schulz,[14] Boulton and colleagues,[4] and Parry and Floberg[11] presented cases with focal weakness of the anterior abdominal wall. The electrodiagnostic features were reported by Massey,[10] Sun and Streib,[17] and Kitka and colleagues.[8]

CLINICAL FEATURES

There is general agreement that focal truncal radiculoneuropathy, as is true for diabetic proximal lower limb neuropathy (diabetic amyotrophy), is usually encountered in middle or later life. It occurs in patients with types 1 and 2 DM. It may affect individuals of either sex, but mainly men; all seven patients reported by Stewart[16] were male. It can be the presenting feature in type 2 DM. The onset of the sensory symptoms is often relatively sudden, but the condition may evolve over weeks or months before maximal severity is reached. Recurrent episodes may occur, sometimes as many as six.[16]

The predominant symptom is pain, which may be aching or burning in quality. Superimposed lancinating stabs may occur. The pain often has a girdlelike distribution around the lower thoracic or abdominal wall, but it can be more diffuse and may be experienced in the back. It is usually unilateral but can be bilateral at the same dermatomal level. The pain is characteristically worse at night and may be associated with cutaneous hyperesthesia so that patients find contact with clothing or bedclothes highly uncomfortable. Patients rather rarely have focal motor weakness, usually on the right side, giving rise to localized bulging of the abdominal wall, at times simulating a hernia.[4, 11] This has been described as a result of other types of pathology.[3, 5] Generalized weakness has also been observed.[16]

The onset of the symptoms may be associated with profound weight loss, sometimes amounting to as much as 18 kg[6, 17] or even 30 kg (Table 34.1, Case 1).

TABLE 34.1   CLINICAL DETAILS OF CASES OBSERVED PERSONALLY*

Case	Age (y)	Sex	Diabetes Type and Duration	Site of Pain	HbA$_{1c}$ (%)	Diabetic Retinopathy	Weight Loss (kg)	Diabetic Treatment	Treatment	Recovery (mo)
1	57	M	Type 2, 4 y	R flank T6–10	6.3	0	30	Metformin, glibenclamide	Tricycl, TENS	3
2	60	M	Type 2, 7 y	L flank, T6–10	8.0	Background, laser later	10	Glibenclamide	Tricycl, CBZ	3
3	55	M	Type 2, 3 mo	R flank, T8–10	10.1	None at onset, laser 5 y later	15	Glibenclamide, metformin	Tricycl, MST	6
4	61	M	Type 2, 7 y	R flank T7–12	11.0	0	5	Diet	Tricycl	6
5	70	M	Type 2, presentation	R + L flanks T9–12	8.1	0	12	Diet	Tricycl, CBZ	12
6	54	M	Type 2, 6 y	R flank T10–12	8.0	0	10	Humulin S, Humulin I	TENS, capsaicin	Under follow-up

*Chandhuri KR, Wren DR, Werning D, Watkins PJ. Unilateral abdominal muscle herniation with pain: A distinctive variant of diabetic radiculopathy. Diabet Med 1997; 14:803.
HbA$_{1c}$, glycated hemoglobin; Tricycl, tricyclic antidepressants; TENS, transcutaneous electrical nerve stimulation; CBZ, carbamazepine; MST, morphine sulphate.

Examination may reveal no abnormal signs or may demonstrate cutaneous sensory impairment and hyperesthesia (allodynia and hyperpathia) in the region of the pain. The pattern of sensory loss is highly variable.[16] The territory of several adjacent main mixed spinal nerves may be affected, leading to a complete unilateral or bilateral dermatomal pattern that may be symmetrical or asymmetrical. More frequently, the loss is restricted either to the distribution of the ventral or dorsal rami of the spinal nerves or branches of these nerves in varying combinations of their distributions (Figs. 34.1 to 34.3). Focal weakness of the abdominal muscles may be evident, with local-

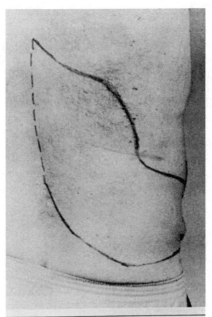

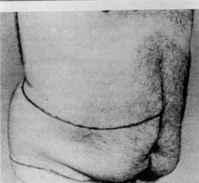

■ **Figure 34.2** Same patient as in Figure 34.1. In his third episode, bilateral but asymmetric sensory abnormality developed. In the upper and midthoracic region, the sensory disturbance affects the distribution of the dorsal rami only, whereas lower down, the entire T9–T11 dermatomes on the right and T7–T12 on the left are involved. The patient also had diffuse laxity of the abdominal wall muscles that was of recent onset. (From Stewart JD. Diabetic truncal neuropathy: Topography of the sensory deficit. Ann Neurol 1989; 25:233–238.)

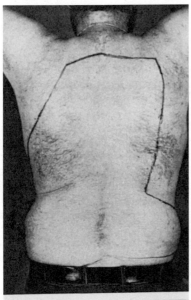

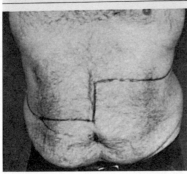

■ **Figure 34.1** Diabetic truncal polyradiculoneuropathy. The area of abnormal sensation on the abdominal wall in the patient's second attack has been outlined. Posteriorly, the area of sensory loss is confined to the distribution of the dorsal rami; in the lower abdomen the entire distributions of several adjacent spinal nerves (T6–T11) are involved. (From Stewart JD. Diabetic truncal neuropathy: Topography of the sensory deficit. Ann Neurol 1989; 25:233–238.)

ized (Figs. 34.3 and 34.4) or generalized (Fig. 34.2) bulging of the anterior abdominal wall, evident when the patient is standing or attempting to sit up without using the upper limbs. Signs of concomitant proximal lower limb motor neuropathy may be present, but distal symmetrical sensory polyneuropathy can be absent. Movements of the spine usually have no effect on the pain.

The natural history of diabetic truncal radiculoneuropathy is usually one of spontane-

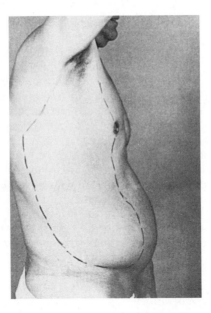
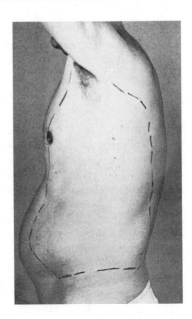

■ **Figure 34.3** Diabetic truncal radiculoneuropathy. The extensive and almost symmetric areas of sensory abnormality that developed in this patient's second episode have been outlined. They involve the territories of many adjacent lateral branches of the T3–T12 intercostal nerves. He also has diffuse bulging of the abdominal wall on the right; this appeared at the time of his first episode. (From Stewart JD. Diabetic truncal neuropathy: Topography of the sensory deficit. Ann Neurol 1989; 25:233–238.)

ous resolution, generally within a matter of some months. In the series of seven patients described by Stewart,[16] the duration of the shortest attacks was 4 months. More rarely, the sensory symptoms can be protracted.

The clinical details for 6 patients observed personally are given in Table 34.1.

ELECTROPHYSIOLOGIC CHANGES

Electromyography using needle electrode sampling may demonstrate denervation potentials in the intercostal muscles, those of the anterior abdominal wall, and the paraspinal muscles at the same level. Electromyographic abnormalities were detected in 15 of the 21 cases docu-

mented by Kitka and colleagues.[8] Conduction studies in the intercostal nerves have not been reported.

Nerve conduction studies may reveal the absence or presence of a coexisting subclinical distal lower limb polyneuropathy or confirm its presence if symptomatic.

ILLUSTRATIVE CASE HISTORY ■ A 57-year-old white man (see Table 34.1, Case 1), with established type 2 DM treated with metformin and glibenclamide, had a 7-month history of right iliac fossa pain extending up to the right subcostal region. This was associated with severe weight loss (30 kg) and subsequent development of bulging of the right flank of his abdomen and cutaneous hypersensitivity over the right subcostal region. On examination, in addition to the signs of a mild distal sensory neuropathy, he had marked bulging of abdominal muscles from right T6 to T10 myotomes, with hyperpathia and mild deviation of the umbilicus to the left (see Fig. 34.4). He had extensive investigations elsewhere to exclude intraabdominal malignancy. Electromyography showed evidence of denervation of the rectus abdominis muscles from T6 to T10 myotomes. Magnetic resonance imaging of the spine was normal, and cerebrospinal fluid was acellular but with a raised protein content (0.6 g/L). He was treated with analgesics, a tricyclic antidepressant, and transcutaneous electrical nerve stimulation. His

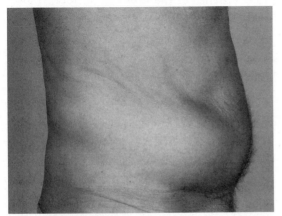

■ **Figure 34.4** Diabetic focal truncal radiculoneuropathy showing localized bulging of the lower right abdominal wall.

pain resolved over a period of 6 weeks, he gained weight, and when reviewed 3 months later, his abdominal herniation had virtually disappeared.

DIFFERENTIAL DIAGNOSIS

In patients with an acute onset of focal truncal pain, herpes zoster will enter into the initial differential diagnosis. The occurrence of girdlelike pain, particularly in the rarer bilateral cases, will raise the possibility of spinal root compression, although in diabetic radiculoneuropathy the pain is rarely aggravated by spinal movement or by coughing, sneezing, etc. If there is concomitant weight loss, the question of occult malignancy with spinal secondary deposits will arise. If doubt exists, spinal imaging and other appropriate studies should be undertaken. When the pain affects the thorax or the abdominal wall more diffusely, intrathoracic or intra-abdominal disease may be suspected, again necessitating appropriate screening investigation. If such investigations are negative and if positive confirmation by electromyography cannot be obtained, follow-up is essential.

PATHOGENESIS

No studies on the underlying pathology are available. Some investigators, such as Schulz[14] and Longstreth and Newcomer,[9] have favored a radiculopathy. Support for this view has been adduced by the finding of denervation in the paraspinal muscles that are innervated by the dorsal primary rami derived from the spinal nerves. Nevertheless, without histologic proof, it is not possible to state whether the lesions responsible for the motor involvement are in the anterior spinal roots, the mixed spinal nerves, their posterior or anterior primary rami, or their branches. Moreover, not all cases show evidence of denervation in the paraspinal muscles.[17] In these, the lesions could be located more peripherally in the intercostal or subcostal nerves. For the sensory loss, it is clear from the careful mapping of the sensory abnormality by Stewart[16] that the lesions must at times be confined to the posterior primary rami of the spinal nerves and, at others, to the intercostal nerves or their branches.

The abrupt onset in some cases may favor an ischemic basis, as has been proposed for diabetic amyotrophy[12] but, if so, the simultaneous involvement of several contiguous dermatomes[17] requires explanation. As suggested by Stewart,[16] the occlusion of a single intercostal artery, if it supplied several truncal nerves, could produce ischemic damage in these nerves at the same point along their course.

The coexistence of some instances of diabetic truncal radiculoneuropathy with proximal lower limb diabetic neuropathy has been noted by Schulz,[14, 15] Longstreth and Newcomer,[9] and Sun and Streib[17] and was evident in one of Garland's[7] original cases of diabetic amyotrophy. This suggests that similar underlying mechanisms may be present in the two syndromes. The findings by Said and colleagues[13] of inflammatory changes, including vasculitis, in the intermediate cutaneous nerve of the thigh in patients with proximal lower limb diabetic neuropathy (see Chapter 35) therefore raises the possibility that a similar pathogenesis may at times be involved in diabetic truncal polyradiculoneuropathy. Histologic verification would unfortunately be difficult short of autopsy study.

TREATMENT

Because the course of diabetic truncal radiculoneuropathy is usually one of spontaneous recovery, treatment of the pain (see Chapter 28) and the establishment of effective glycemic control is all that is necessary. The pain can be intense. If it is considered that an inflammatory mechanism may be possible, in cases with severe or prolonged symptoms the question of immunomodulatory or immunosuppressive therapy, such as with corticosteroids, making certain that glycemic control is maintained, or with high-dose intravenous human immunoglobulin, perhaps deserves consideration. The use of cytotoxic drugs could not be supported in the absence of the histologic demonstration of an inflammatory process, particularly in view of the generally favorable prognosis of this condition. In those patients with associated proximal lower limb involvement, biopsy of the intermediate cutaneous nerve of the thigh[13] could be undertaken.

References

1. Asbury AK. Focal and multifocal neuropathies of diabetes. *In* Dyck PJ, Thomas PK, Asbury AK, et al (eds): Diabetic Neuropathy. Philadelphia, WB Saunders, 1987, p 45.
2. Bastron JA, Thomas JE. Diabetic polyradiculopathy: Clinical and electromyographic findings in 105 patients. Mayo Clin Proc 1981; 56:725.
3. Billet FPJ, Ponssen H, Veenhuizen D. Unilateral paresis of the abdominal wall: A radicular syndrome caused

by herniation of the L1-L2 disc? J Neurol Neurosurg Psychiatry 1989; 52:678.

4. Boulton AJM, Angus E, Ayyar DR, et al. Diabetic thoracic polyradiculopathy presenting as an abdominal swelling. BMJ 1984; 289:798.

4a. Chaudhuri KR, Wren DR, Werning D, Watkins PJ. Unilateral abdominal muscle herniation with pain: A distinctive variant of diabetic radiculopathy. Diabet Med 1997; 14:803.

5. Daffner KR, Saver JI, Biber MP. Lyme polyradiculoneuropathy presenting as increasing abdominal girth. Neurology 1990; 40:373.

6. Ellenberg M. Diabetic truncal mononeuropathy: A new clinical syndrome. Diabetes Care 1978; 1:10.

7. Garland H. Diabetic amyotrophy. BMJ 1955; 2:1287.

8. Kitka DG, Breuer AC, Wilbourn AJ. Thoracic root pain in diabetes: The spectrum of clinical and electromyographic findings. Ann Neurol 1982; 11:80.

9. Longstreth GF, Newcomer AD. Abdominal pain caused by diabetic radiculopathy. Ann Intern Med 1977; 86:166.

10. Massey EW. Diabetic truncal mononeuropathy: Electromyographic evaluation. Acta Diabetol Lat 1980; 17:269.

11. Parry GJ, Floberg J. Diabetic truncal neuropathy presenting as an abdominal hernia. Neurology 1989; 39:1488.

12. Raff M, Sangalang V, Asbury AK. Ischemic mononeuropathy multiplex associated with diabetes mellitus. Arch Neurol 1968; 18:487.

13. Said G, Goulon-Goeau C, Lacroix C, et al. Nerve biopsy findings in different patterns of proximal diabetic neuropathy. Ann Neurol 1994; 35:559.

14. Schulz A. Diabetische Radiculopathie der unteren Thorakalsegmente mit Bauchdeckenparesen. Verh Dtsch Ges Inn Med 1966; 72:1171.

15. Schulz A. Brennende Schmerzen an Rumpf und Oberschenkel mit Bauchdeckenparesen. Dtsch Med Wochenschr 1972; 97:1568.

16. Stewart JD. Diabetic truncal neuropathy: Topography of the sensory deficit. Ann Neurol 1989; 25:233.

17. Sun SF, Streib EW. Diabetic thoracoabdominal neuropathy: Clinical and electrodiagnostic features. Ann Neurol 1981; 9:75.

18. Watkins PJ. Natural history of the diabetic neuropathies. Q J Med 1990; 77:1209.

19. Watkins PJ. Clinical observations and experiments in diabetic neuropathy. Diabetologia 1992; 35:2.

20. Waxman SG, Sabin TD. Diabetic truncal polyneuropathy. Arch Neurol 1981; 38:46.

21. Wessely P, Schnaberth G. Kasuistischer Beitrag zu einer seltenen Lokalisation diabetischer Neuropathie. Wien Klin Wochenschr 1973; 85:710.

Chapter 35

Proximal Diabetic Neuropathy

Gerard Said • *P. K. Thomas*

INTRODUCTION

Early descriptions of diabetic neuropathy recognized cases in which asymmetrical lower limb weakness was the presenting feature. These were first documented in 1890 by Bruns,[8] Buzzard,[9] and Charcot.[12] Similar cases were described by Root and Rogers in 1930[35] and by Alderman[1] in 1938. Garland and Taverner[25] focused attention on the syndrome as a separate entity. Because some of their patients had extensor plantar responses, the condition was referred to as *diabetic myelopathy.*[25] Subsequently, Garland[22–24] introduced the noncommittal title *diabetic amyotrophy* because he considered that the nature of the underlying pathology was not satisfactorily established. Electrodiagnostic[15, 27, 31] and neuropathologic[34, 39] studies later demonstrated that the syndrome represented a proximal motor neuropathy, often referred to as diabetic femoral neuropathy.[10, 16, 26] The distribution of the weakness suggested that the lumbosacral plexus is also involved. Asbury[2] advocated the term *proximal diabetic neuropathy* in view of the ambiguities associated with the designation diabetic amyotrophy and drew a distinction between asymmetrical cases of acute or subacute onset and symmetrical cases with gradual evolution.

CLINICAL FEATURES

All series have commented that the disorder typically occurs in older patients with type 2 diabetes mellitus (DM) and that it is more frequent in males. It may develop at any stage of diabetes and it is not uncommon for it to be the presenting feature in a late-onset case of type 2 DM.[11, 21, 25] Thus, in the series of 27 patients reported by Coppack and Watkins,[16] 24 had type 2 DM and 3 had type 1 DM. The mean age at diagnosis was 62 years (range, 46 to 71 years) in the former and 64 years (range, 33 to 67 years) in the latter. In the 12 cases reported by Casey and Harrison,[11] no patient was younger than 50 years, and 10 were older than 60 years. The male:female ratio in the series of Coppack and Watkins[16] was 16:11.

The major clinical features are pain, muscle weakness and wasting, depression or loss of the knee jerks, and relatively minor sensory changes, although a distal sensory polyneuropathy may coexist. The pain is felt in the thighs and sometimes also in the perineum, buttocks, and lumbar region. It is frequently worse at night and is uninfluenced by movements of the lumbar spine, coughing, sneezing, etc. The weakness predominantly affects the proximal lower limb muscles, particularly the knee extensors and hip flexors and, at times, the hip extensors. The lower leg muscles may also be affected, particularly the anterolateral group, or there may be generalized lower extremity weakness.[23, 41]

Associated sensory changes tend to be slight. Cutaneous hyperesthesia over the thigh was reported in 14 of 27 cases documented by Coppack and Watkins.[16] Others reported tingling and thermal paresthesias. Cutaneous sensory loss over the anterior thigh may be demonstrable.

The disease can begin unilaterally or bilaterally; in the unilateral cases it may then develop on the opposite side, at times within weeks.[25, 28, 33, 35] Relapses may occur, sometimes after an interval of some years, but this is unusual.[4, 16, 25] A tendency for spontaneous recovery was commented on in the early descriptions.[21, 22, 24] Casey and Harrison[11] reported that not all cases recover fully. Of their 12 patients, 3 recovered fully, 4 achieved a good functional result, and 5 showed significant residual functional disability. Root and Rogers[35] and Fry and associates[21] also recorded permanent disability. A longer follow-up review, of up to 14 years, was undertaken by Coppack and Watkins.[16] Recovery in their cases began after a median interval of 3 months (range, 1 to 12 months). Pain was the first symptom to improve, resolution being comparatively rapid, beginning within a few weeks and being almost complete by 12 months. A similar time course was found by Casey and Harrison.[11] Residual discomfort in the patients of Coppack and Watkins[16] took up to 3 years to subside. Motor recovery was satisfactory, and none of their 27 cases showed disabling residual deficits. Seven complained of some persisting weakness, and significant wasting of the thigh was evident in half of the cases. Some patients may slowly develop a distal sensory neuropathy while the proximal motor neuropathy is resolving. In one series, all patients with proximal diabetic neuropathy had clinical or electrophysiologic signs of a distal symmetrical sensory polyneuropathy.[37] It is important to note, for reasons discussed later, that there is usually no clinical, hematologic, or biochemical evidence of an inflammatory process. In all cases, a focal lesion of spinal roots must be excluded by appropriate investigations, such as magnetic resonance imaging of the lower spine.

Proximal upper limb diabetic neuropathy is uncommon. It may develop in patients who have proximal lower limb neuropathy. In the upper limbs the involvement tends to be symmetrical, usually affecting muscles supplied by the C5–6 spinal roots, sparing those innervated by the C7, C8, and T1 roots.[41]

Symmetric Lower Limb Motor Neuropathy. Some authors have described patients with a subacute[42] or insidious[13] onset of proximal lower limb weakness. Asbury,[2] favoring the term *proximal diabetic neuropathy* (PDN), considered that there was a spectrum ranging from asymmetrical cases with a rapid onset to patients with symmetrical proximal weakness of insidious onset. The latter presentation is probably uncommon and has been encountered only rarely by the authors of this chapter.

CLINICAL NEUROPHYSIOLOGY

Needle electrode sampling reveals signs of denervation in affected muscles, with increased insertion activity and spontaneous fibrillation, especially in early cases, and reduced motor unit recruitment. Signs of denervation may be found bilaterally even in cases with weakness restricted to one side. In more severe bilateral cases, there may be evidence of widespread denervation affecting distal leg muscles as well and also those innervated by the lower thoracic spinal roots, indicating an overlap with diabetic truncal radiculoneuropathy (see Chapter 34). In cases of longer duration, motor unit potentials are of increased amplitude, reflecting reinnervation by collateral sprouting from surviving motor axons. At times, the motor action potentials may be polyphasic and of low amplitude, leading to the suspicion of myopathy.[31] Nerve conduction studies indicate axonal loss rather than demyelination.[38] Conduction time is prolonged in the femoral nerve,[14, 15, 31] and the compound muscle action potential in the quadriceps muscles on femoral nerve stimulation is reduced in amplitude. Conclusions concerning the nature of diabetic proximal neuropathy by studying F-wave latencies to distal muscles[13, 42] are difficult to interpret in view of the frequent coexistence of a distal polyneuropathy.[4, 18, 29, 31, 40]

NEUROPATHOLOGY

Muscle biopsy shows evidence of denervation (Fig. 35.1). Nonspecific ultrastructural changes in muscle fibers and thickening and reduplication of the basal lamina around microvessels has been described. In early studies, Bischoff[5] and Locke and colleagues[33] commented on isolated muscle fiber atrophy.

An autopsy study using multiple serial sections[33] concluded that multiple "microinfarcts" were present in nerves to affected muscles. Some of these, it was later realized, were Renaut bodies, a normal structure in peripheral nerve.[3] Others consisted of damage to small bridging fascicles associated with rarefaction of the surrounding epineurium. Unfortunately, sections stained to demonstrate the myelinated fiber population were not included in the report. A single occluded epineurial vessel was found, but the walls of many of the microvessels were found to be thickened. It is of interest that a focal infiltrate of inflammatory cells related to an epineurial vessel was illustrated.

Bradley and associates[7] described a series of six patients with a painful lumbosacral plexopathy associated with an elevated erythrocyte sedimentation rate. Three patients were diabetic. Sural nerve biopsy in all six cases showed axonal degeneration with epineurial arterioles surrounded by inflammatory cells. Unequal fascicular involvement in three of the biopsies suggested an ischemic basis. In none of the patients was there evidence of systemic vasculitis. Five patients received immunosuppressive treatment, and in four the plexopathy improved or arrested. An immunologic basis was assumed, but its nature was obscure.

In a recent morphological study of biopsy specimens of the intermediate cutaneous nerve of the thigh, a sensory branch of the femoral nerve that conveys sensation from the lower third of the anterior aspect of the thigh, a territory commonly involved in PDN, it was found that the pathology of proximal nerves varied with the clinical features of the neuropathy.[37]

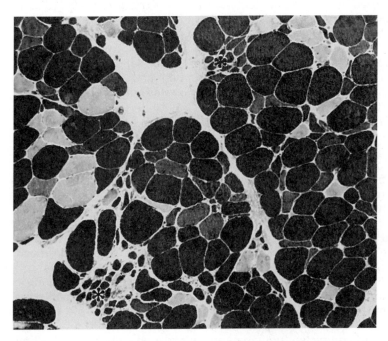

■ **Figure 35.1** A transverse section of quadriceps muscle biopsy specimen, obtained from a patient with proximal diabetic neuropathy, reacted for myosin ATPase at pH 9.4. Type 2 fibers are dark. Changes indicating recent and chronic partial denervation with reinnervation are present with grouped atrophy (*asterisks*) and fiber type grouping, the latter being particularly evident on the right side of the figure. × 120.

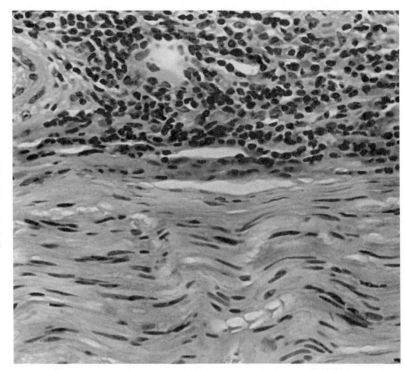

■ **Figure 35.2** Longitudinal section of paraffin-embedded biopsy specimen of the intermediate cutaneous nerve of the thigh of a patient with painful proximal neuropathy of the left lower limb and type 2 diabetes mellitus recently treated with insulin. Note the conspicuous inflammatory infiltration composed of mononuclear cells, around epineurial and perineurial blood vessels. Hematoxylin and eosin; ×250.

In the three patients with the most severe sensory and motor deficit, examination of the biopsy specimen from the intermediate cutaneous nerve of the thigh revealed lesions characteristic of severe nerve ischemia, including total axon loss in the two patients with the most severe deficit, and centrofascicular degeneration of fibers associated with a large number of regenerating fibers in one, following a pattern of axonal loss observed in experimental nerve ischemia. Lesions of nerve fibers coexisted with occlusion of a perineurial blood vessel in one of the patients. In one patient, who developed a rapid, asymmetrical distal sensorimotor deficit shortly after the onset of the proximal deficit, recent occlusion of a perineurial blood vessel and perivascular, perineurial, and subperineurial inflammatory infiltration with mononuclear cells was demonstrated, along with axonal degeneration of the majority of nerve fibers of the superficial peroneal nerve. In the other patients, lesions of nerve fibers and of endoneurial capillaries were similar to those observed in the sural nerve in diabetic patients with symptomatic distal symmetrical sensorimotor polyneuropathy. Mixed, axonal, and demyelinative nerve lesions were associated with increased endoneurial cellularity made up of mononuclear cells that suggested the presence of a low-grade endoneurial inflammatory process in four. More recently, in patients with extremely painful PDN, similar inflammatory lesions were found in biopsies of the intermediate cutaneous nerve of the thigh, with B and T lymphocytes mixed with macrophages (Figs. 35.2 and 35.3). The patients, who were already receiving insulin, became painless within days after performance of the biopsy, without additional treatment, showing that the presence of inflammatory infiltrates did not preclude spontaneous recovery.[38] The presence of epineurial vasculitis in cases of proximal diabetic neuropathy has recently been confirmed by Llewelyn and colleagues.[32a]

The presence of vasculitis and of inflammatory infiltration comes as a surprise in the context of a presumed metabolic neuropathy. The possibility of the development of a superimposed vasculitis of the type observed in polyarteritis nodosa must be considered, even without other signs of polysystemic vasculitis or inflammation, because neuropathy, without clinical or biological signs of inflammation, can be the only manifestation of polyarteritis nodosa.[36] This possibility seems unlikely in the present cases because the morphological features of the vascular lesions did not meet all the histologic criteria of polyarteritis nodosa,

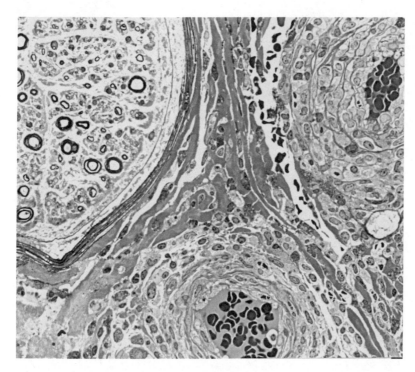

■ **Figure 35.3** Cross section of plastic-embedded biopsy specimen of the intermediate cutaneous nerve of the thigh from the same patient as shown in Figure 35.2 illustrates the inflammatory infiltration around epineurial blood vessels. Note the reduction in the density of myelinated fibers (3380/mm² versus 6980/mm² in a diabetic control) in the adjacent fascicle. In teased fiber preparations, 18% of the fibers showed segmental abnormalities of the myelin sheath, and 17% were at different stages of wallerian degeneration. (From Said G, Elgrably F, Lacroix C, et al. Painful proximal diabetic neuropathy: Inflammatory nerve lesions and spontaneous favorable outcome. Ann Neurol 1997; 41: 662.)

and none of the patients developed other manifestations of vasculitis during up to 5 years of follow-up.

The relationship between the occurrence of inflammatory infiltrates, vasculitis, and diabetes is not clear. Small inflammatory infiltrates have occasionally been encountered in sural nerve biopsy specimens of diabetic patients with a neurologic deficit,[17] in autonomic nerve bundles and ganglia,[19] and in the only detailed autopsy study of a patient with PDN.[34] Lesions of nerve fibers and of blood vessels caused by diabetes may trigger an inflammatory response and a reactive vasculitis in some patients; alternatively, diabetes may make the nerves more susceptible to an intercurrent inflammatory or immune process. In both cases, lesions of epineurial or perineurial blood vessels can result in the ischemic nerve lesions responsible for severe proximal sensory and motor deficits. Conversely, in milder forms, the changes are more reminiscent of those observed in distal symmetrical polyneuropathy.

TREATMENT

Several previous reports have stated that recovery of PDN is more likely to occur if good glycemic control is established, but no controlled trials have been undertaken. Assessment would be difficult in view of the natural tendency of the disorder to spontaneous recovery. The development of PDN in a patient under treatment by hypoglycemic drugs has been taken as an indication to institute insulin therapy. Nevertheless, patients already on insulin treatment can develop proximal diabetic neuropathy, and it may develop shortly after the institution of treatment.[16, 20] Proximal diabetic neuropathy is often very painful. Treatment with analgesics such as acetaminophen and codeine phosphate should be tried first. Tricyclic antidepressants such as imipramine or amitriptyline can help (see Chapter 28). Some authors have suggested the use of immunosuppressive treatment, and occasional patients appear to respond to corticosteroids dramatically. This can be considered in severe forms, but it will necessitate adjustment of diabetic control with insulin in most patients. The spontaneously favorable outcome of PDN in most cases, the cost of treatment with intravenous immunoglobulin, and the disequilibrium induced in diabetic control by corticosteroids must be taken into account before beginning such treatment in patients with PDN. Additionally, patients with PDN are usually referred months after the initial manifestations, which reduces the chance of improvement of weakness after treatment because of the long-standing atrophy of denervated muscles.

CONCLUSION

Proximal diabetic neuropathy constitutes a form of diabetic neuropathy that is distinct from the common distal symmetrical and predominantly sensory polyneuropathy, although the two syndromes may coexist. The basis of PDN is likely to be similar to that of diabetic truncal radiculoneuropathy and the rare instances of proximal upper limb diabetic neuropathy. Diabetic amyotrophy is an acceptable alternative term. The use of the term *femoral neuropathy* has been criticized[41] under the misapprehension that this label has been used to indicate that the condition is an affection of the femoral nerve, whereas the intention was to imply that the femoral region (the thigh) is affected. All cases are not just proximal in distribution because the distal lower limb muscles may also be involved. It is probably not justifiable to separate the acute asymmetrical cases from the rare proximal cases of gradual onset; the latter may represent the summation of multiple bilateral lesions.

Recent histologic studies have demonstrated the presence of inflammatory neural lesions in some cases, raising the possibility of a primary or superimposed immunologic basis for the neuropathy. Proximal diabetic neuropathy has a generally favorable prognosis, and therapy is thus limited to ensuring good glycemic control and treatment of associated pain. In severe cases in which inflammatory changes have been demonstrated on nerve biopsy, the use of immunomodulatory measures can be considered.

References

1. Alderman JE. Anterior neuropathy in diabetics. Arch Neurol Psychiatry 1938; 39:194.
2. Asbury AK. Proximal diabetic neuropathy. Ann Neurol 1977; 2:179.
3. Asbury AK. Renaut bodies: A forgotten endoneurial structure. J Neuropathol Exp Neurol 1981; 32:334.
4. Bastron JA, Thomas JE. Diabetic polyradiculopathy. Mayo Clin Proc 1981;56:725.
5. Bischoff A. Zur diabetische Neuropathie. Stuttgart, Thieme, 1965.
6. Bloodworth JMB Jr, Epstein M. Diabetic amyotrophy: Light and electron microscopic observations. Diabetes 1967; 16:181.
7. Bradley WG, Chad D, Verghese JP, et al. Painful lumbosacral plexopathy with elevated erythrocyte sedimentation rate: A treatable inflammatory syndrome. Ann Neurol 1984; 15:457.
8. Bruns L. Über neuritische Lahmungen beim Diabetes mellitus. Berl Klin Wochenschr 1890; 27:509.
9. Buzzard T. Illustrations of some less known forms of peripheral neuritis, especially alcoholic monoplegia and diabetic neuritis. BMJ 1990; 1:1419.
10. Calverley JR, Mulder DW. Femoral neuropathy. Neurology 1981; 10:963.
11. Casey EB, Harrison MJG. Diabetic amyotrophy: A follow-up study. BMJ 1992; 1:656.
12. Charcot M. Sur un cas de paraplegie diabétique. Arch Neurol (Paris) 1896; 19:318.
13. Chokroverty S. Proximal nerve dysfunction in diabetic proximal amyotrophy. Arch Neurol 1982; 39:403.
14. Chokroverty S, Reyes MG, Rubin FA, et al. The syndrome of diabetic amyotrophy. Ann Neurol 1977; 2:181.
15. Chopra JS, Hurwitz LJ. Femoral conduction in diabetes and chronic occlusive vascular disease. J Neurol Neurosurg Psychiatry 1968; 31:28.
16. Coppack SW, Watkins PJ. The natural history of diabetic femoral neuropathy. Q J Med 1991; 79:307.
17. Costigan DA, Krendel DA, Hopkins LC, et al. Inflammatory neuropathy in diabetes (abstract). Ann Neurol 1990; 28:272.
18. Donovan WH, Sumi SM. Diabetic amyotrophy: A more diffuse process than clinically suspected. Arch Phys Med Rehabil 1976; 57:397.
19. Duchen LW, Anjorin A, Watkins PJ, et al. Pathology of autonomic neuropathy in diabetes mellitus. Ann Intern Med 1980; 92:301.
20. Ellenberg M. Diabetic neuropathy precipitating after institution of diabetic control. Am J Med Sci 1958; 236:466.
21. Fry IK, Hardwick C, Stott GW. Diabetic neuropathy: A survey and follow up of 66 cases. Guy's Hosp Rep 1962; 3:113.
22. Garland H. Diabetic amyotrophy. BMJ 1955; 2:1287.
23. Garland H. Diabetic amyotrophy. *In* Williams D (ed): Modern Trends in Neurology. New York, Paul C Hoeber, 1957, series 2, pp 229–239.
24. Garland H. Neurological complications of diabetes mellitus: Clinical aspects. Proc R Soc Med 1960; 53:137.
25. Garland HT, Taverner D. Diabetic myelopathy. BMJ 1953; 1:1405.
26. Goodman JI. Femoral neuropathy in relation to diabetes mellitus: Report of 17 cases. Diabetes 1954; 3:266.
27. Gilliatt RW, Willison RG. Peripheral nerve conduction in diabetic neuropathy. J Neurol Neurosurg Psychiatry 1962; 25:11.
28. Hirson C, Fienmann EL, Wade HJ. Diabetic neuropathy. BMJ 1956; 1:1409.
29. Isaacs H, Gilchrist G. Diabetic amyotrophy. S Afr Med J 1960; 134:768.
30. Hamilton CR, Dobson HL, Marshall J. Diabetic amyotrophy: Clinical and electron microscopic studies in six patients. Am J Med Sci 1968; 256:81.
31. Lamontagne A, Buchthal F. Electrophysiological studies in diabetic neuropathy. J Neurol Neurosurg Psychiatry 1970; 33:442.
32. Leedman PJ, Davis S, Harrison LC. Diabetic amyotrophy: Reassessment of the clinical spectrum. NZ J Med 1988; 18:768.
32a. Llewelyn JG, Thomas PK, King RMM. Epineurial microvasculitis in proximal diabetic neuropathy. J Neurol 1998; 245:159.
33. Locke S, Lawrence DG, Legg MA. Diabetic amyotrophy. Am J Med 1963; 34:775.
34. Raff MC, Sangalang V, Asbury AK. Ischemic mononeuropathy multiplex associated with diabetes mellitus. Arch Neurol 1968; 18:487.
35. Root HF, Rogers MH. Diabetic neuritis with paralysis. N Engl J Med 1930; 202:1049.
36. Said G, Lacroix-Ciaudo C, Fujimura H, et al. The pe-

ripheral neuropathy of necrotizing arteritis: A clinico-pathological study. Ann Neurol 1988; 23:461.

37. Said S, Goulon-Goeau C, Moulonguet A. Nerve biopsy findings in different patterns of proximal diabetic neuropathy. Ann Neurol 1994; 35:559.

38. Said G, Elgrably F, Lacroix C, et al. Painful proximal diabetic neuropathy: Inflammatory nerve lesions and spontaneous favorable outcome. Ann Neurol 1997; 41:662.

39. Skanse B, Gydell K. A rare type of femoral-sciatic neuropathy in diabetes mellitus. Acta Med Scand 1996; 1:463.

40. Subramony SH, Wilbourn AJ. Diabetic proximal neuropathy: Clinical and electromyographic studies. J Neurol Sci 1982; 3:293.

41. Wilbourn AJ. Diabetic neuropathies. *In* Brown WF, Bolton CF (eds): Clinical Electromyography, ed 2. Boston, Butterworth-Heinemann, 1993, pp 477–516.

42. Williams IR, Mayer RF. Subacute proximal diabetic neuropathy. Neurology 1976; 26:108.

Chapter 36

Diabetic Entrapment and Compression Neuropathies

Asa J. Wilbourn

INTRODUCTION

Many classifications of *diabetic neuropathy*—an umbrella term for all peripheral nervous system (PNS) disorders linked to diabetes mellitus (DM)—include a category of focal mononeuropathies. In the context of diabetic neuropathy, *focal mononeuropathy* has been used to describe cranial neuropathies, radiculopathies, and diabetic amyotrophy as well as isolated lesions of limb peripheral nerves.[46, 48, 104] Focal limb mononeuropathies occurring in diabetic patients often are subdivided into two types: (1) those of abrupt onset, usually considered to be of vascular origin, such as infarctions; and (2) those of more gradual onset, frequently located at common sites of mechanical nerve damage and typically attributed to entrapment or compression.[46, 144] This chapter focuses on limb entrapment/compression mononeuropathies related to DM.

PREVALENCE OF DIABETIC LIMB MONONEUROPATHIES

Surprisingly little information is available regarding the prevalence of diabetic limb mononeuropathies, both in a general population of diabetic patients and in a subpopulation of these patients who were evaluated at various hospitals and clinics. Moreover, much of the published data are severely compromised by problems with definition and by failure to classify the neuropathy into different categories. Sometimes the reasons for inclusion or exclusion appear to be arbitrary and illogical.

Vinik and associates reported that 3% of a sample of 351 patients in their in-patient diabetes clinic had mononeuropathies. In two papers dealing with African populations, they noted that the prevalence of mononeuropathy had been 3.7% and 1.1%. The exact entities included under the category of mononeuropathy were not stated, but radiculopathies and diabetic amyotrophy were specifically excluded.[137] In a retrospective medical record review of a community-based population extending over a 25-year period, Palumbo and colleagues surveyed 995 patients from Olmsted County, MN, and identified 30 (3%) of them who had peripheral nerve fiber disorders other than diabetic symmetrical polyneuropathy. Surprisingly, their "mononeuropathy" category encompassed six patients whose focal disorders usually are not considered to be mononeuropathies—and will not be viewed as such in this chapter—such as cranial neuropathies, radiculopathies, and diabetic amyotrophy. Rather than being included with the mononeuropathies, the 13 instances of carpal tunnel syndrome (CTS) had their own, separate category, and peroneal neuropathies and lateral femoral cutaneous (LFC) neuropathies were assigned to a third category, labeled "other," along with Bell's palsy and alcoholic polyneuropathy. Because anywhere from 2 to 9 of the 11 patients in the last category could have had peroneal or LFC mononeuropathies, when these numbers are added to the 13 patients who had CTS, then 15 to 22 (1.5% to 2.2%) of the 995 patients had limb mononeuropathies.[104] Fry and associates found limb mononeuropathies in 19 of 490 patients (3.8%) they were following in their diabetes clinic.[48] The prevalence of mononeuropathy in these studies (1.1% to 3.8%) is appreciably lower than found by others. Thus, Mulder and associates performed clinical and electrodiagnostic (EDX) examinations of 103 serially evaluated diabetic patients attending metabolic clinics at Mayo Clinic in Rochester, MN, and concluded that 11 patients (11%) had limb mononeuropathies (a 12th patient included in this category had diabetic amyotrophy and is excluded by me from limb mononeuropathies).[98] Asbury and Brown noted, based on unpublished data provided by Brown and Sumner, that compressive mononeuropathies could be detected at entrapment sites by EDX

studies in 25% of patients with type 2 DM.[8] Brown and Greene subsequently reported an even higher prevalence in diabetic patients who had distal symmetrical polyneuropathy (DSPN): "In one unpublished series of 38 patients, we found clinical or electrophysiological evidence of entrapment neuropathy in 40% of all individuals examined."[16] Also of note is that the prevalence figures for focal mononeuropathies occurring in diabetic patients provided by Vinik and coworkers,[137] Palumbo and associates,[104] and Fry and colleagues[48] are low compared with the prevalence of just one type of limb mononeuropathy—CTS—reported by several investigators (see next section).

When the numbers of patients with limb mononeuropathies and those with DSPN are determined among the same group of diabetic patients, it is apparent that mononeuropathies are relatively far less common. Among the 93 to 100 patients in the series of Palumbo and associates, 15 to 22 (16% to 22%) had mononeuropathies, whereas 78 (78% to 84%) had DSPNs.[104] Among the 61 patients in the series of Fry and colleagues who had one or both of these PNS disorders, 19 (31%) had mononeuropathies, and 44 (72%) had DSPN.[48] Finally, among the 42 patients with definite limb nerve abnormalities (excluding one with diabetic amyotrophy) reported by Mulder and associates, 15 (36%) had limb mononeuropathies, and 31 (74%) had DSPNs (4 patients had both).[98] Thus, mononeuropathies occur between one fifth to one third as often as DSPNs do in the diabetic population.

Dyck and colleagues estimated the prevalence of various disorders of peripheral nerve, including limb mononeuropathies, among Rochester, MN, diabetic patients.[41] For a variety of reasons, it is possible to identify a high proportion of patients with DM (by National Diabetes Data Group criteria) in the Rochester population. Of patients with DM, 380 agreed to participate in the Rochester Diabetic Neuropathy Study (RDNS). This is an NIH-sponsored cross-sectional and longitudinal study of the prevalence, incidence, and risk factors for microvascular and macrovascular complications of DM. Because medical records for participating and nonparticipating patients with DM were available, it was possible to assess for bias of selection. In participating patients with DM, clerical and professional patients were overrepresented, but co-morbidity was not significantly different between participants and nonparticipants. Results from the RDNS may, therefore, be representative of diabetic patients of northern U.S. cities with populations predominantly of northern European extraction. The estimate of the prevalence of limb mononeuropathies should be valid because (1) the cohort studied is representative of community patients with DM; (2) all patients were prospectively and comprehensively assessed for limb mononeuropathies by neurologic examination and electrophysiologic studies; (3) mononeuropathies were staged—asymptomatic and symptomatic; (4) test abnormalities were based on study of a healthy subject (HS) cohort (HS-RDNS) and were conservatively set at the 1st or 99th percentile—whichever applied; and (5) the frequency of limb mononeuropathies in the RDNS was compared with that in the HS-RDNS.

The RDNS cohort electrophysiologic evidence of CTS without symptoms (CTS stage 1) was found in 22% of type 1 DM patients and in 29% of type 2 DM patients. Stage 2a was found in 9% of type 1 and 4% of type 2 DM patients. Stage 2b was found in 2% of type 1 DM and 2% of type 2 DM. Symptomatic ulnar neuropathy (UNE) at the elbow (stage 2b UNE) was found in 2% of type 1 DM and 2% of type 2 DM.

HISTORICAL ASPECTS OF DIABETIC LIMB MONONEUROPATHIES

Compression and entrapment neuropathies were probably the last subgroup to have their position secured in the classification of diabetic neuropathy; autonomic neuropathy, for example, was accepted decades earlier.[117] There were several reasons for this delayed recognition.

First, the category of focal mononeuropathy now known to have the highest prevalence among diabetic patients, CTS, did not become a well-defined clinical entity until 1953. That was the year Kremer and coworkers linked acroparesthesias to chronic compression of the median nerve beneath the transverse carpal ligament, thereby providing what is now considered the typical clinical presentation of CTS.[85] Nonetheless, given what is currently known regarding the occurrence of CTS in diabetic patients, it seems incredible that almost none of the early reports, concerned with hundreds of diabetic patients followed over extensive periods of time, mentioned any upper extremity symptoms suggestive of CTS. Thus, in a widely quoted 1936 paper by Jordan, dealing with 226 patients, the only reference to what may have been a patient with CTS is the terse statement, "In case 11,075, there was intractable numbness of the hands."[78] In contrast to the dearth of clinical descriptions suggestive of CTS, the early literature contained many accounts of patients with a symptom complex that would later be designated diabetic amyotrophy (also called proximal diabetic neuropathy, Bruns-Garland syndrome, and diabetic lumbosacral radiculoplexus neuropathy [DLSRPN]). That entity also did not become well defined until 1953; that year, Garland and Taverner "rediscovered" the disorder, which had been described much earlier by Bernard in 1882 and later by Bruns in 1890.[19, 53] However, the level of the neural lesion causing diabetic amyotrophy was uncertain—Garland and Taverner considered it to be a spinal cord disorder in their initial 1953 report[53]—so it is understandable that many investigators were wary of designating it a focal mononeuropathy of DM, even though many others mislabeled it as *diabetic femoral neuropathy*.

Second, many instances of compression and entrapment neuropathy may simply have gone unrecognized because, until relatively recently, the typical situation was as described by Garland in 1960: "Nearly all diabetics are under the care of general physicians, and many attend a diabetic clinic. Because such physicians often have no neurological training and little interest in neurology, they may, and do, overlook neurological abnormalities in the diabetic. . . ."[51] For the same reason, in many of the early papers the descriptions provided of the presumably PNS neurologic disturbances lack specific clinical details, so it is impossible to determine whether they were caused by a focal or a generalized process (such as DSPN). This is especially the case with footdrop, which is mentioned in several articles that neglect to provide information about whether it was strictly unilateral, and therefore likely caused by a peroneal mononeuropathy, or bilateral, in which case it could have been caused by either bilateral peroneal mononeuropathy or DSPN.

Third, whenever many of the early investigators, neurologists and nonneurologists alike, detected a focal PNS disorder in a patient with DM, they doubted that a causal relationship existed between the neural and the metabolic disorder. In 1928, Parker, an experienced neurologist, made the following comments regarding focal diabetic neuropathies: "Besides the peripheral form of diabetic neuritis, there is a form attacking one nerve, the sciatic, femoral, ulnar, and median nerves being involved. This is so rare, however, that it is quite possible that in the cases reported some other factors such as trauma may have been present."[105] Almost 30 years later, Bailey, also a neurologist, expressed a similar view: "The presence of mononeuritis (in persons with DM) should be regarded with suspicion." He observed that focal neurologic deficits in diabetic patients could be caused by independent causes, and he advised physicians to avoid the pitfall of assuming " . . . that one disease capable of causing neurological disorders is likely to be the cause of all neurologic deficits in the patient's lifetime."[10] Similar skepticism was voiced by Garland, in 1960, and for the same reason. He noted that "although palsies of isolated nerves in the limbs" had been ascribed to DM, he had never seen them himself and, therefore, he doubted "their validity." He also cautioned that "in assessing any neurological syndrome, it must always be remembered that diabetes is common, and that the association with neurological syndromes may be accidental."[51]

The refusal of many physicians to attribute focal PNS disorders to underlying DM extended to other types of diabetic neuropathy as well. Garland, for example, also wondered whether many of the reports concerning diabetic autonomic neuropathy were "neurologically valid."[51] Even DSPN had its disbelievers as late as the mid portion of this century. Thus, Hirson and coworkers, in 1953, stated that "although polyneuritis is commonly mentioned as a neurological complication of diabetes, we have not seen any example of the classical sensorimotor symmetrical polyneuritis running a typical course . . . further, we have found in the literature only a single case . . . which satisfied the usual diagnostic criteria." They conceded that 54% of the 100 diabetic patients they were following had abnormalities of the Achilles deep tendon reflexes, along with absence of vibratory and position sense. They contended, however, that even though these were chronic in nature, they were asymptomatic and nonprogressive; for this reason, they labeled them *asymptomatic* neuropathies.[69] Hirson and coworkers' views regarding the existence of DSPN were similar to those expressed by other investigators decades earlier. For example, Kraus stated in 1920 that "peripheral neuritis in diabetes is very rare." He based this opinion on the fact that among 450 diabetic patients with neurologic disorders, selected from nearly 700 followed for 10 years at a metabolic clinic, only a "single case . . . who was also an alcoholic" had a polyneuropathy. He acknowledged that "a group of cases showing objective changes in light touch sensation,

reflexes and with some neuralgia were not uncommon." He attributed these, however, to spinal cord involvement and therefore concluded that these cases "are not neuritis and should not be spoken of as a 'peripheral neuritis.' "[84] In 1931, Murphy and Moxon reported that of the 827 diabetic patients they were following, only 5 (0.6%) had a "neuritis."[99] These authors were expressing the same doubts regarding the existence of DSPN that Joslin had stated in the first edition of his book, *The Treatment of Diabetes Mellitus*, published in 1916: "The most frequent type of neuritis which occurs in diabetes is sciatica . . . which I am inclined to consider . . . as having little causal connection with the disease . . . The type of neuritis almost invariably encountered has occurred in the lower extremities . . . and . . . I am inclined to believe that the poor blood vessels of the lower extremities are the chief offenders."[79]

How the concepts regarding diabetic neuropathy evolved are well illustrated by surveying the first 11 editions of Joslin's textbook, which span a 55-year period between 1916 and 1971. The opinions Joslin expressed in the second through fourth editions of his textbook regarding DSPN were essentially identical to those that appeared in the first edition (1916). Thus, in the fourth edition (1928) the following appears: "Neuritis is most uncommon among my patients. The explanation is simple, because three of the common causes of neuritis (alcoholism, lues, and tuberculosis) have been infrequent. . . . Indeed, primary 'neuritis' in diabetes is usually a misnomer. It is secondary to some form of circulatory obstruction or some form of arthritis. Sciatica is the most common type of neuritis which occurs in diabetes."[80] However, in the fifth edition of the textbook, published just 7 years later in 1935, a completely different view appeared. "Contact with many diabetic patients and careful search for neurological lesions show an extraordinary frequency of neuropathy. Neuritis, paralyses of peripheral nerves . . . are not infrequent. In spite of the association of arteriosclerosis, occasional lues and alcohol, the many neurological lesions in diabetes cannot be explained by such factors."[114] Presumably, this marked reversal of opinion resulted from the chapter on *The Nervous System in Diabetes*, which appeared in that edition, being co-authored by Jordan, who drew heavily on his detailed assessment of 226 diabetic patients, a report of which was to be published the next year.[78]

Little change was apparent in the next two editions (1937, 1940). In the eighth edition

(1946), the authors Bailey and Murray emphasized that DM "has a special predilection for the peripheral nerves" but provided few observations regarding focal mononeuropathies that had not appeared in earlier editions.[11] Root and Kenny, the authors of the ninth edition (1952), stressed that diabetic neuropathy was common; their chapter contained a table showing that of 913 diabetic patients with nervous system disorders seen at one of their hospitals during a 5-year period, 502 (55%) had diabetic neuropathy. Most of the discussion, however, clearly was focused on DSPN. Few statements pertained, or probably pertained, to focal PNS lesions: "complete footdrop, and less frequently, wristdrop, may develop. Rundles reports 10 cases of footdrop and emphasizes that the peroneal nerve is more vulnerable than the tibial, and the ulnar nerve more vulnerable than the radial or median."[113] Essentially, the same views are expressed in the 10th edition, published 7 years later (1959). It is only in the 11th edition, published in 1971, that the concept of diabetic mononeuropathy was finally entrenched. "Any major nerve trunk may be affected. When several nerve trunks are involved simultaneously, the affection is classified as mononeuropathy multiplex. Usually the disorder involves superficially placed nerves such as the ulnar and common peroneal nerve trunks."[92] This chapter was authored by Locke, a neurologist, who also provided a case report of a unilateral common peroneal mononeuropathy occurring in a diabetic patient.[92]

In 1975, Thomas wrote that "After some initial reservations, it is now accepted that isolated peripheral nerve lesions are commoner in diabetic subjects than in the general population . . . virtually any of the peripheral nerve trunks in the limbs may be affected and these frequently occur at common sites of entrapment or external compression."[131] Thomas' view was actually an overstatement; it was not completely accurate then nor is it currently accurate. Thus, although these focal PNS lesions are included in many of the classifications and reviews of diabetic neuropathy,[16, 42, 60, 62, 71, 89, 118, 132, 137, 144] they are not incorporated in all of them. In one 1984 article dealing specifically with classifications of diabetic neuropathy, for example, although mononeuropathies are included, entrapment neuropathies are not mentioned, nor are the peripheral nerves most often affected by them, such as median (at carpal tunnel), ulnar (at elbow), and peroneal (at fibular head).[70] In a still later article, published in 1990, no focal peripheral nerve lesions, including entrapment neuropathies, are mentioned. Although there is a subheading of "mononeuropathies," it concerns only cranial neuropathies and diabetic amyotrophy.[141]

ETIOLOGY OF DIABETIC ENTRAPMENT/COMPRESSION MONONEUROPATHIES

Why focal entrapment and compressive mononeuropathies are more common in diabetic patients—especially those with DSPN—than in the general population is unknown. Several theories have been advanced. Most have focused solely on the increased frequency of CTS in diabetic patients. In 1957, Heathfield was one of the first investigators to attempt to explain the association of DM and CTS. In a series of 80 patients with CTS, diagnosed by their characteristic clinical presentation and their favorable response to wrist splinting, he noted that 3 (3.8%) of them were diabetic, and that he had " . . . seen several others, usually elderly." He attributed these median nerve lesions, however, not to "a diabetic neuropathy," but to coexisting "obesity and osteoarthritis of the wrist."[68] It has been appreciated for decades that obesity is very commonly associated with type 2 DM[79, 143]; Joslin stated in the first edition of his book that the "most common etiological factor . . . (for DM) is obesity."[79] Obesity is also a known predisposing factor for the development of CTS, even more so than underlying DM. Thus, in the study by Cannon and associates, 26.7% of patients with CTS were obese, compared with 12.2% of controls.[21] Of the 313 patients with CTS reported by Cseuz and colleagues, although 36 (11.5%) had DM, 116 (37%) were obese.[29] Dieck and Kelsey found that among 40 women hospitalized for carpal tunnel release, the odds ratio for DM was 2.9, whereas that for a weight gain of 4 kg or greater during the preceding 5 years was 3.7.[35] Nathan and associates studied the hands of several hundred industrial workers on two occasions, 5 years apart, and found slowing of median sensory conduction had a high correlation to weight and body mass index of those persons studied, more so than to job-related factors.[101] Albers and coworkers found a positive correlation between electrophysiologic abnormalities of CTS and body mass index in diabetic patients.[3] de Krom and associates, in a case control study comparing 156 patients with CTS to 473 without CTS, determined that obesity, but not DM, was a risk factor for CTS.[32] Exactly how obesity itself would lead to CTS was unstated in most articles. However, Dieck and Kelsey suggested that fat accumulation in the carpal tunnel could result in compression of the median nerve.[35]

Another possible reason for CTS and other compressive/entrapment neuropathies occurring so frequently in diabetic patients is that DM, by various mechanisms, causes peripheral nerves to be more susceptible to compression. In 1980, Jakobsen and Sidenius demonstrated that slow axonal transport is reduced in nerves of animals with experimentally induced DM.[75] Although they found no abnormalities of fast axonal transport, Dahlin and colleagues subsequently showed that when such nerves are subjected to focal compression, compromise of fast axonal transport occurs at the compression site, to a greater degree than is seen in the nerves of normal control animals. They suggested that several factors may be responsible for diabetic nerves being more susceptible to local compression. These include changes in their microvascular structure, compounded by biochemical disturbances, which could reduce both endoneurial blood flow and oxygen tension.[30] As Dahlin and associates noted, focal compression of normal peripheral nerves causes localized intraneural circulatory changes and increased permeability of endoneurial vessels, abnormalities that could be exaggerated in diabetic nerves. Also, the water content may be increased and the endoneurial space expanded in diabetic nerves. The former could result in the axons absorbing more of the applied pressure; the latter could increase the "diffusion distance for oxygen from the endoneurial capillaries to the axons."[30] Finally, DM probably causes changes in retrograde axonal transport,[30, 75] and this could conceivably "alter the biochemical integrity of the axon," thereby rendering it more susceptible to pressure.[30] It is noteworthy that a generalized increase in susceptibility of diabetic peripheral nerves to local compression was one of the major components of the double-crush hypothesis advanced by Upton and McComas in 1973. They proposed that metabolic disorders such as DM could, via compromise of axoplasmic flow, cause subclinical peripheral nerve entrapments to manifest clinically.[135] This is the theory invoked by Dellon in his proposal that the hand and foot symptoms seen in patients with DSPN are actually caused by a combination of multiple peripheral nerve entrapments and a generalized abnormality of peripheral nerves, rather than the latter alone (see section on Mislabeled Diabetic Limb Mononeuropathies).[33, 34]

Another theory regarding the increased prevalence of entrapment neuropathies in diabetic patients focuses not on the nerves themselves, but on the structures surrounding them.[40] It is known that connected tissue abnormalities, including Dupuytren's disease, palmar flexor tenosynovitis, and limited joint mobility, often are detectable in the hands of patients with DM.[13, 22, 23, 28, 45, 50] Chaudhuri and coworkers showed that CTS is found much more frequently in those patients with type 1 DM who have limited joint mobility of their hands, compared with those who do not. Thus, in 16 diabetic patients with limited joint mobility, 7 (44%) had clinical evidence of CTS and 12 (75%) had electrical evidence, compared with 4 (16%) and 5 (20%), respectively, of the 25 diabetic patients who lacked this complication.[22] Conceivably, alterations in connective tissue in diabetic patients could result in thickening or fibrosis of the flexor synovium within the carpal tunnel, at least in those patients with type 1 DM.[22, 108]

Chaudhuri and associates observed that non-enzymatic "glycosylation is increased in type 1 DM, resulting in alteration of packing, cross-linkage, and turnover of collagen. Increased glycosylation affects collagen degradation, resulting in accumulation of less compliant connective tissue. This ultimately results in fibrosis."[22] Chammas and colleagues noted that the connective tissue proliferation underlying the hand abnormalities that occur with DM may require a "constitutional predilection and a microangiopathy." They reported finding the latter in 14 of 16 patients with type 1 DM who had CTS, and stated: "A significant correlation between the occurrence of CTS and the presence of flexor tenosynovitis and microangiopathy suggests that proliferation of connective tissue and microvascular insufficiency may play a role in the pathogenesis of nerve entrapment."[23] It also has been suggested that lysyl oxidase stimulation, known to occur in type 1 DM, "may be more important than increased glycosylation" in the abnormal accumulation of connective tissue; this enzyme is involved in collagen cross-link formation.[22]

Finally, some investigators, such as Dyck and Giannini, have proposed that a combination of factors may be operative. Thus, "repetitive injury, inflammation, thickening or stiffness of overlying ligaments, tethering of the nerve proximal or distal to the site of compression, increased nerve tissue vulnerability, and occupational and personal behavior patterns might . . . all be involved in (the) pathogenesis" of

TABLE 36.1 COMPARISON OF THREE CORE STUDIES

	Mulder et al.[98]	Fry et al.[48]	Fraser et al.[46]
Diabetic Population Assessed	103	490	Patients of "large diabetes clinic"
Nature of Study	Independent clinical and EDX	Clinical	Clinical with some EDX confirmation
Patient Selection	"Available for EDX and neurological examinations"	"Routine review" of patients	"Patients volunteered symptoms"
Major Focus of Article	Diabetic symmetrical polyneuropathy	Diabetic symmetrical polyneuropathy	Diabetic mononeuropathies
Participation of Neurologists in Study	Performed by neurologists and neurophysiologist	Neurologists consulted	None apparent
EDX Studies Employed	Motor NCS (amps, CVs, latencies) in all 103; NEE in 80	None	Motor NCS CVs "where possible"
Mononeuropathy Diagnosis Based On	"Objective [clinical] evidence"; EDX changes	"Objective [clinical] signs"	"Objective clinical" evidence

NCS, nerve conduction studies; EDX, electrodiagnostic studies; amps, amplitudes; CV, conduction velocity; NEE, needle electrode examination.

focal entrapment/compressive neuropathies occurring so frequently in patients with DM.[39]

In stark contrast to the above views, Rosenbloom and Silverstein, in an article focused on the variety of bone, joint, periarticular tissue and skin abnormalities related to DM, attribute CTS occurring in diabetic patients to DSPN, rather than to nerve compression or entrapment. They base their view, in large part, on the concept that CTS in patients with DM is always: (1) very severe, with end-stage axon loss, resulting in "typical thenar muscular atrophy"; (2) bilateral; (3) accompanied by equally end-stage, axon-loss bilateral ulnar neuropathy, causing "atrophy of intrinsic and hypothenar muscles and contractures involving the metacarpophalangeal and proximal interphalangeal joints of all fingers equally."[116] This theory is quite unlikely to gain widespread acceptance, considering that virtually every part of it is incorrect.

For additional information on this subject, see Chapters 8 and 18.

DIABETIC LIMB MONONEUROPATHIES: PRINCIPAL SOURCE MATERIAL

A great number of publications during the past half-century have been concerned, to various degrees, with diabetic limb mononeuropathies. Nonetheless, extensive perusal of the literature reveals repeated references to just three of them: Mulder and associates (1961),[98] Fry and coworkers (1962),[48] and Fraser and colleagues (1979).[46] Because these serve as much as the source material for diabetic limb mononeuro-

pathies and frequently are referred to in this chapter, they each merit brief discussion; of note is that only one of them (Fraser and associates) is focused primarily on isolated limb lesions (Tables 36.1 to 36.3).

Mulder and Coworkers. Published in 1961, this is considered by many to be the prototypic article concerned with the combined clinical

TABLE 36.2 SPECIFIC TYPES OF DIABETIC MONONEUROPATHY

	Mulder et al.[98]	Fry et al.[48]	Fraser et al.[46]
No. of patients with diabetic neuropathy	43	66	51*
No. of patients with diabetic symmetrical polyneuropathy	31	44	27
No. of patients with cranial neuropathies	0	6	7
No. of patients with diabetic amyotrophy (femoral neuropathy)	1	5†	3
No. of patients with focal limb mononeuropathies (excluding diabetic amyotrophy)	15	19 (12 + 7 CTS)†	41

CTS, carpal tunnel syndrome.

*Patient selection was determined by presence of mononeuropathy.

†Although Fry et al. included 6 patients in this category, one of them had only unilateral proximal upper extremity complaints, probably caused by coincidental neuralgic amyotrophy.

‡For unclear reasons, Fry et al. did not consider CTS as a limb mononeuropathy and provided no information concerning the 7 patients with that disorder.

TABLE 36.3 DETAILS REGARDING THE SPECIFIC TYPES OF FOCAL LIMB MONONEUROPATHIES

	Mulder et al.[98]	Fry et al.[48]	Fraser et al.[46]
No. of patients with limb mononeuropathies (diabetic amyotrophy excluded)	15	19	41
Total no. of limb mononeuropathies	28	23 + *	55
Specific mononeuropathy†			
Median neuropathy (CTS)	9‡ (? 0) ? 9	7 (?) ? 7	15 5 20
Ulnar neuropathy	5‡ (? 0) ? 5	6 1 7	15 8 23
Radial neuropathy	0 (NA) 0	1 (NA) 1	0 (NA) 0
Peroneal neuropathy	13‡ (? 0) ? 13	7 (1) 8	8 (1) 9
Sciatic neuropathy	0 (NA) 0	0 (NA) 0	3 (0) 3
Lateral femoral cutaneous neuropathy	1 (NA) 1	0 (NA) 0	0 (NA) 0

CTS, carpal tunnel syndrome.
*Fry et al. provided no information regarding their 7 patients with CTS, e.g., how many, if any, had bilateral lesions? Did CTS coexist with any other limb mononeuropathies?
†No. of patients with mononeuropathies
  (No. of bilateral lesions)

  Total no. of lesions in series
‡Mulder et al. implied that all 15 patients had unilateral limb mononeuropathies. Yet, there were a total of 28 lesions among the 15 patients. If none were bilateral, then many patients had two (or more) different limb mononeuropathies in combination; no information is provided on this point.

and EDX assessment of diabetic neuropathies. However, the bulk of it pertained to DSPN. The study group consisted of 103 patients followed in an outpatient diabetic clinic "who were available" for EDX and clinical neurologic evaluations during the course of the study. Clinical and EDX assessments were performed independently on each patient. For clinical diagnosis, objective evidence of a PNS disorder was required. On EDX examination, all patients underwent motor nerve conduction studies (NCSs), with amplitudes, latencies, and conduction velocities (CVs) assessed. Eighty patients also underwent a needle electrode examination (NEE).[98] Sensory NCSs were not performed; the publication that described their clinical use, by Gilliatt and Sears, appeared in 1958, probably during the period when Mulder and colleagues were collecting their data.[56] Of the 43 diabetic patients who had unequivocal evidence of PNS lesions, 31 had DSPN, although, "by chance," it was not a "major difficulty" in any of them. Four of the patients with DSPN had superimposed focal mononeuropathies, and an additional 12 patients had limb mononeuropathies alone.[98] If the one patient with diabetic amyotrophy, mislabeled *femoral neuropathy*, is excluded from the group of 16 patients with mononeuropathies, then among the remaining 15 patients there were a total of 28 individual peripheral nerve lesions (see Table 36.3). Unfortunately, few details were provided about this group of patients. Although it was implied that none of them had bilateral lesions, the numbers (i.e., 15 patients with a total of 28 lesions) indicate that almost all of them must have had two separate mononeuropathies. Consequently, if none had bilateral lesions (such as bilateral CTS), then most had combinations of two (or more) focal mononeuropathies (such as unilateral CTS plus unilateral peroneal neuropathy). Yet, no information was provided regarding exactly which nerves were affected in any of the 15 patients. Moreover, the discussion shifts, sometimes confusingly, between the 12 patients with mononeuropathy alone and the 16 patients in all with mononeuropathies (including the 4 who had an associated DSPN). In spite of its limitations, this is apparently the only one of the three articles that was written by physicians skilled in the diagnosis of PNS disorders.[98]

Fry and Associates. Published in 1962, this is probably the least known of the three articles, because it was in a journal (*Guy's Hospital Report*) that did not have as wide a circulation as those in which the other two appeared. The study group consisted of 66 patients with various types of diabetic neuropathy, "obtained from the routine review of 490 patients attending" a diabetic clinic. Assessments consisted solely of clinical examinations—EDX studies were not performed—and only those "patients with objective signs of involvement of the nervous system" were included; those "with symptoms alone" were not. Similar to that by Mulder and colleagues, this report dealt principally with DSPN; two thirds of the patients had that type of diabetic neuropathy.

Six patients were reported to have diabetic amyotrophy, which was a separate category. However, one of the six had only unilateral shoulder complaints, probably the result of a coincidental neuralgic amyotrophy. There were 18 patients "with isolated nerve lesions," but this category included 6 patients with cranial neuropathies and excluded 7 patients with CTS, of which no details (such as unilateral or bilateral presentation) were provided. Of the 19 patients with focal limb neuropathies, including CTS, there was 1 patient with bilateral ulnar neuropathy plus, curiously, what was very likely another neuralgic amyotrophy (see section on Mislabeled Diabetic Limb Mononeuropathies). The number of individual peripheral nerves affected in the 19 patients cannot be determined accurately because no information was provided regarding whether the CTS patients had unilateral or bilateral lesions. Depending on this point, the total number of limb mononeuropathies in the 19 patients ranged from 23 (if all 7 CTS were unilateral) to 30 lesions (if all were bilateral). The authors of this publication presumably were not neurologists, but they did acknowledge the services of neurologic colleagues for assessing many of their patients, "particularly cases of amyotrophy and isolated nerve lesions."[48]

Fraser and Coworkers. Published in 1979, this is the only one of the three articles concerned principally with diabetic mononeuropathies (as opposed to DSPN). The study group consisted of 51 patients who, during a 3-year period in a large diabetic clinic, had "volunteered symptoms suggestive of mononeuropathy involving one or more peripheral or cranial nerves. No attempt was made to actively screen the clinic population." The diagnosis was arrived at by clinical examination "and confirmed, where possible," by EDX studies. However, the latter consisted only of motor NCS distal latencies and CVs; motor NCS amplitudes were not recorded and neither sensory NCSs nor NEE were performed. Of the 51 patients, 7 had cranial neuropathies and 3 had diabetic amyotrophy mislabeled as femoral neuropathy. When these were excluded, there were 41 patients with a total of 55 peripheral nerve lesions. Throughout the article, the number of patients with PNS disorders, and not the total number of nerves involved, was discussed, but the latter can be calculated. It is unclear whether neurologists wrote or contributed to this publication, which originated from diabetic and medicine departments.[46]

DIABETIC ENTRAPMENT/ COMPRESSION MONONEUROPATHIES

General Observations

Entrapment and compressive mononeuropathies occurring in diabetic patients who are not afflicted with DSPN have the same clinical and EDX features as those occurring in nondiabetic populations, and typically they are diagnosed with the same degree of relative ease. A major clinical exception is CTS, because of its ubiquity and marked tendency to be bilateral. Whenever patients with bilateral CTS have coexisting bilateral S1 root compression, with the latter most often caused by lumbar canal stenosis, the resulting clinical presentation (sensory complaints in the distal portion of all four extremities) is readily misinterpreted as evidence of a generalized DSPN. This is particularly likely to occur when the physicians involved are not neurologists, or when they have a tendency to consider all neurologic symptoms occurring in diabetic patients as being caused by DM. The clinical presentation in these situations becomes even more muddled whenever bilateral ulnar neuropathy at the elbow segment (UNE) occurs in association with the bilateral CTS, which happens with some frequency in diabetic patients. This confusing situation is especially common among elderly diabetic patients, in whom both CTS and lumbar canal stenosis occur with relatively high frequencies. The EDX examination can be of considerable assistance in the majority of these instances, by demonstrating that independent PNS disorders—bilateral CTS (sometimes with bilateral UNE) and bilateral S1 radiculopathy—coexist.[144]

Whenever entrapment and compressive mononeuropathies are superimposed on DSPN, particularly when they are present bilaterally and more than one type occurs simultaneously, they can serve as a formidable confounding factor in both clinical and electrophysiological diagnosis. Whenever bilateral peroneal mononeuropathy at the fibular head (PNFH) is superimposed on a moderate DSPN, for example, the resulting clinical presentation can be mistaken for that caused by a rather severe DSPN alone. A more commonly encountered problem that PNS combinations present, however, is in the interpretation of bilateral hand symptoms: are they caused by DSPN involving the upper extremities, by bilateral CTS (with or without coexisting bilateral UNE), or by a co-mingling of both? Walter-Sack and Zollner feared that the CTS-caused hand symptoms in patients with DSPN could mistakenly be considered a manifestation of the latter. As a result, the CTS in these patients could go unrecognized and, consequently, untreated.[139] Conversely, Leffert was concerned that patients with neurologic disturbances in their hands caused by DSPN would incorrectly be thought to have upper extremity entrapment neuropathies.[91] Unfortunately, he apparently did not appreciate that entrapment neuropathies and DSPN can, and often do, coexist. Certainly, judging by the clinical descriptions provided, the hand symptoms in all eight cases he reported were caused by individual peripheral nerve lesions; the abnormalities were unilateral in five cases, and in all the involved hands they were much too focal (wasting, sensory loss, or both, in the distribution of a median or an ulnar nerve) to be upper extremity manifestations of a diffuse DSPN.[91]

In our experience, bilateral hand symptoms in patients with DSPN are more likely to be caused by bilateral focal mononeuropathies (CTS or CTS plus UNE) than by diffuse DSPN. To ensure proper, prompt treatment for the mononeuropathies and to prevent the DSPN being considered more severe than it actually is (because of the presence of bilateral distal upper extremity symptoms), distinguishing focal causes from a generalized cause of hand symptoms in patients with DSPN is quite important. Until the DSPN is rather severe and appreciably affecting the upper extremity nerves, the EDX examination can materially assist in this differentiation. However, once axon loss is prominent in the distal upper extremities because of the DSPN, the value of the EDX examination in sorting out these various etiologies is markedly diminished (see section on CTS).[144]

Individual Lesions

CARPAL TUNNEL SYNDROME

The clinical disorder known as CTS, the result of chronic entrapment of the median nerve beneath the transverse carpal ligament, was not first well defined until 1953, when the article by Kremer and colleagues was published.[85] Since then, CTS has become universally recognized as being the most common entrapment neuropathy. Moreover, it is the most common entrapment neuropathy, by far, encountered in diabetic patients.

Carpal tunnel syndrome affects women more than men, and typically it is more severe in, or

limited to, the dominant hand. In the majority of instances, CTS has a predictable evolution, in which sensory symptoms predominate until late in the course. Frequently, it begins with painful paresthesias involving the fingers of one or both hands. Any combination of median nerve–innervated fingers can be affected and, rather commonly, patients report that all five fingers are symptomatic, including the ulnar nerve–innervated fifth finger. (Schultz, in 1893, used the term *acroparesthesiae* to describe bilateral burning pins and needles occurring at night in the fingers in middle-aged women. Presumably, he was describing the symptoms of CTS.[115]) When severe, the patient often experiences a deep-seated pain (toothache-like) radiating up the forearm. Usually these symptoms are relieved rather promptly by such maneuvers as the patient shaking the hand or hanging it over the bed. As the disorder progresses, the same symptoms often appear intermittently during the day with hand use. Repetitive flexion and extension movements and prolonged gripping are particularly likely to initiate symptoms. Thus, holding a telephone or the steering wheel of a car, working with tools and many kitchen utensils, and gardening are all notorious triggers for CTS symptoms. In earlier days, wringing clothes after washing them was one of the more common causes for CTS symptoms in women. Eventually, a stage often is reached at which one or more of the median nerve–innervated fingers become permanently numb; that is, epicritic sensation is lost. Because of this, the hands frequently are described as being "clumsy" with use. The patient is unable to button buttons or identify small objects by feel, and may drop objects that she or he is holding. In the most advanced stages, seldom encountered currently, lateral thenar wasting is present, caused by severe denervation of the median nerve–innervated muscles.

Occasionally, few, if any, sensory symptoms occur with CTS, and the patient is first seen with substantial wasting of the lateral thenar muscles. The majority of patients in this category are elderly males.

The clinical diagnosis of CTS depends mainly on obtaining a characteristic history. Once persistent sensory symptoms are present, a deficit to pain or position sense may be demonstrated in the affected fingers. The Phalen test (wrist flexion test) and Tinel sign are the two most widely used provocative tests for diagnosing CTS. With the Phalen test, the patient is asked to hold the forearms vertically (often while resting the elbows on a table) and to allow both hands to drop into complete flexion at the wrist, where they are held for approximately 1 minute. A positive Phalen test consists of the appearance of paresthesias in one or more of the median nerve–innervated fingers, typically within the first 30 seconds after the procedure begins.[109] With the Tinel test, the median nerve is percussed both at the wrist and in the palm, and this produces paresthesias in one or more of the median nerve–innervated fingers. Unfortunately, both tests are plagued with a relatively high incidence of false-positive and false-negative results. With advanced CTS, obvious wasting and weakness of the lateral thenar muscles are detectable on clinical examination.

Carpal tunnel syndrome may be mistaken for several neurologic (such as C7 radiculopathy) and nonneurologic disorders (such as osteoarthritis). Usually, these are readily distinguished from CTS by the clinical examination, supplemented with EDX studies. With C7 radiculopathy, for example, almost invariably ipsilateral interscapular pain is present or has been present, and the finger paresthesias tend to be constant and have no nocturnal exaggeration. Moreover, the ipsilateral triceps reflex is often decreased. Similarly, with osteoarthritis the sensory symptoms in the hand are usually diffuse, and although they are exaggerated with hand use, there typically is no nocturnal exaggeration.[127]

As previously noted, the early literature concerned with diabetic neuropathy was nearly devoid of any descriptions of patients having upper-extremity symptoms that could even remotely be attributed to CTS, a then unknown entity. Even in the 1960s and 1970s, the fact that CTS was by far the most commonly encountered entrapment neuropathy was not apparent. Thus, in the 1961 report by Mulder and associates, when 1 patient with diabetic amyotrophy mislabeled as a "femoral neuropathy" is excluded, there were 15 patients with a total of 28 peripheral nerves involved. Of these, 9 (32%) were CTS, and 13 (46%) were PNFH.[98] Similarly, in the 1962 article by Fry and coworkers, if it is assumed that the CTS reported in 7 of their patients was always unilateral, then in 19 patients there were 23 individual peripheral nerve lesions. Of these, 7 (30%) were CTS, and 8 (35%) were PNFH.[48] In the 1979 publication by Fraser and associates, after 3 diabetic amyotrophies mislabeled as femoral neuropathies are excluded, there were 41 patients who had 55 individual limb mononeuropathies. Although 15 patients had CTS and an equal number had UNE, CTS was bilateral in 5 patients, and UNE was bilateral in 8. Hence, there was a total of 20 (36%) limbs with CTS, but 23 (42%) limbs with UNE.[46]

One of the reasons CTS is encountered so commonly in diabetic patients is its high rate of occurrence in those with DSPN. In our experience, it can be detected, at least in the electromyography (EMG) laboratory, in approximately one third of patients with DSPN who are younger than 60 years and in about two thirds of those older than that age.[144] No other entrapment neuropathy begins to approach these prevalence figures in patients with DSPN.

Diabetes mellitus is one of the three systemic illnesses most commonly associated with CTS, the other two being rheumatoid arthritis and hypothyroidism.[115] Based on almost 20 reports, composed of 40 to 1215 patients, the number of patients with CTS who have coexisting DM ranges from 2.6% to 20% (Table 36.4). If the data from all these are combined, with the exception of one[108] that is nearly a duplicate of one of the others,[107] then of 6647 patients with CTS, 467 (7%) had DM.[14, 29, 32, 35, 38, 44, 45, 49, 65, 68, 72, 73, 86, 90, 93, 107, 108, 126, 149] The percentage range is also wide when the association between CTS and DM is approached from the opposite direction; that is, the number of patients with DM who have coexisting CTS. Among eight series (composed of 64 to 995 patients), anywhere from 1.2% to 20.8% of diabetic patients had coexisting CTS (Table 36.5).[23, 26, 41, 48, 50, 97, 98, 104] It is pertinent to note that the percentage provided by Palumbo and colleagues[104] has been misquoted in several subsequent publications as being 12%, rather than 1.2%.[7, 89, 118] In fact, the 12% mentioned in the report by Palumbo and colleagues actually pertained to those patients with diabetic neuropathy; specifically, the percentage of them (13 of 108, or 12%) who had CTS. As would be expected, DSPN occupied a much greater percentage, 72% (78 of 108), of the total number of those with diabetic neuropathy.[104] If the data from these eight sources are pooled, then of 2652 patients with DM, 153 (5.8%) of them had CTS. Additional evidence linking CTS and DM has been presented by other investigators. Dieck and Kelsey reported a case-control study of adult women hospitalized for surgical treatment of their CTS. Of 40 operated patients, 8 (20%) had DM, and of 1027 control patients, 82 (8%), had DM. Thus, " . . . a history of diabetes . . . was associated with a three-fold [actually 2.5-fold]

TABLE 36.4 PATIENTS WITH CARPAL TUNNEL SYNDROME WHO HAVE COEXISTING DIABETES

Investigators	No. With CTS	No. With DM	Percentage
de Krom et al.[32]	156	4	2.6
Hybbinette/Mannerfelt[73]	400	11	2.8
Doyle/Carroll[38]	100	3	3.0
Heathfield[68]	80	3	3.8
Loong[93]	250	12	4.8
Yamaguchi et al.*[149]	1,215	69	5.7
Kulick et al.[86]	100	6	6.0
Stevens et al.*[126]	1,016	62	6.1
Blodgett et al.[14]	915	59	6.4
Hurst et al.[72]	888	65	7.4
Phalen†[109]	439	33	7.5
Florack et al.[45]	106	8	7.5
Frymoyer et al.[49]	49	4	8.2
Czeuz et al.*[29]	313	36	11.5
Leach/Odom[90]	89	11	12.4
Phalen‡[107]	384	56	14.6
Eversmann/Ritsick[44]	47	7	14.9
Phalen‡[108]	379‡	63‡	16.6‡
Haupt et al.[65]	60	10	16.7
Dieck/Kelsey[35]	40	8	20.0
TOTALS§	6647	467	7.0

*All series from Mayo Clinic, so some patients may appear in more than one report.
†Concerns group of patients seen between November 1947 and August 1964.
‡Concerns the same group of patients—those seen between August 1964 and January 1969—but numbers vary slightly between the two articles. Most important variation: the number of patients with associated DM drops from 63 to 56 between the 1970 and 1972 articles, because "seven additional patients were suspected diabetics, but there was insufficient clinical evidence . . . to establish the diagnosis."
§Numbers from Phalen[108] not included, since they duplicate Phalen.[107]

increase in occurrence of CTS."[35] Stevens and associates found that among 1016 patients diagnosed with CTS during a 20-year period, DM was "the only or the major recognized associated condition" in 62 (6.1%) of them. They calculated the population attributable risk percentage ("a measure of the strength of the association between a risk factor and CTS") and a "standardized morbidity ratio" ("the ratio of the observed number of patients with a condition to the expected number") and found them both to be high for patients with CTS and DM. Regarding the population attributable risk percentage, they determined that DM, along with rheumatoid arthritis and pregnancy, was significantly more frequent among the patients with CTS (4.2% for men and 3.8% for women) than for the general population assessed. Similarly, the standardized morbidity ratio for DM was 2.5 for men and 2.2 for women[126]: "The risk for . . . (CTS) and diabetes

is approximately 2.2 times greater than average in females and 2.5 times greater in males."[7] Dyck and coworkers found that among 341 diabetic patients they studied clinically and in the EMG laboratory, 33% of those with type 1 DM had evidence of CTS—clinical, electrical, or both—although only 11% were symptomatic, whereas 35% of patients with type 2 DM had similar evidence of CTS, but just 6% were symptomatic. They noted that the frequency of EDX findings among the diabetic patients (22% in type 1 DM and 29% in type 2 DM) was significantly " . . . higher than in non-diabetic controls (6%) drawn from the same population (P <0.001)."[41] Gamstedt and colleagues performed a cross-sectional study involving 99 diabetic patients selected at random, and found CTS in 19 (19.2%). They concluded that CTS, as well as other hand abnormalities, was strongly associated with DM.[50] Chammas and associates studied 120 adults with DM (60 with type 1 DM and 60 with type 2 DM) and found that 25 (20.8%) had CTS (16 with type 1 DM and 9 with type 2 DM); in contrast, of 120 nondiabetic controls, only 5 (4.2%) had CTS. Thus, CTS was fivefold more common in their DM group than in their non-DM group. They also demonstrated that Dupuytren's disease, limited joint mobility, and flexor tenosynovitis as well as CTS occurred with significantly higher frequency in the diabetic population than in the control group.[23]

In spite of the many publications linking DM and CTS, several investigators have denied that a cause-effect relationship exists between the two disorders, beginning with Heathfield (1957) just 4 years after CTS was first well described.[68] Even Leach and Odom, who found DM in 11 (12.4%) of their 89 operated CTS

TABLE 36.5 PATIENTS WITH DIABETES MELLITUS WHO HAVE COEXISTING SYMPTOMATIC CARPAL TUNNEL SYNDROME

Investigators	No. With DM	No. With CTS	Percentage
Palumbo et al.[104]	995	12	1.2
Fry et al.[48]	490	7	1.4
Dyck et al.[41]	380	29	7.6
Mulder et al.[98]	103	9	8.7
Mayer[97]	64	7	10.9
Comi et al.[26]	401	45	11.2
Gamstedt et al.[50]	99	19	19.2
Chammas et al.[23]	120	25	20.8
TOTAL	2652	153	5.8

CTS, carpal tunnel syndrome; DM, diabetes mellitus.

patients, dismissed the possibility of a link between the two disorders, stating that " . . . a causal relationship is unlikely." They reasoned, as others have, "that patients with . . . CTS may have associated disease that is unrelated to the syndrome."[90] Moreover, a few studies have supported the lack of a relationship between DM and CTS. Pal and coworkers, after excluding patients having (among other factors) known DM, performed glucose tolerance tests on 42 patients with CTS confirmed in their EMG laboratory. They found impairment of glucose tolerance, consistent with DM, in only 1 patient (2.4%). Because such impairment was expected in between 2% and 5% of their study population, they concluded that there was no evidence of an increased prevalence of DM in their CTS patients.[103] Similarly, de Krom and colleagues performed a case-control study of CTS risk factors among a general population; of the 156 subjects included, only 4 (2.6%) had DM. They concluded that they could not demonstrate that DM was a risk factor for the development of CTS.[32] It is also pertinent to note that DM is not listed among the many causes of CTS in several publications concerned solely with entrapment neuropathies.[31, 100, 124] Most physicians who reject the concept that DM in some manner causes an increased prevalence of CTS do not deny that the two disorders often occur together. However, they consider that the association is probably the result of chance alone, because both entities are relatively common and occur predominantly in the same "over 40 years old" age group.[144] Thus, essentially the same reason is being invoked by those opposed to the link between DM and CTS as was used by the early investigators to reject the connection between DM and all PNS lesions. However, those who currently hold this opinion must deny a considerable body of evidence.

Regarding the relationship of CTS to other aspects of the diabetic state, Fraser and associates found that it was more common in females, as in the nondiabetic population, but detected no consistent relationship between CTS and the age, diabetic treatment, control, or duration of DM.[46] In contrast, both Chaudhuri and coworkers and Gamstedt and coworkers found a positive correlation between CTS and duration of the DM.[22, 50] Dyck and colleagues, referring solely to that subgroup of patients with EDX evidence of CTS, also noted that the focal nerve disorder "was significantly associated with duration" of DM, but found no connection between the gender and age of

the patients and the type of DM present.[41] Albers and associates, also dealing primarily with electrical CTS, found a relationship between the median mononeuropathy and the duration of the DM and, in type 2 DM patients, the sex (more often female) and the body mass index (higher).[3]

The only laboratory procedure of consistent value for confirming the presence of CTS is the EDX examination, specifically, various types of median NCSs. Because CTS, for unknown reasons, characteristically is manifested as demyelinating focal slowing until relatively late in its course, the critical component of the median NCSs are those that measure the speed of conduction along the nerve segment that traverses the carpal tunnel. The first of these to do so was the median motor distal latency, initially reported by Simpson, in 1956.[122] Median sensory NCSs, and thereby the median sensory peak latencies, were introduced in 1958 by Gilliatt and Sears.[56] Because CTS is recognized earlier, both of these median NCSs fail to detect many instances of mild CTS. Because of their relative insensitivity, particularly the median motor distal latencies, a number of additional NCS techniques have been devised. Unlike the routine median motor and sensory NCSs, these are performed solely to detect slowing along the distal segment of the median nerve. These include several different NCSs that share the common label *palmar NCS*, as well as a number of other techniques, such as comparing the median sensory and radial sensory latencies at the same distance, while recording the thumb, and, similarly, comparing the median and ulnar sensory latencies, obtained at the same distance, while recording the fourth finger.[115]

It is pertinent for clinicians to appreciate that because CTS is clinically recognized so early in its course currently, routine median motor and sensory NCSs are not sufficiently sensitive to diagnose it in many cases. Consequently, at least one special NCS should be performed in the EMG laboratory before it is concluded that there is no electrical evidence consistent with CTS.

Typically, the EDX results used to diagnose CTS in diabetic patients who do not have coexisting DSPN are very similar to those used to diagnose CTS in the nondiabetic population. However, when the same upper extremity EDX studies are performed on patients with DSPN, problems in recognition and interpretation can arise. Difficulties are encountered in two separate contexts: (1) in detecting a focal neurogenic abnormality in the presence of a generalized one; therefore, confirming the diagnosis of CTS can become quite problematic; and (2) in interpreting prolonged median distal or peak latencies in those patients who lack clinical changes suggestive of CTS. These difficulties are discussed in the next few paragraphs.

In approximately one third of patients with DSPN, the generalized process is so mild that the EDX changes are essentially limited to the lower extremities.[144] Diagnosing CTS in this group is essentially no different than diagnosing it in diabetic patients not affected by DSPN. However, in the other two thirds of patients with DSPN, the latter is severe enough that it causes abnormalities in the upper extremities as well, that is, the process is detectably diffuse. Depending on the type and severity of the changes caused by the generalized disorder, confirming the presence of a superimposed focal median nerve lesion at the wrist can be easy to impossible. This is because the diagnostic process shifts from detecting absolute EDX abnormalities to seeking relative abnormalities, and then attempting to determine when the latter are significant. Characteristically, the sensory nerve action potentials (SNAPs) are affected before the motor NCSs by DSPN, just as they are with CTS. If the only NCS abnormalities caused by the DSPN are reduced SNAP amplitudes, then it is still possible to recognize that distal conduction slowing is occurring only along the median fibers. However, if the NCS latencies along the distal nerve segments are also prolonged by the DSPN, then the recognition rests on: (1) determining that the distal latencies of all the upper extremity nerves are prolonged, but the median nerve latencies in one or both hands are disproportionately slow; or (2) if the CTS is unilateral, observing that the median distal latencies in the affected limb are substantially prolonged compared to those in the contralateral limb. (There are no established guidelines available for ascertaining exactly when a specific median latency can be designated disproportionately slow or relatively substantially prolonged.) Carpal tunnel syndrome can also be suspected, but not confirmed, if the median motor and sensory NCS responses in one or both limbs are unelicitable while the remaining upper extremity NCS responses (ulnar, motor and sensory; radial sensory) are present, albeit abnormal.[144] Johnson proposed using a variety of comparative studies to diagnose CTS in these patients by comparing (1) the median and ulnar SNAP amplitudes, latencies, and duration, while stimulating/recording from the

fourth finger; (2) the median and radial SNAP amplitudes, latencies, and duration while stimulating/recording from the thumb; (3) the median and ulnar palmar responses, obtained by stimulating in the palm while recording at the wrist; and (4) the antidromic median SNAP amplitudes, latencies, and durations of negative spikes, obtained by stimulating both at the wrist and in the mid-palm. (With the last technique, if the abnormalities are similar on stimulation at both sites, it is assumed that they are caused by the DSPN and not by CTS.[76]) Loong suggested comparing the amplitudes of the median and ulnar SNAPs and determining the "median/ulnar amplitude ratio," to detect CTS in the presence of an underlying DSPN. Under normal circumstances, the median sensory SNAPs are higher in amplitude than the ipsilateral ulnar SNAPs; consequently, when the reverse exists, it suggests a lesion of the median nerve.[93] However, many patients with CTS do not have significant abnormalities of the median SNAP amplitudes; often, the changes are limited to the SNAP latencies. Moreover, such amplitude changes alone never permit localization to a specific site, so the best that can be said if an abnormal median/ulnar amplitude ratio exists is that there is probably a lesion at some point along the median nerve, exact location unknown. It is pertinent to note that all comparative studies become valueless whenever the DSPN is so severe that very substantial axon loss has occurred in the distal upper extremities. In these situations, diagnosing a superimposed CTS by EDX studies becomes impossible; when all or nearly all the median nerve fibers have degenerated, evidence of focal slowing can no longer be detected by any NCS.[144]

A second problem concerning CTS, DSPN, and EDX studies hinges on the fact that prolonged median motor distal latencies and median sensory peak latencies are commonly found in patients with DSPN who have no clinical symptoms suggestive of CTS. Mayer was one of the first to remark on this point. He noted in 1963 that focal motor NCS changes were not detectable in 41 diabetic patients who lacked clinical evidence of DSPN, whereas there was slowing of the median motor distal latency in 16 of 64 (25%) diabetic patients who had DSPN; however, only 7 (11%) of those patients had symptoms of CTS. Thus, only 44% of the 16 patients with EDX changes suggestive of CTS had associated clinical findings.[97] Braddom and colleagues reported in 1977 that of 56 patients with DSPN, 66% had prolonged median motor distal latencies, whereas 61% had prolonged median sensory peak latencies. In contrast, only 6% had prolonged ulnar motor distal latencies, and 43% had prolonged ulnar sensory peak latencies. In their series, prolonged median motor distal latencies were the second most frequent EDX abnormality found, trailing only sural NCS changes (84%).[15] In 1979, Kimura and coworkers used F waves to assess conduction along the entire length of 101 median nerves among 156 diabetic patients; all had clinically mild DSPN, but none had clinical evidence of a superimposed CTS. For comparison purposes, the same studies were also performed on 61 limbs of 44 patients symptomatic with CTS. Kimura and associates found in their diabetic group that there was "considerable delay" of the median motor distal latencies, out of proportion to the more proximal segments. In fact, the EDX findings in the members of the diabetic group, none of whom had symptoms of CTS, were similar to the findings in the CTS group in regard to the slowing along the distal segments of the median motor nerves.[81]

Baba and associates reported seven patients with DSPN, all of whom had, on EDX studies, changes consistent with bilateral CTS; three also had evidence of bilateral UNE, and four had changes suggestive of unilateral UNE. However, none of the seven patients had hand symptoms.[9] Ozaki and colleagues recorded antidromic median and ulnar SNAPs from the fourth finger and performed median and ulnar motor NCS on 49 limbs of 31 diabetic patients, most of whom had symptoms or signs of DSPN, but none with symptoms suggestive of CTS. The results were compared with those obtained in 42 limbs of 21 nondiabetic, age-matched controls. The authors found conduction delay along the distal segment of the median motor and sensory fibers that was more severe than for the corresponding segments of the ulnar nerve.[102] Dyck and associates noted that of 101 patients with type 1 DM, 11 had clinical symptoms of CTS, and an additional 19 had median NCS changes suggestive of that focal PNS disorder. The latter number actually could have been higher, because only 86 of the 101 patients had NCSs. It is conceivable that as many as 34 (19 + 15) of the 101 patients (34%) could have had solely electrical evidence suggestive of CTS. Similarly, of 277 patients with type 2 DM, 18 had clinical symptoms of CTS, whereas 74 had median NCS changes alone. Moreover, 22 of the 277 did not have NCS performed, so it is possible that as many as 96

(74 + 22) of the 277 patients (35%) may have had electrical changes alone consistent with CTS. Thus, up to 34 to 35% of both groups could have had these median NCS findings.[41] Albers and coworkers studied the nondominant hand in 414 patients with mild DSPN who had no or only mild symptoms of CTS and found that 95 (23%) fulfilled their criteria for the diagnosis of median mononeuropathy; most often this consisted of a prolonged median SNAP latency. Even when more stringent criteria were used, 68 (16%) of the patients fulfilled the criteria. The authors noted that patients with these NCS abnormalities had a longer duration of DM and that, among type 2 DM patients, they were more likely to be female and to have a higher body mass index than the remaining type 2 DM patients.[3]

How these electrical changes are to be viewed is somewhat controversial. Albers and associates seem concerned that these represent examples of false-positive EDX studies, whereas Dyck and colleagues refer to them as asymptomatic CTS.[3, 41] The latter approach seems more reasonable. As an analogy, it is not uncommon in high volume EMG laboratories to detect evidence of bilateral CTS on median NCSs in patients who have only unilateral symptoms, with the latter typically involving the dominant hands. To consider the findings in the asymptomatic hands as being false-positive studies, rather than evidence of subclinical lesions, appears illogical. Nathan and associates view median mononeuropathy at the wrist as a "disease" that exists in a "silent form" (electrical CTS changes alone) and an "overt form" (the clinical condition of CTS).[101]

In any case, why there is a greater frequency of electrical evidence of distal median neuropathy in diabetic patients than in nondiabetic control subjects is, as Albers and associates note, unknown. One possibility is that there is an increased susceptibility to focal trauma in patients with DSPN. Another possibility is that patients with DSPN have decreased awareness of CTS symptoms—fewer paresthesias and less pain in association with median nerve compression—than do otherwise normal patients with similar degrees of CTS. However, speaking against both these theories is the fact that Albers and coworkers could not demonstrate an increase in the frequency of asymptomatic distal median neuropathy in proportion to an increase in severity of the underlying DSPN.[3]

Nonsurgical treatments for CTS include wrist splints and cortisone injections into the carpal tunnel. Wrist splints are often quite effective in relieving nocturnal paresthesias. However, they frequently cannot be worn during the day because they interfere with hand use. Cortisone injections into the carpal tunnel often relieve symptoms, either partially or completely. However, the relief usually proves short-lived, and many investigators believe that only a few injections should be given during a period of several months to avoid complications.

Surgery is the definitive treatment for CTS. The transverse carpal ligament is sectioned. This brings symptom relief for the majority of patients. However, in those with fixed sensory deficits in a median nerve distribution, and particularly those with lateral thenar wasting, recovery may be imperfect.

An often-asked question is "How well do diabetic patients with CTS, both with and without coexisting DSPN, respond to surgical release of the transverse carpal ligament?" Gilliatt and Willison, in 1962, were among the first to address this issue, but their limited results were inconclusive. They reported two older-aged diabetic women, both of whom had severe CTS (confirmed by both clinical and EDX examinations) but no evidence of associated DSPN, who responded in markedly different fashions to carpal tunnel release. One patient, "in spite of an apparently successful operation . . . continued to complain of weakness and discomfort in the hand." Studies performed at 3 and 6 months after surgery demonstrated progression of the median neuropathy, to the point that, on the later examination, virtually all the median nerve fibers supplying the thenar eminence had apparently degenerated. Gilliatt and Willison denied that inadequate surgical release was the fault and attributed the continued deterioration of this patient's median nerve to her DM. In contrast, the second patient responded quite favorably to operative release, and after 1 year her EDX studies showed significant improvement. Thus, the lesion in this patient appeared to be "due to mechanical compression, and recovery was not impeded by . . . [her] diabetes."[55]

Concerning diabetic patients who have CTS alone—no DSPN associated—most investigators have harbored some reservations regarding the pace and ultimate degree of recovery that will be experienced after surgery, compared to that realized in patients with idiopathic CTS of the same severity. Thus, Winkleman stated that surgery in these patients "sometimes results in slower or unsatisfactory improvement."[148] Eversman and Ritsick agreed

that the clinical response could be slower, but contended that the recovery of sensory function was ultimately as complete as that seen in nondiabetic patients.[44] Both Haupt and associates and Kulick and colleagues disagreed with the latter. Haupt and associates reported that diabetic patients had a "trend towards less pain relief."[65] Kulick and colleagues stated that DM was one of the "predisposing conditions" that resulted in the failure of operative treatment to bring long-term relief.[86] Cseuz and co-workers' comments on the subject are deceptive. On superficial reading, they imply that the results of carpal tunnel release in diabetic patients are similar to those in nondiabetic patients. However, the qualifiers inserted in the pertinent sentences suggest otherwise. Thus, "satisfactory post-operative recovery" is not "*necessarily* precluded" by advanced DM, and "there was no evidence that . . . (DM) *consistently* worsened the prognosis."[29] Probably the most cautionary views were expressed by Rosenbaum and Ochoa and by Thomas and Thomlinson. According to Rosenbaum and Ochoa, "if the diabetic (CTS) . . . has progressed to the stage of objective motor or sensory deficit, post-operative and neurologic recovery will be less likely than an idiopathic . . . (CTS) of similar severity."[115] Thomas and Tomlinson were somewhat more pessimistic. "Although the symptoms may be relieved by decompressive operations, this does not always occur, and surgical intervention may even aggravate the situation."[132]

Concerning patients who have CTS superimposed on DSPN, opinions are also somewhat varied regarding how satisfactorily they respond to operative treatment. Al-Qattan and associates performed such surgery on 15 patients (20 hands in all) who also had DSPN; they reported that the only poor results occurred in patients in whom focal abnormalities could not be demonstrated on preoperative median NCSs; in these patients, the persistent or worsening symptoms were caused by the DSPN and not by the CTS.[2] Ditmars and Houin concluded that surgery in these patients produced lessening of "night burning and pain," but "numbness persisted in many cases."[36] Clayburgh and colleagues reported that complete relief of symptoms occurred in 72% and partial relief in an additional 20% of 44 patients with diffuse polyneuropathy of various etiologies who underwent carpal tunnel release for superimposed median nerve lesions. However, only 19 of these patients had DSPN, and no specifics were provided concerning this group.[24]

Dobyns, also referring to patients with diffuse polyneuropathy of various etiologies who undergo operative treatment for CTS, observed that " . . . the final level of recovery may not equal the results seen in patients without neuropathy, and the time required to achieve final recovery levels may be longer . . . ."[37] Unfortunately, he also did not provide information related specifically to patients with CTS superimposed on DSPN.

The foregoing discussion emphasizes the need to stage severity of CTS (median neuropathy of the wrist [MNW]). Dyck and associates[41] suggested an approach for staging:

Stage 0: No electrophysiologic or clinical evidence of CTS.

Stage 1: Electrophysiologic findings typical of CTS, but without typical symptoms—patients with carpal ligament section are to be included in this stage.

Stage 2a: Symptoms and findings suggestive of CTS, with or without electrophysiologic findings.

Stage 2b: Symptoms and findings and electrophysiologic findings diagnostic of CTS.

This staging approach is similar to the one Dyck and coworkers[41] introduced for DSPN. Much of the variability of the frequency of CTS would be lessened if this staging approach were used to grade severity of CTS.

ULNAR NEUROPATHY AT THE ELBOW

Ulnar neuropathy at the elbow is the second most common upper-extremity entrapment/compressive neuropathy. Its clinical presentation, EDX features, and surgical treatment are all much more varied than for CTS. Typically, one of the main symptoms, and sometimes the only symptom, of UNE is pain and paresthesias in the fourth and fifth fingers; often this is accompanied by an area of pain or tenderness along the medial aspect of the elbow. Less common presentations include combinations of ulnar sensory and motor abnormalities, with the latter usually manifested as weakness and wasting of the ulnar nerve–innervated hand muscles, particularly the first dorsal interosseous. An uncommon presentation is substantial motor abnormalities in an ulnar nerve distribution, without any appreciable sensory complaints.

Ulnar neuropathy at the elbow can develop in patients with deformities of the elbow joint resulting from remote fractures or other trauma as well as from external pressure being applied to the nerve for prolonged periods, such as during surgery and by chronic "elbow leaners." Compression of the ulnar nerve immediately distal to the ulnar groove, in the cubital tunnel, is said to be a common cause for UNE. The nerve is compressed beneath the edge of the flexor carpi ulnaris aponeurosis, and this compression is aggravated by elbow flexion, because this maneuver causes the aponeurosis to become more constricting. There are a number of other causes for UNE, but in many instances the etiology is unclear.

Ulnar neuropathy at the elbow must be distinguished from cervical intraspinal canal lesions involving the C8 and T1 segments or roots and from lower trunk or medial cord brachial plexopathies. Neither sensory symptoms nor sensory deficits are present with anterior horn cell disorders involving the C8/T1 spinal cord segments; generally, careful clinical examination will reveal that the motor abnormalities are outside the distribution of the ulnar nerve with both cervical intraspinal canal lesions and brachial plexopathies. The EDX examination can help in this regard, as will be discussed later in this section.[127]

Rundles in 1945, was one of the first investigators to link UNE with underlying DM: "With distal involvement of the extremities . . . the ulnar (nerve is) more vulnerable than the radial or median."[117] Although this statement subsequently was quoted in other publications, including the 9th and 10th editions of Joslin's book,[110, 113] no data supporting this assertion were provided. Martin later reported that of the 150 patients with diabetic neuropathy he studied, 2 had UNE; this was the most common upper extremity focal nerve lesion in his experience.[96] In four series concerned with DM, which included between 64 and 490 patients, the percentage of patients with UNE ranged from 1.2 to 4.9%. If the data from these four series are combined, then of 756 patients with DM, 16 (2.1%) had UNE (Table 36.6).[48, 50, 97, 98] In the three core articles dealing with diabetic limb mononeuropathies, the percentage of patients with such lesions having UNE were quite similar: Mulder and associates, 5 of 15 patients (33%); Fry and colleagues, 6 of 19 patients (32%); and Fraser and coworkers, 15 of 41 patients (37%). In these three series, UNE was responsible for 18, 30, and 42% of all focal nerve lesions.[46, 48, 98] In the series by Fraser and colleagues, 10 of 15 patients with UNE were males; in contrast, 13 of 15 cases of CTS were in females. Also, the 15 patients who had UNE

TABLE 36.6 PATIENTS WITH DIABETES MELLITUS WHO HAVE COEXISTING ULNAR NEUROPATHY AT THE ELBOW

Investigators	No. With DM	No. With UNE	Percentage
Fry et al.[48]	490	6	1.2
Gamstedt et al.[50]	99	2	2.0
Mayer[97]	64	3	4.7
Mulder et al.[98]	103	5	4.9
TOTAL	756	16	2.1

(8 bilateral) had all experienced a gradual onset of symptoms, similar to the 15 patients who had CTS, thus suggesting an entrapment/compressive etiology.[46]

Viewed from the reverse aspect—the percentage of patients with UNE who have DM—the results are more variable. In many reports dealing with operated series of UNE, no predisposing metabolic or toxic conditions, including DM, appeared. In others, a variety of predisposing factors, including DM, alcoholism, and cancer, were briefly mentioned.[47, 106, 128, 130] Nonetheless, in six series concerned with operated UNE, which included between 20 to 414 patients, the percentage of patients with underlying DM ranged from 4 to 17.4%. If the data from all six of these studies are combined, then of 773 patients with UNE, 69 (8.9%) also had DM (Table 36.7).[57, 63, 87, 136, 138, 140] Noteworthy is that in the large retrospective series by Warner, encompassing 414 patients, 11.1% (46 patients) had DM, compared with 3% of controls. In that series, DM was determined to be the second highest relative risk factor (RRF = 4.3) for UNE, exceeded only by obesity (RRF = 15).[140] Curiously, despite the fact that UNE has been linked to DM by a number of investiga-

tors, UNE was not included among the various types of limb mononeuropathies sought by Palumbo and associates in their epidemiologic study of the neurologic complications of DM.[104]

An interesting point is that alcoholism appears to rank higher than DM as a predisposing condition for UNE. In several of the operated series reported, none of the patients had DM, whereas between 10 and 33% of them abused alcohol.[1, 43, 94, 95] Moreover, in two of the three reports in which both predisposing factors were present, alcoholism appeared in higher frequency than did DM. Thus, Goldberg and associates detected DM in 3 (6.5%) and alcoholism in 2 (4.3%) of the 46 patients with UNE in their series.[57] Conversely, LaRoux and colleagues found that among their 46 patients, 8 (17%) had DM, whereas 15 (33%) abused alcohol.[87] Similarly, Varughese and associates noted that of their 198 patients with UNE, 8 (4%) had DM, whereas 13 (7%) abused alcohol.[136] In all, of seven reports in which alcohol abuse was reported to be a predisposing condition for UNE, DM also was mentioned in only four of them.[1, 43, 57, 87, 94, 95, 136] Of the 418 patients with UNE in these seven series, 19 (4.5%) had DM, whereas 56 (13.4%) had alcohol abuse as a predisposing condition (Table 36.8). In contrast to the situation with UNE, apparently there has never been a reported series in which alcohol abuse was regarded as being a predisposing factor for CTS.

The EDX examination can assist in diagnosing UNE, a fact first demonstrated regarding the NCSs by Simpson in 1956.[122] However, problems can be encountered. First, some UNEs are so mild that, even though they are

TABLE 36.7 PATIENTS WITH ULNAR NEUROPATHY AT THE ELBOW WHO HAVE COEXISTING DIABETES MELLITUS

Investigators	No. With UNE	No. With DM	Percentage
Varughese et al.[136]	198	8	4.0
Goldberg et al.[57]	46	2	4.3
Wadsworth[138]	20	1	5
Harmon[63]	49	4	8
Warner et al.[140]	414	46	11.1
LaRoux et al.[87]	46	8	17.4
TOTAL	773	69	8.9

UNE, ulnar neuropathy at the elbow; DM, diabetes mellitus.

TABLE 36.8 ARTICLES REPORTING ALCOHOL ABUSE, WITH OR WITHOUT ALSO REPORTING DIABETES MELLITUS, AS A PREDISPOSING CONDITION FOR ULNAR NEUROPATHY AT THE ELBOW

Investigators	No. of Patients	No. (%) With DM	No. (%) With Alcohol Abuse
LaRoux et al.[87]	46	8 (17)	15 (33)
Lugnegard et al.*[95]	33	0 (0)	11 (33)
Ekerot[43]	19	0 (0)	2 (10)
Goldberg et al.[57]	46	3 (7)	2 (4)
Varughese et al.[136]	198	8 (4)	13 (7)
Lugnegard et al.*[94]	44	0 (0)	8 (18)
Adelaar et al.[1]	32	0 (0)	5 (16)
TOTAL	418	19 (4.5)	56 (13.4)

DM, diabetes mellitus.
*Two different series collected over different time periods.

symptomatic (typically manifested as intermittent paresthesias in the ulnar nerve–supplied digits), they cause no detectable EDX abnormalities on either NCS or NEE. Thus, false-negative EDX examinations are far more common with UNE than with CTS. Second, unlike CTS, UNE does not have a single characteristic EDX presentation, because its underlying pathophysiology may not only be demyelinating focal slowing (as is the pathophysiology of most CTS), but also demyelinating conduction block, axon loss causing conduction failure, and various combinations of these.

Third, with pure axon loss lesions, which are responsible for nearly half of all UNEs, EDX localization is poor.[145] One of the problems is the anatomy of the ulnar nerve: it does not lend itself to localization by NEE. Two motor branches arise in the proximal forearm, immediately distal to the ulnar groove, to supply the flexor carpi ulnaris and the flexor digitorum profundus. No further motor branches arise throughout the entire length of the nerve in the forearm. Another problem is that even with axon loss lesions at the elbow, the motor branches supplying the ulnar nerve–innervated forearm muscles often are spared, presumably because the nerve fascicles that contain them are not compromised. Consequently, with UNE causing axon loss, the EDX examination can often demonstrate that the lesion involves the ulnar nerve and the severity of axon loss, but it cannot localize the lesion well.[145] Many of the difficulties are exaggerated with diabetic patients. With pure axon loss lesions, for example, often the EDX findings—low-amplitude ulnar SNAPs, recording/stimulating the fifth finger, and fibrillation potentials in the ulnar nerve–innervated hand muscles—are identical to those seen in an ulnar nerve distribution with moderately severe DSPN. Thus, bilateral UNE, when accompanied by rather severe, bilateral CTS, is easily mistaken for the upper extremity manifestations of DSPN.[144]

Fourth, in the presence of DSPN, diagnosing UNE by detecting focal demyelinating slowing along the elbow segment, which is seen with approximately half of all UNE, may also be difficult. This is because the motor CV along the entire ulnar nerve often is diffusely slow. As a result, as Hawley observed: "Patients with . . . [diffuse DSPN] but no superimposed clinical . . . [UNE] had nearly as much relative slowing across the elbow as patients with . . . [DSPN] and superimposed clinical . . . [UNE]."[66] For this reason, Hawley and Capobianco found it impossible to establish ulnar mo-

tor CV criteria for diagnosing UNE in patients with DSPN.[67]

Thus, for different reasons, UNE causing either axon loss or demyelinating conduction slowing can be difficult to identify in diabetic patients with DSPN.

There is no generally acknowledged treatment approach for UNE. In most instances, conservative therapy is initially tried. This consists of cautioning the patient not to put pressure on the elbow and using an elbow pad for protection. However, in many patients, surgery is ultimately proposed, particularly if the symptoms are progressive. A number of operative procedures are available, including medial epicondylectomy, slitting of the flexor carpi ulnaris aponeurosis, and ulnar nerve transposition. Unfortunately, none of these surgical procedures has proven to be substantially better than the others. Compared with CTS surgery, operations for UNE have been somewhat disappointing.

Concerning surgical results in patients with DM, Goldberg and coworkers reported that among their four patients with predisposing factors (two DM alone, one alcoholism alone, one DM plus alcoholism), the UNE was more severe before surgery and "the recovery was less dramatic."[57] The opinion expressed by Winkleman that surgical treatment of diabetic entrapment neuropathies sometimes is followed by "slower or unsatisfactory" recovery pertains to UNE as well as to CTS.[148]

Although CTS attributable to underlying DM has been the main subject of many articles, UNE related to underlying DM has apparently been the focus of only one. Jones, in 1967, rather unconvincingly attempted to prove, using fragmentary clinical data and inadequate EDX studies, that a unilateral postoperative UNE in a 50-year-old man had progressed from "an initially mild ulnar nerve pressure neuritis . . . to a severe palsy over the course of a year," as a result of his underlying DM.[77]

PERONEAL NEUROPATHY AT THE FIBULAR HEAD

Peroneal neuropathy at the fibular head is the most common lower extremity compressive neuropathy. Unlike CTS and UNE, the clinical presentation of PNFH is remarkably consistent. Almost invariably, footdrop is present, because of compromise of the motor nerve fibers supplying the tibialis anterior muscle. Usually, foot eversion also is weak because of involvement of the motor nerve fibers supplying the peroneus muscles. Pain is quite uncommon with these lesions, and sensory abnormalities characteristically are negative in character rather than positive. Paresthesias usually are not present, but the patient notices a sensory deficit whenever objects touch the skin in the affected area.

Peroneal neuropathy at the fibular head has a number of causes, the most common being external compression, which can occur during general anesthesia; in emaciated, bedridden patients; and in persons who have recently lost weight and cross their legs.

Peroneal neuropathy at the fibular head can be mistaken for a number of other disorders involving the central and peripheral nervous systems. One of the most common is L5 radiculopathy, in which pain is often present in the low back, with peripheral radiation. Moreover, foot inversion, eversion, and dorsiflexion typically are affected because the L5 root, via different peripheral nerves, is primarily responsible for all of these foot movements.

One of the first reports to link PNFH with DM was a single case report by Root, published in 1922. A 69-year-old diabetic woman experienced sudden, painless footdrop caused by compromise of the left peroneal nerve.[112] In a discussion of "multiple peripheral neuritis" a year later, Harris mentions painful peroneal neuropathies occurring in diabetic patients.[64] Root and Rogers, in 1930, described 12 patients with "actual paralysis" of lower extremity muscles, four of whom had footdrop, two bilateral and two unilateral.[111] However, in two of these four patients the footdrop was associated with diabetic amyotrophy and could well have represented "territorial extension" of an L2-L4 diabetic polyradiculopathy to the L5 root, rather than PNFH (see discussion of diabetic amyotrophy).[12, 144] Jordan, in 1936, noted that in a retrospective survey of 111 diabetic patients in whom muscle strength had been recorded, weakness of foot dorsiflexion was present in 31 (30 unilaterally, 1 bilaterally), and in slightly more than half of these, no other muscles were weak. Thus, it seems likely that of the 111 patients, at least 16 (14%) had PNFH. Jordan also provided four case reports of footdrop, including a unilateral lesion first noted after a patient recovered from diabetic coma, and bilateral but short-lived lesions, consisting mostly of sensory symptoms, that developed sequentially (1 week between bouts) as a result of leg crossing in a 55-year-old diabetic.[78] Rundles, in 1945, stated: "With distal involvement of the extremities, the peroneal nerve was more vulnerable than the tibial." He reported that of

125 patients, "complete footdrop was present in ten cases." Unfortunately, he provided no clinical details, so it is impossible to determine whether these represented instances of bilateral PNFH or simply severe DSPN.[117]

Garland and Moorhouse found that of their 19 patients with PNFH, 1 (5%) had DM; nonetheless, they stated: "We do not believe that diabetes is in itself ever an important factor in this condition."[54] Hirson and coworkers observed footdrop in 6 of 50 (12%) hospitalized diabetic patients, unilateral in 4 and bilateral in 2.[69] In Martin's series, reported in 1953, of 150 patients with diabetic neuropathy, footdrop was the most common motor finding; partial or complete footdrop was present in 12 patients (8 unilateral, 4 bilateral). Unfortunately, clinical details regarding these patients were lacking, so it is unclear how many of these cases were manifestations of PNFH.[96] Sullivan, in 1958, described a 59-year-old diabetic woman who, during a 2-day period, became "totally unable to extend her (left) foot or turn it laterally." This weakness was not accompanied by sensory symptoms of any type, including pain. A few weeks later, she developed a left facial mononeuropathy.[129]

Among the three core articles, PNFH figures prominently. In the series by Mulder and associates, PNFH was the single most common mononeuropathy; of the 28 individual PNS lesions, 13 (46%) were of this type.[98] Of the 19 patients in the series by Fry and colleagues, PNFH was also the most common focal limb mononeuropathy, being present in 7 (37%) patients. These were unilateral isolated lesions in four patients, bilateral lesions in 1 patient, and in 2 patients, unilateral PNFH coexisting with other mononeuropathies (1 UNE and 1 radial).[48] In the report by Fraser and associates concerning 41 patients with limb mononeuropathies, there were 9 cases of PNFH (16%), 7 unilateral and 1 bilateral. In contrast to the CTS and UNE found in their patient group, the authors noted that the PNFH was acute in onset, with symptoms of just a few weeks' duration before presentation.[46] Probably the most widely quoted article linking PNFH with DM was the 1969 report by Shahani and Spalding. They described two diabetic women, ages 68 and 80, who developed footdrop, initially unilateral but subsequently bilateral (2 weeks and 13 months apart), that had largely resolved approximately 6 months after the onset in the latest of the two limbs to be affected.[119] A similar case with bilateral, but sequential, onset "some months apart" had been reported earlier by Hirson and coworkers.[69] Lawrence and Locke were possibly the first to report PNFH occurring in children with DM. In 1963, they described two adolescents, a 13-year-old girl and a 14-year-old boy, the former with probable bilateral PNFH, the latter with probable bilateral proximal deep PNFH.[88] Subsequently, Locke provided a case report of a patient with painless left-side footdrop, very probably representing PNFH, that persisted unchanged for at least 3 months.[92]

Relatively few of the publications concerned with diabetic PNFH appeared after EDX studies became widely available. In two of them, peroneal motor NCSs were performed but were focused solely on CVs, and in a third, in which peroneal motor NCS amplitudes were considered, no details were provided.[46, 98, 119] In fact, because clinical weakness is the presenting symptom with nearly all PNFH, the most important motor NCS component is the amplitude of the response. In a large series of PNFH extensively studied in the EMG laboratory by Katirji and Wilbourn, reported in 1988, the pathophysiology at the fibular head consistently was either axon loss (resulting in uniform low amplitude or unelicitable NCS responses), conduction block (producing low amplitude or unelicitable responses on stimulating proximal, but not distal, to the lesion), or a combination of both. Both types of pathophysiology are seen with compressive PNFH, depending on the severity of the lesion. In their series of 103 patients with PNFH, 8 (7.8%) had DM.[81]

Few reports concerned with diabetic PNFH have provided information regarding the subsequent course of the disorder. However, five patients, each with bilateral lesions, were reported to have improved during a period of 6 to 7 months.[78, 88, 119] Apparently, unlike the situation with isolated CTS and UNE, all patients with diabetic PNFH have been treated conservatively. Possible exceptions are those patients with DSPN who have been subjected to multiple limb nerve decompressions, including peroneal nerve decompression at the fibular head, by Dellon (see section on Mislabeled Diabetic Limb Mononeuropathies).[33, 34]

Most cases of PNFH are treated conservatively with a foot brace. The majority are caused by external compression and will ultimately improve spontaneously, if additional pressure on the nerve is prevented.

SCIATIC NEUROPATHY

The majority of patients with sciatic neuropathies have substantial motor and sensory deficits in tibial and peroneal nerve distributions, particularly the latter. Footdrop is very commonly present. In contrast to PNFH, however, pain often is present as well, particularly with those lesions caused by trauma; it is usually most prominent over the dorsum of the foot. The causes for sciatic neuropathy include fractures of the pelvis, hip joint and femur; hip surgery; misplaced gluteal injections; and nerve infarcts. Whenever sciatic neuropathies are attributed to DM, the assumed etiology is ischemia causing a nerve infarct, rather than external compression.

Diabetes mellitus was linked to sciatic neuropathies as early as 1907 by Williamson.[147] Since then, this association has been mentioned, in passing, in several other articles.[25, 46, 59, 92, 121, 133, 141] Nonetheless, almost no detailed descriptions of such cases can be found in the literature. Goodman and associates, in 1955, attributed the footdrop present in two of their patients to sciatic neuropathies, in which the peroneal fibers were more affected than the tibial.[59] However, clinical details were lacking, so their localization to the sciatic nerve, rather than the peroneal nerve, cannot be verified. Sullivan described one patient, a 71-year-old woman, who may have had a painful unilateral sciatic neuropathy involving the peroneal component more than the tibial.[129] The most widely quoted article on diabetic sciatic neuropathy is a brief case report by Jacobs, published in 1958. The 59-year-old diabetic female he described had several features of a left sciatic mononeuropathy; however, there were some changes incompatible with that diagnosis, including diffuse atrophy of the buttocks and weakness of the quadriceps muscle.[74]

Apparently, no cases of diabetic sciatic neuropathy had been reported in which the localization was verified by EDX studies.

LATERAL FEMORAL CUTANEOUS NEUROPATHY

Meralgia paresthetica is a clinical syndrome consisting of pain, paresthesias, and sensory deficit over the lateral aspect of the thigh in the distribution of the lateral femoral cutaneous (LFC) nerve. A number of etiologies for LFC neuropathy have been reported, but in most instances, the cause is undetermined.

Lateral femoral cutaneous neuropathies associated with DM have been briefly mentioned in several articles,[25, 62, 70, 133, 137, 141, 147] but specific instances are very rarely found in the literature. Mulder and coworkers reported that 1 of their

15 patients (6.7%) had an LFC neuropathy.[98] These focal PNS lesions are not mentioned in the articles by either Fry and associates or Fraser and colleagues.[46, 48] The question that arises whenever LFC neuropathies develop in diabetic patients is the same one often proffered when CTS is present in a person with DM: Is the cause DM, or is it obesity?[144] Most LFC neuropathies are treated conservatively for several months because most resolve spontaneously.

RADIAL NEUROPATHY

Radial neuropathies are relatively uncommon. The majority occur at the spiral groove, where the nerve is particularly vulnerable. Similar to PNFH, radial neuropathies have a single characteristic presentation, consisting of wristdrop and fingerdrop, sometimes associated with paresthesias; seldom is pain present in a superficial radial nerve distribution on the radial aspect of the dorsum of the hand. Some of the causes for radial neuropathy include humeral fractures, misplaced deltoid injections, blunt trauma, and particularly external compression.

Lesions of the radial nerve have been considered one type of diabetic compressive mononeuropathy since at least 1945, when they were briefly mentioned in the article by Rundles.[117] Subsequently, they have appeared in lists of peripheral nerves affected by DM.[62, 109, 118, 133, 141, 148] Martin, in 1953, reported seeing one patient with wristdrop, presumably the result of a radial nerve lesion, among his series of 150 diabetic patients (0.6%).[96] Among the three core articles, neither Mulder and associates nor Fraser and coworkers reported any instances of radial neuropathy among their 15 and 41 patients, respectively, with limb mononeuropathies.[46, 98] Fry and coworkers noted, among their 19 patients, 1 (5%) with a radial neuropathy.[48] More recently, Gamstedt and associates detected 1 radial neuropathy in their series of 99 diabetic patients (1%).[50] Nonetheless, to my knowledge, not a single case report of this focal PNS lesion occurring in a diabetic patient has appeared in the literature. Because these lesions characteristically present with weakness (similar to PNFH), on EDX examination the pathophysiology should be either conduction failure caused by axon loss, conduction block, or both; consequently, the radial motor NCS component affected should be the amplitude, not the CV.[17] Radial neuropathies caused by trauma, particularly those resulting from fractures, may require surgical exploration and re-

pair. The majority of radial neuropathies at the spiral groove, however, are treated conservatively because they are caused by external compression.

OBTURATOR NEUROPATHY

Lesions of the obturator nerve are rare. The majority result from pelvic fractures, surgical procedures, obturator hernias, and pelvic neoplasms. Often, the sole symptom is weakness of thigh adduction. The only helpful portion of the EDX examination for diagnosing obturator neuropathy is the NEE; abnormalities are found in the thigh adductor muscles.[127]

Lesions of the obturator nerve attributed to DM have been briefly mentioned in at least two articles.[70, 123] Presumably, no detailed reports of these lesions are present in the literature. One possible reason why obturator neuropathies have been linked to DM is the fact that the muscles innervated by the obturator nerve—the thigh adductor muscles—almost invariably are affected by diabetic amyotrophy. If one assumes that diabetic amyotrophy is caused by a disorder of peripheral nerves, then both the femoral and obturator would have to be involved to yield the typical clinical findings.

MISLABELED DIABETIC LIMB MONONEUROPATHIES

At least three different PNS disorders have erroneously been considered types of diabetic limb mononeuropathies. Two of these are caused by DM; the relationship of the remaining disorder to DM is probably coincidental. These three entities—diabetic amyotrophy, distal lower extremity peripheral nerve involvement with DSPN, and neuralgic amyotrophy—are discussed in this section.

Diabetic Amyotrophy

This uncommon disorder, linked to DM, tends to affect elderly men. It involves one or both proximal lower extremities and often begins abruptly with pain in the back and anterior thigh, soon followed by weakness and wasting of the anterior and medial thigh muscles. Weight loss is often prominent.

This disorder affects nerve fibers derived from the L2-L4 roots. Diabetic amyotrophy was one of the first PNS disorders linked to DM. It has been misidentified repeatedly as a femoral neuropathy for more than 115 years, even though for nearly all of that period it has been known that some of the axons involved are outside the distribution of the femoral nerve.

In a detailed 1913 review of the literature on anterior crural (femoral) neuritis, Byrnes observed that Bernard in 1882 reported "the first case of isolated femoral neuritis occurring in a diabetic." Subsequently, in 1890, Bruns described three additional cases, but the disorder was not "strictly limited to a crural nerve" in all of them.[19] Before the turn of the century, Eichhorst, Williamson, and Buzzard described similar cases, some occurring bilaterally.[18, 19] Between 1900 and 1950, descriptions of a disorder occurring in diabetic patients, manifested as anterior thigh pain and weakness, appeared repeatedly in the literature. Such lesions were briefly mentioned by Williamson in 1907 and Harris in 1923.[64, 147] Of 12 patients reported by Root and Rogers in 1930, all of whom had paralysis attributed to a complication of DM, 8 had this disorder (5 bilaterally and 3 unilaterally).[111] In Jordan's series of 111 patients, 21 had these lesions, 7 in isolation.[78] Diabetic "femoral neuropathies" also were mentioned by Rundles.[117] In 1953, Garland and Taverner redefined this disorder; they initially labeled it "diabetic myelopathy," but 2 years later, Garland changed the name to "diabetic amyotrophy."[51, 52, 53] Also in 1953, both Hirson and Martin and colleagues included case reports of this PNS disorder in their articles on diabetic neuropathy. The latter group described it as being "the most striking component of diabetic neuropathy."[69, 96] Of the three core articles, Mulder and associates reported one "femoral neuropathy" among the 16 patients they viewed as having focal limb mononeuropathies. Fraser and coworkers observed three "femoral neuropathies" among the 44 diabetic patients they considered to have limb mononeuropathies. Fry and colleagues reported finding 5 patients with diabetic amyotrophy, which they grouped in a separate category; if Fry and associates had included these cases with their focal limb neuropathies, as did Mulder and coworkers and Fraser and coworkers, then their number of limb PNS lesions would have totaled 24.[46, 48, 98] (As already noted, Fry and associates reported that 6, rather than 5, of their patients had diabetic amyotrophy, but in 1, abnormalities were limited to one shoulder girdle and were probably caused by a coexisting neuralgic amyotrophy.) "Femoral neuropathies" have been linked to DM in many reviews since then.[27, 60, 62, 70, 92, 118, 121, 123, 141] In one 1990 article dealing with diabetic neuropathies, only femoral neuropa-

thies and ocular palsies are included under the heading "mononeuropathies."[141]

In spite of the numerous publications claiming that DM can cause femoral neuropathy, there is compelling clinical and EDX evidence that "diabetic femoral neuropathies" are extremely rare; most patients designated as having such actually have involvement of obturator as well as femoral nerve fibers, resulting from a more proximal lesion involving the L2-L4 roots, the lumbar plexus, or both.[144] The concept that diabetic amyotrophy represents "diabetic femoral neuropathy" has persisted mainly because of two articles on the subject, neither of which substantiates the reputed relationship. Goodman, in 1954, reported 17 patients with what he labeled "femoral neuropathy," 16 of whom had DM.[58] However, it is obvious from the case histories he provided that such a diagnosis was unjustified in nearly all of them. Only a few of the patients had convincing evidence of femoral nerve fiber involvement, and that small subgroup very probably had diabetic amyotrophy, which had just been described the previous year by Garland and Taverner. Calverly and Mulder, in 1960, reported 19 patients with "femoral neuropathy," 14 of whom had associated DM.[20] Both authors conceded in later publications, however, that in their series they had mislabeled cases of diabetic amyotrophy as femoral neuropathy.[144]

It is pertinent to note that the exact location of the PNS lesion responsible for diabetic amyotrophy remains controversial. Bastron and Thomas's concept that the disorder is a diabetic polyradiculopathy involving the L2-L4 roots appears to be the most attractive concept, because it provides a common explanation for both diabetic amyotrophy and certain other PNS diabetic manifestations; for example, diabetic thoracic radiculopathy is also a diabetic polyradiculopathy, but one affecting the T6–T12 roots; footdrop developing ipsilateral to diabetic amyotrophy is caused by extension of the injurious process from the L2-L4 roots to the L5 root.[12, 144] Other investigators hold different views on the subject, however, as perusal of other chapters in this book demonstrates.

Distal Peripheral Nerve Involvement With Distal Symmetrical Polyneuropathy

Referring to DSPN, Dellon hypothesized that "the majority of symptoms of diabetic neuropathy are due to multiple peripheral nerve entrapments."[34] He postulated that the peripheral nerves in diabetic patients are more susceptible to chronic nerve compression because of their decreased axoplasmic flow and their increased water content (with the latter manifested as "subperineurial and endoneurial edema").[34] Consequently, he suggested that some of the symptoms characteristic of DSPN, particularly the "stocking and glove" distribution of sensory loss, may be caused, at least partly, by compression of multiple peripheral nerves. The latter includes, for the upper extremity, the median nerve at the wrist, the ulnar nerve at the elbow, and the radial sensory nerve in the forearm, and for the lower extremity, the common peroneal nerve at the fibular head, the medial and lateral plantar nerves in the tarsal tunnel, the sural nerve, the lateral cutaneous nerve in the calf, and the deep peroneal nerve at the ankle.[33, 34] Attempting to validate this theory, he decompressed 154 peripheral nerves (51 in the upper extremity, 31 in the lower extremity) in 50 diabetic patients. Symptom improvement reportedly occurred, to varying degrees, in the distribution of the operated nerves: in 100% when the preoperative diagnosis had been "localized entrapment," 80% when preoperatively the diagnosis was "peripheral neuropathy with superimposed entrapment," and 50% when it had been "peripheral neuropathy" (i.e., DSPN). Specifically excluded from surgery were those patients in whom "burning pain" (presumably of the feet) was a prominent symptom. Surgical complications, which apparently affected approximately 25% of the 50 patients, included increased pain in the distribution of the operated nerves and, particularly, problems in wound healing; in one patient, a skin graft ultimately was required.[33]

This hypothesis may have some relevance in regard to the upper extremity symptoms in some patients with DSPN. As already noted, in probably the majority of such patients, entrapment neuropathies (specifically CTS, with or without co-existing UNE) are responsible for upper extremity motor and sensory complaints, rather than DSPN. However, this theory appears to have little merit in explaining the distal lower extremity symptoms typical of DSPN. Characteristically, they not only are in the distribution of multiple peripheral nerves, but they also demonstrate a distal-to-proximal gradient. The concept that multiple peripheral nerve entrapments, each at different limb levels (such as fibular head and ankle), could be responsible for graded sensory changes that

are uniform around the circumference of the distal lower extremity is unlikely to gain wide acceptance. Moreover, this theory denies an extensive body of knowledge that has accumulated regarding the nature of the nerve lesions with generalized polyneuropathies, including DSPN. Finally, from a very practical viewpoint, it seems quite ill-advised to perform surgical decompression procedures on multiple peripheral nerves in limbs that have compromised vascular supplies and impaired healing ability.

Neuralgic Amyotrophy

This disorder, of unknown etiology, consists of the abrupt onset of pain in one or both proximal upper extremities, soon followed by weakness and wasting of various forequarter muscles.

Any link between neuralgic amyotrophy and DM is tenuous. As has been pointed out by many investigators, DM is a common disease, and the presence of any focal mononeuropathy in a diabetic patient may be coincidental.[51, 92, 105, 137] Horowitz has observed: "The question of whether an individual peripheral nerve lesion in an individual diabetic patient is due to diabetes may be unresolvable. . . ."[71] The relationship in which the coincidental occurrence of two disorders appears most applicable is in regard to neuralgic amyotrophy and DM. This association has a surprisingly long history. Althaus, in 1890, reported a 56-year-old diabetic man who experienced a classical bout of neuralgic amyotrophy: "He was suddenly awakened in the night by a severe burning pain in the shoulder . . . . When the pain . . . subsided, the patient found himself unable to raise the arm" because of a total right axillary mononeuropathy. Finding no other apparent reason for this lesion, Althaus attributed it to DM.[5] Many investigators have since referred to this report when stating, possibly inaccurately, that DM can affect any peripheral nerve. Other instances of neuralgic amyotrophy being attributed to DM have appeared in the literature. Martin reported that 1 of the patients in his series "suffered from paralysis of the long thoracic nerve."[96] Interestingly, 2 of the diabetic patients in the series by Fry and colleagues (1962) very probably had coincidental neuralgic amyotrophy. One had experienced the sudden onset of simultaneous axillary, musculocutaneous, suprascapular, and ulnar mononeuropathies in one limb. Another patient, whom the authors grouped with their amyotrophy cases rather than their limb mononeuropathy cases, had a 2-week history of pain, weakness, and wasting confined to one shoulder; the serratus anterior and deltoid muscles (long thoracic and axillary nerves) were "particularly" affected.[48] Williams, in 1981, described a 51-year-old diabetic man with bilateral diabetic amyotrophy who developed pain acutely in his right shoulder, followed subsequently by weakness in the distribution of the axillary, suprascapular, and long thoracic nerves; approximately 6 weeks later, "he experienced a similar severe ache in his left shoulder," with subsequent weakness in the distribution of the axillary and suprascapular nerves. Williams commented on the similarities between diabetic amyotrophy and neuralgic amyotrophy and concluded that DM "appears to play an important and etiological role in some cases of neuralgic amyotrophy." To support his theory, he noted that in some studies concerned with neuralgic amyotrophy, patients with DM "have accounted for up to 14% of the cases discussed."[146] This figure is hardly convincing, however, when it is appreciated that it refers to a series reported by Kennedy and Resch that consisted of only 7 patients with neuralgic amyotrophy, 1 of whom was a diabetic.[82] In a much larger series of 99 patients with neuralgic amyotrophy, reported by Tsairis and associates, in 1972, 5 patients (5%) had DM.[134]

References

1. Adelaar RS, Foster WC, McDowell C. The treatment of cubital tunnel syndrome. J Hand Surg 1984; 9A:90–95.
2. Al-Qattan MM, Manktelow RT, Bowen CVA. Outcome of carpal tunnel release in diabetic patients. J Hand Surg 1994; 19B:626–629.
3. Albers JW, Brown MB, Sima AAF, et al. Frequency of median neuropathy in patients with mild diabetic neuropathy in the early diabetes intervention trial (EDIT). Muscle Nerve 1996; 19:140–146.
4. Albers JW, Brown MB, Sima AAF, et al. Frequency of median mononeuropathy in patients with mild diabetic neuropathy in the early diabetes intervention trial (EDIT). Muscle Nerve 1996; 19:1505.
5. Althaus J. Neuritis of the circumflex nerve in diabetes. Lancet 1890; 1:455–456.
6. Alvine FG, Schurrer ME. Postoperative ulnar-nerve palsy. J Bone Joint Surg Am 1987; 69A:255–259.
7. Asbury AK. Focal and multifocal neuropathies of diabetes. In Dyck PJ, Thomas PK, Asbury AK, et al (eds): Diabetic Neuropathy. Philadelphia, WB Saunders, 1984, pp 45–55.
8. Asbury AK, Brown MJ. Clinical and pathological studies of diabetic neuropathies. In Goto Y, Horiuchi A, Kogure K (eds): Diabetic Neuropathy. Amsterdam, Excerpta Medica, 1982, pp 50–57.
9. Baba M, Ozaki I, Watahihi Y, et al. Focal conduction delay at the carpal tunnel and the cubital fossa in

10. Bailey AA. Neurologic complications associated with diabetes. Diabetes 1955; 4:32–36.
11. Bailey CC, Murray J. The nervous system and diabetes. In Joslin EP, Root HF, White P, et al (eds): The Treatment of Diabetes Mellitus, ed 8. Philadelphia, Lea & Febiger, 1946, pp 557–574.
12. Bastron JA, Thomas JE. Diabetic polyradiculopathy. Mayo Clin Proc 1981; 56:725–732.
13. Beacom F, Gillespie EL, Middleton D, et al. Limited joint mobility in insulin-dependent diabetes: Relationship to retinopathy, peripheral nerve function and HLA status. Q J Med 1985; 56:337–344.
14. Blodgett RC, Lipscomb PR, Hill RW. Incidence of hematologic disease in patients with carpal tunnel syndrome. JAMA 1962; 17:814–185.
15. Braddom RL, Hollis JB, Castell DO. Diabetic peripheral neuropathy: A correlation of nerve conduction studies and clinical findings. Arch Phys Med Rehabil 1977; 58:308–313.
16. Brown MJ, Greene DA. Diabetic neuropathy: Pathophysiology and management. In Asbury A, Gilliatt RW (eds): Peripheral Nerve Disorders. London, Butterworths, 1984, pp 126–153.
17. Brown WF, Watson BV. AAEM Case Report #27: Acute retrohumeral radial neuropathies. Muscle Nerve 1993; 16:706–711.
18. Buzzard T. Illustrations of some less-known forms of peripheral neuritis, especially alcohol monoplegia and diabetic neuritis. BMJ 1890; 1:1419–1420.
19. Byrnes CM. Anterior crural neuritis. J Nerv Ment Dis 1913; 40:758–778, 41:19–31.
20. Calverly JR, Mulder DW. Femoral neuropathy. Neurology 1960; 10:963–967.
21. Cannon LJ, Bernacki EJ, Walter SD. Personal and occupational factors associated with carpal tunnel syndrome. J Occup Med 1981; 23:255–258.
22. Chaudhuri KR, Davidson AR, Morris IM. Limited joint mobility and carpal tunnel syndrome in insulin-dependent diabetes. Br J Rheumatol 1989; 28:191–194.
23. Chammas M, Bousquet P, Renard E, et al. Dupuytren's disease, carpal tunnel syndrome, trigger finger, and diabetes mellitus. J Hand Surg 1995; 20A:109–114.
24. Clayburgh RH, Beckenbaugh RD, Dobyns JH. Carpal tunnel release in patients with diffuse peripheral neuropathy. J Hand Surg 1987; 12A:380–383.
25. Colby AW. Neurologic disorders of diabetes mellitus. Diabetes 1965; 14:424–429, 516–525.
26. Comi G, Lozza L, Galardi G, et al. Presence of carpal tunnel syndrome in diabetics: Effect of age, sex, diabetes duration and polyneuropathy. Acta Diabetol Lat 1985; 22:259–262.
27. Coppack SW, Watkins PJ. The natural history of diabetic femoral neuropathy. Q J Med 1991; 288:307–313.
28. Crisp AJ, Heathcote JG. Connective tissue abnormalities in diabetic mellitus. J R Coll Physicians Lond 1984; 18:132–141.
29. Cseuz KA, Thomas JE, Lambert LH, et al. Long-term results of operation for carpal tunnel syndrome. Mayo Clin Proc 1966; 41:232–241.
30. Dahlin LB, Meiri KF, McLean WG, et al. Effects of nerve compression on fast axonal transport in streptozotocin-induced diabetes mellitus. Diabetologica 1986; 29:181–185.
31. Dawson DM, Hallett M, Millender LH. Entrapment Neuropathies, ed 2. Boston, Little, Brown, 1990.
32. de Krom MCTFM, Kester ADM, Knipschild PG, et al. Risk factors for carpal tunnel syndrome. Am J Epidemiol 1990; 132:1102–1110.

33. Dellon AL. Treatment of symptomatic diabetic neuropathy by surgical decompression of multiple peripheral nerves. Plast Reconst Surg 1992; 89:689–697.

34. Dellon AL. A cause for optimism in diabetic neuropathy. Ann Plast Surg 1988; 20:103–105.

35. Dieck GS, Kelsey JL. An epidemiologic study of carpal tunnel syndrome in an adult female population. Prev Med 1985; 14:63–69.

36. Ditmars DM, Houin HP. Carpal tunnel syndrome. Hand Clin 1986; 2:525–532.

37. Dobyns JH. Carpal tunnel release in patients with peripheral neuropathy. In Gelberman RH (ed): Operative Nerve Repair and Reconstruction. Philadelphia, JB Lippincott, 1991, pp 963–965.

38. Doyle JR, Carroll RE. The carpal tunnel syndrome. Cal Med 1968; 108:263–267.

39. Dyck PJ, Giannini C. Pathologic alterations in diabetic neuropathies of humans: A review. J Neuropathol Exp Neurol 1996; 55:1181–1193.

40. Dyck PJ, Lais AC, Giannini C, et al. Structural alterations of nerve during cuff compression. Proc Natl Acad Sci U S A 1990; 87:9828–9832.

41. Dyck PJ, Kratz KM, Karnes JL, et al. The prevalence by staged severity of various types of diabetic neuropathy, retinopathy and nephropathy in a population-based cohort: The Rochester diabetic neuropathy study. Neurology 1993; 43:817–824.

42. Dyck PJ, Karnes J, O'Brien PC. Diagnosis, staging, and classification of diabetic neuropathy and associations with other complications. In Dyck PJ, Thomas PK, Asbury AK, et al (eds): Diabetic Neuropathy. Philadelphia, WB Saunders, 1987, pp 36–44.

43. Ekerot L. Post-anesthetic ulnar neuropathy at the elbow. Scand J Plast Reconstr Surg 1977; 11:225–229.

44. Eversmann WW, Ritsick JA. Intraoperative changes in motor nerve conduction latency in carpal tunnel syndrome. J Hand Surg 1978; 3A:77–81.

45. Florack TM, Miler RJ, Pellegrini VD, et al. The prevalence of carpal tunnel syndrome in patients with basal joint arthritis of the thumb. J Hand Surg 1992; 17A:624–630.

46. Fraser DM, Campbell IW, Ewing DJ, et al. Mononeuropathy in diabetes mellitus. Diabetes 1979; 28:96–101.

47. Froimson AI, Zahrawi F. Treatment of compression neuropathy of the ulnar nerve at the elbow by epicondylectomy and neurolysis. J Hand Surg 1980; 5:391–395.

48. Fry IK, Hardwick C, Scott CW. Diabetic neuropathy: A survey and follow-up on 66 cases. Guy's Hosp Reports 1962; 111:113–129.

49. Frymoyer JW, Bland J. Carpal-tunnel syndrome in patients with myxedematous arthropathy. J Bone Joint Surg Am1973; 55A:78–82.

50. Gamstedt A, Holm-Glad J, Ohlson CG, et al. Hand abnormalities are strongly associated with the duration of diabetes mellitus. J Intern Med 1993; 234:189–193.

51. Garland H. Neurological complications of diabetes mellitus: Clinical aspects. Proc R Soc Med 1960; 53:137–146.

52. Garland H. Diabetic amyotrophy. BMJ 1955; 2:1287–1290.

53. Garland H, Taverner D. Diabetic myelopathy. BMJ 1953; 1:1405–1408.

54. Garland H, Moorhouse D. Compressive lesions of the external popliteal (common peroneal) nerve. BMJ 1952; 2:1373–1378.

55. Gilliatt RW, Willison RG. Peripheral nerve conduction in diabetic neuropathy. J Neurol Neurosurg Psychiatry 1962; 25:11–18.

56. Gilliatt RW, Sears TA. Sensory nerve action potentials in patients with peripheral nerve lesions. J Neurol Neurosurg Psychiatry 1958; 21:109–118.

57. Goldberg BJ, Light TR, Blair SJ. Ulnar neuropathy at the elbow: Results of medial epicondylectomy. J Hand Surg 1989; 1419:182–188.

58. Goodman JI. Femoral neuropathy in relationship to diabetes mellitus: Report of 17 cases. Diabetes 1954; 3:266–273.

59. Goodman JI, Baumoel S, Frankel L, et al. The Diabetic Neuropathies. Springfield, Ill., Charles C Thomas, 1953.

60. Greene DA, Pfeifer MA: Diabetic neuropathy. In Olefsky JM, Sherwin RS (eds): Diabetes Mellitus: Management and Complications. New York, Churchill-Livingstone, 1985, pp 223–254.

61. Halter JB, Porte D. The clinical syndrome of diabetes mellitus. In Dyck PJ, Thomas PK, Asbury AK, et al (eds): Diabetic Neuropathy. Philadelphia, WB Saunders, 1987, pp 3–26.

62. Harati Y. Diabetic peripheral neuropathies. Ann Intern Med 1987; 107:546–559.

63. Harmon RL. Bilaterality of ulnar neuropathy at the elbow. Electromyogr Clin Neurophysiol 1991; 31:195–198.

64. Harris W. Multiple peripheral neuritis. Proc R Soc Med (Neurology Section) 1923; 16:13–26.

65. Haupt WF, Wintzer G, Schop A, et al. Long-term results of carpal tunnel decompression: Assessment of 60 cases. J Hand Surg [Br] 1993; 18:471–474.

66. Hawley RJ. Frequency of median mononeuropathy in patients with mild diabetic neuropathy in the early diabetes intervention trial (EDIT). Muscle Nerve 1996; 19:1504–1505.

67. Hawley RJ, Capobianco J. Localizing ulnar nerve lesions by motor nerve conduction study. Electromyogr Clin Neurophysiol 1987; 27:385–392.

68. Heathfield KWG. Acroparaesthesiae and the carpal tunnel syndrome. Lancet 1957; 2:663–666.

69. Hirson C, Feinmann EL, Wade HJ. Diabetic neuropathy. BMJ 1953; 1:1408–1413.

70. Hogenhuis LAH, Rose FC. The classification of diabetic neuropathy. Neuroepidemiology 1984; 3:169–181.

71. Horowitz SH. Diabetic neuropathy. Clin Orthopedics 1993; 296:78–85.

72. Hurst LC, Weisberg D, Carroll RE. The relationship of the double crush to carpal tunnel syndrome: An analysis of 1,000 cases of carpal tunnel syndrome. J Hand Surg [Br] 1985; 10:202–204.

73. Hybbinette C-H, Mannerfelt L. The carpal tunnel syndrome: A retrospective study of 400 operated patients. Acta Orthop Scand 1975; 46:610–620.

74. Jacobs EM. Diabetic sciatic neuropathy: Report of a case. Diabetes 1958; 7:493–494.

75. Jakobsen J, Sidenius P. Decreased axonal transport of structural proteins in streptozotocin diabetic rats. J Clin Invest 1980; 66:292–297.

76. Johnson EW. Sixteenth annual AAEM Edward H Lambert lecture: Electrodiagnostic aspects of diabetic neuropathies: Entrapments. Muscle Nerve 1993; 16:127–134.

77. Jones HD. Ulnar nerve damage following general anesthesia: A case possibly related to diabetes mellitus. Anesthesia 1967; 22:471–475.

78. Jordan WR. Neuritic manifestations in diabetes mellitus. Arch Intern Med 1936; 57:307–366.

79. Joslin EP. The Treatment of Diabetes Mellitus. Philadelphia, Lea & Febiger, 1916; 333–334.

80. Joslin EP, Marble HE. Neurological and mental complications. *In* Joslin EP: The Treatment of Diabetes Mellitus, ed 4. Philadelphia, Lea & Febiger, 1928, pp 730–736.

81. Katirji MB, Wilbourn AJ. Common peroneal neuropathy: A clinical and electrophysical study of 116 cases. Neurology 1988; 38:1723–1728.

82. Kennedy WR, Resch JA. Paralytic brachial neuritis. Lancet 1966; 86:459–462.

83. Kimura J, Yamada T, Stevland NP. Distal slowing of motor nerve conduction velocity in diabetic polyneuropathy. J Neurol Sci 1979; 42:291–302.

84. Kraus WM. The clinical involvement of the peripheral nerves in diabetes mellitus. J Nerv Ment Dis 1920; 52:331–333.

85. Kremer M, Gilliatt RW, Golding JSR, et al. Acroparaesthesiae in the carpal tunnel syndrome. Lancet 1953; 2:590–595.

86. Kulick MI, Gordillo G, Javidi T, et al. Long-term analysis of patients having surgical treatment for carpal tunnel syndrome. J Hand Surg [Am] 1986; 11:59–66.

87. LaRoux PD, Ensign TD, Burchiel KJ. Surgical decompression without transposition for ulnar neuropathy: Factors determining outcome. Neurosurgery 1990; 27:709–714.

88. Lawrence DG, Locke S. Neuropathy in children with diabetes mellitus. BMJ 1963; 1:784–785.

89. Layzer RB. Neuromuscular Manifestations of Systemic Disease. Philadelphia, FA Davis, 1985, pp 117–125.

90. Leach RE, Odom JA: Systemic causes of carpal tunnel syndrome. Postgrad Med 1968, August, pp 127–131.

91. Leffert RD. Diabetes mellitus initially presenting as peripheral neuropathy in the upper limb. J Bone Joint Surg Am 1969; 51:1004–110.

92. Locke S. The nervous system and diabetes. *In* Marble A, White P, Bradley RF, et al (eds): Joslin's Diabetes Mellitus, ed 11. Philadelphia, Lea & Febiger, 1971, pp 562–580.

93. Loong SC. The carpal tunnel syndrome: A clinical and electrophysiological study in 250 patients. Clin Exp Neurol 1977; 14:51–65.

94. Lugnegard H, Juhlin L, Nilsson BY. Ulnar neuropathy at the elbow treated with decompression. Scand J Plast Reconstr Surg 1982; 16:195–200.

95. Lugnegard H, Walheim G, Wennberg A. Operative treatment of ulnar nerve neuropathy in the elbow region. Acta Orthop Scand 1977; 48:168–176.

96. Martin MM. Diabetic neuropathy: A clinical study of 150 cases. Brain 1953; 76:594–624.

97. Mayer RF. Nerve conduction studies in man. Neurology 1963; 13:1021–1030.

98. Mulder DW, Lambert EH, Bastron JA, et al. The neuropathies associated with diabetes mellitus. Neurology 1961; 11:275–284.

99. Murphy FD, Moxon GF. Diabetes mellitus and its complications: An analysis of 827 cases. Am J Med Sci 1931; 182:301–311.

100. Nakano KK. The entrapment neuropathies. Muscle Nerve 1978; 1:264–279.

101. Nathan PA, Keniston RC, Myers LD, et al. Obesity as a risk factor for slowing of sensory conduction of the median nerve in industry. J Occup Med 1992; 34:379–383.

102. Ozaki I, Baba M, Matsunaga M, et al. Deleterious effects of the carpal tunnel on nerve conduction in diabetic polyneuropathy. Electromyogr Clin Neurophysiol 1988; 28:301–306.

103. Pal B, Mangion P, Hossain MA. An assessment of glucose tolerance in patients with idiopathic carpal tunnel syndrome. Br J Rheumatol 1986; 25:412–413.

104. Palumbo PJ, Elveback LR, Whisnant JP. Neurologic complications of diabetes mellitus: Transient ischemic attack, stroke, and peripheral neuropathy. Adv Neurol 1978; 19:593–601.

105. Parker HL. Discussion of Wakefield EG: Diabetic neuritis: Presentation of a case. Staff Meet Mayo Clinic 1928; 3:256–258.

106. Perreault L, Drolet P, Farny J. Ulnar nerve palsy at the elbow after general anesthesia. Can J Anesth 1992; 39:499–503.

107. Phalen GS. The carpal tunnel syndrome: Clinical evaluation of 598 hands. Clin Orthop 1972; 83:29–40.

108. Phalen GS. Reflections on 21 years' experience with the carpal tunnel syndrome. JAMA 1970; 212:1356–1367.

109. Phalen GS. The carpal tunnel syndrome: Seventeen years experience in diagnosis and treatment of six hundred fifty-four hands. J Bone Joint Surg Am 1966; 48:211–228.

110. Root HF. The nervous system and diabetes. *In* Joslin EP, Root HF, White P, et al: The Treatment of Diabetes Mellitus, ed 10. Lea & Febiger, Philadelphia, 1959, pp 483–506.

111. Root HF, Rogers MH. Diabetic neuritis with paralysis. N Engl J Med 1930; 202:1049–1053.

112. Root HF. Rare paralyses in diabetes mellitus. Med Clin North Am 1922; 5:1433–1440.

113. Root HF, Kenny AJ. The nervous system and diabetes. *In* Joslin EP, Root HF, White P, et al (eds): The Treatment of Diabetes Mellitus, ed 9. Philadelphia, Lea & Febiger, 1952, pp 469–490.

114. Root HF, Jordan WR. The nervous system and diabetes. *In* Joslin EP (ed): The Treatment of Diabetes Mellitus, ed 5. Philadelphia, Lea & Febiger, 1935, pp 371–383.

115. Rosenbaum RB, Ochoa JL. Carpal Tunnel Syndrome and Other Disorders of the Median Nerve. Boston, Butterworth-Heinemann, 1993.

116. Rosenbloom A, Silverstein JH: Connective tissue and joint disease in diabetic mellitus. Endocrinol Metab Clin North Am 1996; 25:473–483.

117. Rundles RW. Diabetic neuropathy: General review of 125 cases. Medicine 1945; 24:111–160.

118. Said G. Diabetic neuropathy: An update. J Neurol 1996; 243:431–440.

119. Shahani B, Spalding JMK. Diabetes mellitus presenting with bilateral foot-drop. Lancet 1969; 2:930–931.

120. Sherwin RS, Tamborlane WV. Metabolic control and diabetic complications. *In* Olefsky JM, Sherwin RS (eds): Diabetic Mellitus: Management and Complications. Edinburgh, Churchill Livingstone, 1985, pp 1–24.

121. Simpson JA. The neuropathies. *In* Williams D (ed): Modern Trends in Neurology-3. London, Butterworth, 1962, pp 245–291.

122. Simpson JA. Electrical signs in the diagnosis of carpal tunnel and other related syndromes. J Neurol Neurosurg Psychiatry 1956; 19:275–280.

123. Spritz N. Nerve disease in diabetes mellitus. Med Clin North Am 1978; 62:787–798.

124. Staal A. Entrapment neuropathies. *In* Vinkin PJ, Bruyn GW (eds): Handbook of Clinical Neurology, vol 7. Diseases of Nerves, Part 1. Amsterdam, North Holland, 1970, pp 285–325.

125. Staal A. General discussion on pressure neuropathies. *In* Vinkin PJ, Bruyn GW (eds): Handbook of Clinical

Neurology, vol 7. Diseases of Nerves, Part 1. Amsterdam, North Holland, 1970, pp 276–284.

126. Stevens JC, Beard CM, O'Fallon WM, et al. Conditions associated with carpal tunnel syndrome. Mayo Clin Proc 1992; 67:541–548.

127. Stewart JD. Focal Peripheral Neuropathies, ed 2. New York, Raven Press, 1993.

128. Stoelting RK: Postoperative ulnar nerve palsy: Is it a preventable complication? Anesth Analg 1993; 76:7–9.

129. Sullivan JF. The neuropathies of diabetes. Neurology 1958; 8:243–249.

130. Tetro AM, Pichora DR. Cubital tunnel syndrome and the painful upper extremity. Hand Clin 1996; 12:665–677.

131. Thomas PK. Peripheral neuropathy. *In* Matthews WB (ed): Recent Advances in Clinical Neurology-1. Edinburgh, Churchill-Livingstone, 1975, pp 253–283.

132. Thomas PK, Tomlinson DR: Diabetic and hypoglycemic neuropathy. *In* Dyck PJ, Thomas PK, Poduslo JF (eds): Peripheral Neurology, ed 3. Philadelphia, WB Saunders, 1993, pp 1219–1250.

133. Thomas PK, Ward JD, Watkins PJ. Diabetic Neuropathy. *In* Keen H, Jarret J (eds): Complications of Diabetes, ed 2. London, Edward Arnold, 1982, pp 109–136.

134. Tsairis P, Dyck PJ, Mulder DW. Natural history of brachial plexus neuropathy. Arch Neurol 1972; 27:109–117.

135. Upton ARM, McComas AJ. The double crush in nerve-entrapment syndromes. Lancet 1973; 2:359–362.

136. Varughese G, Fourney D, Lai S, et al. Ulnar neuropathy at the elbow: A review of 198 cases treated with anterior transposition or simple decompression. Presented at Canadian Congress of Neurological Sciences 32nd annual meeting, Saskatoon, Canada, June 1997.

137. Vinik AI, Holland MT, Le Beau JM, et al. Diabetic neuropathies. Diabetes Care 1992; 15:1926–1975.

138. Wadsworth TG. The external compression syndrome of the ulnar nerve at the cubital tunnel. Clin Orthoped 1977; 124:189–204.

139. Walter-Sack I, Zollner N. Maskiertes Karpaltunnel-syndrom ber diabetischer. Polyneuropathie Dtsch Med Wochenschr 1980; 105:19–21.

140. Warner MA, Warner ME, Martin JT. Ulnar neuropathy: Incidence, outcome, and risk factors in sedated or anesthetized patients. Anesthesiology 1994; 81:1332–1340.

141. Watkins PJ. Natural history of the diabetic neuropathies. Q J Med 1990; 77:1209–1218.

142. Webber SG. Localized neuritis. Boston Med Surg J 1898; 139:439–440.

143. Wendt LFC, Peck FB. Diabetes mellitus: A review of 1073 cases, 1919–1929. Am J Med Sci 1931; 18:52–65.

144. Wilbourn AJ. Diabetic neuropathies. *In* Brown WF, Bolton CF (eds): Clinical Electromyography, ed 2. Boston, Butterworth-Heinemann, 1993, pp 477–515.

145. Wilbourn AJ. Ulnar neuropathy at the elbow: Electrodiagnostic aspects. *In* Syllabus: 1991 AAEM Course D: Focal Peripheral Neuropathies: Selected Topics. Rochester, Minn, American Association of Electrodiagnostic Medicine, 1991, pp 13–17.

146. Williams AJ. Diabetic neuralgic amyotrophy. Postgrad Med J 1981; 57:450–452.

147. Williamson RT. The symptoms due to peripheral neuritis or spinal lesions in diabetes mellitus. Rev Neurol Psych 1907; 5:550–556.

148. Winkelman AC. Peripheral neuropathy. *In* Kryston LJ, Shaw RA (eds): Endocrinology and Diabetes. New York, Grune & Stratton, 1975, pp 419–426.

149. Yamaguchi DM, Lipscomb PR, Soule EH. Carpal tunnel syndrome. Minn Med 1965; 48:22–33.

Chapter 37

Pathophysiology of Nerve Compression

Caterina Giannini • Peter James Dyck

INTRODUCTION

Nerve injury results from mechanical forces externally applied to a nerve. Penetrating wounds cause discontinuity of nerve sheaths and fibers, whereas blunt forces or steadily applied external pressure lead to nerve compression injury.[48] The time course, severity of impairment, and the outcome are strikingly different between transected and compressed nerves. After transection, nerve fiber regeneration is delayed and faulty.[12, 18, 46] With proximal limb nerve transection, virtually no regeneration to distal limb occurs.[45] Compression lesions of nerve may also cause severe paralysis and sensory loss, but the clinical impairment tends to improve often with complete or almost complete restoration of function.[48] With compression, a variable degree of "nerve fiber damage" ensues, whereas nerve sheath continuity is preserved. Experimental crush injury, an extreme example of nerve compression in which virtually all axons are transected, results in 100% myelinated and unmyelinated fiber degeneration (C Cardone and PJ Dyck, unpublished data, 1990), while nerve sheath continuity, including continuity of basement membrane surrounding single axons, is maintained.[17]

Depending on its degree and duration, acute compression may result in conduction block, which may be rapidly reversible and resolve in minutes after release of pressure; be persistent, but completely reversible in 4 to 6 weeks; or persist longer with virtually complete recovery.[48] The transitory conduction block is attributed to a degree of compression barely sufficient to obliterate the vascular supply and causing a reversible ischemic conduction block. Function of fibers is impaired, but no structural change follows. The more persistent conduction block has been attributed to "pure" segmental demyelination, and only very severe compression has been considered responsible for axonal injury, followed by axonal degeneration. This chapter will focus on degrees of compression injury sufficient to cause nerve fiber damage and analyze its pathophysiologic mechanisms. As we will demonstrate, the view of "pure" categories of nerve fiber injury after compression (as reflected in the old peripheral nerve injury classification distinguishing "neuroapraxia," "axonotmesis," and "neurotmesis"), although appealing as a scheme, represents an oversimplification.[39, 44]

ACUTE COMPRESSION AND ENTRAPMENT

Acute compression (single or repeated) and entrapment (and associated phenomena) injury are the two major categories of compression injury to peripheral nerve. Acute compression may result from the application of a tourniquet at high pressure, for too long or in an improper position around a limb, or from lying in one position without moving for a long time with a limb compressed against bone by a protruding ridge or hard surface. The force is applied to the nerve at one point in time. Entrapment results from a chronic, repeated injury to a nerve lying in a natural anatomical compartment that has become too narrow to allow the normal atraumatic motion of the nerve; for example, median nerve injury in carpal tunnel syndrome. Entrapment is too often incorrectly equated to simple nerve compression.[11]

Mechanisms involved in acute compression and entrapment are only partly similar. In both cases, sheer forces distort the nerve from the outside, but depending on the causing agent, there can be major differences in the magnitude and time course of the compression and therefore in the resulting structural nerve changes. In entrapment injury, the mechanisms involved, because of the persistence and repetition of the injury to the nerve, appear to be more complex than in acute compression and are largely unresolved. In acute compression, increased pressure on the nerve trunk seems to be primarily involved in nerve damage. In entrapment—although repeated degrees of nerve compression, especially during unusual joint activity or position, might contribute to nerve damage—other mechanisms, such as stretching and tethering of the nerve and ischemia, are likely to be involved; their relative contribution, which might be quite variable, remains to be determined.

PATHOPHYSIOLOGY OF NERVE COMPRESSION

Acute compression is a simplified model to study nerve compression. Local compression to a nerve is known to cause nerve fiber damage. Very severe compression may actually result in crush or transection of some or many of the nerve fibers and lead to wallerian degeneration.[11] Recovery of fiber function for fibers that have undergone wallerian degeneration is through fiber regeneration. Minor or intermediate degrees of compression may result in a temporary conduction block in the fibers that is either reversed as soon as the pressure is released or might take a few weeks to recover. When it takes weeks to recover, it is usually attributed to focal fiber demyelination and remyelination and perhaps some fiber regeneration.[48]

In reality, compression of a whole nerve trunk results in a variable combination of injuries to single nerve fibers with coexistence of demyelinating and degenerating fibers in variable proportion. When the majority of the nerve fibers have actually been transected in a nerve trunk, nerve excitability distal to the lesion is lost after some time, signs of denervation develop in the nerve territory, and recovery through nerve regeneration might take months and be incomplete. When the proportion of fibers undergoing wallerian degeneration is minor and most fibers show focal demyelination, early and excellent recovery is expected.

Ischemic Hypothesis

The mechanisms underlying nerve compression injury have usually been attributed to ischemia, mechanical forces, or both. Among the first authors to address the issue of the structural changes of nerve in compression were Denny-Brown and Brenner.[8, 9] In their original studies, these authors analyzed the electrophysiologic and histologic changes induced by direct pressure, either through a mercury bag or a spring clip, and by tourniquet application to the sciatic nerve of cats.[8, 9] Their histologic studies were limited to the use of paraffin sections stained with methods for myelin (osmic acid) and for axons (Gros-Bielschowsky). With these relatively "crude" techniques, they were able to identify changes, primarily "traceable" to the segments of nerve directly compressed and especially at the edges of the compressed segment, as early as 24 to 48 hours after nerve compression. No changes were recognized in any instance at earlier times (as early as 2 hours) after compression. With intermediate degrees of compression, the changes consisted mainly of vacuolation of myelin (at 48 hours), followed by dissolution of myelin and enlargement of nodal gap (paranodal demyelination, at 7 days) that evolved to segmental demyelination and became widespread with time (2 weeks). By day 19, most of the fibers that had lost their myelin sheath appeared to have started remyelinating. The time course of the histologic changes seemed to parallel the time course of evolution and recovery of the conduction block. No appreciable degree of axonal degeneration was noted in most of the cases. At low levels of pressure, fibers of large diameter appeared to be primarily affected, but, with higher degrees of compression, most of the smaller diameter fibers also showed similar histologic changes. The authors attributed these changes to ischemia, because (1) nerve function was known to be dependent on blood supply and perfusion was impaired during compression; (2) excitability or conductivity of the nerve fibers did not change when the nerve was exposed in vitro to high pressures, but in oxygenated chambers, in a condition in which shear forces were eliminated; (3) mechanical distortion of fibers, as caused by stretching, was considered among the possible mechanisms, but discarded, because examination failed to demonstrate any "immediate" change after compression, even after extreme pressures and complete failure of conduction. Nerves in these studies were examined as early as 2 hours after compression.

As we describe in the next section, it now seems unlikely that acute compression produces its structural effects from ischemia; instead, these changes are induced through shear forces, particularly at the edges of the cuff. Direct compression injury explains large-fiber vulnerability better than does ischemia. More recent work does not confirm the view that loss of myelin, with the pattern and time course observed in nerve compression, is a characteristic of ischemic lesions.[21, 22, 32] Experimental models of ischemia produce structural alterations that have a different time course, distribution, and type of fiber changes than those described by Denny-Brown and Brenner.[8, 9] The earliest morphologic alterations that follow microsphere injection develop at 12 hours and progress up to 48 hours. The changes predominate in the centrofascicular areas and consist of dark axons, dark axons with light cores, attenuated axons, demyelinated axons, and vacuolated axons.[33] The three-dimensional arrangements of the abnormalities along the length of a single myelinated fiber entering the ischemic core were subsequently described.[33]

Mechanical Hypothesis

An alternative hypothesis—that mechanical forces were responsible for the structural alterations after compression—was proposed by Ochoa and colleagues.[34, 35] These authors examined the ultrastructural changes in single teased nerve fibers of peroneal nerve of baboon after different degrees of nerve compression (sufficient to cause either persistent conduction delay or conduction block), applied by a pneumatic tourniquet. They found that the main direct pathologic change resulting from the application of a tourniquet was in the area of application and consisted of displacement of the node from its original location and intussusception of myelin into the adjacent paranode, in opposite directions at either end of the cuff. These changes followed compression in minutes (minutes being the earliest time point examined after compression) and persisted. The concentration of the changes at the edges of the cuff was explained by the pressure gradient in the tissue between the parts under the cuff and those beyond the cuff. At a later time (1 to 2 weeks after release of pressure), the resultant redundant loops of myelin overlying the nodes of Ranvier would degenerate and cause paranodal demyelination, ultimately followed by remyelination and formation of intercalated internodes. These changes could not be explained by ischemia. The authors emphasized that even with long periods of application of a tourniquet (up to 3 hours) that caused the nerve to be locally compressed and the limb to be ischemic distal to the tourniquet at the same time, they were unable to produce changes in the distal segment of the nerve. Subsequently, Williams and associates showed that making the leg ischemic before and during a moderate nerve compression did not produce a more severe conduction block or pathologic abnormalities than when the nerve was compressed without having made the leg ischemic.[50] This made it unlikely that ischemia could be responsible for the structural changes observed, although it did not exclude that at high-pressure levels ischemia could still contribute to nerve fiber damage. These authors also noted that there was selective vulnerability of large-diameter fiber to compression, which has been explained in terms of Laplace's law.[43] This states that the tension in the wall of a cylinder is proportional to the difference between internal and external pressure and to the radius of the cylinder ($T = \Delta P \ast R$) and is therefore higher in large diameter fibers compared to small and intermediate fibers.

STRUCTURAL CHANGES DURING ACUTE COMPRESSION

We restudied the structural alterations of nerve during compression by using an experimental model in which the peroneal nerve of rats was compressed using an inflated cuff, 8 mm wide, at different pressures for different times. The structural alterations were stopped by simultaneous perfusion and in situ fixation.[13] In our studies, we confirmed the conception by Ochoa and colleagues that the structural alterations during nerve compression mainly result from mechanical forces, but we found more complex changes taking place simultaneously in the

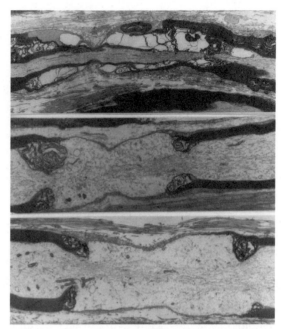

■ **Figure 37.2** Electron micrographs of obscured node (*top;* ×2000) and lengthened nodes (*middle* (×3000) and *bottom* (×3600)) from peroneal nerve of rat compressed at 300 mm Hg for 4 minutes. The obscured node came from peroneal nerve near the edge of the cuff; the lengthened node also came from near the edge of the cuff.

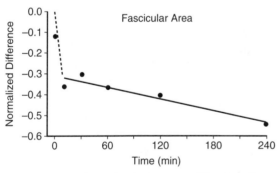

■ **Figure 37.1** Mean fascicular areas (FA) of sections of tissue blocks of peroneal nerve under the cuff expressed as a difference from 1 (the average of the FA of all tissue blocks of the nerve) was calculated for nerves compressed at 150 mm Hg for various times as shown. For the nerve marked 0 time, the compression and the in situ and perfusion fixation began at 0 time, but the structural alterations were actually stopped somewhat later. The point is plotted as if it occurred at 0 time. The change in FA probably has two phases: an initial rapid one and a later slow one. Similar but opposite effects (not shown) were demonstrated for the number of myelinated fibers per mm².

axon and myelin that can explain the further evolution of compression injury.[34, 35]

We observed a series of pressure- and time-related changes that differentially involved the segments under the cuff and at its edges. The first change observed under the cuff is represented by a decrease in fascicular area accompanied by an increase in fiber density. We interpreted this as resulting from expression of endoneurial fluid (Fig. 37.1). Compression of axoplasm with close packing of cytoskeletal elements and organelles, and expression of fluid and/or axoplasm in the adjacent segments, in some fibers to the point of fiber transection, required more pressure and/or time. Under the cuff, internodes also appeared to be lengthened, and nodes of Ranvier appeared to be obscured. At the ultrastructural level, obscured nodes were explained by excessive cleavage of myelin and overlapping of nodes by redundant myelin loops (Fig. 37.2). These changes might in part correspond to the changes described as "intussuscepted" nodes by Ochoa and colleagues,[34, 35] for which we have proposed a somewhat different explanation from that of displacement of node away from the site of compression. At the edges of the cuff, we found an increase in fascicular area, resulting probably from the expression of endoneurial fluid. The main ultrastructural change involving the nodes at this site was represented by "lengthening" of nodes of Ranvier (see Fig 37.2). Lengthened nodes were more frequent and more severe (with gaps of 20 to 50 μm) with increased pressure and/or duration of cuff application. The paranodal myelin was frequently displaced in both directions from the original nodal site, even though the identification of the original nodal site with certainty was often difficult. The axon caliber was enlarged and had a watery appearance, especially in the subplasmalemmal area. We interpreted the lengthening as caused by the displacement of axonal fluid and contents from under the cuff to the adjacent segments, accompanied by detachment of myelin and retraction in both directions from the nodal site. Lengthening of nodes thus corresponded to paranodal demyelination and occurred during compression of a few minutes, frequently at the edges of the cuff, and did not necessarily follow degeneration of redundant loops of myelin.

We also examined by teased fiber preparation the frequency of fiber abnormalities at 1 to 2 weeks after compression both proximally and distally to the compression site. We found that demyelination and axonal degeneration occurred at all pressures and times studied. Demyelination and remyelination were confined to the region of nerve, where the cuff was originally applied. Axonal degeneration was present both at the level of the cuff and distally. The frequency of pathologic abnormalities was in all cases higher under the cuff than distally.

PATHOPHYSIOLOGY OF ENTRAPMENT

Entrapment of a peripheral nerve results from the nerve passing in its course through an anatomical compartment that has become tight.[42] Carpal tunnel syndrome (CTS) or median neuropathy at the wrist (MNW) is the most typical example of this lesion. Although commonly referred to as chronic compression neuropathy, mechanisms involved in entrapment are complex and not fully understood.[3, 24] Pathologic alterations of the ligaments surrounding nerves, such as alterations of the amount and flexibility of the connective tissue, might be a basis for increased pressure on the underlying nerve trunk.[15, 20, 25] A chronic increase in compartmental pressure is observed in CTS, in ad-

dition to repeated nerve injury resulting from restricted gliding of the nerve trunk between tissues in the space.[23, 26, 30, 40] For example, it is calculated that the median nerve at the wrist in normal conditions moves up to 9.6 mm between full flexion and extension of this joint.[26]

Lundborg and Dahlin discuss the complexity of the basic pathophysiology of nerve compression injury and emphasize how in compression a chain of events may set up a vicious cycle that results in nerve injury.[24] Increased pressure on the nerve trunk may deform it and generate a pressure gradient, which tends to redistribute components of compressed tissues toward noncompressed areas with stretching of epineurial and vascular structures (see previous section on acute compression). Edema forms rapidly, mainly in the epineurium, resulting in nerve swelling and increasing the relative discrepancy between the anatomical compartment and its content. Restriction of the normal nerve gliding during movement of the extremities, resulting from narrowing of the anatomical canals or extraneural and intraneural fibrosis, may also result in "nerve irritation," increased pressure on the nerve trunk, and increased nerve edema and swelling. Rapidly, a vicious cycle may be initiated, leading to nerve fiber damage. As described previously, the results of focally increased pressure on nerve fibers depend on duration and amount of pressure.

STRUCTURAL CHANGES OF ENTRAPMENT

Studies of entrapment neuropathies in humans have shown that at the time of surgery or autopsy the nerves appear narrowed at the site of compression, whereas the proximal and to a lesser extent the distal nerve segments are enlarged.[1, 15, 25, 47] In these enlarged segments the endoneurium appears expanded, and nerve fibers are decreased in size and show segmental demyelination and remyelination in the compressed segments.[31, 47] MacKinnon and coworkers, in a series of studies examining the histologic findings in nerves at different sites of entrapment, including superficial radial, ulnar, and tibial nerves, described common progressive changes.[27, 28, 29] Thickening of perineurial and endoneurial microvessels with basement membrane reduplication occurs early, followed by formation of Renaut's bodies, perineurial and epineurial fibrosis, and patchy fiber loss with "thinning" of myelin, probably related to fiber remyelination and regeneration. The increase in number of Renaut's bodies at sites where entrapment is common has been observed at autopsy[19] and can also be induced experimentally.[36] Although Renaut's bodies are frequently described as nerve "cushions" at sites of compression, the mechanism of their formation and their role remain unclear.

Somewhat similar findings have been reported in Morton's neuroma, a lesion developing in a plantar digital nerve, usually in proximity of the bifurcation of the interdigital nerve and likely related to repeated compression injury.[48]

DOUBLE CRUSH SYNDROME

Upton and McComas in 1973 proposed that proximal compression in a nerve trunk may lead to increased vulnerability to compression in the distal segments, a hypothesis widely popularized under the name of "double crush syndrome."[49] This phenomenon was thought to occur more frequently in the upper limbs, where cervical radiculopathy may predispose to development of peripheral nerve compression syndrome. The disturbance of axonal transport, fast and slow components, induced by nerve compression was considered responsible for this phenomenon.[4-6] Interference with axonal transport of both axonal membranes and cytoskeletal elements could result in a "shortage of supplies" to the nerve trunk distally to a site of compression and make the nerve more susceptible to the development of injury from a second site of compression. As an extension of the previous hypothesis, motivated by an impairment of retrograde transport, a "reverse double crush syndrome," resulting in increased susceptibility to proximal compression in a distally compressed nerve, was later thought to occur.[24]

Upton and McComas intended the concept underlying the double crush hypothesis in a broader sense than the one implied by serial sites of compression and suggested that the preexistence of a peripheral neuropathy such as diabetic polyneuropathy could represent a predisposing "conditioning" lesion, a hypothesis largely undemonstrated. Regarding diabetic polyneuropathy, as discussed in the next section, axons do not appear to be more susceptible to compression-induced damage.[10]

NERVE ENTRAPMENT AND DIABETES

It is commonly thought that peripheral nerves at common sites of external pressure, such as the median and ulnar nerves in the carpal and cubital tunnels, the radial nerve in the upper arm, and the peroneal nerve at the fibular head, are more susceptible to compression in subjects with diabetes mellitus, resulting in increased frequency of entrapment neuropathies. In a study of CTS and its associated conditions, diabetes mellitus appears to confer a risk 2.3 times greater than the general population.[41] Similarly, prevalence of CTS was found to be 26.7% and 15% in a population of patients with types 1 and 2 diabetes (n=60, each group) compared to their control population with 3.3% and 5% ($P<0.01$, $P=$nonsignificant).[37] In the Rochester Diabetic Neuropathy Study, the prevalence of symptomatic CTS was low (5% in type 1 and 6% in type 2 diabetes), but a subclinical degree of involvement occurred in approximately one quarter of the diabetic patient population. The frequency of abnormal electrophysiologic findings was significantly higher than in nondiabetic controls from the same patient's population ($P<0.001$).[14] Reasons for this increased susceptibility to entrapment neuropathy remain largely unknown. Nerve fibers per se do not appear to be more vulnerable to compression injury. On the contrary, experimental studies demonstrate a degree of resistance of fibers to axonal degeneration induced by acute compression in streptozotocin-induced diabetic rats compared to controls.[10] Alterations in connective tissue, resulting in changes in the extracellular matrix of vessels, nerve sheaths, and interstitial tissue involving skeleton, joint, and periarticular tissue are thought to contribute to this increased vulnerability.[38] Advanced glycation end products, resulting from nonenzymatic reaction of glucose with proteins, may cause progressive stiffening of connective tissues and might be a basis for increased frequency of entrapment neuropathies.[2]

References

1. Brain WR, Wright A, Dickson A, et al. Spontaneous compression of both median nerves in the carpal tunnel: Six cases treated surgically. Lancet 1947; 1:277.
2. Brownlee M, Cerami A, Vlassara H. Advanced glycosylation end products in tissue and the biochemical basis of diabetic complications. N Engl J Med 1988; 318:1315–1321.
3. Dahlin LB, Danielson N, Ehira T, et al. Mechanical effects of compression of peripheral nerves. J Biomed Eng 1986; 108:120.
4. Dahlin LB, McLean WG. Effects of graded compression on slow and fast axonal transport in rabbit vagus nerve. J Neurol Sci 1986; 82:19.
5. Dahlin LB, Meiri KF, McLean WG, et al. Effects of nerve compression on fast axonal transport in streptozotocin-induced diabetes mellitus. Diabetologia 1986; 29:181.

6. Dahlin LB, Rydevik B, McLean WG, et al. Changes in fast axonal transport during experimental nerve compression at low pressures. Exp Neurol 1984; 84:29.

7. Danta G, Fowler TJ, Gilliatt RW. Conduction block after a pneumatic tourniquet. J Physiol (Lond) 1971; 215:50.

8. Denny-Brown D, Brenner C. Paralysis of nerve induced by direct pressure and by tourniquet. Arch Neurol Psychiatry 1944; 51:1.

9. Denny-Brown D, Brenner C. Lesion in peripheral nerve resulting from compression by spring clip. Arch Neurol Psychiatry 1944; 52:1.

10. Dyck PJ, Engelstad JK, Giannini C, et al. Resistance to axonal degeneration after nerve compression in experimental diabetes. Proc Natl Acad Sci USA 1989; 86:2103.

11. Dyck PJ, Giannini C, Lais AC. Pathologic alterations of nerves. In Dyck PJ, Thomas PK, Griffin JW, et al (eds): Peripheral Neuropathy, ed 3. Philadelphia, WB Saunders, 1993, pp 514–595.

12. Dyck PJ, Lambert EH, Wood MB, et al. Assessment of nerve regeneration and adaptation after median nerve reconnection and digital neurovascular flap transfer. Neurology 1988; 38:1586.

13. Dyck PJ, Giannini C, Lais AC, et al. Structural alterations of nerve during cuff compression. Proc Natl Acad Sci USA 1990; 87:9828.

14. Dyck PJ, Kratz KM, Karnes JL, et al. The prevalence by staged severity of various types of diabetic neuropathy, retinopathy and nephropathy in a population-based cohort: The Rochester Diabetic Neuropathy Study. Neurology 1993; 43:817–824.

15. Feindel W, Stratford J. The role of the cubital tunnel in tardy ulnar palsy. Can J Surg 1958; 1:287.

16. Grundfest H. Effects of hydrostatic pressures upon the excitability, the recovery and the potential sequence of frog nerve. Cold Spring Harb Symp Quant Biol 1936; 4:179.

17. Haftek J, Thomas PK. Electron-microscope observations on the effects of localized crush injuries on the connective tissues of peripheral nerve. J Anat 1968; 103:233.

18. Hawkins GL. Faulty sensory localization in nerve regeneration: An index of functional recovery following suture. J Neurosurg 1948; 5:11.

19. Jefferson D, Neary D, Eames RA. Renaut body distribution at sites of human peripheral nerve entrapment. J Neurol Sci 1981; 49:19.

20. Kerwin G, Williams CS, Seiler JG. The pathophysiology of carpal tunnel syndrome. Hand Clin 1996; 12:243.

21. Korthals JK, Korthals WA, Wisniewski H.M. Peripheral nerve ischemia. Part 2. Accumulation of organelles. Ann Neurol 1978; 4:487.

22. Korthals JK, Wisniewski HM. Peripheral nerve ischemia. Part 1. Experimental model. J Neurol Sci 1975; 24:65.

23. Luchetti R, Schoenhuber R, Alfarano M, et al. Carpal tunnel syndrome: Correlations between pressure measurement and intraoperative electrophysiological nerve study. Muscle Nerve 1990; 13:1164.

24. Lundborg G, Dahlin LB. Anatomy, function and pathophysiology of peripheral nerves and nerve compression. Hand Clin 1996; 12:185.

25. Marie P, Foix C. Atrophie isolee de l'eminence thenar d'origine neuritique, role du ligament annulaire anterieur du carpe dans la pathogenie de la lesion. Rev Neurol (Paris) 1913; 2:647.

26. Millesi H, Zöch G, Rath T. The gliding apparatus of peripheral nerves and its clinical significance. Ann Hand Surg 1990; 9:87.

27. MacKinnon SE, Dellon AL, Daneshvar A. Histopathology of the tarsal tunnel syndrome: Examination of a human tibial nerve. Contemp Orthopaed 1984; 9:43.

28. MacKinnon SE, Dellon AL, Hudson AR, et al. Chronic nerve compression: An experimental model in the rat. Ann Plast Surg 1984; 13:112.

29. MacKinnon SE, Dellon AL, Hudson AR, et al. Chronic human nerve compression: A histological assessment. Neuropathol Appl Neurobiol 1986; 12:547.

30. Nakamichi K, Tachibana S. Restricted motion of the median nerve in carpal tunnel syndrome. J Hand Surg 1995; 20:460.

31. Neary D, Eames RA. The pathology of ulnar compression in man. Neuropathol Appl Neurobiol 1975; 1:69.

32. Nukada H, Dyck PJ. Microsphere embolization of nerve capillaries and fiber degeneration. Am J Pathol 1984; 115:275.

33. Nukada H, Dyck PJ. Acute ischemia causes axonal stasis, swelling, attenuation, and secondary demyelination. Ann Neurol 1987; 22:311.

34. Ochoa J, Danta G, Fowler TJ, et al. Nature of the nerve lesion caused by a pneumatic tourniquet. Nature 1971; 233:265.

35. Ochoa J, Fowler TJ, Gilliatt RW. Anatomical changes in peripheral nerves compressed by a pneumatic tourniquet. J Anat 1972; 113:433.

36. Ortman JA, Sahenk Z, Mendell JR. The experimental production of Renaut bodies. J Neurol 1983; 62:233.

37. Renard E, Jacques D, Chamma M, et al. Increased prevalence of soft tissue hand lesions in type 1 and type 2 diabetes mellitus: Various entities and associated significance. Diabete Metab 1994; 20:513.

38. Rosenbloom AL, Silverstein JH. Connective tissue and joint disease in diabetes mellitus. Endocrinol Metab Clin North Am 1996; 25:473.

39. Seddon HJ. Three types of nerve injury. Brain 1943; 66:237.

40. Seradge H, Jia YC, Owens W. In vivo measurement of carpal tunnel pressure in the functioning hand. J Hand Surg 1995; 20:855.

41. Stevens JC, Beard CM, O'Fallon WM, et al. Conditions associated with carpal tunnel. Mayo Clin Proc 1992; 67:541.

42. Stewart JD, Aguayo AJ. Compression and entrapment neuropathies. In Dyck PJ, Thomas PK, Lambert EH, et al (eds): Peripheral Neuropathy. Philadelphia, WB Saunders, 1984, p 1435.

43. Strain RE, Olson WH. Selective damage of large diameter peripheral nerve fibers by compression: An application of Laplace's law. Exp Neurol 1975; 47:68.

44. Sunderland S. A classification of peripheral nerve injuries producing loss of function. Brain 1951; 74:491.

45. Sunderland S. Nerves and nerve injuries, ed 2. Edinburgh, E&S Livingstone, 1978.

46. Thomas CK, Stein RB, Gordon T, et al. Patterns of reinnervation and motor unit recruitment in human hand muscles after complete ulnar and median nerve section and resuture. J Neurol Neurosurg Psychiatry 1987; 50:259.

47. Thomas PK, Fullerton PM. Nerve fiber size in the carpal tunnel syndrome. J Neurol Neurosurg Psychiatry 1963; 26:520.

48. Thomas PK, Holdorff B. Neuropathy due to physical agents. In Dyck PJ, Thomas PK, Griffin JW, et al (eds): Peripheral Neuropathy. Philadelphia, WB Saunders, 1993, p 990.

49. Upton ARM, McComas AJ. The double crush hypothesis in nerve entrapment syndromes. Lancet 1973; 2:359.

50. Williams IR, Jefferson D, Gilliatt RW. Acute nerve compression during limb ischemia: An experimental study. J Neurol Sci 1980; 46:199.

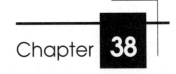

Chapter **38**

Treatment of Diabetic Gastroparesis and Diarrhea

Allison Malcolm • Michael Camilleri

The mainstays of treatment of diabetic gastroparesis are restoration of hydration and nutrition, correction of hyperglycemia, use of prokinetics (e.g., intravenous erythromycin, oral cisapride) to facilitate gastric emptying, and antiemetics (e.g., phenothiazines) for symptom relief. Rarely patients require enteral or parenteral nutrition to restore nutrition effectively.

In patients with chronic diarrhea associated with diabetes, a careful history and focused investigations are essential to identify the causes; osmotic agents in the diet, incontinence due to anal sphincter dysfunction or rectal sensory deficit, and rapid transit are common; bacterial overgrowth appears less frequent on formal testing and should be suspected if there are features of malabsorption. Treatment may include antibiotics, biofeedback and anal sphincter retraining, opioids, clonidine, or specific remedies for rare associated diseases such as celiac sprue.

INTRODUCTION

Fluid and electrolyte imbalance, poor oral intake, and poor nutrient absorption occur in the diabetic patient with significant nausea, vomiting, or diarrhea. Maintenance of adequate hydration, metabolic control, and nutrition are important features of the management of such patients. The Diabetes Control and Complica-

517

tions Trial (DCCT) has demonstrated that tight chronic glycemic control is important in delaying the onset and reducing the progression of diabetic complications such as diabetic neuropathy.[21] Moreover, because acute hyperglycemia alters gastrointestinal function (see Chapter 15), attempts to avoid acute hyperglycemia may improve gastrointestinal symptoms.

DIABETIC GASTROPARESIS

Strategies to manage diabetic gastroparesis differ in the acute and chronic settings. Management involves the use of antiemetics; prokinetic agents; dietary measures to facilitate gastric emptying; nutritional support, including enteral or parenteral nutrition; and rarely surgery. Traditionally, the treatment of diabetic gastroparesis has been focused on treating the motor disorder. However, given the poor correlation between gastric emptying and symptoms and recent evidence that gastric sensation may be enhanced in diabetics with autonomic neuropathy,[59] there has been new interest in other forms of treatment, such as drugs acting on the sensory pathway.

Acute Gastroparesis

Patients with severe symptoms may require hospitalization, no food by mouth, and nasogastric suction. Intravenous fluids should be provided, and metabolic derangements (electrolyte imbalance, uremia, hypoglycemia, or hyperglycemia) should be corrected. Endoscopy may be performed, and if bezoars are present, they may be mechanically disrupted. However, this has rarely been required since the introduction of intravenous erythromycin for acute gastric stasis (see section on erythromycin). Gastric decompression or gastric lavage may be required to drain residual nondigestible particles, especially if acute gastric dilatation is present. An example of acute gastric dilatation is demonstrated in Figure 38.1.

The prokinetic agent of choice in acute gastroparesis with or without bezoar formation is intravenous erythromycin at a dose of 3 mg/kg body weight every 8 hours. This is effective in clearing residue because it induces "dumping" from the stomach by causing highly propulsive gastric contractions.[53] This may be followed with 250 to 500 mg of erythromycin orally 4 times daily once the patient starts to tolerate food.

During the patient's recovery, feeding should initially consist of liquid meals, and

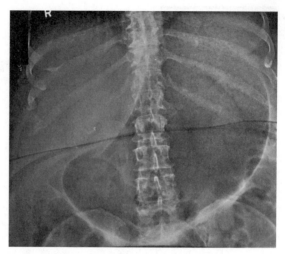

■ **Figure 38.1** Abdominal radiograph of acute gastric dilatation in a diabetic patient.

when these are tolerated, homogenized solids may be added. Frequent monitoring of blood glucose levels and multiple dosing of short-acting insulin are essential during this phase. If there is a poor response to treatment, the stomach may be bypassed with an endoscopically or laparoscopically placed jejunal feeding tube. This may not be appropriate if there is concomitant small bowel dysmotility. Perseverance with conservative measures such as liquidized meals is often rewarded, with resumption of sufficiently rapid gastric emptying to sustain adequate hydration and nutrition. Parenteral nutrition may be required in more severe cases associated with malnutrition. The management of diabetic patients with gastroparesis is outlined in Figure 38.2.

Chronic Gastroparesis

There is a wide range of options for the management of diabetic gastroparesis, although none is ideal (Table 38.1).

DIETARY MEASURES AND NUTRITIONAL SUPPORT

Often a patient may benefit from nonpharmacologic approaches designed to compensate for the motor defect in the stomach. The principles of dietary modification in patients with diabetic gastroparesis include reduction in the size of each meal, reduction of fat and nondigestible fiber-containing foods, and adequate nutritional support with supplemental vitamins and homogenized or liquid meals if required. The

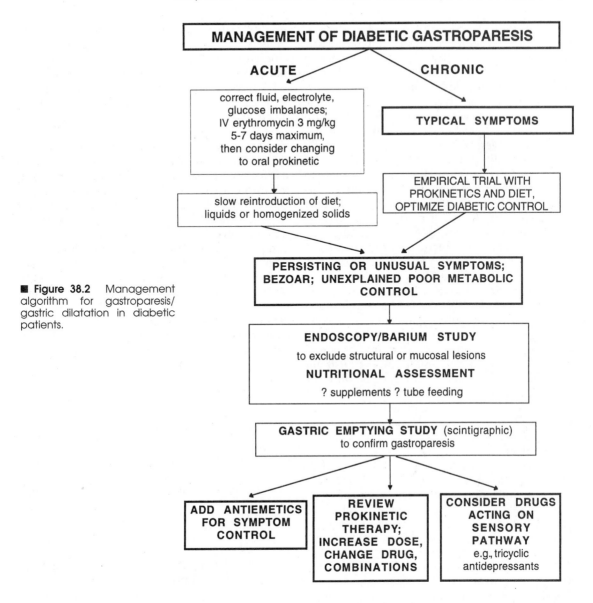

■ **Figure 38.2** Management algorithm for gastroparesis/gastric dilatation in diabetic patients.

rationale for these dietary manipulations include the known deceleration of gastric emptying by fats and high-calorie meals; the need for gastric migrating motor complexes to empty food products that are not susceptible to acid-

peptic digestion or the trituration functions of the distal stomach; and the frequent ability of the gastroparetic stomach to empty liquids and homogenized solids despite the retention and prolonged delay in emptying of larger solid particles.

These recommendations tend to be based on theoretical considerations rather than on clinical trials. However, in one recent study by Hsu and associates[37] eight patients with gastroparesis received either low-fat, normal-fiber diets or normal-fat, low-fiber diets in a randomized order. A normal-fat, low-fiber diet was more effective in alleviating symptoms, suggesting that dietary fiber is more important than fat restriction in controlling symptoms in this

TABLE 38.1 APPROACHES TO THE TREATMENT OF GASTROPARESIS

Dietary manipulation
Optimal glycemic control
Prokinetics and antiemetics
Nutritional support, tube feeding
Surgery and pancreatic transplantation
Agents aimed at treating sensory dysfunction: tricyclic
    antidepressants, fedotozine, serotonin agonists

group of patients. Some early studies showed that a diet that is high in fiber improved diabetic metabolic control or reduced insulin requirements,[4, 64] and therefore high dietary fiber was recommended. More recent data indicate that this may not be the case because metabolic control was not improved with high nondigestible fiber intake, and the issue remains controversial.[10, 47]

Exceptionally, when symptoms are severe and when the motility disorder is limited to the stomach, postpyloric delivery of liquid nutrients may be successful in maintaining nutritional support. A recent study of 26 patients with diabetic gastroparesis showed that jejunostomy tube placement improved overall health, reduced hospital admissions, and improved nausea and vomiting.[30] During follow-up, half of the patients were able to resume full oral intake and have the jejunostomy tube removed. Patients with significant gastric dysmotility may be selected for enteral feeding when the amplitude and patterns of small bowel contractions and small bowel transit are normal. A trial of nasoenteric tube feeding for 48 to 72 hours is wise to ensure that the small bowel can handle an adequate infusion rate, such as 60 mL/hour of iso-osmolar formula. Subsequently, more permanent access to the small bowel may be obtained by advancing an enteric feeding tube through a percutaneously placed gastrostomy[52, 66] or by a surgically placed jejunostomy tube. The surgical tube may be placed during laparoscopy, which is advantageous over the endoscopic placement because it permits examination of the abdominal cavity to exclude mechanical obstruction and to obtain a full-thickness bowel biopsy for diagnostic purposes.[3] This approach is preferred for patients requiring long-term enteral nutrition because it is seldom possible to keep an enteral tube placed via a gastrostomy beyond the angle of Treitz for any significant length of time. Today, most centers advocate the use of a double-lumen feeding tube to allow for suction to prevent reflux or to allow decompression.[8]

The main principle in the choice of formulas for enteric feeding is to use iso-osmolar, nonelemental liquid supplement. High-nitrogen or peptide supplements are not used because they confer no therapeutic advantage, even in the critically ill, hypoalbuminemic patient.[45] Likewise, hydrolysate-based formula has no better side effect profile than that of formula containing intact protein.[64]

Dietary deficiencies of essential vitamins and minerals are frequent in patients with gastroparesis.[48] Diabetic patients who should be considered for total parenteral nutrition include patients with small bowel dysmotility or those who have failed attempts at enteral nutrition at infusion rates required to sustain their fluid, electrolyte, and nutritional requirements. Total parenteral supplementation restores the normal nutritional state in patients with malnutrition.[73] Although there are no documented clinical follow-up studies, this approach may help symptom relief because it avoids the use of the gastrointestinal tract. There is significant morbidity associated with total parenteral nutrition, however, including line sepsis, immune complex glomerulonephritis, biochemical imbalance, liver dysfunction, venous thrombosis, and problems with venous access. These problems are of even greater concern in a diabetic patient who is prone to sepsis, renal failure, electrolyte imbalance, and vascular disease. In cases of coexistent malnutrition, bacterial overgrowth should also be sought and treated.[68]

PROKINETIC DRUGS AND OTHER MEDICATIONS

Table 38.2 outlines the prokinetic drugs used in the treatment of diabetic gastroparesis. The results of subjective and objective effectiveness in several medium- and long-term studies of prokinetic agents in patients with diabetic upper gut stasis were recently reviewed in depth.[12]

Cisapride

Mechanism of Action. Cisapride is a synthetic substituted piperidinyl benzamide[74] with a half-life of 7 to 10 hours. The mechanism of action involves activation of serotonin type 4 receptors on cholinergic neurons, inducing acetylcholine release that in turn stimulates smooth muscle receptors to produce contraction. At therapeutic drug levels, cisapride is devoid of the antidopaminergic side effects that limit the use of metoclopramide (anxiety, dyskinesia, galactorrhea) and of the extraintestinal cholinomimetic actions (excess sweating, bladder instability) that limit the use of bethanechol.[74] Because pretreatment with atropine does not block all the excitatory effects of cisapride, it is thought that there are other mechanisms of action, still to be elucidated.[74]

Use, Dosage, and Side Effects. Several studies have shown the benefit of cisapride in the

TABLE 38.2 PROKINETIC AGENTS FOR DIABETIC GASTROPARESIS

Drug	Mechanism of Action	Dose	Acutely	Chronically
Cisapride	Serotonin agonist stimulates Ach release	5–20 mg 4 times daily, orally	+	+
Erythromycin	Motilin agonist	50–500 mg 4 times daily, orally *or* 3 mg/kg IV	+	–
Metoclopramide	Dopamine antagonist; serotonin agonist	5–20 mg 4 times daily orally, IM, IV, SC	+	+ (side effects)
Domperidone	Dopamine antagonist (peripheral)	5–20 mg 4 times daily orally	+	+

Ach, acetylcholine; IV, intravenous; IM, intramuscular; SC, subcutaneous.

treatment of gastroparesis. Acutely administered cisapride enhances gastric emptying in patients with gastric stasis and has proved effective in the treatment of symptoms of diabetic gastroparesis when administered at a dose of 10 mg 4 times daily for 4 weeks.[36] Other studies have shown improvement of gastric emptying in medium-term trials, but the symptomatic benefit is inconsistent, with only minor trends toward improvement of some symptoms but no improvement in assessment of patient symptoms.[15, 56] Cisapride's long-term efficacy has been demonstrated in open trials with improvement in total symptom score,[1, 2, 38] quality of life,[1] weight gain,[2] objective improvement in electrogastrogram,[57] and improvement in gastric emptying.[2] These findings were not consistent across studies; therefore, the use of long-term cisapride is still somewhat controversial. Its safety profile makes it currently the drug of first choice.

The typical dose of cisapride is 10 to 20 mg 3 times per day, half hour before meals and at bedtime. At this dose, the drug is generally well tolerated. The most common adverse effects reported include transient abdominal cramping, borborygmi, increased stool frequency, and headache. In a Mayo Clinic study, the drug significantly reduced symptoms in about 65% of patients, and there was no evidence of tolerance during 1 year of continuous treatment.[14] Drugs that inhibit the metabolism of cisapride (azole antifungals such as ketoconazole and macrolide antibiotics including erythromycin) may produce cardiac arrhythmias (torsades de pointes, ventricular arrhythmias) in susceptible persons; therefore, these drugs should not be used in combination.

Cisapride is available in tablet and suspension preparation (1 mg/mL), the latter being suitable for use via a gastrostomy or jejunostomy tube or in pediatric patients. It is also very useful in adults in whom the dose needs to be titrated more closely than is possible with the 10 and 20 mg tablets.

Erythromycin

Erythromycin is a macrolide antibiotic distinguished by the presence of a lactone ring.[51] The frequent gastrointestinal side effects of erythromycin have been well known for several years; the drug was introduced into the clinical motility arena by Janssens and colleagues,[39] who demonstrated that acute administration accelerated gastric emptying of solids and increased antral contractions in patients with diabetes, some of whom had evidence of gastric stasis.

Mechanism of Action. Two mechanisms of action have been reported: stimulation of motilin receptors and a cholinergic mechanism.[17, 50] Erythromycin also activates L-type calcium channels, increasing intracellular calcium and causing contraction.[28] The half-life is short (1.5 to 2.5 hours), and drug absorption is formulation dependent. There is a dose-dependent effect on interdigestive gastric motility. A dose of 40 mg induces a phase III–like activity that starts in the stomach. Higher doses (200 mg and 350 mg) induce strong rhythmic contractions in the antrum of maximal frequency (3 per minute), but the contractions do not propagate to the small bowel.[22] In the original study, 200 mg intravenous erythromycin increased the rate of emptying of solids and liquids in patients with diabetes. When patients were treated with oral erythromycin (250 mg at bedtime), the beneficial effect persisted but was less prominent.[39] Erythromycin can stimulate intense contractions of the fundus and antrum, resulting in the dumping of solids out of the stomach.[5] This can be a disadvantage because nontriturated solids, unprepared for chemical digestion, are delivered into the small bowel. On the other hand, this property can be exploited when needed, such as when moving nondigestible solids (bezoars, feeding tubes) into the small bowel from the stomach. Erythromycin may also initiate migrating motor complex activity in the small bowel.

Use, Dosage, and Side Effects. The standard dose used acutely for exacerbations of gastroparesis is 3 mg/kg body weight intravenously every 8 hours. In most patients, it is stopped after 5 to 7 days as intolerance or tachyphylaxis develops. Typical oral doses used are between 200 mg and 500 mg 4 times per day. Erythromycin has been shown to improve gastric emptying of solids[22, 55] and symptoms of gastroparesis[27, 55] when given orally at a dose of between 50 mg and 500 mg 4 times per day for 4 weeks. The long-term efficacy is less clear, and down regulation of the motilin receptor may reduce its efficacy. There is little evidence that it improves symptoms in the long term.[13] Common side effects include nausea, diarrhea, and abdominal cramping, which tend to develop at higher doses. Ototoxicity may occur in patients with renal failure; pseudomembranous colitis is another side effect. Erythromycin inhibits the metabolism of drugs that use the cytochrome P-450 pathway, such as cisapride, quinidine, lovastatin, nifedepine, midazolam, carbamazepine, and others. Ventricular tachycardia has been reported at high doses, but is unlikely at low doses. There is also the theoretical risk of inducing resistant bacterial strains with long-term administration of erythromycin. Other macrolides (not yet approved for prescription) share the prokinetic properties of erythromycin but do not have antibiotic properties.

Metoclopramide
Mechanism of Action. Metoclopramide is a derivative of para-aminobenzoic acid and has a half-life of 2.5 to 5 hours. Metoclopramide antagonizes dopamine at central and peripheral receptor sites, has cholinergic-like effects, possibly through serotonergic receptors ($5HT_3$ and $5HT_4$). It may also act directly on smooth muscle.[43] It acts as an antiemetic and as a prokinetic agent. Given acutely, metoclopramide acts as a prokinetic to enhance gastric emptying, relax the pylorus, and increase jejunal peristalsis.[43] In a double-blind study, metoclopramide improved symptoms, but gastric emptying was not evaluated.[54] In a separate study by

McCallum and associates,[43] there was also improvement in symptoms but no significant effect on gastric emptying. It is thought that much of the drug's symptomatic efficacy is probably because of its central antiemetic effect.

Use, Dosage, and Side Effects. A commonly used dose of metoclopramide is 10 mg 3 times per day before meals. This may be given orally, subcutaneously, intramuscularly, or intravenously. Parenteral metoclopramide has a secondary role after intravenous erythromycin during episodes of severe nausea and vomiting in gastroparetic patients who are unable to tolerate oral medications. At therapeutic doses, central nervous system side effects such as anxiety, restlessness, dizziness, or drowsiness occur in 20% of individuals. Extrapyramidal reactions are less common and are reversible with benztropine. Tardive dyskinesia is rare but may be irreversible. Hyperprolactinemia may occur, leading to galactorrhea, breast tenderness, or menstrual irregularities in females and gynecomastia in males. Because of this side-effect profile, cisapride has now largely supplanted metoclopramide as the first-line oral prokinetic agent.

Domperidone
Mechanism of Action. Domperidone (a benzimidazole derivative) is chemically related to metoclopramide, except that its dopamine antagonism is limited to peripheral dopamine receptors and the chemoreceptor trigger zone that lies outside the blood-brain barrier. The half-life is 8 to 10 hours. Domperidone does not penetrate the blood-brain barrier; consequently, neurologic side effects are rare and less common than with metoclopramide.[35] Galactorrhea resulting from the drug's dopamine-blocking effects on the hypothalamopituitary axis is a recognized side effect. Dry mouth, headache, and diarrhea may also occur. Domperidone has no cholinergic activity but does possess antiemetic and antinausea efficacy.

Use, Dosage, and Side Effects. Typical doses used are 10 to 20 mg 4 times per day orally. It has also been used intravenously and rectally. Acute administration enhances gastric emptying of liquids and solids in diabetic patients with gastroparesis.[35] The long-term effect is less clear. In a study by Koch and coworkers[40] using 20 mg orally 4 times per day, there was no improvement in gastric emptying, but the total symptom scores improved. In another study, the treatment outcome and quality of life were improved with long-term domperidone.[63] As with metoclopramide, it is possible that domperidone's symptomatic efficacy results from its antiemetic properties. This agent is not yet approved by the U.S. Food and Drug Administration.

Octreotide

Octreotide, the long-acting somatostatin analogue, will be discussed primarily in the section on management of diabetic diarrhea. The role of octreotide in the long-term management of gastroparesis is unclear. The rationale for its use, however, is that a subcutaneous dose of 50 μg every 8 hours will induce an interdigestive migrating motor complex–like activity front[38, 65] and hence presumably dump indigestible debris out of the stomach. However, this theoretical action has not been demonstrated in practice.

Combinations

Erythromycin and cisapride should not be used in combination because of the risk of cardiac arrhythmias. There has been little work on the benefit of other combinations. Lehman and Patterson[42] reported that the combination of domperidone and cisapride improved symptoms in gastroparesis except pain, but had no impact on the number of hospital admissions for gastroparesis. Prokinetics may be used simultaneously with antiemetic agents, such as antihistamines and phenothiazines, and may be quite effective in clinical practice. Such combinations have not been formally studied.

Other Agents

If, despite therapy, there are ongoing symptoms, especially abdominal discomfort, a trial of medications aimed at suppressing sensory afferent function may be considered. These drugs include tricyclic antidepressants (such as amitriptyline, 10 to 25 mg twice daily), κ-opioid agonists (such as fedotozine), or serotonin antagonists such as ondansetron, granisetron, or tropisetron. The latter are best reserved for intravenous use in hospitalized patients because of their high cost and unproved efficacy in relief of nausea or vomiting in gastric stasis syndromes unrelated to chemotherapy-induced emesis.

SURGERY

In general, major surgical intervention should be avoided in diabetic gastroparesis. Anecdotal reports of antrectomy with vagotomy, gastrectomy, bypass surgery, and pyloroplasty have demonstrated poor clinical outcome. Jejunostomy tubes, which can be placed laparoscopically, may be helpful for maintenance of nutrition and for decompression to aid in symptom control. Gastric electrical stimulation or "gastric pacing" at the physiological frequency of 3 cycles per minute does not appear to have a significant effect on the gastric myoelectrical activity of gastroparetic patients.[18] Pacing at higher rates may relieve symptoms in some patients, and controlled studies are under way.

PANCREAS TRANSPLANTATION

With the evidence that acute and chronic hyperglycemia can alter gastrointestinal function, it would be expected that the prospect of complete euglycemic control with pancreas transplantation would also improve gastrointestinal symptoms and gastrointestinal function. In a study on 32 patients, Zehr and associates[75] reported 96% of 24 patients with gastrointestinal symptoms improved after a pancreatic transplant. On the other hand, objective evaluation of gastrointestinal motor function revealed conflicting results. Gaber and colleagues[31] studied gastric emptying of solids and gastrointestinal symptoms in 10 patients before and 12 months after combined renal and pancreatic transplantation; symptoms improved significantly, and gastric emptying kinetics improved in the 6 patients who had pretransplant gastric stasis. In a study of 32 patients with diabetes mellitus and end-stage renal failure, Murat and colleagues[46] found that at 6 and 12 months after combined renal and pancreatic transplantation, gastric emptying of solids remained abnormal, but liquid emptying improved significantly. These findings suggest that glycemic control or correction of uremia may normalize the emptying of liquids, whereas impaired emptying of solids and antral hypomotility (which depends on vagal input) persist because the "autovagotomy" is not reversed by the transplantation. The most recent study by Hathaway and coworkers[34] showed improved autonomic and gastric function at 1 year follow-up in patients with pancreas-kidney versus pancreas alone transplantation. This suggests there may be a degree of reversibility of the autonomic dysfunction. Thus, the precise role of pancreatic transplantation in the management of diabetic gastroparesis remains somewhat unclear.

DIABETIC DIARRHEA

As with severe gastroparesis, initial management of the diabetic patient with diarrhea should involve resuscitation with correction of dehydration and electrolyte imbalance, correction of hypoglycemia or hyperglycemia, and nutritional support if required. It is preferable for treatment to be directed at the cause of diarrhea if it can be identified, rather than directed by empirical trials.[68] It is useful to group patients according to their clinical picture: associated malabsorption, associated fecal incontinence, rapid transit diarrhea, and other. If the cause of diarrhea remains unclear, then empirical trials may be considered. Figure 38.3 is a management algorithm for assessment of patients with diabetes and diarrhea.

Diarrhea and Malabsorption

Small bowel bacterial overgrowth is diagnosed preferably by small bowel culture rather than breath tests, which can give false positive or false negative results because of altered transit times.[68] Broad-spectrum oral antibiotics such as tetracycline, cephalosporins, ciprofloxacin, and metronidazole are effective treatments of bacterial overgrowth. Several different regimes are suitable; we suggest using a single antibiotic for 10 to 14 days each month on a rotating basis to avoid development of bacterial resistance.

A gluten-free diet should be implemented

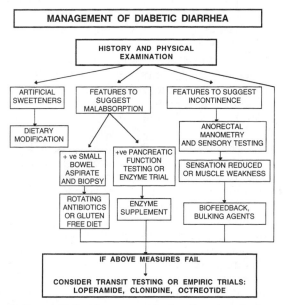

■ Figure 38.3 Management algorithm for diarrhea in diabetes. +ve, positive.

and is likely to improve symptoms in those with coexisting celiac disease.

Pancreatic exocrine insufficiency is rare in diabetes mellitus, but, if documented, pancreatic enzyme supplements should be administered. Pancreatic enzyme supplements may also be tried on an empirical basis if testing of pancreatic function is unavailable. It is important to tell patients to take this supplement before, during, and after each meal and to include supplements with snacks.

Rapid Transit Diarrhea

Antidiarrheal agents such as loperamide or diphenoxylate may be used if diarrhea is associated with documented rapid intestinal transit (Fig. 38.4) or may be used empirically if methods to measure intestinal transit are not readily available and there is no other clear pathogenesis for the diarrhea. Controlled clinical trials, however, are lacking. These drugs are reviewed in this section and are summarized in Table 38.3.

Loperamide

Loperamide is an opioid-like drug that works as an antidiarrheal, retarding small intestinal and colonic transit[20] and thereby increasing the contact time for absorption, particularly by small bowel mucosa. Gastric motor function is minimally affected,[7] which makes this drug suitable for diabetic patients who often have a combination of slow gastric emptying and rapid small bowel transit. Loperamide's main mechanism of action is through binding to peripheral μ-opioid receptors in the gastrointestinal tract,[6] although it may also have an antisecretory role[61] and probably inhibits rectal tone.[49] It is not well absorbed from the gastrointestinal tract, and much of the ingested dose is excreted in stool. It also does not cross the blood-brain barrier and has no abuse potential. A suitable dosage of loperamide is between 2 and 4 mg 3 to 4 times per day. It is also available in a liquid form (5 to 10 mL 3 times per day), which may be administered via a gastrostomy or jejunostomy tube. It may be used either after diarrhea has occurred or before a meal if the patient notices particularly severe exacerbation of diarrhea by meal ingestion.

Codeine

Codeine is an opiate that is available in tablet form and is sometimes used in the treatment of diarrhea. Doses used range between 15 to

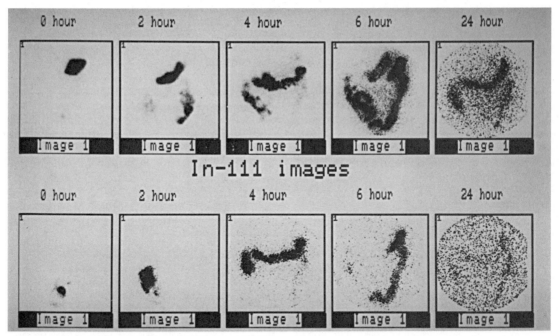

■ **Figure 38.4**   Scintigraphic transit test showing rapid small bowel transit; at 6 hours 100% of the marker has reached the colon (normal, 11 to 70%).

60 mg 4 times per day. Codeine and acetaminophen combinations are not recommended because of the possibility of acetaminophen toxicity.[62] Codeine is largely avoided because of its sedative action and potential for addiction.

Diphenoxylate

Diphenoxylate is less potent than codeine but is sufficient for most cases of diarrhea.[49] Diphenoxylate is well absorbed and is metabolized to the active metabolite diphenoxylic acid.[62] Diphenoxylate is usually available in combination with atropine, which was included to discourage drug abuse by producing anticholinergic side effects if more than 10 tablets are taken. The usual dose is 1 to 2 2.5-mg tablets 4 times per day. Patients should be warned that they may experience difficulty with visual accommodation and may need to avoid driving or handling heavy machinery.

Clonidine

Clonidine is a centrally acting α_2-adrenergic receptor agonist used in the treatment of hypertension. As discussed in Chapter 15, the mechanism of action of clonidine in diabetic diarrhea may be via inhibition of gut motility and by an effect on the enterocyte, resulting in increased fluid absorption and decreased secretion. In a study on three patients with diabetic diarrhea, use of clonidine orally at doses of 0.1 to 0.6 mg twice daily resulted in a

TABLE 38.3   DRUGS USED TO TREAT RAPID TRANSIT DIARRHEA IN DIABETES

Drug	Mechanism of Action	Dose
Loperamide	Opioid; inhibits transit; inhibits rectal tone	2–4 mg 4 times daily, orally
Codeine	Opiate; inhibits transit; increases fluid absorption	15–60 mg 4 times daily, orally
Diphenoxylate	Opioid; inhibits transit; increases fluid absorption	2.5–5 mg 4 times daily, orally
Verapamil	L-type calcium channel blocker; inhibits colonic transit	20–40 mg twice daily, orally
Clonidine	α_2-Adrenergic agonist; inhibits gut motility; reduces intestinal secretions	0.1–0.2 mg orally per day *or* by topical patch
Octreotide	Somatostatin analogue; inhibits transit; decreases intestinal secretion	50–75 μg 2 or 3 times per day subcutaneously

significant decrease in diarrhea.[29] The starting dose should be 0.1 mg twice a day and should be increased by 0.1 mg per dose daily until diarrhea improves or hypotension develops (maximum 0.6 mg/d). Maintenance of adequate hydration is necessary if this drug is being used. The clinical use of clonidine is limited by some of its adverse effects, such as orthostatic hypotension, excessive sedation, and depression.[29, 62] Clonidine skin patches have been reported to control diarrhea without causing hypotension.[58]

Verapamil

Constipation is a well-known side effect of the calcium channel blocker verapamil and occurs in about 6% of patients at therapeutic dosage. Verapamil has no effect on gastric emptying and does not appear to alter small intestinal transit, but it increases colonic transit time.[41] A suitable dosage is 40 mg twice daily but, as with clonidine, hypotension may limit its use.

Octreotide

Octreotide is a long-acting somatostatin analogue that has been proposed as an alternative treatment for chronic diarrhea in diabetic patients refractory to other measures.[24, 67, 72] These are anecdotal reports; no controlled trials are available. Somatostatin inhibits intestinal transit and affects several other gastrointestinal functions, including inhibition of gastric and pancreatic secretion, peptide and hormone secretion (insulin and gastrin), nutrient absorption, intestinal chloride secretion, and mesenteric blood flow.[70]

Octreotide administered as a subcutaneous injection of 50 to 75 μg twice a day retards small bowel transit in healthy controls.[70] At higher doses, inhibition of pancreatic exocrine secretion may aggravate diarrhea, although this effect may diminish in time. Octreotide has also been noted to inhibit gastric antral motility.[70] In view of this, it is unlikely to benefit patients with delayed gastric emptying, but it may be of use in patients with normal or rapid gastric emptying and rapid small bowel transit. Side effects of therapy are rare. There may be a stinging sensation at the site of injection, which may be minimized by warming the drug before injection and injecting slowly.[62] Disturbances of carbohydrate metabolism caused by the inhibition of insulin and glucagon secretion have been infrequent in healthy subjects, but there have been cases of significant hypoglycemia in diabetic patients.[44, 72] Insulin doses may need to be reduced by approximately 25%.[44, 72] There appears to be an increased risk of gallstones presumably because of inhibition of gallbladder contractility.[23]

Fecal Incontinence

The diabetic with fecal incontinence may be managed with biofeedback. The incontinence may be caused by weakness of the internal anal sphincter or by loss of rectal sensation.[71] Biofeedback involves the use of auditory or visual displays of a physiologic process to aid the patient in learning to control this process voluntarily.[9] The biofeedback protocol used differs depending on the cause of the fecal incontinence.

For muscle weakness resulting from pudendal nerve damage, biofeedback involves providing a visual display of anal canal pressures or pelvic floor electromyograms during attempts to contract the sphincter.[9] Abdominal muscle electromyography may be used in the treatment of patients who contract the abdominal muscles when they contract the sphincters. During the biofeedback sessions, patients learn to perform exercises that they can repeat at home and also learn to assess the improvement in sphincter strength. Several sessions are usually required. There are no controlled trials of biofeedback for fecal incontinence resulting from diabetes, but several reports in patients with fecal incontinence of diverse etiologies show improvement in measures of continence,[16, 25] including some with long-term follow-up.[26, 32]

Impaired ability to perceive rectal sensation is a common cause of fecal incontinence in diabetic patients.[11] The protocol for these patients involves distending a balloon in the rectum with a relatively large volume of air that the patient can reliably perceive, and then gradually reducing the volume of air until the patient begins to make mistakes (that is, to miss some distentions). The volume of balloon distention is varied above and below this threshold in an effort to teach the patient to recognize weaker distentions. The patient is instructed to contract the sphincter in response to rectal distention so that this stimulus-response sequence becomes a well-practiced habit. Rates of substantial improvement of continence occur in approximately 67% of patients, including diabetic patients, with fecal incontinence caused by impaired sensation.[9, 11] No long-term data are available.

Miscellaneous Causes of Diarrhea in Diabetes

Bile acid catharsis is a possible cause of diarrhea in diabetic patients. The treatment consists of cholestyramine, up to 16 g/day, which is unfortunately often ineffective.[19, 60] Alternatively, agents that retard small bowel transit, such as loperamide, may facilitate bile acid absorption by the ileum and avoid their cathartic effects in the colon. Incidental causes such as infection or malignancy should also be considered in cases of diabetes and diarrhea without an obvious cause.

SUMMARY AND PROSPECTS

The therapeutic armamentarium for gastroparesis and diarrhea in patients with diabetes has increased significantly in the past decade, with a variety of pharmacologic approaches that are not limited to modulation of the cholinergic nervous system. In the future, we anticipate that the introduction of nonantibiotic motilinomimetic agents (from the macrolide family of drugs) will provide an alternative strategy to stimulate gastric emptying. Understanding visceral afferents that convey sensation to conscious perception or the vomiting center will lead us to use other agents, such as serotonin antagonists or κ-opioid agonists to provide symptom relief. More widespread application of biofeedback and selection of patients with lack of sensation rather than those with paralyzed sphincters will lead to effective use of biofeedback in incontinent patients. Finally, we anticipate that the role of acute hyperglycemia will be clarified, and as diabetic control is managed more closely, this may result in improvement in some gastrointestinal symptoms. The lack of reversibility of autonomic denervation leaves us with little hope that pancreatic transplantation will have any significant impact on gastrointestinal complications once they have developed. Hence, gastroenterologists, endocrinologists, and neurologists must interact to optimize patient management when gastrointestinal symptoms arise.

References

1. Abell TL, Camilleri M, DiMagno EP, et al. Long-term efficacy of oral cisapride in symptomatic upper gut dysmotility. Dig Dis Sci 1991; 36:616.
2. Abell TL, Camilleri M, Hench VS. Gastric electromechanical function and gastric emptying in diabetic gastroparesis. Eur J Gastroenterol Hepatol 1991; 3:163.
3. Albrink MH, Foster J, Rosemurgy AS, et al. Laparoscopic feeding jejunostomy: Also a simple technique. Surg Endosc 1992; 6:259.
4. Anderson JW, Zeigler JA, Deakins DA, et al. Metabolic effects of high-carbohydrate, high-fiber diets for insulin-dependent diabetic individuals. Am J Clin Nutr 1991; 54:936.
5. Annese V, Janssens J, Vantrappen G, et al. Erythromycin accelerates gastric emptying by inducing antral contractions and improved antroduodenal coordination. Gastroenterology 1992; 102:823.
6. Awouters F, Megens A, Verlinden M, et al. Loperamide: Survey of studies on mechanism of its antidiarrheal activity. Dig Dis Sci 1993; 38:977.
7. Basilisco G, Bozzani A, Camboni G, et al. Effect of loperamide and naloxone on mouth-to-caecum transit time evaluated by lactulose hydrogen breath test. Gut 1985; 26:700.
8. Baskin WN. Advances in enteral nutrition techniques. Am J Gastroenterol 1992; 87:1547.
9. Bassotti G, Whitehead WE. Biofeedback as a treatment approach to gastrointestinal tract disorders. Am J Gastroenterol 1994; 89:158.
10. Bruttomesso D, Biolo G, Inchiostro S, et al. No effects of high-fiber diets on metabolic control and insulin-sensitivity in type I diabetic subjects. Diabetes Res Clin Pract 1991; 13:15.
11. Buser WD, Miner PB Jr. Delayed rectal sensation with fecal incontinence: Successful treatment using anorectal manometry. Gastroenterology 1986; 91:1186.
12. Camilleri M. Appraisal of medium- and long-term treatment of gastroparesis and chronic intestinal dysmotility. Am J Gastroenterol 1994; 89:1769.
13. Camilleri M. The current role of erythromycin in the clinical management of gastric emptying disorders. Am J Gastroenterol 1993; 88:169.
14. Camilleri M, Balm RK, Zinsmeister AR. Symptomatic improvement with one-year cisapride treatment in neuropathic chronic intestinal dysmotility. Aliment Pharmacol Ther 1996; 10:403.
15. Camilleri M, Malagelada J-R, Abell TL, et al. Effect of six weeks of treatment with cisapride in gastroparesis and intestinal pseudoobstruction. Gastroenterology 1989; 96:704.
16. Cerulli MA, Nikoomanesh P, Schuster MM. Progress in biofeedback conditioning for fecal incontinence. Gastroenterology 1979; 76:742.
17. Chaussade S, Michopoulos S, Sogni P, et al. Motilin agonist erythromycin increases human lower esophageal sphincter pressure by stimulation of cholinergic nerves. Dig Dis Sci 1994; 39:381.
18. Chen JD, Schirmer BD, McCallum RW. Serosal and cutaneous recordings of gastric myoelectrical activity in patients with gastroparesis. Am J Physiol 1994; 266:G90.
19. Codon JR, Suleman MI, Fan YS, et al. Cholestyramine and diabetic post-vagotomy diarrhoea. BMJ 1973; 4:423.
20. Corbett CL, Thomas S, Read NW, et al. Electrical detector for breath hydrogen determination: Measurement of small bowel transit time in normal subjects and patients with the irritable bowel syndrome. Gut 1982; 22:836.
21. Crofford OB. Diabetes control and complications. Annu Rev Med 1995; 46:267.
22. Desautels SG, Hutson WR, Christial PE, et al. Gastric emptying response to variable oral erythromycin dosing in diabetic gastroparesis. Dig Dis Sci 1995; 40:141.
23. Dowling RH, Hussaini SH, Murphy GM, et al. Gallstones during octreotide therapy. Digestion 1993; 54:107.

24. Dudl RJ, Anderson DS, Forsythe AB, et al. Treatment of diabetic diarrhea and orthostatic hypotension with somatostatin analogue SMS 201-995. Am J Med 1987; 83:584.

25. Enck P. Biofeedback training in disordered defecation: A critical review. Dig Dis Sci 1993; 38:1953.

26. Enck P, Daublin G, Lubke HJ, et al. Long-term efficacy of biofeedback training for fecal incontinence. Dis Colon Rectum 1994; 37:997.

27. Erbas T, Varoglu E, Erbas B, et al. Comparison of metoclopramide and erythromycin in the treatment of diabetic gastroparesis. Diabetes Care 1993; 16:1511.

28. Farrugia G, Rich A, Rae JL, et al. Calcium currents in human and canine jejunal circular smooth muscle cells. Gastroenterology 1995; 109:707.

29. Fedorak RN, Field M, Chang E. Treatment of diabetic diarrhea with clonidine. Ann Intern Med 1985; 102:197.

30. Fontana RJ, Barnett JL. Severe refractory diabetic gastroparesis: What is the utility of jejunostomy tube placement? A long-term retrospective review of 26 patients. Gastroenterology 1995; 108:A599.

31. Gaber AO, Oxley D, Karas J, et al. Changes in gastric emptying in recipients of successful combined pancreas-kidney transplants. Dig Dis Sci 1991; 9:437.

32. Guillemot F, Bouche B, Gower-Rousseau C, et al. Biofeedback for the treatment of fecal incontinence: Long-term clinical results. Dis Colon Rectum 1995; 37:997.

33. Haruma K, Wiste JA, Camilleri M. Effect of octreotide on gastrointestinal pressure profiles in health and in functional and organic gastrointestinal disorders. Gut 1994; 35:1064.

34. Hathaway DK, Abell T, Cardoso S, et al. Improvement in autonomic and gastric function following pancreas-kidney versus kidney alone transplantation and the correlation with quality of life. Transplantation 1994; 57:816.

35. Horowitz M, Harding PE, Chatterton BE, et al. Acute and chronic effects of domperidone on gastric emptying in diabetic autonomic neuropathy. Dig Dis Sci 1985; 30:1.

36. Horowitz M, Maddox A, Harding PE, et al. Effect of cisapride on gastric and esophageal emptying in insulin-dependent diabetes mellitus. Gastroenterology 1987; 92:1899.

37. Hsu JJ, Lee ST, Glena RC, et al. Gastroparesis syndrome: Nutritional sequelae and the impact of dietary manipulation of symptoms. Gastroenterology 1995; 108:A17.

38. Hyman PE, Di Lorenzo C, McAdams L, et al. Predicting the clinical response to cisapride in children with chronic intestinal pseudo-obstruction. Am J Gastroenterol 1993; 88:832.

39. Janssens J, Peeters T, Vantrappen G, et al. Improvement of gastric emptying in diabetic gastroparesis by erythromycin. N Engl J Med 1990; 322:1028.

40. Koch KL, Stern RM, Stewart WR, et al. Gastric emptying and gastric myoelectrical activity in patients with diabetic gastroparesis: Effect of long-term domperidone treatment. Am J Gastroenterol 1989; 84:1069.

41. Krevsy B, Maurer AH, Niewiarowski T, et al. Effect of verapamil on human intestinal transit. Dig Dis Sci 1992; 37:919.

42. Lehman KA, Patterson DJ. Does combination prokinetic therapy benefit patients with refractory diabetic gastroparesis? Gastroenterology 1995; 108:A636.

43. McCallum RW, Ricci PA, Rakatansky H, et al. A multicenter placebo-controlled clinical trial of oral metoclopramide in diabetic gastroparesis. Diabetes Care 1983; 6:463.

44. Mourad FH, Gorard D, Thillainayaham AV, et al. Effective treatment of diabetic diarrhoea with somatostatin analogue, octreotide. Gut 1992; 33:1578.

45. Mowatt-Larsen CA, Brown RO, Wojtysiak SL, et al. Comparison of tolerance and nutritional outcome between a peptide and a standard enteral formula in critically ill hypoalbuminemic patients. J Parenter Enteral Nutr 1992; 16:20.

46. Murat A, Pouliquen B, Cantarovich D, et al. Gastric emptying improvement after simultaneous segmental pancreas and kidney transplantation. Transplant Proc 1992; 24:855.

47. Nuttall FQ. Dietary fiber in the management of diabetes. Diabetes 1993; 42:503.

48. Ogorek CP, Davidson L, Fisher RS, et al. Idiopathic gastroparesis is associated with a multiplicity of severe dietary deficiencies. Am J Gastroenterol 1991; 86:423.

49. Palmer KR, Corbett CL, Holdsworth CD. Double-blind cross-over study comparing loperamide, codeine and diphenoxylate in the treatment of chronic diarrhea. Gastroenterology 1980; 79:1272.

50. Peeters T, Matthijs G, Depoortere I, et al. Erythromycin is a motilin receptor agonist. Am J Physiol 1989; 257:G470.

51. Peeters TL. Erythromycin and other macrolides as prokinetic agents. Gastroenterology 1993; 105:1886.

52. Ponsky JL, Gauderer MW, Stellato TA, et al. Percutaneous approaches to enteral alimentation. Am J Surg 1985; 149:102.

53. Prather CM, Camilleri M, Thomforde GM, et al. Gastric axial forces in experimentally delayed and accelerated gastric emptying. Am J Physiol 1993; 264:G928.

54. Ricci DA, Saltzman MB, Meyer C, et al. Effect of metoclopramide in diabetic gastroparesis. J Clin Gastroenterol 1985; 7:25.

55. Richards RD, Davenport K, McCallum RW. The treatment of idiopathic and diabetic gastroparesis with acute intravenous and chronic oral erythromycin. Am J Gastroenterol 1993; 88:203.

56. Richards RD, Valenzuela JA, Davenport KG, et al. Objective and subjective results of a randomized, double-blind, placebo-controlled trial using cisapride to treat gastroparesis. Dig Dis Sci 1993; 38:811.

57. Rothstein RD, Alavi A, Reynold JC. Electrogastrography in patients with gastroparesis and effect of long-term cisapride. Dig Dis Sci 1993; 38:1518.

58. Sacerdote A. Topical clonidine for diabetic diarrhea (letter). Ann Intern Med 1986; 105:139.

59. Samsom M, Salet GA, Roelofs JM, et al. Compliance of the proximal stomach and dyspeptic symptoms in patients with type I diabetes mellitus. Dig Dis Sci 1995; 40:2037.

60. Scarpello JH, Hague RV, Cullen DR, et al. The ^{14}C-glycocholate test in diabetic diarrhoea. BMJ 1976; 2:673.

61. Schiller LR, Santa Ana CA, Morawski SG, et al. Mechanism of the antidiarrheal effect of loperamide. Gastroenterology 1984; 86:1475.

62. Schiller LR. Anti-diarrhoeal pharmacology and therapeutics. Aliment Pharmacol Ther 1995; 9:87.

63. Shifflett J, McCallum RW. Long-term efficacy, treatment outcome and quality of life in patients receiving chronic domperidone therapy for gastroparesis. Gastroenterology 1995; 108:A35.

64. Simpson HC, Simpson RW, Lousley S, et al. A high carbohydrate leguminous fibre diet improves all aspects of diabetic control. Lancet 1981; 1:1.

65. Soudah HC, Hasler WL, Owang C. Effect of octreotide on intestinal motility and bacterial overgrowth in scleroderma. N Engl J Med 1991; 325:1461.

66. Stellato TA. Endoscopic intervention for enteral access. World J Surg 1992; 16:1042.
67. Tsai ST, Vinik AI, Brunner JF. Diabetic diarrhea and somatostatin (letter). Ann Intern Med 1986; 104:894.
68. Valdovinos MA, Camilleri M, Zimmerman BR. Chronic diarrhea in diabetes mellitus: Mechanisms and an approach to diagnosis and treatment. Mayo Clin Proc 1993; 68:691.
69. Viall C, Porcelli K, Teran JC, et al. A double-blind clinical trial comparing the gastrointestinal side effects of two enteral feeding formulas. J Parenter Enteral Nutr 1990; 14:265.
70. von der Ohe MR, Camilleri M, Thomforde GM, et al. Differential regional effects of octreotide on human gastrointestinal motor function. Gut 1995; 36:743.
71. Wald A, Tunuguntla K. Anorectal sensorimotor dysfunction, faecal incontinence and diabetes mellitus. N Engl J Med 1984; 310:1282.
72. Walker JJ, Kaplan DS. Efficacy of the somatostatin analog octreotide in the treatment of two patients with refractory diabetic diarrhea. Am J Gastroenterol 1993; 88:765.
73. Warner E, Jeejeebhoy KN. Successful management of chronic intestinal pseudo-obstruction with home parenteral nutrition. J Parenter Enteral Nutr 1985; 9:173.
74. Wiseman LR, Faulds D. Cisapride: An updated review of its pharmacology and therapeutic efficacy as a prokinetic agent in gastrointestinal motility disorders. Drugs 1994; 47:116.
75. Zehr PS, Milde FK, Hart LK, et al. Pancreatic transplantation: Assessing secondary complications and life quality. Diabetologia 1991; 34:S138.

Chapter **39**

Treatment of Diabetic Sexual Dysfunction and Cystopathy

Claire C. Yang • William E. Bradley

INTRODUCTION

The standard treatments for diabetic sexual dysfunction and cystopathy include medical and surgical options. In male sexual dysfunction, the goals of treatment are to restore an erection rigid enough for sexual intercourse and to recover sperm for purposes of fertility in instances of ejaculatory disturbances. Female sexual dysfunction has not been found to be more prevalent in the diabetic population as compared with nondiabetic women, and treatment is based on psychological and sex therapy. In the treatment of cystopathy, the goal is to assure the patient a continent manner to store urine, release it efficiently at regular intervals, minimize urinary symptoms, and avoid infection. Selection of a treatment for genitourinary complications of diabetes should take into consideration the patient's physical and cognitive abilities.

ERECTION

Based on the patient's etiologies for sexual dysfunction and treatment goals, an appropriate treatment can be instituted from a broad range of options (Table 39.1). Several of the treatments pose special considerations for the diabetic patient. Very rarely do the treatments for sexual dysfunction improve sensory loss or hy-

TABLE 39.1 TREATMENT OPTIONS FOR MALE SEXUAL DYSFUNCTION

Erectile dysfunction
    Psychological counseling/sex therapy
    Medical treatment
        Medication changes
        Hormone replacement
        Oral medications
        Experimental preparations
    Vacuum constriction device
    Penile injection therapy
    Intraurethral therapy
    Vascular intervention
    Penile prosthesis
Ejaculatory dysfunction
    Medications
    Sperm retrieval
        Post-ejaculate catheterization
        Electroejaculation
        Vas/epididymis/testis aspiration

peresthesia, and with the more invasive measures, sensory problems may be aggravated.

Psychological Counseling and Sexual Therapy

Approximately 10% of diabetic males complaining of impotence are reported to have primarily psychogenic impotence, based on comprehensive psychological and physiologic testing.[51, 61] When the erectile dysfunction is confirmed by nocturnal penile tumescence testing, this percentage is even smaller. In one study, only 6% of men with type 2 diabetes mellitus (DM) were found to have pure psychogenic impotence, and all patients with type 1 DM were found to have organic causes.[39] Affective factors can also exacerbate organic impotence, with 50% of impotent diabetic men demonstrating abnormalities on psychological assessment.[12] In these men, psychological treatment for them and their partners can be helpful in regaining sexual health. A description of psychological methods is beyond the scope of this chapter, and the reader is referred to other sources.[26, 47, 60]

Medical Treatment

The causes of impotence in the diabetic are primarily neurologic and vascular, and if the pathology is not severe, medical treatment can be effective. The following treatments involve drugs whose systemic effects impact on erectile function.

Medication Changes. Many medications are known to cause or exacerbate male sexual dysfunction.[17] Antihypertensive preparations are the most commonly used medications associated with impotence, and in many instances, changing from one class of drug to another may result in improved erectile capacity. Antidepressants are also commonly associated with impotence; however, trazodone has demonstrated efficacy in restoring erectile function in patients who are switched from other antidepressants.[45] If use of a particular medication is temporally related to the onset of sexual dysfunction, a change in the patient's drug regimen should be attempted, in consultation with the patient's primary physician.

Hormone Replacement. The primary effect of testosterone replacement on sexual function in the hypogonadal male is to improve libido and secondarily, to improve potency.[31] Testosterone replacement is indicated only in those patients who have documented hypogonadism, after pituitary dysfunction has been eliminated as a cause. As noted in a previous chapter, hypogonadism is an uncommon cause of impotence in the diabetic population. Intramuscular injection of testosterone cypionate 200 mg every 2 to 3 weeks is one of the most commonly used preparations, and new transdermal forms of testosterone are being used with increasing frequency. Oral formulations are not well absorbed from the gastrointestinal tract and are associated with liver enzyme abnormalities. The fear that testosterone replacement will increase a patient's risk for prostate disease has not been substantiated[13, 16]; however, a digital rectal exam and prostate-specific antigen test are recommended in older men before starting replacement therapy.

Oral Medications. Yohimbine is a presynaptic α_2-receptor blocker that decreases outflow of blood from the corporeal tissue and may have a central nervous system effect to increase libido. The drug is contraindicated in renal insufficiency. A dose of 5.4 mg 3 times daily has been effective in improving erectile function in some patients,[58] but the overall outcomes data for yohimbine indicate that it has marginal efficacy.[44]

Trazodone has been known to cause priapism, and it was this observation that led to its use for treatment of erectile dysfunction. Its mechanism of action is thought to be secondary to α-adrenergic antagonist properties[1] as well as its antiserotonergic effects. Dosages ranging from 50 mg at night to 50 mg 3 times daily have been effective in restoring erectile function,[30] but the drug has not been found to be efficacious in older patients or men with long-standing impotence.[34] Side effects are minimal at these low dosages, but they can include dizziness, lightheadedness, and somnolence.

Experimental Preparations. A burgeoning area of research is the development of oral medications to induce erections "on demand," in contrast to the existing medications for erectile function that require long-term use. The drugs have demonstrated efficacy in psychogenic impotence and now are being tested in organic impotence.

Sildenafil is a selective inhibitor of type 5 cyclic guanosine monophosphate phosphodiesterase (cGMP), which is found in corporal tissue. Inhibition of this phosphodiesterase enhances the effects of neurotransmitters such as nitric oxide to cause relaxation of the sinusoidal tissue, resulting in penile tumescence.[11] Clinical trials of this oral preparation are under way in Europe and the United States. Apomorphine is a dopaminergic agonist with centrally acting effects resulting in erections.[32, 56] Preliminary studies have demonstrated an improvement in erectile function caused by psychogenic impotence.[24]

Oral medications used for the treatment of diabetic neuropathies may also prove beneficial in the management of impotence (see section on Therapy of Diabetic Cystopathy–Pharmacologic Agents).

Vacuum Constriction Device

The vacuum constriction device (VCD) is a mechanical method of creating an erect penis; this device is noninvasive and requires no medication. It consists of a plastic cylinder, a vacuum pump, and an elastic constriction band. The cylinder is placed over the penis, and a mechanical pump creates a vacuum within the cylinder, drawing blood into the erectile tissue. The pump is either hand- or battery-operated (Fig. 39.1). When the penis achieves maximal engorgement, the constriction band, which is mounted on the open end of the cylinder, is transferred to the base of the erect penis to hold blood in the corpora and maintain the erection. Because the band creates penile ischemia, it may be left on for no longer than half an hour at a time. The device can be reused after the penis is allowed to detumesce.

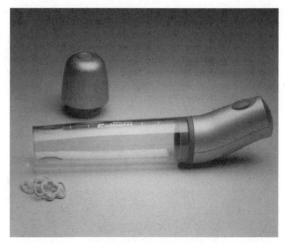

■ **Figure 39.1** Battery-operated vacuum constriction device. Pressing a button on the pump at the end of the cylinder creates a vacuum within the cylinder, drawing blood into the erectile tissue of the penis. When an adequate erection has developed, a constriction band is unloaded from the proximal end of the cylinder and constricts the base of the penis. This contains the blood within the penis, maintaining a rigid erection for sexual activity. (Esteem ErecAid® System; courtesy of Osbon Medical Systems, Augusta, Georgia.)

The majority of impotent men are successfully able to use the VCD. The VCD is safe with minimal side effects when used appropriately. Persons in whom the device may not be effective are obese men who have a significant suprapubic fat pad that buries the penis and those with limited hand function. An overall effectiveness rate has been reported at 60 to 70%.[3, 44] Patients who are unsatisfied with this method cite ecchymosis, lack of spontaneity, and the cumbersome use of the cylinder and pump as their reasons for discontinuing use. Penile injury has been described in persons with insensate genitals who have left the constriction band on for extended periods.

Penile Injection Therapy

Penile injection therapy or intracorporeal therapy has been used widely throughout the world since the mid-1980s.[62] The medications used are vasoactive substances that act within the penis to decrease the penile vascular resistance, allowing blood to enter the erectile tissues.[37] Effective to some degree in most patients, intracorporeal injections work best in men with neurologic or psychogenic impotence. This type of treatment is not recommended in men with severe psychiatric disease, poor manual dexterity or eyesight, and morbid obesity and is contraindicated in men with an existing penile prosthesis.

The most commonly used vasoactive substances are prostaglandin E_1 (PGE_1) (alprostadil), papavarine, and phentolamine.[37, 49] The first two have been used individually, and all three have been used in varying combinations. Combination use was introduced to decrease the amount of individual medication needed, thus avoiding some of the toxicity of each drug. Recently, the U.S. Food and Drug Administration approved PGE_1 for penile injection therapy. The safety profile of PGE_1, with a lower incidence of associated priapism and fibrosis, has made it the first-line drug for injection therapy as recommended by the American Urological Association Clinical Guidelines Panel.[44]

The method of penile injection uses a small-gauge needle and syringe, such as that used for administration of insulin. The appropriate dose of medication is determined through titration to achieve a rigid erection adequate for intercourse, lasting 30 to 60 minutes. Patients with primarily neurogenic impotence, such as young men with diabetes, typically require less medication than those patients with a vascular basis of impotence. The medication is injected at the base of the penis on the lateral aspect to avoid underlying nerves and vessels (Fig. 39.2). An erection develops within 5 to 10 minutes. Alternate sides of the penis are used with each injection, and use of this treatment should be limited to twice a week to avoid intracorporeal fibrosis.

Patient satisfaction with this treatment has been good in long-term follow-up. Approximately 80% of intrapenile injection users continue with treatment, although initial acceptance rates of this mode of treatment has been reported at 50%.[20] Reasons for dissatisfaction include pain, inconvenience, loss of efficacy, and lack of sexual interest.

Side effects of this method include priapism, penile pain, and plaque formation (fibrosis), and the incidence varies with each particular medication. Priapism is a prolonged erection and occurs in 1 to 4% of all penile injection users.[20] It should be treated within 4 to 6 hours, typically with corporal irrigation and infusion of sympathomimetic agents to induce detumescence. Penile pain is the most common side effect of penile injection therapy[38] and may occur at the injection site or along the shaft of the penis after an erection begins. Persistent pain may lead to cessation of treatment. Plaque formation or fibrosis is scarring that results in response to the trauma of injection as well as in response to the medication itself. The duration of treatment is directly related to the incidence of fibrosis,[33] and plaque formation is a relative indication to discontinue treatment. A case of penile necrosis caused by fulminant infection of the corpora from an intrapenile shot has been described, occurring in a diabetic patient.[54] Anticoagulated patients may experience local hematoma formation.

Intraurethral Therapy

The Food and Drug Administration recently approved the use of intraurethral PGE_1. It has been demonstrated to be effective in 65% of impotent patients with varying etiologies.[48] The PGE_1 acts in the same manner as with the penile injections; the method of drug delivery is through transurethral absorption into the corpora. The drug pellet is inserted into the penile urethra through an applicator, with a resultant erection occurring within 10 to 20 minutes (Fig. 39.3). Its appeal lies in its nonin-

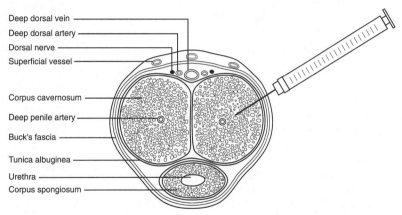

■ **Figure 39.2** Cross section of penis demonstrating penile injection therapy for erectile dysfunction. Vasoactive medications are dispensed into the corpora cavernosa, decreasing penile vascular resistance. Increased blood flow into the penis results in penile tumescence and rigidity.

Deep dorsal vein
Deep dorsal artery
Dorsal nerve
Superficial vessel
Corpus cavernosum
Deep penile artery
Buck's fascia
Tunica albuginea
Urethra
Corpus spongiosum

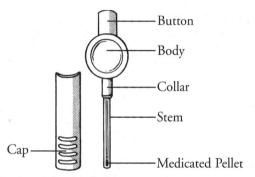

■ **Figure 39.3** Intraurethral alprostadil for erectile dysfunction. The applicator is inserted into the urethral meatus. Pressing the button at the tip of the applicator dispenses the alprostadil pellet into the urethra. The patient then sits, stands, or walks to facilitate blood flow into the penis as the medication diffuses into the corpora cavernosa. (MUSE; courtesy of VIVUS, Inc., Menlo Park, California. Drawing by Phoebe Gloeckner.)

vasive application, as compared with intrapenile injection. Urethral pain and dizziness are the most common side effects, and priapism and penile fibrosis are not reported to be significant complications. Long-term data on efficacy and satisfaction are not yet available at this time.

Vascular Intervention

Vascular surgery for treatment of impotence continues to be a subject of debate, and its role in treating diabetic impotence is limited.[14] The success of arterial and venous procedures range from 31 to 80%, and these inconsistent results have led the American Urological Association Clinical Guidelines Panel on Erectile Dysfunction to recommend that vascular surgery be considered investigational and performed only in a research setting.[44] Arterial revascularization has the best success rate in the young man with pelvic trauma and vascular injury with resultant impotence.

Penile Prosthesis

Penile prostheses were initially used in the 1960s and have been a standard option of impotence treatment ever since. The first penile prosthetic devices were rigid and semirigid devices, with the first inflatable models introduced in 1973.[55] Many modifications have been made in the last two decades, resulting in improved prosthesis durability and biocompatibility. At the time of its introduction, penile prosthesis implantation was one of the only

treatments for impotence. With the current array of nonsurgical options, a surgical implant now is generally reserved for patients after they have tried less invasive methods for treatment of erectile dysfunction.

The semirigid, or malleable, and inflatable penile prostheses are the two major types of devices in use today. The semirigid models are solid silicone cylinders containing a metal or plastic interlocking component system, allowing it to be malleable yet maintain a fixed position. These cylinders are placed within the corpora cavernosa. The penis is bent downward when not in use, and straightened for sexual activity. The inflatable models consist of a pump, a reservoir, and inflatable rods that are interconnected by tubing. Fluid transfers between the components to achieve an erect or flaccid state. The pump is placed in the scrotum, and the reservoir is placed behind the rectus muscle, although in some models, the pump and the reservoir are combined into one piece for scrotal placement (Fig. 39.4). Placement of the rods or cylinders results in obliteration of most of the erectile tissue within the corpora cavernosa; thus, other methods of impotence treatment will not be successful after prosthesis implantation.

Reported patient satisfaction rates for all types of prostheses range from 70 to 90%, and partner satisfaction ranges from 60 to 80%.[36] One early study of diabetic men who had pe-

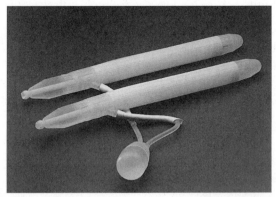

■ **Figure 39.4** Inflatable penile prosthesis, with reservoir and pump combined into one piece. The two cylinders are placed into the corpora cavernosa and the pump/reservoir is placed into the scrotum. The cylinders are inflated by squeezing the pump, which transfers fluid from the reservoir to the cylinders. Deflation is achieved by bending the cylinders at mid-shaft, which breaks the one-way valve and allows the fluid back into the reservoir. (Ambicor™ Penile Prosthesis; courtesy of American Medical Systems, Inc., Minnetonka, Minnesota.)

nile prosthesis implants (mostly noninflatable) reported an overall satisfaction rate of more than 80% in patients and partners.[6] Reasons for dissatisfaction included inadequate penile length or girth, change in penile sensation, and lack of concealment.

Complications of implants can be significant, including infection, erosion, and mechanical failure. In these instances, removal or replacement of part or all of the device is indicated. The incidence of mechanical failure has decreased with improvements in the prostheses, but the long-term reoperation rate is difficult to track because of the rapid, ongoing introduction of new models of penile implants. Mechanical failure rates are lower with the less intricate, semirigid devices, but these are more prone to erosion. The current models of prostheses can be expected to have a 5% incidence of long-term mechanical failure, with the majority of reoperations occurring in the first 5 years after implantation.[36] Certain patients are at greater risk for developing a prosthetic infection, including those with type 1 DM who have a history of urinary tract infections or other infections[36] or those with poor glucose control as measured by glycosylated hemoglobin.[10] However, with careful patient selection, diabetics in general have not been found to have a higher reoperation rate in several large series of implants,[43, 50, 66] but the most severe complications have been reported in diabetics.[7] Diabetics have a high rate of prosthesis infection (18%) with revisions.[66] Erosion of part of the device can occur because of ischemia or infection. A common cause of ischemia is the prolonged use of a large-diameter Foley catheter in the patient with a penile prosthesis,[41] resulting in urethral erosion. Another point of erosion is at the glans. Replacement may be possible after prosthesis removal and healing has occurred, generally after several months. Some patients experience prolonged periods of penile pain because of an oversized device, which may require prosthesis removal or replacement. Silicone particle shedding and migration from penile implants has been described, but no systemic silicone-induced disorder from such a device has been reported.[5]

The most common causes of impotence in men are neurologic, vascular, psychological, and endocrine. There frequently is more than one etiology for the dysfunction, as is seen in the diabetic male. With organic impotence, there may be a significant psychological overlay to the patient's situation, and this should be addressed as well.

EJACULATION

If ejaculatory dysfunction is caused by failure of seminal emission or retrograde ejaculation (lack of bladder neck closure during perineal muscle contraction), sympathomimetic medications can assist in antegrade ejaculation. Commonly used preparations include ephedrine, pseudoephedrine, and imipramine, which are taken 60 minutes before engaging in sexual activity. Brompheniramine has also been reported to be effective in diabetics for ejaculatory dysfunction.[52] If ejaculatory dysfunction is a result of peripheral sensory neuropathy and erectile dysfunction, then increasing genital stimulation, such as with a vibrator, may be helpful.

Diabetic men with ejaculatory dysfunction wishing to achieve pregnancy with their partner have several options for sperm retrieval if the treatments listed above are unsuccessful.

1. Collection of sperm from postejaculate urine is possible in retrograde ejaculation. The bladder is catheterized and filled with a buffered solution before sexual activity. After ejaculation, the urine is collected and centrifuged to separate the sperm, which are then used for intrauterine insemination or other assisted reproduction techniques. This is not possible without seminal emission.
2. Electroejaculation has been used in diabetic patients with absent seminal emission.[44] Emission is induced by a transrectal probe that delivers an electrical discharge to the prostate and male adnexa and the semen is then milked out of the urethra. This procedure may require regional or general anesthesia.
3. Vasal or epididymal sperm aspiration is an operation performed under local anesthesia in which the vas deferens is opened close to the testis and cannulated with a small catheter.[9] Gentle irrigation with a buffered solution and aspiration of the fluid can retrieve sperm for assisted reproduction techniques. Other methods of retrieving sperm directly from the testis are currently under investigation.[64]

FEMALE SEXUAL DYSFUNCTION

Sexual dysfunction as a complication of DM in women has been controversial. Because of the lack of a standardized, objective evaluation of female sexual function, the evaluation of the female diabetic relies on questionnaire data.

Aspects of the female sexual response include libido, sexual arousal, vaginal lubrication, and orgasmic capacity. In contrast to the relatively high incidence of male diabetic sexual dysfunction, several studies report that female patients with type 1 DM do not experience significantly more sexual incapacity than nondiabetic controls,[19, 27, 53] although one study reported a higher incidence of anorgasmia.[29] Ellenberg reports that there was no correlation between female diabetic sexual dysfunction and the presence of peripheral neuropathy or other diabetic sequela.[19] The apparent difference in the rates of sexual dysfunction in diabetic males and females when compared with controls is surprising, but may be attributed to gender-related psychological differences with regard to sexual behavior and satisfaction.[19, 27] Although necessary in men, specific physiologic responses are not essential for sexual gratification in women. Treatment of female sexual dysfunction depends heavily on psychological counseling and sex therapy.

Because fertility is not directly related to sexual responses in women, reproductive capacity in female diabetics will not be addressed in this chapter. The reader is referred to standard obstetric texts.

THERAPY OF DIABETIC CYSTOPATHY

Treatments for diabetic cystopathy are directed at providing the patient with a continent, infection-free lower urinary tract with minimal urinary symptoms and an appropriate method of urine drainage (Table 39.2). Patients with mild forms of cystopathy who have urinary complaints are treated with noninvasive measures.

TABLE 39.2 TREATMENT OPTIONS FOR DIABETIC CYSTOPATHY

Behavioral management
   Timed voiding
   Double voiding
   Physical therapy
Clean intermittent catheterization
Urine collection devices
   Condom catheters
   Indwelling catheters
Pharmacologic management
   α-Adrenergic blocking agents
   Experimental treatments
Surgical procedures
   Prostatectomy
   Bladder suspension
   Pancreas transplantation

Severe cystopathy requires some form of catheter drainage of urine. New developments in treating diabetes and its neuropathic sequelae may have potential benefit to diabetics with cystopathy.

Behavioral Management

One of the most important and perhaps least appreciated treatment modalities is behavioral modification. Timed voiding can be used by diabetic patients with poorly sensate or insensate bladders. They are instructed to attempt urination every 4 to 6 hours, whether they have the sensation to void or not. Double voiding is another maneuver in which patients with known large postvoid residual volumes are told to attempt urination 5 to 10 minutes after initially urinating. Both these techniques are aimed at preventing accumulation of large bladder volumes in the poorly sensate bladder, to avoid overdistension and possibly preserve detrusor contractility. Using the Valsalva maneuver to empty the bladder should not be encouraged because this can contribute to pelvic floor relaxation, with subsequent bladder, uterine, and enteric prolapse in women and inguinal hernia development in men. Physical therapy to strengthen pelvic floor muscles are helpful in men and women with symptoms of stress urinary incontinence,[28] after overflow incontinence has been ruled out.

Clean Intermittent Catheterization

Clean intermittent catheterization (CIC) was popularized by Lapides in 1972 and is now a common and valuable tool in diabetic bladder hygiene.[35] The concept of CIC is based on the importance of efficient bladder emptying, despite possible bacterial entry into the urinary system. Intermittent catheterization bypasses the sequela of long-term, chronic catheterization while also maintaining low bladder pressure, totally evacuating bladder contents, and allowing the patient voluntary control of urine elimination. Often, commencement of CIC results in amelioration of irritative symptoms (e.g., frequency, nocturia, incontinence) caused by large, residual urine volumes. Patients are instructed to catheterize on a schedule that drains volumes between 450 and 500 mL or less, which is the approximate normal adult bladder capacity. Typically, anticholinergic medications are not needed in the diabetic patient to suppress residual detrusor activity. Most patients can perform CIC provided they have adequate cognitive ability and manual dexterity and physical agility to position themselves for catheterization. The use of a mirror can assist the female learning the technique. Catheter care requires cleaning the reusable catheters with soap and water after each use, followed by air drying. Maintaining clean technique is the objective, because sterile procedure is generally unmanageable for long-term use.

Complications are few, but include occasional urinary tract infections, urinary tract trauma during catheterization (usually during the learning curve), and bladder stone formation, typically a result of the introduction of small foreign bodies, for example, lint or hair, into the bladder. Bacteriuria and pyuria are common and generally should not be treated unless the patient is experiencing symptoms, such as fever, dysuria or pain, or incontinence. There is no demonstrable benefit from suppressive antibiotics in patients who perform CIC.[42] Frequent urinary tract infections (versus colonization or bacteriuria) can be caused by improper catheterization technique or a sign of another problem, such as urolithiasis.

Urine Collection Devices

Condom catheters are often used for urine collection in patients who are unable to do self-catheterization. For the catheters to be used most effectively, the patient's bladder must be able to empty reasonably well, which is often not the case in diabetic cystopathy. They have a theoretical benefit of not being indwelling, but they still are associated with chronic bacteriuria from the high concentration of organisms at the urethral meatus.[22] Condom catheter use in a patient with a poorly emptying bladder puts him at high risk for recurrent urinary tract infections.

Indwelling catheters, either urethral or suprapubic, are used frequently in diabetic patients, particularly those who are in urinary retention and are unable to care for themselves. Although the complications of chronic catheterization are well known, a large number of patients tolerate them well. Catheter care includes monthly catheter changes, securing the catheter to the patient's leg to avoid unnecessary movement or traction, having a one-way valve on the drainage bag to prevent drained urine from refluxing, and copious fluid intake to minimize sediment accumulation in the bladder.

Pharmacologic Agents

In diabetic patients with only mild cystopathy and intact sensation, treatment of urinary symptoms follows the same guidelines as for nondiabetic patients. However, the physician must be aware of the possibility for progression of the neuropathic process, and annual follow-up in patients with detrusor dysfunction to assess bladder emptying must be maintained. In diabetic men, obstructive and irritative voiding symptoms can be diminished by the use of α-adrenergic blocking agents. This may improve bladder emptying as well.

The evidence in humans that the peripheral innervation of the urinary detrusor is cholinergically mediated is convincing. Hence, bethanechol, a cholinergic agonist,[4] has been used extensively in the past for the treatment of detrusor areflexia in such neurologic diseases as diabetic autonomic neuropathy. An oral dosage of several hundred milligrams a day has been suggested from its use in the clinical setting. However, the lack of drug metabolism data, the absence of randomized trials, and the impression that bethanechol is relatively ineffective in correcting an impaired detrusor reflex[65] have discouraged continued use of the drug. No other medications are available to resuscitate the denervated bladder.

Aldose reductase inhibitor therapy, although providing improvement in diabetics with peripheral neuropathy, has been shown to have minimal, if any, effect in the treatment of diabetic cystopathy, although there were some beneficial effects on other manifestations of diabetic autonomic neuropathy.[23] Anecdotal reports of improvement in erectile function suggest that this treatment may be beneficial in diabetic impotence.[25] Further investigation is needed to determine its indication for use in autonomic dysfunction.[21, 57] Strict maintenance of the blood glucose concentration in a normal range has been shown to slow the progression of diabetic sequelae, such as retinopathy,[63] and probably has a beneficial effect on bladder function as well.

Nerve growth factor (NGF) is suspected of playing a role in diabetic neuropathy. Recent work suggests that systemic administration of NGF may prevent or reverse neuropathy by providing NGF directly to its receptors on dorsal root ganglion cell bodies,[2] bypassing the retrograde axonal transport defect present in diabetes. At the time of this writing, NGF is entering phase III clinical trials, and the patients most likely to benefit from this therapy would be those who are at risk for small-fiber diabetic neuropathy.[18] Because erectile and bladder function involve autonomic fibers, NGF may have a significant impact on the genitourinary sequelae of diabetes.

Surgical Management

Prostatectomy. A transurethral prostatectomy can be performed in men with mild forms of diabetic cystopathy who also have evidence for bladder outlet obstruction caused by benign prostatic hyperplasia. This method of decreasing outlet resistance may allow the patient to empty his bladder more effectively, but detrusor contractility must be confirmed with cystometry before operation or the patient may still experience urinary retention postoperatively.

Bladder Suspension Procedures. In diabetic women with or without cystopathy, urinary incontinence may be present. If pharmacologic measures and physical therapy or pelvic floor strengthening exercises (Kegel exercises) fail to improve the urine leak and overflow incontinence has been ruled out, then a bladder suspension procedure may be indicated to treat stress urinary incontinence. Women with cystopathy should be counseled that they are at higher risk for urinary retention and may require CIC after the operation.

Pancreas Transplantation. Although pancreas transplantation is not considered a treatment for diabetic cystopathy, there does appear to be an arrest of the progression of bladder dysfunction postoperatively.[15] Diabetic cystopathy has been reported to improve in patients after pancreas transplantation in one study,[40] but this result may be caused by improved detrusor mechanics within the stabilized hormonal milieu rather than nerve regeneration. Before transplantation, the diabetic patient should be screened for cystopathy.[67] Queries about voiding habits and symptoms and urine flow and postvoid residual measurements should be obtained initially, and cystometry or urodynamics should be performed as indicated. The presence of cystopathy and even total detrusor failure does not preclude transplantation,[59] particularly if the patient can perform CIC. Postoperative urethrovesical irritation caused by metabolic derangements and pancreatic enzymes draining into the bladder is managed initially by catheter drainage and then with copious fluid intake and frequent voids.

CONCLUSION

Standard management options for the genitourinary sequelae of DM provide the patient with a functional substitute for diminished sexual or urinary capacity. Some of the newer treatments for diabetic neuropathy, which is the primary cause of these problems, may improve or reverse the dysfunction. Continued research in the area of genitourinary innervation, particularly using electrophysiologic techniques to identify neuropathy in the genitourinary tract, will contribute to improved understanding of the neuropathology of diabetes and, subsequently, improved therapies.

References

1. Abber JC, Lue TF, Luo J, et al. Priapism induced by chlorpromazine and trazodone: Mechanism of action. J Urol 1987; 137:1039.
2. Apfel SC, Arezzo JC, Brownlee M, et al. Nerve growth factor administration protects against experimental diabetic sensory neuropathy. Brain Res 1994; 634:7.
3. Baltaci S, Aydos K, Kosar A, et al. Treating erectile dysfunction with a vacuum tumescence device: A retrospective analysis of acceptance and satisfaction. Br J Urol 1995; 76:757.
4. Barrett DM. The effect of oral bethanechol chloride on voiding in female patients with excessive residual urine: A randomized double-blind study. J Urol 1981; 126:640.
5. Barrett DM, O'Sullivan DC, Malizia AA, et al. Particle shedding and migration from silicone genitourinary prosthetic devices. J Urol 1991; 146:319.
6. Beaser RS, Van der Hoek C, Jacobson AM, et al. Experience with penile prostheses in the treatment of impotence in diabetic men. JAMA 1982; 248:943.
7. Bejany DE, Perito PE, Lustgarten M, et al. Gangrene of the penis after implantation of penile prosthesis: Case reports, treatment recommendations and review of the literature. J Urol 1993; 150:190.
8. Bemelmans BLH, Meuleman EJH, Doesburg WH, et al. Erectile dysfunction in diabetic men: The neurological factor revisited. J Urol 1994; 151:884.
9. Berger RE, Muller CH, Smith D, et al. Operative recovery of vasal sperm from anejaculatory men: Preliminary report. J Urol 1986; 135:948.
10. Bishop JR, Moul JW, Sihelnik SA, et al. Use of glycosylated hemoglobin to identify diabetics at high risk for penile periprosthetic infections. J Urol 1992; 147:386.
11. Boolell M, Gepi-Attee S, Gingell JC, et al. Sildenafil, a novel effective oral therapy for male erectile dysfunction. Br J Urol 1996; 78:257.
12. Buvat J, Lemaire A, Buvat-Herbaut M, et al. Comparative investigations in 26 impotent and 26 nonimpotent diabetic patients. J Urol 1985; 133:34.
13. Cooper CS, MacIndoe JH, Perry PJ, et al. The effect of exogenous testosterone on total and free prostate specific antigen levels in healthy young men. J Urol 1996; 156:438.
14. DePalma RG, Olding M, Yu GW, et al. Vascular inter-

ventions for impotence: Lessons learned. J Vasc Surg 1995; 21:576.

15. Dmochowski RR, Littlejohn J, Cox C, et al. Stability of bladder function two years following simultaneous pancreas kidney transplantation. Trans Proc 1995; 27:3127.

16. Douglas TH, Connelly RR, McLeod DG, et al. Effect of exogenous testosterone replacement on prostate-specific antigen and prostate-specific membrane antigen levels in hypogonadal men. J Surg Oncol 1995; 59:246.

17. Drugs that cause sexual dysfunction: an update. Med Lett 1992; 34:73.

18. Dyck PJ. Nerve growth factor and diabetic neuropathy. Lancet 1996; 348:1044.

19. Ellenberg M. Sexual aspects of the female diabetic. Mt Sinai J Med 1977; 44:495.

20. Fallon B. Intracavernous injection therapy for male erectile dysfunction. Urol Clin North Am 1995; 22:833.

21. Guigliano D, Marfella R, Quatraro A, et al. Tolrestat for mild diabetic neuropathy: A 52-week, randomized, placebo-controlled trial. Ann Intern Med 1993; 118:7.

22. Golji H. Complications of external condom drainage. Paraplegia 1987; 19:189.

23. Green A, Jaspan J, Kavin H, et al. Influence of long-term aldose reductase inhibitor therapy on autonomic dysfunction of urinary bladder, stomach and cardiovascular systems in diabetic patients. Diabetes Res Clin Prac 1987; 4:67.

24. Heaton JPW, Morales A, Adams MA, et al. Recovery of erectile function by the oral administration of apomorphine. Urology 1995; 45:200.

25. Jaspan JB, Herold K, Bartkus C. Effects of sorbinil therapy in diabetic patients with painful peripheral neuropathy and autonomic neuropathy. Am J Med 1985; 79(suppl 5A): 24.

26. Jefferson TW, Glaros A, Spevack M, et al. An evaluation of the Minnesota Multiphasic Personality Inventory as a discriminator of primary organic and primary psychogenic impotence in diabetic males. Arch Sex Behav 1989; 18:117.

27. Jensen SB. The natural history of sexual dysfunction in diabetic women: A 6-year follow-up study. Acta Med Scand 1986; 219:73.

28. Kegel AH. Physiologic therapy for urinary stress incontinence. JAMA 1951; 146:915.

29. Kolodny RC. Sexual dysfunction in diabetic females. Diabetes 1971; 20:557.

30. Kurt U, Ozkarde H, Altug U, et al. The efficacy of anti-serotoninergic agents in the treatment of erectile dysfunction. J Urol 1994; 152:407.

31. Kwan M, Greenleaf WJ, Mann J, et al. The nature of androgen action on male sexuality: A combined laboratory-self report study on hypogonadal men. J Clin Endocrinol Metab 1983; 57:557.

32. Lal S, Laryea E, Thavundayil JX, et al. Apomorphine-induced penile tumescence in impotent patients: Preliminary findings. Prog Neuropsychopharmacol Biol Psychiatry 1987; 11:235.

33. Lakin MM, Montague DK, VanderBrug-Medendorp S, et al. Intracavernous injection therapy: Analysis of results and complications. J Urol 1990; 143:1138.

34. Lance R, Albo M, Costabile RA, et al. Oral trazodone as empirical therapy for erectile dysfunction: A retrospective review. Urology 1995; 46:117.

35. Lapides J, Diokno AC, Silber SJ, et al. Clean, intermittent, self-catheterization in the treatment of urinary tract disease. J Urol 1972; 107:458.

36. Lewis RW. Long-term results of penile prosthetic implants. Urol Clin North Am 1995; 22:847.

37. Lue TF, Tanagho EA. Physiology of erection and pharmacologic management of impotence. J Urol 1987; 137:829.

38. Lugg J, Rajfer J. Drug therapy for erectile dysfunction. AUA Update Series 1996, Lesson 36, vol 15, p 290.

39. Maatman TJ, Montague DK, Martin LM. Erectile dysfunction in men with diabetes mellitus. Urology 1987; 29:589.

40. Martin X. Improvement of diabetic vesicopathy after pancreatic transplantation. Trans Proc 1995; 27:2441.

41. McClellan DS, Masih BK. Gangrene of the penis as a complication of penile prosthesis. J Urol 1985; 133:862.

42. Mohler JL, Cowen DL, Flanigan RC. Suppression and treatment of urinary tract infection in patients with an intermittently catheterized neurogenic bladder. J Urol 1987; 138:336.

43. Montague DK. Periprosthetic infections. J Urol 1987; 138:68.

44. Montague DK, Barada JH, Belker AM, et al. Clinical guidelines panel on erectile dysfunction: Summary report on the treatment of organic erectile dysfunction. J Urol 1996; 156:2007.

45. Nelson RP. Nonoperative management of impotence. J Urol 1988; 139:2.

46. Ohl D. Electroejaculation. Urol Clin North Am 1993; 20:181.

47. Osborne D. Psychologic evaluation of impotent men. Mayo Clin Proc 1976; 51:363.

48. Padma-Nathan H, Hellstrom WJG, Kaiser FE, et al. Treatment of men with erectile dysfunction with transurethral alprostadil. N Engl J Med 1997; 336:1.

49. Porst H. The rationale for prostaglandin E_1 in erectile failure: A study of worldwide experience. J Urol 1996; 155:802.

50. Radomski SB, Herschorn S. Risk factors associated with penile prosthesis infection. J Urol 1992; 147:383.

51. Sarica K, Arikan N, Serel A, et al. Multidisciplinary evaluation of diabetic impotence. Eur Urol 1994; 26:314.

52. Schill WB. Pregnancy after brompheniramine treatment of a diabetic with incomplete emmision failure. Arch Androl 1990; 25:101.

53. Schreiner-Engel P, Schiavi RC, Vietorisz D, et al. Diabetes and female sexuality: A comparative study of women in relationships. J Sex Marital Ther 1985; 11:165.

54. Schwartzer JU, Hofmann R. Purulent corporeal cavernositis secondary to papavarine-induced priapism. J Urol 1991; 146:845.

55. Scott FB, Bradley WE, Timm GW. Management of erectile impotence: Use of implantable inflatable prosthesis. Urology 1973; 2:80.

56. Segraves RT, Bari M, Segraves K, et al. Effect of apomorphine on penile tumescence in men with psychogenic impotence. J Urol 1991; 145:1174.

57. Sundkvist G, Armstrong FM, Bradbury JE, et al. Peripheral and autonomic nerve function in 259 diabetic patients with peripheral neuropathy treated with ponalrestat or placebo for 18 months. J Diabetes Complications 1992; 6:123.

58. Susset JG, Tessier CD, Wincze J, et al. Effect of yohimbine hydrochloride on erectile impotence: A double-blind study. J Urol 1989; 141:1360.

59. Taylor RJ, Mays SD, Grothe TJ, et al. Correlation of preoperative urodynamic findings to postoperative complications following pancreas transplantation. J Urol 1993; 150:1185.

60. Tiefer L, Schuetz-Mueller D. Psychological issues in diagnosis and treatment of erectile disorders. Urol Clin North Am 1995; 22:767.

61. Veves A, Webster L, Chen TF, et al. Aetiopathogenesis and management of impotence in diabetic males: Four years experience from a combined clinic. Diabetic Med 1995; 12:77.

62. Virag R. Intracavernous injection of papavarine for erectile failure. Lancet 1982; 2:938.

63. Wang PH, Lau J, Chalmers TC. Meta-analysis of effects of intensive blood-glucose control on late complications of type I diabetes. Lancet 1993; 341:1306.

64. Watkins W, Bourne H, Nieto F, et al. Testicular aspiration of sperm for intracytoplasmic sperm injection: A novel treatment for ejaculatory failure on the day of oocyte retrieval. Fertil Steril 1996; 66:660.

65. Wein AJ, Malloy TR, Shofer F, et al. The effects of bethanechol chloride on urodynamic parameters in normal women and in women with significant residual urine volumes. J Urol 1980; 124:397.

66. Wilson SK, Delk JR. Inflatable penile implant infection: Predisposing factors and treatment suggestions. J Urol 1995; 153:659.

67. Yang CC, Rohr MC, Assimos DG. Pretransplant urologic evaluation. Urology 1994; 43:169.

Index

Note: Page numbers in *italics* refer to illustrations; numbers followed by t indicate tables; numbers followed by n indicate notes.

ISBN 0-7216-6182-3

90038